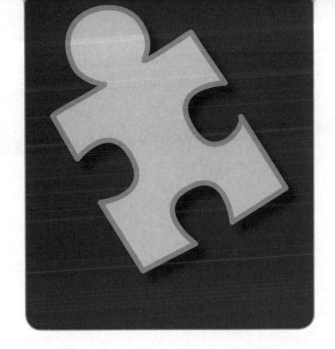

Textbook of
Physical Diagnosis

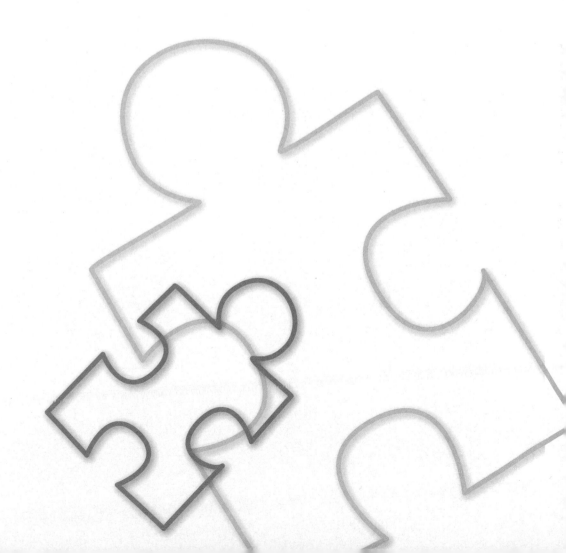

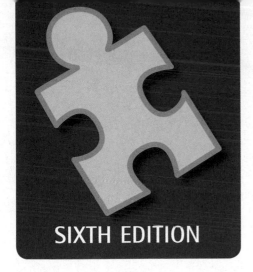

SIXTH EDITION

Textbook of Physical Diagnosis

History and Examination

Mark H. Swartz, MD, FACP

Professor of Medicine
State University of New York (SUNY)
Downstate College of Medicine
Brooklyn, New York

Adjunct Professor of Medicine
New York Medical College
Valhalla, New York

Professor of Medical Sciences
New York College of Podiatric Medicine
New York, New York

Director
C3NY — Clinical Competence Center
  of New York
New York, New York

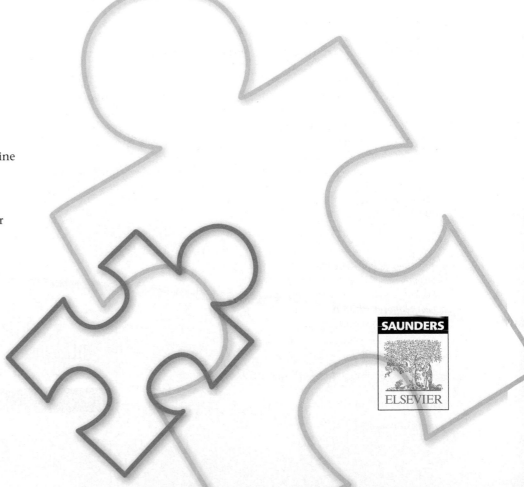

SAUNDERS

ELSEVIER

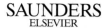

SAUNDERS
ELSEVIER

1600 John F. Kennedy Blvd.
Ste 1800
Philadelphia, PA 19103-2899

Textbook of Physical Diagnosis   ISBN: 978-1-4160-6203-5

Notice

Neither the Publisher nor the Author assume any responsibility for any loss or injury and/or damage to persons or property arising out of or related to any use of the material contained in this book. It is the responsibility of the treating practitioner, relying on independent expertise and knowledge of the patient, to determine the best treatment and method of application for the patient.

The Publisher

Previous editions copyrighted

Library of Congress Cataloging-in-Publication Data

Swartz, Mark H.
    Textbook of physical diagnosis : history and examination / Mark H Swartz. – 6th ed.
    p. ; cm.
    Includes bibliographical references and index.
    ISBN 978-1-4160-6203-5
    1. Physical diagnosis–Textbooks. I. Title.
    [DNLM: 1. Diagnosis. 2. Medical History Taking. 3. Physical Examination. WB 200 S973t 2010]
    RC76.S95 2010
    616.07'54–dc22
                                                                 2008029911

Acquisitions Editor: James Merritt
Developmental Editor: Christine Abshire
Publishing Services Manager: Linda Van Pelt
Project Manager: Sharon Lee
Design Direction: Lou Forgione

Printed in the United States of America

Last digit is the print number: 9 8 7 6 5 4 3 2 1

One of the essential qualities of the clinician is interest in humanity,
*for the secret in the care **of** the patient is in caring **for** the patient.*

Francis Weld Peabody (1881–1927)

To **Vivian Hirshaut, MD,**
*my wife, my life's companion and my best friend, for her
love, support, and understanding;*

To **Talia H. Swartz, MD, PhD,**
my wonderful and devoted daughter;

To the memory of my parents, **Hilda** *and* **Philip;**

and

To my **students,** *from whom I am always learning.*

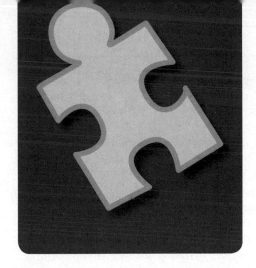

Preface to the Sixth Edition

Textbook of Physical Diagnosis: History and Examination has been written for students of health care who are learning to communicate effectively with patients, to examine patients, and to assess their medical problems. Although 20 years have passed since the publication of the first edition, this text still offers a unique approach to physical diagnosis. By discussing pathophysiology of disease and emphasizing the humanistic element of health care, I attempt to show the importance of the "old-fashioned" doctor's approach to the patient. "The *primary* aim of this textbook," as stated in the Preface to the First Edition, "is to provide a framework for the clinical assessment of the patient in a *humanistic* manner." The book, then and now, focuses on the patient: his or her needs, problems, and concerns.

The history and physical examination must not be seen as procedures performed by a robot but rather as a process that requires interpersonal awareness as well as technical skill. In this era of extraordinary advances in diagnostic modalities, procedures and tests have been emphasized, while the importance of the history and physical examination has been minimized. It is well known, however, that among the most valuable and least costly medical evaluations are the history and physical examination. This book focuses on how to offer the best medical care through the art of interviewing and physical examination.

The Sixth Edition represents a major revision based on a complete review of the field of physical diagnosis. The chapters have been reviewed and modified where appropriate. Extensive changes have been made to the pediatric chapter and to the chapter on the pregnant patient. As times change, so do standards of physical diagnosis. Therefore, several of the tests indicated in the previous editions have been either modified or eliminated. The bibliography has been updated. This edition includes a new chapter on the focused history and physical examination, since this skill is so important today with the introduction of the USMLE Step 2CS examination.

Another feature of this edition is the inclusion of a DVD-ROM that contains step-by-step demonstrations of the complete physical examination of the man and of the breast and pelvic examinations of the woman. The DVD-ROM, playable on your computer as well as on a DVD player, also illustrates the pediatric examinations of the newborn and of the toddler, as well as a new section on the neurologic evaluation of the toddler. Using standardized patients, the DVD-ROM shows history-taking with an adolescent and her mother, as well as interviewing techniques regarding sensitive topics with a geriatric patient. These sensitive topics include a discussion of advance directives (i.e., health care proxy determination and living wills), a mental status examination of a patient with cognitive impairment, and a scenario showing how to give bad news. In addition, this new edition also contains scenarios demonstrating the focused history and physical examination of a young man with abdominal pain, counseling a woman about health-related issues, and a demonstration of a pediatric telephone consultation. The DVD-ROM coupled with the textbook provide a comprehensive clinical reference for the understanding of the organization and fluidity of the complete assessment of the patient.

The book is richly illustrated with over 900 photographs and line art. Many of the original black-and-white images demonstrating the techniques of the examination have been replaced with color images captured from the DVD-ROM videos.

In addition, this Sixth Edition includes an accompanying website on Student Consult, which is an online interactive learning platform presenting a collection of over 50 Elsevier textbook titles with a wide array of ancillary materials. The website features fully searchable text; integration links that will seamlessly connect the user to additional and related content in other Student Consult titles; an image library, with figures that can be easily downloaded into PowerPoint; and supplementary material such as audio clips. Users can gain access to the online version of this book by going to www.studentconsult.com and entering the unique PIN code provided on the inside front cover of this book.

The health care provider of today must be able to synthesize basic pathophysiology with humanistic medical care. As the medical profession continues to be under great scrutiny, we must emphasize an empathetic approach to patient care, recognizing the role of culture in illness and using modern technology only to *enhance* our clinical assessment, not to replace it. We must always remember that a patient is a *person* suffering from disease.

I hope that you will find this Sixth Edition of *Textbook of Physical Diagnosis: History and Examination* to be reader-friendly, comprehensive, and an exciting addition to your library.

Mark H. Swartz, MD, FACP

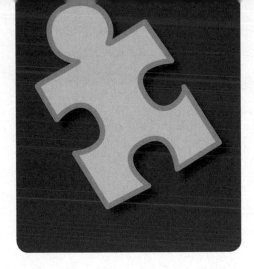

Acknowledgments

I wish to acknowledge all of my professional colleagues and friends who have supported and guided me in writing this Sixth Edition. I express my heartfelt thanks to the following people, without whose assistance I could not have brought this book to a reality:

To all my teachers, students, and patients who have taught me so much about medicine.

Special thanks to the following people who have helped in reviewing chapters for this edition:

Jerry A. Colliver, PhD
Former Director of Statistics and Research
Consulting and Professor of Medical
  Education (1981–2007)
Southern Illinois University School of Medicine
Springfield, Illinois

Margaret Clark Golden, MD
Clinical Associate Professor of Pediatrics
Director, Third Year Pediatric Clerkship
Department of Pediatrics
State University of New York (SUNY)
Downstate College of Medicine
Brooklyn, New York

Mark Kosinski, DPM
Professor of Medicine
New York College of Podiatric Medicine
New York, New York
Instructor of Surgery
New York Medical College
Valhalla, New York

Robert Kushner, MD
Professor of Medicine
Northwestern University Feinberg School
  of Medicine
Chicago, Illinois

Robert W. Marion, MD
Professor of Pediatrics and Obstetrics
  and Gynecology
Ruth L. Gottesman Professor of
  Child Development
Director of the Children's Evaluation
  and Rehabilitation Center
Co-Director, Medical Student Education,
  Department of Pediatrics
Albert Einstein College of Medicine
Co-Chief, Section of Genetics, and Director,
  Center for Congenital Disorders
Children's Hospital at Montefiore
Bronx, New York

Mimi McEvoy, RN, CPNP, MA
Assistant Professor of Pediatrics
Albert Einstein College of Medicine
Bronx, New York

Joanna F. Shulman, MD
Assistant Professor of Obstetrics and
  Gynecology
Director, Third Year OB/GYN Clerkship
Department of Obstetrics, Gynecology &
Reproductive Science
Mount Sinai School of Medicine
New York, New York

Talia H. Swartz, MD, PhD
Department of Internal Medicine
Mount Sinai Medical Center
New York, New York

And to the following people who helped in previous editions:

James R. Bonner, MD
Dennis W. Boulware, MD
University of Alabama School of Medicine
Birmingham, Alabama

Gabriele Chryssanthou, CO
New York, New York

Tracie L. DeMack
University of Chicago School of Medicine
Chicago, Illinois

Ethan D. Fried, MD
Columbia University College of Physicians
  and Surgeons
New York, New York

Sheldon Jacobson, MD
Mount Sinai School of Medicine
New York, New York

Peter B. Liebert, MD
Mount Sinai School of Medicine
New York, New York

Meryl H. Mendelson, MD
Mount Sinai School of Medicine
New York, New York

And finally, special thanks:

To Wendy Beth Jackelow, who has artistically illustrated all editions of this book.

To Frederick S. Bobrow for his tireless efforts to expertly produce the DVD-ROM in this book, as well as the DVD-ROM and CD-ROM in earlier editions.

To Margaret Clark Golden, MD, for all of her time and help in preparing the pediatric and adolescent portions of the DVD-ROM. Dr. Golden wishes to acknowledge with thanks Dr. Robert Louis Gatson, who taught her what it means to be a pediatrician.

To Ella-Jean L. Richards-François, MD, for preparing the adolescent history portion of the DVD-ROM.

To Joan Kendall, Meg Anderson, Lily Burd, Tom Pennacchini, Sandra Parris, and Lane Binkley, who were the remarkable actors portraying the patients in the DVD-ROM.

To the many employees at Elsevier for their expert assistance and cooperation. In particular, I would like to acknowledge the help of James Merritt, my editor, and the production team of Christine Abshire, Sharon Lee, Lou Forgione, David Rushing, and Lisa Damico, whose efforts have been critical in the planning, production, design, media, and marketing of this edition.

And finally to my wife, Vivian Hirshaut, for her personal support, endless patience, and understanding. Without her boundless affection, indefatigable help, sustained devotion, and encouragement, this book could never have come to fruition.

Mark H. Swartz, MD, FACP

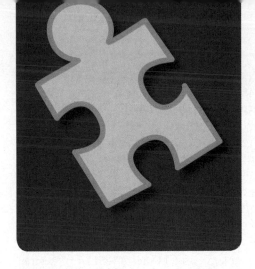

Photograph Credits

A photograph makes a concept or disease entity more understandable and easier to recognize. As the well-known proverb says, *"A picture is worth a thousand words."* I wish to acknowledge with deep gratitude the following colleagues who have graciously allowed me to use slides from their own teaching collections to help illustrate this Sixth Edition.

Brian M. Kabcenell, DMD
Rye Dental Associates, PC
Rye, New York
(Figure 12-37A)

Mark Kosinski, DPM
New York College of Pediatric Medicine
New York, New York
(Figure 10-58)

The following individuals were kind enough to contribute their slides to previous editions:

J. Daniel Arbour, MD
Marc Blouin, DEC, OA
Andrew H. Eichenfield, MD
Stephen A. Estes, MD
Neil A. Fenske, MD
Raul Fleischmajer, MD
Peter T. Fontaine, CRA, EMT
Howard Fox, DPM
Alan Friedman, MD
Bechara Y. Ghorayeb, MD
Alejandra Gurtman, MD
Michael Hawke, MD
Donald E. Hazelrigg, MD
Gregory C. Hoffmeyer
Anthony Iorio, DPM, MPH
Brian M. Kabcenell, D.M.D.
Michael P. Kelly

Karen Ann Klima, BA, CRA, COMT
Mark A. Kosinski, DPM
William Lawson, MD
Alan B. Levine, DC
Thomas P. Link, CRA
Harry Lumerman, DDS
Bryan C. Markinson, DPM
Michael A. Rothschild, MD
Donald Rudikoff, MD
Ben Serar, M.A., CRA
Deborah L. Shapiro, MD
Michael Stanley
Arthur Steinhart, DPM
Phillip A. Wackym, MD
Joseph B. Walsh, MD
Katherine Ward, DPM

I wish to acknowledge with thanks the authors and publishers of the following books for permission to reprint figures from their texts:

4–7: Redrawn from Wensel LO (ed): Acupuncture in Medical Practice. Reston, Virginia, Reston Publishing Co., Appleton & Lange, 1980.

5–2, 5–5ABC, 5–6, 5–7A, 5–9AB, 5–10AB, 5–11AB: From Morgan SL, Weinsier RL: Fundamentals of Clinical Nutrition, 2nd ed. St. Louis, Mosby, 1998.

5–7B, 5–8, 8–6B, 8–8, 8–16AB, 8–26B, 8–29, 8–43, 8–48, 8–58, 8–59, 8–61, 8–64B, 8–65, 8–70, 8–71, 8–73, 8–75, 8–78, 8–81, 8–82, 8–87, 8–88, 8–90, 8–99, 8–102, 8–104, 8–106, 8–109, 8–112, 12–13, 12–50, 14–15, 15–2, 18–8, 18–9, 18–10, 18–14A, 18–15, 18–17, 18–34, 19–15, 19–34, 20–65A, 20–72, 24–29, 24–50, 24–51, 24–52, 24–55, 24–57: From Callen JP, Paller AS, Greer KE, et al: Color Atlas of Dermatology, 2nd ed. Philadelphia, WB Saunders, 2000.

8–6A, 8–28, 8–32, 8–35, 8–44, 8–51, 8–60, 8–72, 8–74, 8–91, 8–98, 8–101, 8–103, 8–105, 8–108, 11–20, 12–25, 14–13, 15–16, 16–5, 16–13, 18–16, 18–36, 18–37, 24–54: From Callen JP, Greer KE, Hood AF, et al: Color Atlas of Dermatology. Philadelphia, WB Saunders, 1993.

8–9, 8–10, 8–39, 8–40, 8–115, 8–116, 8–117, 19–6, 19–7, 19–8: From Hordinsky MK, Sawaya ME, Scher RK: Atlas of Hair and Nails. Philadelphia, Churchill Livingstone, 2000.

8–67, 8–92, 8–93B to E, 8–94AB, 8–100, 10–27: From Friedman-Kien AE, Cockerell CJ (eds): Color Atlas of AIDS, 2nd ed. Philadelphia, WB Saunders, 1996.

8–86, 8–111, 14–14, 17–5, 20–64: From Lebwohl MG (ed): Atlas of the Skin and Systemic Disease. New York, Churchill Livingstone, 1995.

8–107: From Jordon RE: Atlas of Bullous Disease. Philadelphia, Churchill Livingstone, 2000.

8–119, 8–120: Photographs courtesy of the Centers for Disease Control (CDC).

8–121: Photo courtesy of Public Health Image Library (PHIL) ID #3. Source: CDC/Cheryl Tyron.

8–122: Photo courtesy of Public Health Image Library (PHIL) ID #284. Source: CDC/James.

9–14: From Wallace C, Siminoski K: The Pemberton sign. Ann Intern Med 125:568, 1996.

10–19, 10–20, 10–25, 10–30, 10–31, 10–42, 10–47, 10–54, 10–59, 10–65B, 10–92, 10–94, 10–102, 10–122, 10–124, 10–136: From Kanski JJ, Nischal KK: Ophthalmology: Clinical Signs and Differential Diagnosis. St. Louis, Mosby, 2000.

10–28, 10–43A, 10–48, 10–49, 10–56, 10–63, 10–68B, 13–7, 13–8, 17–14: From Mir MA: Atlas of Clinical Diagnosis. London, WB Saunders, 1995.

10-32, 10-33, 10-55: From Kanski JJ, Nischal KK: Ophthalmology: Clinical Signs and Differential Diagnosis. London, Mosby, 2002.

12–3, 12–4, 12–18, 12–34, 12–37A, 12–43, 12–47, 12–48, 12–49, 12–57, 24–42: From Eisen D, Lynch DP: The Mouth: Diagnosis and Treatment. St. Louis, Mosby, 1998.

12–12, 24–7, 24–11, 24–27, 24–31, 24–53: From Cohen BA: Atlas of Pediatric Dermatology. London, Wolfe Publishing, 1993.

12–27, 12–58: From Silverman S: Color Atlas of Oral Manifestations of AIDS, 2nd ed. St. Louis, Mosby–Year Book, 1996.

18-7, 19–32, 19–33: From Korting GW: Practical Dermatology of the Genital Region. Philadelphia, WB Saunders, 1980.

18–11, 18–12, 18–41, 19–9, 19–10, 19–11, 19–13, 24–9: From Leibowitch M, Staughton R, Neill S, et al: An Atlas of Vulval Disease: A Combined Dermatological, Gynecological and Venereological Approach, 2nd ed. London, Mosby, 1997.

18–40: From Bolognia JK, Jorizzo JL, Rapini RP: Dermatology. London, Mosby, 2003.

20–23: From Baran R, Dawber RPR, Tosti A, Haneke E: A Text Atlas of Nail Disorders: Diagnosis and Treatment. St. Louis, Mosby, 1996.

20–65B: From Nzuzi SM: Common nail disorders. Clin Podiatr Med Surg 6:273, 1989.

20–78: From Kosinski MA, Stewart D: Nail changes associated with systemic disease and vascular insufficiency. Clin Podiatr Med Surg 6:295, 1989.

24–6, 24–12, 24–13, 24–14, 24–17, 24–19, 24–20, 24–21, 24–26, 24–27, 24–29, 24–31, 24–33, 24–40: From Shah BR, Laude TA: Atlas of Pediatric Clinical Diagnosis. Philadelphia, WB Saunders, 2000.

24–42B: From Zitelli B, Davis H: Atlas of Pediatric Physical Diagnosis, 4th ed. Philadelphia, Mosby, 2002.

26–3: From Henry MC, Stapleton ER: EMT Prehospital Care, 2nd ed. Philadelphia, WB Saunders, 1997.

27–3: Redrawn from Fagan TJ: Nomogram for Bayes' theorem. N Engl J Med 293:257, 1975. Copyright 1975 Massachusetts Medical Society. All rights reserved.

27–5, 27–6: Redrawn from Sackett DL, Haynes RB, Guyatt GH, et al (eds): Clinical Epidemiology: A Basic Science for Clinical Medicine, 2nd ed. New York, Little, Brown & Co., 1991.

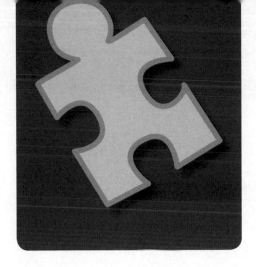

Contents

SECTION 4: Putting the Data to Work

CHAPTER 1

The Interviewer's Questions

What is spoken of as a "clinical picture" is not just a photograph of a man sick in bed;
it is an impressionistic painting of the patient surrounded by his home, his work,
his relations, his friends, his joys, sorrows, hopes and fears.

Francis Weld Peabody (1881–1927)

Basic Principles

Good communication skills are the foundation of excellent medical care. Even with the exciting new technology that has appeared since 2000, communicative behavior is still paramount in the care of patients. Studies have shown that good communication improves health outcomes by resolving symptoms and reducing patients' psychological distress and anxiety. Technologic medicine cannot substitute for words and behavior in serving the ill. The quality of patient care depends greatly on the skills of interviewing, because the relationship that a patient has with a physician is one of the most extraordinary relationships between two human beings. Within a matter of minutes, two strangers—the patient and the healer—begin to discuss intimate details about a person's life. Once trust is established, the patient feels at ease discussing the most personal details of the illness. Clearly, a strong bond, a therapeutic alliance, has to have been established.

The main purpose of an interview is to gather all basic information pertinent to the patient's illness and the patient's adaptation to illness. An assessment of the patient's condition can then be made. An experienced interviewer considers all the aspects of the patient's presentation and then follows the leads that appear to merit the most attention. The interviewer should also be aware of the influence of social, economic, and cultural factors in shaping the nature of the patient's problems. Other important aspects of the interview are educating the patient about the diagnosis, negotiating a management plan, and counseling about behavioral changes.

Any patient who seeks consultation from a clinician needs to be evaluated in the broadest sense. The clinician must be keenly aware of all clues, obvious or subtle. Although body language is important, the spoken word remains the central diagnostic tool in medicine. For this reason, the art of speaking and listening continues to be the central part of the doctor-patient interaction. Once all the clues from the history have been gathered, the assimilation of those clues into an ultimate diagnosis is relatively easy.

Communication is the key to a successful interview. The interviewer must be able to ask questions of the patient freely. These questions must always be easily understood and adjusted to the medical sophistication of the patient. If necessary, slang words describing certain conditions may be used to facilitate communication and avoid misunderstanding.

Health care providers are increasingly treating patients across language barriers. For any patient who speaks a language other than that of the clinician, it is important to seek the

Conducting an Interview

Getting Started

The diagnostic process begins at the first moment of meeting. You should be dressed appropriately, wearing a white coat with your name badge identifying you as a member of the health-care team. Patients expect this standard of professional attire. Casual attire may signify condescension.

Introduce yourself, greet the patient by last name, make eye contact, shake hands firmly, and smile. You may wish to say something like

> *"Good morning, Mr. Smith; I'm Mary Jones, a medical student at the ... School of Medicine. I've been asked to interview and examine you in the next hour."*

Alternatively, you may say,

> *"Good morning, I'm Mary Jones; are you Mr. Smith?* [Pause and wait for answer.] *I am a medical student at the ... School of Medicine. I've been asked to interview and examine you in the next hour."*

or

> *"Good morning, I'm Mary Jones; please tell me how to pronounce your name?* [Pause and wait for answer.] *I am a medical student at the ... School of Medicine. I've been asked to interview and examine you in the next hour."*

or

> *"Good morning, I'm Mary Jones, are you Mr. Smith? Did I pronounce your name correctly?* [Pause and wait for answer.] *I am a medical student at the ... School of Medicine. I've been asked to interview and examine you in the next hour."*

The term *student doctor* should generally be avoided because patients may not actually understand this term; they may hear only the word *doctor*. The introduction also includes a statement of the purpose of the visit. The welcoming handshake can serve to relax the patient.

It is appropriate to address patients by their correct titles—Mr., Mrs., Dr., Ms.—unless they are adolescents or younger. A formal address clarifies the professional nature of the interview. Name substitutes such as "dear," "honey," or "grandpa" are *not* to be used. If you are not sure about the pronunciation, ask the patient how to say his or her name correctly.

The patient may address an interviewer as Ms. Jones, for example, or might elect to use the interviewer's first name. It is not correct for an interviewer to address the patient by his or her first name, because this changes the professional nature of this first meeting.

If the patient is having a meal, ask whether you can return when he or she has finished eating. If the patient is using a urinal or bedpan, allow privacy. Do not begin an interview in this setting. If the patient has a visitor, you may inquire whether the *patient* wishes the visitor to stay. Do not assume that the visitor is a family member. Allow the patient to introduce the person to you.

The interview can be helped or hindered by the physical setting in which the interview is conducted. If possible, the interview should take place in a quiet, well-lit room. Unfortunately, most hospital rooms do not afford such luxury. The teaching hospital with four patients in a room is rarely conducive to good human interactions. Therefore, make the best of the existing environment. The curtains should be drawn around the patient's bed to create privacy and minimize distractions. You may request that the volume of neighboring patients' radios or televisions be turned down. Lights and window shades can be adjusted to eliminate excessive glare or shade. Arrange the patient's bed light so that the patient does not feel as if he or she is under interrogation.

You should make the patient as comfortable as possible. If the patient's eyeglasses, hearing aids, or dentures were removed, ask whether the patient would like to use them. It may be useful to use your stethoscope as a hearing aid for hearing-impaired patients. The ear tips are placed in the ears of the patient, and the diaphragm serves as a microphone. The patient may be in a chair or lying in bed. Allow the patient the choice of position. This makes the patient

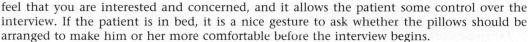

feel that you are interested and concerned, and it allows the patient some control over the interview. If the patient is in bed, it is a nice gesture to ask whether the pillows should be arranged to make him or her more comfortable before the interview begins.

Normally, the interviewer and patient should be seated comfortably at the same level. Sometimes it is useful to have the patient sitting even higher than the interviewer to give the patient the visual advantage. In this position, the patient may find it easier to open up to questions. The interviewer should sit in a chair directly facing the patient to make good eye contact. Sitting on the bed is too familiar and not appropriate. It is generally preferred that the interviewer sit at a distance of about 3 to 4 feet from the patient. Distances greater than 5 feet are impersonal, and distances closer than 3 feet interfere with the patient's "private space." The interviewer should sit in a relaxed position without crossing arms across the chest. The crossed-arms position is not appropriate because this body language projects an attitude of superiority and may interfere with the progress of the interview.

If the patient is bedridden, raise the head of the bed, or ask the patient to sit so that your eyes and the patient's eyes are at the same level. Avoid standing over the patient. Try to lower the bed rail so that it does not act as a barrier to communication, and remember to put it back up at the conclusion of the session.

Regardless of whether the patient is sitting in a chair or lying in bed, make sure that he or she is appropriately draped with a sheet or robe.

Once the introduction has been made, the interview may begin with a general, open-ended question, such as "What medical problem has brought you to the hospital?" or "I understand you are having ... Tell me the problem." This type of opening remark allows the patient to speak first. The interviewer can then determine the patient's *chief complaint:* the problem that is regarded as paramount. If the patient says, "Haven't you read my records?" it is correct to say, "No, I've been asked to interview you without any prior information." Alternatively, the interviewer could say, "I would like to hear your story in your own words."

Patients can determine very quickly if you are friendly and personally interested in them. You may want to establish rapport by asking them something about themselves before you begin diagnostic questioning. Take a few minutes to get to know the patient. If the patient is not acutely ill, you may want to say, "Before I find out about your headache, tell me a little about yourself." This technique puts the patient at ease and encourages him or her to start talking. The patient usually talks about happy things in his or her life rather than the medical problems. It also conveys your interest in the patient as a person, not just as a vehicle of disease.

The Narrative

Novice interviewers are often worried about remembering the patient's history. However, it is poor form to write extensive notes during the interview. Attention should be focused more on what the person is saying and less on the written word. In addition, by taking notes, the interviewer cannot observe the facial expressions and body language that are so important to the patient's story. A pad of paper may be used to jot down important dates or names during the session.

After the introductory question, the interviewer should proceed to questions related to the chief complaint. These should naturally evolve into questions related to the other formal parts of the medical history, such as the present illness, past illnesses, social and family history, and review of body systems. Patients should largely be allowed to conduct the narrative in their own way. The interviewer must select certain aspects that require further details and guide the patient toward them. Overdirection is to be avoided, because this stifles the interview and prevents important points from being clarified.

Small talk is a useful method of enhancing the narrative. Small talk is neither random nor pointless, and studies in conversation analysis indicate that it is actually useful in communication. It has been shown that during conversations, the individual who tells a humorous anecdote is the one who is in control. For example, if an interviewer interjects a humorous remark during an interview and the patient laughs, the interviewer is in control of the conversation. If the patient does not laugh, the patient may take control.

Be alert when a patient says, "Let me ask you a hypothetical question" or "I have a friend with ...; what do you think about ...?" In each case, the question is probably related to the patient's own concerns.

A patient often uses utterances such as "uh," "ah," and "well" to avoid unpleasant topics. It is natural for a patient to delay talking about an unpleasant situation or condition.

Pauses between words, as well as the use of these words, provide a means for the patient to put off discussing a painful subject.

When patients use vague terms such as "often," "somewhat," "a little," "fair," "reasonably well," "sometimes," "rarely," or "average," the interviewer must always ask for clarification: "What does *sometimes* mean?" "How often is *often?*" Even terms such as "dizzy," "weak," "diarrhea," and "tired" necessitate explanation. Precise communication is always desirable, and these terms, among others, have significant variations in meaning.

The interviewer should be alert for subtle clues from the patient to guide the interview further. There are a variety of techniques to encourage and sustain the narrative. These guidelines consist of verbal and nonverbal facilitation, reflection, confrontation, interpretation, and directed questioning. These techniques are discussed later in this chapter.

The Closing

It is important that the interviewer pace the interview so that adequate time is left for the patient to ask questions and for the physical examination. About 5 minutes before the end of the interview, the interviewer should begin to summarize the important issues that were discussed.

By the conclusion of the interview, the interviewer should have a clear impression of the reason why the patient sought medical help, the history of the present illness, the patient's past medical history, and the patient's social and economic position. At this time, the interviewer may wish to say, "You've been very helpful. I am going to take a few notes." If any part of the history needs clarification, this is the time to obtain it. The interviewer may wish to summarize for the patient the most important parts of the history to help illuminate the important points made.

If the patient asks for an opinion, it is prudent for the novice interviewer to answer, "I am a medical student. I think it would be best to ask your doctor that question." You have not provided the patient with the answer that he or she was seeking; however, you have not jeopardized the existing doctor-patient relationship by possibly giving the wrong information or a different opinion.

At the conclusion, it is polite to encourage the patient to discuss any additional problems or to ask any questions: "Is there anything else you would like to tell me that I have not already asked?" "Are there any questions you might like to ask?" Usually, all possible avenues of discussion have been exhausted, but these remarks allow the patient the "final say." At this time, the interviewer can thank the patient and tell him or her that the physical examination will begin.

Basic Interviewing Techniques

The successful interview is smooth and spontaneous. The interviewer must be aware of subtleties and be able to pick up on these clues. The successful interviewer sustains the interview. Several techniques can be used to encourage someone to continue speaking, and this section discusses those interviewing techniques. Each of them has its limitations, and not all of them are used in every interview.

Questioning

The secret of effective interviewing lies in the art of questioning. The wording of the question is often less important than the tone of voice used to ask it. In general, questions that stimulate the patient to talk freely are preferred.

Open-Ended Questions

Open-ended questions are used to ask the patient for general information. This type of question is most useful in beginning the interview or for changing the topic to be discussed. An open-ended question allows the patient to tell his or her story spontaneously and does not presuppose a specific answer. It can be useful to allow the patient to "ramble on." Examples of open-ended questions are the following:

"What kind of medical problem are you having?"

"How has your health been?"

"Are you having stomach pain? Tell me about it."

"Tell me about your headache."

"How was your health before your heart attack?"

"Can you describe your feelings when you get the pain?"

"I'm curious about ..."

Too much rambling, however, must be controlled by the interviewer in a sensitive but firm manner. This freedom of speech should obviously be avoided with overtalkative patients, whereas it should be used often with silent patients.

Direct Questions

After a period of open-ended questioning, the interviewer should direct the attention to specific facts learned during the open-ended questioning period. These *direct questions* serve to clarify and add detail to the story. This type of question gives the patient little room for explanation or qualification. A direct question can usually be answered in one word or a brief sentence; for example:

"Where does it hurt?"

"When do you get the burning sensation?"

"How do you compare this pain with your ulcer pain?"

Care must be taken to avoid asking direct questions in a manner that might bias the response.

Symptoms are classically characterized according to several dimensions or elements, including *bodily location, quality, quantity, chronology, setting, precipitating* (and *palliating*) *factors*, and *associated manifestations*. These elements may be used as a framework to clarify the illness. Examples of appropriate questions follow.

Bodily Location

"Where in your back do you feel pain?"

"Can you tell me where you feel the pain?"

"Do you feel it anywhere else?"

Onset (Chronology)

"When did you first notice it?"

"How long did it last?"

"Have you had the pain since that time?"

"Then what happened?"

"Have you noticed that it is worse during your menstrual period?"

Precipitating Factors

"What makes it worse?"

"What seems to bring on the pain?"

"Have you noticed that it occurs at a certain time of day?"

"Is there anything else besides exercise that makes it worse?"

"Does exercise increase the shortness of breath?"

"Does stress precipitate the pain?"

Palliating Factors

"What do you do to get more comfortable?"

"Does lying quietly in bed help you?"

"Does rest help?"

"Does aspirin help the headache?"

"Does eating make it better?"

Quality

"What does it feel like?"

"Can you describe the pain?"

"What do you mean by a 'sticking pain'?"

"Was it sharp (pause), dull (pause), or aching?"

"When you get the pain, is it steady, or does it change?"

Radiation

"When you get the pain in your chest, do you feel it in any other part of your body at the same time?"

"When you experience your abdominal pain, do you have pain in any other area of your body?"

Severity

"What do you mean by 'a lot'?"

"How many sanitary napkins do you use?"

"How many times did you vomit?"

"What kind of effect does the pain have on your work?"

"How does the pain compare with the time you broke your leg?"

"Can you fall asleep with the pain?"

"How has the pain affected your lifestyle?"

"On a scale from 1 to 10, with 10 the worst pain you can imagine, how would you rate this pain?"

Temporal

"Does it ever occur at rest?"

"Do you ever get the pain when you are emotionally upset?"

"Where were you when it occurred?"

"Does the pain occur with your menstrual cycle?"

"Does it awaken you from sleep?"

"Have you noticed any relationship of the pain to eating?"

Associated Manifestations

"Do you ever have nausea with the pain?"

"Have you noticed other changes that happen when you start to sweat?"

"Before you get the headache, do you ever experience a strange taste or smell?"

The mnemonic *O-P-Q-R-S-T*, which stands for *o*nset (chronology), *p*recipitating (or *p*alliative), *q*uality, *r*adiation, *s*everity, and *t*emporal, is useful in helping the interviewer remember these important dimensions of a symptom.

Question Types to Avoid

There are several types of questions that should be avoided. One is the *suggestive* question, which provides the answer to the question. For example:

"Do you feel the pain in your left arm when you get it in your chest?"

A better way to ask the same question would be as follows:

"When you get the pain in your chest, do you notice it anywhere else?"

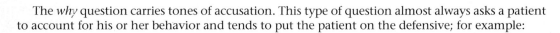

The *why* question carries tones of accusation. This type of question almost always asks a patient to account for his or her behavior and tends to put the patient on the defensive; for example:

"Why did you stop taking the medication?"

"Why did you wait so long to call me?"

The answers to such questions, however, are important. Try rephrasing as *"What is the reason ...?"* The "why" question is useful in daily life with friends and family, with whom you have a relationship different from that with your patients; do not use it with patients.

The *multiple* or *rapid-fire* question should also be avoided. In this type of question, there is more than one point of inquiry. Don't barrage the patient with a list of questions. The patient can easily get confused and respond incorrectly, answering no part of the question adequately. The patient may answer only the last inquiry heard; for example:

"Have you had night sweats, fever, or chills?"

"How many brothers and sisters do you have, and has any one of them ever had asthma, heart disease, pneumonia, or tuberculosis?"

The other problem with multiple questions is that you may think you have asked the question, but the patient has answered only part of it. For example, in the first inquiry just mentioned, the patient may answer "No" to indicate "no chills," but if you ask about the symptoms separately, you might find out that the patient does have a history of night sweats.

Questions should be concise and easily understandable. The context should be free of *medical jargon*. Frequently, novice interviewers try to use their new medical vocabularies to impress their patients. They may sometimes respond to the patient with technical terms, leaving the patient feeling confused or put down. By using medical jargon, the interviewer distances himself or herself from the patient. This use of technical medical terms is sometimes called *doctorese* or *medicalese*. For example,

"You seem to have a homonymous hemianopsia."

"Have you ever had a myocardial infarction?"

"We perform Papanicolaou smears to check for carcinoma in situ."

"I am going to order a CBC with differential."

"The MUGA scan shows that you have congestive heart failure."

Medical terminology, as a rule, should not be used in conversations with patients. Technical terms scare patients who are unfamiliar with them. Every medical and nursing student understands the term *heart failure*, but a patient might interpret it as failure of the heart to pump—that is, cardiac standstill, or death. Although patients should be given only as much information as they can handle, adequate explanations must always be provided. A partial explanation can leave the patient confused and fearful. Conversely, patients may try to use medical terms themselves. Do not take these terms at face value; ask patients to describe what they mean. For example, some patients may use "heart attack" to describe angina, "stroke" to describe a transient ischemic attack, "spells" to describe dizziness, or "water pills" or "heart pills" when referring to their medication.

A *leading* or *biased* question carries a suggestion of the kind of response for which the interviewer is looking. For example, "You haven't used any recreational drugs, have you?" suggests that the interviewer disapproves of the patient's use of drugs. If the patient has used recreational drugs, he or she may not admit it under this line of questioning. Instead, ask, "Do you use recreational drugs?" Questions should be asked in the positive or affirmative mode, not the negative. Questions asked in the affirmative or positive mode convey a nonjudgmental approach and encourage the patient to answer more candidly without the fear of being blamed for an action.

It is also incorrect to ask, "You don't have diabetes, do you?" or "You haven't been wheezing, have you?" Instead, the interviewer should ask in the positive affirmative mode, "Do you have diabetes?" or "Have you been wheezing?" A leading question may also invite a particular answer. For example, "Did you notice that the pain came on after you vomited?"

In addition to avoiding certain types of questions, the interviewer should avoid certain situations. For example, patients may respond to a question in an unexpected manner, resulting in a period of unexpected silence. This "stumped silence" can be interpreted by the patient in a variety of ways. The interviewer must be able to respond quickly in such instances, even if it means broaching another topic.

False reassurances restore a patient's confidence but ignore the reality of the situation. Telling a patient that "surgery is always successful" clearly discounts the known morbidity and mortality rates associated with it. The patient *wants* to hear such reassurance, but it may be false.

If a patient suggests that a test not be performed, perhaps because of an underlying fear of the test, the interviewer should never respond by stating, "I'm the doctor. I'll make the decisions." The interviewer should recognize the anxiety and handle the response from that point of view. He or she should ask the patient, "What are your concerns about taking the test?"

If a patient appears overweight, ask first whether there has been any change in the patient's weight before asking whether he or she has tried to lose weight. The patient may have lost 30 pounds already but is still overweight.

Finally, assume nothing about patients' knowledge of their disease, their sexual orientation or experiences, their education, their family, or their knowledge of illness in general. People come from different backgrounds and have different beliefs based on culture, religion, and experience. It is incorrect to assume that if a medicine has been prescribed for an illness, the patient is taking it correctly or actually taking it at all. Do not even presume that a patient is happy or sad about an event in his or her life or in the lives of friends and family. It is much safer to ask questions in the following manner:

"How do you feel about it?"

"What do you know about ...?"

"How often do you take this medication?"

"How do you remember to take this medication?"

"How does that make you feel?"

Silence

This technique is most useful with silent patients. Silence should never be used with over-talkative patients, because letting them talk continuously would not allow the interviewer to control the interview. This difficult type of communication, when used correctly, can indicate interest and support. Silence on the part of the patient can be related to hostility, shyness, or embarrassment. The interviewer should remain silent, maintaining direct eye contact and attentiveness. The interviewer may lean forward and even nod. After no more than 2 minutes of silence, the interviewer may say,

"What are you thinking about?"

"You were saying ...?"

"These things are hard to talk about."

"You were about to say ...?"

If the patient remains silent, another method of sustaining the interview must be chosen.

The interviewer must use silence when the patient becomes overwhelmed by emotion. This act allows the patient to release some of the tension evoked by the history and indicates to the patient that it is acceptable to cry. Handing the patient a box of tissues is a supportive gesture. It is inappropriate for the interviewer to say, "Don't cry" or "Pull yourself together," because these statements imply that the patient is wasting the interviewer's time or that it is shameful to show emotions.

It is important to use silence correctly. An interviewer who remains silent, becomes fidgety, reviews notes, or makes a facial expression of evaluation will inhibit the patient. The patient may perceive the frequent use of silence by the interviewer as aloofness or a lack of knowledge.

Facilitation

Facilitation is a technique of verbal or nonverbal communication that encourages a patient to continue speaking but does not direct him or her to a topic. A common verbal facilitation is "Uh huh." Other examples of verbal facilitations include "Go on," "Tell me more about that," "And then?" and "Hmm."

An important nonverbal facilitation is nodding the head or making a hand gesture to continue. Moving toward the patient connotes interest. Be careful not to nod too much, as this may convey approval in situations in which approval may not be intended.

Often, a puzzled expression can be used as a nonverbal facilitation to indicate, "I don't understand."

Confrontation

Confrontation is a response based on an observation by the interviewer that points out something striking about the patient's behavior or previous statement. This interviewing technique directs the patient's attention to something of which he or she may or may not be aware. The confrontation may be either a statement or a question; for example:

> *"You look upset."*
>
> *"Is there any reason why you always look away when you talk to me?"*
>
> *"You're angry."*
>
> *"You sound uncomfortable about it."*
>
> *"What is the reason you are not answering my questions?"*
>
> *"You look as though you are going to cry."*

Confrontation is particularly useful in encouraging the patient to continue the narrative when there are subtle clues given. By confronting the patient, the interviewer may enable the patient to explain the problem further. Confrontation is also useful to clarify discrepancies in the history.

Confrontation must be used with care; excessive use is considered impolite and overbearing. If correctly used, however, confrontation can be a powerful technique. Suppose a patient is describing a symptom of chest pain. By observing the patient, you notice that there are now tears in the patient's eyes. By saying sympathetically, "You look very upset," you are encouraging the patient to express emotions.

Interpretation

Interpretation is a type of confrontation that is based on inference rather than on observation. The interviewer interprets the patient's behavior, encouraging the patient to observe his or her own role in the problem. The interviewer must fully understand the clues the patient has given before he or she can offer an interpretation. The interviewer must look for signs of underlying fear or anxiety that may be indicated by other symptoms, such as recurrent pain, dizziness, headaches, or weakness. Once these underlying fears have been discovered, the patient may be led to recognize the inciting event during future interviews. Interpretation frequently opens previously unrecognized lines of communication. Examples are the following:

> *"You seem to be quite happy about that."*
>
> *"Sounds as if you're scared."*
>
> *"Are you afraid you've done something wrong?"*
>
> *"I wonder whether there's a relation between your dizziness and arguments with your wife."*

Interpretation can demonstrate support and understanding if used correctly.

Reflection

Reflection is a response that mirrors or echoes that which has just been expressed by the patient. The tone of voice is important in reflection. The intonation of the words may indicate entirely different meanings. For example:

Patient: I was so sick that I haven't worked since October 2006.

Response: Haven't worked since 2006?

In this example, the emphasis should be on "2006." This asks the patient to describe the conditions that did not allow him or her to work. If the emphasis is incorrectly placed on "worked," the interviewer immediately puts the patient on the defensive, implying, "What did you do with your time?" Although often very useful, reflection can hamper the progress of an interview if used improperly.

Support

Support is a response that indicates an interest in or an understanding of the patient. Supportive remarks promote a feeling of security in the doctor-patient relationship. A supportive response might be "I understand." An important time to use support is immediately after a patient has expressed strong feelings. The use of support when a patient suddenly begins to cry strengthens the doctor-patient relationship. Two important subgroups of support are *reassurance* and *empathy*.

Reassurance

Reassurance is a response that conveys to the patient that the interviewer understands what has been expressed. It may also indicate that the interviewer approves of something the patient has done or thought. It can be a powerful tool, but false reassurance can be devastating. Examples of reassurance are the following:

"That's wonderful! I'm delighted that you started in the rehabilitation program at the hospital."

"You're improving steadily."

"That's great that you were able to stop smoking."

The use of reassurance is particularly helpful when the patient seems upset or frightened. Reassurance must always be based on fact.

Empathy

Empathy is a response that recognizes the patient's feeling and does not criticize it. It is understanding, not an emotional state of sympathy. The empathetic response is saying, "I hear what you're saying." The use of empathy can strengthen the doctor-patient relationship and allow the interview to flow smoothly. Examples of empathy are the following:

"I'm sure your daughter's problem has given you much anxiety."

"The death of someone so close to you is hard to take."

"I guess this has been kind of a silent fear all your life."

"You must have been very sad."

"I know it's not easy for you. I'm delighted to see that you're trying to eat everything on your tray."

"That's wonderful that you have stopped smoking."

The last two examples illustrate an important point: giving credit to patients to encourage *their* role in their own improvement.

Empathetic responses can also be nonverbal. An understanding nod is an empathetic response. In certain circumstances, placing a hand on the shoulder of an upset patient

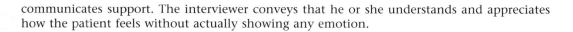

communicates support. The interviewer conveys that he or she understands and appreciates how the patient feels without actually showing any emotion.

Transitions

Transitional statements are used as guides to allow the patient to understand better the logic of the interviewer's questioning and for the interview to flow more smoothly from one topic to another. An example of a transitional statement might be, after learning about the current medical problem, the interviewer's statement "Now I am going to ask you some questions about your past medical history." Other examples while the history is documented might be, "I am now going to ask you some questions about your family" and "Let's talk about your lifestyle and your activities in a typical day." Usually, the line of questioning being pursued is obvious to the patient, so transitions are not always needed. On occasion, however, a transitional statement such as "I am now going to ask you some routine questions about your sexual history" may bridge to this area comfortably for both the patient and interviewer. Avoid phrases such as "personal habits" or "personal history," because these expressions send the message of what the interviewer considers these habits to be; the patient may be more open to discuss this area and may not consider it "personal." Other words to be avoided include "like" or "have to" ("I would now like to ask you some questions about your sexual habits" or "I now have to ask you some questions about your sexual habits").

Format of the History

The information obtained by the interviewer is organized into a comprehensive statement about the patient's health. Traditionally, the history has been obtained by using a *disease-oriented* approach emphasizing the disease process that prompted the patient to seek medical advice. For example, a patient may present with shortness of breath; the interview would be conducted to ascertain the pathologic causes of the shortness of breath.

An alternative approach to obtaining the history is a *patient-oriented* one. This entails evaluating the patient and his or her problems more holistically. By using this approach, the health-care provider can elicit a more complete history, keeping in mind that other symptoms (e.g., pain from arthritis, weakness, depression, anxiety) may have an impact on the patient's shortness of breath. For example, if a patient has arthritis and cannot walk, shortness of breath may manifest as less severe than if the patient were able to walk and experienced shortness of breath with minimal activity. In this way, the entire patient is taken into account.

The major traditional sections of the history, with some patient-oriented changes, are as follows:

- Source and reliability
- Chief complaint
- History of the present illness and debilitating symptoms
- Past medical history
- Health maintenance
- Occupational and environmental history
- Biographic information
- Family history
- Psychosocial and spiritual history
- Sexual, reproductive, and gynecologic history
- Review of systems

Source and Reliability

The source of information is usually the patient. If the patient requires a translator, the source is the patient and the translator. If family members help in the interview, their names should be included in a single-sentence statement. The reliability of the interview should be assessed.

Chief Complaint

The chief complaint is the patient's brief statement explaining why he or she sought medical attention. It is the answer to the question, "What is the medical problem that brought you to the hospital?" In the written history, it is frequently a quoted statement of the patient, such as

"Chest pain for the past 5 hours."

"Terrible nausea and vomiting for 2 days."

"Headache for the last week, on and off."

"Routine examination for school."

Patients sometimes use medical terms. The interviewer must ask the patient to define such terms to ascertain what the patient means by them.

History of Present Illness and Debilitating Symptoms

The history of the present illness refers to the recent changes in health that led the patient to seek medical attention at this time. It describes the information relevant to the chief complaint. It should answer the questions of what, when, how, where, which, who, and why.

Chronology is the most practical framework for organizing the history. It enables the interviewer to comprehend the sequential development of the underlying pathologic process. In this section, the interviewer gathers all the necessary information, starting with the first symptoms of the present illness and following its progression to the present day. To establish the beginning of the present illness, it is important to verify that the patient was entirely well before the earliest symptom. Patients often do not remember when a symptom developed. If the patient is uncertain about the presence of a symptom at a certain time, the interviewer may be able to relate it to an important or memorable event; for example: "Did you have the pain during your summer vacation?" In this part of the interview, mainly open-ended questions are asked because these afford the patient the greatest opportunity to describe the history.

In the patient-centered evaluation, the interviewer must determine whether any debilitating symptoms are also present and what impact they have on the patient. These symptoms include pain, constipation, weakness, nausea, shortness of breath, depression, and anxiety.

Pain is one of the most debilitating symptoms and has traditionally been underrecognized. Unrelieved pain is very common and is one of the most feared symptoms of illness. Surveys indicate that 20% to 30% of the U.S. population experiences acute or chronic pain, and it is the most common symptom experienced by hospitalized adults. More than 80% of patients with cancer and more than two thirds of patients dying of noncancer illnesses experience moderate to severe pain. There are approximately 75 million episodes of acute pain per year resulting from traumatic injuries and surgical procedures. Acute pain is caused by trauma or medical conditions, is usually brief, and abates with resolution of the injury. Chronic pain persists beyond the period of healing or is present for longer than 3 months.

The effect of pain on the quality of life is important to understand. Untreated or undertreated pain impairs physical and psychological health, functional status, and quality of life. In particular, pain may produce unnecessary suffering; decrease physical activity, sleep, and appetite, which further weakens the patient; may increase fear and anxiety that the end is near; may cause the patient to reject further treatment; may diminish the ability to work productively; may diminish concentration; may decrease sexual function; may alter appearance; and may diminish the enjoyment of recreation and social relationships. In addition, pain has been associated with increased medical complications, increased use of health-care resources, decreased patient satisfaction, and unnecessary suffering. In the United States, the economic costs of undertreated pain approach $80 billion per year in treatment, compensation, and lost wages.

Because of health-care providers' lack of knowledge about analgesics, negative attitudes toward the use of pain control, and lack of understanding about addiction, and because of drug regulations and the cost of effective pain management, patients often suffer unnecessarily from inadequate pain control. A study of medical inpatients and the use of narcotic analgesics revealed that 32% of patients were continuing to experience "severe" distress despite the analgesic regimen, and 41% were in "moderate" distress. Breitbart and colleagues (1996) also revealed that pain was dramatically undertreated in ambulatory patients with acquired immunodeficiency syndrome (AIDS). Of patients experiencing severe pain, only 7.3% received opioid analgesics at the recommended doses. Approximately 75% with severe pain received no opioid analgesics at all. The Study to Understand Prognoses and Preferences for Outcomes and Risks of Treatment (SUPPORT) (1995) indicated that 50% of conscious patients who died in a hospital suffered "moderate-severe" pain during their last week of life.

Cleeland and associates (1997) reported that members of ethnic minority groups are likely to receive inadequate treatment for pain. Their study showed that minority patients were three times more likely to be undertreated for pain. Sixty-five percent of minority patients did not receive guideline-recommended analgesic prescriptions. Latino patients reported less pain relief than did African-American patients. Morrison and colleagues (2000) investigated the availability of commonly prescribed opioid analgesics in pharmacies in New York City. They found that 50% of a random sample of pharmacies surveyed did not stock sufficient medications to treat patients with severe pain adequately. Pharmacies in predominantly nonwhite areas were less likely to stock opioid analgesics than were pharmacies in predominantly white neighborhoods.

Whatever the cause of pain, health-care providers must ask repeatedly about the presence of pain and the adequacy of its control:

"Are you having pain?"

"Have you had pain in the past week?"

"Tell me where your pain or pains are located."

"How has the pain affected your life?"

"Are you satisfied with your pain control?"

"Tell me a little more about your pain."

It is often useful with geriatric patients to say, "Many people have pain. Is there anything you want to tell me?" In cognitively impaired patients, the interviewer should ask about the real-time assessment of pain: pain now, *not* pain in the past 3 days.

Patients must be able to assess pain with easily administered rating scales and should document the efficacy of pain relief at regular intervals after the initiation or modification of treatment. In addition, it is vital to teach patients and their families how to promote effective pain management at home. The interviewer should ask patients to quantify their pain and should try using some form of pain rating scale. There are four commonly used ones:

- Simple Descriptive Pain Intensity Scale
- 0–10 Numeric Pain Intensity Scale
- Visual Analog Scale
- Face Scale

These scales are illustrated in Figure 1-1.

Past Medical History

The past medical history consists of the overall assessment of the patient's health before the present illness. It includes all of the following:

- General state of health
- Past illnesses
- Injuries
- Hospitalizations
- Surgery
- Allergies
- Immunizations
- Substance abuse
- Diet
- Sleep patterns
- Current medications
- Complementary and alternative therapies

As an introduction to the past medical history, the interviewer may ask, "How has your health been in the past?" If the patient does not elaborate about specific illnesses but says only "Excellent" or "Fair," for example, the interviewer might ask, "What does 'excellent' mean to

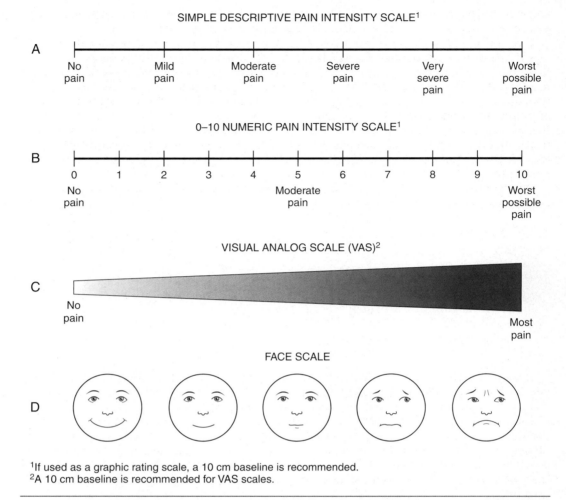

SIMPLE DESCRIPTIVE PAIN INTENSITY SCALE[1]

A

| No pain | Mild pain | Moderate pain | Severe pain | Very severe pain | Worst possible pain |

0–10 NUMERIC PAIN INTENSITY SCALE[1]

B

0   1   2   3   4   5   6   7   8   9   10

No pain   Moderate pain   Worst possible pain

VISUAL ANALOG SCALE (VAS)[2]

C

No pain   Most pain

FACE SCALE

D

[1]If used as a graphic rating scale, a 10 cm baseline is recommended.
[2]A 10 cm baseline is recommended for VAS scales.

Figure 1-1 Examples of pain scales. *A*, Simple Descriptive Pain Intensity Scale. *B*, 0–10 Numeric Pain Intensity Scale. *C*, Visual Analog Scale. *D*, Face Scale.

you?" Direct questioning is appropriate and allows the interviewer to focus on pertinent points that need elaboration.

The record of *past illnesses* should include a statement of childhood and adult problems. Recording childhood illnesses is obviously more important for pediatric and young adult interviewees. All patients should nevertheless be asked about measles, mumps, whooping cough, rheumatic fever, chickenpox, polio, and scarlet fever. Older patients may respond, "I really don't remember." It is important to remember that a diagnosis given to the interviewer by a patient should never be considered absolute. Even if the patient was evaluated by a competent clinician in a reputable medical center, the patient may have misunderstood the information given.

The patient should be asked about any *prior injuries* or accidents: "Have you ever been involved in a serious accident?" The type of injury and the date are important to record.

All *hospitalizations* must be indicated, if not already described. These include admissions for medical, surgical, and psychiatric illnesses. The interviewer should not be embarrassed to ask specifically about psychiatric illness, which *is* a medical problem. Interviewer embarrassment inevitably leads to patient embarrassment and reinforces the "shame" associated with psychiatric illness. Student interviewers should learn to ask direct questions in a sensitive manner. The interviewer might ask, "Have you ever been in therapy or counseling?" or "What nervous or emotional problems have you had?"

All *surgical procedures* should be specified. The type of procedure, date, hospital, and surgeon's name should be documented, if possible.

All *allergies* should be described. These include environmental, ingestible, and drug-related reactions. The interviewer should seek specificity and verification of the patient's allergic response. "How do you know you're allergic?" "What kind of problem did you have when you took …?" The symptoms of an allergy (e.g., rashes, itching, anaphylaxis) should be clearly indicated.

It is important to determine the *immunization history* of all patients. Tetanus and diphtheria immunity is present in fewer than 25% of adults, and fewer than 25% of targeted groups receive influenza vaccines yearly. Tetanus and diphtheria are preventable, and the current recommendation is to use the combined toxoid whenever either immunization is considered. Any patient who has never received this toxoid receives an initial injection and follow-up doses at 1 month and 6 to 12 months. A booster dose is required every 10 years.

All patients with chronic cardiovascular, pulmonary, metabolic, renal, or hematologic disorders and patients with immunosuppression should be vaccinated yearly against influenza. Patients older than 65 years should also receive the vaccine.

Indications for the pneumococcal polysaccharide vaccine are similar to those for the influenza vaccine. In addition, patients with multiple myeloma, lymphoma, alcoholism, cirrhosis, and functional or anatomic asplenia should receive the vaccine. This vaccine usually provides lifelong immunity. Revaccination every 6 years is necessary only in asplenic patients, because they are at high risk for pneumococcal infection.

Hepatitis A is one of the most common vaccine-preventable infections acquired during travel. Hepatitis A is a liver disease caused by the hepatitis A virus. Hepatitis A can affect anyone and is transmitted by the fecal-oral route. In the United States, hepatitis A can occur in situations ranging from isolated cases of disease to widespread epidemics. Good personal hygiene and proper sanitation can help prevent hepatitis A. Vaccines are also available for long-term prevention of hepatitis A virus infection in persons 12 months of age and older. The first dose of hepatitis A vaccine should be administered as soon as travel to countries with high or intermediate endemicity is considered. One month after receiving the first dose of monovalent hepatitis A vaccine, 94% to 100% of adults and children have protective concentrations of antibody. The final dose in the hepatitis A vaccine series is necessary to promote long-term protection. Immune globulin is available for short-term prevention of hepatitis A virus infection in individuals of all ages.

Hepatitis B vaccine should be given to all health-care providers, staff of institutions for developmentally disabled patients, intravenous drug abusers, patients with multiple sexual partners, hemodialysis patients, sexual partners of hepatitis B carriers, and patients with hemophilia. Complete immunization necessitates three injections: an initial one and follow-up doses at 1 month and at 6 to 12 months. Booster doses are not required. For best results, persons at high risk of exposure (especially medical, dental, and nursing students) should receive immunization before possible exposure.

Haemophilus influenzae type B vaccine is now used routinely in children to prevent invasive *H. influenzae* diseases. In 2005, *H. influenzae* type B (Hib) was estimated to have caused 3 million cases of serious disease, notably pneumonia and meningitis, and 450,000 deaths in young children. Meningitis and other serious infections caused by Hib disease can lead to brain damage or death. Hib disease is preventable by immunizing all children younger than 5 years with an approved Hib vaccine. Several Hib vaccines are available. The general recommendation is to immunize children with a first dose at 2 months of age and to follow with additional doses according to the schedule for the vaccine being used. Three to four doses are needed, depending on the brand of Hib vaccine used. Hib vaccine should never be given to a child younger than 6 weeks, because this might reduce his or her response to subsequent doses.

Between 1991 and 1992, there was a 75% decrease in the number of cases of measles, mumps, and rubella (MMR), presumably because of the use of the MMR vaccine. This vaccine is now typically given in childhood, but it should also be given to adult health-care providers who have not had the diseases. Because the vaccine contains a live virus, it should not be given to pregnant patients, those with generalized malignancies, those receiving steroid therapy, those with active tuberculosis, or those receiving antimetabolites.

The Advisory Committee on Immunization Practices (ACIP) annually reviews the recommended Adult Immunization Schedule to ensure that the schedule reflects the current recommendations for the licensed vaccines. It is advisable for the health-care worker to review these guidelines regularly. The current recommendations at the time of this publication may be found at *www.cdc.gov/mmwr/pdf/wk/mm5641-Immunization.pdf.*

A careful review of any *substance abuse* by the patient is included in the past medical history. Substance abuse includes cigarette smoking and the use of alcohol and recreational drugs. In the United States in 2007, an estimated 46 million people were smokers. About 23%

of men and 19% of women smoke. As many as 30% of all deaths related to coronary heart disease in the United States each year are attributable to cigarette smoking; the risk is strongly dose-related. Smoking also nearly doubles the risk of ischemic stroke. Smoking acts synergistically with other risk factors, substantially increasing the risk of coronary disease. Smokers are also at increased risk for peripheral vascular disease, cancer, chronic lung disease, and many other chronic diseases. Cigarette smoking is the single most alterable risk factor contributing to premature morbidity and mortality in the United States, accounting for approximately 430,000 deaths annually.

The interviewer should always ask whether the patient smokes and for how long: "Do you use nicotine in any form: cigarettes, cigars, pipes, chewing tobacco?" A *pack-year* is the number of years a patient has smoked cigarettes multiplied by the number of packs per day. A patient who has smoked two packs of cigarettes a day for the past 25 years has a smoking history of 50 pack-years. If the patient answers that he or she does not smoke now, the interviewer should inquire whether the patient ever smoked.

It has been estimated that the incidence of hazardous alcohol drinking in the United States ranges from 4% to 5% among women and 14% to 18% among men. In primary care settings, the prevalence rates range from 9% to 34% for hazardous drinking. Although studies have shown the beneficial effects of moderate alcohol consumption (one to two drinks daily), these effects are lost at higher doses. Heavy alcohol consumption is associated with many medical problems (e.g., hypertension, decreased cardiac function, arrhythmias, hemorrhagic stroke, ischemic stroke, liver disease, increased risk of breast cancer), as well as behavioral and psychiatric problems. According to the American Psychiatric Association and the National Institute on Alcohol Abuse and Alcoholism, "moderate drinking" for men is defined as less than two drinks per day; for women and persons older than 65 years, it is defined as less than one drink per day.

The history of alcohol consumption and dependency should be integrated into the general history immediately after the interviewer inquires about less threatening subjects such as smoking. It is easy to miss alcohol dependency unless specific direct questions are asked. It is acceptable to broach the topic of alcoholism by asking, "Please tell me about your drinking of alcohol." The interviewer should focus not on the quantity of alcohol consumed but rather on the adverse effects of drinking. By asking, "How much do you drink?" the interviewer may put the patient on the defensive. This type of question may also create an unnecessary power struggle between patient and interviewer. Ask instead, "How much *can* you drink?" which puts the patient and interviewer in a position of alliance. Most individuals who drink heavily also underestimate the quantities they consume. The interviewer can often learn more about the quantity of alcohol consumed by asking about the patient's feelings and interpersonal relationships than by asking directly about the amount. The interviewer should determine whether the patient drives while intoxicated, has suffered amnesia of events that occurred during drinking, neglects or abuses his or her family, and has missed work as a result of alcohol consumption.

Ewing and Rouse (1970) developed the CAGE questionnaire as a formal screening instrument to help identify patients in primary care with alcohol problems. The acronym *CAGE* helps the interviewer remember the four clinical interview questions that focus on the social and behavioral aspects of alcohol problems. Once it is established that a patient drinks alcohol, the following questions should be asked:

> *"Have you ever felt you should **C**ut down on your drinking?"*
>
> *"Have people **A**nnoyed you by criticizing your drinking?"*
>
> *"Have you ever felt bad or **G**uilty about your drinking?"*
>
> *"Have you ever taken a drink first thing in the morning (**E**ye-opener) to steady your nerves or get rid of a hangover?"*

Since its introduction, the CAGE questionnaire has been shown to be one of the most efficient and effective screening devices for detecting alcoholism. In a primary care setting, CAGE scores of 2 (two positive responses) have a sensitivity of 77% to 94% and a specificity of 79% to 97% for a current diagnosis of alcohol abuse. One positive CAGE response has a sensitivity of 21% to 71% and a specificity of 84% to 95%. The history of alcohol consumption and dependency can be further assessed by using the sets of questions referred to by the acronyms *HALT*, *BUMP*, and *FATAL DT*.

The HALT questions are as follows:

*"Do you usually drink to get **H**igh?"*

*"Do you drink **A**lone?"*

*"Do you ever find yourself **L**ooking forward to drinking?"*

*"Have you noticed whether you seem to be becoming **T**olerant of alcohol?"*

The BUMP questions are as follows:

*"Have you ever had **B**lackouts?"*

*"Have you ever used alcohol in an **U**nplanned* way?"*

*"Do you ever drink alcohol for **M**edicinal† reasons?"*

*"Do you find yourself **P**rotecting‡ your supply of alcohol?"*

The final acronym reminds the interviewer about other major associations with alcoholism. The FATAL DT questions are as follows:

*"Is there a **F**amily history of alcoholic problems?"*

*"Have you ever been a member of **A**lcoholics Anonymous?"*

*"Do you **T**hink you are an alcoholic?"*

*"Have you ever **A**ttempted or had thoughts of suicide?"*

*"Have you ever had any **L**egal problems related to alcohol consumption?"*

*"Do you ever **D**rive while intoxicated?"*

*"Do you ever use **T**ranquilizers to steady your nerves?"*

These questions provide the interviewer with a useful, thoughtful, and organized approach to the interview strategy designed to identify patients with a drinking problem.

In the late stages of alcoholism, a person may suffer delirium tremens (DTs). DTs are completely different from the hallucinations that occur in the earlier stages of alcoholism. During hallucinations, the patient may see or hear "things." DTs occur 24 to 96 hours after withdrawal from alcohol; occasional patients hallucinate or have convulsions, but all patients tremble. DTs are the most severe form of withdrawal and are fatal in one of every four cases.

The interviewer must ask all patients about the use of other drugs. People who use recreational drugs often engender negative feelings or anger in the interviewer. These feelings are almost unavoidable. The interviewer must not allow these feelings to interfere with empathetic interviewing. A useful way of approaching the topic of recreational drugs is to ask,

"Have you ever used drugs other than those required for medical reasons?"

"Do you use drugs other than those prescribed by a physician?"

"Have you abused prescription drugs?"

If the answer to any of these questions is affirmative, the interviewer should determine the types of drugs used, the routes of administration, and the frequency of use. In contrast to alcohol abusers, drug abusers are more likely to magnify their use. The interviewer must ask all patients with a history of drug abuse the following questions:

"What type of drugs do you use?"

"At what age did you start using drugs?"

---

*Drink more than you intended or have an additional drink after you decided you had had enough.
†As a cure for anxiety, depression, or the "shakes."
‡Buying enough alcohol just in case "company" arrives.

"What was your period of heaviest use?"

"What is your recent pattern of use?"

"Are larger doses necessary to get the same effect now?"

"What do you feel when you take the drug?"

"Have you ever tried to quit? What happened?"

"Have you ever had any convulsions after taking the drug?"

"Do you use more than one drug at a time?"

"Do you use drugs on a continuous basis?"

"Have you been in trouble at work because of drug use?"

"Have you ever had withdrawal symptoms as a result of your use of drugs?"

It is important to use simple words and expressions when inquiring about recreational drugs. It may also be more appropriate to use slang than to use more formal terms. For example, "Do you ever shoot up or snort coke?" may be better understood than "Have you ever taken cocaine intravenously or by insufflation?" With experience, the interviewer acquires relevant knowledge about recreational drugs. Knowing the local street names for drugs can be as important as knowing the pharmacologic effects and may provide a means of better communication. It should be recognized that these street names are often different from place to place and change from time to time. Appendix A (Commonly Abused Drugs) lists their street names and the major symptoms and signs associated with each of them.

It should also be recognized that *any* medication can be abused. Drugs such as propranolol and metoprolol (beta blockers used in the treatment of hypertension) are not usually considered recreational drugs. They are, however, frequently abused by the acting community to relieve performance anxiety, or stage fright.

In questioning a patient about *diet*, it is useful to ask the patient to describe what he or she ate the day before, including all three meals plus any snacks. How many fish meals does he or she have each week? What is the proportion of red meat in the diet in comparison with fish or poultry? How much saturated fat is there in the diet? Does the patient add salt when he or she cooks, and does he or she add salt at the table? Has his or her diet changed recently? What kinds of foods does the patient like or dislike, and why? Are there any food intolerances? Does the patient eat foods with a high fiber content, such as whole-grain breads and cereals, bran, fresh fruits, and vegetables? Does the patient eat high-fiber snack foods (which include sesame bread sticks, date-nut bread, oatmeal cookies, fig bars, granola bars, and corn chips)? What is the consumption of sodium? Pickled foods, cured meats, snack foods, and prepared soups have a high sodium content. The consumption of caffeine-containing products such as coffee, tea, cola sodas, and chocolate is important to determine. Caffeine ingestion may produce a variety of symptoms, including heart palpitations, fatigue, lightheadedness, headaches, irritability, and many gastrointestinal symptoms (see Chapter 5, Assessment of Nutritional Status, for a detailed description). The interviewer should also ascertain the amount of exercise the patient gets.

It is important to know a patient's *sleep patterns* because this may provide information about the patient's psychological problems. Sleep-related complaints such as insomnia and excessive daytime somnolence impair the lives of 20% to 50% of Americans. More than 60% of patients with psychiatric problems complain of disturbed sleep patterns. Eighty percent of patients with depression complain of disturbed sleep. The most common problem in patients with post-traumatic stress disorder is disturbed sleep; more than 50% of patients with chronic pain experience sleep problems. An estimated 200,000 automobile accidents a year are caused by excessive sleepiness on the part of drivers; 20% of drivers report that they have fallen asleep behind the wheel. The following questions should be asked:

"When do you go to bed?"

"Do you have trouble falling asleep?"

"Do you stay asleep the whole night, or do you awaken in the middle of the night, unable to go back to sleep?"

"Do you go to bed only when sleepy?"

"Do you adhere to a regular waking time?"

All current medications should be noted. The following questions should be asked:

"Do you use any prescription medications?"

"Do you use any over-the-counter medications?"

"Do you use any herbal medications or vitamins?"

"Do you use any recreational drugs?"

If possible, the patient should show the interviewer the bottles and demonstrate how the medications are taken. The interviewer should note whether the patient is taking them according to the directions on the bottle. Frequently, patients consider over-the-counter medications such as vitamins, laxatives, antacids, or cold remedies not worth mentioning; the interviewer should ask specifically about each of these types of drugs. The interviewer should determine the type of contraception used, if any, and whether a woman has used or uses birth control pills.

The use of *alternative therapies* is extremely common, as discussed in Chapter 4, Understanding Complementary and Alternative Medicine. The patient and the health-care provider must be comfortable with how questions about these therapies are asked. Avoid using the terms *other therapies, unorthodox therapy*, or *unconventional medicine*. These labels may be perceived as judgmental and could inhibit free discussion. You might start by saying, "Many patients frequently use other kinds of therapy when they have the symptoms you described. Have you used or thought about using massage, herbs, chiropractic, acupuncture, vitamin, or other different therapies for your problem or for any other reasons?"

Health Maintenance

Clinicians can play a key role in the identification and management of medical, social, and psychiatric problems. Counseling skills include building a supportive therapeutic relationship with the patient and family. A patient's family is often helpful in confirming the diagnosis and developing the treatment plan. Health maintenance consists of three main areas: disease detection, disease prevention, and health promotion.

Ask patients whether they have regular doctors and routine medical checkups. When was their last dental examination? Do they get their eyes checked periodically? Are they aware of their cholesterol levels? Do they do anything for exercise? If the patient is a woman, does she see a gynecologist regularly? Does she perform breast self-examination? When were her last mammogram and her last Pap smear obtained? If the patient is a man, does he perform routine testicular self-examination?

Tobacco use is probably the main avoidable cause of morbidity and mortality in the world. It is responsible for more than 450,000 deaths each year from cancer, heart disease, stroke, and chronic obstructive lung disease in the United States alone. Despite this fact, however, tobacco use is still prevalent. The Centers for Disease Control and Prevention estimates that 25% of all Americans still smoke and that more than 3000 children and adolescents become regular users every day. It is estimated that the cost of medical care for tobacco-related illness in the United States is more than $50 billion annually, and the cost of lost productivity and forfeited wages due to disability is an additional $50 billion per year. Despite these staggering statistics, health-care providers often fail to treat tobacco use effectively. Health-care providers have unique access to patients who use tobacco, and yet studies show that fewer than half of individuals who use tobacco reported being urged to quit by their physicians.

Health-care providers must determine and document the tobacco use status of all patients. If patients use tobacco, they should be offered smoking cessation treatment at every office visit. It has been shown that a discussion of only 3 minutes per visit can be effective. More intensive treatment with other medical therapies, social support, and other specific skills is more effective in producing long-term results. At the time of this writing, in addition to nicotine replacement products (i.e., nicotine patches, nicotine gum, nicotine lozenge, nicotine nasal spray, and nicotine inhaler), another drug has been introduced to help someone quit smoking.

Varenicline (Chantix) is non-nicotine prescription medicine specifically developed to help adults quit smoking. Varenicline, approved by the U.S. Food and Drug Administration (FDA) in 2006, contains no nicotine, but it targets the same receptors that nicotine does. It is believed to block nicotine from these receptors. It is the only prescription treatment of its kind at this time. Studies have demonstrated that at the end of 12 weeks of varenicline therapy, 44% of patients were able to quit smoking. It also helped reduce the urge to smoke.

It has been also been demonstrated, however, that there are times when patients are unreceptive or even resentful if the issue is broached. According to the "stages of change" model, success is most likely when the health-care provider is sensitive to the patient's stage. Stage 1 is the precontemplation stage in which the smoker is in denial about the hazards of smoking and is not willing to stop. Stage 2 is the contemplation stage, when the patient acknowledges a willingness to quit but has not determined when that will occur. Stage 3 is the action stage during which the patient has prepared for a change, is engaged in changing behavior, and has a plan for smoking cessation. Stage 4 is the maintenance stage during which the health-care provider needs to encourage the patient about the experience of quitting. Stage 5 is the relapse. Smokers generally make three or more attempts to quit smoking before permanent success is achieved.

Patients should be told in clear, strong language that it is in their best interest to quit smoking. Say, "I think that it is important for you to quit smoking, and I will help you. I need you to know that quitting smoking is the most important thing you can do to protect your current and future health."

Also remember to ask the questions about alcohol consumption discussed in the previous section.

Counseling is very important, but interviewers must remember that a patient must *want* to change his or her behavior. If he or she does not, interviewers should indicate to the patient that they will provide support when the patient is ready.

Finally, do not forget to ask all patients whether they wear seat belts in cars or use helmets if they ride bicycles or motorcycles.

Occupational and Environmental History

The occupational and environmental history concerns exposure to potential disease-producing substances or environments. Occupational exposures account for an estimated 50,000 to 70,000 deaths annually in the United States. More than 350,000 new cases of occupational disease are recognized each year. These diseases can involve every organ system. Because they often mimic other diseases, occupational diseases may be incorrectly ascribed to some other cause. One of the important barriers to the accurate diagnosis of occupational and environmental diseases is the long latency between exposure and appearance of the illness.

Many occupational diseases have been well described over the years: malignant mesothelioma in workers exposed to asbestos; cancer of the bladder in workers exposed to aniline dye; malignant neoplasms of the nasal cavities in woodworkers; pneumoconiosis in coal miners; silicosis in sandblasters and quarry workers; leukemia in those exposed to benzene; hepatic angiosarcoma in workers exposed to vinyl chloride; byssinosis in cotton industry workers; skin cancer in those chronically exposed to the sun, such as sailors; ornithosis in bird breeders; toxic hepatitis in solvent users and workers in the plastics industry; and chronic bronchitis in individuals exposed to industrial dusts. It has been shown that there is an association between sterility in men and women and exposure to certain pesticides and an association between dementia and exposure to certain solvents.

The environment is also responsible for significant morbidity and mortality rates. Lead, radon, pesticides, and air pollution cause illness and death. Examples include Chernobyl, with its widespread high levels of radiation; Minamata Bay in Japan, with its mercury poisoning; Hopewell, Virginia, with its poisoning pesticide chlordecone; and Bhopal, India, where a leak at an industrial plant exposed hundreds of thousands of people to toxic methyl isocyanate gas. In India, thousands died shortly after exposure, and more than 200,000 people have suffered illness from the gas. The long-range effects of these agents have yet to be determined.

A careful occupational and environmental history is the most effective means of properly diagnosing occupational and environmental diseases. It is important to inquire about all occupations and the duration of each. The history should include more than just a listing of jobs. The duration and precise activities must be ascertained. The use of protective devices and cleanup practices, as well as work in adjacent areas, must also be determined. The job title (e.g., electrician, machine operator) is important, but actual exposure to hazardous materials may not be reflected in these descriptions. Industrial work areas are complex, and it is important to ascertain the actual location of work in relation to other areas in which hazardous materials are used. It is well known that just living near areas of industrial toxins is linked to the development of disease many years later. It is therefore relevant to inquire whether the patient resides or ever resided near mines, farms, factories, or shipyards. The following questions regarding occupational and environmental exposure should be asked of all patients:

"What type of work do you do?"

"How long have you been doing this work?"

"Describe your work."

"Are you exposed to any hazardous materials? Do you ever use protective equipment?"

"What kind of work did you do before you had your current job?"

"What was your wartime employment, if any?"

"Where do you live? For how long?"

"Have you ever lived near any factories, shipyards, or other potentially hazardous facilities?"

"Has anyone in your household ever worked with hazardous materials that could have been brought home?"

"What types of hobbies do you have? What types of exposures are involved?"

"Do you now have, or have you previously had, environmental or occupational exposure to asbestos, lead, fumes, chemicals, dusts, loud noise, radiation, or other toxic factors?"

Attention must be paid to any temporal relationship between the onset of illness and toxic exposure in the workplace. Did the symptoms start after the patient began a new job? Did the symptoms abate during a vacation and then recur when the patient resumed work? Were the symptoms related to the implementation of any new chemical or process? Is there anyone else at work or are there any neighbors with a similar illness?

Biographic Information

Biographic information includes the date and place of birth, sex, race, and ethnic background.

Family History

The family history provides information about the health of the entire family, living and dead. Pay particular attention to possible genetic and environmental aspects of disease that might have implications for the patient. Determine the age and health of all the immediate family members. If a family member is deceased, record the age of the person and the cause of death. It is important to inquire how a family member's illness affects the patient psychologically.

It is important to inquire where the patient's parents were born. Where were the grandparents born? In what setting, urban or rural, did the patient grow up? In what country did the parents grow up? If the patient was born in another country, at what age did he or she come to the United States? Does the patient maintain contact with other family members? Was the original family name changed? If the patient is married, is the spouse of the same ethnic background as the patient? What is the patient's native language?

The answers to these questions provide valuable information as a heritage assessment.

Psychosocial and Spiritual History

The psychosocial history includes information on the education, life experiences, and personal relationships of the patient. This section should include the patient's lifestyle, other people living with the patient, schooling, military service, religious beliefs (in relation to the perceptions of health and treatment), and marital or significant-other relationships. You can start by asking one of the following questions:

"Tell me a little about yourself: your background, education, work, family."

"Who are the important people in your life?"

"What do you do for fun?"

"How do you feel about the way your life is going?"

A statement regarding the patient's knowledge of symptoms and illness is important. Has the illness caused the patient to lose time from work? What kind of insight does the patient have with regard to the symptom? Does he or she think about the future? If so, how does it look? An excellent question that can elicit a vast amount of information is "What is your typical day like?"

A spiritual history provides information about what gives meaning to the patient's life. Spirituality helps patients cope with serious illnesses, debilitation, and dying. This part of the medical history provides excellent insight into the patient's spiritual needs and belief systems. Meditation and prayer can complement medical care. Spirituality can offer hope to those with chronic disease and may even provide new meaning to their suffering. Several studies have revealed the beneficial effect of spirituality with regard to stress reduction, recovery from illness, mitigation of pain, and faster recovery from surgery. Puchalski and Romer (2000) suggested that a spiritual history might begin with an introductory question such as

"Do you consider yourself spiritual or religious?"

"How important are these beliefs to you, and do they influence how you care for yourself?"

Sexual, Reproductive, and Gynecologic History

The sexual history has traditionally been part of the psychosocial history or review of systems. However, because the sexual, reproductive, and gynecologic history is so vital for the complete evaluation of the patient, these histories are now considered a separate part of the interview.

There are several reasons for documenting a sexual history. Sexual drive is a sensitive indicator of general well-being. Anxiety, depression, and anger may relate to sexual dysfunction; however, many physical symptoms can lead to sexual problems. In addition, it is critical to identify risk behaviors. A well-documented sexual history enables the examiner to establish norms of sexuality for the patient. Opening up the interview to issues of sexuality allows the interviewer to educate the patient about human immunodeficiency virus (HIV)–related illnesses, sexually transmitted diseases, and pregnancy prevention. It is an excellent opportunity to provide useful information to the patient.

It is important to ask about sexual activity in children, as well as in older adults. Child abuse is very common, and the interviewer must identify it as early as possible. Interviewers must not assume that a senior citizen is sexually inactive. Sexuality is a part of normal life, and many older adults enjoy sexual contact.

Tailor your questions and terms to each specific interview. Can vernacular terms be used in the interview? Patients and interviewers may fear the use of these terms because of their emotional charge. Sometimes patients, because of embarrassment about using these terms, may try to express their symptoms with inaccurate medical terminology. Often the use of street language leads to a more relaxed and informative discussion, especially with younger adults.

The interviewer must inquire about sexual relationships in a nonjudgmental manner. Direct questions regarding oral and anal sex, sexual contacts, and sexual problems are very important. Patients are frequently less inhibited than are novice interviewers when discussing sexual behavior. If a patient's sexual preference is in doubt, the term *partner* rather than a gender-specific term is appropriate. There is no easy way to ask about sexual preference, but it is vital to know. Asking the patient whether he or she has had any contact with individuals with AIDS or AIDS-related illness is appropriate. The term *homosexual* as an adjective for gender (e.g., "homosexual man") should be avoided.

There are several general questions that can help broach the topic of sexual activity. In general, the best way to introduce the sexual history is to say, "Now I am going to ask you some questions about your sexual health and practices." Because the question, "Are you sexually active?" can be ambiguous, it is better to ask, "Have you ever had intimate physical contact with anyone?" If the answer is "Yes," the next question should be "Did that contact include sexual intercourse?" The interviewer should also then ask, "Are your partners male, female, or both?"

It is not acceptable to ask whether the person has "had sex" or is "sexually active," because there is great variability in the way individuals define these phrases. In one study, 599 college students attending a major midwestern university were asked, "Would you say you 'had sex' with someone if the most intimate behavior you engaged in was ... (mark 'yes' or 'no' for each behavior)." There were 11 items on the list, including "deep kissing," "oral contact on your breasts/nipples," "you touch other's genitals," "oral contact with other's genitals," and "penile-vaginal intercourse." Although 99.7% agreed that penile-vaginal intercourse qualified as "had sex," 19% did not believe that penile-anal intercourse meant "had sex." Only 40% felt that they "had sex" if oral-genital contact was their most intimate behavior. The study suggests that Americans hold widely divergent opinion about what behaviors do and not constitute having "had sex." Therefore, a better question to ask is "What is the most intimate physical contact you have had with someone else?"

Some of the following questions about specific sexual behaviors and satisfaction may also be helpful in acquiring a sexual history:

> *"Are you having any sexual problems?"*

> *"Are you satisfied with your sexual performance?" "Do you think your partner is?" If not, "What is unsatisfactory to you (or your partner)?"*

> *"Have you had any difficulty achieving orgasm?"*

> *"How frequently does it occur that your partner desires sexual intercourse and you do not?"*

> *"Are there any questions pertaining to your sexual performance that you would like to discuss?"*

> *"Most people experience some disappointment in their sexual function. Can you tell me what disappointments you might have?"*

> *"Many people experience what others may consider unusual sexual thoughts or wish to perform sexual acts that others consider abnormal. We are often bothered by these thoughts. What has been your experience?"*

> *"Do you have protected sex?"*

> *"Have you ever had a sexually transmitted disease?"*

> *"Have you been tested for HIV?" If yes, "What was the result?"*

Asking a patient "How many sexual partners do you have or have you had?" is rather intrusive and does not help very much. It is much better to determine whether a person routinely uses protection with condoms, if appropriate. It is true, however, that studies have shown that the more sexual partners a woman has had, the greater is the chance that she will develop cervical carcinoma.

It is less appropriate to ask "What activities and positions does your sexual contact include?" than to ask specifically about oral-genital, penile-vaginal, or penile-anal contact tailored specifically to the individual patient.

Health-care providers, regardless of their sexual orientation, must provide the highest standard of care to all patients. They must reconcile their own fears and prejudices about homosexuality. In 1978, only one third of Americans believed that they knew a gay man or lesbian; in 1996, about two thirds of Americans reported that they knew someone who was gay or lesbian. Despite this fact, there is a significant degree of homophobia in society. By definition, *homophobia* is the "irrational fear of, aversion to, or discrimination against homosexuality or homosexuals." The medical and psychological effects of homophobia can pose a significant health hazard to gay or lesbian patients and can be detrimental to establishing a strong doctor-patient relationship. If a gay or lesbian patient senses this discrimination, he or she may become alienated from the health-care system and not use standard screening modalities, thus risking higher mortality and morbidity from disease. One study revealed that 98% of gay and lesbian patients believed that it was medically important to inform their physicians of their sexual orientation, but 64% believed that in doing so, they risked receiving substandard care. In the same study, 88% of the patients reported that their physicians made disparaging remarks about gay and lesbian patients. Because homophobia is widespread in society, a gay or lesbian patient should have the confidence to speak candidly with his or her physician.

Domestic violence, rape, child abuse, sibling violence, and *elder abuse* are rampant and have reached staggering proportions. Of all domestic violence victims, 90% to 95% are women, and the perpetrators are mostly men. An estimated 2 million to 4 million American women are victims of domestic violence yearly. The violence is often a combination of physical, sexual, and psychological abuse, and the signs and symptoms may be subtle or obvious. It is therefore important to ask all patients whether they have ever been emotionally, physically, or sexually abused.

Much of the violence against women is perpetrated by their intimate partners or in relationships that are commonly protective, such as that of father and daughter. U.S. Department of Justice studies indicate that a woman is more likely to be raped, assaulted, or murdered by a male partner or ex-partner than by a stranger. Up to 45% of abused women are beaten during pregnancy. Four percent of all male homicide victims are killed by spouses or female partners. As many as one per seven women seen in emergency departments has symptoms related to abuse. A national survey indicated that more than 2 million women are severely beaten by their male partners each year. It is recognized that such violence is vastly underreported; the actual number of cases is probably double the number reported. Clinicians frequently treat the injuries only symptomatically and often fail to recognize the abuse. According to the *Washington Post*, the rate of rape in the United States increased fourfold from 1981 to 1991, in comparison with the overall crime rate. It has been estimated that 60% to 80% of all college women have been sexually assaulted by dates or friends.

Although many women who are victims of abuse do not volunteer any information, they often discuss the incidents if asked simple, direct questions in a nonjudgmental way and in a confidential setting. Be aware of the possibility of domestic violence in any woman with multiple medical visits for sexual dysfunction, chronic pelvic pain, fatigue, chest pain, gastro-intestinal disturbances, headaches, depression, anxiety, panic attacks, eating disorders, substance abuse, suicidal attempts, and abdominal pain.

Because the perpetrator often accompanies the victim to the interview, ask any other person present to leave while you speak to the patient. Begin with the following direct question: "Since domestic violence is so common, I've begun to ask about it routinely. At any time, has your partner hit, kicked, or otherwise hurt or frightened you?" If the patient answers in the affirmative, encourage her to talk about it. Alternatively, you may ask, "Do you feel safe in your relationship?" Always listen nonjudgmentally to encourage the patient to continue talking about the episode. Showing support is very important. A statement such as "You are not alone" or "Help is available for you" shows empathy. It is crucial to assess the danger to the patient as quickly as possible before she leaves the medical facility. If the patient is in imminent danger, determine whether she can stay with friends or family. A shelter for battered women may be an alternative. Finally, provide the patient with the telephone number of the local domestic violence hotline.

If the patient answers "no" to your introductory query and you suspect some form of domestic violence, be aware of the clinical findings that may indicate abuse:

- Injury to head, neck, breasts, abdomen, or genitals
- Multiple injuries
- Delay in seeking treatment
- Unusual explanation for the injury
- Injury during pregnancy
- Chronic pain syndrome
- Psychological distress
- A partner who seems overly protective

Any of these injuries must have a plausible explanation. If there is none, it is appropriate to ask further questions, but the partner must not be present. You might say, "It looks as if you've been hurt. Can you tell me how it happened?" Another approach could be "Sometimes when people feel the way you do, it's because they may have been abused. Is this happening to you?" Even if a patient is in an abusive setting and she fails to acknowledge it once you have provided an opportunity, allow her to return to discuss it at a later date. Serious injury and homicide often result once a person attempts to leave an abusive partner. Allow her to make the decision to leave. You will have indicated your support.

In 1986, more than 1.5 million children nationwide were reported as abused, an increase of 74% since 1980. Reports of childhood sexual abuse have tripled since 1980, to more than 350,000 cases per year. A history of childhood sexual abuse is nearly always associated with enduring physical and psychological sequelae. There are many somatic disorders that may result after abuse. These include eczema, sleep disorders, sexual dysfunction, substance abuse, eating disorders, headaches, "mystery" pain, depression, asthma, and a wide variety of phobias. Health-care providers have an ethical and legal responsibility to report all cases of suspected child abuse and to protect the child from further abuse. Any injury that cannot be adequately explained should raise concern about either nonaccidental injury or neglect. Injuries to the skin are seen in 90% of abused children (see Figure 24-32). Multiple injuries in various stages of healing almost always indicate repeated beatings.

Male rape is also on the rise. According to the District of Columbia Rape Crisis Center, one of every seven boys in the United States is raped before 18 years of age. Most male rape victims are raped by other men, in the sense that they are forced to submit to anal intercourse, masturbation of the offender, oral sex, or other sex acts. Information about male rape is scarce because male victims, like their female counterparts, feel humiliation and shame and are reluctant to report it. Many men believe that if they have been raped by another man, it implies that the victim has homosexual tendencies.

The *reproductive and gynecologic history* obtains information about a woman's age at menarche, regularity of menstrual flow, and duration of periods. In addition, the number of pregnancies, number of deliveries, number of abortions (spontaneous or induced), and complications of pregnancies are included in this part of the history. It is also vital to determine whether the woman was exposed to diethylstilbestrol (DES) through her mother's use during pregnancy. This is particularly important in any woman born before 1975. Other important questions are discussed in Chapter 19, Female Genitalia.

In the reproductive history for a man, it is important to inquire about sexual interest, function, satisfaction, and any sexual problems. Has the man been unable to procreate? If so, is he aware of the reason? Other questions for men are discussed in Chapter 18, Male Genitalia and Hernias.

Review of Systems

The *review of systems* summarizes in terms of body systems all the symptoms that may have been overlooked in the history of the present illness or in the medical history. By reviewing the list of possible symptoms in an orderly manner, the interviewer can specifically check each system and uncover additional symptoms of "unrelated" illnesses not yet discussed. The review of systems is best organized from the head down to the extremities, and the questions can be asked while the physical examination of that body area is being examined. Patients are told that they are going to be asked whether they have ever had a particular symptom and should answer "yes" or "no." If they answer in the affirmative, further direct questioning is appropriate. The interviewer need not repeat questions that were previously answered, unless clarification of the data is necessary.

Table 1-1 is the review of systems, about which questions should be asked of all patients. The questions should be understandable to the patient. For example, a question regarding paroxysmal nocturnal dyspnea should be asked in this manner:

> *"Do you ever awaken in the middle of the night with sudden shortness of breath or sudden difficulty in breathing?"*

Each of the organ- and system-specific chapters that follow discusses the review of symptoms in more detail. Hints about specific questioning and pathophysiologic features of the symptoms are also provided.

Sometimes, a patient may answer all the questions in the affirmative. If the interviewer detects that this is occurring, it may be useful to ask a question about a physiologically impossible condition. For example, if a patient answers "yes" when asked, "Do your stools glow in the dark?" the interviewer should not continue with the review of systems. The interviewer can state in the written history or in the verbal presentation that "the patient has a positive review of systems."

Because the goal of the medical history is to acquire as much information about each illness as possible, other specific questions related to the particular patient may be indicated. Look at the patient shown in Figure 1-2. Note the large jaw and nose. If you saw such a patient, you

Table 1–1 Review of Systems

General
- Usual state of health
- Fever
- Chills
- Usual weight
- Change in weight
- Weakness
- Fatigue
- Sweats
- Heat or cold intolerance
- History of anemia
- Bleeding tendencies
- Blood transfusions and possible reactions
- Exposure to radiation

Skin
- Rashes
- Itching
- Hives
- Easy bruising
- History of eczema
- Dryness
- Changes in skin color
- Changes in hair texture
- Changes in nail texture
- Changes in nail appearance
- History of previous skin disorders
- Lumps
- Use of hair dyes

Head
- "Dizziness"
- Headaches
- Pain
- Fainting
- History of head injury
- Stroke

Eyes
- Use of eyeglasses
- Current vision
- Change in vision
- Double vision
- Excessive tearing
- Pain
- Recent eye examinations
- Pain when looking at light
- Unusual sensations
- Redness
- Discharge
- Infections
- History of glaucoma
- Cataracts
- Injuries

Ears
- Hearing impairment
- Use of hearing aid
- Discharge
- "Dizziness"
- Pain
- Ringing in ears
- Infections

Nose
- Nosebleeds
- Infections
- Discharge
- Frequency of colds
- Nasal obstruction
- History of injury
- Sinus infections
- Hay fever

Mouth and Throat
- Condition of teeth
- Date of most recent dental appointment
- Condition of gums
- Bleeding gums
- Frequent sore throats
- Burning sensation of tongue
- Hoarseness
- Voice changes
- Postnasal drip

Neck
- Lumps
- Goiter
- Pain on movement
- Tenderness
- History of "swollen glands"
- Thyroid trouble

Chest
- Cough
- Pain
- Shortness of breath
- Sputum production (quantity, appearance)
- Tuberculosis
- Asthma
- Pleurisy
- Bronchitis
- Coughing up blood
- Wheezing
- Most recent x-ray film
- Most recent test for tuberculosis
- History of bacille Calmette-Guérin (BCG) vaccination

Cardiac
- Chest pain
- High blood pressure
- Palpitations
- Shortness of breath with exertion
- Shortness of breath when lying flat
- Sudden shortness of breath while sleeping
- History of heart attack
- Rheumatic fever
- Heart murmur
- Most recent electrocardiogram
- Other tests for heart function

Vascular
- Pain in legs, calves, thighs, or hips while walking
- Swelling of legs
- Varicose veins
- Thrombophlebitis
- Coolness of extremity
- Loss of hair on legs
- Discoloration of extremity
- Ulcers

Breasts
- Lumps
- Discharge
- Pain
- Tenderness
- Self-examination

Gastrointestinal
- Appetite
- Excessive hunger
- Excessive thirst
- Nausea
- Swallowing
- Constipation
- Diarrhea
- Heartburn
- Vomiting
- Abdominal pain
- Change in stool color
- Change in stool caliber
- Change in stool consistency
- Frequency of bowel movements
- Vomiting blood
- Rectal bleeding
- Black, tarry stools
- Laxative or antacid use
- Excessive belching
- Food intolerance
- Change in abdominal size
- Hemorrhoids
- Infections
- Jaundice
- Rectal pain
- Previous abdominal x-ray films
- Hepatitis
- Liver disease
- Gallbladder disease

Urinary
- Frequency
- Urgency
- Difficulty in starting the stream
- Incontinence
- Excessive urination
- Pain on urination
- Burning sensation
- Blood in urine
- Infections
- Stones
- Bed-wetting
- Awakening at night to urinate
- History of retention
- Urine color
- Urine odor

Male Genitalia
- Lesions on penis
- Discharge
- Erectile dysfunction
- Pain
- Scrotal masses
- Hernias
- Frequency of intercourse
- Ability to enjoy sexual relations
- Fertility problems
- Prostate problems
- History of venereal disease and treatment

Female Genitalia
- Lesions on external genitalia
- Itching
- Discharge
- Date of most recent Pap smear and result
- Pain on intercourse
- Frequency of intercourse
- Birth control methods
- Ability to enjoy sexual relations
- Fertility problems
- Hernias
- History of venereal disease and treatment
- History of diethylstilbestrol (DES) exposure
- Age at menarche
- Interval between periods
- Duration of periods
- Amount of flow
- Date of last period
- Bleeding in between periods
- Number of pregnancies
- Abortions
- Term deliveries
- Complications of pregnancies
- Description(s) of labor
- Number of living children
- Menstrual pain
- Age at menopause
- Menopausal symptoms
- Postmenopausal bleeding

Musculoskeletal
- Weakness
- Paralysis
- Muscle stiffness
- Limitation of movement
- Joint pain
- Joint stiffness
- Arthritis
- Gout
- Back problems
- Muscle cramps
- Deformities

Neurologic
- Fainting
- "Dizziness"
- "Blackouts"
- Paralysis
- Strokes
- "Numbness"
- Tingling
- Burning sensation
- Tremors
- Loss of memory
- Psychiatric disorders
- Mood changes
- Nervousness
- Speech disorders
- Unsteadiness of gait
- General behavioral change
- Loss of consciousness
- Hallucinations
- Disorientation

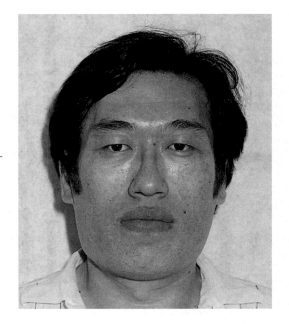

Figure 1–2 Acromegaly: facial characteristics.

might try to determine when the facial changes occurred. In such a case, you could ask the man whether he has noticed a change in his hat or baseball cap size and when he first noticed it.

Look at Figure 1-3, in which the right hand of the same patient (on the right) is compared with the right hand of a normal individual. Asking about a change in glove size would be useful with this particular patient. It would be appropriate to inquire whether there has been a change in shoe size as well.

A useful bit of information may be an old photograph of the patient to help determine when the suspected changes occurred. Compare Figure 1-2 with the photograph in Figure 1-4 (of the same patient taken 20 years earlier). Notice the bulging forehead and the prominent jaw in the later photograph. The patient has acromegaly, a condition of abnormal, excess growth hormone secreted by a pituitary tumor. The changes are insidious, occurring over many years. The photograph was helpful in determining the changes in bone and soft tissue structure.

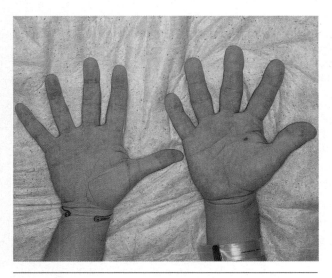

Figure 1–3 Acromegaly: characteristics of hands. Note the stubby fingers of the patient on the right, compared with the fingers of a normal hand on the left.

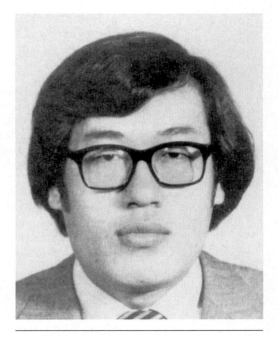

Figure 1–4 Photograph of the patient shown in Figure 1-2, taken 20 years earlier. Compare the facial features (i.e., nose and chin) in the two photographs.

Concluding Thoughts

A medical history must be dynamic. Every history is different. All patients are asked the standard questions, but each patient should be evaluated individually. There is no limit to the questions to be asked.

The *written history* is a permanent, legal document of the patient's health history. The information that is recorded must be accurate and objective. On the basis of all the information gleaned from the patient's history, the interviewer carefully summarizes all the data into a readable format. Anything that is written in a patient's record could be presented to a court of law. Only objective data should be included. Opinions or statements about previous care and therapy must be avoided.

By convention, when the review of systems is stated or written, all symptoms that the patient has experienced are indicated first. Symptoms never experienced are indicated afterward. The *pertinent positive symptoms* are symptoms that have possible relevance to the present illness. *Pertinent negative symptoms* are symptoms that are not present but are often related to the present illness.

If information in the review of systems has been described previously—in the history of present illness, for example—it is correct to indicate under the systems review of that symptom, "see history of present illness."

As you proceed with the interview, you may sense that it is not going well. Is the patient comfortable? Is there a language barrier? Did you say or do something to interfere with the rapport? Is the patient intimidated? Is the patient concerned about confidentiality? Is the patient reluctant to talk in the presence of family members? Is the patient able to express his or her feelings? These issues reflect just a few of the common reasons for lack of progression of an interview. If you can alleviate the problems, do so. Perhaps interviewing the patient on another day but using the same approach will be more successful.

The key to success in an interview is the ability to put the patient at ease. To do so, the interviewer must be relaxed. What techniques are available to the interviewer and patient to relax? One useful approach is the visualization of color; for example, if the interviewer were to say, "Close your eyes and visualize the color blue," the patient would feel a definite response in body as well as in mind. If the patient were then to let that image dissolve, take a few breaths, close the eyes again, and visualize the color red, he or she would notice that the response to this color is quite different. Red creates a different state of mind than do blue, green, yellow, and so forth.

Whether this is entirely a result of psychological association is irrelevant to this discussion. The point is that because people respond strongly to color, interviewers can influence the state of mind of patients and themselves by suggesting an atmosphere of color that calms, warms, cheers, cools, and so forth, depending on what is called for in the situation. Because color can help a patient relax, it can have beneficial effects on blood pressure, heart rate, and other bodily functions.

The same is true of the visualization of environments that are pleasant, beautiful, and peaceful. Having the patient take a few moments, with eyes closed, to imagine himself or herself in a garden or a quiet pine forest can substantially lessen nervousness and tension. The connection between relaxation and health is becoming more widely understood and accepted. According to studies in behavioral medicine, the practice of meditation has a beneficial effect in the treatment of hypertension, some heart problems, depression, and anxiety, among other illnesses.

Many visualization techniques are far from new. In the Tibetan approach to medicine, a system that developed between the 4th and 12th centuries, there is a direct connection between the state of a person's mind and the state of his or her health.

In the next chapter, the patient's responses to the questions are investigated, and the influence of background and age on those responses is observed.

Bibliography

Abrahm JL: Management of pain and spinal cord compression in patients with advanced cancer. ACP-ASIM End-of-Life Care Consensus Panel. American College of Physicians–American Society of Internal Medicine. Ann Intern Med 131:37, 1999.

Acute Pain Management Guideline Panel: Acute Pain Management: Operative or Medical Procedures and Trauma. Clinical Practice Guideline (AHCPR publication no. 92-0032). Rockville, Md, Agency for

Health Care Policy and Research, Public Health Service, U.S. Department of Health and Human Services, 1992.

Adams RM: Occupational Skin Disease, 3rd ed. Philadelphia, WB Saunders, 1999.

Adler G, Buie DH: The misuses of confrontation with borderline patients. Int J Psychoanal Psychother 1:109, 1972.

Advisory Committee on Immunization Practices (ACIP) Centers for Disease Control and Prevention (CDC): Update: Prevention of hepatitis A after exposure to hepatitis A virus and in international travelers. Updated recommendations of the Advisory Committee on Immunization Practices (ACIP). MMWR Morb Mortal Wkly Rep 56(41):1080, 2007.

Alpert EJ, Cohen S (eds): Educating the nation's physicians about family violence and abuse. Acad Med 72(Suppl):Svi, 1997.

Barrier PA: Domestic violence. Mayo Clin Proc 73:271, 1998.

Bauer HM, Mooney D: California's mandatory reporting of domestic violence injuries: Does the law go too far or not far enough? West J Med 171:118, 1999.

Benson H, Klipper MZ: The Relaxation Response, New York, Wing Books, 1975.

Bernstein J: Conversations in public places. J Commun 25:85, 1975.

Billings JA, Stoeckle JD: The Clinical Encounter: A Guide to the Medical Interview and Case Presentation, 2nd ed. St. Louis, Mosby, 1999.

Bird B: Talking with Patients, Philadelphia, JB Lippincott, 1973.

Bradley KA, Bush KR, McDonell MB, et al: Screening for problem drinking: Comparison of CAGE and AUDIT. Ambulatory Care Quality Improvement Project (ACQUIP). Alcohol Use Disorders Identification Test. J Gen Intern Med 13:379, 1998.

Breitbart W, Rosenfeld BD, Passik SD, et al: The undertreatment of pain in ambulatory AIDS patients. Pain 65:243, 1996.

Brown BL, Strong WJ, Rencher AC: Perceptions of personality from speech: Effects of manipulation of acoustical parameters. Acoust Soc Am J 54:29, 1973.

Buchwald D, Caralis PV, Gany F, et al: The medical interview across cultures. Patient Care 27:141, 1993.

Buckman R: How to Break Bad News: A Guide for Health Care Professionals, Baltimore, Johns Hopkins University Press, 1992.

Bush B, Shaw S, Cleary P, et al: Screening for alcohol abuse using the CAGE questionnaire. Am J Med 83:231, 1987.

Centers for Disease Control and Prevention: Annual smoking-attributable mortality, years of potential life lost, and productivity losses—United States, 1997–2001. MMWR Morb Mortal Wkly Rep 54(25): 625, 2005.

Centers for Disease Control and Prevention: Cigarette smoking among adults—United States, 1993. MMWR Morb Mortal Wkly Rep 43(50):925, 1994.

Centers for Disease Control and Prevention: Physician and other health-care professional counseling of smokers to quit—United States, 1991. MMWR Morb Mortal Wkly Rep 42(44):854, 1993.

Centers for Disease Control and Prevention: Recommended adult immunization schedule—United States. October 2007–September 2008. MMWR Morb Mortal Wkly Rep 56(Q1),, 2007.

Chafetz ME: No patient deserves to be patronized. Med Insight 2:68, 1970.

Cherpitel CJ: Performance of screening instruments for identifying alcohol dependence in the general population, compared with clinical populations. Alcohol Clin Exp Res 22:1399, 1998.

Clark WD: The medical interview: Focus on alcohol problems. Hosp Pract 11:59, 1985.

Cleeland CS, Gonin R, Baez L, et al: Pain and treatment of pain in minority patients with cancer. The Eastern Cooperative Oncology Group Minority Outpatient Pain Study. Ann Intern Med 127:813, 1997.

Cleeland CS, Gonin R, Hatfield AK, et al: Pain and its treatment in outpatients with metastatic cancer. N Engl J Med 330:592, 1994.

Coulehan JL, Platt FW, Egener B, et al: "Let me see if I have this right...": Words that build empathy. Ann Intern Med 135:221, 2001.

Council on Scientific Affairs, American Medical Association: Violence against women: Relevance for medical practitioners. JAMA 267:3184, 1992.

Culliton BJ: Doctor, are you there? Am J Med 109:602, 2000.

Eisenberg DM: Advising patients who seek alternative medical therapies. Ann Intern Med 127:61, 1997.

Ende J, Rockwell S, Glasgow M: The sexual history in general medicine practice. Arch Intern Med 144:558, 1984.

Ewing JA: Detecting alcoholism: The CAGE questionnaire. JAMA 252:1905, 1984.

Ewing JA, Rouse BA: Identifying the hidden alcoholic. Presented at the 29th International Congress on Alcohol and Drug Dependence, Sydney, Australia, February 3, 1970.

Faust S, Drickey R: Working with interpreters. J Fam Pract 22:131, 1986.

Fields R: Drugs in Perspective: A Personalized Look at Substance Use and Abuse, 4th ed. Boston, McGraw-Hill, 2001.

Fiellin DA, Reid MC, O'Connor PG: Outpatient management of patients with alcohol problems. Ann Intern Med 133:815, 2000.

Fiellin DA, Reid MC, O'Connor PG: Screening for alcohol problems in primary care: A systematic review. Arch Intern Med 160:1977, 2000.

Fiore AE: Hepatitis A Transmitted by Food. Clin Infect Dis 38:705, 2004.

Foley KM: The treatment of cancer pain. N Engl J Med 313:84, 1985.

Francis V, Korsch BM, Morris MJ: Gaps in doctor-patient communication. N Engl J Med 280:535, 1969.

Goldman RH, Peters JM: The occupational and environmental health history. JAMA 246:2831, 1981.

Haffner L: Translation is not enough: Interpreting in a medical setting. West J Med 157:255, 1992.

Hart CL, Smith GD, Hole DJ, et al: Alcohol consumption and mortality from all causes, coronary heart disease, and stroke: Results from a prospective cohort study of Scottish men with 21 years of follow up. BMJ 318:1725, 1999.

Henningfield JE: Nicotine medications for smoking cessation. N Engl J Med 333:1196, 1995.

Herdman R, Hewitt M, Laschober M: Smoking-Related Deaths and Financial Costs: Office of Technology Assessment Estimates for 1990. Washington, DC, U.S. Congress, Office of Technology Assessment, 1993.

Holland JC, Passik S, Kash KM, et al: The role of religious and spiritual beliefs in coping with malignant melanoma. Psychooncology 8:14, 1999.

Jewell ME, Jewell GS: How to assess the risk of HIV exposure. Am Fam Physician 40:153, 1989.

Landrigan PJ, Baker DB: The recognition and control of occupational disease. JAMA 266:676, 1991.

Larsen KM, Smith CK: Assessment of nonverbal communication in the patient-doctor relationship. J Fam Pract 12:48, 1981.

Leppala JM, Paunio M, Virtamo J, et al: Alcohol consumption and stroke incidence in male smokers. Circulation 100:1209, 1999.

Levinson W: Physician-patient communication: A key to malpractice prevention. JAMA 272:1619, 1994.

Levinson W, Gorawara-Bhat R, Lamb J: A study of patient clues and physician responses in primary care and surgical settings. JAMA 284:1021, 2000.

Levinson W, Roter DL, Mullooly JP, et al: Physician-patient communication: The relationship with malpractice claims among primary care physicians and surgeons. JAMA 277:553, 1997.

Marks RM, Sachar EJ: Undertreatment of medical inpatients with narcotic analgesics. Ann Intern Med 78:173, 1973.

Marvel MK, Epstein RM, Flowers K, et al: Soliciting the patient's agenda: Have we improved? JAMA 281:283, 1999.

Matthews D, Hingson R: Improving patient compliance: A guide to physicians. Med Clin North Am 61:879, 1977.

Mayfield D, McLeod G, Hall P: The CAGE questionnaire: Validation of a new alcoholism screening instrument. Am J Psychiatry 131:1121, 1974.

McEwen BS: Protective and damaging effects of stress mediators. N Engl J Med 338:171, 1998.

Meier DE, Morrison RS, Cassel CK: Improving palliative care. Ann Intern Med 127:225, 1997.

Molyneux A: Nicotine replacement therapy. BMJ 328:454, 2004.

Morrison RS, Wallenstein S, Natale DK, et al: "We don't carry that"—failure of pharmacies in predominantly nonwhite neighborhoods to stock opioid analgesics. N Engl J Med 342:1023, 2000.

Mutsch M, Spicher VM, Gut C, et al: Hepatitis A virus infections in travelers, 1988–2004. Clin Infect Dis c42:490, 2006.

Myerscough PR: Talking with Patients: A Basic Clinical Skill, Oxford, UK, Oxford University Press, 1992.

National Institutes of Health: The Physician's Guide to Helping Patients with Alcohol Problems (NIH publication no. 95-3769). Rockville, Md, U.S. Department of Health and Human Services, 1995.

Neufeld B: SAFE questions: Overcoming barriers to the detection of domestic violence. Am Fam Physician 53:2575, 1996.

Newman LS: Occupational illness. N Engl J Med 333:1128, 1995.

O'Hanlan KA, Cabaj RP, Schatz B, et al: A review of the medical consequences of homophobia with suggestions for resolution. J Gay Lesbian Med Assoc 1:25, 1997.

Ong LML, de Haes JCJM, Hoos AM, et al: Doctor-patient communication: A review of the literature. Soc Sci Med 40:903, 1995.

Peabody FW: The care of the patient. JAMA 88:877, 1927.

Platt FW, Gasper DL, Coulehan JL, et al: "Tell me about yourself": The patient-centered interview. Ann Intern Med 134:1083, 2001.

Platt FW, Gordon GH: Field Guide to the Difficult Patient Interview, Philadelphia, Lippincott Williams & Wilkins, 1999.

Post SG, Puchalski CM, Larson DB: Physicians and patient spirituality: Professional boundaries, competency, and ethics. Ann Intern Med 132:578, 2000.

Puchalski CM, Romer AL: Taking a spiritual history allows clinicians to understand patients more fully. J Palliat Med 3:129, 2000.

Rosenstock L, Cullen M: Textbook of Clinical Occupational and Environmental Medicine, 2nd ed. Philadelphia, WB Saunders, 1994.

Roter D, Stewart M (eds): Communication with Medical Patients. Newbury Park, CA, Sage, 1989.

Samet JH, Rollnick S, Barnes H: Beyond CAGE: A brief clinical approach after detection of substance abuse. Arch Intern Med 156:2287, 1996.

Sanders SA, Reinisch JM: Would you say you "had sex" if…? JAMA 281:275, 1999.

Sargent JD, DiFranza JR: Tobacco control for clinicians who treat adolescents. CA Cancer J Clin 53:102, 2003.

Schatz B, O'Hanlan K: Anti-Gay Discrimination in Medicine: Results of a National Survey of Lesbian, Gay and Bisexual Physicians. San Francisco, Gay and Lesbian Medical Association, 1994.

Schenker Y, Lo B, Ettinger KM, et al: Navigating language barriers under difficult circumstances. Ann Intern Med 149:264, 2008.

Sloan RP, Bagiella E, Powell T: Religion, spirituality, and medicine. Lancet 353:664, 1999.

Smith WR, Penberthy LT, Bovbjerg VE, et al: Daily assessment of pain in adults with sickle cell disease. Ann Intern Med 148:94, 2008.

Spiro II: What is empathy and can it be taught? Ann Intern Med 116:843, 1992.

Steiner JF, Earnest MA: The language of medication-taking. Ann Intern Med 132:926, 2000.

Suchman AL, Markakis K, Beckman HB, et al: A model of empathic communication in the medical interview. JAMA 277:678, 1997.

SUPPORT Principal Investigators: A controlled trial to improve care for seriously ill hospitalized patients. The Study to Understand Prognoses and Preferences for Outcomes and Risks of Treatment (SUPPORT). JAMA 274:1591, 1995.

Tomlinson J, Milgrom ET: Taking a sexual history. West J Med 170:284, 1999.

Tonstad S, Tonnesen P, Hajek P, et al: Effect of maintenance therapy with varenicline on smoking cessation: A randomized controlled trial. JAMA 296:64, 2006.

Travis LB, Rabkin CS, Brown LM, et al: Cancer survivorship—genetic susceptibility and second primary cancers: Research strategies and recommendations. J Natl Cancer Inst 98(1):15, 2006.

U.S. Department of Health and Human Services: The Health Consequences of Smoking: A Report of the Surgeon General. Atlanta, GA: U.S. Department of Health and Human Services, Centers for Disease Control and Prevention, National Center for Chronic Disease Prevention and Health Promotion, Office on Smoking and Health, 2004.

Vertosick FT: Why We Hurt: The Natural History of Pain, New York, Harcourt, 2000.

Victor JC, Surdina TY, Suleimenova SZ, et al: Person-to-person transmission of hepatitis A virus in an urban area of intermediate endemicity: Implications for vaccination strategies. Am J Epidemiol 163:204, 2006.

Zhang U, Kreger B, Dorgan JF, et al: Alcohol consumption and the risk of breast cancer: The Framingham Study revisited. Am J Epidemiol 149:93, 1999.

Zimmerman GL, Olsen CG, Bosworth MF: A "stages of change" approach to helping patients change behavior. Am Fam Physician 61:1409, 2000.

CHAPTER 2

The Patient's Responses

It is our duty to remember at all times and anew that medicine is not only a science, but also the art of letting our own individuality interact with the individuality of the patient.

Albert Schweitzer (1875–1965)

Responses to Illness

Health is characterized by a state of well-being, enthusiasm, and energetic pursuit of life's goals. Illness is characterized by feelings of discomfort, helplessness, and a diminished interest in the future. Once patients recognize that they are ill and possibly face their own mortality, a series of emotional reactions occurs, including anxiety, fear, depression, denial, projection, regression, anger, frustration, withdrawal, and an exaggeration of symptoms. These psychological reactions are general and are not specific to any particular physical illness. Patients must learn to cope not only with the symptoms of the illness but also with life as it is altered by the illness.

Conflict is an important medical and psychological concept to understand. Patients live with conflict. What is conflict? Conflict exists when a patient has a symptom and wants to have it evaluated by a member of the health-care team, but the patient does not want to learn that it represents a "bad" disease process. Conflict is very widespread in medical practice. It is very common for patients to be seen by a physician and at the very end of the consultation, the patient may state, "Oh doctor, there is one other thing that I wanted to tell you!" That information is often the most important reason for that patient to have sought consultation. Patients with an acute myocardial infarction often suffer chest pain for several weeks before the actual event. They convince themselves that it is indigestion or musculoskeletal pain; they do not seek medical attention because they do not want to receive a diagnosis of coronary heart disease. The health-care provider must be able to identify conflict, which is often a precursor of denial, to facilitate care of the patient.

Anxiety

Anxiety is a state of uneasiness in which the patient has a sense of impending danger. It is the fundamental response to stress of any kind, such as separation, injury, social disapproval, or decreased self-esteem. Anxiety and fear are common reactions to the stress of illness. The terms *anxiety* and *fear* are often used interchangeably. There are, however, two important differences. First, fear tends to be specific and is triggered by a specific event or object; in contrast, anxiety tends to be more diffuse, often occurring without a specific trigger. Second, fear is more acute and tends to appear rapidly, whereas anxiety develops more slowly and takes longer to resolve. The feelings of loss of control, guilt, and frustration contribute to the patient's emotional reaction. Illness makes patients feel helpless. Recognizing the body's mortality leads patients

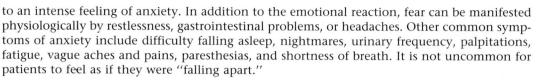

to an intense feeling of anxiety. In addition to the emotional reaction, fear can be manifested physiologically by restlessness, gastrointestinal problems, or headaches. Other common symptoms of anxiety include difficulty falling asleep, nightmares, urinary frequency, palpitations, fatigue, vague aches and pains, paresthesias, and shortness of breath. It is not uncommon for patients to feel as if they were "falling apart."

The young man who has been stricken with a heart attack feels helpless. As he lies in his intensive care unit bed, he begins to recognize that he really is mortal. The patient believes that he must be dependent on everyone and everything: the nurse, the doctor, the intravenous line, even the monitor. His anxiety, based on helplessness, is a normal response to his illness. His sudden illness and the threat of possible death oppose his belief that he is indestructible.

A 72-year-old man who has lived alone for years since his wife's death is admitted to a hospital for a transurethral prostatectomy. He is anxious that he may become dependent on his children. He may be more threatened by his fear of dependency than by the illness itself.

The hospitalized patient who is brought to the radiology department for a routine chest x-ray film and is forced to wait for 2 hours for a transporter to bring her back to her room suffers anxiety. She is angry that she has been left waiting and perhaps has missed some visitors, but she says nothing. Her anxiety is based on the fear of expressing anger to the nurses and staff members on the floor. She believes that if she were to express her anger, the hospital personnel might interfere with her medical care.

Some hospitalized patients cannot accept the love and care expressed by family or friends. This inability to accept tenderness is a common source of anxiety. Such patients feel threatened by these affectionate acts because they serve to reinforce their dependency.

All patients who are admitted to a hospital experience anxiety. The patients must put their most important commodity, their lives, into the hands of a group of strangers who may or may not be competent to assume responsibility for the patients' survival.

It is most important for the interviewer to identify the causes or roots of a patient's fear or anxiety, as well as to acknowledge the existence of the patient's feelings without expressing judgment. Whenever possible, the interviewer should provide some information to allay the patient's fear or anxiety.

Depression

Depression is a term used to describe a chronic state of lowering of mood. Some patients have a predilection for depression, but depression is a common state, occurring in more than 20% of all patients with major illnesses, particularly cancer.

Depression is a psychological reaction to the loss of health, a loved one, or one's own self-esteem. Certain degrees of depression probably accompany every chronic illness. There are many types of depression; reactive, neurotic, manic, melancholic, and agitated are only a few types. In general, patients with depression have pessimistic tones in speech and a downcast facial expression. They may express feelings of futility and self-accusation. They respond to questions with brief answers. Their speech is slow; their volume is low; their pitch is monotonous. Depressed patients feel inadequate, worthless, and defeated. They also suffer profound feelings of guilt. A remark such as "You look sad" invites these patients to talk about their depression. Crying can relieve severe depressive feelings, even if only momentarily, and thus enables patients to continue their story. Although crying may be brought on by patients' concern for their own illness, crying usually occurs when patients think of an illness or death of a loved one or of a potential loss. They often have much hostility and resentment and suffer from rejection and loneliness. Self-accusative and self-deprecating delusions can occur in severely depressed patients. When these delusions are present, the feelings of worthlessness are so overwhelming that patients may believe that suicide is the only way out.

For example, a 23-year-old law student is engulfed by anxiety when he learns that he has acquired immunodeficiency syndrome (AIDS). When his friends and family learn of the illness, he is immediately excluded from all relationships. He has extreme feelings of guilt. His depression is worsened when he learns that his university has asked him to discontinue his studies. He is found later hanged in his parents' attic. His only way of coping with his illness has been through suicide.

Depression may be the most common reaction to illness, as well as the most frequently overlooked. The most important diagnostic symptoms of depression are the following:

- Markedly diminished interest or pleasure in almost all activities
- Insomnia

- Change in appetite or weight
- Fatigue or loss of energy
- Agitation
- Feelings of guilt or worthlessness
- Decreased ability to think or concentrate
- Thoughts of death or suicide

Interviewers must not ignore any talk of suicide. If patients bring up suicidal thoughts, interviewers must get the assistance of someone experienced in the field.

Denial

Denial consists of acting and thinking as if a part of reality is not true. Denial is one of the most common psychological mechanisms of defense and can occur in both patients and health-care providers. Denial is often an emotional response to inner tension and prevents a painful conflict from producing overt anxiety. It is actually a form of self-deception. Denial is often observed in patients with terminal illnesses or with chronic, incurable diseases. In general, the more acute the illness, the greater is the patient's acceptance; the more insidious, the greater the denial.

A patient dying slowly from cancer can observe his or her weight decreasing and the side effects of medications. Frequent visits to the hospital for chemotherapy or radiation therapy confirm the severity of the illness; yet, in spite of all this, the patient may continue to deny the illness. He or she makes plans for the future and talks about the time when he or she will be cured. Denial is the psychological mechanism that keeps this patient going. The interviewer should not confront the patient's denial despite its apparent absurdity. Telling such a patient to "face the facts" is cruel. Breaking down denial in such a patient serves only to add to the dying patient's misery. However, the patient's family must understand and accept the poor prognosis.

Denial can sometimes obstruct proper medical care. A woman presents to a breast clinic with an orange-sized mass in one breast. The mass has already started to ulcerate, with a resultant foul-smelling infection. When asked how long she has had the mass, she responds that she noticed it "just yesterday." It is often best to interview a reliable informant when the patient with denial is recognized.

Figure 2-1 illustrates another example of the tragic sequelae of denial. This man has a basal cell carcinoma of the face. As is discussed in Chapter 8, The Skin, basal cell carcinomas are very slow growing and rarely metastasize; they are locally invasive. Had the patient sought medical attention when the lesion first appeared (and was very small), he would have been totally cured. A person's denial can be so deep that it prevents him or her from seeing reality and seeking medical attention. It is therefore important for the health-care provider to be sensitive to this very powerful psychological mechanism. For another example of denial, see the unfortunate patient depicted in Figure 16-8.

Projection

Projection is another common defense mechanism by which people unconsciously reject an unacceptable emotional feature in themselves and "project" it onto someone else. It is the major mechanism involved in the development of paranoid feelings. For example, hostile patients may say to interviewers, "Why are you being so hostile to me?" In reality, such patients are projecting *their* hostility onto the interviewers.

Patients commonly project their anxieties onto doctors. Patients who use projection are constantly watching a doctor's face for subtle signs of their own fears. For example, a 42-year-old woman with a strong family history of death from breast cancer has intense fears of developing the disease. During the inspection portion of the physical examination, the patient may be watching the clinician's face for information. If the clinician frowns or makes some type of negative gesture, the patient may interpret this as "The doctor sees something wrong!" The clinician may have made this expression thinking about the amount of work still to be done that day or what type of medication to prescribe for another patient. The patient has projected her anxiety onto the clinician. The clinician must be aware of these silent "conversations."

In some instances, projection may have a constructive value, saving the patient from being overwhelmed by the illness.

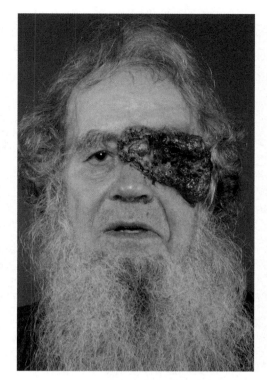

Figure 2–1 A portrait of denial. This man has a locally invasive basal cell carcinoma.

Regression

Regression is a common defense mechanism by which the patient with extreme anxiety attempts unconsciously to return to earlier, more desirable stages of development. During these periods, the individual enjoyed full gratification and freedom from anxiety. Regressed patients become dependent on others and free themselves from the complex problems that have created their anxiety.

For example, consider a middle-aged married man who has recently been told that he has inoperable lung cancer that has already spread to his bones. He is stricken with grief and intense anxiety. There are so many unanswered questions. How long will he live? Will his last months be plagued with unremitting pain? How will his wife be able to raise their young child by herself? How will she manage financially without his income? By regression, the patient can flee this anxiety by becoming childlike and dependent. The patient becomes withdrawn, shy, and often rebellious; he now requires more affection.

A teenager learns that the cause of his 6-month history of weakness and bleeding gums has been diagnosed as acute leukemia. He learns that he will spend what little time he has left in the hospital undergoing chemotherapy. His reaction to his anxiety may be regression. He now needs his parents at his bedside around the clock. He becomes more desirous of his parents' love and kisses. His redevelopment of enuresis (bed-wetting) is part of his psychological reaction to his illness.

A 25-year-old woman with inflammatory bowel disease has had many admissions to hospitals for exacerbations of her disease. She fears the future and the possibility that a cancer may have already started to develop. She is engulfed by a feeling of terror and apprehension. She fears that some day she may require a colostomy and that she will be deprived of one of her most important functions: bowel control. She acts inappropriately, has temper tantrums, and is indecisive. Her dependency on her parents is a manifestation of regression.

Responses to the Interviewer

Much of the enjoyment of medical practice comes from talking with patients. Each patient brings a challenge to the interviewer. Just as there are no two identical interviews, there are no two people who would interview the same patient in the same manner. This section describes a few characteristically troubling patient "types" and indicates some strategies for how the interview may be modified in each case.

Many of the patients to be described can arouse intensely negative feelings in the interviewer; as such, these patients have been collectively called "the hateful patient." The interviewer should recognize these feelings and deal with them directly so that they do not interfere with the interaction. The interviewer must recognize early in the interaction the general characteristics of these patient types so that he or she can facilitate the interview appropriately.

A variety of pejorative labels have unfortunately been given to many of these patient types. The labels serve only to reduce the interviewer's stress through the use of humor. This humor is demeaning to patients and can ultimately prevent them from receiving the proper medical care they deserve.

The Silent Patient

Some patients have a lifelong history of shyness. Some of these individuals lack self-confidence. They are very concerned about their self-image and do not want to say or do the wrong thing. These patients are easily embarrassed. Other individuals become hostile or silent as fear of illness develops. Many silent patients are seriously depressed, which may be a primary response as a result of the illness itself or a secondary response to it. These patients commonly have many of the other signs of depression, as seen in their attitude, facial expressions, and posture. The use of open-ended questions with these patients is usually of little value. Carefully directed questioning may yield some of the answers.

The Overtalkative Patient

The overtalkative patient presents a challenge to the novice interviewer. These patients dominate the interview; the interviewer can hardly get a word in. Every question gets a long answer. Even the answers to "yes-no" questions seem endless. There is usually an aggressive quality to this patient's communications. Every answer is overdetailed. A courteous interruption followed by another direct question helps focus on the subject of the interview. The use of open-ended questions, facilitations, or silence is to be avoided because these techniques encourage such a patient to continue speaking. If all else fails, the interviewer should try to relax and accept the problem.

The Seductive Patient

One of the most difficult types of patients for the novice to interview and examine is the seductive patient. In many ways, it is more difficult to deal with the seductive patient than with a hostile patient. Many of these patients have one of the personality disorders (e.g., histrionic, narcissistic) and harbor fantasies of developing an intimate relationship with their physician. These patients are often attractive and tend to be flashy in the way they dress, walk, and talk. They commonly offer inappropriate compliments to the interviewer to gain his or her attention. The patients are frequently emotionally labile. Not uncommonly, these patients expose themselves physically early in the interview. The interviewer may elect to cover the patient, but usually this is unsuccessful, as the patient may expose him/herself again. It is difficult for the interviewer to cope with his or her own feelings when he or she is attracted to such a patient. The feeling of attraction is a natural one, and the interviewer must accept it. However, the interviewer must always maintain a strictly professional demeanor. Empathy and reassurance must be kept to a minimum because these supportive techniques stimulate further fantasies in the patient. The interviewer must always maintain professional distance. It may be necessary to say, "Thank you for your nice compliments, but in order for me to help you, we must keep our relationship strictly professional. I hope you understand." If necessary, the interviewer should get the advice of someone he or she trusts.

The Angry Patient

Angry, obnoxious, or hostile patients are common. Some make demeaning comments or are sarcastic, whereas others are demanding, aggressive, and blatantly hostile. Some hostile patients may remain silent during most of the interview. At other times, they may make inappropriate remarks that are condescending to the novice or even to the experienced clinician. The interviewer may feel resentment, anger, threatened authority, impatience, or frustration. Reciprocal hostility should be avoided, for a power struggle can develop.

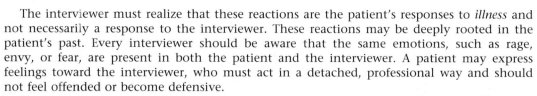

The interviewer must realize that these reactions are the patient's responses to *illness* and not necessarily a response to the interviewer. These reactions may be deeply rooted in the patient's past. Every interviewer should be aware that the same emotions, such as rage, envy, or fear, are present in both the patient and the interviewer. A patient may express feelings toward the interviewer, who must act in a detached, professional way and should not feel offended or become defensive.

Students of the health-care professions may have been taught that they must like their patients to treat them appropriately. Ambivalence in the interviewer can be a problem. Health-care providers must treat patients medically correctly and with respect, but in fact it is not necessary to like the patient in order to provide good care. Because of their illness, patients may have feelings of loss of control, threatened authority, and fear. Their anger is the mechanism by which they attempt to handle their fears. Once interviewers gain this insight and become aware of their own feelings, they can better treat such patients. Interviewers must accept and restrain their own negative feelings toward the patients so that their professional judgment is not distorted. Interviewers' awareness of their own anxieties and feelings aids in conducting a more productive interview. Conscious expression of the interviewer's own feelings in a frank and noninsulting manner facilitates the interviewing process. Regulation and control of the interviewer's feelings is the goal.

Confrontation may be a useful technique for interviewing such patients. By saying, "You sound very angry," the interviewer allows patients to vent some of their fears. Another confrontational approach is to say, "You're obviously angry about something. Tell me what you think is wrong." Maintain equanimity and avoid becoming defensive. If at the beginning of the interview the patient is angry, try to calm the patient. Proceed slowly with questioning, avoid interpretations, and ask questions that are confined to the history of the present illness.

The Paranoid Patient

The paranoid patient constantly asks, "Why are you asking me that? Do I have...?" When the interviewer asks the many questions in the review of systems, the patient responds, "Who told you about that?" Paranoid patients think there is some devious plan and that people are constantly talking about them. The patients' suspiciousness can sometimes be handled by the interviewer's saying, "These are routine questions that I ask all my patients." Reassurance tends to be threatening to these patients and should not be used because it tends to produce more suspicion. The patient's delusion is beyond reason. The interviewer should therefore complete the questioning and not try to convince such patients about their false ideations. Avoidance of any anger by the interviewer is of paramount importance.

The Insatiable Patient

Insatiable patients are never satisfied. They have many questions, and despite adequate explanations, they feel that the interviewer has not answered all their questions. They tend to be very sensitive, anxious individuals. These patients are best handled with a firm, noncondescending approach. A definite closing statement is helpful, such as "We have reached the end of our time for today, but I will be back." Alternatively, the interviewer could say, "We have reached the end of our time for today. I will refer your concerns to Dr. ____."

The Ingratiating Patient

The ingratiating patient attempts to please the interviewer. Such patients believe that they must provide the "right" answers to satisfy the interviewer. They think that if they answer a question in a way that arouses the disapproval of the interviewer, the interviewer will abandon them. Intense feelings of possible rejection are present in this type of patient. The interviewer must recognize that anxiety is the cause of the patient's behavior and should try not to respond to that behavior. The interviewer should recognize the patient's tendency of trying to please and should stress to the patient how important it is to be accurate.

The Aggressive Patient

Many aggressive patients have a personality disorder. Such patients are easily irritated and often fly into a rage when dealing with the normal stresses of daily life. They are domineering and try to control the interview. However, if allowed to have their way, they may be quite pleasant. Frequently, aggressive patients have intense dependency needs that they cannot consciously handle. These patients mask the primary problem by becoming aggressive and hostile to disguise their anxiety and feelings of inadequacy and inferiority. Aggressive patients are difficult to interview. The interviewer must try carefully to avoid areas provoking anxiety early in the interview. Once a rapport is established, the interviewer may attempt to delve into the deeper areas. In general, aggressive patients refuse any type of psychotherapy.

The Help-Rejecting Patient

Help-rejecting patients are usually not hostile. They describe having been seen by many "expert" physicians for help and often tell interviewers that no one can find out what is wrong with them. They return again and again to the doctors' offices, indicating that the physicians' suggestions "didn't work." Commonly, when a symptom appears relieved, another suddenly appears. These patients use their symptoms to enhance their relationship with their doctors. Such patients are often very depressed, although they may deny it. They believe that they have made many self-sacrifices and have had countless disappointments, which they attribute to their "illness." The best approach to these individuals is strong emotional support and gentle reasoning. Despite the need for psychiatric help, these patients usually refuse to accept it.

The Demanding Patient

The demanding patient makes demands of everyone: the physician, the nurse, the student, the aide. These patients use intimidation and guilt to force others to take care of them. They view themselves as being neglected and abused. They may have outbursts of anger toward physicians, who may fear for their own reputations. A power struggle may result. Inform the patient that it is good that he or she came in and that you will do everything possible to help.

The Compulsive Patient

Compulsive patients are concerned about every detail of their lives. These patients pride themselves on their ability to solve all problems, but when their health deteriorates, they lose their composure because they cannot deal with ambiguity or uncertainty. They deny their feelings of anger and anxiety, and projection is a common reaction to their illness. In dealing with the compulsive patient, the interviewer must provide very detailed and specific information to the patient in a straightforward manner. The patient should be allowed as much control as possible, and all the possibilities discussed should be explained clearly.

The Dependent Patient

The dependent patient finds life difficult without the help of others. The other persons provide the necessary support, both emotional and physical. If this support is removed, the patient feels hurt and deserted and demands even more help. When dependent persons become ill, they imagine that their illness will lead to loss of their support groups. Thus, dependent patients need to be cared for most closely. Sometimes, however, these patients can take advantage of a compassionate health-care provider by demanding enormous amounts of time. Be as direct as possible when informing such patients of the appropriate limits without leaving them rejected. The interviewer might say, "You've given me a lot to think about. I do have to leave now. Please don't feel I'm rejecting you. I'll be back later to discuss some of your other problems."

The Masochistic Patient

The masochistic, or self-defeating, patient goes through life suffering. Although these patients need to continue to suffer mentally, they do not seek physical abuse or pain. The masochistic patient is dedicated to a life of self-sacrifice. In contrast to other types of patients, this type adapts well to illness and, in fact, may feel threatened by recovery. Thus, such patients often frustrate physicians. The goal for these patients is to be able to function despite their problems. Interviewers should not promise cures because this creates more problems for the patient and the health-care provider.

The Borderline Patient

Borderline patients are defined as individuals with a personality disorder who have an instability in their personal relationships, engage in impulsive behavior, and have unstable moods. Intense, fluctuating emotions of love and hate are typical of borderline patients. They need emotional support because they are constantly threatened by people and circumstances. It is often very difficult to develop a good doctor-patient relationship with borderline patients because the swings of affect are rapid. Borderline patients are always afraid, but this fear may be masked by outbreaks of anger. These patients are best handled with reassuring words.

Influence of Background and Age on Patient Response

Although disease is universal, patients respond to their illnesses differently. A particular question asked of different patients is answered in a style that is governed by the patient's ethnic background, emotions, customs, age, medical history, social history, and family history. These factors determine the way in which a patient perceives and responds to a question. This section illustrates the importance of understanding a patient's background as an aid to better communication. The important influence of ethnic and cultural background on the patient response is discussed at length in Chapter 3, Caring for Patients in a Culturally Diverse Society.

The Child Who Is Ill

Children tend always to be "on guard." Ill children are especially vulnerable and wary. First, they are taken from their "friendly" home environment. Second, doctors, nurses, and students are constantly staring at them with a wide variety of facial expressions. Many older children believe that the physician has some sort of "magical eye" that can see through them and know everything about them. This all adds up to a frightening experience for youngsters. Frequently, tests that cause discomfort may have to be performed by those "people in white." The health-care provider becomes a symbol of danger and pain.

When the physicians, nurses, or technicians take the youngster for a test, the child experiences his or her greatest fear: separation from parents. This separation produces intense fear and anxiety, manifested by wailing, irritability, and aggressive behavior. The child's fear is that he or she will not see his or her parents again. This fear may actually be subconscious. Health-care providers should explain to the child, if old enough, that they know why the child is crying and should assure the child that he or she will see his or her parents soon. Parents should be urged to talk to their children, informing them that the doctor is going to help them. The parents should be careful *not* to indicate that the doctor will *not* hurt the child, because if the child has pain as a result of a test, the child-parent relationship may be jeopardized. The parent should be encouraged to stay with the child in the hospital as long as possible and even sleep in the child's room at night, if permitted. Studies have shown that when parents are permitted to stay with their children, the recovery is quicker and there is less emotional trauma. An important part of caring for children is talking to the parents. If the parents understand the situation, they can do much to help the doctor-child relationship.

Disabled children, like disabled adults, are extremely apprehensive of the atmosphere in the hospital. It reminds them of previous experiences. The interviewer must take time to play with the child while talking to the parent or the person accompanying the child. Complimenting the youngster with statements such as "How pretty you are" or "What a nice outfit you're wearing" seems to foster good will. These children crave love, affection, and attention. The parent has to be reassured that the staff members are reliable and caring. This will give the parent peace of mind. If a child wishes to keep a favorite toy or blanket, there should be no restrictions. Separation from home and family is a terrible experience for any child, but it is even more so for disabled children, who function better in familiar surroundings.

The Aged Patient

The aged patient requires a lot of attention. Depression is prevalent among elderly persons. Aged patients must frequently cope with the loss of loved ones and other important persons in their life. They are also stressed by changes in their own self-images and the way they are perceived by others. Deterioration in bodily function also contributes to depression in aged patients.

A patient's depression may be so severe that he or she may consider suicide a reasonable alternative to living with a severe chronic illness or living alone after the death of a spouse. Among this bereaved population, more deaths within the first 4 years after the spouse's death result from suicide than from all other causes.

The interviewer must never assume that older patients' complaints are natural for their age. People do not die of old age; they die of illnesses. Most of these patients are alert and capable of independent living. The ones who are unable to care for themselves are usually accompanied by a family member or an attendant. The interviewer must obtain as much information as possible from these sources. The interviewer should also refrain from using patronizing mannerisms that belittle the individual. A friendly, respectful approach reassures the patient. Aged patients should be advised about everything that will be done to them. This makes patients confident that there will be no unpleasant surprises. Because of advanced age, such patients may be afraid of dying. Those who are afraid should be reassured that everything possible will be done to make them better. Many people survive an illness because of their desire to live and therefore fight to stay alive. Overzealous reassurance is not appropriate for all aged patients; many regard death as a reasonable outcome.

The Widowed Patient

Many widowed patients come to the hospital alone, with the thought that because their spouses are gone, nobody cares about them. They may be suffering from depression as a result of loneliness. The interviewer should inquire gently whether there are any children, relatives, or friends who can be contacted or will come to visit. Such a patient may be at odds with his or her children and may prefer that the children not know that the patient has entered a hospital. In other cases, the family may live far away. The patients do not want their family to worry, so they do not tell the family. In these cases, it is advisable for the clinician to alert the social worker to the particular situation. Volunteers visiting the patient, as well as members of the clergy, can bring soothing counsel. A warm handshake and reassurance are effective ways of putting this patient in a relaxed state of mind. Many widowed patients are quite active. The clinician should not presume that all widowed individuals are isolated.

The Patient with Post-traumatic Stress Disorder

Although the effects of natural calamities and their aftermaths have been recognized since the time of ancient Greece, it is only since 1980 that the American Psychiatric Association included post-traumatic stress disorder (PTSD) in its handbook of psychiatric disorders, the *Diagnostic and Statistical Manual of Mental Disorders*, third edition (*DSM-III*). One of the first descriptions of PTSD was made by the Greek historian Herodotus. In 490 BCE, he described an Athenian soldier who suffered no injury in the Battle of Marathon but became permanently blind after witnessing the death of a fellow soldier. Health-care providers are only beginning to recognize the enormous toll that trauma can take in personal suffering and functional impairment. PTSD may also have an impact on future generations through effects on parental (or guardian) behavior and competence.

For many years, PTSD was considered only a wartime affliction. During World War I, PTSD was called "shell shock," and during World War II, it was referred to as "combat fatigue." After the Vietnam War, it was often mistakenly called the "post-Vietnam syndrome." It has been estimated that 15% of 500,000 veterans of the Vietnam War are affected with PTSD. These patients have a variety of symptoms, including nightmares, sleep disturbances, avoidance reactions, guilt, intrusive memories, and dissociative flashbacks. In addition, as much as 9% to 10% of the U.S. population may have some form of PTSD. Almost 18% of 10 million women who were victims of physical assault have PTSD. Studies have shown that PTSD develops in 2% of people exposed to any type of accident, 30% of those exposed to a community disaster, 25% of those who have experienced traumatic bereavement, 65% of those experiencing nonsexual assault, 85% of battered women in shelters, and 50% to 90% of those who were raped. Of all psychiatric disorders, PTSD poses one of the greatest challenges to the health-care provider because of its complexity and variability of signs and symptoms.

In 1987, the revised *DSM-III* (*DSM-III-R*) defined PTSD as including traumatic events that were "outside the range of usual human experience and that would be markedly distressing to almost anyone." PTSD is a normal reaction to an abnormal amount of stress. Although trauma

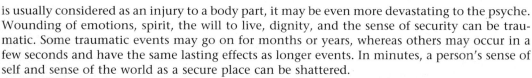

is usually considered as an injury to a body part, it may be even more devastating to the psyche. Wounding of emotions, spirit, the will to live, dignity, and the sense of security can be traumatic. Some traumatic events may go on for months or years, whereas others may occur in a few seconds and have the same lasting effects as longer events. In minutes, a person's sense of self and sense of the world as a secure place can be shattered.

One problem with the *DSM-III-R* description is that it fails to recognize the importance of the subjective appraisal of the event; this includes the ethnocultural aspects of PTSD. The 1994 edition, *DSM-IV*, lists PTSD as the only diagnosis that identifies the origin of symptoms from external events rather than from within the individual. All the following *DSM-IV* criteria must be met to make a diagnosis of PTSD:

- Experience of a traumatic event
- Experience of the trauma
- Evidence of numbing or other avoidance behavior
- Exhibition of signs of hyperarousal
- Evidence of symptoms for at least 1 month
- Experience of difficulties at home, work, or in other important areas of life as a result of the symptoms

Life is filled with many crises, such as losing a parent or being robbed. Although these events can be stressful, they are not considered "traumatic." A *traumatic event* is defined as an unusual occurrence that is not part of normal human experience and that evokes extreme helplessness, fear, and despair. Examples of traumatic events include a natural catastrophe, such as a tornado, hurricane, volcano, earthquake, fire, landslide, or flood; a human catastrophe, such as war, concentration camps, refugee camps, sexual assault, physical assault, or other forms of victimization; witnessing a death, rape, torture, or beating; a suicide of a family member or close friend; and any exposure to danger of one's own safety and life.

Experiencing the trauma can take many forms, including dreams, flashbacks, or situations that remind the person of the traumatic event. While dreaming, the person may shout, shake, or thrash about the bed. Although the person may awake suddenly, he or she may not remember the nightmare, but the intense emotion may persist for long periods.

Psychic or emotional numbing is a form of self-protection against unbearable emotional pain. After the event, the individual may experience periods of feeling emotionally dead or numb. That person may have great difficulty in expressing tenderness or loving feelings. *Avoidance behavior* is another important aspect of PTSD. People with PTSD often feel alienated and apart from others. They may lose interest in activities that once gave them pleasure. Others are unable to remember certain aspects of the traumatic event.

Hyperarousal symptoms include difficulty in falling or staying asleep, irritability, outbursts of anger, difficulty in concentration, overprotectiveness of oneself or others, and an exaggerated startle response. People who were abused in a bed commonly experience insomnia. People with an exaggerated startle response may jump at loud noises or if someone touches them on the back.

Duration of symptoms is variable, but according to the official diagnostic criteria for PTSD, the symptoms must endure at least 1 month.

The last criterion relates to the *impact of the psychic trauma on lifestyle*. Survivors of human-engendered catastrophes, in general, suffer longer than survivors of natural catastrophes. In addition, the devastating effects of emotional trauma may be influenced by exposure of the individual to one or more traumatic events. Rape is traumatic, but multiple rapes are even more traumatic. Do the person's symptoms interfere with his or her ability to work, study, socialize, or maintain healthy familial relationships?

Many trauma-related disorders have been recognized and include brief reactive psychosis, multiple personality disorder, dissociative fugue, dissociative amnesia, conversion disorder, depersonalization disorder, dream anxiety disorder, summarization disorder, borderline personality disorder, and antisocial personality disorder. Many other trauma-related disorders have been postulated. These disorders and the trauma that may precede them are indicated as follows:

- *Brief reactive psychosis:* any one or more events that would be stressful to anyone
- *Multiple personality disorder:* abuse or other childhood emotional trauma
- *Dissociative fugue:* severe psychologically stressful event such as marital quarrels, military conflict, natural disaster, or personal rejection
- *Dissociative amnesia:* severe psychologically stressful event such as the tragic death of a loved one, abandonment, or a threat of personal injury

- *Conversion disorder:* extreme psychologically stressful event such as warfare or a recent tragic death of a loved one
- *Depersonalization disorder:* severe stressful event such as military combat or an automobile accident
- *Dream anxiety disorder:* any major life stress, depression, substance abuse, or substance withdrawal
- *Somatization disorder:* early childhood abuse
- *Borderline personality disorder:* early childhood trauma
- *Antisocial personality disorder:* early childhood abuse

Learned helplessness syndrome is a condition that is frequently seen in trauma survivors, commonly women and children; prisoners of war; concentration camp survivors; refugee camp survivors; or other tortured survivors. The name developed from animal experiments by Seligman (1967, 1975). Animals subjected to electric shocks and unable to escape despite their attempts would sink into listlessness and despair. Later, they were reshocked, but although trained to press a lever to stop the shocks, the animals made no effort to do so. The animals had learned to be helpless. It has been postulated that there is an adrenal neurotransmitter problem in animals and humans exposed to severe, repeated traumatic events that may serve as the biologic basis for the hyperarousal and numbing phases of PTSD.

Although almost any symptom can result from PTSD, some of the more common ones are as follows:

- Eating disorders
- Anger or rage
- Self-condemnation
- Self-mutilation
- Depression
- Self-hatred
- Suicidal thoughts
- Homicidal thoughts
- Headaches
- Backaches
- Chronic gastrointestinal problems
- Worsening or activation of chronic medical problems (e.g., diabetes, hypertension)
- Drug abuse
- Overworking
- Self-isolation

The Holocaust is a classic example of a tragic, traumatic event that inflicted significant, permanent changes in the victims' physical and psychological responses to stress. Holocaust survivors have complex problems that have affected their lives for more than 60 years. They are *survivors;* therefore, they never stopped fighting for survival. They are especially frightened of becoming sick because, in the past, to survive meant to be in good health; the alternative was to face doom. These patients are afraid of losing control of their lives, as well as losing their dignity.

Patients who are Holocaust survivors may have many psychosomatic complaints commonly related to the gastrointestinal tract. Chest pain, often relieved by belching, may be related to frequent air swallowing. These patients experience vivid dreams and nightmares. They are suspicious and do not trust people readily because they suffered so much in the past. The interviewer must be especially kind and understanding. The majority of the survivors of the Nazi concentration camps are now 85 to 90 years of age, and many suffer from PTSD. Many suffer from severe depression, panic attacks, and anxiety. The interviewer must be careful when asking about family history and background. Most survivors lost entire families; many lost their first spouse and children. The psychological wounds are deep, and anything can trigger an outpouring of grief. It is frequently difficult to find out anything about the family medical history because the patients' parents and grandparents might have been killed at early ages. These patients should be reassured that they will be treated gently and competently. They, like all patients with PTSD, must be assured of security. Feeling safe is the highest priority in their lives.

It has become clear that individuals need not be present at a catastrophic event to experience stress symptoms. The terrorist attacks that shook the United States on September 11, 2001, were immediately broadcast on television screens around the world. The events and their aftermath were shown in graphic detail repeatedly after the attacks.

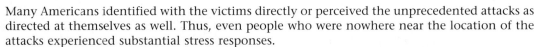

Many Americans identified with the victims directly or perceived the unprecedented attacks as directed at themselves as well. Thus, even people who were nowhere near the location of the attacks experienced substantial stress responses.

In a study published in the *New England Journal of Medicine* shortly after the attacks, 90% of the adults surveyed reported experiencing, to at least some degree, one or more symptoms of stress, and 44% of the adults reported a substantial level of at least one symptom of stress (Schuster et al, 2001). Although those closest to the sites of attack had the most substantial stress, respondents throughout the country, from large cities to small communities, reported stress symptoms: 36% of respondents more than 1000 miles from the World Trade Center reported substantial stress reactions, in comparison with 60% of those within 100 miles of the site. Among respondents who lived south of Canal Street in Manhattan (i.e., near the World Trade Center), the prevalence of PTSD was 20% after the attacks, in comparison with 4% before the tragic event. The article notes that more than 130,000 Manhattan citizens suffered from PTSD, depression, or anxiety after the attacks. Other studies have shown that children who were exposed solely through television to such horrifying events as these attacks, the Challenger disaster, the Oklahoma City bombing, and the Gulf Wars experienced trauma-related stress reactions.

Five to 8 weeks after the attack on the World Trade Center, a random telephone survey was conducted to estimate the prevalence of increased cigarette smoking, alcohol consumption, and marijuana use among residents of Manhattan (Vlahov et al, 2002). Among 988 persons included, 28.8% reported an increase in use of any of these three substances, 9.7% reported an increase in smoking, 24.6% reported an increase in alcohol consumption, and 3.2% reported an increase in marijuana use. Persons who increased smoking of cigarettes and marijuana were more likely to experience PTSD than were those who did not (24.2% vs. 5.6% for cigarettes; 36.0% vs. 6.6% for marijuana). The study was repeated 6 months later, and the increases were sustained, suggestive of potential long-term health consequences as a result of such disasters.

The Sick Physician

Perhaps the most difficult of all patients to care for is the sick physician. The anxiety of sick physicians should not be underestimated. The expression "A little knowledge is a dangerous thing" applies to the sick physician. Every medical or nursing student goes through the "student syndrome," which is the suspicion that he or she has been stricken with the disease about which he or she is learning. Imagine the anxiety that occurs when the physician actually is stricken. In addition to anxiety about health, there is the new role identification of being the patient. Physicians feel helpless and have great difficulty divorcing themselves from the role of physician. They constantly ask what the electrocardiogram shows and for the results of blood tests. They may suggest additional tests or may even disagree with the tests that have been ordered. The novice interviewer should provide ample time for the sick physician to express fears and anxieties. With the interviewer's support, sick physicians eventually recognize and accept their new role as patient.

Influence of Disease on Patient Response

Just as background and age govern a patient's response, so do the patient's present illness and past medical illnesses. This section illustrates the influence of disease on the type of response.

The Disabled Patient

Disabled patients may come to the hospital with great apprehension and mistrust. They are usually familiar with the shortcomings of hospitals because they have probably been hospitalized for painful tests or surgery. They may be burdened with an inferiority complex and may feel unattractive. The interviewer must take all this into consideration and assure patients that everything will be done to make them comfortable. The interviewer must sort out the emotional problems of disabled persons from the physical ones that brought them to the hospital. A friendly smile or a few kind words can encourage these patients to cooperate, thereby securing a better doctor-patient relationship.

Many disabled people have developed their own routines that work for them. They often do not want medical personnel to impose their way of doing something if the patient's way works.

Patients with a hearing impairment need to be treated differently from other disabled patients. Sit directly in front of these patients to allow them to benefit from lip reading. Make sure that the lighting in the room is correct so that your face is well illuminated. It is important to speak slowly with appropriate gestures and expressions to punctuate the question. Ask these patients whether it is necessary for you to speak louder. If a patient wears a hearing aid, speaking louder may not be necessary. If all else fails, the use of written questions can be helpful.

Another special type of disabled patient is the visually impaired patient. Because the patient with limited or no vision has no reference for you in the room, it is useful for you to occasionally touch the patient on the arm or shoulder. This can be done instead of the more standard nonverbal facilitations, which are of no value in this patient.

The severely mentally retarded patient must be accompanied by a family member or guardian to provide a proper history.

The Patient with Cancer

The patient with cancer has five major concerns: loss of control, pain, alienation, mutilation, and mortality. Loss of control makes this patient feel helpless. The knowledge of something growing uncontrolled within a patient's body creates frustration, fear, and anger. Suffering with pain is one of the most feared aspects of cancer. The feeling of alienation stems from the reactions of people around the patient.

Fears of mutilation are common among patients with cancer. The fear of being perceived as lacking "wholeness" contributes to depression and anxiety. The young woman with breast cancer who requires a mastectomy fears that she will be rejected as no longer being a complete woman. Supportive family members are the key in reassuring this patient that they will love her just as they have before her surgery. A diagnosis of cancer makes a patient aware of mortality and leads to intense fear of unremitting pain.

Family members and friends often express grief before death occurs. Resentment and anger may be directed toward the patient with cancer. Physicians often harbor feelings of inadequacy about these patients and have difficulty speaking with them. The patients are thus rejected by their own physician. The physician is afraid that the patient may ask some questions, perhaps about death, that the physician cannot handle. The physician must recognize his or her emotional and behavioral reaction and be realistic about the limitations of medical science.

The interviewer should allow the patient to vent anxieties and should promote dialogue. Listening to the patient enhances the doctor-patient relationship.

The Patient with AIDS

Patients with AIDS are fearful for their lives and of being stigmatized as a member of an undesirable group. The fear and misunderstanding common in high-risk groups result in delays in medical treatment. Denial is the important factor in most of these patients. The patient may have an intense fear of physicians, nurses, students, and paramedical personnel, who may have strong emotions related to this disease and its risk groups. The patient's fear is paralleled by the anxiety of the hospital workers who have to treat an individual with this disease. Their fear of contracting the disease, even by casual contact, is formidable. These fears are also present among the patient's friends and family, who often banish the patient from all activities. The patient may have been fired from a job because the employer is afraid of catching the disease. There is an unsympathetic rejection of patients with AIDS. They suffer emotional turmoil, which contributes to intense anxiety, hostility, and depression.

The interviewer should be as supportive as possible without giving false reassurances. The patients should be given as many facts as appropriate, and the staff members tending to them must be educated about the disease.

The Dysphasic Patient

The dysphasic patient has an impairment of speech and cannot arrange words correctly. Dysphasia is usually caused by a cerebral lesion, such as a stroke. The degree of dysphasia can vary enormously and can be as extensive as almost complete aphasia. Although patients may appear relatively unresponsive, they may be totally aware of all conversation. Therefore, all discussions conducted in the presence of such patients must be undertaken with the assumption that the patient can understand. Before the interview, the interviewer may give

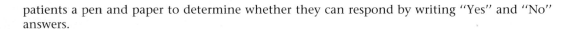

patients a pen and paper to determine whether they can respond by writing "Yes" and "No" answers.

The Psychotic Patient

Psychotic patients have an impairment of their reality-testing abilities. They have a gross inability to communicate effectively. They may also suffer from hallucinations, delusions, or feelings of persecution. Psychotic patients cannot deal with their fear. They are constantly struggling with the ever-changing demands of their environment. It is most important to recognize the psychotic patient early and remain as calm as possible. If the patient has had violent episodes, make sure assistance is standing by.

In general, interviewing psychotic patients presents a difficult task for the inexperienced interviewer. Some of these patients tend to be inarticulate and preoccupied with fantasies, whereas others are reasonably lucid. The symptoms and signs of their psychosis are not usually evident at first assessment. There are several clues to the existence of a psychosis. Interviewers should pay particular attention to the speech pattern and its organization. Is there a jumble of ideas? Psychotic patients are easily distracted, and the interviewer must constantly remind them of the subject. These patients fail to complete any chain of thought and cannot follow any idea to completion. They can have bizarre impressions about their bodies. They may complain that they have noticed that one arm has recently shortened or that their external genitalia have suddenly shrunk or enlarged. In addition, they may have evidence of an inappropriate affect; for example, a patient may laugh while telling about the death of a friend or relative.

A special type of psychotic personality disorder is found in patients with *Munchausen's syndrome*. Such patients are the classic hospital malingerers. They are pathologic liars and travel from clinician to clinician, from hospital to hospital. They complain of a wide variety of symptoms and, in fact, *create* signs of illness to seek an advantage. Their histories are well rehearsed, and they have a masochistic perpetuation of self-injury. For example, the patient with Munchausen's syndrome may actually prick the skin under a fingernail so that it will not be obvious, drop some blood into the urine, and call the clinician, stating that there is blood in the urine. These patients frequently seek out painful diagnostic and therapeutic procedures. At times, they may even undergo unnecessary surgical procedures.

The Demented or Delirious Patient

Demented patients have lost previously acquired intellectual function, most typically memory. Delirious patients have a disorder of consciousness that does not allow them to interact correctly with the surroundings. Demented patients frequently become more confused when taken out of their normal environment, especially at night. The term *sundowning* is used in such circumstances. Fear is common in both types of patients. In interviewing these patients, clinicians must try to be sensitive to their emotions as much as possible, and above all, try to allay their fears. Interviewers must be particularly aware of questions that may be possibly threatening to the patient.

Patients with an organic mental syndrome present a special problem. At times, these patients seem lucid; at other times, they are disoriented with regard to person, place, or time. If the patient is able to answer some of the questions, the interviewer should record the answers. The same questions should be asked again later to determine whether the patient will respond similarly. These patients have defects in attention span, memory, and abstract thought. Interviewers should be alert to inconsistent and slow, hesitant responses. On occasion, patients may interject some humor to try to cover up for their difficulty in memory. A careful mental status examination indicates the problem. It may be useful to remind the patient of your name and tell him or her that you will ask for the name in a few minutes. Frequently, such patients have forgotten it. Furthermore, the histories these patients give may not be reliable.

The Acutely Ill Patient

The acutely ill patient merits prompt attention. In these situations, a concise history and physical examination are in order. A careful history of the present and past illnesses must be taken expeditiously so that the diagnosis may be made and treatment begun. It may be appropriate in this setting to interview the patient while performing the physical examination; time is of the essence. However, patients who are acutely ill may respond to questions more slowly than normal because of pain, nausea, or vomiting. Be considerate of their problems, and allow them time to answer questions. After a patient's condition has been stabilized, there will be time to go back and take a more complete history.

The Surgical Patient

Patients faced with a surgical procedure may be frightened despite a calm appearance. They may feel helpless and out of control. The fear of anesthesia, disfigurement, disability, or death is always present. The fear of not awakening from the anesthesia can be devastating. When they awaken, will they find that their body is no longer "whole"? Did the surgeon find something that was not expected? These patients fear the unknown. A question about the surgeon's ability is an expression of the patient's anxiety. Often, patients have tests and are told the results are normal "except" for a small area: they will need surgery to "check it out." This lack of communication by the surgeon adds to the patient's anxiety. A surgeon's schedule is frequently erratic. Surgery may be delayed or postponed, which adds to the surgical patient's anxiety and anger. Many possible communication difficulties exist. The best way to avoid the unnecessary anxiety-provoking situations is to maintain open communication among the patient, the physician, and the patient's family. In the postoperative period, the patient's relief over having lived through surgery may be displayed in a variety of ways. The patient may be apathetic and show a general lack of interest or may be moody, irritable, aggressive, angry, or tearful. Subconsciously, patients may wish to harm the surgeon for "cutting" into their bodies, whereas consciously they want to thank the surgeon. This dichotomy may be the root of the anger so commonly seen in postoperative patients. In other patients, depression may be seen as a result of the loss of part of the body. The best example of this is the "phantom limb." Patients who have undergone an amputation of a leg frequently claim sensation in their lost limb. Some of this may be physiologic, but certainly some of the phantom leg pain is related to depression. The caring interviewer should allow the patient time to release these tensions and feelings of loss.

The Alcoholic Patient

Alcoholic patients are both physiologically and psychologically dependent on alcohol. Most of the time, interviewers conduct the sessions when the patient is not inebriated. Excessive drinking is often an attempt to deaden feelings of guilt and failure. The more patients drink, the more they are abandoned by their family and friends. They feel castigated and alone. They are left to their only "friend": alcohol. They are often ready to talk, and their account of their drinking habits may be interesting. Alcoholic patients generally have a low opinion of themselves. They may even be upset about their persistent drinking habits. Their hatred of themselves may be a manifestation of a self-destructive wish. Alcoholic patients may also have fears about sexual inadequacy or homosexuality. It is not easy to open up such topics because these patients are likely to respond explosively. The sensitive interviewer should approach these issues in a manner that is neither condescending nor moralistic.

The Psychosomatic Patient

Just as physical illness can produce psychological problems, so can psychological problems create physical ailments. The intimate interaction of the mind and body is clearly demonstrated in the psychosomatic disorder.

Psychosomatic patients express emotional discomfort and distress in the form of bodily symptoms. They may be totally unaware of the psychological stress in their lives or the relationship of stress to the symptoms.

There are many ways of dealing with psychosomatic patients. First, identify the disorder: Do not miss the possible diagnosis of an affective or anxiety disorder. Treatment of somatization is directed toward teaching the patient to cope with the psychological problems. Be aware that somatization operates unconsciously; the patient really is suffering. Above all, the patient should *never* be told that his or her problem is "in your head." Anxiety, fear, and depression are the main psychological problems associated with psychosomatic illness. The list of associated common symptoms and illnesses is long and includes chest pain, headaches, peptic ulcer disease, ulcerative colitis, irritable bowel syndrome, nausea, vomiting, anorexia nervosa, urticaria, tachycardia, hypertension, asthma, migraine, muscle tension syndromes, obesity, rashes, and dizziness. Answers to an open-ended question such as "What's been happening in your life?" often provide insight into the problems.

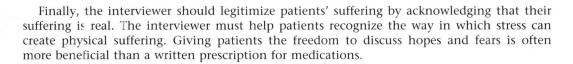

Finally, the interviewer should legitimize patients' suffering by acknowledging that their suffering is real. The interviewer must help patients recognize the way in which stress can create physical suffering. Giving patients the freedom to discuss hopes and fears is often more beneficial than a written prescription for medications.

The Dying Patient

Few patients are as conscious of taking up a clinician's time as those who have less time remaining. Dying patients may initially have many questions, but as time goes by, they ask less and less of their health-care providers.

Many health-care providers have a dread of death that is so intense that they behave irrationally. They avoid patients who are dying or those with incurable diseases. The emotional needs of the dying patients may be largely ignored. Many patients have a greater fear of the process of dying than of death itself. The fear of living as a chronically ill patient can be almost as intolerable as (and often more so than) the fear of death.

Dying patients suffer from the pain, nausea, or vomiting caused by the disease or treatment. They may be rejected by their families, hospital staff members, or even their own physicians. Many patients have strong feelings of anger, guilt, resentment, and frustration: "Why me?" "It should have been diagnosed earlier." They may envy healthy individuals. They may deny their imminent death; this is the first stage of dying. Not uncommonly, a dying patient is interviewed and does not tell the interviewer about the illness. Even when asked specifically about the disease, the patient may deny any knowledge of having a fatal disease. This mechanism of denial allows the patient to cope with life as it is. Each person faces death differently. Some can deal with it head-on; others cannot. Some approach it with fear and tears, whereas others grow to accept it as an inevitable event. Given sufficient time and the necessary understanding, most dying patients can arrive at the final stage of dying: acceptance. This stage is characterized by apathy and social withdrawal. Counselors specifically trained in the grieving process are often helpful to the patient, family, and health-care providers.

Once a patient has come to grips with the fact that he or she has a terminal disease, the patient may ask, "Am I going to die?" The interviewer cannot answer this question as asked, and so he or she should then ask the patient, "What are you afraid of?" The patient may then indicate that he or she is afraid of dying in pain or dying alone. The interviewer can answer these questions by saying that he or she will do everything possible to make sure that the patient will not have pain or that they or their associates will be with the patient throughout duration of the illness.

The dying patient needs to speak with someone. The clinician should be alert for subtle clues that the patient wishes to discuss the topic of death. For example, if a patient remarks that his "wife is well provided for," it is correct to pursue this point by making an interpretive statement such as, "I sense that you are very worried about your illness." Although the conversation that ensues might be emotionally draining for the interviewer, the interviewer must allow the dying patient to speak. Sometimes the most appropriate response to an expression of grief is a thoughtful period of silence.

Bibliography

Adelman RD, Greene MG, Charon R: Issues in physician-elderly patient interaction. Ageing Soc 11:127, 1991.

Adler G: The physician and the hypochondriacal patient. N Engl J Med 304:1394, 1981.

American Psychiatric Association: Diagnostic and Statistical Manual of Mental Disorders, 3rd ed. Washington, DC, American Psychiatric Press, 1980.

Cassem NH, Hackett TP: Psychological aspects of myocardial infarction. Med Clin North Am 61:711, 1977.

Catalano RA, Kessell ER, McConnell W, et al: Psychiatric emergencies after the terrorist attacks of September 11, 2001. Psychiatr Serv 55:163, 2004.

Cousins N: Anatomy of an illness (as perceived by the patient). N Engl J Med 295:1458, 1976.

Davidson JRT, Foa EB (eds): Posttraumatic Stress Disorder: *DSM-IV* and Beyond. Washington, DC, American Psychiatric Press, 1993.

Galea S, Ahern J, Resnick H, et al: Psychological sequelae of the September 11 terrorist attacks in New York City. N Engl J Med 346:982, 2002.

Gorlin R, Zucker HD: Physician's reactions to patients: A key to teaching humanistic medicine. N Engl J Med 308:1057, 1983.

Groves JE: Taking care of the hateful patient. N Engl J Med 298:883, 1978.

Hahn SR, Feiner JS, Bellin EH: The doctor-patient-family relationship: A compensatory alliance. Ann Intern Med 109:884, 1988.

Kraut AM: Healers and strangers: Immigrant attitudes toward the physicians in America—a relationship in historical perspective. JAMA 263:1807, 1990.

Kübler-Ross E: On Death and Dying, New York, Macmillan, 1969.

Lipsett DR: Medical and psychological characteristics of "crocks." J Psychiatry Med 1:15, 1970.

Matsakis A: I Can't Get Over It: A Handbook for Trauma Survivors, 2nd ed. Oakland, Calif, New Harbinger, 1996.

Mezzich JE, Kleinman A, Fabrega H Jr, et al (eds): Culture and Psychiatric Diagnosis: A *DSM-IV* Perspective, Washington, DC, American Psychiatric Press, 1996.

Pandya A, Weiden PJ: Trauma and disaster in psychiatrically vulnerable populations. J Psychiatr Pract 7:426, 2001.

Pynoos RS (ed): Posttraumatic Stress Disorder: A Clinical Review. Lutherville, Md, Sidran Press, 1994.

Rainwater L: The lower class: Health, illness, and medical institutions. In Millon T (ed): Medical Behavioral Science, Philadelphia, WB Saunders, 1975.

Sansone RA, Sansone LA: Borderline personality disorder: Office diagnosis and management. Am Fam Physician 44:194, 1991.

Schuster MA, Stein BD, Jaycox LH, et al: A national survey of stress reactions after the September 11, 2001, terrorist attacks. N Engl J Med 345:1507, 2001.

Seligman MEP: Helplessness: On Depression, Development, and Death. San Francisco, CA, W.H. Freeman, 1975.

Seligman MEP, Maier SF: Failure to escape traumatic shock. J Exp Psych 74:1, 1967.

Smith RC: Somatization disorder: Defining its role in clinical medicine. J Gen Intern Med 6:168, 1991.

Stern M, Pascale L, Ackerman A: Life adjustment postmyocardial infarction. Arch Intern Med 137:1680, 1977.

U.S. Department of Commerce, Bureau of the Census: 1990 Census. Washington, DC, U.S. Government Printing Office, 1990.

Vlahov D, Galea S, Ahern J, et al: Sustained increased consumption of cigarettes, alcohol, and marijuana among Manhattan residents after September 11, 2001. Am J Public Health 94:253, 2004.

Vlahov D, Galea S, Resnick H, et al: Increased use of cigarettes, alcohol, and marijuana among Manhattan, New York, residents after the September 11th terrorist attacks. Am J Epidemiol 155:988, 2002.

Waxman HS: The patient as physician. Ann Intern Med 126:656, 1997.

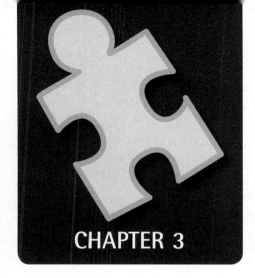

CHAPTER 3

Caring for Patients in a Culturally Diverse Society

What the scalpel is to the surgeon, words are to the clinician ... the conversation between doctor and patient is the heart of the practice of medicine.

Philip A. Tumulty, MD (1912–1989)

The cultural aspects of physical diagnosis and medicine are becoming increasingly important. By the middle of the 21st century, the majority of the population in the United States will no longer be white. It is imperative that all health-care professionals understand the dimensions and complexities of caring for individuals of culturally diverse backgrounds in the United States. Equally important is the provider's knowledge of the cultural and socioeconomic factors that affect the patient's access to and use of health-care resources. When treating recent immigrants, clinicians must be aware that their attitudes toward illness and treatment may be very different from those of the indigenous population. Second-generation immigrants may have yet a different appreciation.

The United States is home to one of the most ethnically and culturally heterogeneous populations in the world. There are more than 100 ethnic groups and 400 tribes of Native Americans in the United States, each with diverse practices and beliefs. This chapter provides some relevant issues of cultural diversity in health care and is intended to sensitize the health-care provider to the impact of cultural diversity on health-care delivery. This chapter is not comprehensive, because not all groups are represented; no culture was intentionally omitted. The chapter is divided into two main sections: (1) a discussion of some general considerations in delivery of health care in a multicultural society and (2) selected cross-cultural perspectives.

The names used to identify various groups change with time. Within a cultural group, there are variations as to how its members identify themselves and what name they prefer. The names of cultural groups often grow out of ethnic and ideologic movements.

The examples of health-care practices in this chapter illustrate *traditional* cultural differences. However, not all patients of a certain group hold that group's traditional beliefs. Many patients who are now second- or third-generation Americans may not follow these practices but may know of them from parents or grandparents. Caution should also be taken to avoid stereotyping the patient by race, lifestyle, cultural or religious backgrounds, economic status, or level of education; this is detrimental to establishing a solid doctor-patient relationship. The health-care provider must recognize that there is also great variability within cultures. The following is intended not to stereotype or label any particular group but rather to teach how to recognize common cultural characteristics to understand better the needs of patients.

General Considerations

According to the 2000 census, 281.4 million people were counted in the United States, a 13.2% increase from the 1990 census population of 248.7 million. The population growth of 32.7 million people between 1990 and 2000 represents the largest census-to-census increase in American history. The previous record increase was 28.0 million people between 1950 and 1960, primarily as a result of the post–World War II baby boom.

Of the 281.4 million people, 211.4 million (75.1%) were white; 34.6 million (12.3%) were African American, or black; 10.2 million (3.6%) were Asian; 2.4 million (0.9%) were Native Americans (American Indian, Inuit and Inupiat, and Aleut); and 398,835 (0.1%) were Native Hawaiian and other Pacific Islanders. "White" individuals are people whose origins are in any of the original peoples of Europe, the Middle East, or North Africa. This includes individuals who indicated their race(s) as "white" or their original nationality as English, Italian, French, Dutch, Scottish-Irish, Scottish, Irish, Swedish, Norwegian, Spanish, German, Italian, Polish, Lebanese, Near Easterner, or Arab. The members of the Asian community are Chinese, Filipino, Asian Indian, Japanese, Korean, Vietnamese, and other Asian. The actual numbers are probably several million higher, given that many people are uncounted because of their undocumented status (i.e., no immigration papers) and inadequate census counts.

There were 35 million people (12.5% of the total population) of Hispanic/Latino origin, who constitute a multicultural diverse group. The federal definition of Hispanic/Latino is "a person of Cuban, Mexican, Puerto Rican, South or Central American, or other Spanish culture or origin regardless of race." Among the Hispanic/Latino population, 66.1% were of Mexican origin; 14.5% were Central and South American; 9.0% were Puerto Rican; 4.0% were Cuban; and the remaining 6.4% were of other Hispanic origins. The United States now ranks sixth in the world in terms of the numbers of Latinos residing within its borders.

There have been significant changes in the U.S. population since the 1950s: the white majority has been shrinking and aging, whereas the Hispanic/Latino, African American, Asian American, and Native American populations are young and growing. It has been projected that by the year 2010, there will be a decrease in white youth by 3.8 million and an increase in nonwhite youth by 44 million.

Language can be a significant barrier to good health care. According to the 2000 census, there are more than 15 million people in the United States who have "limited English proficiency."[*] More than 5% of the populations of California, New York, Texas, New Mexico, and Hawaii have limited English-language skills.

Race, Culture, and Ethnicity

Race, as defined by *Merriam-Webster's Collegiate Dictionary*, 10th edition, is a "class or kind of people unified by community of interests, habits, or inherited physical characteristics" (p. 959). The term *culture* has a broad meaning; it refers to the unifying beliefs of any group of people of similar religion, values, attitudes, ritual practices, family structure, language, or mode of social organization. Culture provides values that are shared by members of a specific society or a social group within a society. Culture socializes its members on how to perceive the world, how to behave in the world, and how to experience the world emotionally. Elements that represent cultural values and notions include language, social or familial roles, and beliefs about the universe, the nature of good and evil, appropriate dress, eating and hygienic habits, manners, and food. Culture pervades lives and shapes human identity. All personal experiences and norms are perceived through the culture from which they emerge. It shapes human perception of reality and influences societal forms of conduct. Different cultures reinforce different behaviors; what is acceptable in one culture may be considered deviant in another.

Cultural values determine, in part, how a patient should behave. This includes the types of acceptable treatment, type of follow-up permitted, and who will make the decisions. From the medical point of view prevalent in the United States, the clinician and the patient make the decisions, but when a patient's family exerts great influence, the situation can be very different. In some traditional cultures, the family takes over this role for the patient.

---

[*]"Limited English proficiency" is a term used by the U.S. Department of Health and Human Services to define the portion of the population that is non–English speaking or limited-English speaking.

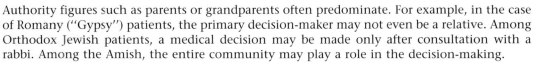

Authority figures such as parents or grandparents often predominate. For example, in the case of Romany ("Gypsy") patients, the primary decision-maker may not even be a relative. Among Orthodox Jewish patients, a medical decision may be made only after consultation with a rabbi. Among the Amish, the entire community may play a role in the decision-making.

Ethnicity is a cultural group's sense of identification associated with the group's common social and cultural heritage. The *Harvard Encyclopedia of American Ethnic Groups* defines ethnicity as "a common geographical origin, language, religious faith, and cultural ties (e.g., shared traditions, values, symbols, literature, music, and food preferences)."

Disease, Illness, and Health

The terms *disease* and *illness* are often used interchangeably. Medical sociologists and cultural anthropologists, however, make a distinction. The word *disease* refers to a disorder in which there is a change from normal in the body's structure or function, involving one or more organs of the body. *Illness* is the subjective distress felt by the patient and by those close to the patient, rather than the actual state of ill health. The patient's culture often determines how the patient interprets, explains, responds to, and deals with a disease. It also influences when a patient will seek health-care decisions and from whom. Members of some cultures try to "normalize" their symptoms, maintaining that symptoms in a certain age group are not abnormal. Affected members might say that they have experienced the symptoms before and that therefore the symptoms are normal for them. Other cultures dictate immediate care even if symptoms are minimal. According to some cultures, to be ill is a punishment or curse, whereas according to others, to be ill is to be weak, irresponsible, or unmasculine. For many patients in the United States, the clinician is only one of many health-care providers and often not the first. Some patients are likely to consult a healer from their own culture before seeking consultation from a Western-trained clinician. Two patients from different cultures may react differently to the same disease or symptoms. Thus, treating illness, rather than treating disease, requires the health-care provider to have not only a broad understanding of medicine but an understanding of the patient's cultural background.

Health, as defined in *The Random House Dictionary of the English Language*, is "the general condition of the body or mind with reference to soundness and vigor." It is often defined more abstractly as the "absence of disease." In some cultures, health is viewed as the freedom from evil. Other cultures regard health as day and illness as night. By extrapolation, health reflects light and clean, and illness reflects dark and dirty. These depictions form the basis of the beliefs of many cultures, which are discussed later in this chapter.

Culture and Health

It is crucial for any health-care provider to have an appreciation for cross-cultural family values, language, norms, religion, and political ideology. An estimated 80% to 90% of all self-recognized episodes of illness are managed exclusively outside a formal health-care system. Traditional healers, mediums, self-help groups, and religious practitioners provide a substantial proportion of this health care.

Within the United States, there are many culturally distinct groups. Even within these groups, there are many variables such as educational achievement, socioeconomic class, generational status, and political relationship between the country of origin and the United States. All these factors contribute to establishing the dynamic reality of an ethnic group. Being in a low socioeconomic bracket appears to be a strong predictor that ethnicity will influence the behavior of such patients, regardless of whether they are newly arrived or native born. The following factors are other predictors of behavioral ethnicity:

- Emigration from rural areas
- Frequent return visits to the native area
- Lack of formal education
- Immigration to the United States at an older age
- A major difference in dress or diet from the surrounding population

Newly arrived immigrants often experience prejudice; the toll on their psyche may be a heavy one. But cultural change is not limited merely to immigration. Moving around in the same country or changing professions may also result in *culture shock*. The new culture may be viewed as unempathetic, cruel, and critical. The newcomer may experience frustration, irritability, fatigue, loss of flexibility, and an inability to communicate feelings to others.

Distrust, paranoid tendencies, depression, anxiety, and physical and psychosomatic illnesses may develop. It is therefore necessary to include a patient's and family's immigrational and migrational history in the evaluation of the patient because the family is the carrier of ethnic traits and identity.

Cross-cultural marriages can offer the best and worst of both worlds. The reconciliation of different norms and traditions may provide an enriching experience, but a clash of different cultural traits may lead to strained relations among spouses and families.

The influence of ethnicity and culture on health and health-belief practices has long been recognized as a result of the presence of racially related diseases and syndromes, as well as societal predispositions to illness. It is very important to inquire about patients' perceptions of their symptoms and illness. To understand better the cultural influences on a patients' medical problem, Lipkin and colleagues (1995) suggested several questions for eliciting patients' explanations for their symptoms or health-belief practices:

"What do you call your problem?"

"What causes your problem?"

"Why do you think it started when it did?"

"How does it work—what is going on in your body?"

"What kind of treatment do you think would be best for this problem?"

"How has this problem affected your life?"

"What frightens or concerns you most about this problem and treatment?"

The answers to these questions provide insight into the hopes, aspirations, and fears of the patient.

Genetic Diseases

The simultaneous manifestation of two or more forms or alleles of a gene in a population is a genetic polymorphism. Certain genetic polymorphic states, such as blood groups, are strongly associated with disease. As early as 1953, an association of blood group A with gastric carcinoma was recognized. The causal relationship of hemoglobin S to sickle cell anemia is well known. Thalassemia comprises more than 50 genetic disorders characterized by ineffective erythropoiesis that leads to severe anemia, fever, hyperuricemia, and skeletal deformities. The association of these disorders with Mediterranean background has been established. The human leukocyte antigen gene complex and the many diseases associated with it continue to receive attention. Table 3-1 summarizes some specific diseases on the basis of geographic distribution and ethnic populations.

Traditional Medical Beliefs

People interpret traditional medical beliefs about the body's shape and size, inner structure, and functions in terms of their cultural background. To illustrate various cultural beliefs about body functions, consider that patients often ascribe their symptoms to blood that is "too thin," "too thick," "too little," or "too slow." Blood can be used as an index of an emotional state (blushing); a personality type ("cold-blooded" or "hot-blooded"); a kinship ("blood is thicker than water"); a diet ("thin blood"); or a social relationship ("bad blood between people"). "Bad blood" is also frequently used to refer to syphilis.

As another example of the cultural beliefs about blood, consider views about menstruation. A study in 1977 by Snow and Johnson evaluated the views of inner-city women in a public clinic in Michigan. Many of the 40 women interviewed felt that menstruation was a method of ridding the body of impurities that could cause illness or poison the body. Many of these women believed that when the uterus was "open" during menstrual flow, they were vulnerable to disease. They also believed that it was only at this time that a woman could become pregnant. At all other times in the menstrual cycle, the uterus was "closed," and pregnancy was impossible. Another common fear among the women was that of impeded menstrual flow. They feared that stoppage might cause a backup of poison and hence a stroke, cancer, or sterility. This fear may be a reason why these women avoid the use of certain methods of contraception, such as intrauterine devices and diaphragms.

Table 3-1 Geographic and Ethnic Distributions of Specific Diseases

Specific Disease	Highest Incidence	Specific Disease	Highest Incidence
Cancer of the skin	Eastern Australia	Ischemic heart disease	North America South America Europe Finland
Cancer of the cheek	Southern India, New Guinea		
Cancer of the nasopharynx	Southeast Asia, Kenya		
Cancer of the esophagus	Northern France (Brittany) South Africa Eastern Zimbabwe Western Kenya East of the Caspian Sea	Hypertension	Japan Taiwan
		Venous thrombosis	North America South America Europe
Cancer of the stomach	Japan Korea Eastern Finland Mountain region of Colombia Eastern Zaire Southwest Uganda	Varicose veins	North America
		Diabetes	North America South America Europe
		Urinary bladder stones	Rural Thailand
Cancer of the colon	North America Western Europe	Multiple sclerosis	Northern United States Northern Europe
Cancer of the liver	Sub-Saharan Africa	Rosacea	Great Britain, especially Scotland
Burkitt's lymphoma	Africa (10° north and south of equator)	Vogt-Koyanagi-Harada syndrome	Japan Italy
Appendicitis	North America South America Europe	Takayasu's disease	Japan
		Lactase deficiency	Greece Jewish people African Americans Thailand Eskimos Japan
Diverticular disease	North America Western Europe Australia New Zealand		
Hemorrhoids	North America South America Europe	Choroideremia	Northern Finland
		Abetalipoproteinemia	Ashkenazi Jews
Cholelithiasis	Southwestern United States Sweden	Glycosphingolipidoses Gaucher's disease Niemann-Pick disease Tay-Sachs disease	Ashkenazi Jews
Stenosing duodenal ulcer	Southern India Eastern Zaire	Familial Mediterranean fever	Sephardic Jews Armenians

Another belief about menstruation was studied by Skultans (1970) in two groups of women from a small mining village in South Wales, U.K. One group of women felt that menstruation was a process by which the body "cleansed" itself; the longer the period or greater the blood loss, the better. These women regarded menstruation as normal and essential to a healthy life. In contrast, another group of women from the same mining town viewed menstruation as damaging to their overall health; they feared that the blood loss was threatening to their health and welcomed the thought of menopause.

Finally, Ngubane (1977) described the beliefs of South African Zulu women about menstruation. They felt that menstruating women had a "contagious pollution" that was deleterious to other living creatures and to the natural world. A man's virility would be reduced if he had sexual relations with a menstruating woman. Crops would be ruined and cattle would die if menstrual blood came in contact with them. In some of these African communities, menstruating women are isolated from the community because of their "dangerous pollution."

Although food is a source of nutrition, it plays many roles and is deeply embedded in almost all aspects of everyday life. Some foods eaten in one society are forbidden in others. Each culture has its own rules of food preparation and of how it is served and how it should be eaten.

Every culture defines foods that are edible and those that are not. In France, frogs' legs and snails are delicacies, whereas in the nearby United Kingdom, they are rarely eaten. Some foods are considered sacred and others are prohibited. Food abstentions occur during the Jewish fast of Yom Kippur and the Muslim fast of Ramadan. Orthodox Hindus are forbidden to kill or eat any animal, especially the cow. However, milk or milk products may be consumed because they do not require the death of the animal. Orthodox followers of Islam and Judaism are prohibited from eating pork products. Only the meat from mammals that chew their cud and that have cloven hoofs is edible, provided that the animal was slaughtered ritually: according to *halal* (Islam) or *kosher* (Jewish) law. Kosher law dictates that meat and milk products are never eaten together. In Sikhism, pork is allowed, but never beef. Rastafarians are generally vegetarians, and alcohol is strictly forbidden.

Some cultural groups in the Islamic world, the Indian subcontinent, Latin America, and China believe in the "hot-cold theory" of disease. This belief, which is intuitive and common throughout Latin America, states that the body is regulated by hot and cold "humors." The belief stems from Hippocratic humoral theories brought to this hemisphere in the 16th and 17th centuries by the Spanish and Portuguese. Health is the balance of these hot and cold body fluids. Illness is defined by a humoral imbalance of these forces. All mental states, illnesses, and natural and supernatural forces are grouped into hot and cold categories. Foods, herbs, and medications are also classified as hot or cold and serve to restore the body to its natural balance. Although it may seem that the system is based on temperature, the thermal state in which the foods or medications are taken is not important. Certain types of herbal tea, served hot, are considered cold, whereas cold beer, because of its alcoholic content, is considered hot. In the hot-cold theory of disease, conditions that are hot, such as ulcer disease, constipation, pregnancy, diarrhea, and rashes, should be balanced and treated with cold foods, such as coconut, avocado, sugar cane, and lima beans. Menstruating or postpartum women who believe in the hot-cold theory may avoid certain "cold" vegetables and fruits because these fruits are liable to clot their "hot" menstrual blood, impeding its flow, making it flow backward into the body and thus causing nervousness or insanity. Cold illnesses, such as arthritis or joint pains, are treated with hot therapy, such as aspirin, iron tablets, penicillin, chili peppers, chocolate, evaporated milk, onions, garlic, or cinnamon.

Consider the following. A patient may be on diuretic therapy and require potassium supplementation. The clinician may advise the patient to eat foods high in potassium, such as oranges or bananas. If the patient acquires an upper respiratory infection, which is a cold disease, he or she may stop eating these fruits, which are classified as cold, because eating them will only worsen the imbalance. This belief should be recognized because it contributes significantly to whether a patient does or does not adhere to therapy. Problems can arise when a clinician prescribes a "hot" medication for a "hot" disease or a "cold" medication for a "cold" disease. The hot-cold theory is even more complex in that the assignment of the "hot" or "cold" qualities varies from culture to culture. It is often difficult for the health-care provider to remember the various hot-cold combinations. If a Hispanic/Latino patient has these beliefs, the clinician should ask Hispanic/Latino colleagues on the medical team or the patient and family directly about these combinations. Inquiring respectfully about the patient's culture can be effective in enhancing doctor-patient relationships. To achieve maximum therapeutic benefits for patients who believe in the hot-cold theory of disease, the health-care provider is advised to work within its framework, if possible, in prescribing medicines and diet. He or she should try to consult medical colleagues, nurses, and social workers who share the patient's background.

Belief in *witchcraft* as a cause of illness is widespread. In the Hispanic/Latino population, terms such as *mal puesto, mal de ojo, mal artificial, brujería, hechicería*, and *enfermedad endañada* are used to describe the "illness of damage": someone has done something to cause injury, illness, or death. *Mal de ojo*, or evil eye, is believed to result from excessive respect or love from another person, especially toward newborn children. A recurring theme in witchcraft belief is that animals are present in the body and are introduced by magical means. Almost always, the offending animal is a reptile, insect, or amphibian. These animals have been dried and pulverized, sprinkled onto food, and reconstituted in the body of the victim. Symptoms are often described as animals crawling over the body or wriggling throughout the intestines. The belief is that this is a magical expression of friends, relatives, or strangers wishing bad luck to come to an individual. A *hex* is an evil spell, a misfortune, or a case of bad luck that one person can impose on another. Magical oils, incenses, religious items, and candles may be used to repel the evil. In the Hispanic/Latino community, a *botánica*, or religious artifact shop, sells many of these items. The shopkeeper serves as a consultant on health and related issues. Figures 3-1 and 3-2, taken in the Otto Chicas Rendon *Botánica* on 116th Street in New York City, depict examples of such shops. Often, the entrance to a *botánica*, as shown in Figure 3-1, shows predominant Roman Catholic imagery.

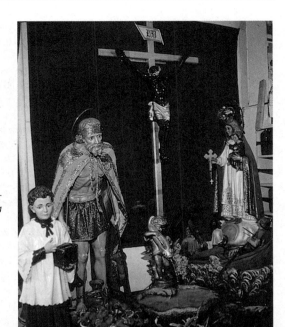

Figure 3–1 Entrance to Otto Chicas Rendon *Botánica* on 116th Street, New York City.

Candles, flowers, plants, and bowls of coconut and molasses frequently surround the Christian statues. The influence of Christianity, as well as of the African and Arabic cultures, is apparent in the idols shown in Figure 3-2. As of mid-2004, there were more than 750 *botánicas* listed in the business telephone books in the United States, of which there were more than 95 in Manhattan. There are probably many more that are not listed.

Very often, patients who believe they are victims of witchcraft do not seek medical attention from a clinician. Certain members of their community may be consulted to chant special prayers and incantations to cure the illness. At other times, they may require exorcism or some other dramatic therapy to drive the illness out of the body. Other common "cures" include turpentine, kerosene, mothballs, and carbon tetrachloride.

Culture and Response to Pain

The sociocultural variations in physical pain expression are important to recognize. Pain is a complex phenomenon for both the patient and the health-care provider, influenced as much

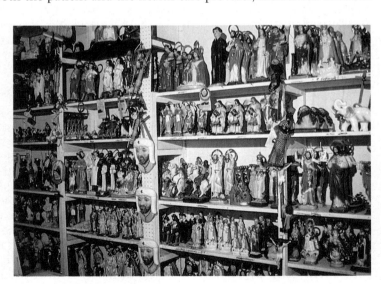

Figure 3–2 Idols in a *botánica*.

by personal values and cultural traditions as by physiologic injury and disease. Multiple factors influence the perception and expression of pain. Pain is an important form of biofeedback and is essential, as a warning signal, for survival. The experience of physical pain, however, has three components: (1) a person's sensation of pain, (2) a person's tolerance for pain, and (3) a person's expression of pain. Health-care providers must rely on the pain sufferer to describe the symptom of pain, the sum of these three components. The last of the three is culturally mediated.

Some studies have indicated that there may be cultural variations in the tolerance for pain as well. In some cultures, the complaints of pain are rewarded with increased attention and comforting behavior. Individuals of Hispanic/Latino background or from the Middle East or Mediterranean areas commonly voice their pain with great emotion. Some believe that they must openly express their pain; if they do not, they may aggravate their illness. In contrast, Southeast Asian, Asian-Indian, Japanese, and Native American patients believe that emotional control is extremely important. Their cultures encourage stoicism; these people rarely openly express or even indicate the presence of pain, unless it is extremely severe. In many instances, the ability to withstand great pain is a sign of manhood, reliability, and moral uprightness.

The anthropologist Zborowski (1952) studied pain in four groups of male patients in a veterans' hospital. Third-generation Americans generally expressed pain with little emotional behavior and became withdrawn from their friends. Italian and Jewish men were very expressive and preferred to be with others while in pain. Irish men endured pain as a private event and neither sought any medication for it nor wanted to socialize with others. These generalizations about cultural responses to pain must be used cautiously and not become the basis of stereotyping.

It is also important for the health-care provider to recognize that many patients from Southeast Asian and Native American cultures frequently express their illness through altered states of consciousness such as trances and hallucinations. The clinician who is unaware of this type of presentation may incorrectly diagnose it as some form of psychosis.

Ethnicity and Pharmacotherapy

It is increasingly recognized that there are ethnic differences in the response to pharmacologic agents. For example, in psychopharmacology, new research has begun to provide insight concerning the biologic mechanisms that underlie this differential response. Data have been accumulated about the ethnic differences in drug metabolism, as well as the plasma proteins that bind psychotropic agents. Several ethnic differences in drug metabolism appear to be related to different genetic forms in the drug-metabolizing cytochrome P-450 enzyme system. It has been demonstrated that a high percentage of Asians and African Americans have an enzyme form that metabolizes drugs at a much slower rate; in individuals with this form, potentially toxic blood levels of drugs may develop after administration of standard doses of certain psychotropic agents. Some Chinese herbs, such as ginseng and muscone, have been shown to have potent stimulating effects on cytochrome enzymes; other herbs substantially inhibit the activities of these enzymes. It is therefore important to determine the serum levels of drugs in a patient in whom an atypical response has developed. Other studies have shown that Asian and Hispanic/Latino patients with schizophrenia require lower doses of neuroleptic agents, such as chlorpromazine, than do white patients. Asian patients are also more likely to exhibit the extrapyramidal side effects of the neuroleptic agents than are white patients.

Cross-Cultural Differences in Morbidity and Mortality Rates

It is important to be aware of the considerable cultural diversity in patterns of morbidity and mortality rates in the United States. Some patterns may be purely genetic, as in Tay-Sachs disease among persons of Ashkenazi Jewish (Eastern European) descent or sickle cell anemia among African Americans. The pattern of health for African Americans is very different from that of their white counterparts. The average life expectancy for African Americans is 69.6 years of age, in comparison with 75.9 years of age for white persons. This may in part be related to a higher infant mortality rate among African Americans. The incidence of hypertension and its consequences is much higher in African Americans than in white persons. African-American men die from cerebrovascular accidents at almost twice the rate of white men. In addition, death from coronary artery disease in African-American women is more common than in white women. Diabetes is 35% more common among African Americans than among the white population. Many African Americans, like members of other ethnic groups, have had negative experiences with the Western medical system. The perception of a judgmental or impersonal attitude in a white health-care provider may contribute to a fear or distrust of the traditional health-care system. As a result of this lack of trust, many African-American patients seek alternative medical treatment.

People of Hispanic/Latino descent (Mexican Americans, Puerto Ricans, and Cuban Americans) are the fastest-growing minority in the United States. Many are at increased risk for alcoholism, cirrhosis, hypertension, specific cancers, and tuberculosis. The incidences of diabetes and cancers of the gallbladder, liver, pancreas, cervix, and stomach are higher among Hispanic/Latino people than in the general population. Cervical and stomach cancers occur more than twice as often in Hispanic/Latino people as among non-Hispanic/Latino whites. There is also an increased incidence of acute promyelocytic leukemia in the Hispanic/Latino population. Within this group, the Puerto Ricans have the poorest health. This may be related to the fact that many older patients do not trust conventional medicine or health-care providers or that migrant people are often forced to live in areas of crowding and poor sanitation.

The rate of tuberculosis among Chinese Americans is higher than in the general population. In fact, the incidence of tuberculosis is more than 40 times higher among Southeast Asians than among the non-Asian population. Both first- and second-generation Chinese Americans have a greater incidence of coronary artery disease than do Asian Chinese, presumably because of differences in diet and stress in the United States. The Japanese and Koreans have the highest incidence of gastric cancer, presumably related to diet and their high consumption of salt. The incidence of liver cancer is more than 12 times higher among the Chinese, Japanese, and Koreans than within the non-Asian population. Hepatitis B is also more common in Southeast Asians.

Native Americans have one of the highest morbidity and mortality rates; their death rate is 30% higher than that of the general population in the United States. This risk may be linked to the fact that Native Americans are one of the most disadvantaged ethnic groups in the United States. They have a high incidence of fetal alcohol syndrome and fetal alcohol effects. In addition, the incidence of congenital adrenal hyperplasia is greater in Native Americans than in the white population.

Traditional Healing Systems

Traditional, or *folk*, *healers* still play a large role in medicine in industrialized societies. Each culture has its own healers: spiritual healers, mediums, herbalists, shamans, fire doctors, medicine men, astrologists, occult healers, bone setters, lay midwives, and leg lengtheners are only a few. Meditation, prayer, massage, exercise, relaxation techniques, acupuncture, acupressure, hypnosis, imagery, therapeutic touch, martial arts, and herbs are important therapeutic modalities of many of these healers. Spiritual healing is widespread. Christian Science healing, started in 1879 in Boston, teaches that those who follow Jesus must follow him in healing, which is done through the mind.

The Hispanic/Latino groups call their traditional healers by different names, such as the Mexican-American *curanderos* (male) or *curanderas* (female) and *parteras*, Puerto Rican *espiritistas*, and Cuban *santeros*. The Haitian voodoo healers, Inuit and African shamans,* Hawaiian *kahunas*, and Navaho singers are also important folk healers for their ethnic groups. It is crucial for the health-care provider to respect patients who follow these practices and to encourage them to express their need for these providers without shame or fear. The health-care provider should discuss with the patients how to combine the help of these providers and medical therapy.

In addition to the natural healing traditions, there are many magical-religious traditions. As stated previously, religion plays a major role in one's perception of illness. The "evil eye" is one of the oldest and most widespread of all superstitions. The nature of the evil eye is defined differently by different groups, but it is generally accepted that an evil eye causes a sudden injury or illness that may be prevented or cured by rituals or symbols. The afflicted person may or may not know the source of the evil eye. There are several traditional practices used in the protection of health; they include wearing objects, such as charms, that protect the wearer.

---

*The *shaman* is a medicine man or priest. He cures illness, directs communal sacrifices, and escorts the souls of the dead to the other world. He accomplishes these tasks by his power to leave his body at will during a trancelike state. A person becomes a shaman by inheriting the shamanistic profession or by election by a supernatural agency. Most self-made shamans are regarded as weaker than those who inherit the profession. The shaman who is born to his role is said to have more bones or teeth than others.

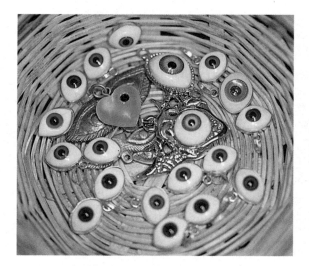

Figure 3–3 Eye beads to protect from the "evil eye."

Figure 3-3 is a photograph that was taken in a *botánica;* it shows eye bead charms that are worn on a string or chain around the neck, wrist, or waist to protect an individual. The blue eye bead is commonly worn by Greeks to ward off the evil eye. The *mal occhio* is worn by people of Italian descent; the *mano milagroso* by Mexicans; the *mano negro* by Puerto Rican babies; the *hamsa,* or Hand of God, by Jews; the *ayn* by the Arabic cultures; the Thunderbird by Hopi Indians; knotted hair or fragments of the Koran by people of South Asia; and red ribbons by Eastern European Jews. The Chinese wear jade to protect them from disease. When the green or red jade object discolors or turns brownish, it is replaced because it is assumed that the person has been exposed to an evil eye or other disease. Figure 3-4 shows several jade bracelets and charms. This photograph was taken in a Chinese jewelry shop in San Francisco's Chinatown.

Various traditional cultures use food substances to protect health. Many people eat raw garlic or onions or wear them around their necks to prevent disease. Members of Greek, Italian, and Native American ethnic groups may hang onion and garlic in their homes for protection. Chicken soup, a Jewish remedy, has long been thought to protect health and speed recovery. *Nervo forza* is a Guatemalan vitamin tonic commonly used in Central America. Traditional Chinese eat "1000-year-old" eggs to prevent illness. The most famous of all Chinese herbs is *ginseng* (*Panax schinseng*), which is derived from the root of a plant

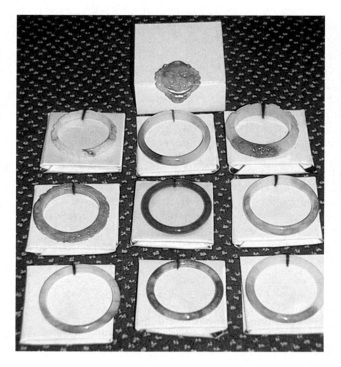

Figure 3–4 Jade bracelets and charms.

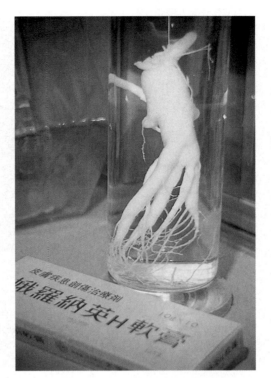

Figure 3–5 Ginseng root.

resembling a human figure. A typical ginseng root appears in Figure 3-5. Ginseng has been revered for thousands of years as a general panacea. Known as an "adaptogen," ginseng has many medicinal purposes; it naturally "adapts" the vital functions of the human system to compensate for adverse conditions such as stress, malnutrition, and the deterioration associated with aging. Ginseng is a slightly bitter root that is used to promote secretion of bodily fluids, and it is recommended by Chinese health practitioners to treat more than 25 medical problems. It is commonly used for anemia, indigestion, impotence, and depression, as well as for replenishing energy and improving sleep. By "building the blood" and stimulating vital organ energies, it is intended to balance the *yin* and *yang* (described later in this chapter) throughout the body. Ginseng must be prepared in earthenware and not in metal because metal destroys its healing properties. Ginseng is contraindicated in patients with excess heat. A bowl of ginseng roots and other ginseng preparations are shown in Figure 3-6.

Finally, many religious objects are worn to protect individuals from disease. The Virgin of Guadalupe is the patron saint of Mexico. It is believed that she protects people and their homes from the evil eye. Her image is pictured on medallions. In the Roman Catholic tradition, there are many saints who are concerned with specific illnesses. People may wear medals with the

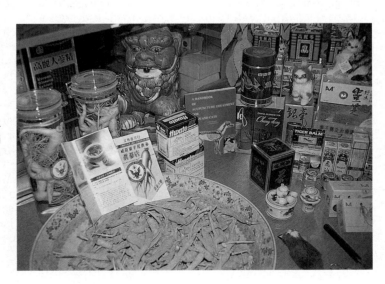

Figure 3–6 Bowl of ginseng roots and other ginseng products.

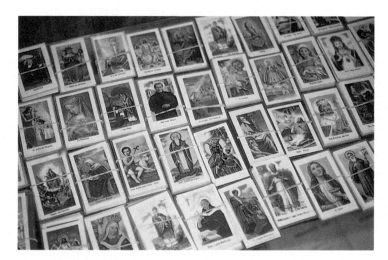

Figure 3–7 Holy cards.

name and the image of the saint on them to prevent the development of a problem. Figure 3-7 shows holy cards with the pictures of saints. These pictures are used to cure and protect individuals from disease. *Gris-gris* are symbols of voodoo; they may take a variety of forms and be used either to protect or harm a person.

Specific Cross-Cultural Perspectives

In this section, some cross-cultural perspectives, including some common beliefs regarding health and illness, are examined. This section also discusses some strategies that can be applied to improving care of patients. The intention is to sensitize the reader to the vast differences among the major ethnic groups in the United States. It is beyond the scope of this book to include all ethnic groups; the reader is referred to the Bibliography at the end of this chapter.

A note about socioeconomic status: Any patient in a low socioeconomic bracket is concerned with maintaining dignity and autonomy, and this should never be compromised in the eyes of the clinician. In addition, a respectful attitude is necessary in attaining a patient's confidence and trust. Patients who are poor may fear that they may not be treated respectfully. Addressing the patient by the appropriate title, such as Dr., Miss, Ms., Mr., or Mrs., is important.

African Americans

African Americans constitute a heterogeneous ethnic group, and therefore it is impossible to make generalizations because there is no prototypical African-American patient. They live in all areas of the United States and are represented in every socioeconomic group, with a disproportionate number living in poverty. As a result, in many inner-city populations, lack of access to quality health care has particular deleterious consequences for many of them. One alarming result is that many preventable diseases often progress to life-threatening stages. Some diseases, such as diabetes mellitus and hypertension, are highly prevalent among African Americans. Consequently, when examining an African-American patient, regardless of socioeconomic status, the clinician should screen for these diseases and educate both the patient and the patient's family. Because of media stereotyping, African Americans may react negatively to a general screening for human immunodeficiency virus (HIV) or substance abuse. Clinicians need to approach this with sensitivity and reserve this testing for the segment of the African-American community that is at risk.

In Africa, illness has traditionally been attributed to several causes, primarily to demons and evil spirits. Beliefs regarding the role of spirits in causing disease may persist.

It is particularly important to investigate dietary patterns in the African-American patient. Certain ethnic foods, such as rice, plantain, yams, and okra, have deep cultural roots and should not be eliminated from the diet, if possible. Other ethnic foods, such as collards and turnips that are often heavily seasoned with salt and cured meat, may pose a health problem. Without the salt, these foods are wholesome parts of a diet. The eating of Argo starch has a

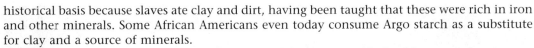

historical basis because slaves ate clay and dirt, having been taught that these were rich in iron and other minerals. Some African Americans even today consume Argo starch as a substitute for clay and a source of minerals.

As culture defines health and illness, it also defines acceptable health-care and treatment practices. All cultures offer home remedies as part of self-care. For some African Americans, the following is a partial list of home remedies:

- Poultices to fight infection
- Herbal teas
- Hot lemon tea with honey for colds
- Hot toddies for colds and congestion
- Raw onions placed on the feet in cases of fever
- The white membrane from a raw egg placed over a boil to bring it to a head
- Hot camphorated oil and mustard plaster on the chest for chest congestion
- Garlic placed on an ill person or in the person's room to remove evil spirits

Hispanic/Latino People

The fastest-growing minority group in the United States comprises the Spanish-speaking peoples from various parts of the western hemisphere: Puerto Rico, Cuba, the Dominican Republic, Mexico and other Central American countries, and South America. The Latinos residing in the United States are one of the youngest of the ethnic groups. In Census 2000, 35.7% of people in the Hispanic/Latino group were younger than 18 years of age. Demographers have predicted, on the basis of the Latinos' young age, their high fertility rate, and their migratory patterns, that by 2010 they would become the largest ethnic group in the United States, accounting for 42% of the population. Although bonded by a common language and grouped together by their Spanish surnames, the Latino group has great heterogeneity and diversity in its many different traditions. Although Spanish has no dialects, many words may carry different meanings for various Latino groups, depending on their community of origin. The prevention of illness is a common practice frequently accomplished with praying, keeping relics in the home, and wearing religious amulets or medals. Figure 3-8 shows some religious amulets; Figure 3-9 shows a variety of rosaries and good-luck beads hanging in the foreground and magical oils and elixirs in the background. These photographs were taken in a *botánica* in New York City.

Latinos, like other traditional groups, are known for having a close-knit family unit, *la familia*. Latino families have strong ties and have maintained many of the qualities of the extended family system. They may have a great fear of being hospitalized and thus being separated from their families. Those who speak only Spanish are concerned that they will not be able to communicate with the medical personnel when help is needed. They have a sense of obligation toward each other and are expected to be responsible for all members of the family. It is not uncommon for a 90-year-old patient who speaks no English to be accompanied to the hospital by his or her children, grandchildren, great-grandchildren, and even great-

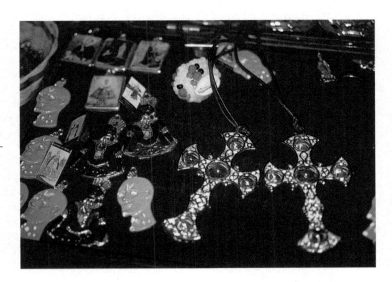

Figure 3–8 Religious amulets.

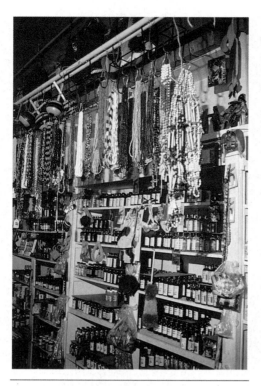

Figure 3–9 Beads, rosaries, and magic oils.

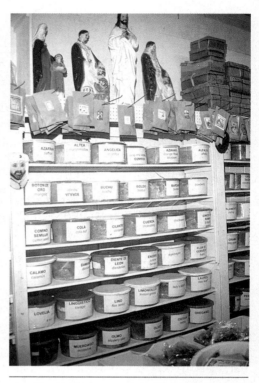

Figure 3–10 Dried exotic herbs and teas in a *botánica*.

great-grandchildren. Decision-making is likewise a family matter. Never pressure the patient into making a decision; allow the patient time to discuss an issue with his or her family.

It is common for first- and second-generation Hispanic/Latino U.S. residents, as for many other immigrant groups, to regard health-care institutions with a certain amount of distrust. When caring for a Hispanic/Latino patient, the clinician must consider the family as well. Some Hispanic/Latino people (more often the elderly, recent immigrants, and the less educated) still believe in *curanderos* or *curanderas, espiritistas,* or *santeros*, who are the holistic, family folk practitioners and spiritual counselors. These spiritualists believe that illness is caused by an intentional act of God, supernatural forces, or the ill will of others, and they emphasize healing through religious or medical ceremonies, potions, and amulets. They use a variety of *yerbas* (herbs, especially teas), charms, massages, and magical rituals. *Limpias,* or cleansing, is performed by passing an unbroken egg or selected herbs tied together over the body of the ill person. These healers do not advertise but are well known throughout their individual communities and play an important role in Hispanic/Latino health care. A *yerberia* or *botánica* is a community resource for purchasing traditional remedies and charms. Figure 3-10 shows containers with dried exotic herbs and teas. Again, the Christian and Arabic influences are evident.

Patients are often fearful of discussing these health-care practices with clinicians. For this reason, when they feel trusting enough to do so, it is important that the health-care provider receive this information in a respectful manner. Try to work with the belief. Because many herbal remedies are pharmacologically active, it may be necessary to ask the patient not to consume them simultaneously with pharmaceuticals. There is usually a close, personal relationship between the patient and the healer. By using medical knowledge and adapting it to the patient's beliefs, you can gain the patient's confidence and encourage cooperation.

Candles play an important role in traditional healing. The votive candles are for specific deities or saints or for specific requests, such as money, love, health, and success. The candles are lit, and prayers are recited. Figure 3-11 shows some of the candles for sale in a *botánica*.

Two important values in the Latino culture are *respeto* and *dignidad*. *Respeto* is demonstrated to a Hispanic/Latino patient when the health-care provider dresses in the traditional garb of the profession expected by the Latino patient and communicates an interest in his or her life and health. Hispanic/Latino people also enjoy a brief social conversation before a discussion of their illness. This helps to develop a sense of *confianza,* or trust.

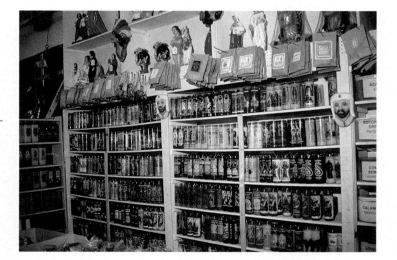

Figure 3-11 Votive candles.

The belief in *Santería* originated more than 400 years ago in Cuba out of traditions of the African Yoruba people from Nigeria and Benin. These people were transported to Cuba to work as slaves on sugar plantations. From Cuba, this religious cult spread to the neighboring islands and to the United States; it arrived in New York in the late 1940s. *Santería* blends elements of West African beliefs with Roman Catholicism. Once a ghetto religion, *Santería* has a growing following among middle-class professionals, including white persons, African Americans, Latinos, and Asian Americans. The followers believe in one Supreme Being but also in African divinities known as *orishas*, each of which represents a human characteristic, such as power, or an aspect of nature, such as thunder. Each of these deities is worshiped in the image of a Catholic saint. There are several *orishas* related to health problems: the *orisha* Chango is linked to Saint Barbara,* who is the god of thunder, lightning, and violent death; *orisha* Bacoso, with Saint Christopher (infections); and *orisha* Ifa, with Saint Anthony (fertility). Statues of saints or deities are commonly purchased for the home.

Figures 3-2 and 3-12 show some religious statues sold in a *botánica*. The believers pray to these idols to intervene with God to improve their lives and obtain blessings. Many of these idols are used for prayers for health. Notice the African elements blended with Catholicism in the idols. The seated figure with the red tie is Maximón, a Guatemalan believed to have powers for producing health, tranquility, protection, happiness, wealth, and improved sexual performance. The standing figure in the black suit to the right is the Venezuelan physician Dr. José Gregorio Hernandez Cisnero. He was known for his health-related miracles, and patients pray

---

*St. Barbara's father was struck by lightning as he beheaded her for her faith.

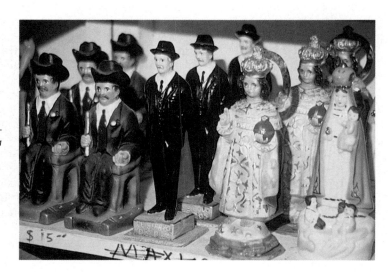

Figure 3–12 Religious *Santería* statues.

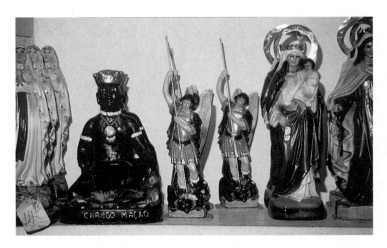

Figure 3–13 The orisha Chango on the left.

to him for health. The figure in the reddish-pink and gold robe with the crown is the famous statue of Baby Jesus of Prague, known in Spanish as *El Niñito Jesus de Prague* (also, *Atacha*). Figure 3-13 shows the orisha Chango.

There is a very structured hierarchy in the practice of *Santería*. In charge is the *babalow;* next is the *presidente*, the head medium; and the third practitioner is the *santero*. The *santero*, an important, respected member of the Latino community, is said to possess the magical power of the *orishas*, known as *ache*. Ritual devotions involving African rhythms and dancing; offerings of food and animal sacrifice; divination with shells, bones, and eggs; trancelike states; and other rites are thought to reveal the sources of problems and to help in their resolution. During the ritual, the *santero* dresses in white robes with beaded necklaces and bracelets. *Santería* can be practiced in homes, parks, storefronts, or basements.

La partera or *la comadrona* is the traditional midwife or birth attendant in the Latino culture. These women are described as warm, caring, and cooperative. Their role is to give advice to pregnant women, to treat pregnant women for illnesses with herbs and massages, and to be in attendance during labor and delivery. The women offer both emotional and instrumental support during and after childbirth. Most *parteras* have birthing rooms in their homes.

There are several traditional, or *culture-bound*, illnesses of the Latinos. A culture-bound illness is one that is culturally defined. It may or may not have an equivalent from a Western medical perspective. Emotional trauma and strong emotions are recognized throughout Latin America as causes of illness. Conditions such as *mal de ojo, empacho, ataque de nervios, susto, male aire*, and *caida de mollera* are examples of Latino culture-bound syndromes.

*Mal de ojo,** or evil eye, is the result of dangerous imbalances in social relationships; illness is blamed on the "strong glance" of an envious person. Fever, sleeplessness, and headaches are common symptoms. *Empacho*, or upset stomach, occurs when a Latino patient is psychologically stressed during or immediately after eating. The main symptom is a feeling of a "ball in the stomach" associated with abdominal pain. *Ataque de nervios* is manifested by a sudden outburst of shouting or swearing, accompanied by a variety of symptoms that include dyspnea, chest tightness, memory loss, trembling, sense of heat, palpitations, dizziness, and paresthesias; it may be accompanied by, or caused by, hyperventilation. It is often seen when the patient is confronted with stressful life events, such as an accident, an acute severe illness, a funeral, or a death. During the episode, the person may fall to the ground with convulsions or lie motionless. An *ataque de nervios* may progress to *susto*, which is a prolonged condition that a patient experiences after having been exposed to a traumatic event. The patient is depressed, lacks interest in living, is withdrawn, and has a disruption of eating and hygienic habits. *Susto*, a nonkinetic fugue state, is a common stress reaction and may be described in part as a state of disorientation and confusion. Ritual prayers and herbal remedies are the common treatment. *Mal aire*, or bad air, is said to cause pain, facial twitching, and paralysis in children. Mothers are concerned that their young children will develop *mal aire* when exposed to cold air. It is therefore important to keep Latino children covered during an examination. *Caida de mollera*, or fallen fontanelle, affects infants; the fontanelle is displaced from its normal position at the top of the head. Diarrhea and restlessness are associated symptoms. It is important to reiterate

*Also used by some groups to refer to actual eye disease.

that beliefs in folk healing cannot be generalized to all Latinos. These traditional beliefs vary from generation to generation and depend largely on the extent of assimilation into the mainstream culture.

Asian Americans

Asian Americans place much emphasis on obligation, authority, and honor. Those who have disgraced their families consequently suffer guilt. This guilt can be transformed into psychosomatic disease, which is common in this culture. Asian-American patients rarely complain of pain. They may suffer with it, but their complaints are few. If the health-care provider suspects that a patient is having pain, it is fitting to ask whether pain is present. In general, after being asked, the patients acknowledge the pain. Older-generation Chinese individuals tend not to display emotions openly to strangers, nor do they usually accept any type of comforting physical contact, such as touching a shoulder or hand, as a form of empathy. In contrast to the Chinese or Japanese, in the Korean culture touching is common among men and women. In fact, it is far more common than in Western cultures.

Titles are important in communicating with the Japanese patient, as with other groups. The family name is usually written first. Bowing is very common and indicates respect; it is used when greeting and leaving. Avoiding eye contact, particularly with older Japanese patients, demonstrates respect. Another aspect of dealing with Japanese or Korean patients relates to the "yes-no" question and the infrequent use of the word "no." Most older Japanese and Korean persons believe that to answer "no" puts an individual on the defensive. Therefore, they may answer "yes," meaning that they understand, not necessarily answering in the affirmative to the question. Nodding the head generally indicates attentiveness of the Japanese patient and not necessarily agreement. With some Japanese patients, as in other cultures, giggling is often a sign of embarrassment. Interviewers require patience and may need to proceed more slowly when questioning the Asian patient about intimate information, such as sexual behavior. It is generally best to avoid humor when interviewing a Japanese patient, especially an older patient.

Many Asian Americans believe in traditional medicine and distrust Western medicine. The "hot-cold" theory of disease is still accepted by some Asian Americans. Another example of the balancing of internal forces is seen in the Chinese belief in *yin* and *yang*. Everything in the world consists of both *yin* and *yang* forces. *Yin* is dark, female, and negative; *yang* is light, male, and positive. The key to good health is the balance between *yin* and *yang*; Chinese herbs and acupuncture help restore this balance. A common problem among Chinese patients is related to medication. According to traditional Chinese medicine, one dose of an herbal remedy usually "cures" an illness. Prescriptions of Western medications may require multiple doses over longer periods. Chinese patients may have difficulty in complying with this schedule. It is the clinician's responsibility to explain carefully this difference in "medical" therapy.

Figure 3-14 is a picture taken in a traditional herbal pharmacy in San Francisco; it shows jars containing medicinal Chinese herbs. Deer antlers, mercury, turtle shells, bull testicles,

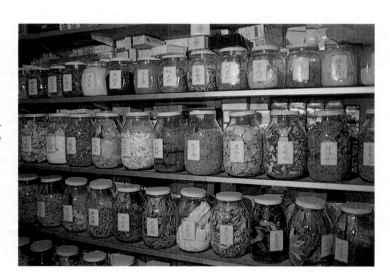

Figure 3–14 Medicinal Chinese herbs.

snake meat, seahorses, and rhinoceros horns are other popular Chinese cures. The interviewer must respect the patient's belief and, by attempting to understand it, is equipped to provide better care.

Many Chinese and Vietnamese persons, like other people, have an intense fear of being admitted to a Western hospital. This anxiety stems from the language barrier, inability to find a translator, fear of isolation from the family, different practices, and even food; many Southeast Asian persons are lactose intolerant. The health-care provider must explain in detail the plan of treatment to the patient and the family members. If an interpreter is needed, the provider must ensure that the interpreter speaks the same dialect.

As in other traditional cultures, Asian Americans have several important culture-bound syndromes: *hwa-byung, taijin kyofusho, hsieh-ping, amok, wagamama, shinkeishitsu*, and *koro*. *Hwa-byung* is a common, multiple somatic and psychological disorder, seen usually in married Korean women. Epigastric pain is the presenting symptom; it is feared that the pain will lead to death, and associated symptoms include insomnia, dyspnea, palpitations, and muscle aches. It often appears that anger is the precipitating cause. *Taijin kyofusho* is a syndrome in Japanese patients in which the patients complain that their body parts or functions are offensive to others. *Hsieh-ping* is a trancelike state in which Chinese patients believe themselves to be possessed by a dead relative or friend whom they have offended. *Amok*, which afflicts Malay men, is a sudden spree of violent attacks on people, animals, and objects. *Wagamama*, seen in Japanese patients, manifests with apathetic childish behavior with emotional outbursts. *Shinkeishitsu* is a form of severe anxiety and obsessional neurosis seen in young Japanese patients. *Koro*, a name of Malay origin, is a delusional condition seen in Southeast Asian and Chinese male patients; the patient suddenly grasps his penis, fearing that it will retract into his abdomen and ultimately cause his death. Family members are frequently called on to hold the penis. This disorder may continue for several days. The condition may be linked to another associated belief called "semen anxiety," in which the patient feels that he has a deficiency of semen, which is believed to be a fatal condition.

Asian Indians

Asian Indians are people from India, Pakistan, Nepal, Bangladesh, and Sri Lanka. Although most Asian Indians speak English well, some idioms may produce confusion. The most common religious groups among Asian Indians are Hindus, Muslims, and Sikhs. Hindus believe that life is a circle, continuous, without a beginning or end. There is also a strong belief in astrology. The Hindu family is a very strong unit, and health-care decisions are commonly made by the senior members of the family. The cow is considered sacred; eating beef or veal, therefore, is strongly prohibited.

Muslims follow the teachings of Mohammed and Islam. The main principles of Islam are generosity, fairness, respect, cleanliness, and honesty. The consumption of alcohol, pork, and lard is strictly prohibited. Sex education and cremation are also commonly forbidden. Older Muslim patients may have a fatalistic attitude, which can interfere with compliance with medical therapy. Many Muslim women wear a veil over their head when in the presence of men outside the family and prefer female health-care providers. In some cases, if a patient's husband is present, a male clinician may be allowed to examine her.

Sikhism started in the 15th century in northern India. Sikhs believe in a single God and in reincarnation. Baptized Sikhs do not cut their hair and do not smoke or drink alcohol; many are vegetarians. A traditional Sikh greeting, similar to that of other Asian Indians, is with the palms of the hands pressed together in front of the chest. Women generally do not shake hands, and eye contact may be considered disrespectful.

The Asian-Indian population relies heavily on a wide-ranging pharmacopeia. Remedies can come from almost any natural substance. *Ayurvedic medicine* is an ancient Indian medical system; it teaches that imbalance in the body humors results in illness. Treatment is to restore the balance. Although Western medicine is recognized in India, it is estimated that there are nearly 4000 people for every Western-taught physician.

It is important for the clinician to recognize that taste and food are important parts of Asian-Indian beliefs. Each taste is believed to have special properties: sweet increases phlegm and appeases hunger and thirst; acid increases salivation and improves digestion; salt purifies the blood; pungent food provokes the appetite; bitter food also stimulates the appetite and clears the complexion. The study of medicines is more important than the study of illness; the traditional healer deals with symptoms and usually ignores the disease.

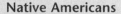

Native Americans

Native Americans constitute a heterogeneous group that comprises more than 400 federally recognized nations. American Indians, Aleuts, and Inuits (and Inupiats)* are the largest groups of Native Americans. The traditional belief about health is that it reflects living in total harmony with nature and having the ability to survive under dire circumstances. People must treat their bodies with respect. Many Native Americans believe that there is a reason for every illness; illness is the price paid for something bad that had occurred or will occur. Several tribes associate illness with evil spirits. Illness may also result from breaking a taboo or the attack of a ghost or witch.

The traditional healer is the medicine man or woman. Often, the medicine man or woman uses meditation and crystal balls. On occasion, the medicine man or woman uses the root of jimsonweed to produce a trance to enable him or her to treat the patient better. The cause of illness is diagnosed by three types of divination: motion of the hand, star gazing, and listening. Chanting is a major part of the process. Many Native Americans also believe in witchcraft. Herbal remedies and an act of purification are major steps to curing illness.

Two important problems among Native Americans are alcohol abuse and domestic violence. Alcohol abuse is a critical health problem that is widespread and immeasurably costly to the Native American community. In historical, traditional Native American homes, alcohol abuse was not common. Currently, domestic violence is a major problem, and it is frequently related to alcohol abuse. The rate of suicide is also high among this population. In addition, there is a higher proportion of postnatal deaths among Native Americans, presumably because the women have inadequate prenatal care.

The Jewish People

Approximately 6 million Jewish people live in the United States. There are two large groups: the *Ashkenazim*, whose origins can be traced to Eastern or Northern Europe, and the *Sephardim*, whose origins are from the Mediterranean countries or the Iberian Peninsula. The majority of the Jews in the United States follow the Ashkenazi traditions. The Ashkenazim are linked linguistically through Yiddish, and the Sephardim are linked by Ladino, Spanish, Portuguese, French, or Arabic.

In the United States, there are three main divisions of the Jewish people, based on adherence to traditional practices and interpretation of Jewish law: Orthodox, Conservative, and Reform. Although most Jews dress indistinguishably from others, many Orthodox individuals observe Jewish law by covering their heads with a skullcap called a *yarmulke* or *kippah*. Many married Orthodox women cover their heads with hats, wigs, or kerchiefs. Because of tradition, men and women are commonly separated in social situations. Another division of Jewish people is the *Hasidim*. This group broke off from mainstream Judaism in the 17th century in order to serve God without the necessity for immersion in religious study that was the standard in the Eastern European Jewish community at that time. Hasidim usually wear 17th century-type black robes or suits with black hats. The men twirl their hair into ringlets at the sides of their face. Hasidim are generally passionate about their worship and adhere strictly to the biblical laws. These laws include restrictions regarding permissible foods (*kosher* laws, or *Kashrut*[†]) and forbidden foods (pork products or shellfish).

The Sabbath (*Shabbat* or *Shabbos*) is a strictly observed day of rest. When scheduling appointments, be aware of the Sabbath and do not schedule tests or clinic visits from Friday afternoon until after Saturday evening. Many religious Jews do not use anything electrical on the Sabbath. Therefore, when visiting a religious Jewish person in the hospital, an interviewer may find that the rooms are dark because the patient and his or her family are not allowed to turn on the lights; the interviewer, however, may turn them on. Despite the many rules of

---

*The Eskimo people are identified by place of residence. The Eastern Eskimos live from eastern Greenland to northern Alaska. The Western Eskimos live to the west of Alaska: the Bering Sea, St. Lawrence Island, and the northern Pacific. The term *Eskimo* is now thought to be unflattering. Speakers of the Eastern Eskimo language call themselves *Inuit*, on the basis of the *Inuit* language they speak. Although the term *Inuit* has been used to describe all Eskimos, it is appropriate only for those speaking the eastern language. In Alaska, the Eskimo people call themselves *Inupiat*, on the basis of the Inupiat dialect of the Inuit language. The Western Eskimos are now referred to as *Yupik,* on the basis of the language they speak.

[†]The rules of the kosher diet mandate the exclusion of shellfish and pork products. Dairy products may not be eaten with meat products. In addition, only fish with scales and fins and only certain types of meat from animals with a cloven hoof and that chew the cud can be eaten.

Orthodox Judaism, health always comes first. Even on fasting days, pills may be taken, and ill and elderly persons, as well as children, are permitted to eat.

Many Jewish holidays are not marked on calendars. The health-care provider should ask the patient about them when scheduling tests, to determine whether holidays will conflict with appointments. Many Jewish people may want to consult their rabbi before having a certain test performed or taking some form of medication. This should not be misconstrued as a mistrust of the health-care provider; it is often culturally motivated.

There are several genetic conditions that appear more frequently in the Jewish population. These include Tay-Sachs disease, Gaucher's disease, Bloom's syndrome, ataxia-telangiectasia, Creutzfeldt-Jakob disease, familial Mediterranean fever, Glanzmann's thrombasthenia, pemphigus vulgaris, polycythemia vera, and Niemann-Pick disease.

When an Orthodox Jew dies, the body is never left alone from the time of death until burial; Orthodox friends and family pray around the body. The body is not embalmed, and the burial is usually within 24 hours. One exception to this rule would be if the death occurred on a Friday evening (the Sabbath); the burial would then be on Sunday. Autopsies usually are not allowed unless approved by the family's rabbi.

The primary group targeted for annihilation in World War II was the Jewish people. Because of these experiences, Jewish patients, especially the older generation and older immigrants, may manifest greater discomfort, fear, and anxiety when confined in a hospital and when decisions are made about them. For more information, refer to the discussion of post-traumatic stress disorder in Chapter 2, The Patient's Responses.

International Society for Krishna Consciousness

An important, small, originally Indian group in the United States is the International Society for Krishna Consciousness. Its members believe in four rules of conduct: (1) no eating of meat, fish, or eggs; (2) no illicit sex; (3) no intoxicants; and (4) no gambling. They believe that the body is ruled by passion and the soul by serenity. The Krishna lifestyle is strictly regulated, and illness should never interfere with these activities. Followers seek medical assistance only when they are extremely ill.

Romanies

The tradition of the Romanies (or "Gypsies") poses important health-care problems. According to the Romany culture, the sources of all disease are demons, the evil eye, breaking taboos, and the fear of disease itself. Several Romany treatments involve transferring disease symbolically to another person or object. In general, Romanies turn to organized health care only during times of crisis. They do not hesitate to come to the hospital for serious illness; often, the extended family or entire tribe may accompany the patient. Preventive medicine and follow-up care are rarely used. Romany women are extremely reluctant to expose their bodies to male health-care providers.

In order to protect their anonymity, Romanies are reluctant to identify themselves as such, often use assumed names, and may not provide truthful answers to non-Romany interviewers. Once a trusting relationship with a health-care provider has been established, however, many Romanies feel more inclined to rely on that individual.

Concluding Thoughts

Health-care professionals cannot be expected to know everything about each culture; rather, it is important that they know it is important to keep in mind cultural considerations in the treatment process and the doctor-patient relationship. This chapter has introduced the health-care provider to some aspects of several diverse cultures. Ideally, the clinician can be better prepared for the challenges of caring for patients in this multicultural society.

Bibliography

Aday LA: At Risk in America—The Health and Health Care Needs of Vulnerable Populations in the United States. San Francisco, Jossey-Bass, 1993.
Adler NE, Boyce WT, Chesney MA, et al: Socioeconomic inequities in health: No easy solution. JAMA 269:3140, 1993.

Association of State and Territorial Health Officials: ASTHO bilingual health initiative: Report and recommendations. Washington, DC, Office of Minority Health, 1992.

Bigby JA (ed): Cross-Cultural Medicine. Philadelphia, American College of Physicians, 2003.

Blackhall LJ, Murphy ST, Frank G, et al: Ethnicity and attitudes toward patient autonomy. JAMA 274: 820, 1995.

Brooks T: Pitfalls in communication with Hispanic and African-American patients: Do translators help or harm? J Natl Med Assoc 84:941, 1992.

Buchwald D, Caralis PV, Gany F, et al: Caring for patients in a multicultural society. Patient Care 15: 105, 1994.

Carrese JA, Rhodes LA: Western bioethics on the Navajo reservation: Benefit or harm? JAMA 274:826, 1995.

Cohen MR, Doner K: The Chinese Way to Healing: Many Paths to Wholeness. New York, Perigee, 1996.

D'Avanzo CE: Barriers to health care of Vietnamese refugees. J Prof Nurs 8:245, 1992.

Fadiman A: The Spirit Catches You and You Fall Down: A Hmong Child, Her American Doctors, and the Collision of Two Cultures. New York, Farrar, Straus, and Giroux, 1997.

Galanti G: An introduction to cultural differences. West J Med 172:335, 2000.

Goston L: Informed consent, cultural sensitivity, and respect for persons. JAMA 274:844, 1995.

Grieco EM, Cassidy RC: Overview of Race and Hispanic Origin: Census 2000 Brief. C2KBR/01-1, Census 2000. Washington, DC, U.S. Census Bureau, 2001.

Haffner L: Translation is not enough. West J Med 157:255, 1992.

Hartog J, Hartog EA: Cultural aspects of health and illness behavior in hospitals. West J Med 139:106, 1983.

Helman CG: Culture, Health and Illness, 2nd ed. London, Wright, 1990.

Herrera J, Lawson W (eds): Cross-Cultural Issues in Psychopharmacology. Mt Sinai J Med 63:283, 1996.

Hodgkinson HL: A Demographic Look at Tomorrow. Washington, DC, Institute for Educational Leadership, 1992.

Kaptchuk TJ: The Web That Has No Weaver: Understanding Chinese Medicine. Chicago, Congdon & Weed, 1983.

Lipkin M, Putnam SM, Lazare A (eds): The Medical Interview: Clinical Care, Education, and Research. New York, Springer-Verlag, 1995.

McIvor RJ: Making the most of interpreters. Br J Psychiatry 165:268, 1994.

Mezzich JE, Kleinman A, Fabrega H Jr, et al (eds): Culture and Psychiatric Disorder: A DSM-IV Perspective. Washington, DC, American Psychiatric Press, 1996.

Mollina CW, Aguirre-Molina M (eds): Latino Health in the U.S.: A Growing Challenge. Washington, DC, American Public Health Association, 1994.

Morrison T, Conaway WA, Borden GA: Kiss, Bow, or Shake Hands. Holbrook, Mass, Adams Media, 1994.

Murray RH, Rubel AJ: Physicians and healers: Unwitting partners in health care. N Engl J Med 326:61, 1992.

Ngubane H: Body and Mind in Zulu Medicine. London, Academic Press, 1977.

Nilchaikowit T, Jill JM, Holland JC: The effects of culture on illness behavior and medical care: Asian and American differences. Gen Hosp Psychiatry 15:41, 1993.

Nwanna GI: Do's and Don'ts Around the World: A Country Guide to Cultural and Social Taboos and Etiquette: Asia. Baltimore, World Travel Institute, 1998.

Nwanna GI: Do's and Don'ts Around the World: A Country Guide to Cultural and Social Taboos and Etiquette: Europe. Baltimore, World Travel Institute, 1998.

Nwanna GI: Do's and Don'ts Around the World: A Country Guide to Cultural and Social Taboos and Etiquette: South America. Baltimore, World Travel Institute, 1998.

Nwanna GI: Do's and Don'ts Around the World: A Country Guide to Cultural and Social Taboos and Etiquette: The Caribbean. Baltimore, World Travel Institute, 1998.

Nwanna GI: Do's and Don'ts Around the World: A Country Guide to Cultural and Social Taboos and Etiquette: The Middle East. Baltimore, World Travel Institute, 1998.

O'Connor BB: Healing Traditions. Philadelphia, University of Pennsylvania Press, 1995.

Penny CA: Interpretation for Inuit patients essential element of health care in eastern Arctic. CMAJ 150:1860, 1994.

Perry MJ, Mackun PJ: Population Change and Distribution: Census 2000 Brief. C2KBR/01-2, Census 2000. Washington, DC, U.S. Census Bureau, 2001.

Post LF, Blustein J, Gordon E, et al: Pain: Ethics, culture, and informed consent to relief. J Law Med Ethics 24:348, 1996.

Ramakrishna J, Weiss MG: Health, illness, and immigration: East Indians in the United States. West J Med 157:265, 1992.

Reid D: The Shambhala Guide to Traditional Chinese Medicine. Boston, Shambhala Publications, 1996.

Sisty-LePeau N: Oral healthcare and cultural barriers. J Dent Hyg 67:156, 1993.

Skultans V: The symbolic significance of menstruation and the menopause. Man 5:639, 1970.

Snow LF: Folk medical beliefs and their implications for care of patients: A review based on studies among black Americans. Ann Intern Med 81:82, 1974.

Snow LF, Johnson SM: Modern-day menstrual folklore. JAMA 237:2736, 1977.

Spector RE: Cultural Diversity in Health and Illness, 4th ed. Stamford, Conn, Appleton & Lange, 1996.

Thernstorm S (ed): Harvard Encyclopedia of American Ethnic Groups. Boston, Relknar Press. 1980.

Therrien, M, Ramirez RR: The Hispanic Population of the United States: Population Characteristics: March 2000. Current Population Reports, P20-535, Census 2000. Washington, DC, US Census Bureau, 2001.

Todd KH, Samaroo N, Hoffman JR: Ethnicity as a risk factor for inadequate emergency department analgesia. JAMA 269:1537, 1993.

Trill MD, Holland J: Cross-cultural differences in the care of patients with cancer: A review. Gen Hosp Psychiatry 15:21, 1993.

Tumulty P: What is a clinician and what does he do? N Engl J Med 283:20, 1970.

U.S. Census Bureau: Census 2000 Current Population Survey. Washington, DC, U.S. Census Bureau, 2000.

U.S. Census Bureau: Census 2000 Redistricting, Public Law 94-171. Washington, DC, U.S. Census Bureau, 2000.

U.S. Department of Health and Human Services: Healthy People 2000: National Health Promotion and Disease Prevention Objectives—Special Population Objectives. Washington, DC, U.S. Department of Health and Human Services, 1989.

Watt IS, Howel D, Lo L: The health care experience and health behavior of the Chinese: A survey based in Hull. J Public Health Med 15:129, 1993.

Woloshin S, Bickell NA, Schwartz LM, et al: Language barriers in medicine in the United States. JAMA 273:724, 1995.

Zborowski M: Cultural components in response to pain. J Soc Issues 8:16, 1952.

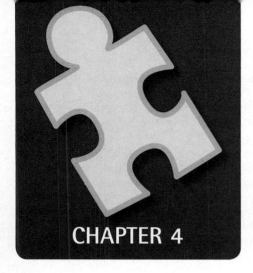

CHAPTER 4

Understanding Complementary and Alternative Medicine

The natural healing force within each of us is the greatest force in getting well.

Hippocrates (460–377 BCE)

General Considerations

Studies have shown that the frequency of use of complementary or alternative medical therapy in the United States is far greater than previously reported. These therapies include relaxation techniques, imagery, chiropractic, massage, spiritual healing, herbal medicine, acupuncture, homeopathy, folk remedies, and prayer, to name a few. It has been estimated that 42% of the American population uses at least one of these and other alternative healing methods to satisfy their medical needs. The most common users of complementary and alternative therapy are the more affluent people, women, those better educated, individuals born after 1950, and those who are concerned about emotional stress and the environment. The most common therapies were relaxation techniques (18%), massage (12%), herbal medicine (10%), and megavitamin therapy (9%). The perceived efficacy of these therapies ranged from 76% (hypnosis) to 98% (energy healing). The number of visits to providers of this health care is greater than the number of visits to all primary care medical doctors nationwide. More than 70% of these patients never mention using alternative therapy to their clinicians. Out-of-pocket expenditures of more than $34 billion per year in the United States are an apparent testament to a widely held belief that complementary and alternative medicine therapies have benefits that outweigh their costs. This figure is in contrast to the $12.8 billion spent out of pocket annually for all hospitalizations in the United States.

One of the reasons why patients seek complementary and alternative therapies may be a failure in the doctor-patient relationship. Health-care providers often fail to discuss the use of these therapies because they lack adequate knowledge in this area and have poor insight into the cultures and beliefs of those who practice complementary and alternative medicine (CAM). To many health-care providers, "alternative medicine" entails the threat of displacing conventional medicine for the sake of unproven therapies. It may lack organization and the rigorous, scientific standards of Western, evidence-based medicine. The response of the health-care providers ranges from outright dismissal of the practices to a gradual recognition that their extensive use can no longer be ignored. A lack of communication and knowledge in this area may also prove to be detrimental to the patient because the use of some forms of these therapies, if unsupervised, may be dangerous.

There has been an increasing interest throughout the world in the use of natural ingredients for health, especially tea. Tea is the world's second most popular beverage after water. Green tea accounts for approximately 20% of all tea consumed. It has been claimed that overall health of the body, especially the oral cavity, can be maintained by the consumption of green tea. Green tea is not fermented; therefore, it contains polyphenols that are inactivated in the fermentation process of black tea production. Green tea has been consumed in East Asia, where its benefits have been claimed for centuries. Green tea polyphenols possess antioxidant and antiviral properties that account for its benefits; these benefits have been touted to include lowering blood pressure, lowering cholesterol, stabilizing blood glucose, inhibiting bacterial growth, and blocking many carcinogenic agents. Polyphenols have been shown to inhibit the growth of *Streptococcus mutans*, the major etiologic bacterium associated with dental caries, and *Porphyromonas gingivalis*, the bacterium associated with periodontal disease.

In April 1995, the National Center for Complementary and Alternative Medicine (NCCAM) of the National Institutes of Health (NIH) defined CAM as "a broad domain of healing resources that encompasses all health systems, modalities, and practices and their accompanying theories and beliefs, other than those intrinsic to the politically dominant health system of a particular society or culture in a given historical period." This group of diverse medical and health-care systems, practices, and products is not currently part of conventional (i.e., allopathic) medicine, although some conventional medical practitioners (those with an MD, DO, or other health-related degrees) are also practitioners of CAM. The CAM marketplace is currently valued at $24 billion or more, and the growth rate is close to 15% per year. Since the inception of the NCCAM, Congress has provided almost $550 million to promote CAM and CAM research. In fiscal year 2004, the funding for NCCAM was $117.7 million.

In December 1995, the American Medical Association (AMA) passed the resolution "Unconventional Medical Care in the United States." The AMA encourages NCCAM to determine by objective scientific evaluation the efficacy and safety of practices and procedures of unconventional medicine and encourages its members to become better informed regarding the practices and techniques of alternative or unconventional medicine.*

What is CAM? **Complementary medicine,** such as aromatherapy, is used *in conjunction with* conventional medicine: for example, to lessen a patient's postoperative discomfort. **Alternative medicine,** such as some herbal medicines, is used *instead of* conventional medicine to treat cancer. Alternative therapies include, but are not limited to, the following disciplines: folk medicine, herbal medicine, diet fads, homeopathy, faith healing, new age healing, chiropractic, acupuncture, naturopathy, reflexology, massage, and music therapy. **Integrative medicine** combines conventional medical and CAM therapies for which there is some scientific evidence of safety and effectiveness, regardless of their origin.

The purpose of this chapter is to educate the reader about CAM. Medical schools in the United States are now including courses in which CAM is taught, but 80% of medical students polled have indicated that they would like more information. Because 29 health-care insurance companies in the United States now cover CAM therapies and 67% of health maintenance organizations now offer at least one form of CAM, it is crucial for health-care providers to become more cognizant about these therapies. In the future, there will be more well-designed, randomized, controlled studies that will provide answers to many of today's questions regarding CAM.

Classifications of Complementary and Alternative Medicine

The NCCAM has classified CAM therapies into five major but overlapping categories:

1. Alternative medical systems
2. Mind-body interventions
3. Biologically based therapies
4. Manipulative and body-based methods
5. Energy therapies

---

*Policies of House of Delegates-I-95; H-480.973; BOT Rep. 15-A-94, Reaffirmed and Modified by Sub. Res. 514, I-95.

Each meridian has an entry and exit point; energy enters through the entry point and flows through to the exit point. There are 12 primary meridians of the body, each running vertically, bringing *qi* and the other four essential substances to specific parts of the body. No part of the body is without *qi*; a blockage causes an imbalance in the flow of the life force. In Figure 4-2, a male model demonstrates where the meridians and acupuncture sites are indicated. Figure 4-3*A* depicts the clinician placing an acupuncture needle in the buttocks of a man with sciatica; Figure 4-3*B* shows all the needles in position.

Shen is the energy, unique to human life, that is responsible for the spirit, consciousness, emotions, and thoughts. It is associated with the force of human personality. *Jing* is the fluid that is the basis of reproduction and development. *Xue* (pronounced "schwhey") moves in the same channels as *qi* and is similar to blood but is produced by food, refined in the spleen, and transported to the lungs, where nutritive *qi* turns it into *xue*. *Jin-ye* is all fluids other than *xue*. It includes sweat, urine, saliva, mucus, bile, and gastric juice. These five essential substances constitute the basis for the Chinese traditional medical system.

Acupuncture is used for prevention and treatment of disease and for maintenance of health by manipulating the flow of *qi* and *xue*, or body fluids, through the body channels. Although most Western clinicians have heard of acupuncture, few understand it. The Chinese have used acupuncture for more than 6000 years to stimulate or awaken the natural power within the body. It is estimated that there are 9 to 12 million treatments a year in the United States. Acupuncture involves the use of nine fine needles, each with a specific purpose. There are as many as 2000 specific points, each 3 mm in diameter, along the meridian lines on the skin into which these needles can be inserted. Most acupuncturists use only 150 of these points. The Chinese have different names for each acupuncture point. Examples of the classic needles,

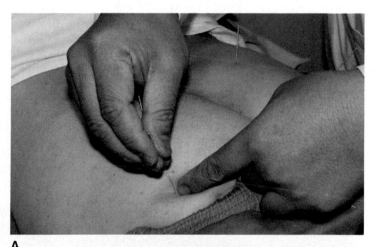

A

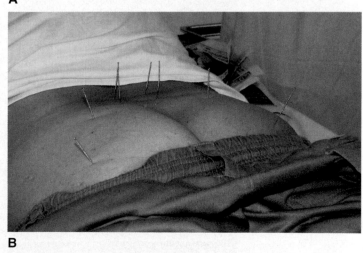

B

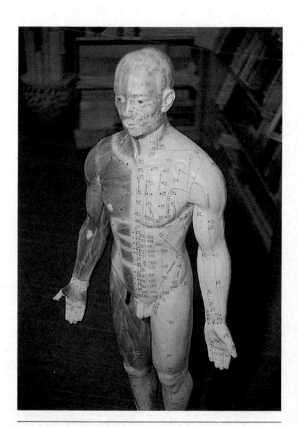

Figure 4–2 Meridians and acupuncture sites on male model.

Figure 4–3 Acupuncture. *A,* Physician inserting needles into a patient with sciatica. *B,* Needles in position.

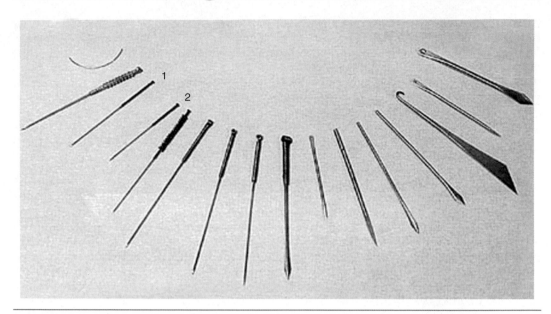

Figure 4–4 Classic acupuncture needles. 1 and 2, Thin filiform needles most commonly used in the United States.

which also include scalpel and lancet-like instruments, are shown in Figure 4-4. The needles marked "1" and "2" are the most commonly used needles. The needles act as antennae to direct *qi* to organs of the body. At other times, the needles may drain *qi* when it is excessive.

Acupuncture has been used to treat illnesses from childhood to old age. Figure 4-5 depicts an acupuncture tray with supplies. While lecturing in Taiwan, I had the good fortune to visit the China Medical College in Taichung, where there is a special department for patients who wish to obtain traditional Chinese medical treatment. The child shown in Figure 4-6*A* was brought in by his mother, who stated that her son was having symptoms of a cold; the man in Figure 4-6*B* was complaining of sinus problems; and the older woman in Figure 4-6*C* was complaining of headaches. Figure 4-6*D* is the foot of the child shown in Figure 4-6*A*.

Ear acupuncture, known as *auriculotherapy*, is practiced by traditional Chinese acupuncturists for the diagnosis and therapy of organ system disharmony. This technique, however,

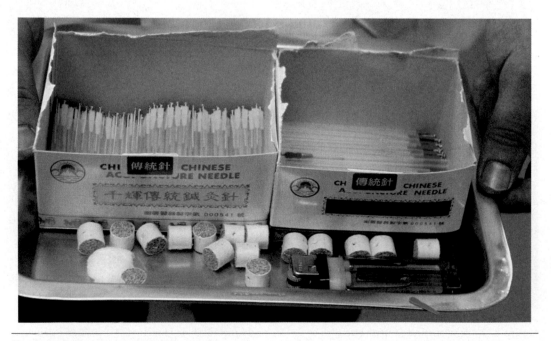

Figure 4–5 Acupuncture supplies.

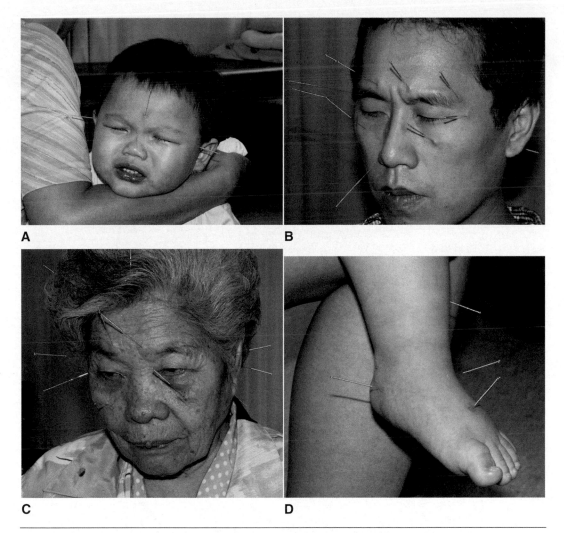

Figure 4-6 Acupuncture. *A,* Child with upper respiratory infection, under treatment. *B,* Man with sinus headache, under treatment. *C,* Woman with headache, under treatment. *D,* Foot of child with upper respiratory infection shown in *A.*

did not develop in China. A French physician, Paul Nogier, introduced this concept in 1958. Figure 4-7 shows the acupuncture sites of the ear. Auriculotherapy is based on the concept that there are specific parts of the ear that can be related to specific parts of the body and its functions. Although the specificity of ear acupuncture points has never been clearly demonstrated, most acupuncturists agree that ear acupuncture has a calming effect. Indeed, the most frequently cited ear point used in treatments is called *shenmen,* or spirit gate. The *Handbook of Chinese Auricular Therapy* (Chen and Cui, 1997) states of this point that "It is used in numerous diseases of the neuropsychiatric system . . . . The application of this point is fairly extensive and flexible, covering no less than 30 kinds of diseases or ailments."

Moxibustion is a specific form of acupuncture in which herbs are burned to stimulate specific acupuncture sites. If a disease fails to respond to traditional acupuncture, moxibustion is used. Moxa leaves (*Artemisia chinensis*) are either rolled into a cigar-shaped stick or pulverized and made into a cone. The moxa stick is lit, and the glowing end is held over the vital spot to be treated; the cone is placed on the skin over the acupuncture site and ignited, letting it burn slowly near the skin, as shown in Figure 4-8*A.* Often, the rolled moxa cone is placed on the end of an acupuncture needle and then lit to enhance the acupuncture therapy; this is shown in Figure 4-8*B* in a patient complaining of lower back pain. Moxibustion is used for conditions in which there is an excess of *yin* and is contraindicated for heat and excess *yang* disharmonies.

In 1997, the NIH convened a panel of independent experts to review the clinical studies of acupuncture. The panel noted that the results of several studies, many sponsored by the NIH, were unclear because of design, sample size, and other factors, complicated by difficulties in

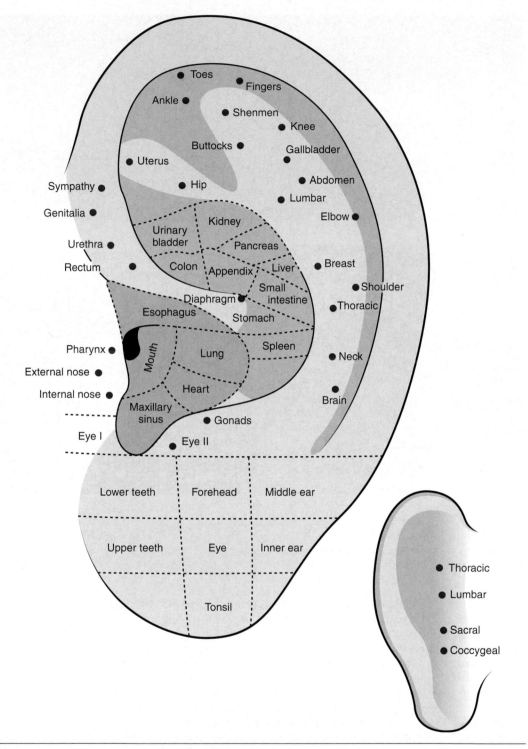

Figure 4–7 Acupuncture sites of the ear.

the use of appropriate control subjects. The panel did agree that acupuncture has been shown to be effective for relief of the following:

1. Adult postoperative nausea and vomiting
2. Nausea and vomiting secondary to chemotherapy
3. Postoperative dental pain

The panel determined that acupuncture may be useful as an adjunct treatment, as an acceptable alternative, or as part of a comprehensive management program for addiction, stroke

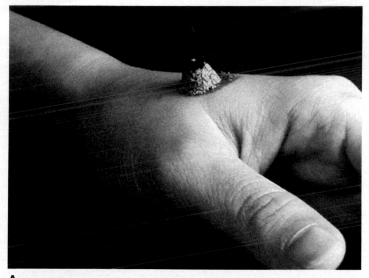

Figure 4—8 Moxibustion. *A,* Moxibustion cone. *B,* Moxibustion and acupuncture therapy in a patient with low back pain.

A

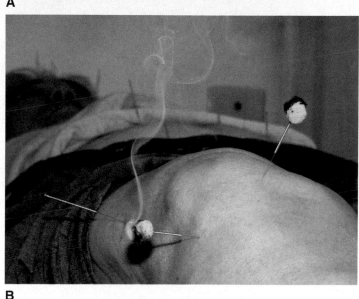

B

rehabilitation, headache, menstrual cramps, tennis elbow, fibromyalgia, myofascial pain, osteoarthritis, low back pain, carpal tunnel syndrome, and asthma. Further research is likely to uncover additional areas in which acupuncture interventions is useful.

Traditional Chinese Medicine

There are many traditional medical practices. Of particular note are the Chinese, Ayurvedic, and Greek systems of healing. Owing to the limitations of space in this chapter, one traditional system of healing, Chinese medicine, which has influenced so many other systems, is considered.

With more than 10 million people, the Asian and Pacific Islander group represents the third largest minority group in the United States. The Chinese approach to healing is a rich and complex tradition. It emphasizes the importance of promoting balance and harmony in body, mind, and spirit and has become the foundation for many other traditional medical systems. Chinese medicine had its origins more than 2500 years ago and is still in use to treat millions of people in China and throughout the world. As a result, to the traditional Chinese healers, allopathic medicine is new and experimental.

Chinese medicine is based on the idea that the human system is a microcosmic mirror of the macrocosmic universe. This means that no one thing can exist without the existence of the others. Each person is subject to the same laws that govern the stars, the planets, the trees, and the land. *Tao*, sometimes translated as "the infinite origin," is the single unified source from which all life and the entire universe originated; it is the way to ultimate reality. To follow the laws of nature is to be blessed with good health, long life, and good fortune. Because nature is the most enduring manifestation of *tao*, much of the traditional terminology of Chinese medicine is derived from natural phenomena, such as fire and water, wind and heat, and dryness and dampness. When the elements in the human body remain in balance, "fair weather" is said to prevail in the body, and the human is well both physically and mentally.

Tao created two opposing forces, *yin* and *yang*, which are the opposites that combine to create everything in the world. *Yin* is a force of darkness and is associated with such qualities as femininity, cold, rest, passivity, emptiness, introverted, and negative energy. *Yang* is a force of brightness and is associated with masculinity, heat, stimulation, activity, excitement, vigor, fullness, extroverted, and positive energy. Table 4-1 lists the aspects of *yin* and *yang* polarity.

There are two main concepts in traditional Chinese medicine. The first is that the occurrence of disease represents a failure in preventive health care. The second is that health is a responsibility shared equally by the patient and clinician. According to a Chinese proverb, "The superior physician teaches his patients how to stay healthy." In traditional Chinese medicine, the clinician treats the patient as a whole system rather than dealing with separate parts, as is common in Western medicine. An important belief is that the mind is engaged to

Table 4–1 Aspects of *Yin* and *Yang* Polarity

Aspect	Yin	Yang
Cosmic bodies	Earth Moon	Sun
Energy condition	Passive Mentality active Asleep Weak Empty Deficient Cold	Aggressive Physically active Awake Strong Full Excessive Hot
Time of day	Night	Day
Season	Fall Winter	Spring Summer
Magnetic pole	Negative	Hot
Speed	Slow	Fast
Body location	Interior Lower torso Lower extremities Feet Right side Back Exterior	Upper torso Upper extremities Head Left side Front
Gender	Female	Male
Numbers	Even	Odd
Distance	Near	Far
Relative moisture	Very moist, saturated	Dry
Quality of light	Dark	Light
Acid/base	Alkaline	Acid
Speed	Slow	Fast
Metabolism	Anabolism	Catabolism
Psychic type	Contemplative Introverted Gentle	Active Extroverted Robust

control and guide energy to heal and repair the body. Chinese medicine is a system of preserving health and curing disease that treats the mind, body, and spirit as a whole.

Whereas the Western clinician starts with a symptom and tries to search for the cause of a specific disease, the traditional Chinese clinician directs his or her attention to the whole patient and forms a "pattern of disharmony." This pattern describes the situation of "imbalance" in the patient's body. The traditional Chinese clinician asks not "Which *A* is causing *B?*" but "What is the relationship between *A* and *B?*" The patterns of disharmony provide the framework for therapy. In Chinese medicine, a person does not catch the flu; a person develops a disharmony. If a patient requires an antibiotic, herbs or acupuncture may be used to dispel the disharmony. Regardless of the ailment, the mind, body, and spirit must be treated as a whole. Healing is achieved by rebalancing *yin* and *yang* and restoring harmony in the whole person.

The traditional Chinese clinician inspects a patient in four stages: looking, listening or smelling, asking, and touching. Inspection of the tongue and palpation of the pulse are the two most important examinations. The tongue is believed to be the clearest indicator of the nature of the disharmony. The Chinese recognize more than 100 different conditions of internal energy imbalance, based on the color and texture of the tongue "fur." The condition of the five major organ-energy systems is evaluated according to their corresponding areas on the tongue. These systems are the kidneys, liver, spleen, lungs, and heart.

In traditional Chinese medicine, pulse diagnosis is evaluated at the radial artery. It is believed that disharmonies of the body leave a specific impression on the pulse. Figure 4-9 depicts an early description, from a scroll, of pulse diagnosis. There are at least 28 specific types of pulse abnormalities. The pulse is evaluated by placing subtle pressure by the three middle fingers on three points on the radial pulse. When the pulse is strong and regular, the person is considered to be in good health. The traditional Chinese clinician can evaluate six organs on each wrist.

The Chinese have used iron balls for health since the Ming Dynasty (1368–1644). The balls, originally solid, today are hollow with a sounding plate inside them. Each pair consists of one that produces a high tone and the other a low tone. The iron balls are believed to enhance the user's health and well-being. By moving the iron balls with the fingers, various acupuncture points on the hand are stimulated, resulting in increased circulation of vital energy and blood to the internal organs. Those who use these balls believe that, with daily use, the brain can be kept in good health with improved memory, fatigue will be relieved, and life will be prolonged.

Another major concept in traditional Chinese medicine is the *five element theory*, also known as the *five phases* (*wu xing*). This theory is an attempt to classify phenomena in terms of five quintessential processes represented by wood, fire, earth, metal, and water. Each phase has

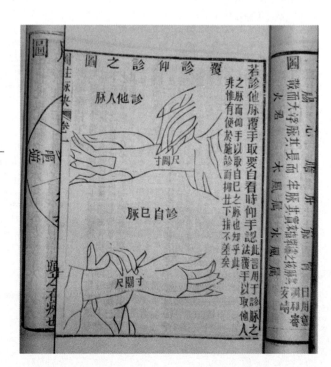

Figure 4–9 Ancient Chinese description of pulse diagnosis.

Table 4-2 Somatic Associations of the Five Phases

	Wood	**Fire**	**Earth**	**Metal**	**Water**
Taste	Sour	Bitter	Sweet	Pungent	Salty
Yin organ	Liver	Heart	Spleen	Lungs	Kidney
Yang organ	Gallbladder	Small intestine	Stomach	Colon	Urinary bladder
Orifice	Eyes	Tongue	Mouth	Nose	Ears
Tissue	Tendons	Blood vessels	Flesh	Skin	Bones

qualities and functions that describe the various processes in the body and their interactions with the environment. The phases are as follows:

- *Wood:* proper and straight; characterizes the liver, gallbladder, anger, sour taste, and windy weather
- *Fire:* ascending and blooming; characterizes the heart, small intestine, joy, bitter taste, and hot weather
- *Earth:* solid and quiet; characterizes the spleen, stomach, melancholy, sweet taste, and damp weather
- *Metal:* firm and strong; characterizes the lung, colon, grief, pungent taste, and dry weather
- *Water:* inward and clear; characterizes the kidney, urinary bladder, fear, salty taste, and cold weather

Traditional Chinese healers use this theory to diagnose and treat illness. Often plotted on a circle, the five phases show a unity in the world and in the body. Many conditions correspond to the five phases. Table 4-2 lists some of the medically relevant associations.

In addition to acupuncture, acupressure and massage are also important aspects of the traditional Chinese healing arts. Acupressure, or *dian hsueh*, is the forerunner of the Japanese technique called *shiatsu*. Acupressure is the technique of transferring energy from the therapist's body directly into the patient's system by pressing thumb and hands into the patient's vital areas. Acupressure involves the application of deep pressure to the same points along the channels used in acupuncture. Once a point is located, rotating pressure is applied for 10 to 15 seconds, released, and then repeated as often as the therapist believes necessary. Massage (*tui na*), in contrast, focuses primarily on the muscle masses, ear, abdomen, foot, and spine. Massage offers the energy of acupuncture, the serenity of meditation, and spiritual refreshment. *Tui na* stimulates circulation and energy within the body, activates and drains the lymph, tones the muscles, and enhances nerve function.

Tui na therapy is accompanied by cupping, a technique called *ba guan*, in which glass or bamboo cups containing small amounts of alcohol are applied to the areas of disease and the alcohol is ignited, creating a vacuum inside. The underlying tissue swells up, and the vacuum pressure draws out heat, damp, or wind energies. This technique has been adapted by many other ethnic groups. Figure 4-10 shows the glass cups and a modern suction device for their application.

Chinese herbal therapy encompasses eight methods: sweating, vomiting, purging, harmonizing, warming, removing, supplementing, and reducing. There are 5767 herbal remedies known in traditional Chinese medicine, fewer than 10% of which are commonly used currently. Through clinical experience, Chinese medicine recognizes that each herbal remedy has an affinity for a particular meridian or organ. If an illness is caused by heat, cooling with herbal therapy is used; if caused by a deficiency, drugs that restore are used. In a manual of Chinese herbal remedies, each herb is listed as to the part of the plant used (P), the taste and nature (T&N), the meridian or organ affected (M), the actions (Act), the amount and form of use (A&F), and the cautions and contraindications (C&C). For example*:

- *Acorus gramineus* (Japanese sweet flag)
- Shichangpu
- P: Root stalk
- T&N: Acrid; slightly warm

---

*Adapted from Warner and Fan (1996).

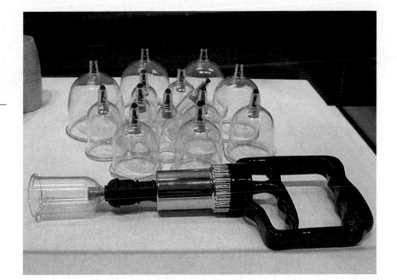

Figure 4–10 *Ba guan* (cupping) devices.

- M: Heart, liver, spleen
- Act: To open ostia and conduits, to eliminate sputum, to regulate *qi*, to mobilize blood, to disperse wind, to excrete dampness
- A&F: 3 to 6 g (fresh 9 to 24 g) as decoction, pill, or powder
- C&C: Waning *yin* with waxing *yang*, restlessness with diaphoresis, cough, vomiting of blood, spontaneous semen emission

The photograph in Figure 4-11 was taken in a traditional Chinese herbal pharmacy in San Francisco's Chinatown. Note the prescription written in Chinese, which is necessary to purchase these herbal medications. Figure 4-12 shows the modern herbal pharmacy at the China Medical College in Taichung, Taiwan. Figure 4-13 shows an automated prescription for herbal medications.

The use of medicinal herbs is prevalent and growing. The health-care provider must be cognizant of the commonly used herbs and their benefits and limitations. Some herbs can interfere with prescribed medications and with surgery. Bleeding is a common problem. Certain antioxidants may interfere with chemotherapy. The use of medicinal herbs in the West goes back to the days of Paracelsus (1493–1541), who said, "The dose determines the poison." More clinical trials of safety and efficacy of medicinal herbs are needed to help understand the active ingredients and herb actions.

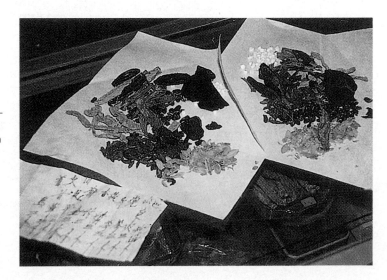

Figure 4–11 Herbal Chinese medications, with prescription in lower left.

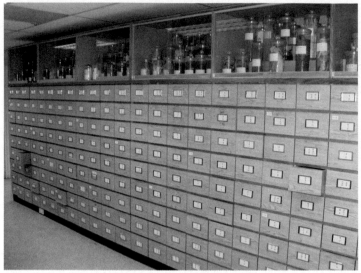

A

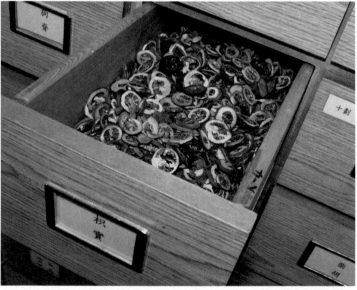

B

Figure 4–12 *A* and *B*, Modern herbal pharmacy at China Medical College in Taichung, Taiwan.

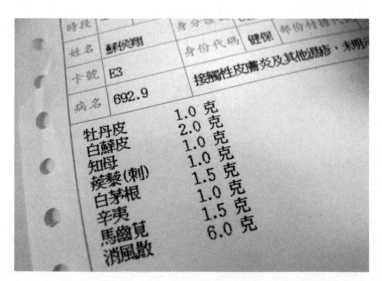

Figure 4–13 Computer-generated herbal medication prescription.

Concluding Thoughts

CAM therapies have long played a key role in health care. Most health-care providers have failed to recognize the magnitude of these forms of healing. Many of the therapies, however, are not based on any sound medical knowledge. Some have been derived from ethnic and folk traditions, semireligious cults, metaphysical movements, and health-care groups who rebel against technology and the perceived impersonality of 21st-century medical care. Unfortunately, marketing terms such as "miracle cure," "new discovery," and "satisfaction guaranteed" attract patients looking for cures for diseases for which there are no cures. "Purify," "detoxify," and "energize" sound impressive, but they are often used to cover up the lack of scientific proof of efficacy. Finally, clinicians must advise patients that the word *natural* does not always mean that the therapy is safe, and these products may have druglike effects that may be deleterious to their health and have dangerous interactions with prescribed medications. Therefore, clinicians should look for solid scientific studies. A lack of solid evidence does not always mean these treatments do not work, but it does mean they have not been proven effective.

This chapter has introduced the health-care provider to the richness of several of these CAM therapies. Ideally, the health-care provider is better prepared to deal with patients of diverse backgrounds who use CAM and with the challenges of caring for those patients in U.S. society. The provider must be open-minded with regard to these therapies and able to incorporate alternative and complementary therapies into Western medicine. All health-care providers must become familiar with CAM practices, the efficacies of the various practices, and the potential risks and benefits from their use.

Bibliography

Acupuncture. NIH Consensus Statement 15(5):1, 1997.

Ang-Lee MK, Moss J, Yuan CS: Herbal medicines and perioperative care. JAMA 286:213, 2001.

Barnes PM, Powell-Griner E, McFann K, et al: Complementary and alternative medicine use among adults: United States, 2002. CDC Advance Data 343:1, 2004.

Cardini F, Weixin H: Moxibustion for correction of breech presentation: A randomized controlled trial. JAMA 280:1580, 1998.

Chen K, Cui Y: Handbook of Chinese Auricular Therapy. Beijing, Foreign Languages Press, 1997.

Chenot JF, Becker A, Leonhardt C, et al: Use of complementary alternative medicine for low back pain consulting in general practice: A cohort study. BMC Complement Altern Med 7(1):42, 2007.

Cherkin D, Deyo RA, Battie M, et al: A comparison of physical therapy, chiropractic manipulation, and provision of an educational booklet for the treatment of patients with low back pain. N Engl J Med 339:1021, 1998.

Cohen MR, Doner K: The Chinese Way to Healing: Many Paths to Wholeness. New York, Perigee, 1996.

Deihl DL, Kaplan G, Coulter I, et al: Use of acupuncture by American physicians. J Altern Complement Med 3:119, 1997.

De Smet PA: Herbal remedies. N Engl J Med 347:2046, 2002.

Eisenberg DM: Advising patients who seek alternative medical therapies. Ann Intern Med 127:61, 1997.

Eisenberg DM, Davis RB, Ettner SL, et al: Trends in alternative medicine use in the United States, 1990–1997: Results of a follow-up national survey. JAMA 280:1569, 1998.

Eisenberg DM, Kessler RC, Foster C, et al: Unconventional medicine in the United States: Prevalence, costs, and patterns of use. N Engl J Med 328:246, 1993.

Ernst E: The role of complementary and alternative medicine. BMJ 321:1133, 2000.

Freund PES, McGuire MB: Health, Illness, and the Social Body: A Critical Sociology, 2nd ed. Englewood Cliffs, NJ, Prentice-Hall, 1995.

Gray CM, Tan AW, Pronk NP, et al: Complementary and alternative medicine use among health plan members: A cross-sectional survey. Eff Clin Pract 5:17, 2002.

Hager M (ed): Education of Health Professionals in Complementary/Alternative Medicine. New York, Josiah Macy, Jr. Foundation, 2001.

Hypericum Depression Trial Study Group: Effect of *Hypericum perforatum* (St. John's wort) in major depressive disorder: A randomized controlled trial. JAMA 287:1807, 2002.

Kaptchuk TJ, Eisenberg DM: Medical pluralism in the United States. Ann Intern Med 135:189, 2001.

Kaptchuk TJ, Eisenberg DM: Varieties of healing: a taxonomy of unconventional healing practices. Ann Intern Med 135:196, 2001.

Kessler DA: Cancer and herbs. N Engl J Med 342:1742, 2000.

Kessler RC, Davis RB, Foster DE, et al: Long-term trends in the use of complementary and alternative medical therapies in the United States. Ann Intern Med 135:262, 2001.

Kjellgren A, Bood SA, Axelsson K, et al: Wellness through a comprehensive Yogic breathing program—A controlled pilot trial. BMC Complement Altern Med 7(1):43, 2007.

Leach RA: The Chiropractic Theories: A Synopsis of Scientific Research, 2nd ed. Baltimore, Williams & Wilkins, 1986.

MacPherson H: Fatal and adverse events from acupuncture: Allegation, evidence, and the implications. J Altern Complement Med 5:47, 1999.

Marcus DM: How should alternative medicine be taught to medical students and physicians? Acad Med 76:224, 2001.

Maxion-Bergemann S, Wolf M, Bornhöft G, et al: Complementary and alternative medicine costs—a systematic literature review. Forsch Komplementärmed 13(2):42, 2006.

McLaughlin C, Hall N: Secrets of Reflexology. East Sussex, U.K, Dorling Kindersley, 2002.

Monte T: World Medicine: The East-West Guide to Healing Your Body. New York, GP Putnam's Sons, 1993.

National Center for Complementary and Alternative Medicine: NCCAM Funding: Appropriations History. 2004. Available at: *http://nccam.nih.gov/about/appropriations/*; accessed June 2, 2008.

Niggemann B, Gruber C: Side-effects of complementary and alternative medicine. Allergy 58:707, 2003.

Novey DW: Clinician's Complete Guide to Complementary Medicine. St. Louis, CV Mosby, 2000.

Oschman JL: Energy Medicine: The Scientific Basis. Edinburgh, Churchill Livingstone, 2000.

Reginster JY, Deroisy R, Rovati LC, et al: Long-term effects of glucosamine sulfate on osteoarthritis progression: A randomized, placebo-controlled clinical trial. Lancet 357:251, 2001.

Rubik B: The biofield hypothesis: Its biophysical basis and role in medicine. J Altern Complement Med 8:703, 2002.

Sharma HM, Triguna BD, Chopra D: Maharishi Ayur-Veda: Modern insights into ancient medicine. JAMA 265:2633, 1991.

Shen J, Wenger N, Glaspy J, et al: Electroacupuncture for myeloablative chemotherapy-induced vomiting: A randomized controlled trial. JAMA 284:2755, 2000.

Warber SL, Gordon A, Gillespie BW, et al: Standards for conducting clinical biofield energy healing research. Altern Therap Health Med 9(3):A54, 2003.

Warner JW, Fan MD: A Manual of Chinese Herbal Medicine: Principles and Practice for Easy Reference. Boston, Shambhala Publications, 1996.

White House Commission on Complementary and Alternative Medicine Policy: Interim Progress Report. Washington, DC, White House Commission on Complementary and Alternative Medicine Policy, 2001.

White LB, Foster S: The Herbal Drugstore. Emmaus, PA, Rodale, 2000.

Yamashita H, Tsukayama H, White AR, et al: Systematic review of adverse events following acupuncture: The Japanese literature. Complement Therap Med 2:98, 2001.

Young JH: The development of the Office of Alternative Medicine in the National Institutes of Health, 1991–1996. Bull Hist Med 72:279, 1998.

CHAPTER 5

Assessment of Nutritional Status*

One must eat to live, and not live to eat.

Jean Baptiste Molière (1622–1673)

Nutrition is one of the most important factors involved in an individual's health and disease, because it affects almost every system. It has been shown that dietary habits contribute importantly to the pathogenesis of many of the major causes of death in the United States.

One of the most challenging nutritional problems in the United States today is obesity. Between 1980 and 2004, the prevalence of obesity doubled among adults. About 97 million adult Americans are overweight or obese. Today, more than 20% of adolescents are overweight. Approximately one third of the American population and more than half of African-American women are overweight.

Obesity is a risk factor for many diseases, including hypertension, coronary artery disease, diabetes, osteoarthritis, cancers of the breast and endometrium, and hepatobiliary disease. There is an increased awareness of obesity, but it remains a major problem. The overall cost to society of obesity is estimated to be more than $100 billion per year.

Malnutrition is also a problem in the United States. Surveys have shown that among general medical and surgical admissions to hospitals, approximately 50% of the patients suffer from some form of malnutrition. Approximately 25% may actually have functional disease related to it, and 10% may have evidence of advanced malnutrition. Malnutrition is a problem that targets a number of specific populations, including elderly persons who live alone, chronically ill patients, adolescents who eat and diet erratically, and patients with recently diagnosed cancer, because chemotherapeutic and radiation therapeutic protocols may promote nutritional problems. Even obese patients may suffer from malnutrition, most commonly secondary to catabolic stress.

Health-care providers have a unique opportunity to educate patients and help modify their behavior. More than half of these health-promoting behaviors are nutrition related. They include balancing caloric intake to match energy expenditure, limiting salt consumption, reducing cholesterol intake, taking vitamins, and decreasing dietary fat consumption. The health-care professional must have a firm understanding of clinical nutrition and its impact on health and illness. A patient's ability to recover from an illness or from surgery depends, in many cases, on his or her past and current nutritional status. Adequate protein-calorie nutrition is important for wound healing, recovery from infection, and responsiveness to

*This chapter was written in collaboration with Robert F. Kushner, MD, Professor of Medicine at Northwestern University Feinberg School of Medicine, Chicago.

treatment, and protein-calorie malnutrition may be a factor in development of decubitus ulcers and wound disruption. Five of the leading causes of death in this country—heart disease, cancer, stroke, diabetes mellitus, and atherosclerosis—are diet related. Therefore, knowing what patients eat, the nutritional adequacy of their diets, and their clinical nutritional status is a necessary component of physical diagnosis.

This chapter focuses on the aspects of the history and physical examination that constitute a nutritional assessment. At present, there is no standardized set of dietary history questions or method for assessing nutritional status. Rather, nutritional assessment requires the integration of information obtained from the medical history and physical examination. Throughout this chapter, nutritionally focused questions and examples of diet-related diseases are provided to assist in building history-taking and physical examination skills. The chapter begins with a review of the medical history and physical examination, demonstrating the integration of nutritionally focused information. Then it covers the nutritional assessment of select patient groups, followed by some pathophysiologic correlations.

Medical History

Chief Complaint

Often the chief complaint is directly related to the patient's nutrition, which may affect treatment and prognosis. The most commonly voiced nutritional concerns are "loss of appetite," "weight loss," and "weakness." Changes in dietary intake and in weight are among the earliest signs of medical problems. These complaints should prompt a detailed inquiry about diet and related symptoms in the history of present illness.

History of Present Illness

After asking the patient to describe the symptoms or medical problem that caused him or her to seek medical attention, begin to explore any diet-disease relationship that may exist. The following self-directed questions should guide your inquiry:

- *Does nutrition contribute to the cause, severity, or treatment of the illness?* For example, type 2 diabetes is most often seen among obese patients and is diet responsive. Inquiry should be made into the patient's body weight history and diet, including calorie content, pattern and types of foods eaten, and relationship to blood glucose levels.
- *How has the illness affected the patient's diet and nutritional status?* For example, a patient with dysphagia from esophageal cancer typically experiences increasing difficulty swallowing solid foods, occasional vomiting, weight loss, and reduced muscle strength.
- *Does the patient see a relationship between diet and disease?* For example, is a patient with hypercholesterolemia aware that consumption of dietary saturated fats, *trans*-fatty acids, and cholesterol raises blood cholesterol, whereas intake of dietary fiber lowers blood cholesterol?
- *Was the patient ever advised to follow a special diet or use other nutritional therapy, such as defined formula supplements, tube feedings, or intravenous (parenteral) nutrition? What were the particular aspects of this therapy? What was the patient's understanding of how the treatment works? What was the patient's understanding of its potential efficacy?* For example, a patient with celiac disease must learn to follow a strict gluten-free diet to control the disease. The patient must become knowledgeable of sources of gluten in the diet, how to read food labels, and how to make dietary substitutions. This requires guidance from a registered dietitian.

Body Weight History

Body weight is a global indicator for overall health. Any weight loss is a good general indication of the severity or systemic nature of the presenting symptoms, whether they are acute or chronic. Both low body weight and unintentional weight loss have been shown to be predictive of increased morbidity and mortality. Although the cause of weight loss is often linked to the presenting medical problem, often no identifiable physical cause is apparent. In all cases,

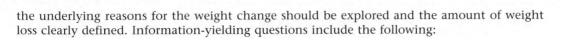

the underlying reasons for the weight change should be explored and the amount of weight loss clearly defined. Information-yielding questions include the following:

"Has your weight changed, either up or down, over the past several weeks or months?" If so, *"In what way?"*

"How much weight did you lose or gain?"

"What was your weight before the symptoms started?"

"Over what period of time did you experience the weight loss or gain?"

"How was your appetite over this time?"

"Do you know what may have contributed to your change in weight?"

Rapid weight gain is often an indicator of fluid retention and may be accompanied by edema or ascites. Common diseases associated with rapid weight gain include congestive heart failure, liver disease, and renal disease. In contrast, rapid weight loss usually signifies loss of body tissue, unless the patient has been undergoing therapeutic diuresis (in which case the patient would report markedly increased urination) or is experiencing dehydration (in which case the patient would report decreased fluid ingestion, dry mouth, weakness, and dizziness). If the patient has experienced weight loss, it is useful to think in terms of the percentage of weight lost over a specific time frame. To convert absolute pounds into percentage lost, the following simple equation is used:

$$\text{\% weight change} = [(\text{usual weight} - \text{current weight})/\text{usual weight}] \times 100$$

Significant involuntary weight loss is generally defined as more than 5% of usual weight during the preceding 6 months or 10% or more within the year. When a patient has experienced weight loss, it is useful to direct your questions toward the underlying causes. There are four physiologic categories for weight loss: (1) decreased caloric intake, (2) malabsorption or maldigestion, (3) impaired metabolism or increased requirements, and (4) increased losses or excretion (Table 5-1).

Past Medical History

As patients list their past illnesses, the health-care provider should consider the role of nutrition or diet in the cause or treatment. Common diet-related diseases include cardiovascular disease (coronary artery disease, peripheral vascular disease, cerebrovascular disease), hypertension, diabetes, hyperlipidemia, some forms of cancer, and gastrointestinal (GI) diseases. In addition to asking how the illness was diagnosed and what treatment was rendered, ask the patient whether he or she received dietary counseling or altered his or her diet in response to the diagnosis. Try to ascertain the patient's understanding of the role that diet plays in the condition.

Past Surgical History

All surgical procedures should be recorded in this section, along with serious surgical complications such as draining fistulas, abscesses, open wounds, and chronic blood loss. These complications often lead to malnutrition and the need for specialized nutritional support, including enteral and parenteral feedings. If the patient is currently in the postoperative period, you should consider the role of nutritional support in the recovery process and how the particular surgery has altered the patient's dietary habits and requirements. For example, a patient with a total gastrectomy needs to alter his or her diet to reduce simple sugars, eat multiple small meals each day, and receive supplemental vitamin B_{12} and iron to maintain good nutritional health.

Medications

The medication history should include both prescription and over-the-counter medications. Because complementary and alternative therapies have become popular, many patients take vitamins, minerals, herbs (Table 5-2), and other dietary supplements that they may not mention without prompting. A thorough review of alternative therapy use should be a standard

Table 5–1 Physiologic Categories Associated with Weight Loss

Category	Symptoms	Diseases
Decreased caloric intake	Loss of appetite (anorexia) or early fullness (satiety) Change in taste, dry mouth, or sore mouth and tongue Difficulty chewing or swallowing Nausea or vomiting Inability to feed self or obtain food Self-imposed diet	Social isolation, depression Dysmotility Gingivitis, poor dentition Gastroparesis Obstruction (esophageal, gastric, or intestinal) Anorexia nervosa Cancer
Maldigestion/malabsorption	Diarrhea Fatty, malodorous stools Change in bowel habits Food particles in stool	Pancreatic insufficiency Radiation enteritis Crohn's disease Short bowel syndrome Lactose intolerance Celiac disease
Impaired metabolism/increased requirements	Fever Increased or decreased appetite	Acquired immunodeficiency syndrome (AIDS) Pneumonia, sepsis Major surgery or trauma Hyperthyroidism Chronic hepatic, renal, or pulmonary disease Pregnancy and growth
Increased losses/excretion	Draining fistulas or open wounds Diarrhea Increased urination Excessive vomiting	Burns Occult gastrointestinal bleeding (iron loss) Hemodialysis Diabetes (glucosuria)

Table 5–2 Commonly Used Herbs and Their Side Effects

Herb	Common Use	Side Effect and Interaction
Echinacea	Treatment and prevention of upper respiratory infections, common cold	Rash, pruritus, dizziness
St. John's wort	Treatment of mild to moderate depression	Gastrointestinal upset, photosensitivity
Gingko biloba	Treatment of dementia	Mild gastrointestinal distress, headache; may have anticoagulant effects
Garlic	Treatment of hypertension, hypercholesterolemia, atherosclerosis	Gastrointestinal upset, gas, reflux, nausea, allergic reaction, antiplatelet effects
Saw palmetto	Treatment of benign prostatic hyperplasia	Uncommon
Ginseng	General health promotion, energy	High doses: diarrhea, hypertension, insomnia, nervousness
Goldenseal	Treatment of upper respiratory infections, common cold	Diarrhea, hypertension, vasoconstriction
Aloe	Topical application for dermatitis, herpes	Possible delay in wound healing after topical application; diarrhea and hypokalemia with oral use
Siberian ginseng	Similar to those of ginseng	May alter digoxin levels
Valerian	Treatment of insomnia, anxiety	Fatigue, tremor, headache, paradoxical insomnia

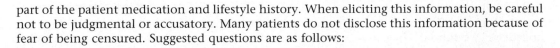

part of the patient medication and lifestyle history. When eliciting this information, be careful not to be judgmental or accusatory. Many patients do not disclose this information because of fear of being censured. Suggested questions are as follows:

"Are you taking any vitamins, minerals, herbs, or other dietary supplements, either prescription or over-the-counter?" If so, *"What is the dosage?"*

"What is the reason you are taking the supplement?"

"Have you experienced any side effects or benefits from the supplements?"

"Is anybody monitoring you, such as your doctor, nutritionist, or herbalist?"

"What is your consumption of grapefruit and grapefruit juice?"

Drugs and nutrients interact in many ways to affect both nutritional status and the effectiveness of drug therapy. Drugs may influence nutritional status by several physiologic mechanisms: altering food intake (through changes in appetite, nausea, altered taste sensations), producing malabsorption (through alterations in intestinal mucus, motility, or pH; competition with nutrients for absorption sites; binding of bile acids), or modifying excretion (through renal tubular reabsorption or secretion). Drug-induced nutrient deficiencies usually develop slowly and are more likely in patients who use drugs chronically, especially the elderly. Other risk factors include high drug dosages, multiple drug dosages, multiple drug regimens, poor diets, and marginal nutrient stores. Table 5-3 lists examples of drug interactions and nutrient metabolism.

Studies by Bailey and associates (1998) revealed possible drug interactions involving grapefruit and grapefruit juice (fresh or frozen) with several common medications used to treat

Table 5–3 Drug Interactions and Nutrient Metabolism

Drug Class and Examples	Nutrients Affected
Antacids	
Aluminum hydroxide	Phosphorus
Magnesium trisilicate	Iron
Antibiotics	
Tetracyclines	Calcium, magnesium, iron, vitamin B_{12}
Neomycin, kanamycin	Fat-soluble vitamins, vitamin B_{12}
Sulfasalazine	Folate
Anticonvulsants	
Phenobarbital, phenytoin	Calcium, vitamin D, folate
Hypolipidemics	
Cholestyramine, colestipol	Fat and fat-soluble vitamins
Cytotoxic agents	
Methotrexate	Folate
Laxatives	
Mineral oil	Water, electrolytes, fat, and fat-soluble vitamins
Antituberculotics	
Isoniazid	Pyridoxine (vitamin B_6)
Anticoagulants	
Warfarin	Vitamin K
Analgesics	
Aspirin, nonsteroidal anti-inflammatory drugs	Iron
Diuretics	
Thiazides, furosemide	Potassium, magnesium, calcium, zinc
Antineoplastic agents	
Cisplatin	Potassium, magnesium

high blood pressure, anxiety, depression, cancer, gastroesophageal reflux disease, erectile dysfunction, angina, convulsions, and human immunodeficiency virus infection/acquired immunodeficiency syndrome. In general, the grapefruit or its juice tends to increase the drug's effect. The advisory also cautioned that sour oranges and tangelos may also interfere with medication blood levels. Other citrus fruits were considered safe. The study stated that as little as one 8-oz (0.26-mg) glass of grapefruit juice could increase the blood drug level and the effects could last for 3 days or more.

Allergies and Food Intolerances

In addition to asking about allergies to medications and environmental allergens, the interviewer should inquire about allergies and intolerances to food. The most common allergenic foods among adults are peanuts, tree nuts, shellfish, fish, eggs, soy, wheat, and milk. The first four foods listed may cause life-threatening reactions. If the patient states that he or she has a food allergy, the interviewer should ask what happens when those foods are eaten. Allergic symptoms may affect the respiratory tract (rhinorrhea, sneezing, wheezing, chest tightness, laryngeal edema), skin (urticaria, angioedema, pruritus, erythematous macular rash), or GI tract (nausea, vomiting, diarrhea, abdominal cramping).

A food allergy needs to be differentiated from food intolerance. Symptoms of food intolerance are usually confined to the GI tract and may be acute or chronic. Upper GI tract symptoms of belching and bloating may be due to aerophagia (swallowing air during the ingestion of food or drink), which is commonly associated with smoking, eating rapidly or talking while eating, chewing gum and hard candy, or ingesting carbonated beverages. Chronic lower GI tract symptoms of bloating, cramping, flatulence, or diarrhea may result from the ingestion of sugar substitutes (sorbitol, xylitol) or fructose, high fiber intake, or lactase deficiency. Of these potential causes, lactose intolerance is the most common, affecting 25% of the population in the United States and up to 80% of African Americans. In lactose-intolerant individuals, symptoms occur after the consumption of products containing lactose, including milk, cheese, ice cream, yogurt, and some processed foods.

Social History

Multiple social factors affect the dietary and nutritional status of patients. For example, low socioeconomic status, low fixed income, homelessness, or lack of access to a variety of food choices may contribute to nutritional deficiencies. Chronic alcoholism and recreational drug use are two additional conditions that put people at high nutritional risk. The patient's attitudes about food and nutrition, as well as religious observances, also determine eating patterns and the selection or avoidance of specific foods. This information is important to note and document.

Lifestyle Habits

The lifestyle habits section of the medical history includes the dietary history, physical activity history, alcohol use, and smoking history. Questions related to alcohol use and smoking are discussed in Chapter 1, The Interviewer's Questions.

Dietary History

The dietary history provides information about the patient's food habits, diet, and any counseling he or she may have received. Depending on the patient's medical problems, the dietary history may be brief or comprehensive. It is often difficult to obtain accurate information about a patient's diet because of variability, general lack of focus on what is eaten, and forgetfulness. For this reason, the primary goal is to obtain a qualitative description of eating patterns and the foods and beverages that are habitually chosen, along with any dietary changes that occurred over the course of the illness. Three methods are commonly used: a 24-hour intake recall, a typical day, and food frequency.

A 24-hour intake recall is used extensively and may be broached as follows: "Please tell me what you had to eat and drink for the entire day yesterday. Could you start with the first item you had to eat or drink and bring me through the entire day? I would also like to know the times you ate and the amounts." The advantage of this method is that patients can usually remember what they ate over the course of one recent day. The disadvantage is that one particular day may not adequately depict the patient's usual diet, especially if there has been a recent change.

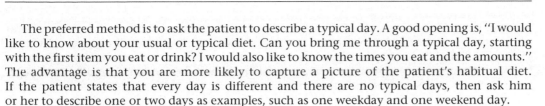

The preferred method is to ask the patient to describe a typical day. A good opening is, "I would like to know about your usual or typical diet. Can you bring me through a typical day, starting with the first item you eat or drink? I would also like to know the times you eat and the amounts." The advantage is that you are more likely to capture a picture of the patient's habitual diet. If the patient states that every day is different and there are no typical days, then ask him or her to describe one or two days as examples, such as one weekday and one weekend day.

The third method is *food frequency*. This refers to how often the patient consumes specific food groups or nutrients and about other dietary practices. Examples of questions are "How often do you eat fruits and vegetables: daily, every few days, weekly, or rarely?" and "When you do eat them, how many servings do you choose?" The same qualitative questions can be extended to the consumption of dairy products, whole-grain breads and cereals, red meats, visible fats, and so forth. Examples of other informative questions for taking a dietary history are as follows:

"What are your favorite foods and snacks?"

"Are you following any special diet (diabetic, low sodium, low fat, kosher, vegetarian, low protein, commercial)?" If so, *"What does this diet entail?"*

"How often are meals home cooked? Who prepares the meals?"

"What sort of fats or oils (if any) do you use in cooking?"

"How often do you eat out or order food in?" (Meals prepared outside the home are generally higher in calories, fat, and sodium.)

"How is food usually prepared (baked, broiled, fried, boiled, steamed, poached)?"

Targeted disease-focused questions should be asked, depending on the patient's medical history. For example, if the patient has *osteoporosis*, you would probe for the consumption of calcium-containing foods, such as milk, cheese, sardines, and greens. For a patient with *hypercholesterolemia* or *coronary artery disease*, you would ask about the intake of saturated fats, whole dairy products, egg yolks, fried foods, tropical oils, and fiber sources. For a patient with *diabetes mellitus*, you would ask whether meals and snacks are timed to correspond with insulin injections, whether the patient follows the American Diabetes Association food group exchange system and counts carbohydrate grams, and whether the patient knows symptoms of hypoglycemia and how to treat it.

Patients should be asked whether they read nutrition labels and, if they do not, instructed how to read them. Since May 1994, nutritional labeling has been required for almost all foods. There are now uniform definitions for the terms "free," "low," "light," "reduced," "high," "lean," "extra lean," and so forth. The current food label, known as *Nutrition Facts*, allows individuals to choose healthier foods more easily. Nutrition labeling provides the "% Daily Value," which shows how a food fits into the overall daily diet. This value is based on a 2000-calorie diet and informs the individual whether the food is high or low in the specific nutrient. These labels must include serving size, total calories, calories from fat, total fat, saturated fat, cholesterol, sodium, total carbohydrate, dietary fiber, sugars, and protein. The % Daily Value of four key vitamins and minerals (vitamin A, vitamin C, calcium, and iron) is also mandatory on these labels. Information about other vitamins and minerals is optional. Information about thiamine, riboflavin, and niacin is no longer necessary because deficiencies of these vitamins are rare in the United States. The % Daily Value is only a guide; if a patient eats more than 2000 calories a day, the food would contribute a lower % Daily Value to the diet.

The Institute of Medicine of the National Academies recommends that the following guidelines be used daily for achieving a healthful diet:

Carbohydrates: 45% to 65% of calories

Fat: 20% to 35% (<10% saturated fat)

Trans fat: no more than 1% total body calories

Protein: 10% to 35% of calories

Sodium: 1.5 g (3.8 g of salt)

Cholesterol: no more than 300 mg each day

Fiber: women need 21 to 25 g/day; men need 30 to 38 g/day

Most individuals on a balanced diet consume foods that contain all the vitamins and minerals they need. Some individuals, however, might benefit from vitamin supplementation. These individuals include habitual dieters, ill patients (especially those with loss of appetite or impaired absorption), pregnant or lactating women, infants consuming formula, some vegetarians, elderly patients, and patients with anorexia nervosa.

Physical Activity

Both nutrition and regular physical activity play an important role in the overall health of the individual. It is recommended that all adults perform at least 30 minutes of moderately intense physical activity 5 days a week. There are many benefits to regular physical activity: increasing physical fitness; building and maintaining healthy bones, muscles, and joints; improving endurance and muscle strength; lowering the risk of certain diseases (e.g., diabetes, cardiovascular disease, colon cancer); controlling blood pressure; promoting and improving a sense of well-being; reducing feelings of anxiety and depression; and managing weight problems.

Always ask patients about their current level of physical activity and functioning. Some helpful questions include the following:

"What is the most physically active thing you do in the course of the day?"

"How do you spend your working day and leisure time?"

"What types of physical activity do you enjoy? How often do you do them?"

"Do you exercise regularly?" If so, *"What exercises do you do regularly? How often?"*

"What gets in the way of you consistently doing physical activity?"

"How many hours of TV do you watch every day?"

"How many hours are you at a computer or desk every day?"

"Do you belong to (and attend) a health club or exercise classes?"

Review of Systems

The review of systems section is a reexamination of the patient's history by organ system. This section should include a general statement about the patient's body weight history and appetite if such a statement is not included in the history of present illness or the past medical history.

Physical Examination

Vital Signs

Along with recording the patient's heart rate, pulse, blood pressure, and temperature, you should also routinely record the patient's height and weight. Height and weight, although not typically considered true "vital signs," provide significant information about the patient's overall health status and are frequently used for medication dosing. Height and weight should be measured, if possible, although estimated measurements are better than no values at all. If values are estimated, you should record these as *reported* rather than *measured* values. Body weight varies with hydration status and the presence of clothing or wet dressings. Conditions that affect fluid balance such as renal failure or congestive heart failure also affect body weight.

The nutritional status of the patient based on height and weight is interpreted by the *body mass index* (BMI). BMI is an international designation of relative weight for stature and is a more reliable index of obesity than are the older height-weight tables. It is calculated in one of the two following ways:

- **BMI** = weight (kg)/height (meters)^2
- **BMI** = weight (pounds)/height (inches)^2 × 703

BMI	19	20	21	22	23	24	25	26	27	28	29	30	31	32	33	34	35
Height (inches)							Body Weight (pounds)										
58	91	96	100	105	110	115	119	124	129	134	138	143	148	153	158	162	167
59	94	99	104	109	114	119	124	128	133	138	143	148	153	158	163	168	173
60	97	102	107	112	118	123	128	133	138	143	148	153	156	163	168	174	179
61	100	106	111	116	122	127	132	137	143	148	153	158	164	169	174	180	185
62	104	109	115	120	126	131	136	142	147	153	158	164	169	175	180	186	191
63	107	113	118	124	130	135	141	146	152	158	163	169	175	180	186	191	197
64	110	116	122	128	134	140	145	151	157	163	169	174	180	186	192	197	204
65	114	120	126	132	138	144	150	156	162	168	174	180	186	192	198	204	210
66	118	124	130	136	142	148	155	161	167	173	179	186	192	198	204	210	216
67	121	127	134	140	146	153	159	166	172	178	185	191	198	204	211	217	223
68	125	131	138	144	151	158	164	171	177	184	190	197	203	210	216	223	230
69	128	135	142	149	155	162	169	176	182	189	196	203	209	216	223	230	236
70	132	139	146	153	160	167	174	181	188	195	202	209	216	222	229	236	243
71	136	143	150	157	165	172	179	186	193	200	208	215	222	229	236	243	250
72	140	147	154	162	169	177	184	191	199	206	213	221	228	235	242	250	258
73	144	151	159	166	174	182	189	197	204	212	219	227	235	242	250	257	265
74	148	155	163	171	179	186	194	202	210	218	225	233	241	249	256	264	272
75	152	160	168	176	184	192	200	208	216	224	232	240	248	256	264	272	279
76	156	164	172	180	189	197	205	213	221	230	238	246	254	263	271	279	287

BMI	36	37	38	39	40	41	42	43	44	45	46	47	48	49	50	51	52	53	54
58	172	177	181	186	191	196	201	205	210	215	220	224	229	234	239	244	248	253	258
59	178	183	188	193	198	203	208	212	217	222	227	232	237	242	247	252	257	262	267
60	184	189	194	199	204	209	215	220	225	230	235	240	245	250	255	261	266	271	276
61	190	195	201	206	211	217	222	227	232	238	243	248	254	259	264	269	275	280	285
62	196	202	207	213	218	224	229	235	240	246	251	256	262	267	273	278	284	289	295
63	203	208	214	220	225	231	237	242	248	254	259	265	270	278	282	287	293	299	304
64	209	215	221	227	232	238	244	250	256	262	267	273	279	285	291	296	302	308	314
65	216	222	228	234	240	246	252	258	264	270	278	282	288	294	300	306	312	318	324
66	223	229	235	241	247	253	260	266	272	278	284	291	297	303	309	315	322	328	334
67	230	236	242	249	255	261	268	274	280	287	293	299	306	312	319	325	331	338	344
68	236	243	249	256	262	269	276	282	289	295	302	306	315	322	328	335	341	348	354
69	243	250	257	263	270	277	284	291	297	304	311	318	324	331	338	345	351	358	365
70	250	257	264	271	278	285	292	298	306	313	320	327	334	341	348	355	362	369	376
71	257	265	272	279	286	293	301	308	315	322	329	338	343	351	358	365	372	379	386
72	265	272	279	287	294	302	309	316	324	331	338	346	353	361	368	375	383	390	397
73	272	280	288	295	302	310	318	325	333	340	348	355	363	371	378	386	393	401	408
74	280	287	295	303	311	319	328	334	342	350	358	365	373	381	389	396	404	412	420
75	287	295	303	311	319	327	335	343	351	359	367	375	383	391	399	407	415	423	431
76	295	304	312	320	328	336	344	353	361	369	377	385	394	402	410	416	426	435	443

Figure 5–1 Body mass index (BMI) table. To find a specific BMI, (1) look down the left column to find the height (measured in inches); (2) look across that row and find the weight; and (3) look to the top of the column to find the number that is the BMI.

The advantage of BMI is that it is relatively easy to calculate and can be readily used for comparisons between women and men and persons of different heights. BMI can easily be determined from tables, as shown in Figure 5-1.

A disadvantage of using BMI is that it does not directly measure body composition and therefore may yield a spurious interpretation. For example, a malnourished patient with excessive fluid retention may be miscategorized as having a healthy BMI, or a muscular body builder may be classified as obese. A person with a BMI less than 18.5 kg/m^2 is considered underweight; a person with a BMI between 18.5 and 25.0 is considered to have a healthy weight; a person with a BMI between 25.1 and 29.9 is considered overweight; and a person with a BMI of 30 and above is considered obese.

Table 5–4 Common Manifestations of Nutritional Deficiencies

Site	Sign	Deficiency
Skin	Dry and scaly, cellophane appearance	Protein (see Fig. 5-5)
	Flaking dermatitis	Zinc (see Fig. 5-11)
	Follicular hyperkeratosis	Vitamin A (see Fig. 5-6)
	Pigmentation changes	Niacin (see Fig. 5-10)
	Petechiae	Vitamin C (see Fig. 5-8)
	Purpura	Vitamin C (see Fig. 5-8), vitamin K
	Pallor	Iron, vitamin B_{12}, folate
Eyes	Night blindness	Vitamin A
	Conjunctiva pallor	Iron, vitamin B_{12}, folate
Mouth	Angular stomatitis	Riboflavin, pyridoxine, niacin
	Cheilosis (dry, cracking, ulcerated lips)	Riboflavin, pyridoxine, niacin
	Glossitis	Riboflavin, niacin, B vitamins, iron, folate (see Fig. 5-9)
	Bleeding gums	Vitamin C (see Fig. 5-7), riboflavin
Muscles	Interosseous muscle atrophy, squaring off of shoulders, poor hand grip and leg strength	Protein, calories (see Fig. 5-5)

Appearance

A description of the patient's general appearance is always found at the beginning of the physical examination report; for example, "On examination, Ms. B. is a well-developed, thin, white female." Other nutritionally descriptive terms are as follows:

- Emaciated
- Cachectic
- Malnourished
- Thin/slim
- Underweight
- Normal weight
- Fit
- Overweight
- Obese
- Edematous

Nutrition-oriented aspects of the physical examination focus on the skin, eyes, mouth, skeletal muscle, and fat stores. The skin provides an excellent barometer of clinical nutrition and is accessible to the health-care provider in its entirety. Chronic wasting associated with loss of subcutaneous fat from calorie or protein deficiency results in a fine wrinkling of the skin. Easy bruising may result from vitamin deficiencies. In areas of the skin where sebaceous glands are dense, such as the nasolabial folds, neck, cheeks, and forehead, a deficiency of essential nutrients may result in disturbance of their secretory function and blockage of their ducts with plugs of dried sebum. Around hair follicles, there may be accumulations of keratin associated with vitamin and fatty acid deficiencies. Edema may result from protein deficiencies. This occurs as a consequence of low plasma albumin and a reduced oncotic pressure. Excessive skin pigmentation may also be seen. In deficiencies of niacin or tryptophan, increased pigmentation occurs in areas of skin exposed to the sun. Changes in the hair and nails are also common in nutritional deficiencies. Blindness may result from vitamin A deficiency. Fissuring of the lips is indicative of riboflavin deficiency. The tongue may be large in iodine or niacin deficiency. Some of the more common physical signs of nutritional deficiency are listed in Table 5-4.

Special Populations

Obese Patients

According to the National Health and Nutrition Examination Survey (NHANES) 2005–2006, 65.7% of adult Americans, representing nearly 100 million individuals, are classified as overweight or obese (defined as a BMI of 25 kg/m^2 or higher). Among the general population, 35% are considered overweight (BMI of 25 to 29.9), and 30.7% are considered obese (BMI of 30 or higher). Thus, obesity represents the most significant diet-related health problem encountered by health-care professionals.

There are several lifestyle factors that may predispose to obesity. When calorie intake continuously exceeds requirements, obesity results. The converse is likewise true. Fewer than 1% of all cases of obesity are related to neuroendocrine causes, and these conditions rarely cause massive obesity. These syndromes include hypothyroidism, hypopituitarism, adrenocortical excess, polycystic ovary syndrome, and hypothalamic tumors or other damage to this part of the brain, as well as some rare inherited conditions. Prader-Willi syndrome is a rare chromosomal microdeletion syndrome associated with childhood massive obesity, mental retardation, and failure of sexual development. A patient with Prader-Willi syndrome and morbid obesity is pictured in Figure 5-2.

Obesity-Focused History

An obesity-focused history should include a chronologic history of the patient's weight, identifying age at onset, description of weight gain, and inciting events. For women, weight gain often occurs during adolescence, pregnancy, child-rearing years, and menopause. For many patients, weight gain occurs with smoking cessation or other changes in lifestyle, such as changes in marital status, occupation, or housing. The patient's history may be suggestive of, as already mentioned, several endocrinologic causes for weight gain. With the exception of polycystic ovary syndrome, these conditions are uncommon causes of obesity. Several medications are known to cause weight gain as an unintended side effect. The most common drug groups are antidepressants (tricyclic agents and mirtazapine), lithium, antipsychotics (phenothiazines, butyrophenones, olanzapine, clozapine, and risperidone), anticonvulsants (valproic acid, carbamazepine), steroid hormones (corticosteroid derivatives, megestrol acetate, estrogen), and antidiabetics (insulin, sulfonylureas, thiazolidinediones).

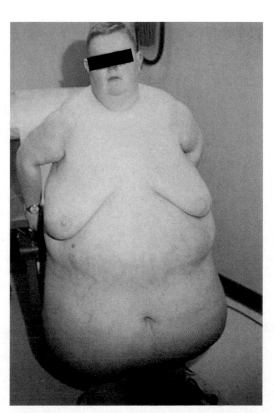

Figure 5–2 Patient with Prader-Willi syndrome.

When a patient's weight history is documented, it is important to be sensitive. Many patients feel discriminated against because of their obesity or feel ashamed and frustrated about not being able to control their weight. The following questions should be considered part of an obesity-focused history:

> *"When did you first consider yourself overweight or have a weight problem?"*
>
> *"Do you remember what you weighed when you were in high school? College? Your 20s, 30s, and so forth?"*
>
> *"What was your lowest weight as an adult?"*
>
> *"What was your highest weight as an adult?"*
>
> *"Were there any particular life events that caused you to gain weight, such as pregnancy, stopping smoking, changing jobs, getting a divorce, and so forth?"*
>
> *"Did you experience weight gain after taking any medication?"* If so, *"Which medication, and how much weight did you gain?"*

In addition to characterizing the chronologic history of the patient's weight, it is important to appreciate what impact the obesity has had on the patient. Obesity may affect the physical and mental health functioning of the patient, both of which are important aspects of quality of life. Physical effects of obesity include difficulties with mobility, such as bending, kneeling, and stair climbing; mental health effects may include low self-esteem, poor body image, shame, and social isolation. You should also ascertain whether the patient participated in any weight management programs in the past and what the response to treatment was. You can obtain this information through the following questions:

> *"How does your body weight affect you?"*
>
> *"Is there anything that you cannot do because of your weight?"*
>
> *"Does your weight affect your own sense of self-worth?"*
>
> *"Have you participated in any weight management programs in the past?"* If so, *"What were they, and how did you respond?"*

Obesity-Focused Physical Examination

According to the most recent National Heart, Lung, and Blood Institute (1998) guidelines, assessment of risk status according to overweight and obesity is based on the patient's BMI, waist circumference, and existence of comorbid conditions.

Being overweight or obese substantially increases the risk of morbidity and mortality from hypertension, type 2 diabetes mellitus, dyslipidemia, coronary artery disease, stroke, gallstones, osteoarthritis, respiratory problems (including sleep apnea), several cancers, and the metabolic syndrome, which is a clustering of risk factors for cardiovascular disease and diabetes. Factors characteristic of this syndrome are abdominal obesity, elevated triglyceride levels, low high-density lipoprotein cholesterol level, raised blood pressure, and impaired fasting blood glucose. Excess abdominal fat, a hallmark of the metabolic syndrome, can be clinically defined as a waist circumference greater than 40 inches (102 cm) in men and greater than 35 inches (88 cm) in women. To measure waist circumference, a horizontal mark is drawn just above the upper-most lateral border of the iliac crest. A cloth or metal tape is then placed in a horizontal plane around the abdomen at the level of the mark (Fig. 5-3). The measurement is made at a normal minimal respiration. An increased waist circumference can indicate increased risk even at a healthy weight. In contrast, waist circumference is less useful as an independent marker of medical risk when the BMI is greater than 35. Table 5-5 lists the classification of weight status and risk of disease.

The physical examination process for patients with obesity is identical to that for other adult patients, with the exception of specific measures to determine the obesity category (height, weight, and waist circumference) and the use of an appropriate blood pressure cuff. A bladder cuff that is not the appropriate width for the patient's arm circumference can cause a systematic error in blood pressure measurement; if the bladder is too narrow, the pressure will be overestimated and lead to a false diagnosis of hypertension. The most frequent error in measuring blood pressure is "miscuffing," with undercuffing large arms accounting for

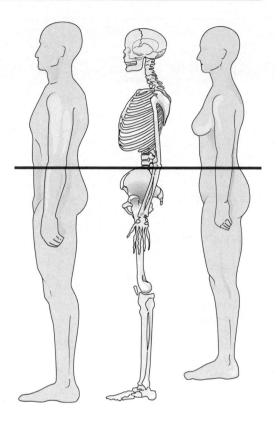

Figure 5–3 Measuring tape position for determining abdominal circumference.

84% of the ''miscuffings.'' To avoid errors, the ''ideal'' cuff should have a bladder length that is 80% and a width that is at least 40% of arm circumference (a length-to-width ratio of 2:1). Therefore, a large adult cuff (16 × 36 cm) should be chosen for patients with mild to moderate obesity (or arm circumference of 14 to 17 inches [36 to 43 cm]) while an adult thigh cuff (16 × 42 cm) must be used for patients whose arm circumferences are greater than 17 inches.

When the interviewer completes the review of systems section of the history and performs the physical examination, it is important to have a high index of suspicion for obesity-related diseases. Clinically, obesity affects at least nine organ systems. Obesity has been linked with an increased risk of breast and endometrial cancers in women. The mechanism is thought to be

Table 5–5 Classification of Weight Status and Risk of Disease

		Risk of Disease*	
Classification	**Body Mass Index**	**Women: ≤35 inches (88 cm); Men: ≤40 inches (102 cm)**	**Women: >35 inches (88 cm); Men: >40 inches (102 cm)**
Underweight	<18.5	—	—
Healthy weight	18.5–24.9	—	—
Overweight	25.0–29.9	↑	↑↑
Obesity	30.0–34.9	↑↑	↑↑↑
Obesity	35.0–39.9	↑↑↑	↑↑↑
Extreme obesity	≥40	↑↑↑↑	↑↑↑↑

*Waist circumference is measured just above the iliac crest. An increased waist circumference may indicate increased disease risk even at a normal weight.
Adapted from National Institutes of Health and National Heart, Lung, and Blood Institute: Clinical Guidelines on the Identification, Evaluation, and Treatment of Overweight and Obesity in Adults. Rockville, Md, U.S. Department of Health and Human Services, Public Health Service, 1998.

Table 5–6 Review of Obesity-Related Organ Systems

Cardiovascular
  Hypertension
  Congestive heart failure
  Cor pulmonale
  Varicose veins
  Pulmonary embolism
  Coronary artery disease
  Atrial fibrillation
Endocrine
  Metabolic syndrome
  Type 2 diabetes mellitus
  Dyslipidemia
  Polycystic ovary syndrome/androgenicity
  Amenorrhea/infertility/menstrual disorders
Musculoskeletal
  Hyperuricemia and gout
  Immobility
  Osteoarthritis (knees and hips)
  Low back pain
Psychologic
  Depression/low self-esteem
  Body image disturbance
  Social stigmatization
Integumentary
  Striae distensae (stretch marks)
  Stasis pigmentation of legs
  Lymphedema
  Cellulitis
  Intertrigo, carbuncles
  Acanthosis nigricans/skin tags

Respiratory
  Dyspnea
  Obstructive sleep apnea
  Hypoventilation syndrome
  Pickwickian syndrome
  Asthma
Gastrointestinal
  Gastroesophageal reflux disease
  Nonalcoholic fatty liver disease
  Cholelithiasis
  Hernias
  Colon cancer
Genitourinary
  Urinary stress incontinence
  Obesity-related glomerulopathy
  End-stage renal disease
  Hypogonadism (male)
  Breast and uterine cancer
  Pregnancy complications
Neurologic
  Stroke
  Idiopathic intracranial hypertension
  Meralgia paresthetica

related to increased circulating estrogens as a consequence of increased conversion of androgens to estrogens in adipose tissue. Obesity increases the risk of gallstone formation by increasing gallbladder volume and bile stasis. Increased cholesterol production is also thought to play a role. Degenerative joint disease is seen in obese individuals more frequently than in persons of normal weight. Regardless of whether it is a causative factor, osteoarthritis aggravates joint symptoms. A positive association has been noted between serum triglyceride and low-density lipoprotein cholesterol levels and obesity. High-density lipoprotein cholesterol level tends to be lower in patients with obesity. The pickwickian, or obesity-ventilation, syndrome is characterized by marked obesity, somnolence, periodic apnea (transient cessation of breathing), chronic hypoxemia (deficient oxygenation of the blood), hypercapnia (carbon dioxide retention), and polycythemia (increased number of red blood cells). Table 5-6 lists the symptoms and diseases that are directly or indirectly related to obesity. Although individuals vary, the number and severity of organ-specific comorbid conditions usually rise with increasing levels of obesity.

Malnourished Patients

Malnutrition is associated with slower wound healing, increased number of medical complications, longer length of hospital stay, higher health-care costs, and increased mortality rate. By performing a nutritionally focused history and physical examination, you can identify individuals who are at high nutritional risk or are malnourished. Key elements from the history and physical examination were reviewed earlier in this chapter.

The *Subjective Global Assessment* (SGA) provides an integration of historical and physical examination data to arrive at an evaluation of the patient's nutritional status. As shown in Figure 5-4, five features of the history and eight features of the physical examination are combined to assess risk. The historical features are weight loss, changes in dietary intake, significant GI symptoms, functional status or energy level, and metabolic demand of the patient's underlying disease state. Physical findings are scored as normal (0), mild (1+), moderate (2+), or severe (3+), and include depletion of subcutaneous fat in the chest and triceps, muscle wasting in the quadriceps and deltoid muscles, and the presence of edema or ascites.

Select appropriate category with a checkmark, or enter numerical value where indicated by a "#".
A. History
    1. Weight change and height
       Overall loss in past 6 months; Amt. = # _____ kg; % loss = # _____ Height – # _____ cm
       Change in past 2 weeks: _____ increase, _____ no change, _____ decrease.
    2. Dietary intake change (relative to normal)
       _____ No change.
       _____ Change _____ duration = # _____ weeks.
       Type: _____ suboptimal solid diet, _____ full liquid diet,
       _____ hypocaloric liquids, _____ starvation.
       Supplement: (circle) nil, vitamin, minerals, # _____ frequency/week.
    3. Gastrointestinal symptoms (that persisted for > 2 weeks)
       _____ none, _____ nausea, _____ vomiting, _____ diarrhea, _____ anorexia.
    4. Functional capacity
       _____ No dysfunction (e.g., full capacity).
       _____ Dysfunction: duration # _____ weeks.
       Type: _____ working suboptimally, _____ ambulatory, _____ bedridden.
    5. Disease and its relation to nutritional requirements
       Primary diagnosis (specify) _____
       Metabolic demand (stress): _____ no stress, _____ low stress, _____ moderate
       stress, _____ high stress.
B. Physical (for each trait specify: 0 = normal, 1+ = mild, 2+ = moderate, 3+ = severe)
    # _____ Loss of subcutaneous fat (triceps, chest)   # _____ Ascites
    # _____ Muscle wasting (quadriceps, deltoids, temporalis)   # _____ Mucosal lesions
    # _____ Ankle edema   # _____ Cutaneous lesions
    # _____ Sacral edema   # _____ Hair change
C. SGA rating (select one)
    _____ Well nourished.
    _____ Moderately (or suspected of being) malnourished.
    _____ Severely malnourished.

Figure 5–4 Subjective Global Assessment (SGA). (From Jeejeebhoy KN: Clinical and functional assessments. In Shils ME, Olson JA, Shike M [eds]: Modern Nutrition in Health and Disease, 8th ed. Philadelphia, Lea & Febiger, 1994, p 805.)

On the basis of the history and physical examination findings, patients are ranked according to the following three categories: A, good nutrition; B, moderate or suspected malnutrition; and C, severe malnutrition. Weight loss, poor dietary intake, loss of subcutaneous tissue, muscle wasting, and functional impairment are considered the most significant factors. These nutritional categories can be used to classify the severity of nutritional risk and the need for intervention. In addition, a low BMI, generally less than 19, should be considered an important predictor of mortality in a hospitalized patient. Figure 5-5 depicts three patients with protein-energy malnutrition, or deficiency of macronutrients. Note the severe loss of subcutaneous fat reserves and muscle mass and the prominence of the bones.

Impairment of function secondary to loss of body protein and energy reserves is the most important component of the assessment of nutritional status. You can evaluate function while performing the physical examination and by watching the patient's activity. You can assess grip strength by asking the patient to squeeze your index and middle fingers hard for at least 10 seconds. You can assess respiratory muscle function by asking the patient to exhale quickly or cough deeply. Shortness of breath may be noted at rest. You can assess leg muscle strength by asking the patient to push his or her legs and feet against your hand and by watching the patient ambulate.

Elderly Patients

Elderly people represent a diverse group who are at specific risk for a variety of nutritional problems. These problems are caused by a combination of environmental, social, and economic factors and are compounded by numerous physiologic changes that occur at different rates as individuals age. The *Nutrition Screening Initiative*, a multidisciplinary effort to promote nutrition screening and better nutritional care in America's health-care system, has identified the following risk factors associated with poor nutritional status in older Americans: inappropriate food intake, poverty, social isolation, dependency or disability, acute or chronic diseases or conditions, and chronic medication use.

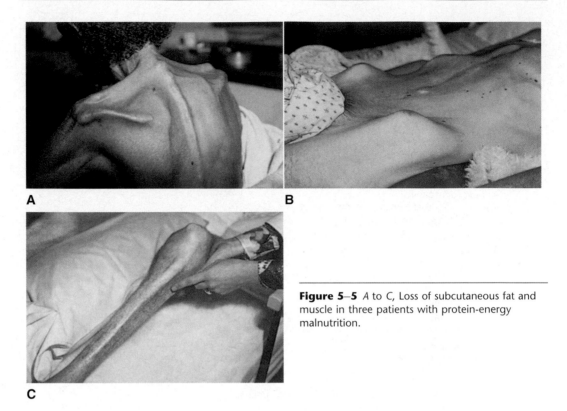

A   **B**

C

Figure 5–5 *A* to *C*, Loss of subcutaneous fat and muscle in three patients with protein-energy malnutrition.

These factors have been incorporated into a risk factor checklist with the acronym **DETERMINE,** which identifies several warning signs for individuals at risk for poor nutritional status:

- **D**isease: Any disease can cause the patient to change the way he or she eats or make it hard to eat, cook, or shop. Confusion or memory loss can make it hard for people to remember what or how to eat. Depression can lead to changes in appetite, energy level, and weight.
- **E**ating poorly: This may involve eating too little or too much, drinking too much alcohol, or not eating the foods needed for health every day. A diminished sense of taste and smell can decrease appetite and influence food choices. Many elderly people have a decreased ability to taste salt, which results in the liberal salting of foods. A reduced sense of smell may make it difficult for an elderly person to detect whether food has spoiled. Elderly patients should be advised to read all dates stamped on food products.
- **T**ooth loss or mouth pain: Some people do not eat well because they have lost teeth or have problems with their mouth, teeth, or gums.
- **E**conomic hardship: When a patient has very little money to spend on food, he or she may not eat enough food or may eat foods that do not have enough vitamins, minerals, or calories to stay healthy. The individual may buy prepackaged or convenience foods that are typically high in sodium, potassium, and sugar.
- **R**educed social contact: Cooking and eating alone are hard. Some people who live alone do not feel like shopping for or preparing the food they need. Loss of a spouse, retirement, or social isolation can lead to loneliness, depression, and lack of motivation to eat.
- **M**ultiple medications or drugs: Drugs and other medications can depress the appetite and alter nutrient absorption and excretion. Drugs can further alter the sense of taste and smell, change the secretion of saliva, irritate the stomach, and cause nausea. Some drugs can contribute directly to dietary deficiencies; for example, antacids absorb folic acid and calcium, laxatives absorb fat-soluble vitamins, and aspirin increases the excretion of folic acid.
- **I**nvoluntary weight loss or gain.
- **N**eed for assistance with self-care.
- **E**lderly years: older than 80 years.

Specific nutritional interventions are vital components of the health-care delivery system for elderly patients. The elderly person may overeat as a way of coping with feelings of loneliness. Some of these individuals, however, can be overweight but malnourished; their diet consists of cake and candy, which are high in calories but low in nutrients. The National Institute on Aging suggests that the daily diet for the geriatric population include the following:

- Two servings of milk or dairy products low in lactose (3 cups per day)
- Two servings of high-protein foods ($5-5\frac{1}{2}$ ounces per day)
- Four servings of fruit and vegetables, including a citrus fruit and a dark green leafy vegetable ($2-2\frac{1}{2}$ cups per day)
- Four servings of bread or cereal products (3 ounces per day)

Clinicopathologic Correlations

There are myriad vitamin and trace element deficiencies, and it is beyond the scope of this book to describe them. There are, however, several worth considering.

Vitamin A, a fat-soluble vitamin, is an integral component of rhodopsin and iodopsin, the light-sensitive proteins in the rods and cones of the retina. A deficiency of vitamin A is associated with follicular hyperkeratosis and night blindness. Figure 5-6 illustrates a patient with vitamin A deficiency and follicular hyperkeratosis.

Vitamin C, or ascorbic acid, is a biologic antioxidant and free radical scavenger. The biosynthesis of bile acids, collagen, and norepinephrine, as well as the normal functioning of the hepatic oxygenase system, depends on these antioxidant properties. Vitamin C deficiency is rarely found in the United States. The classic deficiency state is known as *scurvy*. It is characterized by depression, fatigue, and widespread abnormalities in connective tissue. Oral lesions (including inflamed gingiva), petechiae, hemorrhage, impaired wound healing, hyperkeratosis, and bleeding into body cavities are commonly seen. Figure 5-7 depicts marked periodontal disease in two patients with scurvy. Figure 5-8 illustrates perifollicular purpura and ecchymoses in a patient with vitamin C deficiency.

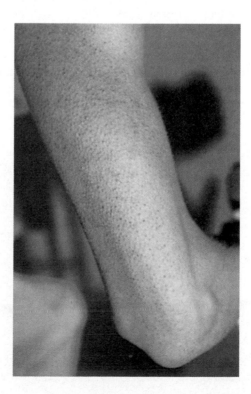

Figure 5–6 Effects of vitamin A deficiency.

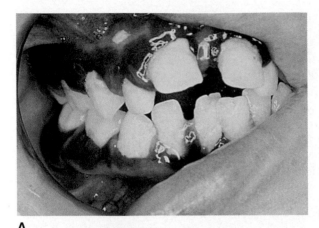

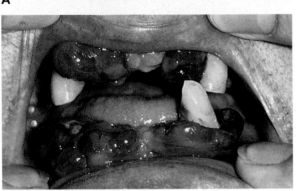

A

Figure 5—7 *A* and *B*, Marked periodontal disease in two patients with vitamin C deficiency.

B

Folate is required for the synthesis of nucleotides and the metabolism of several amino acids. The inhibition of folate metabolism in bacteria and in cancer cell growth is the mechanism of action of the sulfonamide antibiotics and chemotherapeutic agents such as methotrexate and 5-fluorouracil. Folate deficiency is seen in women of childbearing age and in alcoholic patients. It manifests with a megaloblastic anemia reflecting ineffective DNA synthesis. Depapillation of the tongue and diarrhea are common findings. Figure 5-9*A* depicts the classic glossitis of folate deficiency in an alcoholic patient; Figure 5-9*B* illustrates the patient's tongue after folate replacement.

Niacin, a B-complex vitamin, is required as a coenzyme to form nicotinamide adenine dinucleotide or nicotinamide adenine dinucleotide phosphate. There are more than 200 enzymes that require the active coenzyme forms of niacin as electron acceptors or hydrogen donors. The classic deficiency of niacin is *pellagra*. It is seen in populations in China, Africa, and India,

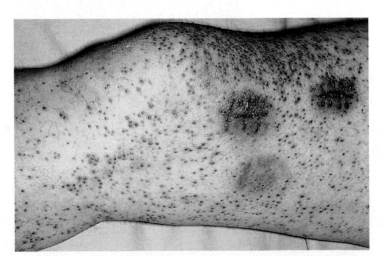

Figure 5—8 Perifollicular purpura and ecchymoses caused by vitamin C deficiency.

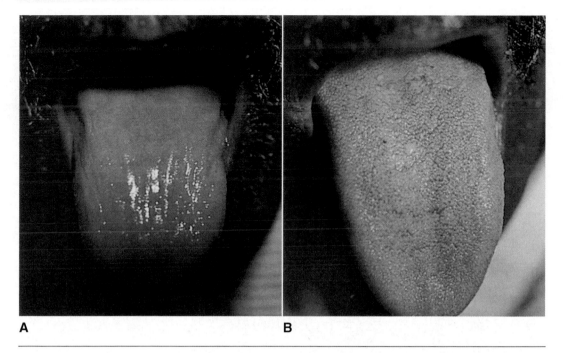

A   B

Figure 5–9 Tongue of a patient with folate deficiency. *A*, Before folate therapy. *B*, After folate therapy.

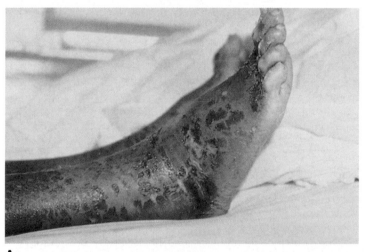

A

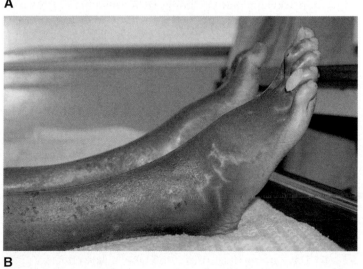

B

Figure 5–10 Legs and feet of a patient with niacin deficiency. *A*, Before niacin therapy. *B*, After niacin therapy.

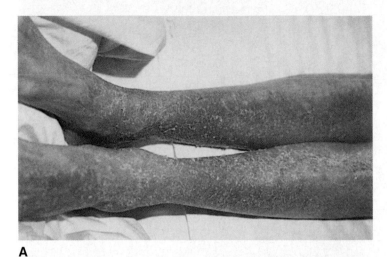

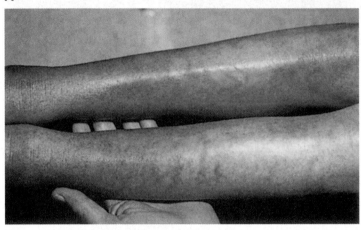

A

B

Figure 5–11 Legs of a patient with zinc deficiency. *A*, Before zinc therapy. *B*, After zinc therapy.

where rice is the major source of energy. The most common symptoms are diarrhea, dementia, and pigmented dermatitis in sun-exposed areas. Glossitis, stomatitis, vertigo, and burning paresthesias are also common. Figure 5-10*A* illustrates marked pigmented dermatitis secondary to niacin deficiency in an alcoholic patient; Figure 5-10*B* depicts the skin of the same patient after replacement therapy.

Zinc is a trace element needed for a variety of metabolic processes. It is a component of more than 100 enzymes, including DNA polymerase, RNA polymerase, and transfer RNA synthetase. Zinc deficiency is associated with growth retardation and hypogonadism in children. In adults, infertility, poor wound healing, diarrhea, and dermatitis are frequent symptoms. Figure 5-11*A* illustrates a widespread scaling dermatitis secondary to zinc deficiency in a patient with fat malabsorption; Figure 5-11*B* illustrates the patient's skin after treatment with zinc.

Concluding Thoughts

The public is fascinated with weight reduction and is quick to buy books on fad diets, drugs to suppress appetite, and cures for disease. Most of these do little for patients except cost them money. Instead, a good health-care provider should inform patients how to eat healthily. Any good diet should accomplish the following:

- Include a wide variety of foods to ensure adequate amounts of all essential nutrients
- Educate the person about proper nutrition
- Be based on sound biochemical facts
- Have no medical risks or metabolic side effects

- Be economical
- Be adaptable to a variety of lifestyles

For health-care providers, dealing with patients who are following diets of questionable nutritional value requires tact and skill. Your success often depends more on how you meet the patient's emotional needs than on your academic credentials. Always be informed about contemporary fad diets and cures. Discuss them openly with the patients; never condemn them out of your ignorance or unwillingness to learn about them.

Nutritional assessment does not stand alone as a separate process; it must be integrated into the entire history and physical examination. The depth of the assessment and the information recorded depend on the patient's specific medical problems. This chapter has provided the framework for integrating key nutrition-related questions and considerations into patient evaluations.

Bibliography

Bailey DG, Malcolm J, Arnold O, et al: Grapefruit juice-drug interactions. Br J Clin Pharmacol 46:101, 1998.

Barrocas A, Belcher D, Champagne C, et al: Nutritional assessment: Practical approaches. Clin Geriatr Med 11:675, 1995.

Bauer BA: Herbal therapy: What a clinician needs to know to counsel patients effectively. Mayo Clin Proc 75:835, 2000.

Casper RC: Recognizing eating disorders in women. Psychopharmacol Bull 34:267,1998.

Eisenberg DM: Advising patients who seek alternative medical therapies. Ann Intern Med 127:61, 1997.

Gazewood JD, Mehr DR: Diagnosis and management of weight loss in the elderly. J Fam Pract 47:19, 1998.

Grapefruit juice interactions with drugs. Med Lett Drugs Ther 37(955):73-4, 1995.

Grundy SM, Brewer B, Cleeman JI, et al: Definition of metabolic syndrome: Report of the National Heart, Lung, and Blood Institute/American Heart Association conference on scientific issues related to definition. Circulation 109:433, 2004.

Hark L, Deen D: Taking a nutrition history: A practical approach for family physicians. Am Fam Physician 59:1521, 1999.

Hark L, Morrison G (eds): Medical Nutrition and Disease: A Case-Based Approach, 3rd ed. Malden, Mass, Blackwell Science, 2003.

Haskell WL, Lee IM, Pate RR, et al: Physical activity and public health: Updated recommendation for adults from the American College of Sports Medicine and the American Heart Association. Med Sci Sports Exerc 39:1423, 2007.

Herbert V, Subak-Sharpe GJ, Kasden TS (eds): Total Nutrition: The Only Guide You'll Ever Need. New York, St. Martin's Press, 1995.

Joshipura KJ, Hu FB, Manson JE, et al: The effect of fruit and vegetable intake on risk for coronary heart disease. Ann Intern Med 134:1106, 2001.

Kriepe RE: Eating disorders among children and adolescents. Pediatr Rev 16:370, 1995.

Kushner RF: Roadmaps for Clinical Practice: Case Studies in Disease Prevention and Health Promotion-Assessment and Management of Adult Obesity: A Primer for Physicians. Chicago, American Medical Association, 2003. Available at: *www.ama-assn.org/ama/pub/category/10931.html*; accessed June 3, 2008.

Kushner RF, Roth JL: Assessment of the obese patient. Endocrinol Metab Clin North Am 32:915, 2003.

Lankisch PG, Gerzmann JF, Lehnick D: Unintentional weight loss: Diagnosis and prognosis. The first prospective follow-up study from a secondary referral centre. J Int Med 249:41, 2001.

Manson JE, Willett WC, Stampfer MJ, et al: Body weight and mortality among women. N Engl J Med 333:677, 1995.

Marcoe K, Juan W, Yamini S, et al: Development of food group composites and nutrient profiles for the My Pyramid food guidance system. J Nutr Edu Behav 38:S93, 2006.

Maskalyk J: Grapefruit juice: Potential drug interactions. CMAJ 167:279, 2002.

Mehler PS: Diagnosis and care of patients with anorexia nervosa in primary care settings. Ann Intern Med 134:1048, 2001.

Morgan JF, Lacey JH: The SCOFF questionnaire: A new screening tool for anorexia nervosa. West J Med 172:164, 2000.

Morgan SL, Weinsier RL: Fundamentals of Clinical Nutrition, 2nd ed. St. Louis, Mosby, 1998.

National Health and Nutrition Examination Survey (NHANES), 2005–2006. Available at: *www.cdc.gov/nchs/about/major/nhanes/nhanes2005-2006/nhanes05_06.htm*; accessed June 3, 2008.

National Institutes of Health and National Heart, Lung, and Blood Institute: Clinical Guidelines on the Identification, Evaluation, and Treatment of Overweight and Obesity in Adults. Rockville, Md: U.S. Department of Health and Human Services, Public Health Service, 1998.

National Institutes of Health, National Heart, Lung, and Blood Institute (NHLBI), and North American Association for the Study of Obesity (NAASO): Practical Guide to the Identification, Evaluation, and

Treatment of Overweight and Obesity in Adults. NIH publication no. 00-4084. Bethesda, Md, National Institutes of Health, 2000.

Newton JM, Halstead CH: Clinical and functional assessment of adults. In Shils ME, Olson JA, Shike M, et al (eds): Modern Nutrition in Health and Disease, 9th ed. Baltimore, Williams & Wilkins, 1999.

Ogden CL, Carroll MD, McDowell MA, et al: Obesity among adults in the United States—no statistically significant change since 2003–2004. NCHS data brief no 1. Hyattsville, Md: National Center for Health Statistics, 2007.

Pennachio DL: Drug-herb interactions: How vigilant should you be? Patient Care 15:41, 2000.

Pickering TG, Hall JE, Appel LJ, et al: Recommendations for blood pressure measurement in humans and experimental animals: Part 1: Blood pressure measurement in humans: A statement for professionals from the Subcommittee of Professional and Public Education of the American Heart Association Council on High Blood Pressure Research. Circulation 111:697, 2005.

Pleis JR, Lethbridge-Çejku M: Summary health statistics for U.S. adults: National Health Interview Survey, 2006. National Center for Health Statistics. Vital Health Stat 10:235, 2007.

Popkin BM, Siega-Riz AM, Haines PS: A comparison of dietary trends among racial and ethnic subgroups in the United States. N Engl J Med 335:716, 1996.

Reife CM: Involuntary weight loss: Common medical problems in ambulatory care. Med Clin North Am 70:299, 1995.

Stallings VA, Yaktine AL (eds): Nutrition Standards for Foods in Schools: Leading the Way Toward Healthier Youth, Washington, DC, National Academies Press, 2007.

U.S. Department of Health and Human Services and U.S. Department of Agriculture: Dietary Guidelines for Americans, 6th ed. Washington, DC, U.S. Government Printing Office, 2005.

Walsh BT, Devlin MJ: Eating disorders: Progress and problems. Science 280:1387, 1998.

Wynder EL, Stellman SD, Zang EA: High fiber intake: Indicator of a healthy lifestyle. JAMA 275:486, 1996.

CHAPTER 6

Putting the History Together

The doctor may also learn more about the illness from the way the patient tells the story than from the story itself.

James B. Herrick (1861–1954)

In the first few chapters, the interviewer's questions and the patient's responses were discussed. In this chapter, these materials are put together to shape a mock interview.

In the ensuing interview, note the way in which the interviewer allows the patient to speak and how the various techniques are incorporated. The footnotes refer to the type of technique used or to some other important aspects of the interview.

Interview of Mr. John Doe

Mr. John Doe, the patient, is lying comfortably in a two-bed room in St. Catherine's Hospital. He is a white man, is slightly obese, and is in his mid-40s. Mr. Doe is watching television. The interviewer enters the room, wearing a white coat.

	(Interviewer smiles and extends hand for a firm handshake)
Interviewer:	Good morning, I'm Susan Smith, a second-year medical student. Are you Mr. Doe?
	(Pause; interviewer watches for response)
Interviewer:	I've been asked to interview and examine you today.
	(Patient smiles, appearing friendly)
Patient:	Dr. James, my resident, told me you'd be coming to see me.
	(Interviewer draws curtain around bed; pulls up a chair at the patient's bedside and sits down; legs crossed, arms in lap)
Interviewer:	Would you mind if we turn off the TV?
	(Patient turns off television)
Patient:	Not at all.
Interviewer:	How are you today?
Patient:	OK. No pain for the past 2 days.

Interviewer:	What was the problem that brought you to the hospital, Mr. Doe?*
Patient:	I've been having terrible chest pain for the past 6 months ....
	(pause)
Patient:	I guess I should start at the beginning. . . . About 4 years ago, I started having this strange sensation in my chest. It wasn't pain exactly . . . it was a dull aching discomfort. I didn't pay any attention to it. I guess I should have. . . . Well, anyway, I was able to go to work, play tennis, and have fun. Occasionally when I had an argument at work, I would get this sensation.
	(looking sad)
Patient:	My wife never knew anything about it. I never told her. No one knew. I didn't want to upset them. Then all of a sudden on July 15, 2008, it happened.
	(silence)
Interviewer:	It happened?†
Patient:	Yeah. I had my first heart attack.‡ I was playing tennis when I got this awful pain. I never had anything like that before. I was just getting ready to serve when this pain hit me. All I could do was lie down on the court. My partner ran over to me, and all I remember was that pain. . . . I woke up in Kings Hospital.
	(pause)
Patient:	They told me I lost consciousness and was taken to the hospital by ambulance. I remember that when I came to in the hospital, I still had the pain. I was there for 2 weeks.
Interviewer:	How did you feel when you left the hospital?
Patient:	I really felt fine. No more chest pain. My doctor there had given me some pills and said I would be fine.§
Interviewer:	Then what happened?¶
Patient:	I went back to work after about 3 weeks. I really felt great!
	(smiles)
Interviewer:	What type of work do you do?
Patient:	I'm a lawyer.
Interviewer:	You mentioned that this was your first heart attack. Have you had others?
Patient:	Unfortunately. . . .
	(looking down)
Patient:	Yes.
Interviewer:	Tell me about it.¶¶
	*(leaning forward**)*
Patient:	Six months later, I had my second attack.
	(pause)

---

*Inquiring about the chief complaint by using an open-ended question.
†This is an example of reflection.
‡The patient is now telling the history of the current illness.
§Possibly false reassurance from the physician, or the patient heard what he wanted to hear.
¶Interviewer continues obtaining information with another open-ended question about the current illness.
¶¶An example of verbal facilitation.
**An example of nonverbal facilitation.

Interviewer:	What were you doing?
Patient:	Playing tennis.
	(silence)
Patient:	This time I don't remember anything . . . not even the pain. I remember being on the court and waking up in the intensive care unit of Kings Hospital. They said I had a massive heart attack and had some irregularity of my pulse that made me faint. But I left the hospital in 3 weeks feeling much better. I went back to work after 3 weeks at home.
Interviewer:	Did you have any tests while you were in the hospital?
Patient:	No. . . .
	(pause, hand over mouth)
Patient:	The doctor just gave me some pills to strengthen my heart and for the irregularity.
	(silence for 10 seconds)
Interviewer:	Your silence makes me think that you want to tell me something.*
Patient:	I should have listened to him.
	(pause, shaking head)
Interviewer:	To whom?
Patient:	My doctor suggested after my first heart attack that I should have cardiac catheterization. I told him that I was fine, I didn't need it. Even after my second attack, I didn't listen to him.
	(pause)
Patient:	I hope it's not too late.
Interviewer:	Too late?
Patient:	Yeah. That's why I'm here. I'm going to have the cardiac catheterization tomorrow. Emily finally convinced me to have it.
	(pause)
Patient:	I've really not been able to do anything for the past 6 months.
	(pause, looking down)
Patient:	I had to give up my work at the office. Sure, they still call me for advice, but it's not the same.
	(pause, almost tearful)
Patient:	The commuting by car just got to me.
	(pause)
Patient:	My son and his friends yelling around the house.
	(longer pause)
Patient:	I just can't take it anymore.
Interviewer:	What did your doctor tell you about the test?†
Patient:	The doctor told me if I have some blockage, he'll operate or fix it with a balloon or a type of Roto-Rooter. Will I be normal again?
	(pause)

---

*An example of confrontation.
†Inquiring about the patient's understanding of the test.

Interviewer:	After the study, your doctor will be in the best position to answer that question.*
	(pause)
Interviewer:	Tell me about the pain you've been having.
Patient:	It seems I have the pain all the time. I can hardly walk up the stairs at home without getting the pain.
Interviewer:	What's the pain like now?
Patient:	It's an awful tightness, like a vise. . . .
	(closes fist over chest[†])
Patient:	Right here.
Interviewer:	When you get the pain, do you feel it anywhere else?
Patient:	Yeah. It goes straight to my back and my left arm. . . . The arm feels so heavy.
Interviewer:	Are there any other times when you get the pain?
Patient:	It seems I get it with the slightest effort or emotion.
Interviewer:	Do you get the pain during sexual intercourse?
Interviewer:	I had to stop even that 6 months ago. I'd get the pain just when I'm about to come . . . and . . . and . . . I'd have to stop.
Interviewer:	Have you had any difficulty breathing?
Patient:	When I get the pain, I get short of breath.
Interviewer:	Do you ever get short of breath without the pain?
Patient:	I find I just can't walk far any more without getting winded.
Interviewer:	How many level blocks can you walk now without getting short of breath?
Patient:	About one block.
Interviewer:	How much could you walk 6 months ago?
Patient:	I guess about two to three blocks.
Interviewer:	Since your heart attack, have you had any skipped beats or fluttering of your heart?
Patient:	No, never.
Interviewer:	Has anyone ever told you that your cholesterol or fats in your blood were high?[‡]
Patient:	No.
Interviewer:	Have you ever smoked?
Patient:	I stopped after my first heart attack.
Interviewer:	That's great that you stopped smoking. How much did you smoke?
Patient:	About two packs a day.
Interviewer:	For how long?
Patient:	Oh . . . since I was about 18.

---

*The interviewer does not want to give false reassurances. Therefore, she chooses not to answer the question directly. Notice how the interviewer gets the narrative back on course.

[†]This example of body language has been termed *Levine's sign.* It is discussed in Chapter 14, The Heart.

[‡]The interviewer is now starting to ascertain whether the patient has any risk factors for coronary artery disease.

Interviewer:	May I ask your age?*
Patient:	I'm 42.
Interviewer:	Have you ever had high blood pressure?
Patient:	Yep. . . . My doctor gave me some medications for it, but . . . but . . . I never refilled the pills after they ran out. . . . I felt fine.
Interviewer:	Do you know how high your pressure was?†
Patient:	Not really.
Interviewer:	Do you have diabetes?
Patient:	Thank goodness, I don't. . . . My father does, though. . . . He's been pretty sick lately. . . . He's got some sort of a problem with his eyes. The doctor said that it's from his diabetes. He's going to see a specialist in a couple of weeks. . . . He's had a lot of problems. He broke his hip a few years ago when he was walking our dog. Some big guy came pulling a cart out of the supermarket and knocked my father over. He was hospitalized for several weeks because he really couldn't take care of himself. His hip is fine now. He would. . . .
Interviewer:	(interrupting) I'm glad his hip is well healed. Is there anyone else in your family who has diabetes?‡
Patient:	No.
Interviewer:	Anyone else in your family who's had a heart attack?
Patient:	I think my mother's father died of a heart attack.
Interviewer:	How old was he?
Patient:	About 75.
Interviewer:	What about your mother?§
Patient:	She died when she was age 64 . . . right after my first heart attack. She had stomach cancer. She really suffered. . . . I guess it's a blessing.
Interviewer:	Do you have any brothers or sisters?
Patient:	My sister is 37 and she's fine. . . .
Interviewer:	Any other siblings?
Patient:	My brother is 45. . . . He had a heart attack when he was 40.¶
Interviewer:	Do you have any children?
Patient:	One boy who's 15.
Interviewer:	How's your son's health?
Patient:	No problem, except he's a little overweight.
Interviewer:	Are you married?¶¶

---

*Notice that the interviewer has just now decided to ask the patient's age.

†Notice that the interviewer ignores the statement that the patient didn't take his medications. Questioning the patient "Why not?" would only put the patient on the defensive.

‡Notice that the patient was beginning to ramble. The interviewer politely interrupted and redirected the interview. She is now inquiring about the family history.

§Notice that the interviewer does not assume anything about the mother's well-being or health. Because the patient approached the family's health history, the interviewer is now directing her questions to that history.

¶Notice that the patient did not mention his brother when first asked about other family members with heart attacks or when asked about other brothers or sisters. The patient did not even acknowledge his brother's cardiac problem.

¶¶Notice that the interviewer does not assume that Mr. Doe is married *now*, even though he referred to his wife at the beginning of the interview and has acknowledged "Emily." "Emily" may not be his wife.

Patient:	To a great gal. Emily's the one who convinced me to have the test.*
Interviewer:	Does anyone in your family have high blood pressure?
Patient:	No.
Interviewer:	Asthma?
Patient:	No.
Interviewer:	Tuberculosis?
Patient:	No.
Interviewer:	Birth defects or congenital diseases?
Patient:	Not that I know of.
Interviewer:	Have you ever been hospitalized here at St. Catherine's Hospital?
Patient:	No.†
Interviewer:	Have you ever been hospitalized at any time other than for your heart attacks?
Patient:	I had my appendix taken out when I was 15.
Interviewer:	Do you remember the surgeon's name and the hospital?
Patient:	I think it was a Dr. Meyers at Booth Memorial Hospital. We were living in Rochester.
Interviewer:	Any other operations?
Patient:	No.
Interviewer:	Have you ever been hospitalized for any other reason?‡
Patient:	No, what do you mean?
Interviewer:	Just a routine question. Do you have any allergies?
Patient:	No.
Interviewer:	How was your health as a child?
Patient:	I guess OK. I had the usual sore throats and earaches that most kids get.
Interviewer:	Did anyone ever tell you that you had rheumatic fever?§
Patient:	No.
Interviewer:	Did you have any of these illnesses¶: chickenpox? measles? diphtheria? polio? mumps? whooping cough?
	(Patient shakes head "no")
Interviewer:	Do you take any medications?
Patient:	Just atenolol and isosorbide dinitrate.
Interviewer:	Do you know the dosages?

---

*In this case, "Emily" is the patient's wife. It is extremely important for the patient to identify family members. The interviewer must never make an assumption that another person with the patient or described in the history is related to the patient.

†Had the patient answered in the affirmative, the interviewer would have asked when, and the patient's record would have been reviewed later.

‡The interviewer is specifically asking about nonmedical hospitalizations (e.g., for psychiatric reasons). This type of question is not offensive. If the patient has had such admissions to hospitals, he can usually describe them at this time. If not, as in this case, watch how the interview progresses. (Notice how the interviewer continues directly with the next question.)

§This question can follow nicely after the history of sore throats.

¶The interviewer slowly asks about each illness, after which she pauses for the patient to respond.

Patient:	I take 50 mg of atenolol once daily and 10 mg of isosorbide dinitrate four times a day.
Interviewer:	Do you think the medications help you?
Patient:	I guess so. I think I feel better with them.
Interviewer:	Any other medications?
	(pause)
Patient:	Nitroglycerin . . . when I get the pain.
Interviewer:	How long does the nitroglycerin take to work?
Patient:	Real quickly.
Interviewer:	How long is that?
Patient:	About 4 to 5 minutes.
Interviewer:	Do you take any other medications?
	(pause)
Interviewer:	Over-the-counter medicine? herbal medicines? anything else?
Patient:	(thinks for a moment) I take Chlor-Trimeton when I get a cold . . . but that's about it.
Interviewer:	Have you ever had any other health problems?
Patient:	No.
Interviewer:	Any problems with your liver? kidneys? stomach? lungs?*
	(Patient shakes head "no")
Interviewer:	How's your appetite?
Patient:	Pretty good. I haven't been real hungry lately.
Interviewer:	Starting with breakfast yesterday, what did you eat?
Patient:	Toast, coffee, and juice for breakfast. . . .
	(pause)
Patient:	A ham sandwich with a Tab for lunch. . . .
	(pause)
Patient:	Oh, yeah, blueberry pie for dessert. . . .
	(pause)
Patient:	And . . . uh . . . steak with a baked potato and salad for dinner.
Interviewer:	Any snacks between meals?
Patient:	I had a cupcake with milk before I went to bed.
Interviewer:	Do you eat fish?
Patient:	Sometimes.
Interviewer:	How often?†
Patient:	Maybe. . . .
	(pause)

---

*Because this patient has demonstrated so much denial, the interviewer wishes to ask specifically about diseases of the major organs. Each question is asked slowly, and the interviewer pauses after each question, waiting for a response.

†The interviewer is not satisfied with qualitative statements. She pursues each question to quantify as best as possible.

Patient: Once every 2 weeks. I enjoy shrimp, but I know it's not good for me.*

Interviewer: Have you had any weight change recently?

Patient: I lost about 10 pounds in the past 3 months. . . .

                  (pause)

Patient: But I wanted to. . . .

Interviewer: Were you on a diet?

Patient: No . . . not exactly . . . I just haven't been too hungry lately.

Interviewer: How well do you sleep?†

Patient: Like a baby. . . .

                  (pause)

Patient: Although I've been getting up pretty early recently.

Interviewer: Mmmm?

Patient: Yeah . . . recently I go right to sleep . . . but seem to get up about 3 in the morning . . . and can't go back to sleep. . . .

                  (pause)

Patient: I guess I've got a lot on my mind. . . .

                  (pause, looking down, hand to mouth)

Interviewer: You seem depressed.‡

                  (Patient pauses)

Patient: I guess I am. . . . What's going to happen to me? I really want to live. . . .

                  (beginning to cry)

Patient: I've been so stupid. . . .

                  (pause)

Patient: My kid's only 15. . . . He's a great kid. . . . He needs me. . . . What's the test gonna show? I hope I can have the surgery or the balloon to get relief from this pain.§

                  (Interviewer is silent, handing a box of tissues to the patient)¶

                  (Patient is sobbing, trying to control his emotions)

Patient: I'm sorry. . . . I can't help it. . . .

                  (wiping his tears)

Patient: I guess we'll have to wait till tomorrow.

Interviewer: I just have a few more questions for you. Do you drink alcohol?

                  (Patient shakes his head "no")

Patient: Just socially . . . one drink . . . maybe after work, sometimes.

Interviewer: Do you ever feel that you have a need for a drink as the day goes on?

---

*Despite the fact that he knows that shrimp is not as healthy as fish, he still eats it. This is further denial of his illness.

†The interviewer has now picked up some other somatic element of depression and will now pursue it.

‡An example of an interpretation.

§The interviewer could have elected to ask the patient his reactions if surgery cannot be performed. How will he face life? Is there a possibility of suicide? The interviewer chose not to create further anxiety at this time.

¶An example of empathetic support. The interviewer cannot answer the patient's questions, but she allows the patient to express his emotions. She is, in essence, saying, "I'm with you."

Patient:	Yeah . . . I sure do!
Interviewer:	Have you ever felt the need to cut down on your drinking?
Patient:	No.
Interviewer:	Have people annoyed you by criticizing your drinking?
Patient:	Never . . . but my wife doesn't like me drinking.
Interviewer:	Have you ever felt bad or guilty about your drinking?
Patient:	Yeah. . . . Once about 10 years ago my friend's father made some wine. . . . We got really drunk . . . it was terrible . . . but never again!
Interviewer:	Do you drink in the morning?
Patient:	Never.
Interviewer:	Do you ever drive while intoxicated?
Patient:	No! That's suicide.
Interviewer:	Do you drink coffee or tea?
Patient:	About three cups of coffee a day at work. I have tea only when I'm sick with a cold.
Interviewer:	Have you ever used recreational drugs?
Patient:	I've tried pot a couple of times . . . never did anything to me. . . . Nothing else.
Interviewer:	What's your usual day like?*
Patient:	Before I stopped working at the office, I got up about 5:30, dressed, and was at my desk in the office by 7:30. I usually left the office about 7 and got home by 8:15. We'd have dinner, and I'd be in bed by 11:30, after the news.
Interviewer:	Sounds like you have a pretty busy day.
Patient:	Yeah. . . . I enjoy my work . . . or at least I used to.
Interviewer:	How long have you been working with your present office?
Patient:	I started right after law school. I guess I've been there . . . about . . . 17 years. I'm one of the senior partners.
	(pause)
Patient:	I was just promoted . . . A lot of good that will do now.
Interviewer:	Congratulations on your promotion! I now have several questions to ask you. You can answer just "yes" or "no" to each.†
	(pause)
Interviewer:	Have you had any recent fevers?
Patient:	No.
Interviewer:	Chills?
Patient:	No.
Interviewer:	Sweats?
Patient:	No.
Interviewer:	Rashes?
Patient:	No.
Interviewer:	Changes in your hair or nails?

---

*Interviewer is inquiring about the patient's lifestyle and psychosocial history.
†The interviewer now begins asking the *review of systems*. She asks about each symptom. If the patient answers in the affirmative, further questioning is appropriate.

Patient:	No.
Interviewer:	Headaches?
Patient:	Rarely, about once every 2 to 3 months.
Interviewer:	For how long have you been having headaches?
Patient:	Years . . . I guess about 20 to 25 years.
Interviewer:	Can you describe them to me?
Patient:	That's hard. They're right here.
	(pointing to the center of his forehead)
Patient:	They last about 1 to 2 hours.
Interviewer:	What relieves them?
Patient:	Usually aspirin.
Interviewer:	Have you noticed a change in the pattern or severity of your headaches?
Patient:	No.
Interviewer:	Have you had any head injuries?
Patient:	Never.
Interviewer:	Have you ever fainted?
Patient:	No.
Interviewer:	Do you have any problems with. . . .*
	(The interviewer completes the review of systems)
Interviewer:	Is there anything else you would like to tell me that I haven't asked about?
Patient:	No . . . you've certainly been very thorough.
Interviewer:	Let's summarize your history briefly to make sure I have the details correct before I proceed with your physical examination. This is your first time here at St. Catherine's Hospital. You had your first heart attack on July 15, 2008, while playing tennis. You were hospitalized in Kings Hospital for 2 weeks. Your second heart attack was 6 months later. You were again hospitalized in Kings Hospital. Your medications since then have been atenolol, 50 mg once daily, and isosorbide dinitrate, 10 mg four times a day. Because of a worsening of your chest pain and an increase in your shortness of breath in the past 6 months, you're now being admitted for cardiac catheterization. Is that correct, Mr. Doe?
Patient:	Exactly!
Interviewer:	Do you have any questions for me before I begin your physical examination?
Patient:	No . . . I can't think of any.
	(The interviewer stands up, sets up the equipment on the night table, and goes to the sink to wash her hands. The physical examination then commences.)
	(Interviewer concludes the physical examination)
Interviewer:	I want to thank you for your time.
Patient:	Well . . . what do you think? Will I make it?

---

*The interviewer continues through the entire review of systems, asking further questions when necessary.

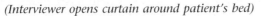

(Interviewer opens curtain around patient's bed)

Interviewer: I'm now going to meet with my preceptor. Afterward, we'll be back to discuss your medical condition.*

Written History of Mr. John Doe

The preceding interview has revealed much about this 42-year-old lawyer. Superficially, he is a patient with coronary artery disease. Just as important as his physical illness is his emotional reaction to it. As the interview progressed, the interviewer recognized that the patient is frightened and anxious. What will happen "after tomorrow"? Will he be a candidate for balloon angioplasty? Can it be performed? Is he a good candidate for bypass surgery? Will he live? The anxiety from these questions has resulted in his depression, which must be dealt with as well.

The written history is a summary of the information obtained during the interview. It is usually written after the interview and the physical examination have been completed. The following is an example of the written history of Mr. Doe, based on the preceding interview.

Chief Complaint: "Chest pain for the past 6 months."

History of Current Illness: This is the first St. Catherine's Hospital admission for Mr. John Doe, a 42-year-old lawyer with coronary artery disease. His history dates back to approximately 4 years before admission, when he started to experience a vague discomfort in his chest. He describes it as "a dull ache," provoked by emotional upsets at work. He suffered his first heart attack on July 15, 2008, while playing tennis. He was hospitalized for 3 weeks in Kings Hospital. After 3 weeks at home, he returned to work. Six months later, he suffered his second heart attack, again while playing tennis. He was again hospitalized at Kings Hospital and was told that he had "irregularity" of his heart. He was started on some medications for this irregularity. The patient denies any palpitations since then.

Over the past 6 months, the patient has had increasing chest pain with radiation down his left arm despite atenolol, 50 mg daily, and isosorbide dinitrate, 10 mg qid.† The patient's chest pain is produced by exercise, emotion, and sexual intercourse. The patient takes nitroglycerin as needed, with relief within 5 minutes. One-block dyspnea on exertion is also present. This has worsened in the past 6 months, before which he could walk two to three blocks. The patient's risk factors for coronary artery disease include a history of untreated hypertension, a 40-pack-year history of smoking (2 packs per day for 20 years), and a brother with a myocardial infarction at the age of 40 years. The patient's brother is now 45 years of age. The patient denies any history of diabetes or hyperlipidemia. At his physician's and wife's request, he has entered the hospital for elective cardiac catheterization. The patient has a significant denial of his illness and a secondary depression.‡ Although cardiac catheterization was suggested after the patient's first heart attack, he refused to accept it until this admission.

Past Medical History: The patient was hospitalized at age 15 years for an appendectomy in Booth Memorial Hospital in Rochester, New York. The surgery was performed by a Dr. Meyers. The only other hospitalizations were for the patient's two heart attacks, as indicated previously. The patient is predominantly a red meat eater with little fish in his diet. Recently, presumably owing to depression, there has been a loss of appetite with a 10-pound weight loss. The patient admits to a sleeping problem. He falls asleep normally but awakens early and cannot go back to sleep. His only medications are indicated in the history of current illness. There is no history of renal, hepatic, pulmonary, or gastrointestinal disease. There is no history of allergy.

Family History: The patient's father is 75 years of age and has a history of diabetes. He apparently has some ocular problem related to diabetes. The patient's mother died at age 64 years from stomach cancer. The patient's older brother, as mentioned previously, is

---

*By indicating to the patient that the interviewer and her preceptor will be back, the patient is less likely to press the interviewer for her opinion at this time. The interviewer should never provide an answer at this point. False reassurances can be dangerous.

†The abbreviation *qid* means four times a day.

‡Notice that the history of the current illness summarizes all the information related to the current illness chronologically, regardless of when the information was obtained during the interview.

45 years of age and has coronary artery disease. The patient has a younger sister who is 37 years of age and is well. There is no history of congenital disease. The patient is married and has a 15-year-old son, who is well.

Psychosocial History: The patient is a ''type A'' personality. He admits to having a need to drink alcohol occasionally after work. He drinks coffee about three times a day. He has used only marijuana on rare occasions, and he denies the use of other recreational drugs.

Review of Systems: There is a 20- to 25-year history of headaches without any recent change in their pattern or severity. The patient denies any head injury. There is. . . .* There is no history of claudication.† The remainder of the review of systems is noncontributory.‡

---

*The review of systems would then indicate any of the other symptoms that may be present.

†Notice that the positive symptoms are indicated first. The important, or pertinent, negative symptoms are then listed. A pertinent negative symptom in this patient is the lack of claudication. Coronary artery disease is often associated with peripheral vascular disease. The absence of a major symptom of peripheral vascular disease, claudication, makes claudication in this patient a pertinent negative symptom. Chapter 15, The Peripheral Vascular System, provides a further discussion of pertinent positives and negatives.

‡This statement indicates that none of the other symptoms is either present or contributes to the patient's current illness.

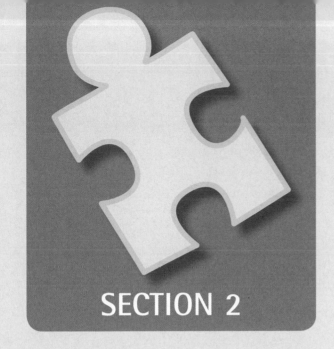

SECTION 2

The Science of the Physical Examination

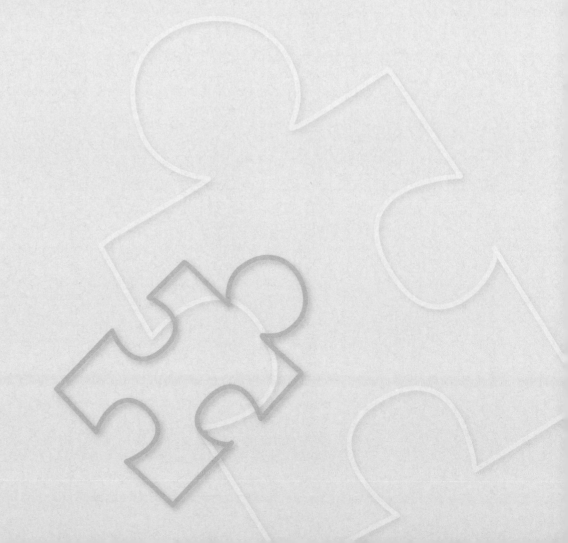

CHAPTER 7

The Physical Examination

Don't touch the patient—state first what you see; cultivate your powers of observation.

Sir William Osler (1849–1919)

The Basic Procedures

In the previous chapters, the general rules for mastering the art of taking the history were discussed. The specific skills necessary to perform a proper physical examination are discussed in this chapter. The four principles of physical examination are as follows:

1. Inspection
2. Palpation
3. Percussion
4. Auscultation

To achieve competence in these procedures, the student must, in the words of Sir William Osler, "teach the eye to see, the finger to feel, and the ear to hear." The ability to coordinate all this sensory input is learned with time and practice.

Even though examiners do not use all these techniques for every organ system, they should think of these four skills before moving on to the next area to be evaluated.

Inspection

Inspection can yield an enormous amount of information. Proper technique requires more than just a glance. Examiners must train themselves to look at the body by using a systematic approach. All too often, the novice examiner rushes to use the ophthalmoscope, stethoscope, or otoscope before the naked eyes have been used for inspection.

An example of what is meant by "teaching the eye to see" can be demonstrated in the following exercise. Read the sentence in the box. Then count the number of "f's" in the sentence.

> Finished files are the result of years of scientific study combined with the experience of years.

How many did you count? The answer is given in a footnote at the end of this chapter. This example clearly shows that eyes have to be trained to see.*

---

*This test has been circulated widely in the medical community. The original writer is unknown.

While taking the history, the examiner should observe the following aspects of the patient:

- General appearance
- State of nutrition
- Body habitus
- Symmetry
- Posture and gait
- Speech

The *general appearance* includes the state of consciousness and personal grooming. Does the patient look well or sick? Is he or she comfortable in bed, or does he or she appear in distress? Is the patient alert, or is he or she groggy? Does he or she look acutely or chronically ill? The answer to this last question is sometimes difficult to determine from inspection, but there are some useful signs to aid the examiner. Poor nutrition, sunken eyes, temporal wasting, and loose skin are associated with chronic disease. Does the patient appear clean? Although the patient is ill, he or she does not have to appear unkempt. Is his or her hair combed? Does he or she bite fingernails? The answers to these questions may provide useful information about the patient's self-esteem and mental status.

Inspection can evaluate the *state of nutrition.* Does the patient appear thin and frail? Is the patient obese? Most individuals with chronic disease are *not* overweight; they are cachectic. Long-standing ailments such as cancer, hyperthyroidism, or heart disease can result in a markedly wasted appearance. See Chapter 5, Assessment of Nutritional Status.

The *body habitus* is useful to observe, because certain disease states are more common in different body builds. The asthenic, or ectomorphic, patient is thin, has poor muscle development and small bone structure, and appears malnourished. The sthenic, or mesomorphic, patient is the athletic type with excellent development of the muscles and a large bone structure. The hypersthenic, or endomorphic, patient is a short, round individual with good muscle development but frequently has a weight problem.

Because the outward appearance of the body is *symmetric,* any asymmetry should be noted. Many systemic diseases provide clues that can be uncovered on inspection. For example, an obvious unilateral supraclavicular swelling or a less obvious unilateral miotic pupil is a clue that can aid the examiner in reaching a final diagnosis. A left supraclavicular swelling in a 61-year-old man may represent an enlarged supraclavicular lymph node and could be the only sign of gastric carcinoma. A miotic pupil in a 43-year-old woman may be a manifestation of interruption of the cervical sympathetic chain by a tumor of the apex of the lung. The recent onset of a left-sided varicocele in a 46-year-old man could be related to a left hypernephroma.

The patient is usually in bed when introduced to the examiner. If the patient were walking about, the examiner could use this time to observe the patient's *posture* and *gait.* The ability to walk normally involves coordination of the nervous and musculoskeletal systems. Does the patient drag a foot? Is there a shuffling gait? Does the patient limp? Are the steps normal?

The examiner can learn much about the patient from his or her *speech patterns.* Is the speech slurred? Does the patient use words appropriately? Is the patient hoarse? Is the voice unusually high or low in pitch?

Is the patient oriented to person, place, and time? This can easily be evaluated by asking the patient, "Who are you?" "Where are you?" "What is the date, season, or month?" and "What is the name of the president of the United States?" These questions certainly do not have to be asked at the beginning, but they should be asked at some time during the interview and examination. These questions provide an insight into the mental status of the patient. The mental status examination is discussed further in Chapter 21, The Nervous System.

The examiner must be able to recognize the cardinal signs of inflammation: swelling, heat, redness, pain, and disturbance of function. Swelling results from edema or congestion in local tissues. Heat is the sensation resulting from an increased blood supply to the involved area. Redness is also a manifestation of the increased blood supply. Pain often results from the swelling, which exerts increased pressure on the nerve fibers. Because of the pain and swelling, a disturbance of function may occur.

Palpation

Palpation is the use of touch to determine the characteristics of an organ system. For example, an abnormal impulse may be palpated in the right side of the chest and could be related to an ascending aortic aneurysm. A pulsatile mass palpated in the abdomen might be an

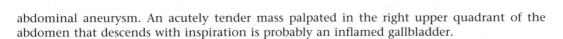

abdominal aneurysm. An acutely tender mass palpated in the right upper quadrant of the abdomen that descends with inspiration is probably an inflamed gallbladder.

Percussion

Percussion relates to the tactile sensation and sound produced when a sharp blow is struck to an area being examined. This provides valuable information about the structure of the underlying organ or tissue. A difference from normal sensation may be related to fluid in an area that normally does not contain fluid. Collapse of a lung changes the percussion note, as does a solid mass in the abdomen. Percussion that produces a dull note in the midline of the lower abdomen in a man probably represents a distended urinary bladder.

Auscultation

Auscultation involves listening to sounds produced by internal organs. This technique furnishes information about an organ's disease process. The examiner is urged to learn as much as possible from the other techniques before using the stethoscope. This instrument should corroborate the signs that were suggested by the other techniques. To examine the heart, chest, and abdomen, auscultation should be used, not alone, but together with inspection, percussion, and palpation. Listening for carotid, ophthalmic, or renal bruits can provide lifesaving information. The absence of normal bowel sounds could indicate a surgical emergency.

Preparation for the Examination

The physical examination usually begins after the history has been documented. You should have a portable case designed to contain all the necessary equipment, which includes the items listed in Table 7-1.

Place the equipment on the patient's night table or bed stand. By laying out all the tools, you are less likely to forget to perform a specific examination. It is preferable to use daylight for illumination because skin color changes may be masked by artificial light. The patient's curtains should be closed for privacy at the start of the interview.

Before examining the patient, wash your hands, preferably while the patient is watching. Washing with soap and water is an effective way to reduce the transmission of disease. Be sure to lather for 10 seconds or more. If soap and water is not available, it is also acceptable to use an alcohol-based hand hygiene product unless there is visible soiling.

The patient should be wearing a gown that opens at the front or back. Pajamas are also acceptable. It is most important to consider the comfort of the patient. You should allow the patient the use of pillows if requested. This is one of the few relationships in which individuals are willing to expose themselves to a stranger after only brief contact.

It is important that you become facile in each organ system examination. Incorporate the individual evaluations into the complete examination with the least amount of movement

Table 7–1 Equipment for Physical Examination

Required	**Optional**	**Available in Most Patient Care Areas**
Stethoscope	Nasal illuminator[†]	Sphygmomanometer
Oto-ophthalmoscope	Nasal speculum	Tongue blades
Penlight	Tuning fork: 512 Hz	Applicator sticks
Reflex hammer		Gauze pads
Tuning fork: 128 Hz		Gloves
Safety pins*		Lubricant gel
Tape measure		Guaiac card for occult blood
Pocket visual acuity card		Vaginal speculum

*A new pin should be used for each patient as a precaution against transmission of the human immunodeficiency and hepatitis viruses. As an alternative, a broken wooden applicator stick may be used.

[†]Attachment for the otoscope handle.

of the patient. Regardless of age, patients tire quickly when asked to "sit up," "lie down," "turn on your left side," "sit up," "lie down," and so on. You should perform as much of the examination as possible with the patient in one position. It is also important that the patient never be asked to sit up in bed without support for any extended period.

By convention, the examiner stands to the *right* of the patient as the patient lies in bed. The examiner uses the right hand for most maneuvers of the examination. It is common practice that even left-handed individuals learn to perform the examination from the right side, using the right hand. Each of the subsequent chapters on organ systems discusses the placement of hands.

Although it is necessary for the patient to disrobe completely, the examination should be carried out by exposing only the areas that are being examined at that time, without undue exposure of other areas. When a woman's breast is examined, for example, it is necessary to check for any asymmetry by inspecting both breasts at the same time. After inspection has been completed, you may use the patient's gown to cover the breast not being examined. The examination of the abdomen may be done discreetly by placing a towel or the bed sheet over the genitalia. Examination of the heart with the patient in the supine position may be performed with the right breast covered. Respecting the patient's privacy goes a long way in establishing a good doctor-patient relationship.

While performing the physical examination, you should continue speaking to the patient. You may wish to pursue various parts of the history, as well as tell the patient what is being done. You should refrain from comments such as "That's good" or "That's normal" or "That's fine" in reference to any part of the examination. Although this is initially reassuring to the patient, if you fail to make such a statement during another part of the examination, the patient will automatically assume that there is something wrong or abnormal.

The following chapters discuss the individual organ system examinations. Chapter 22, Putting the Examination Together, then summarizes a method of combining all the individual evaluations into one smooth, continuous examination.

Health-Care Infection Control Practices

Students and clinicians are frequently exposed to patients with hepatitis or acquired immunodeficiency syndrome. Clinicians' fear of these diseases often interferes with the development of a good doctor-patient relationship. Once clearly defined procedures are implemented to ensure the safety of health-care workers, this fear can be better handled.

Several precautionary guidelines have been established by both the Centers for Disease Control and Prevention and the Occupational Safety and Health Administration. These guidelines should be followed routinely by all health-care workers whenever there is a possibility of exposure to potentially infectious materials such as blood or other body fluids:

1. The use of gloves should provide adequate protection when the physical examination is performed or when blood-soiled or body fluid–soiled sheets or clothing are handled.
2. Gloves should be worn when any individual with exudative lesions or weeping dermatitis is examined.
3. When a procedure is performed, fluid-resistant gowns, masks, and eye covers should be worn if the patient's body fluids may be splattered or aerosolized.
4. Hands or other contaminated skin surfaces should be washed thoroughly and immediately if accidentally soiled with blood or other body fluids.
5. All sharp items, such as needles, scalpel blades, and other pointed items, must be handled with extraordinary care to prevent injuries.
6. To prevent needle-stick injuries, needles should *not* be recapped. They should be disposed in clearly marked puncture-resistant containers.
7. If mouth-to-mouth contact is necessary, mouthpieces, resuscitation bags, or other ventilatory devices should be used.
8. Blood and other body fluid specimens should be handled with gloves.
9. Areas that have been soiled with blood or other body fluids should be cleaned and decontaminated with an appropriate disinfectant.
10. All reusable items should be processed in accordance with current recommendations. The level of disinfection or sterilization is based on the specific tissues that the item contacted.

11. If a sharps injury or exposure to blood or body fluid occurs, the injured or exposed area should be cleansed immediately, and if mucous membranes are exposed, they should be irrigated thoroughly with water. The incident should be reported and the exposed person referred *promptly* for management and counseling. Time is of the essence.

12. All health-care providers who have direct contact with patients should complete the hepatitis B vaccine series. In certain populations, testing for immunity before vaccination may be indicated. Typical preemployment/Student Health Service screening includes a purified protein derivative (for tuberculosis) and various serologic testing, including testing for hepatitis B virus.

A patient may be in isolation or on special precautions, which indicates that he or she is suffering from a contagious disease, such as tuberculosis or varicella-zoster virus infection or is colonized with a multidrug-resistant organism. Health-care providers should consult the institutional infection control manual for guidelines regarding restrictions on entry into the patient's room and on protective attire.

It is also the responsibility of all health-care workers not to transmit disease to their patients. If they have a lesion on their hands, they should wear gloves; if they have a cold, they should cover their nose and mouth; if they are sick, they should consider deferring patient contact.

Goal of the Physical Examination

The goal of the physical examination is to obtain valid information concerning the health of the patient. The examiner must be able to identify, analyze, and synthesize the accumulated information into a comprehensive assessment.

The validity of a physical finding depends on many factors. Clinical experience and reliability of the examination techniques are most important. False-positive or false-negative results reduce the precision of the techniques. Variance can occur when techniques are performed by different examiners, with different equipment, on different patients. The concepts of validity and precision are discussed further in Chapter 27, Diagnostic Reasoning in Physical Diagnosis.

Unconscious bias is an important concept to understand. It is well known that unconscious bias in an examiner can influence the evaluation of a physical finding. For example, in patients with rapid atrial fibrillation, the ventricular rate is irregular and varies from 150 to 200 beats per minute. The radial pulse rate is significantly lower, owing to a pulse deficit (explained in Chapter 14, The Heart). If examiners record the apical heart rate first, they find that the rate varies from 150 to 200 beats per minute. If they then check the radial pulse, they detect a faster pulse rate than if they had measured the radial pulse first. The first observation, therefore, biases the second observation. Alternatively, if examiners determine the radial pulse first and the heart rate second, the apical heart rate appears slower, but the chance of bias is lower because observer error is less at the apex (Chalmers, 1981).

It is important to review the concepts of sensitivity and specificity. *Sensitivity* is the frequency of a positive result of a test or technique in individuals with a disease or condition. *Specificity* is the frequency of a negative result of a test or technique in individuals without a disease or condition. Sensitivity and specificity refer to properties of the test or technique, whereas the health-care provider is interested in properties or characteristics of the patient, which are characterized by the predictive values. The *positive predictive value* is the frequency of disease in patients with positive test results. The *negative predictive value* is the frequency of lack of disease in patients with negative test results. The question, "What is the possibility that a woman with a stony-hard breast mass has cancer?" addresses the positive predictive value. Predictive value depends on the prevalence of disease in the respective population, as well as the sensitivity and specificity of the test. In an individual from a population with a low prevalence of disease, a positive test result still yields a low positive predictive value.

For example, eliciting the presence of shifting dullness is a highly sensitive technique for detecting ascites. Thus, an examiner who does not detect shifting dullness in the abdomen of a patient can be reasonably sure that this negative finding rules out ascites. In contrast, the finding of microaneurysms in the macular area of the retina is a highly specific finding for diabetes. Thus, an examiner who finds microaneurysms at the macula can be reasonably confident that this finding confirms diabetes, because normal individuals without diabetes do not have macular microaneurysms; that is, the finding of microaneurysms at the macula has a high degree of specificity. Unfortunately, a technique is rarely both very sensitive and very specific. Several techniques must be applied together to make an appropriate assessment.

In summary:

1. A technique or test with high sensitivity can be used confidently to rule out disease for a patient with a negative finding.
2. A technique or test with high specificity can be used confidently to confirm disease for a patient with a positive finding.

These concepts are discussed in more detail in Chapter 27, Diagnostic Reasoning in Physical Diagnosis.

Useful Vocabulary

The vocabulary of medicine is difficult and broad. Memorizing a term is less useful than being able to determine the meaning by understanding its etymology, or roots. The spelling of terms will also be easier.

Listed here are some general prefixes, roots, and suffixes that are important to understand. At the end of each chapter in Section 2 is a list of terminology for that area of the body. The following list should not be memorized at this time. It should be referred to in conjunction with the lists in subsequent chapters.

Prefix/Root/Suffix	Pertaining to	Example	Definition
ab-	away from	**ab**duction	Away from the body
ad-	toward	**ad**duction	Toward the body
aden-	gland	**aden**opathy	Glandular disease
an-	without	**an**osmia	Without the sense of smell
aniso-	unequal	**aniso**coria	Unequal pupils
asthen-	weak	**asthen**opia	Eye fatigue
contra-	against; opposite	**contra**lateral	Pertaining to the opposite side
diplo-	double	**diplo**pia	Double vision
duc-	lead	ab**duc**tion	Turning outward
dys-	bad; ill	**dys**uria	Painful urination
eso-	in	**eso**tropia	Eye deviated inward
eu-	good; advantageous	**eu**pnea	Easy breathing
exo-	out	**exo**tropia	Eye deviated outward
hemi-	half	**hemi**plegia	Paralysis of one side of the body
hydro-	water	**hydro**philic	Readily absorbing water
hyper-	beyond; greater than normal	**hyper**emia	Excess of blood
hypno-	sleep	**hypno**tic	Inducing sleep
hypo-	below	**hypo**dermic	Below the skin
idio-	separate; distinct	**idio**pathic	Of unknown cause
infra-	below	**infra**hyoid	Below the hyoid gland
intra-	within	**intra**cranial	Within the skull

Prefix/Root/Suffix	Pertaining to	Example	Definition
ipsi-	self	**ipsi**lateral	Situated on the same side
iso-	equal	**iso**tonic	Equal tension
leuko-	white	**leuko**cyte	White blood cell
lith-	stone	**lith**otomy	Incision of an organ to remove a stone
macro-	larger than normal	**macro**cephaly	Abnormally large head
micro	smaller than normal	**micro**cephaly	head size smaller than normal
neo-	new	**neo**plasm	Abnormal new growth
pedia-	child	**pedia**trics	Branch of medicine treating diseases of children
peri-	around	**peri**cardium	Sac around heart
poly-	many	**poly**cystic	Many cysts
presby-	old	**presby**opia	Impairment of vision as a result of advancing age
retro-	situated behind	**retro**bulbar	Behind the eye
soma-	body	**soma**tic	Pertaining to the body
sten-	narrowed	**sten**osis	Narrowed
trans-	through	**trans**urethral	Through the urethra
-dynia	pain	cephalo**dynia**	Headache
-ectomy	removal of	append**ectomy**	Removal of the appendix
-gnosis	recognition	stereo**gnosis**	Recognizing an object by touch
-gram	something written	myelo**gram**	X-ray film of the spinal cord
-ism	state; condition	gigant**ism**	State of abnormal overgrowth
-itis	inflammation of	col**itis**	Inflammation of the colon
-kinesia	movement	brady**kinesia**	Abnormal slow movement
-lysis	dissolution	hemo**lysis**	Liberation of hemoglobin into solution
-malacia	softening	osteo**malacia**	Softening of bones
-megal-	enlargement	cardio**megaly**	Cardiac enlargement
-mycosis	fungus	blasto**mycosis**	A specific fungal infection
-oid	resembling	human**oid**	Resembling a human

Continued

Useful Vocabulary—cont'd

Prefix/Root/Suffix	Pertaining to	Example	Definition
-ologist	specialist in study of	cardi**ologist**	A specialist in heart disease
-oma	tumor; growth	fibr**oma**	A tumor of fibrous tissue
-osis	diseased state	endometri**osis**	Disease state of abnormally located uterine tissue
-otomy	cutting; incision	gastr**otomy**	Incision of the stomach
-pathy	disease	uro**pathy**	Disease of the urinary tract
-phobia	fear; pain; intolerance	photo**phobia**	Abnormal intolerance of light
-plasty	repair	valvulo**plasty**	Surgical repair of a valve
-plegia	paralysis	hemi**plegia**	Paralysis of one half of the body
-ptosis	drooping	blepharo**ptosis**	Drooping eyelids
-rrhagia	hemorrhage	oto**rrhagia**	Hemorrhage from the ear
-rrhaphy	suture; repair	hernio**rrhaphy**	Repair of a hernia
-rrhexis	rupture	gastro**rrhexis**	Rupture of stomach
-scope	instrument for	ophthalmo**scope**	Instrument for examination of the eye
-spasmos	spasm	blepharo**spasm**	Twitching of the eyelids
-stom-	opening	ileo**stom**y	Surgical creation of an opening into the ileum
-tome	cut	micro**tome**	An instrument for cutting thin slices

Bibliography

Advisory Committee on Immunization Practices: Recommended immunization schedule: United States, October 2007–September 2008. Ann Intern Med 147:725.

Bolyard EA, Tablan OC, Williams WW, et al: Guideline for infection control in health care personnel, 1998. Infect Control Hosp Epidemiol 19:493, 1998.

Centers for Disease Control and Prevention. Recommended adult immunization schedule—United States. October 2007–September 2008. MMWR Morb Mortal Wkly Rep 56(Q1), 2007.

Chalmers TC: The clinical trial. Milbank Mem Fund Q 59:324, 1981.

Panlilio AL, Cardo DM, Grohskopf LA, et al: Updated U.S. Public Health Service guidelines for the management of occupational exposures to HIV and recommendations for postexposure prophylaxis. MMWR Morb Mort Wkly Rep 54(RR-9):1, 2005.

Siegel JD, Rhinehart E, Jackson M, et al: 2007 Guideline for isolation precautions: Preventing transmission of infectious agents in healthcare settings. June 2007. (Available at: *http://www.cdc.gov/ncidod/dhqp/pdf/isolation2007.pdf*; accessed June 5, 2008.)

There are six "f's" in the sentence in the box. Go back and count them. Most individuals count only three, neglecting to include the "f's" in the three instances of "of."

CHAPTER 8

The Skin

What is the hardest of all? That which you hold the most simple; seeing with your own eyes what is spread out before you.

Johann Wolfgang von Goethe (1749–1832)

General Considerations

The skin, which is the largest organ of the body, is one of the best indicators of general health. Even a person without medical training is capable of detecting changes in skin color and texture. The trained examiner can detect these changes and at the same time evaluate more subtle cutaneous signs of systemic disease.

Diseases of the skin are common. Approximately one third of the population in the United States has a disorder of the skin that warrants medical attention. Nearly 8% of all adult outpatient visits are related to dermatologic problems. Nonmelanoma skin cancers, basal cell carcinomas, and squamous cell carcinomas are by far the most common malignancies that occur in the United States. One of every three new cancers is a skin cancer, and the vast majority are basal cell carcinomas. About 80% of the new skin cancer cases are basal cell carcinoma, 16% are squamous cell carcinoma, and 4% are melanoma. The American Cancer Society estimates that there are more than 65,000 new cases of basal cell carcinoma annually. Most of these cases occur on the head and neck, which is evidence of the importance of sun exposure as a causative stimulus. Squamous cell carcinoma, the second most common skin cancer after basal cell carcinoma, afflicts more than 200,000 Americans each year. Although in most of these patients the cancer is treated and cured, skin cancer still causes more than 5000 deaths a year.

The incidence of malignant melanoma is rising at a rate faster than that of any other tumor; it has more than tripled among white persons between 1980 and 2004. It was estimated that there were approximately 59,940 new cases of melanoma in 2007: 33,910 in men and 26,030 in women. There were 8110 total deaths estimated in 2007 from melanoma. In 2007, the lifetime risk of developing melanoma (invasive and in situ) for all races was 2.76%; in white persons, the lifetime risk was 3.15%, and in African Americans, it was 0.11%. In 2006, invasive melanoma was the fifth most common cancer diagnosed in men and the sixth most common cancer in women. Six of every seven deaths from skin cancer in the United States are caused by melanoma. The incidence of melanoma has increased 7% per year since the early 1990s. The reasons for this are unclear, but excessive sun exposure is a major factor.

Early detection and treatment of malignant melanoma, as with most cancers, offers the best chance of a cure. Both basal cell carcinoma and squamous cell carcinoma have a better than 95% cure rate if detected and treated early. Among patients with a superficial melanoma (<0.76 mm in depth), the survival rate is more than 99%, whereas among those with a larger lesion (>3.64 mm in depth), the 5-year survival rate is only 42%. The external nature of melanoma gives the examiner an opportunity to detect these small, curable lesions.

The most important function of the skin is to protect the body from the environment. The skin has evolved in humans to be a relatively impermeable surface layer that prevents the loss of water, protects against external hazards, and insulates against thermal changes. It is also actively involved in the production of vitamin D. The skin appears to have the lowest water permeability of any naturally produced membrane. Its barrier to invasion retards potentially noxious agents from entering the body and causing internal damage. This barrier protects against many physical stresses and prohibits the invasion of microorganisms. By observing patients with extensive skin problems, such as burns, clinicians can appreciate the importance of this organ.

Structure and Physiology

The three tissue layers of the skin, depicted in Figure 8-1, are as follows:

- Epidermis
- Dermis
- Subcutaneous tissue

The *epidermis* is the thin, outermost layer of the skin. It is composed of several layers of keratocytes, or keratin-producing cells. Keratin is an insoluble protein that provides the skin with its protective properties. The *stratum corneum* is the outermost layer of the epidermis and serves as a major physical barrier. The stratum corneum is composed of keratinized cells, which appear as dry, flattened, anuclear, and adherent flakes. The *basal cell layer* is the deepest layer of the epidermis and is a single row of rapidly proliferating cells that slowly migrate upward, keratinize, and are ultimately shed from the stratum corneum. The process of

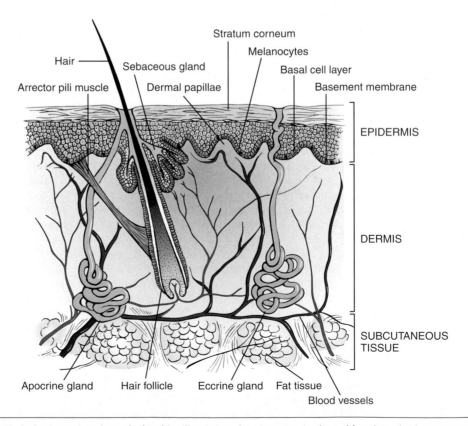

Figure 8–1 Cross section through the skin, illustrating the structures in the epidermis and subcutaneous tissues.

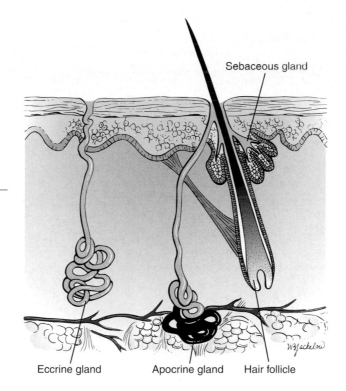

Figure 8–2 Types of sweat glands.

maturation, keratinization, and shedding takes approximately 4 weeks. The cells of the basal layer are intermingled with melanocytes, which produce melanin. The number of melanocytes is approximately equal in all people. Differences in skin color are related to the amount and type of melanin produced, as well as to its dispersion in the skin.

Beneath the epidermis is the *dermis*, which is the dense connective tissue stroma forming the bulk of the skin. The dermis is bound to the overlying epidermis by finger-like projections that project upward into the corresponding recesses of the epidermis. In the dermis, blood vessels branch and form a rich capillary bed in the dermal papillae. The deeper layers of the dermis also contain the hair follicles with their associated muscles and cutaneous glands. The dermis is supplied with sensory and autonomic nerve fibers. The sensory nerves end either as free endings or as special end organs that mediate pressure, touch, and temperature. The autonomic nerves supply the arrector pili muscles, blood vessels, and sweat glands.

The third layer of the skin is the *subcutaneous tissue*, which is composed largely of fatty connective tissue. This highly variable adipose layer is a thermal regulator, as well as a protection for the more superficial skin layers from bone prominences.

The sweat glands, hair follicles, and nails are termed *skin appendages*. The evaporation of water from the skin by the sweat glands provides a thermoregulatory mechanism for heat loss. Figure 8-2 illustrates the types of sweat glands.

Within the skin, there are 2 to 3 million small, coiled *eccrine glands*. The eccrine glands are distributed over the body surface and are particularly profuse on the forehead, axillae, palms, and soles. They are absent in the nail beds and in some mucosal surfaces. These glands are capable of producing more than 6 L of watery sweat in 1 day. The eccrine glands are controlled by the sympathetic nervous system.

The *apocrine glands* are larger than the eccrine glands. The apocrine glands are found in close association with hair follicles but tend to be much more limited in distribution than are the eccrine glands. The apocrine glands occur mostly in the axillae, the areolae, the pubis, and the perineum. They reach maturity only at puberty, secreting a milky, sticky substance. Apocrine glands are adrenergically mediated and appear to be stimulated by stress.

The *sebaceous glands* are also found surrounding hair follicles. The sebaceous glands are distributed over the entire body; the largest glands are found on the face and upper back. They are absent on the palms and soles. Their secretory product, sebum,

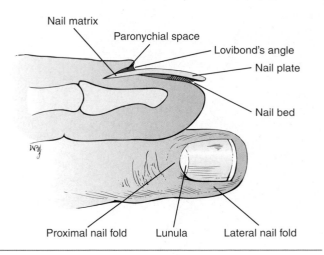

Figure 8-3 Structural relations of the nail: cross section and from above.

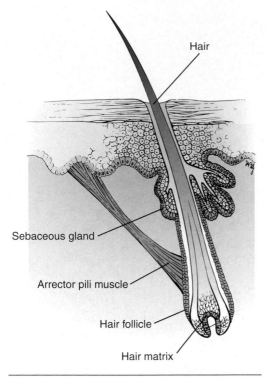

Figure 8-4 The hair follicle and its surrounding structures.

is discharged directly into the lumen of the hair follicle, where it lubricates the hair shaft and spreads to the skin surface. Sebum consists of sebaceous cells and lipids. The production of sebum depends on gland size, which is directly influenced by androgen secretion.

Nails protect the tips of the fingers and toes against trauma. They are derived by keratinization of cells from the nail matrix, which is located at the proximal end of the nail plate. The nail plate consists of the nail root embedded in the posterior nail fold, a fixed middle portion, and a distal free edge. The whitish nail matrix of proliferating epithelial cells grows in a semilunar pattern. It extends outward past the posterior nail fold and is called the *lunula*. The structural relationships of the nail are shown in Figure 8-3.

A *hair shaft* is a keratinized structure that grows out of the hair follicle. Its lower end, called the *hair matrix*, consists of actively proliferating epithelial cells. The cells at this end of the follicle, along with those of the bone marrow and gut epithelium, are the most rapidly growing dividing cells in the human body. This is the reason that chemotherapy causes hair loss, along with anemia, nausea, and vomiting. Visible hair is present over the entire body surface except on the palms, soles, lips, eyelids, glans penis, and labia minora. In apparently hairless areas, the hair follicles are small, and the shafts produced are microscopic. Hair follicles show conspicuous morphologic and functional heterogeneity. Follicles and their developing shafts differ from location to location in shaft length, color, thickness, curl, and androgen sensitivity. Some follicles, those in the axilla and inguinal areas, are very sensitive to androgens, whereas others in the eyebrow are insensitive. The arrector pili muscles attach to the follicle below the opening of the sebaceous gland. Contraction of this muscle erects the hair and causes "goose bumps." The structure of a hair follicle is shown in Figure 8-4.

Review of Specific Symptoms

The main symptoms of disease of the skin, hair, and nails are the following:

- Rash or skin lesion
- Changes in skin color

- Itching (pruritus)
- Changes in hair
- Changes in nails

Rash or Skin Lesion

There are some important points to clarify when a patient is interviewed about a new rash or skin lesion. The specific time of onset and location of the rash or skin lesion are critical. A careful description of the first lesions and any changes is vital. The patient with a rash or skin lesion should be asked the following questions:

"Was the rash initially flat? raised? blistered?"

"Did the rash change in character with time?"

"Have there been new areas involved since the rash began?"

"Does the rash itch or burn?"

"Is the lesion tender or numb?"

"What makes the rash better? worse?"

"Was the rash initiated by sunlight?"

"Is the rash aggravated by sunlight?"

"What kind of treatment have you tried?"

"Do you have any joint pains? fever? fatigue?"

"Does anyone near you have a similar rash?"

"Have you traveled recently?" If so, *"To where?"*

"Have you had any contact with anyone who has had a similar rash?"

"Is there a history of allergy?" If so, *"What are your symptoms?"*

"Do you have any chronic disease?"

Note whether the patient has used any medications that may have changed the nature of the skin disorder.

Inquire whether the patient uses any prescription medications or over-the-counter drugs. Ask specifically about aspirin and aspirin-containing products. Patients can suddenly develop a reaction to medications that they have taken for many years. Do not ignore a long-standing prescription. Has the patient had any recent injections or taken any new medications? Does the patient use "recreational" drugs? Ask the patient about the use of soaps, deodorants, cosmetics, and colognes. Has the patient changed any of these items recently?

A family history of similar skin disorders should be noted. The effect of heat, cold, and sunlight on the skin problem is important. Can there be any contributing factor, such as occupation, specific food allergies, alcohol, or menses? Is there a history of gardening or household repair work? Has there been any contact with animals recently? The interviewer should also remember to inquire about psychogenic factors that may contribute to a skin disorder.

Determine the patient's occupation, if it is not already known. Ascertain avocational and recreational activities. This information is important even if the patient has been exposed to chemicals or similar agents for years. Manufacturers frequently change the basic constituents without notifying the consumer. It may also take years for a patient to become sensitized to a substance.

Changes in Skin Color

Patients may complain of a *generalized* change in skin color as the first manifestation of an illness. Cyanosis and jaundice are examples of this type of problem. Determine whether the patient is aware of any chronic disease that may be responsible for these changes. *Localized* skin color changes may be related to aging or to neoplastic changes. Certain medications can also be responsible for skin color changes. Inquire whether the patient is taking or has recently taken any medications.

Pruritus

Pruritus, or itching, may be a symptom of a generalized skin disorder or an internal illness. Ask any patient with pruritus the following questions:

> *"When did you first notice the itching?"*
>
> *"Did the itching begin suddenly?"*
>
> *"Is the itching associated with any rash or lesion on your body?"*
>
> *"Are you taking any medications?"*
>
> *"Has there been any change in the sweating or dryness of your skin?"*
>
> *"Have you been told that you have a chronic illness?"*
>
> *"Have you traveled recently?"* If so, *"To where?"*

Diffuse pruritus is observed in biliary cirrhosis and in cancer, especially lymphoma. Pruritus in association with a diffuse rash may be dermatitis herpetiformis. Determine whether the pruritus has been associated with a change in perspiration or dryness of the skin, because either of these conditions may be the cause of the pruritus.

Changes in Hair

Inquire whether there has been a loss of hair or an increase in hair. Ascertain any changes in distribution or texture. If there have been changes, ask the following questions:

> *"When did you first notice the changes?"*
>
> *"Did the change occur suddenly?"*
>
> *"Is the hair loss symmetric?"*
>
> *"Has the change been associated with itching? fever? recent stress?"*
>
> *"Are you aware of any exposure to any toxins? commercial hair compounds?"*
>
> *"Have you changed your diet?"*
>
> *"What medications are you taking?"*

Changes in diet and medications are frequently responsible for changes in hair patterns. Hypothyroidism is frequently associated with loss of the lateral third of the eyebrows. Vascular disease in the legs often causes hair loss on the legs. Alternatively, ovarian and adrenal tumors can cause an increase in body hair.

Changes in Nails

Changes in nails may include splitting, discoloration, ridging, thickening, or separation from the nail bed. Ask the patient the following questions:

> *"When did you first notice the nail changes?"*
>
> *"Have you had any acute illness recently?"*
>
> *"Do you have any chronic illness?"*
>
> *"Have you been taking any medications?"*
>
> *"Have you been exposed to chemicals at work or at home?"*

Fungal disease causes thickening of the nail. Clues to systemic disease may be found by close examination of the proximal nail fold, the lunula, the nail bed, the nail plate,

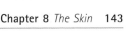

and the hyponychium. Acute illnesses are associated with lines and ridges in the nail bed and nail. Medications and chemicals are notorious for causing nail changes.

General Suggestions

All patients should be asked whether there have been any changes in moles, birthmarks, or spots on the body. Determine any color changes, irregular growth, pain, scaling, or bleeding. Any recent growth of a flat, pigmented lesion is relevant information.

All patients should be asked whether there are any red, scaly, or crusted areas of skin that do not heal. Has the patient ever had skin cancer? If the patient has had skin cancer, further questioning regarding the body location, treatment, and description is appropriate.

Impact of Skin Disease on the Patient

Diseases of the skin play a profound role in the way the affected patient interacts socially. If located on visible skin surfaces, long-standing skin diseases may actually interfere with the emotional and psychologic development of the individual. The attitude of a person toward self and others may be markedly affected. Loss of self-esteem is common. The adult with a skin disorder often faces limitation of sexual activity. This disruption of intimacy can foster or increase hostility and anxiety in the patient. Skin is a sensitive marker of an individual's emotions. It is known that blushing can reflect embarrassment, sweating can indicate anxiety, and pallor or "goose bump" skin may be associated with fear.

Patients with rashes have always evoked feelings of revulsion. Rashes have been associated with impurity and evil. Even today, friends and family may reject the individual with a skin disease. Patients with skin that is red, oozing, discolored, or peeling are rejected not only by family members but perhaps even by their physicians. At other times, skin lesions cause others to stare at the patient, which causes further discomfort. Some skin disorders may be associated with such extreme physical or emotional pain that marked depression may result and, on occasion, lead to suicide.

Skin diseases are often treated palliatively. Because numerous skin disorders have no cure, many patients go through life helpless and frustrated, as do their physicians.

The role of anxiety as a natural stressor in producing rashes is frequently observed. Stress tends to worsen certain skin disorders, such as eczema. This creates a vicious cycle, because the rash then exacerbates the anxiety. Rashes are common symptoms and signs of psychosomatic disorders.

Clinicians should discuss these anxieties with the patient in an attempt to break the cycle. The interviewer who tries to elicit the patient's feelings about the disease allows the patient to "open up." The fears and fantasies can then be discussed. The examiner should also be comfortable in touching the patient for reassurance. This tends to improve the doctor-patient relationship because the patient has a lesser sense of isolation.

Physical Examination

The only equipment necessary for the examination of the skin is a penlight. The examination of the skin consists of only two steps:

- Inspection
- Palpation

The examination of the skin depends on inspection, but palpation of a skin lesion must also be performed. Although most skin lesions are not contagious, it is prudent to wear gloves to evaluate any skin lesion. This is especially true because of the prevalence of skin disease associated with human immunodeficiency virus (HIV) infection. Palpation of a lesion helps define its characteristics: texture, consistency, fluid, edema in the adjacent area, tenderness, and blanching.

The patient and the examiner must be comfortable during the examination of the skin. The lighting should be adjusted to produce the optimal illumination. Natural light is preferable. Even in the absence of complaints related to the skin, a careful examination of the skin must be performed on all patients because the skin may provide subtle clues of an underlying systemic illness. Examination of the skin may be performed as a separate system approach, or, preferably, the skin should be examined when the other parts of the body are evaluated.

General Principles

The examiner should be suspicious of any lesion that the patient describes as having increased in size or changed in color. The development of any new growth warrants attention.

When examining the skin, the clinician initially determines the general aspects of the skin: the *color, moisture, turgor,* and *texture* of the skin.

Any *color* changes, such as cyanosis, jaundice, or pigmentary abnormalities, should be noted.

Red vascular lesions may be either extravasated blood into the skin, known as *petechiae* or *purpura*, or malformed elements of the vascular tree, known as *angiomas*. When pressure is applied by a glass slide over an angioma, it blanches. This is a useful test to differentiate an angioma from petechiae, which do not change when pressure from a glass slide is applied.

During the physical examination, inspect all pigmented lesions and be aware of the "ABCD" warning signs associated with malignant melanoma:

- **A**symmetry of shape
- **B**order irregularity
- **C**olor variation
- **D**iameter larger than 6 mm

Asymmetry means that half the lesion appears different from the other half. *Border irregularity* describes a scalloped or poorly circumscribed contour. The *color variation* refers to shades of tan and brown, black, and sometimes white, red, or blue. A *diameter* larger than 6 mm, which is the size of a pencil eraser, is considered a danger sign for melanoma.

The clinician should remember this axiom in dermatology: "There are more errors made by not looking than by not knowing."

Excessive *moisture* may be seen in normal individuals, or it may be associated with fevers, emotions, neoplastic diseases, or hyperthyroidism. Dryness is a normal aging change, but it may also be seen in myxedema, nephritis, and certain drug-induced states. Look for excoriations, which might indicate the presence of pruritus as a clue to an underlying systemic illness.

When palpating the skin, evaluate its *turgor* and *texture*. Tissue turgor provides a mechanism for estimating the patient's general state of hydration. If the skin over the forehead is pulled up and released, it should promptly reassume its normal contour. In a patient with decreased hydration, this response is delayed.

It is often difficult for the inexperienced examiner to evaluate the texture of the skin because texture is a qualitative parameter. Softness has occasionally been likened to the texture of skin over a baby's abdomen. "Soft"-textured skin is seen in secondary hypothyroidism, hypopituitarism, and eunuchoid states. "Hard"-textured skin is associated with scleroderma, myxedema, and amyloidosis. "Velvety" skin is associated with Ehlers-Danlos syndrome.

Examination with Patient Seated

When the patient is seated, examine the hair and the skin on the hands and upper extremities.

Inspect the Hair

The hair and scalp are evaluated for any lesions. Is alopecia or hirsutism present? Pay attention to the pattern of distribution and texture of hair over the body. In certain diseases, such as hypothyroidism, the hair becomes sparse and coarse. In contrast, patients with hyperthyroidism have hair that is very fine in texture. Loss of hair occurs in many conditions: anemia, heavy metal poisoning, hypopituitarism, and some nutritional disease states, such as pellagra. Increased hair patterns are seen in Cushing's disease, Stein-Leventhal syndrome, and several neoplastic conditions, such as tumors of the adrenal glands and gonads.

Inspect the Nail Beds

Evaluation of the nails can provide important clues about diseases. The nails may be affected in many systemic and dermatologic conditions. Nail-bed changes are usually not pathognomonic for a specific disease. Disorders stemming from renal, hematopoietic, or hepatic conditions may be evident from the nails. The nails should be inspected for shape, size, color, brittleness, hemorrhages underneath, transverse lines or grooves in the nail or nail bed, and an increased

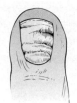
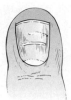

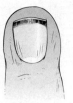

Beau's lines   Mees' bands   Lindsay's nails   Terry's nails

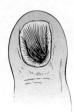
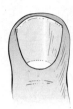
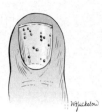

Koilonychia   Clubbing   Psoriasis

Figure 8–5 Common nail findings associated with medical diseases.

white area of the nail bed. Figure 8-5 illustrates some typical nail changes associated with medical diseases.

Beau's lines are transverse grooves or depressions parallel to the lunula. They are often associated with infections (typhus, acute rheumatic fever, malaria, acquired immunodeficiency syndrome [AIDS]); nutritional disorders (protein deficiency, pellagra); circulatory problems (myocardial infarction, Raynaud's disease); dysmetabolic states (diabetes, hypothyroidism, hypocalcemia); digestive diseases (diarrhea, enterocolitis, chronic pancreatitis, sprue); drugs (chemotherapy agents); operations; and alcoholism. Beau's lines are caused by conditions that cause the nail to grow slowly or even cease to grow for short intervals. The point of arrested growth is seen as a transverse groove in the nail. These lines are most commonly seen in the thumbnails and toenails. Figure 8-6*A* shows a patient's fingers with Beau's lines on the nails. Figure 8-6*B* shows Beau's lines in the toenails of a patient who had undergone major surgery 5 months earlier.

On occasion, a white transverse line or band results from poisoning or an acute systemic illness. These lines, called *Mees' bands*, are historically associated with chronic arsenic poisoning. These lines or bands are also parallel to the lunula. By measuring the width of the line and approximating nail growth at 1 mm per week, the examiner may be able to determine the duration of the antecedent acute illness. Figure 8-7 shows the fingernails of a patient who had received chemotherapy several weeks earlier.

Lindsay's nails are also called "half-and-half nails." The proximal portion of the nail bed is whitish, whereas the distal part is red or pink. Chronic renal disease and azotemia are commonly associated with this type of nail abnormality. Figure 8-8 shows Lindsay's nails secondary to chronic renal failure.

Terry's nails are white nail beds to within 1 to 2 mm of the distal border of the nail. These nail findings are most commonly associated with cirrhosis, hypoalbuminemia, chronic congestive heart failure, and adult-onset diabetes mellitus. Figure 8-9 shows classic Terry's nails.

Splinter hemorrhages are formed by extravasation of blood from longitudinal nail bed blood vessels into adjacent troughs. Splinter hemorrhages are very common. It has been estimated that up to 20% of all hospitalized patients have splinter hemorrhages. Their presence is most often related to local, light trauma, but these hemorrhages are commonly associated with systemic disease. Classically associated with subacute bacterial endocarditis, splinter hemorrhages may also be seen in leukemia, vasculitis, infection, rheumatoid arthritis, systemic lupus erythematosus, renal disease, liver disease, and diabetes mellitus, among other diseases. Splinter hemorrhages are depicted in Figure 8-10.

Is *koilonychia* present? Koilonychia, or "spoon nail," is a dystrophic state in which the nail plate thins and a cuplike depression develops. Spoon nails are most commonly associated with iron-deficiency anemia but may be seen in association with thinning of the nail plate from any cause, including local irritants. Figure 8-11 shows a normal fingernail in comparison with koilonychia secondary to iron-deficiency anemia.

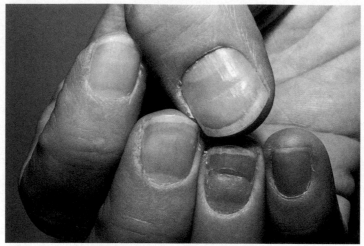

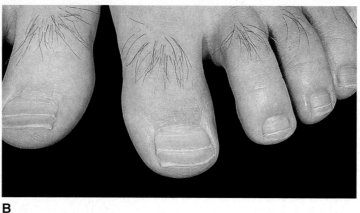

A

Figure 8–6 Beau's lines. *A,* Fingernails. *B,* Toenails.

B

Inspect the Nails for Clubbing

The angle between the normal nail base and finger is about 160°, and the nail bed is firm. The angle is referred to as *Lovibond's angle*. When clubbing develops, this angle straightens out to greater than 180°, and the nail bed, when palpated, becomes spongy or floating. As clubbing progresses, the base of the nail becomes swollen, and Lovibond's angle greatly exceeds 180°. The nail has a bullous shape with exaggerated longitudinal and horizontal curvatures. A fusiform enlargement of the distal digit may also occur. In Figure 8-12, a normal finger is compared with a finger with nail clubbing.

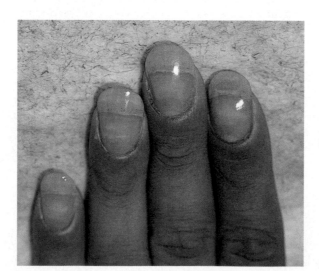

Figure 8–7 Mees' bands.

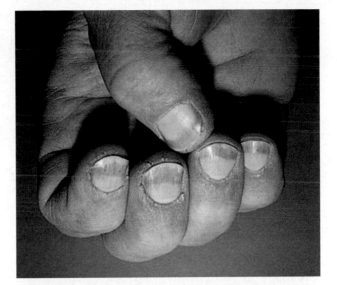

Figure 8–8 Lindsay's nails.

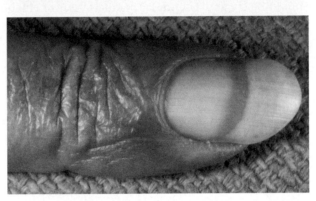

Figure 8–9 Terry's nails.

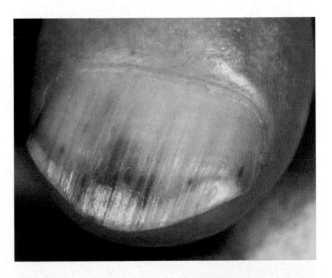

Figure 8–10 Splinter hemorrhages.

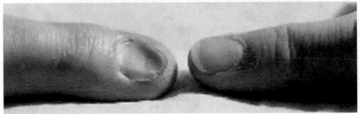

Figure 8–11 Koilonychia.

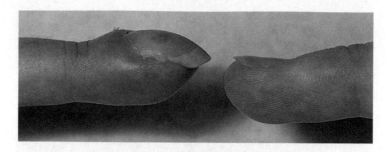

Figure 8–12 Late-stage clubbing.

To examine for clubbing, the patient's finger is placed on the pulp of the examiner's thumbs, and the base of the nail bed is palpated by the examiner's index fingers. Figure 8-13 illustrates the technique for assessing whether early clubbing is present.

Clubbing of the nails is most commonly acquired but may be inherited as an autosomal dominant trait. When acquired, clubbing is associated with congenital cyanotic heart disease, cystic fibrosis, and acquired pulmonary disease. The most common acquired pulmonary cause is bronchogenic carcinoma. In a patient with chronic obstructive pulmonary disease who manifests clubbing, other causes, including bronchiectasis or bronchogenic carcinoma, should be sought. The initial manifestation of clubbing is a softening of the tissue over the proximal nail fold.

Inspect the Nails for Pitting

Pitting of the nails is commonly associated with psoriasis and psoriatic arthropathy. Involvement of the nail bed and nail matrix by psoriasis causes the nail plate to be thickened and pitted. Nail involvement occurs in about 50% of all patients with psoriasis. Multiple pits in the nail are produced by discrete psoriatic foci in the nail matrix. Minor degrees of pitting are also seen in persons with no other skin complaints. Pitting rarely occurs in toenails. Psoriatic nail pitting is shown in Figure 8-14; Figure 8-15 illustrates a cross section of pitting. Figure 8-16*A* shows psoriatic nail lesions in another patient. Notice the characteristically dystrophic nail changes caused by subungual hyperkeratosis. Figure 8-16*B* is a close-up of a typical nail with psoriatic changes.

Inspect the Skin of the Face and Neck

Evaluate the eyelids, forehead, ears, nose, and lips carefully. Evaluate the mucous membranes of the mouth and nose for ulceration, bleeding, or telangiectasis. Is the skin at the nasolabial fold and mouth normal?

Inspect the Skin of the Back

Examine the skin of the patient's back. Are any lesions present?

Examination with Patient Lying Down

Inspect the Skin of the Chest, Abdomen, and Lower Extremities

Ask the patient to lie down so that you can complete the examination of the skin. Inspect the skin of the chest and abdomen. Pay particular attention to the skin of the inguinal and

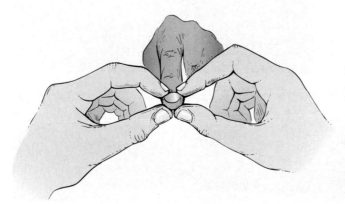

Figure 8–13 Technique for assessing whether clubbing is present.

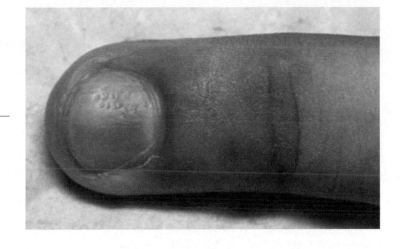

Figure 8–14 Psoriasis: nail pitting.

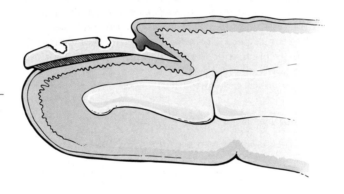

Figure 8–15 Cross section of nail pitting.

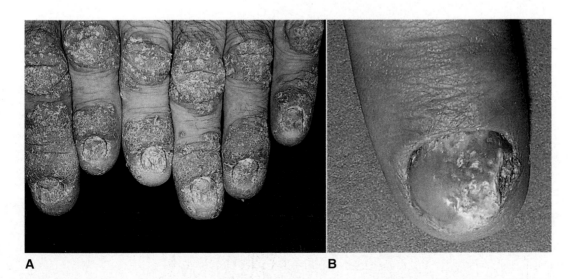

A

B

Figure 8–16 *A* and *B,* Psoriatic nail lesions.

genital area. Inspect the pubic hair. Elevate the scrotum. Inspect the perineal area. Evaluate the pretibial areas for the presence of ulcerations or waxy deposits.

Examine the feet and soles carefully for any skin changes. Spread the toes in order to evaluate the webs between them thoroughly.

Ask the patient to roll onto the left side so that you may examine the skin on the back, gluteal, and perianal areas.

Description of Lesions

If a skin lesion is found, it should be classified as a *primary* or *secondary* lesion, and its shape and distribution should be described. Primary lesions arise from normal skin. They result from anatomic changes in the epidermis, dermis, or subcutaneous tissue. The primary lesion is the most characteristic lesion of the skin disorder. Secondary lesions result from changes in the primary lesion. They develop during the course of the cutaneous disease.

The first step in identifying a skin disorder is to characterize the appearance of the primary lesion. In the description of the skin lesion, the clinician should note whether the lesion is flat or raised and whether it is solid or contains fluid. A penlight is often useful to determine whether the lesion is slightly elevated. If a penlight is directed to one side of a lesion, a shadow forms according to the height of the lesion.

The location of the lesion on the body is important. Therefore, the distribution of the eruption is crucial in making a diagnosis. It may be rewarding to inspect a patient's clothing when contact dermatitis or pediculosis (infestation with lice) is suspected. On occasion, occupational exposure may leave traces of contamination with oils or other materials that may be visible on the clothing and help in the assessment.

The three specific criteria for a dermatologic diagnosis are based on *morphology, configuration*, and *distribution*, morphology being the most important. The purpose of the following section is to acquaint the reader with the morphologic features of the primary and secondary lesions and the vocabulary associated with them.

Primary and Secondary Lesions

To facilitate reading, the primary lesions are listed here with regard to being flat or elevated and solid or fluid-filled (Figs. 8-17 to 8-20). There is no "standard" size of a primary lesion. The dimensions indicated are only approximate. The secondary lesions are grouped according

Primary Skin Lesions: Nonpalpable, Flat		
Lesion	**Characteristics**	**Examples**
Macule	Smaller than 1 cm	Freckles, moles
Patch	Greater than 1 cm	Vitiligo, café au lait spots

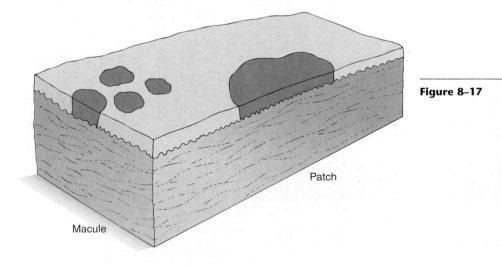

Figure 8–17

Patch

Macule

Primary Skin Lesions: Palpable, Solid Mass

Lesion	Characteristics	Examples
Papule	Smaller than 1 cm	Nevus, wart
Nodule	1-2 cm	Erythema nodosum
Tumor	Greater than 2 cm	Neoplasms
Plaque	Flat, elevated, superficial papule with surface area greater than height	Psoriasis, seborrheic keratosis
Wheal	Superficial area of cutaneous edema	Hives, insect bite

Figure 8–18

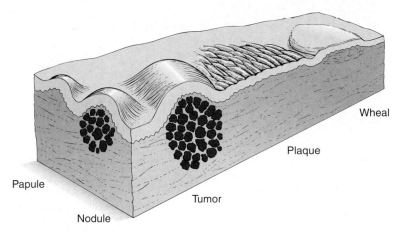

Primary Skin Lesions: Palpable, Fluid Filled

Lesion	Characteristics	Examples
Vesicle	Smaller than 1 cm; filled with serous fluid	Blister, herpes simplex
Bulla	Greater than 1 cm; filled with serous fluid	Blister, pemphigus vulgaris
Pustule	Similar to vesicle; filled with pus	Acne, impetigo

Figure 8–19

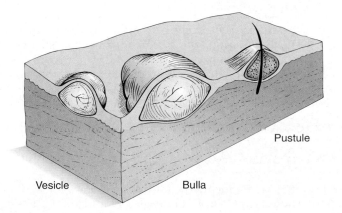

Special Primary Skin Lesions

Lesion	Characteristics	Examples
Comedo	Plugged opening of sebaceous gland	Blackhead
Burrow	Smaller than 10 mm, raised tunnel	Scabies
Cyst	Palpable lesion filled with semiliquid material or fluid	Sebaceous cyst
Abscess	A specific type of primary lesion with localized accumulation of purulent material in the dermis or subcutis; in general, the accumulation is so deep that the pus is not visible from the skin's surface	
Furuncle	A specific type of primary lesion that is a necrotizing form of inflammation of a hair follicle	
Carbuncle	A coalescence of several furuncles	
Milia	Tiny, keratin-filled cysts representing an accumulation of keratin in the distal portion of the sweat gland	

Figure 8–20

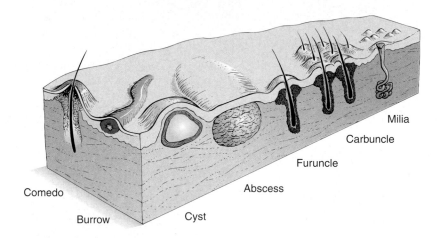

to their occurrence below or above the plane of the skin (Figs. 8-21 and 8-22). Other important lesions are shown and described in Figure 8-23.

Configuration of Skin Lesions

It is not essential for the examiner to make a definitive diagnosis of all skin disease. A careful description of the lesion, the pattern of distribution, and the arrangement of the lesion often points to a group of related disease states with similar manifesting dermatologic signs (e.g., confluent macular rashes, bullous diseases, grouped vesicles, papular rashes on an erythematous base). For example, grouped urticarial lesions with a central depression are suggestive of insect bites. Figure 8-24 lists the terms used to describe the configurations of lesions.

Clinicopathologic Correlations

Skin disorders are frequently perplexing to the examiner. When an examiner sees a rash, the common thought is "Where do I begin?" All too often, the examiner may become frustrated

Secondary Skin Lesions Below the Skin Plane

Lesion	Characteristics	Examples
Erosion	Loss of part or all of the epidermis; surface is moist	Rupture of a vesicle
Ulcer	Loss of epidermis and dermis; may bleed	Stasis ulcer, chancre
Fissure	Linear crack from epidermis into dermis	Cheilitis, athlete's foot
Excoriation	A superficial linear, or "dug out," traumatized area, usually self-induced	Abrasion, scratch mark
Atrophy	Thinning of skin with loss of skin markings	Striae
Sclerosis	Diffuse or circumscribed hardening of skin	

Figure 8–21

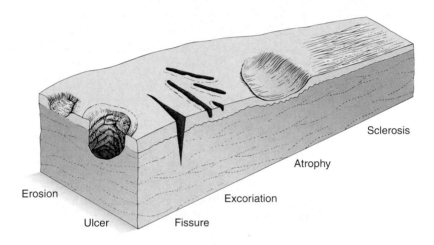

Secondary Skin Lesions Above the Skin Plane

Lesion	Characteristics	Examples
Scaling	Heaped-up keratinized cells; exfoliated epidermis	Dandruff, psoriasis
Crusting	Dried residue of pus, serum, or blood	Scabs, impetigo

Figure 8–22

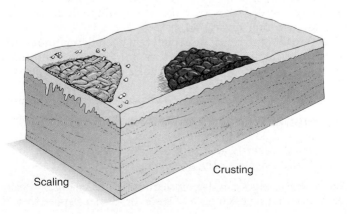

Vascular Skin Lesions

Lesion	Characteristics	Examples
Erythema	Pink or red discoloration of the skin, secondary to dilatation of blood vessels, that blanches with pressure	
Petechiae	Reddish-purple; nonblanching; smaller than 0.5 cm	Intravascular defects
Purpura	Reddish-purple; nonblanching; greater than 0.5 cm	Intravascular defects
Ecchymosis	Reddish-purple; nonblanching; variable size	Trauma, vasculitis
Telangiectasia	Fine, irregular dilated blood vessels	Dilatation of capillaries
Spider angioma	Central red body with radiating spider-like arms that blanch with pressure to the central area	Liver disease, estrogens

Miscellaneous Skin Lesions

Lesion	Characteristics	Examples
Scar	Replacement of destroyed dermis by fibrous tissue; may be atrophic or hyperplastic	Healed wound
Keloid	Elevated, enlarging scar growing beyond boundaries of wound	Burn scars
Lichenification	Roughening and thickening of epidermis; accentuated skin markings	Atopic dermatitis

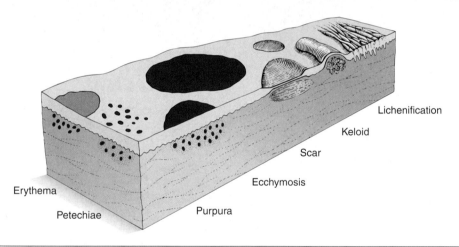

Figure 8–23

and not even attempt to make a diagnosis. Dermatologic terms are complicated, and the names of dermatologic disorders may be intimidating. Often the descriptions of skin disorders in textbooks are more confusing than helpful.

There are more than 2500 separately named dermatologic diagnoses. Most of these diseases occur in low frequencies; only 10 to 15 common conditions constitute about 50% of all dermatologic diagnoses. If the 50 most common conditions were considered, a diagnosis could be rendered for over 95% of all patients.

In approaching a skin lesion, the examiner must do the following:

1. First, identify the primary lesion.
2. Second, identify its distribution.
3. Third, identify any associated findings.
4. Fourth, consider the age of the patient.

Skin diseases evolve and their manifestations change. A lesion may evolve from a blister to an erosion, from a vesicle to a pustule, or from a papule to a nodule or tumor.

Descriptive Dermatologic Terms

Lesion	Characteristics	Examples
Annular	Ring-shaped	Ringworm
Arcuate	Partial rings	Syphilis
Bizarre	Irregular or geographic pattern *not* related to any underlying anatomic structure	Factitial dermatitis
Circinate	Circular	
Confluent	Lesions that run together	Childhood exanthems
Discoid	Disc-shaped without central clearing	Lupus erythematosus
Discrete	Lesions that remain separate	
Eczematoid	An inflammation with a tendency to vesiculate and crust	Eczema
Generalized	Widespread	
Grouped	Lesions that are clustered together	Herpes simplex
Iris	Circle within a circle; a bull's-eye lesion	Erythema multiforme
Keratotic	Horny thickening	Psoriasis
Linear	In lines	Poison ivy dermatitis
Multiform	More than one type of shape of lesion	Erythema multiforme
Papulosquamous	Papules or plaques associated with scaling	Psoriasis
Reticulated	Lacelike network	Oral lichen planus
Serpiginous	Snakelike, creeping	Cutaneous larva migrans
Telangiectatic	Relatively permanent dilatation of the superficial blood vessels	Osler-Weber-Rendu disease
Universal	Entire body involved	Alopecia universalis
Zosteriform*	Linear arrangement along a nerve distribution	Herpes zoster

*Also known as *dermatomal.*

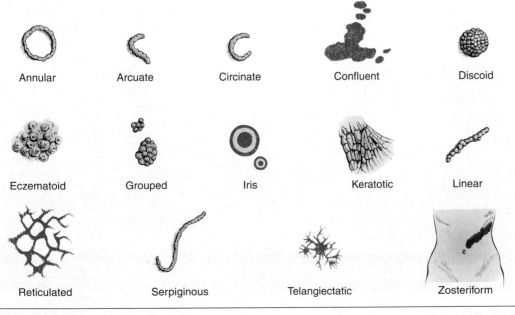

Annular   Arcuate   Circinate   Confluent   Discoid

Eczematoid   Grouped   Iris   Keratotic   Linear

Reticulated   Serpiginous   Telangiectatic   Zosteriform

Figure 8–24

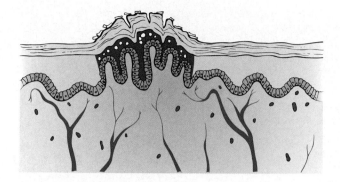

Figure 8–25 Cross section through a wart. Note the thickened epidermis and hyperkeratosis.

There are many common skin disorders or lesions with which the examiner should be familiar. Illustrated in the figures in this chapter are examples of some of these conditions; these cross-sectional diagrams illustrate the locations of these abnormalities in the skin and the involvement of the various skin layers in the pathogenesis of the conditions. The text describes the primary lesions.

A *common wart* is a common, benign growth usually caused by an infection of an epidermal cell by a virus. These firm nodules with rough, keratinous surfaces range in size from pinhead to pea size and can coalesce to form an extensive bed. There is vacuolation of the epidermis with scaling and an upward growth of the dermal papilla. Figure 8-25 illustrates a cross section through a wart. Two examples of finger warts are pictured in Figure 8-26.

Warts can also occur on the soles of the feet (*plantar verruca*), where they have a distinctive appearance because of constant pressure. They are very painful owing to the constant pressure, which forces the keratinous material into the deeper tissue. An example of a plantar wart on the heel is shown in Figure 8-27*A*. Notice the keratotic lesion with a yellow center, within which are visible areas of multiple red to black dots that represent hemorrhage from the tips of the dermal papillae. Classically, there is interruption of the normal skin lines as well. Figure 8-27*B* shows the excised lesion. Notice the depth of the lesion when viewed horizontally. Because warts are in the epidermis, excision just to the level of the dermis is sufficient for complete removal with minimal to no scarring.

A *squamous cell carcinoma* is a malignant neoplasm of keratocytes in the epidermis and is locally invasive into the dermis. The tumor results in a scaling, crusting nodule or plaque that can ulcerate and bleed. Squamous cell carcinoma is a potentially dangerous lesion that can infiltrate the surrounding structures and metastasize to lymph nodes and other organs. The causes include ultraviolet radiation, x-radiation, polycyclic hydrocarbons (e.g., tar, mineral oils, pitch, and soot), mucosal diseases (e.g., lichen planus and Bowen's disease), scars, chronic

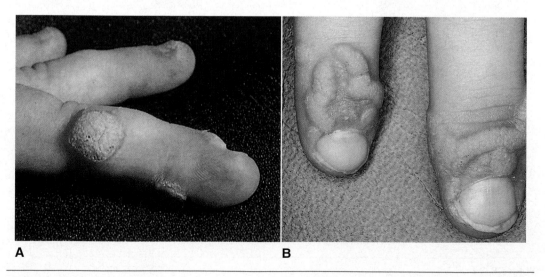

A   **B**

Figure 8–26 *A* and *B*, Warts.

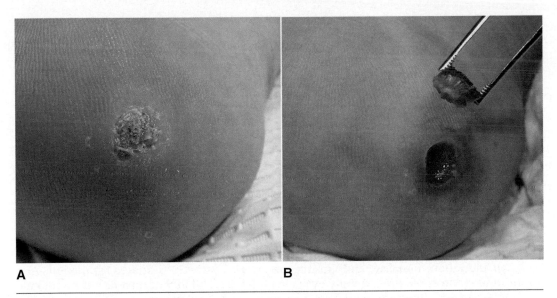

A   B

Figure 8–27 Plantar wart. *A,* Note the keratotic lesion with the yellow center and areas of hemorrhage within. *B,* After excision.

skin disorders, genetic diseases (e.g., albinism and xeroderma pigmentosum), and human papillomavirus. The tumor develops predominantly on areas of skin exposed to sunlight. The latency from carcinogenic exposure to the development of the tumor may be as long as 25 to 30 years. Two examples of squamous cell carcinoma of the skin are pictured in Figure 8-28. Notice that the lesions are ulcerated with firm, raised indurated margins. Figure 11-11 also shows a patient with a squamous cell carcinoma and a malignant melanoma of the ear lobule. A squamous cell carcinoma on the lip of another patient is pictured in Figure 8-29. Notice the round, centrally ulcerating tumor. Figure 8-30 illustrates a cross section through a squamous cell carcinoma.

A *basal cell carcinoma* is a malignant neoplasm of the basal cells of the epidermis and is the most common skin malignancy. The epidermis is thickened, and the dermis may be invaded by the malignant basal cells. It may manifest as a lesion with a pearly, rolled, well-defined margin and a central ulcerated depression. Although sunlight is an important etiologic factor, basal cell carcinomas are almost always seen on the face and rarely in other sun-exposed areas. They are slow-growing tumors and rarely metastasize, in contrast to squamous cell carcinomas.

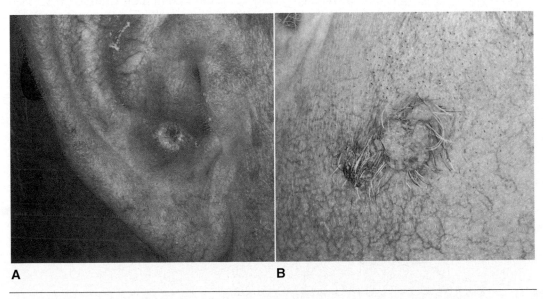

A   B

Figure 8–28 Squamous cell carcinoma of the skin. *A,* Ear. *B,* Face.

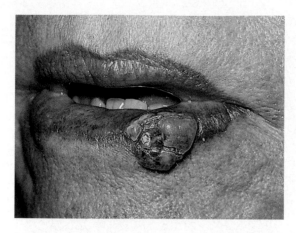

Figure 8–29 Squamous cell carcinoma of lip.

They are locally invasive, and when located near the eye or nose, they may invade the cranial cavity. If ulceration, bleeding, and crusting occur, a *rodent ulcer* is said to be present. Any nonhealing lesion should be carefully evaluated for the possibility of a basal cell carcinoma. Figures 8-31 to 8-33 illustrate the typical features of a basal cell carcinoma.

A *melanoma* is a malignant neoplasm of the melanocytes of the epidermis. If untreated or unrecognized, a melanoma progresses to fatal metastases. Most melanomas have a prolonged superficial, or horizontal, growth phase in which there is a progressive lateral expansion. With time, the melanoma enters the vertical, or deep, phase by penetrating into the dermis, and metastatic spread may occur.

Malignant melanomas are the most common malignancy seen by dermatologists. The incidence of malignant melanoma is increasing faster than that of any other form of malignancy. Most melanomas have atypical pigmentation in the epidermis, such as shades of red, white, gray, blue, brown, and black, all in a single lesion. There are four types of malignant melanoma: lentigo maligna melanoma, superficial spreading melanoma, nodular malignant melanoma, and acral-lentiginous malignant melanoma. Figure 8-34 shows the typical features of a lentigo maligna melanoma on the face. The lentigo maligna melanoma is seen frequently in the geriatric population. This type of melanoma has a prolonged horizontal growth phase and appears in areas of sun-exposed, sun-damaged skin. The superficial spreading variety (Fig. 8-35) is the most common type of melanoma (70% of all melanomas). Typically, an irregularly colored plaque has sharp notches and variegation of pigment. If it is diagnosed early, the prognosis is excellent, with a 5-year survival rate of 95%. Figure 8-36 illustrates a cross section through a melanoma. Vertical growth and deep invasion follow the spreading phase of superficial malignant melanomas. Figure 8-37 shows another superficial spreading melanoma that has developed vertical growth. The nodular melanoma is the second most common type, seen in approximately 15% of cases of melanoma. Unlike the superficial spreading type, these melanomas are usually black, brown, or dark blue and tend to grow rapidly for months.

Melanomas occur predominantly in white individuals and have a predilection for the back in men and women and for the anterior tibial areas in women. In general, lesions on the back, axillae, neck, and scalp (the so-called BANS area) tend to have a worse prognosis than do melanomas on the extremities. A great contrast between the risk of acquiring melanoma and basal or squamous cell carcinoma is that basal and squamous cell carcinomas occur more

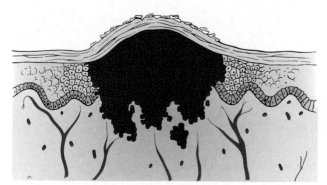

Figure 8–30 Cross section through a squamous cell carcinoma. Note the invasion into the dermis.

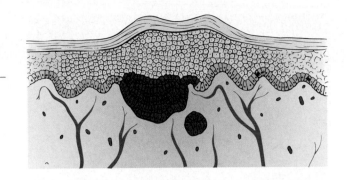

Figure 8–31 Cross section through a basal cell carcinoma.

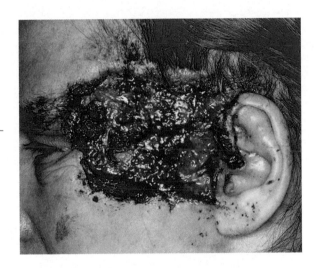

Figure 8–32 Basal cell carcinoma (rodent ulcer).

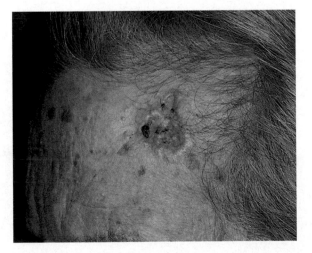

Figure 8–33 Basal cell carcinoma. Notice the rolled, well-defined margin.

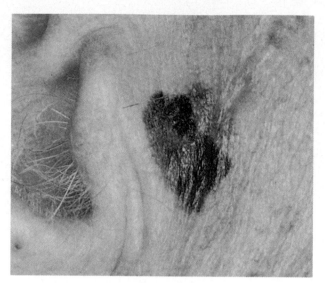

Figure 8–34 Lentigo maligna melanoma.

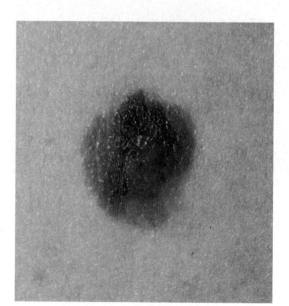

Figure 8–35 Superficial spreading malignant melanoma.

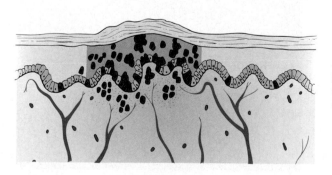

Figure 8–36 Cross section through a melanoma. Note the nests of melanoma cells in the dermis.

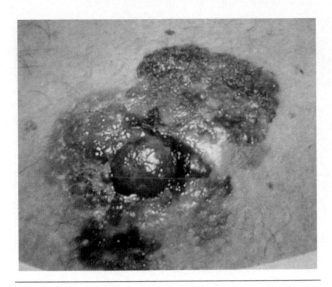

Figure 8–37 Superficial spreading malignant melanoma with vertical growth.

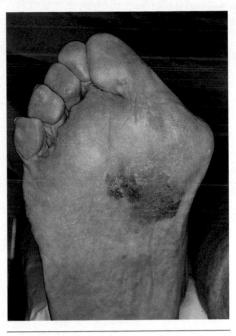

Figure 8–38 Acral-lentiginous melanoma.

frequently in individuals who are exposed to constant sunlight, such as sailors and agricultural workers. Melanomas occur more often in rather fair-skinned individuals who experience brief, intense sun exposure, such as that occurring during vacations in the southern latitudes.

Fewer than 5% of all melanomas occur in the African-American population. The acral-lentiginous melanoma is the most common form in African Americans and occurs on the palms, soles, and nail beds. These melanomas have a short superficial growth phase and an early vertical growth phase and, as such, are associated with a poor prognosis. An acral-lentiginous melanoma on the sole of an African-American patient is pictured in Figure 8-38.

Malignant melanoma of the nail apparatus represents 2% to 3% of all melanomas in white individuals and about 20% in dark-skinned individuals. The most common pathologic type is the acral-lentiginous melanoma. It is frequently diagnosed in the sixth decade; women are affected more often than men. The thumb and the great toe are the most common sites. Figure 8-39 shows a classic malignant melanoma of the nail, with a wide longitudinal band and the variegated colors. Figure 8-40 shows a malignant melanoma of the nail bed. Notice that the band width is wider at the base than at the tip, indicating a rapidly growing lesion.

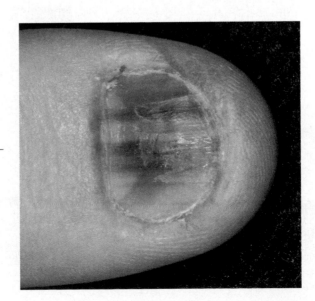

Figure 8–39 Melanoma of the nail.

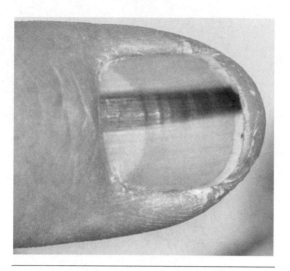

Figure 8–40 Melanoma of the nail bed.

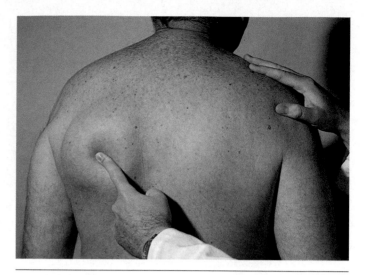

Figure 8–41 Lipoma of the back.

A *lipoma* is a benign growth of subcutaneous fat and has a rubbery appearance. The epidermis is normal. Frequently, an encapsulated lipoma may grow to a very large size and elevate the overlying dermis and epidermis, as shown in Figure 8-41; a cross section through a lipoma is illustrated in Figure 8-42. The examiner can easily push into the soft tissue tumor. Another example of a lipoma is shown on the arm of the patient in Figure 8-43.

Café au lait spots are patch lesions that are well circumscribed and brownish. They may occur as a solitary birthmark in up to 10% of the normal population. The café au lait macule or patch results from an increased number of functionally hyperactive melanocytes. Multiple café au lait patches in a patient may suggest neurofibromatosis. Figure 8-44 shows a café au lait patch in a patient with neurofibromatosis.

A *neurofibroma* is a tumor produced by a focal proliferation of neural tissue in the dermis. The epidermis is normal. Neurofibromas may appear as papules or nodules. Cutaneous neurofibromas are soft in consistency. Neurofibromatosis is a disorder in which multiple neurofibromas are present, sometimes as many as several hundred. Although the tumors are benign, the occurrence of these space-occupying lesions may produce severe disfigurement or neurologic disease. Other dermatologic features of neurofibromatosis include multiple café au lait patches and axillary freckling. Figure 8-45 shows several neurofibromas in a patient with

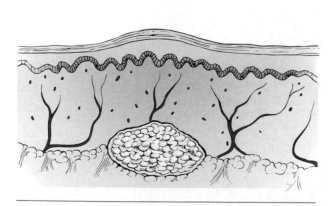

Figure 8–42 Cross section through a lipoma.

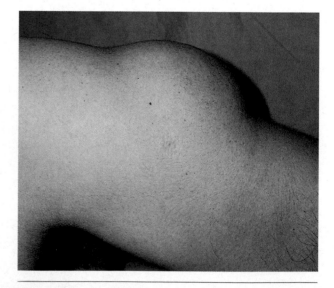

Figure 8–43 Lipoma of the arm.

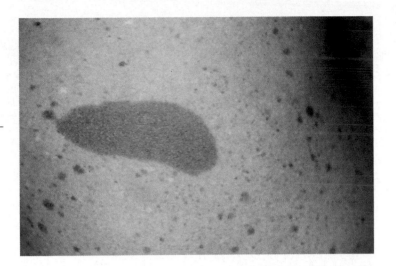

Figure 8–44 Café au lait spot in a patient with neurofibromatosis.

neurofibromatosis; a cross-sectional view is illustrated in Figure 8-46. Figure 8-47 shows axillary freckling (Crowe's sign) in a patient with neurofibromatosis. Figure 8-48 shows multiple neurofibromas on the face of another patient with neurofibromatosis.

Contact dermatitis is an inflammatory reaction of the skin that is precipitated by contact with an irritant or allergen, such as detergents, acids, alkali, plants, medicines, and solvents. Vesicles in the epidermis and perivascular inflammation result. Figure 8-49 shows contact dermatitis in reaction to poison ivy; the area is illustrated in cross section in Figure 8-50. The characteristic linear distribution of papules, vesicles, and bullae is visible on this patient's calf where the leaves of the plant touched the leg. The distribution of the bullous lesions together with their location is strongly suggestive of the diagnosis, which was confirmed by biopsy.

Psoriasis is one of the most common noninfectious skin disorders. It is frequently inherited and often chronic, and it, too, may affect the joints and nails. The rash is characterized by well-defined, slightly raised, hyperkeratotic (scaling) plaques. If the lesion is scratched, small bleeding points appear, which is a specific sign of the disease. The lesions are frequently symmetric and can be extremely itchy. The stratum corneum thickens, and erythematous plaques with silvery scales result. Within the dermis, there is capillary proliferation with perivascular inflammation. The lesions are characteristically located on the elbows, knees, scalp, and intergluteal cleft. Figure 8-51 shows the typical, symmetric lesions on the knees of an affected patient. Figure 8-52 shows the classic scaling lesions at the intergluteal cleft of another patient. Figure 8-53 illustrates a cross section through an area of psoriasis (see also Fig. 8-15). Figure 8-54 shows psoriasis of the scalp. The lesions commonly extend beyond the hair-bearing areas onto the adjacent skin. Surprisingly, this lesion rarely results in hair loss. Figure 8-55 shows severe, diffuse psoriasis involving more than 85% of the body of a 56-year-old man. This patient suffered from persistent itching, burning, and bleeding with psoriasis for more than 35 years. Psoriasis may produce several nail changes. Pitting of the nail has already been

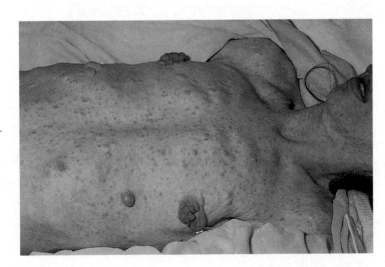

Figure 8–45 Multiple neurofibromas in a patient with neurofibromatosis.

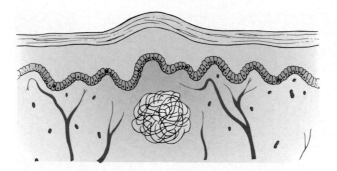

Figure 8–46 Cross section through a neurofibroma. Note that the tumor is a well-delimited mass of loosely packed neural elements.

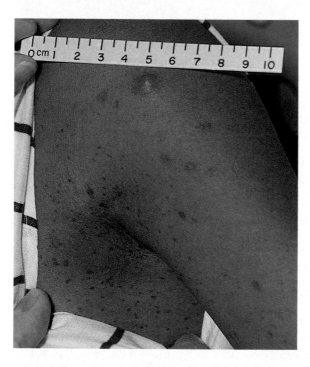

Figure 8–47 Neurofibromatosis: axillary freckling (Crowe's sign).

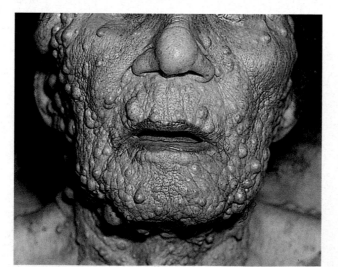

Figure 8–48 Multiple neurofibromas on the face of a patient with neurofibromatosis.

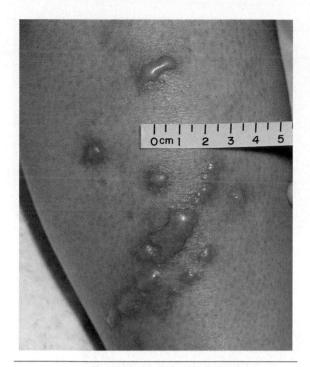

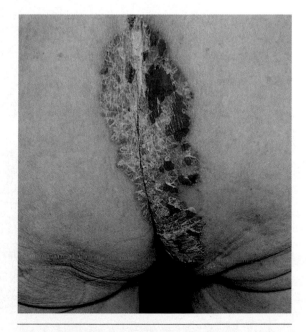

Figure 8–50 Cross section through an area of contact dermatitis. Note the perivascular inflammation in the dermis, as well as the vesicles and bullae in the epidermis.

Figure 8–49 Contact dermatitis: poison ivy reaction.

discussed (see Fig. 8-14). There are several other nail changes: oily patches, onycholysis, subungual hyperkeratosis, and splinter hemorrhages.

Tinea corporis is "ringworm" infection. Fungal infections of the skin produce a scaling, erythematous patch, often with a reddened, raised, serpiginous border. The term *tinea* indicates the fungal cause, and the second word denotes the area of the body involved: *tinea corporis* is infection in the body; *tinea pedis*, in the foot; *tinea faciale*, in the face; *tinea barbae*, in the beard and moustache area in men; *tinea cruris*, in the groin; and *tinea capitis*, in the head. In all cases, the epidermis is thickened, and the stratum corneum is infiltrated with fungal hyphae.

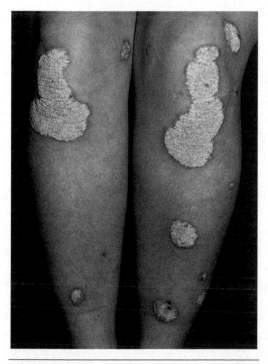

Figure 8–51 Psoriatic lesions on the knees.

Figure 8–52 Psoriatic lesions on the intergluteal cleft.

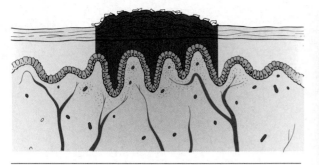

Figure 8–53 Cross section through an area of psoriasis. Note the area of hyperkeratosis.

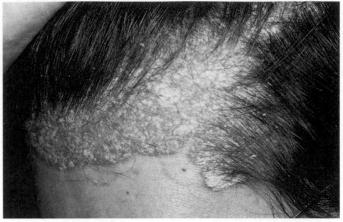

Figure 8–54 Psoriasis of the scalp.

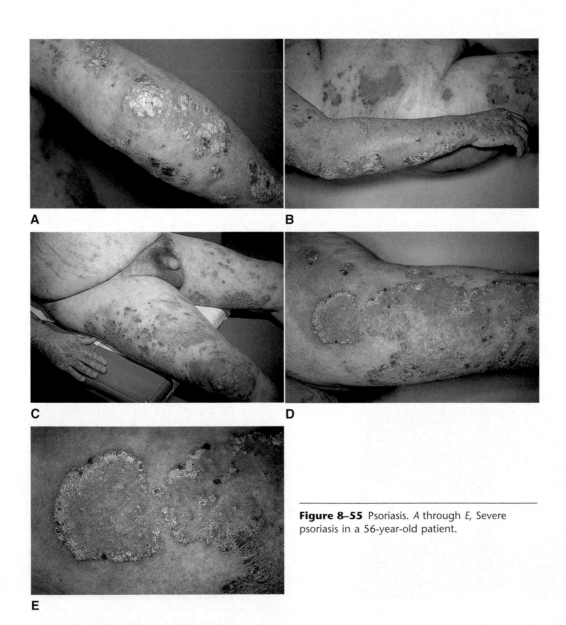

A

B

C

D

E

Figure 8–55 Psoriasis. *A* through *E,* Severe psoriasis in a 56-year-old patient.

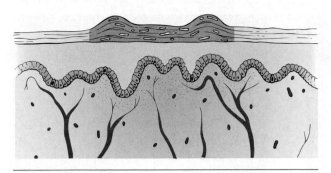

Figure 8–56 Cross section through an area of tinea corporis. Note the thickened stratum corneum, which is infiltrated by the fungus.

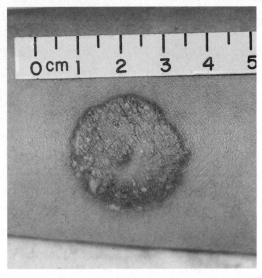

Figure 8–57 Tinea corporis.

The underlying dermis displays mild inflammation. Figures 8-56 and 8-57 illustrate the classic annular lesion of tinea corporis with its raised erythematous border and central clearing. Another example of tinea corporis is pictured in Figure 8-58. Tinea faciale in a child is pictured in Figure 8-59. Tinea cruris is pictured in Figure 8-60. This common pruritic lesion is seen commonly in young men; it is unusual in women. It spreads outward from the groin, down the thigh, leaving postinflammatory pigmentation. The advancing border is well defined, red, scaly, and slightly raised. If untreated, the eruption can spread onto the lower abdomen, as shown, and the buttocks. The foot of a patient with tinea pedis is pictured in Figure 8-61. Notice the maceration with erosions and scaling.

Pityriasis rosea is a common, acute, self-limiting inflammatory disease of unknown cause that usually occurs during the spring. The generalized eruption is preceded by a "herald patch," which is a single lesion resembling that of tinea corporis. In several days, the generalized eruption appears. Papulosquamous plaques appear over the trunk and rarely on the face and distal extremities. Although patients may complain of mild itching, they feel quite well. The full-blown picture develops slowly over 5 to 10 days and lasts for approximately 3 to 6 weeks. Slight hyperkeratosis of the epidermis with moderate dermal perivascular infiltration occurs. Figure 8-62 shows a herald patch and the characteristic lesions of pityriasis

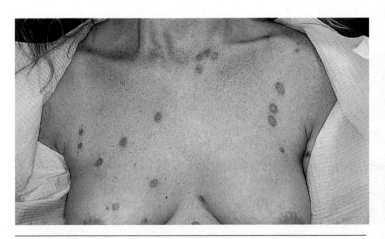

Figure 8–58 Tinea corporis.

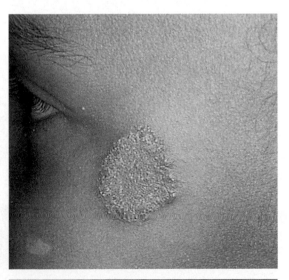

Figure 8–59 Tinea faciale.

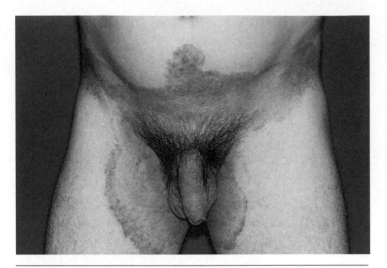

Figure 8–60 Tinea cruris.

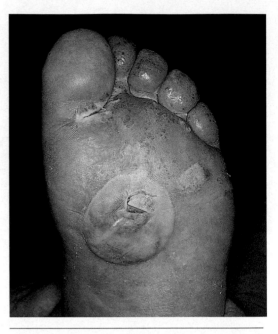

Figure 8–61 Tinea pedis.

rosea; Figure 8-63 illustrates a cross-sectional view. Notice the delicate scale at the border of the annular lesion. Secondary syphilis may manifest with a similar eruption. It is therefore important to order a serologic test for syphilis in any individual with pityriasis rosea.

Herpes zoster, or shingles, is an intraepidermal vesicular eruption occurring in a dermatomal distribution. Bullae and multinucleated giant cells are present in the epidermis, with perivascular inflammation of the dermis. The condition is caused by activation of the varicella-zoster virus. Groups of vesicles and bullae on erythematous bases are present along the distribution of peripheral nerves. Severe pain often precedes the eruption. Figure 8-64 shows herpes zoster lesions along the T3 distribution in two patients. Usually, the distribution occurs along the spinal or cranial nerves, but it can become generalized, as pictured in Figure 8-65; Figure 8-66 illustrates a cross section. Figure 8-67 is a close-up photograph of the typical vesicles on an erythematous base in a dermatomal distribution.

Herpesvirus infections are frequently encountered in patients with HIV infection; approximately 25% to 50% of these patients have some form of herpetic disease during the course of their illness. Herpesvirus infections are thought to be predictive of future progression from HIV

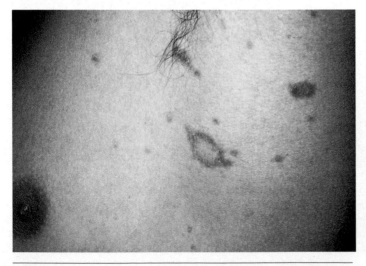

Figure 8–62 Pityriasis rosea. Note the herald patch.

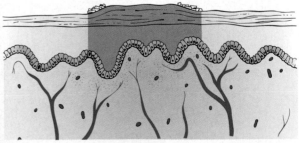

Figure 8–63 Cross section through a lesion of pityriasis rosea.

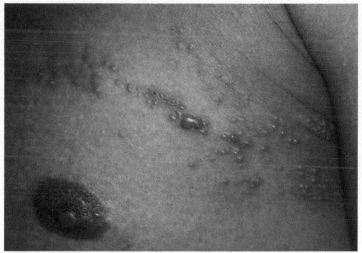

A

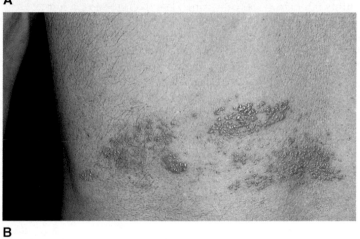

B

Figure 8–64 *A* and *B*, Herpes zoster lesions in T3 distribution.

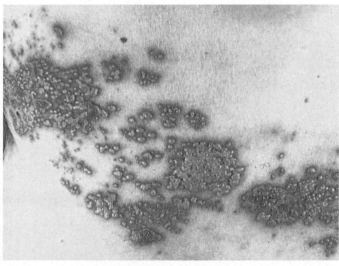

Figure 8–65 Herpes zoster, generalized.

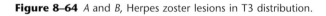

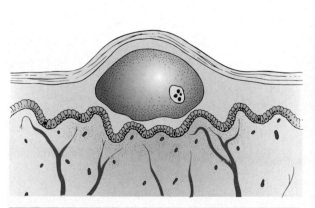

Figure 8–66 Cross section through one of the vesicles in herpes zoster. Note the large epidermal bullae with the classic multinuclear cells.

Figure 8–67 Herpes zoster vesicles.

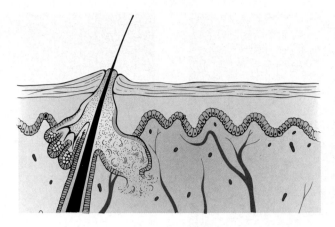

Figure 8–68 Cross section through an area of acne. Note the rupturing of the sebaceous gland in the dermis as a result of a plugged hair follicle, which results in dermal inflammation.

infection to AIDS; the rate of this association with progression is 23% at 2 years and up to 73% at 6 years. When CD4$^+$ T cell counts fall below 100 cells/mm^3, the likelihood of a herpesvirus infection approaches 95%. Herpes zoster infections may be severe and fulminant in immuno-compromised patients, such as in the patient shown in Figure 10-58.

Acne is a pustular disease affecting the hair follicles and sebaceous glands. In this condition, pustules, papules, and comedones are the primary lesions. There are collections of intradermal and intrafollicular neutrophils. Within the dermis, the hair follicle is occluded by a collection of keratin, sebum, and inflammatory cells. The hair follicle often ruptures into the dermis as a result of increasing pressure, which leads to further dermal inflammation (Figs. 8-68 to 8-71).

Tinea versicolor is a common superficial, noninflammatory, noncontagious fungal skin infection of young adults occurring most often during the summer. Pregnancy, warm climate, corticosteroids, and debilitation seem to be predisposing factors. Persons older than 40 years are rarely affected. The lesion consists of very fine, scaly patches that coalesce as they enlarge. The hypopigmented lesions are frequently seen on seborrheic areas of the body: the neck, the upper trunk, the upper arms, the shoulders, and, on occasion, the groin. The lesions are usually

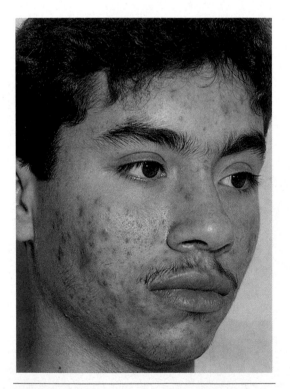

Figure 8–69 Acne.

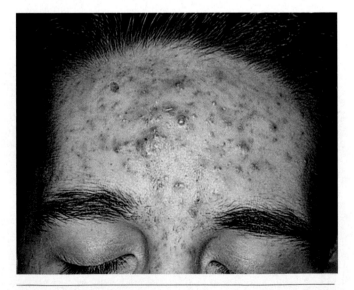

Figure 8–70 Acne.

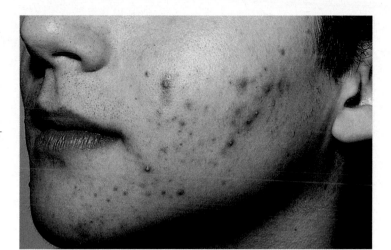

Figure 8–71 Acne.

asymptomatic but may be mildly pruritic. Figure 8-72 shows the back of a patient with the classic hypopigmented patches of tinea versicolor. Figure 8-73 shows another patient with tinea versicolor.

A *ganglion cyst* is a chronic, painless lesion on the dorsum of the wrist or ankle. It results from leakage of synovial fluid through the tendon sheath of the capsule of the joint. This fluid eventually becomes encapsulated, and a cyst results. Figure 8-74 shows a ganglion in the wrist, the typical location.

A *spider angioma* is a common pale red lesion, usually less than 2 cm in diameter, with a pulsating, central arteriole, often raised, surrounded by erythema and radiating "legs." If pressure is exerted on the central body, blanching of the spider's legs occurs. These benign lesions are commonly seen on the face, neck, arms, and upper trunk; they are rarely seen on the lower extremities. Although seen in normal individuals, spider angiomas are found more commonly in pregnant women and in patients with liver disease or vitamin B deficiency. These angiomas frequently become more evident during various times of a woman's menstrual cycle. Figure 8-75 shows a spider angioma on the face of a young woman. Notice the central arteriole with the peripheral blush.

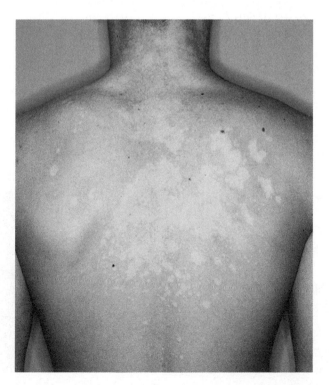

Figure 8–72 Tinea versicolor.

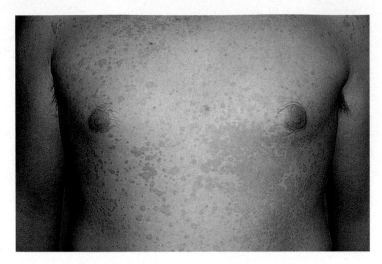

Figure 8–73 Tinea versicolor.

Vitiligo consists of patches of lightened skin resulting from decreased melanin pigmentation. Vitiligo is essentially a large macule that is totally depigmented. The epidermis manifests a complete absence of pigment, whereas the dermis is normal. Vitiligo can occur in any area, but it is commonly found on the neck, knees, elbows, and back of the hands. Figure 8-76 shows extensive vitiligo on the face and neck; a cross section is shown in Figure 8-77. Diffuse vitiligo is pictured in Figure 8-78.

Urticaria is a common condition. The primary lesion is the wheal, or hive. In urticaria, the epidermis is normal. The dermis demonstrates papillary edema. Inflammatory cells may be found surrounding dilated blood vessels. Itching is a common complaint. There are several mechanisms for the development of urticaria, which include both immunologic and nonimmunologic causes. Regardless of the cause, the common factor is the release of substances, such as histamine, that change the vascular permeability and produce dermal edema. Figure 8-79 shows urticaria, and Figure 8-80 depicts the cross section.

Erythema multiforme is an immunologic reaction in the skin triggered by various causative agents, including viruses, bacteria, drugs, and x-radiation. In many cases, the agent cannot be identified. As the name implies, the condition includes a variety of lesions: papules, bullae, plaques, and "target lesions." Target lesions are the diagnostic lesions and have three zones of color: A central, tense bulla, or dark area, is surrounded by a zone of relative pallor that is rimmed by a thin area of erythema. Typically, target lesions are seen on the palms and soles (Fig. 8-81). The epidermis is usually normal. In the dermis, there is a subepidermal separation with inflammatory cells in the papillary dermis. Penicillin and sulfonamides are the drugs most commonly implicated as the cause of this condition. The most severe form of erythema multiforme involves the mucous membranes and is called *Stevens-Johnson syndrome*. The classic skin lesions of erythema multiforme are shown in Figures 8-82 and 8-83; Figure 8-84 illustrates a cross-sectional view.

Scabies is a common, intensely pruritic skin disorder caused by a mite, *Sarcoptes scabiei* var. *hominis.* The female mite burrows into the stratum corneum of the skin and lays her eggs.

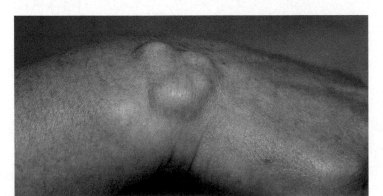

Figure 8–74 Ganglion cyst.

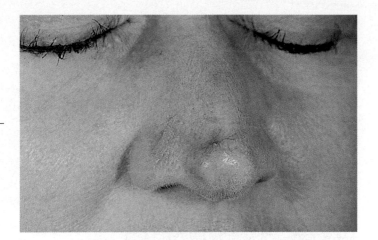

Figure 8–75 Spider angioma.

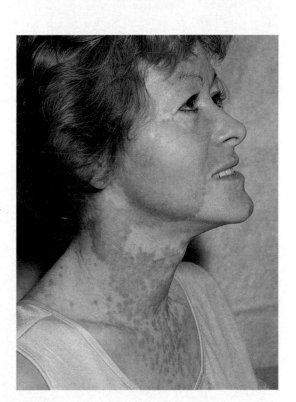

Figure 8–76 Vitiligo.

Figure 8–77 Cross section through an area of vitiligo. Note the absence of melanocytes and skin pigment.

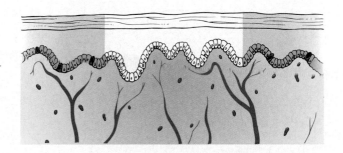

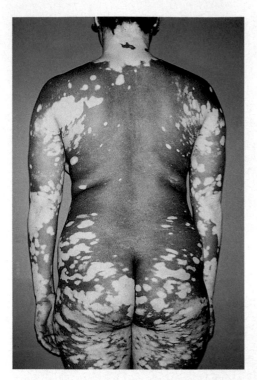

Figure 8–78 Diffuse vitiligo.

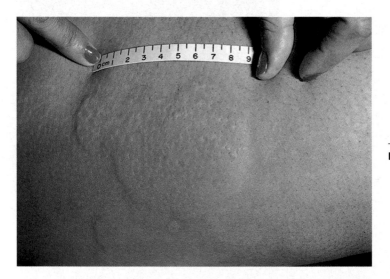

Figure 8–79 Urticaria.

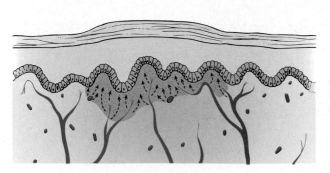

Figure 8–80 Cross section through an area of urticaria.

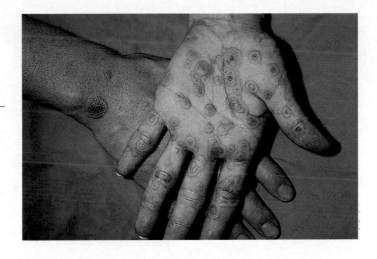

Figure 8–81 Target lesions on palms and hands in a patient with erythema multiforme.

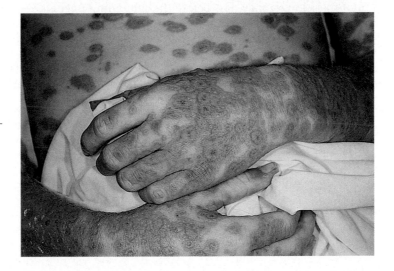

Figure 8–82 Erythema multiforme.

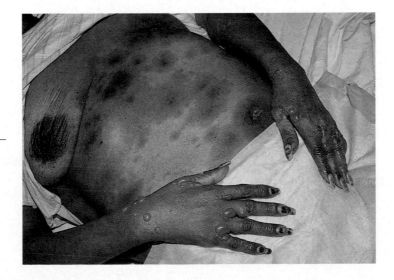

Figure 8–83 Erythema multiforme.

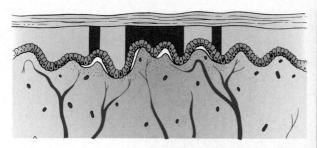

Figure 8–84 Cross section through an area of erythema multiforme. Note the separation of the epidermis from the dermis.

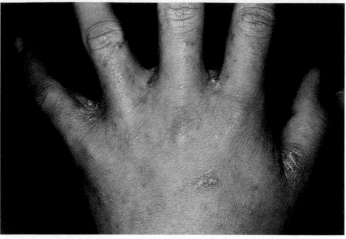

Figure 8–85 Scabies.

A month or longer may pass before the symptom of generalized pruritus develops. The diagnostic physical sign is the burrow, which is a serpiginous, palpable track about 1 cm in length that may end in a papule, nodule, or tiny vesicle. The adult female mite is present in the burrow. The extremely pruritic rash of scabies has a predilection for the web spaces of the fingers and toes, as well as the groin. The buttocks are also frequently involved, as are the genitals of men and the nipples of women. A generalized papular or urticarial eruption may ensue after localized scabies infection. The presence of papules on the genitalia in a patient with intense pruritus should raise the strong suspicion of scabies. Outbreaks of scabies are common in population groups in which HIV infection is prevalent. Figure 8-85 shows the hand of a patient with scabies. Notice the classic eruption between the fingers. Figure 18-16 shows another patient with scabies; the papular rash in the groin and on the penis is clearly seen.

Norwegian scabies is a rare, highly infectious form of scabies that is often seen in immunosuppressed patients and patients with psychiatric illness; recently, this form of scabies has been seen in patients with AIDS. It is characterized by very thick, white hyperkeratotic scales containing thousands of mites. The dorsal aspects of the hands, the feet, and the extensor surfaces of the elbows and knees are commonly involved. Figure 8-86 shows the hand of a patient with Norwegian scabies. Figure 8-87 shows the diffuse lesions of Norwegian scabies in another patient.

Pyoderma gangrenosum is a cutaneous condition consisting of large, tender, necrotic ulcers having a violaceous, overhanging edge with a purulent base. The lesions are most frequently seen on the face, lower legs, and abdomen. Although most often associated with inflammatory

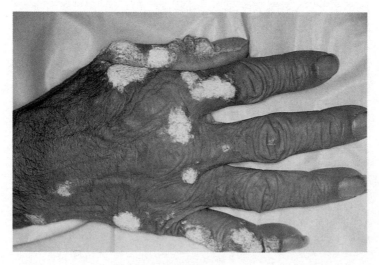

Figure 8–86 Norwegian scabies.

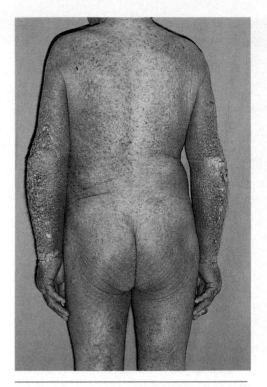

Figure 8–87 Norwegian scabies.

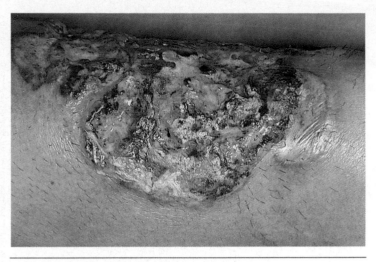

Figure 8–88 Pyoderma gangrenosum of the shin.

bowel disease, this condition is also seen in association with various blood dyscrasias (especially multiple myeloma), chronic active hepatitis, rheumatoid arthritis, systemic lupus erythematosus, and acute leukemias. Approximately 10% of all patients with ulcerative colitis, however, have cutaneous manifestations, especially pyoderma gangrenosum. The skin lesions of pyoderma gangrenosum are closely linked to the bowel disease; exacerbations of bowel symptoms are associated with extension of existing lesions or development of new ones. Removal of the diseased bowel often leads to improvement in the cutaneous manifestations. Figure 8-88 shows the classic shin lesions of pyoderma gangrenosum in a patient with regional enteritis. See also Figure 17-6, which shows another patient with an exacerbation of ulcerative colitis and pyoderma gangrenosum of the shin.

Insect bites are common and should always be considered when a patient complains of a pruritic rash. Papules, vesicles, and wheals amid excoriations suggest the diagnosis. Papules in a grouped or linear arrangement on an arm or face suggest bedbug bites. These insects, which live in crevices in furniture, shun the light and feed at night on exposed areas of the body. They bite and then move around only to bite again. Figure 8-89 shows the linear papules on the arm of a patient who was bitten by bedbugs. Figure 8-90 shows another patient with persistent erythematous papules as a result of bedbug bites. Flea bites were the cause of the pruritic eruption on the feet of the patient shown in Figure 8-91. Notice the excoriations. The lower legs and feet are common sites for flea bites.

Kaposi's sarcoma (KS) is a neoplasm characterized by dark blue–purple macules, papules, nodules, and plaques. The classic form of the disease is a rare, slow-growing neoplasm occurring mostly on the lower extremities, especially the ankles and soles, of elderly men of Mediterranean or Jewish eastern European descent. The male-to-female ratio is 10:1 to 15:1, and the majority of patients are 60 to 80 years of age. Figure 8-92 shows a large reddish-colored plaque, which was slow-growing, on the sole of the foot of a 60-year-old man of eastern European origin.

Currently, KS is the most frequent neoplasm occurring in patients with AIDS. Approximately 35% of patients with AIDS who acquired the disease by sexual contact are affected, as opposed to approximately 5% of patients whose infection was acquired from intravenous drug use. Overall, 24% of all patients with AIDS develop this rapidly progressive form of the disease, also known as the epidemic HIV-associated form. The widely disseminated lesions are present on the legs, trunk, arms, neck, and head. They start as light-colored papules or nodules and coalesce into larger, darker lesions. Unlike the classic form, the epidemic

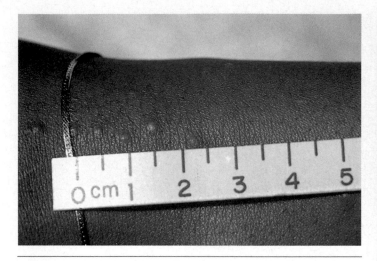

Figure 8–89 Bedbug bites.

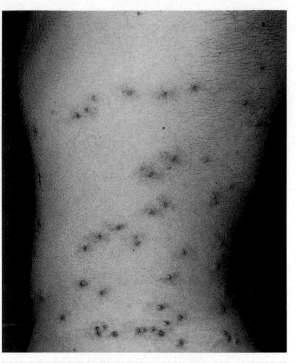

Figure 8–90 Bedbug bites.

HIV-associated form is commonly associated with visceral involvement, frequent oral lesions, and lymphadenopathy. The average length of patient survival from the onset of the disease is 18 months. The skin lesions of epidemic HIV-associated KS are shown in Figure 8-93. Figure 8-93*A* shows the typical lesions on the arm and chest; Figure 8-93*B* shows the widely disseminated plaque lesions varying in color from dark red to violet; Figure 8-93*C* shows a violaceous lesion on the lateral aspect of the lower eyelid; Figure 8-93*D* shows a large confluent plaque of KS on the hard palate; Figure 8-93*E* shows a purplish-red, nodular lesion of KS on the gingiva and an infiltrative, violaceous lesion of the nose.

Figure 8-94 demonstrates the rapidity of the growth of epidemic KS. The initial manifestation (Fig. 8-94*A*) on the back of a 36-year-old gay man was only a few macular lesions of KS; a follow-up photograph, taken only 6 months later, shows the widely disseminated, purplish plaques of KS (Fig. 8-94*B*).

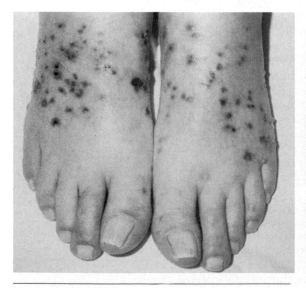

Figure 8–91 Flea bites.

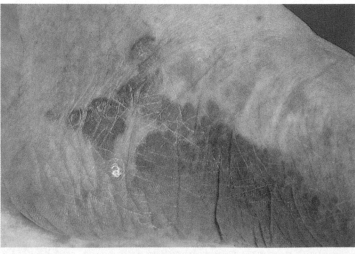

Figure 8–92 Kaposi's sarcoma: a classic plaque.

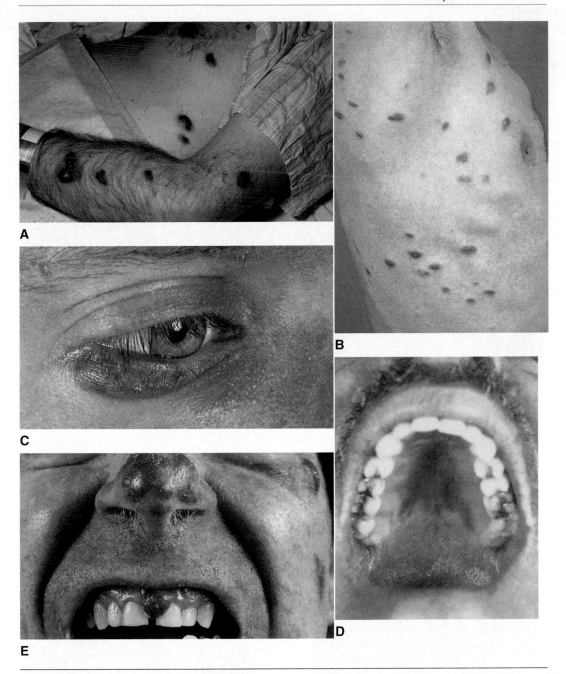

Figure 8–93 Kaposi's sarcoma: epidemic human immunodeficiency virus (HIV) associated. *A* and *B*, Plaque lesions. *C*, Violaceous lesion affecting the lateral lower eyelid. *D*, Confluent plaque on the hard palate. *E*, Nodular lesion on the gingiva and the nose.

Scleroderma, also known as *progressive systemic sclerosis*, is an important rheumatic disease characterized by hardening of the skin. Vascular changes occur with visceral involvement and involve the microvessels and small arteries. The onset of the disease is often heralded by the development of Raynaud's phenomenon, which is discussed in Chapter 15, The Peripheral Vascular System. The cutaneous manifestations of scleroderma involve tightening of the skin, especially on the face and hands. As a result of tendon contractures, flexion of the fingers results. The fingers of a patient with scleroderma are shown in Figure 8-95; notice that the skin is bound tightly and obscures the superficial vasculature. Skin lines are absent. Figure 8-96 shows the face of the same patient. Notice the tightening and wrinkling of the skin around her mouth and the fixed, expressionless countenance as a result of flattening of the nasolabial folds. The patient had great difficulty in opening her mouth. The skin around the mouth has many furrows radiating outward, creating a mouselike appearance known as *mauskopf*.

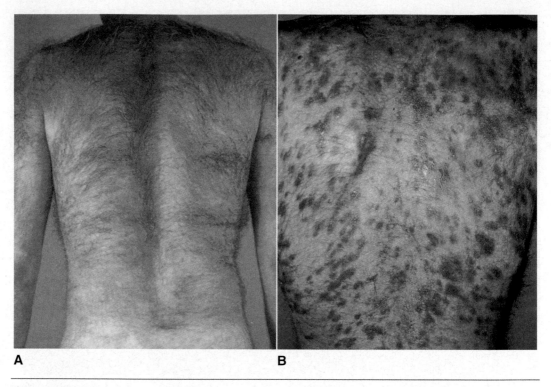

A   B

Figure 8–94 *A,* Early lesions of Kaposi's sarcoma on the back. *B,* Follow-up photograph, 6 months later, showing rapid development of purplish plaques of Kaposi's sarcoma.

Erythema nodosum is a common reaction associated with streptococcal infections, sarcoidosis, tuberculosis, inflammatory bowel diseases, and fungal diseases. It is infrequently associated with rheumatic disorders. Patients, primarily young women, seek medical attention after the appearance of extremely painful, erythematous nodules on the lower legs, especially over the anterior tibia. The lesions range in size from 1 cm to several centimeters in diameter. The lesions can then coalesce and spread over the entire leg. The lesions of erythema nodosum begin to regress after 1 to 2 weeks. As they disappear, they undergo a series of characteristic color changes: bright erythema to shades of purple, yellow, and green. Figure 8-97 shows the

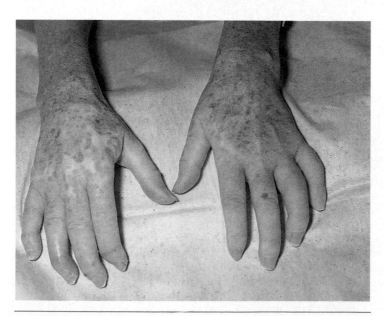

Figure 8–95 Scleroderma: hands.

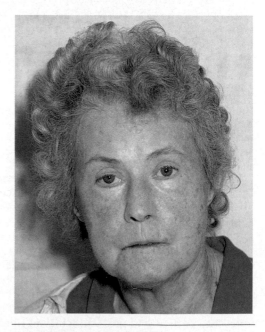

Figure 8–96 Scleroderma: face.

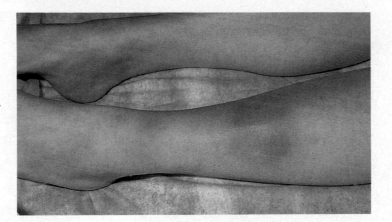

Figure 8–97 Erythema nodosum.

early lesions of erythema nodosum in a 33-year-old woman in whom sarcoidosis was diagnosed 3 months later.

Lichen planus is a relatively common skin disorder of unknown cause. The primary lesion is a polygonal, shiny, flat-topped papule with a violaceous hue. The pruritic lesions can be seen on any part of the body but have a predilection for the front of the wrists and forearms, the backs of the hands, the ankles, the shins, the genitalia, and the lumbar areas. The lesions range in size from 2 mm to more than 1 cm. Figure 8-98*A* shows the characteristic rash on the arm. Fine reticulated scales are visible (see Fig. 8-98*B*). Oral lesions are seen in 50% of all patients with lichen planus and consist of a white, lacy network on the buccal mucosa. On occasion, involvement of the mouth may be the only manifestation of lichen planus. The patient usually experiences severe pain as the lesions ulcerate. Figure 12-15 depicts lichen planus of the buccal mucosa. Lichen planus may also involve the genitalia. Figure 8-99 shows lichen planus of the penis. Note the reticular markings on the penis. Figure 18-10 depicts another case of lichen planus of the penis. Note again the fine reticular markings.

Seborrheic dermatitis is a papulosquamous disorder associated with epidermal hyperplasia and scaling. The lesions have a greasy-looking scale in a seborrheic distribution: scalp, eyebrows, nasolabial fold, perioral area, midchest, and groin. Seborrheic dermatitis is one of the most common skin conditions associated with HIV infection; it is estimated that 85% of patients infected with HIV have this skin lesion at some time. In some patients, the development of seborrheic dermatitis is the first sign of HIV infection. Figure 8-100 shows the typical greasy scales of seborrheic dermatitis on the face of a patient with AIDS.

Seborrheic warts are common, benign skin tumors, seen in light-skinned individuals; they occur more frequently with advancing age. Also known as *seborrheic keratosis* (Fig. 8-101), seborrheic warts may be solitary or multiple lesions. They occur in any area of the body exposed to ultraviolet light. The lesions are well defined and raised and have a fissured surface. The lesions result from a failure of keratinocytes to mature normally, which produces an accumulation of immature cells in the epidermis. Sometimes the lesions may be pedunculated. A similar condition known as *dermatosis papulosis nigra* is seen in African Americans. Figure 8-102 is a close-up photograph of the characteristic appearance of a seborrheic wart.

A *keloid* is a hyperproliferative response of fibrous tissue to injury, inflammation, or infection. It has a smooth appearance with a shiny surface and is raised and firm to palpation. It is more commonly seen in dark-skinned individuals. The lesion characteristically spreads beyond the site of the initiating factor. Figure 8-103 shows an extensive keloid on the shoulder.

Nevi are common, localized abnormalities of the skin that may be present at birth or appear within the first few decades of life. Sometimes called "moles," nevi may arise from almost any area of the skin. They are well defined, with a smooth surface and a round shape (Fig. 8-104). Hair may sometimes project from the surface. A *strawberry nevus* is a vascular tumor or hemangioma that occurs shortly after birth and is red and raised. These grow rapidly and are often seen on the face of a child. They may bleed and ulcerate. Fortunately, most strawberry nevi involute by 6 or 7 years of age. Figure 24-8 shows a strawberry nevus in a child. Figure 24-9 shows a hemangioma in another child.

Blistering, or vesiculobullous, diseases of the skin are rare but important to recognize. *Pemphigus vulgaris*, *pemphigus vegetans*, and *bullous pemphigoid* are autoimmune diseases that affect skin and mucosal surfaces. Pemphigus vulgaris is a vesiculobullous disease of

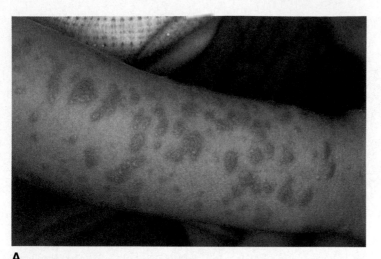

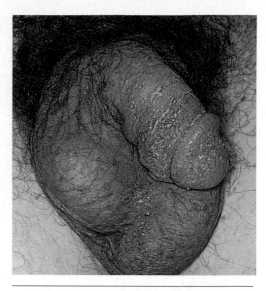

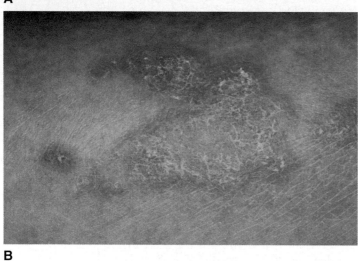

Figure 8–99 Lichen planus of the penis.

Figure 8–98 *A* and *B,* Lichen planus. Notice the fine reticulated white scales.

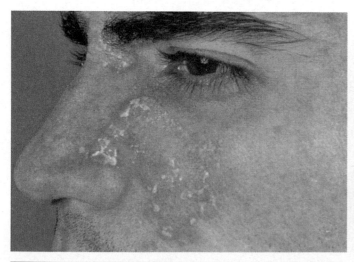

Figure 8–100 Seborrheic dermatitis.

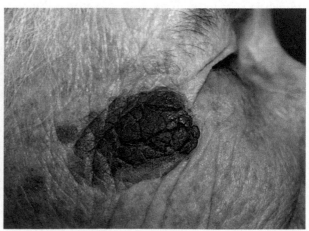

Figure 8–101 Seborrheic keratosis.

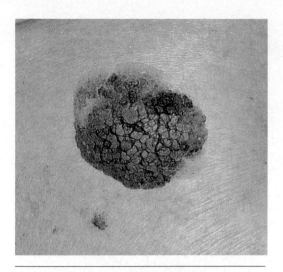

Figure 8–102 Seborrheic wart, close-up.

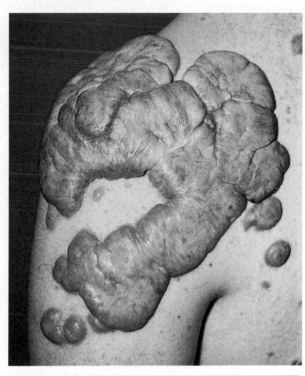

Figure 8–103 Keloid.

middle age, seen more commonly in Jewish people. The lesions are superficial, flaccid blisters that break easily, leaving the skin denuded and eroded. The broken bullae may crust but do not heal spontaneously. These lesions are nonpruritic but are painful. The disease is caused by the production of antibodies to the intercellular junctions of the epidermis. The defective junctions lead to the formation of traumatic fissures and bullae. Figure 8-105*A* shows pemphigus vulgaris and broken bullae. Figure 8-105*B* shows pemphigus vegetans. The lesions may be present on any area of the skin, especially the trunk, umbilicus, intertriginous areas, and scalp. The lesions are frequently found in the mucous membranes of the oral cavity, pharynx, and genitalia. Figure 8-106 shows pemphigus vegetans of the lips.

Bullous pemphigoid is a blistering disorder seen more frequently in elderly patients. It is more common than pemphigus vulgaris. There is no racial predilection, and the disease is not

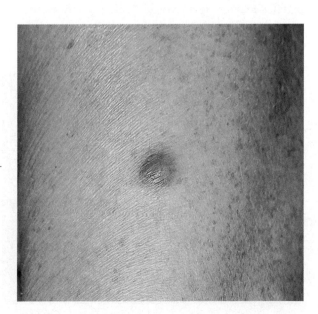

Figure 8–104 Blue nevus.

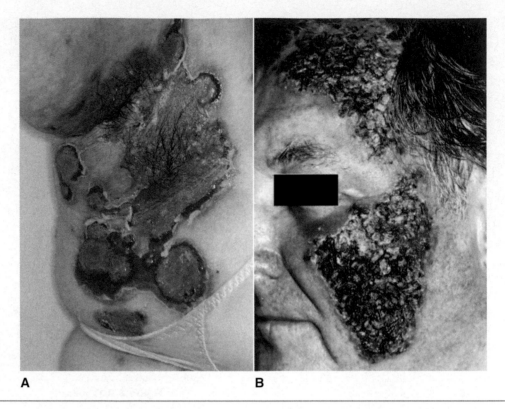

A   B

Figure 8–105 *A* and *B,* Pemphigus vulgaris. *B,* A vegetative form sometimes called *pemphigus vegetans.*

as serious as pemphigus. The lesions are intensely pruritic, tense bullae often on an erythematous base and are symmetric on the limbs, inner aspects of the arms, thighs, and trunk. Oral and mucosal lesions are rarer than those of pemphigus. Figure 8-107 depicts generalized bullous pemphigoid. Figure 8-108 shows bullous pemphigoid in another patient. Notice the tense bullae, which help differentiate this disease from pemphigus. Figure 8-109 is a close-up photograph of the tense bullae of bullous pemphigoid in yet another patient.

Atopic dermatitis, a form of eczema, is a common disease associated with other atopic diseases such as asthma and allergic rhinitis. It is characterized by itchy, dry, inflamed skin. The symptoms of atopic dermatitis often begin at a young age. Infants and young children may have eczematous patches on the face, scalp, and extensor surfaces of the extremities. These patches may erode and ooze. Scaling erythematous plaques often develop. As the child grows older, the atopic dermatitis begins to involve the flexural areas such as the neck, antecubital

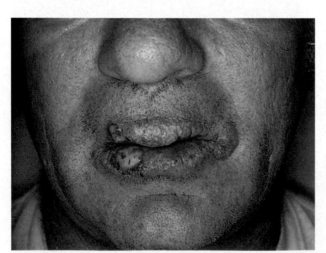

Figure 8–106 Pemphigus vegetans of the lips.

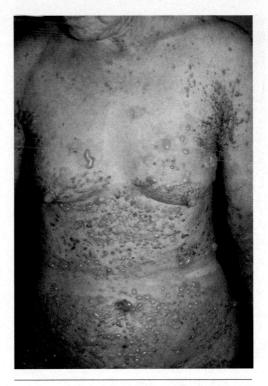

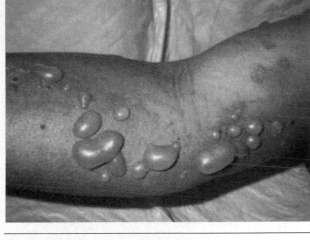

Figure 8–108 Bullous pemphigoid.

Figure 8–107 Bullous pemphigoid.

fossae, and popliteal fossae. The pruritic lesions result in excoriations; thickening and lichen-ification of the skin with increased skin markings are common. In the adult, oozing, weeping, and excoriated plaques may become generalized. Although the pathogenesis of atopic derma-titis is unknown, many patients have elevated levels of serum immunoglobulin E. Since the 1970s, the incidence of atopic dermatitis has increased from 4% to 12%; the reasons are unclear. Immune dysregulation appears to play an important role in atopic dermatitis. Up to 50% of children with atopic dermatitis may have evidence of a food sensitivity. Emotional stressors do not cause atopic dermatitis but do exacerbate the symptoms. Figure 8-110 shows classic lesions of atopic dermatitis in the axilla. Figure 8-111 shows atopic dermatitis in another patient. Notice the oozing lesions and excoriations.

Lyme disease is an infection caused by the spirochete *Borrelia burgdorferi* that is transmitted by the usually asymptomatic bite of certain ticks of the genus *Ixodes*. Lyme borreliosis occurs in northeastern, mid-Atlantic, north-central, and far western regions of the United States. Erythema migrans is the clinical, distinctive hallmark of Lyme disease. It is a dynamic lesion

Figure 8–109 Bullous pemphigoid; close-up of tense bullae.

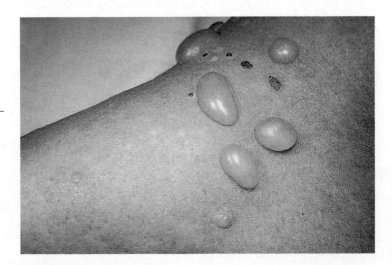

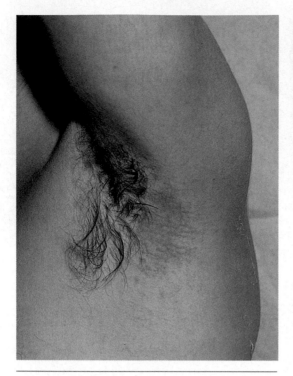

Figure 8–110 Atopic dermatitis.

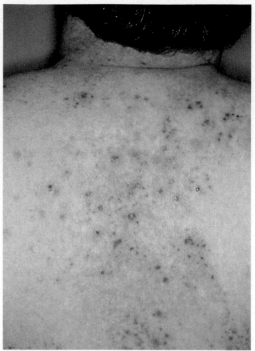

Figure 8–111 Atopic dermatitis.

whose appearance can change dramatically over a period of days. The rash is recognized in 90% of patients with objective evidence of *B. burgdorferi* infection. The erythema begins as a red macule or papule at the site of the tick bite that occurred 7 to 10 days earlier. The rash expands as an annular erythematous plaque as the spirochetes spread centrifugally through the skin. Central clearing may or may not be present. Local symptoms of pruritus or tenderness are hardly noticeable. Systemic symptoms are common and include fatigue (54%), myalgia (44%), arthralgia (44%), headache (42%), fever and chills (39%), and stiff neck (35%). Neurologic symptoms are also common. The most common sign is regional lymphadenopathy (23%). Figures 8-112 and 8-113 show the classic erythema migrans of Lyme disease. Note the central lesion in Figure 8-113, which was the area of the tick bite.

As indicated previously in this chapter, there are many cutaneous manifestations of AIDS. Three of these common lesions are shown on the face of a patient with AIDS in Figure 8-114. The umbilicated, white papules on and around the lips, nose, and cheek are lesions of molluscum contagiosum. The verrucous papule on the upper lip is a wart. The violaceous lesions of KS are present on the lips and chin.

Fungal infections of the nails and hair are very common. The main fungi responsible for hair and nail diseases are dermatophytes of the genera *Trichophyton*, *Microsporum*, and

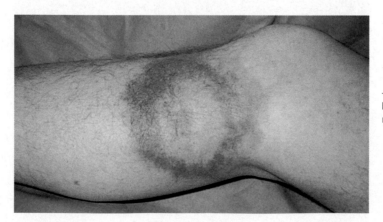

Figure 8–112 Erythema migrans of Lyme disease.

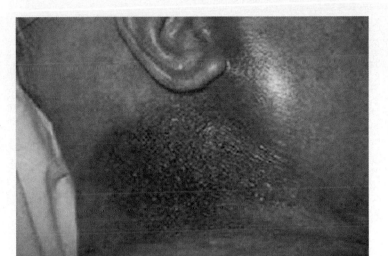

Figure 8–119 Anthrax. Note the early lesion and marked edema.

The inhalation, or pulmonary, form of anthrax usually occurs 1 to 60 days after exposure, although longer incubation periods can follow milder degrees of exposure. During the initial stage of the disease, nonspecific, influenza-like symptoms are common: myalgias, cough, low-grade fever, nonproductive cough, malaise, nausea, vomiting, chills, sweating, headache, and shortness of breath. Usually there follows a period of 1 to 3 days of improvement and then the rapid progression of high fever, severe respiratory distress, and cardiovascular collapse, often leading to shock and death within 24 to 36 hours. Massive mediastinal adenopathy occurs often. Person-to-person spread is not a significant risk because the main lesions are in the mediastinal lymph nodes and surrounding tissue. The mortality rate is 90% to 100% among untreated patients but 30% to 50% if patients are treated, depending on how quickly treatment with antibiotics is initiated.

B. anthracis is susceptible to common antibiotics, including ciprofloxacin, penicillin G, or tetracyclines.

Smallpox is a severe, highly contagious, febrile viral disease caused by a DNA virus of the orthopoxvirus genus. These viruses are among the largest and most complex of all viruses. There is an incubation period of 10 to 12 days after exposure. The illness begins with the symptoms of fever, fatigue, and myalgias. A distinctive erythematous, vesicular rash, centrifugal in distribution, then develops over the next 1 to 2 days, with the lesions appearing early on the face (Fig. 8-121) and arms, with relative sparing of the trunk. As the disease progresses, lesions appear on the trunk. The lesions are uniform in their stage of development and are often umbilicated (Fig. 8-122). After approximately 2 weeks, the lesions form crusts, which fall

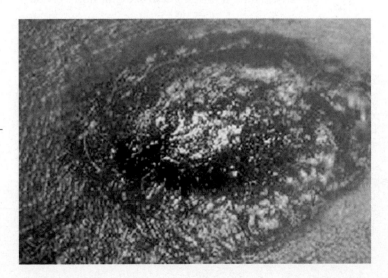

Figure 8–120 Anthrax. Note the black eschar.

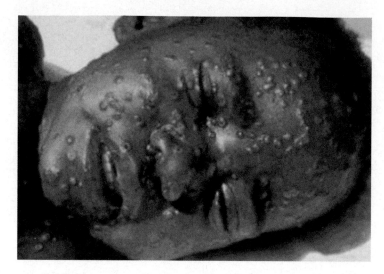

Figure 8–121 Smallpox. Note the uniform stage of development of the vesicles.

away after 3 to 4 weeks. The case-fatality rate is 30% to 40% or more. The last naturally occurring case of smallpox was in 1977 in Somalia. In 1980, the World Health Organization officially declared that smallpox was eradicated worldwide as a result of a global vaccination program. Although smallpox was long feared as one of the most devastating infectious diseases, its potential for devastation today is far greater than ever before. In a now highly susceptible, mobile population, medically ignorant of this infection once considered eradicated, smallpox could spread widely and rapidly throughout the world. The presence of even one case would constitute an international health emergency.

Plague is caused by a gram-negative, non–spore-forming bacillus, *Yersinia pestis*. Natural human infection usually follows the bite of an infected flea and is less commonly caused by droplet spread from a person or cat with pneumonic plague. Plague occurs in three forms: bubonic, pneumonic, and septicemic. In the case of pneumonic plague, after an incubation period of 1 to 6 days, there is the fulminant onset of high fever, chills, extreme malaise, headache, and myalgias. Within 24 hours, cough with hemoptysis occurs. Dyspnea rapidly develops, and respiratory and cardiovascular collapse ensue. The mortality rate is 100% if the disease is untreated and could be as high as 50% even with treatment.

In the bubonic form of plague, sudden flulike symptoms develop after an incubation period of 2 to 8 days. At about the same time, the patient notices the presence of an oval, elevated, 1-to 10-cm, firm, nonfluctuant mass associated with intense pain in the enlarged regional lymph nodes, known as a *bubo*. Gangrene of the extremities is one of the common manifestations of plague, accounting for the name of the "Black Death" throughout the ages. The mortality rate is 50% to 60% if the disease is untreated. Treatment for all forms of plague is with streptomycin, doxycycline, or ciprofloxacin.

The typical distribution of lesions in six common skin disorders is shown in Figure 8-123.

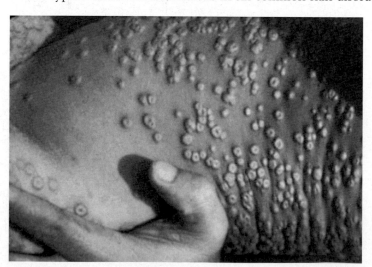

Figure 8–122 Smallpox. Note the umbilicated lesions on the trunk.

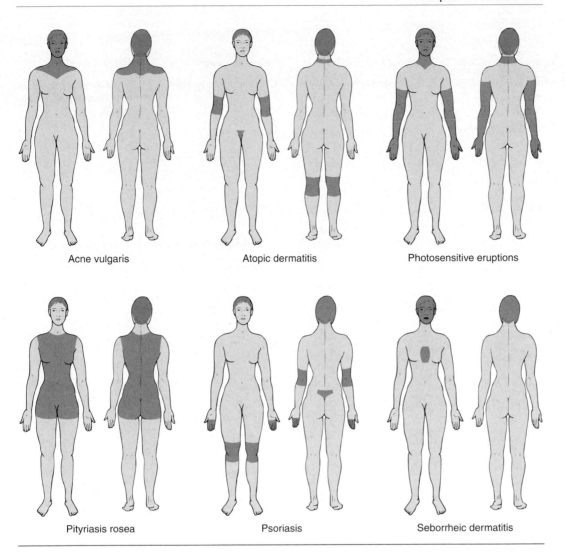

Acne vulgaris Atopic dermatitis Photosensitive eruptions

Pityriasis rosea Psoriasis Seborrheic dermatitis

Figure 8–123 Typical distributions of common skin conditions.

Table 8-1 describes the differential diagnosis of common maculopapular diseases. Table 8-2 lists the differentiation of some common eczematous disorders and gives some special hints about their causes derived from the history. Table 8-3 provides information for a differential diagnosis of the vesiculobullous diseases. Table 8-4 classifies some of the common benign tumors by color. Table 8-5 lists some of the common allergens associated with contact dermatitis. Table 8-6 lists the important differences between chickenpox and smallpox.

Table 8–1 Common Maculopapular Diseases*

Characteristic	Psoriasis	Pityriasis Rosea	Tinea Versicolor	Lichen Planus	Seborrheic Dermatitis
Color	Dull red	Pinkish-yellow	Reddish-brown	Violaceous	Pinkish-yellow
Scale	Abundant	Fine, adherent	Fine	Shiny, adherent	Greasy
Induration†	1+	0	0	1+	1+
Face lesions	Rare	Rare	Occasional	Rare	Common
Oral lesions†	0	0	0	2+	0
Nail lesions†	4+	0	0	Rare	0

*See Figures 8-14, 8-51, 8-52, 8-54, 8-55, 8-62, 8-72, 8-73, 8-98, 8-100, and 12-15.
†0, rarely seen; 1+, occasionally seen; 2+, frequently seen; 4+, nearly always associated.

Table 8–2 Common Eczematous Diseases*

Characteristic	Contact Dermatitis	Atopic Dermatitis	Neurodermatitis	Stasis Dermatitis
History	Acute, localized to specific area	History in patient or family member of asthma, hay fever, or eczema	Chronic, in same areas, associated with anxiety	Varicosities, past history of thrombophlebitis or cellulitis
Location	Areas of exposure to allergen	Eyelids, groin, flexural areas	Head, lower legs, arms	Lower legs

*See Figures 8-49, 8-110, 8-111, and 15-2.

Table 8–3 Vesiculobullous Diseases*

Characteristic	Pemphigus Vulgaris	Dermatitis Herpetiformis	Epidermolysis Bullosa†	Bullous Pemphigoid
Age of patient	40-60 years	Children and adults	Infants and children	60-70 years
Initial site	Oral mucosa	Scalp, trunk	Extremities	Extremities
Lesions	Normal skin at margins	Erythematous base	Bullae produced by trauma	Normal skin at margins
Sites	Mouth, abdomen, scalp, groin	Knees, sacrum, back, elbows	Hands, knees, elbows, mouth, toes	Trunk, extremities
Groupings‡	0	4+	1+	0
Weight loss	Marked	None	None	Minimal
Duration	1 or more years	Several years	Normal lifetime	Months to years
Pruritus‡	0	4+	0	±
Oral pain‡	4+	0	±	±
Palms/soles involved	No	No	Yes	Yes
Typical lesion	Flaccid bullae	Grouped vesicles	Flaccid vesicles	Tense bullae

*See Figures 8-105, 8-106, 8-107, 8-108, and 8-109.
†Refers to a group of inherited diseases.
‡0, rarely seen; 1+, occasionally seen; 4+, nearly always associated; ±, sometimes present.

Table 8–4 Common Benign Tumors by Color

Color	Benign Tumor
Skin color	Warts (see Figs. 8-26 and 8-27) Cysts Keloids (see Fig. 8-103) Nevi (see Fig. 8-104)
Pink or red	Hemangiomas (see Figs. 24-8 and 24-9) Keloids (see Fig. 8-103)
Brown	Seborrheic keratoses (see Fig. 8-101) Nevi (see Fig. 8-104) Lentigines (see Fig. 8-101) Dermatofibromas (see Fig. 8-48)
Tannish-yellow	Xanthomata (see Figs. 14-12 to 14-15) Xanthelasma (see Fig. 14-18) Warts (see Fig. 8-26A) Keloids (see Fig. 8-103)
Dark blue or black	Seborrheic keratoses (see Fig. 8-101) Hemangiomas (see Figs. 24-8 and 24-9) Blue nevi (see Fig. 8-104) Dermatofibromas (see Fig. 8-48)

Table 8–5 Allergens Associated with Contact Dermatitis

Location	Possible Allergen
Scalp	Hair dyes Shampoos Tonics
Eyelids	Eye makeup Hair sprays
Neck	Aftershave lotions Perfumes Soaps Washing agents Nickel jewelry
Trunk	Clothing Washing agents
Axillae	Deodorants Soaps
Genitalia	Soaps Contraceptives Deodorants Washing agents
Feet	Shoes Sneakers Deodorants Socks Washing agents
Hands	Nickel jewelry Soaps Dyes Plants

Table 8–6 Important Differences Between Chickenpox and Smallpox

Characteristics	Chickenpox	Smallpox
Onset of symptoms	Begin with rash	Begin 2-4 days before rash
Rash	Evenly distributed all over body	More dense on face, head, arms, and legs (centrifugal distribution)
Presence on palms and soles	Almost never	Common
Development into other lesions	Rapidly into vesicles (less than 24 hours)	Slowly into pustules (7-14 days)
Time frame of lesions	New lesions form and scab at different times	Lesions form and go through their stages at the same time
Nature of lesions	Pruritic but relatively soft	Painful and hard
Patient appears extremely ill and moribund	Rarely	Commonly

Useful Vocabulary

Listed here are the specific roots that are important to understand the terminology related to diseases of the skin.

Root	Pertaining to	Example	Definition
kerat(o)-	horny	***kerat*oma**	Horny growth
derm(a)-	skin	***derma*titis**	Inflammation of the skin
trich(o)-	hair	***trich*oid**	Resembling hair
seb(o)-	sebum	***sebo*rrhea**	Excess flow of sebum
hidr(o)-	sweat	***hidr*adenitis**	Inflammation of sweat glands
onych(o)-	nails	***onycho*mycosis**	Disease of the nails caused by fungus

Writing Up the Physical Examination

Listed here are examples of the writeup for the examination of the skin.

- There are oval plaques with well-defined borders and silvery scales symmetrically present on the elbows, knees, scalp, and gluteal cleft. The plaques in the scalp are along the hairline. The scales are large. Examination of the nails reveals pitting of the nail plates. The hair is of normal texture.
- There is an annular lesion 3-4 cm in diameter on the right forearm. Scale is present on the narrow (1- to 2-mm), raised, erythematous border. The central area is slightly hypopigmented. The hair and nails are unremarkable.
- There is a linear bullous eruption along the lateral aspect of the left leg. The eruption consists of bright red edematous papules and bullae. There are no lesions on the palms or soles or in the mouth.
- A wide variety of lesions are seen on the face, shoulders, and back. The predominant lesions are pustules on an inflammatory base. Many pustules are present, and several have become confluent over the chin and forehead. Open and closed comedones are present on the face, especially along the nasolabial folds. Inflammatory papules are present on the lower cheeks and chin. Large abscesses and ulcerated cysts are present over the upper shoulder areas. Numerous scars are present over the face and upper back.
- A diffuse erythematous maculopapular rash is present on the trunk. Some excoriations are present over the shoulders and chest. The hair and nails are unremarkable.
- Examination of the skin reveals several types of lesions. The main lesions are small papules in the antecubital and popliteal fossae. The papules in some areas have become confluent, and plaques are present. On the dorsum of the feet, eczema is present with erythema, weeping, crusting, and scaling. Lichenification of the anogenital area, especially the scrotum, is present.
- The skin is slightly cool and dry. Scattered lentigines are present over the trunk. The hair is very fine and soft. There is loss of the lateral one third of the eyebrows. No nail abnormalities are present.

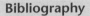

Bibliography

Adams RM: Occupational Skin Disease, 3rd ed. Philadelphia, WB Saunders, 1999.

Ali I, Dawber R: Hirsutism: Diagnosis and management. Hosp Med 65:293, 2004.

Aly R, Maibach HI: Atlas of Infections of the Skin. New York, Churchill Livingstone, 1999.

Callen JP, Paller AS, Greer KE, et al: Color Atlas of Dermatology, 2nd ed. Philadelphia, WB Saunders, 2000.

Cancer Facts & Figures. Atlanta, American Cancer Society, 2007.

DevCan: Probability of developing or dying of cancer software, version 5.1. Statistical Research and Applications Branch, National Cancer Institute, 2003. Available at *http://srab.cancer.gov/devcan*; accessed June 6, 2008.

Fawcett RS, Linford S, Stulberg DL: Nail abnormalities: Clues to systemic disease. Am Fam Physician 69:1417, 2004.

Freedberg IM, Eisen AZ, Wolff K, et al (eds): Fitzpatrick's Dermatology in General Medicine, 5th ed. New York, McGraw-Hill, 1999.

Friedman-Kien AE, Cockerell CJ: Color Atlas of AIDS, 2nd ed. Philadelphia, WB Saunders, 1996.

Habif TP: Clinical Dermatology: A Color Guide to Diagnosis and Therapy, 4th ed. Philadelphia, Mosby, 2004.

Hordinsky MK, Sawaya ME, Scher RK: Atlas of Hair and Nails. Philadelphia, Churchill Livingstone, 2000.

Jemel A, Tiwari R, Murray T, et al: Cancer Statistics, 2004. CA Cancer J Clin 54:8, 2004.

Jordan RE: Atlas of Bullous Disease. New York, Churchill Livingstone, 2000.

Lebwohl MG: Atlas of the Skin and Systemic Disease. New York, Churchill Livingstone, 1995.

Mandell GL, Fekety R (eds): Atlas of Infectious Diseases, vol 8: External Manifestations of Systemic Infections. Philadelphia, Churchill Livingstone, 1997.

Mandell GL, Mildvan D (eds): Atlas of Infectious Diseases, vol 1: AIDS, 2nd ed. Philadelphia, Churchill Livingstone, 1997.

Nadelman RB, Wormer GP: Lyme borreliosis. Lancet 352:557, 1998.

Safai B, Johnson KG, Myskowski PL, et al: The natural history of Kaposi's sarcoma in the acquired immunodeficiency syndrome. Ann Intern Med 103:744, 1985.

Stone DR, Gorbach SL: Atlas of Infectious Diseases. Philadelphia, WB Saunders, 2000.

CHAPTER 9

The Head and Neck

A lady, aged twenty, became affected with some symptoms which were supposed to be hysterical .... After she had been in this nervous state about three months it was observed that her pulse had become singularly rapid .... She next complained of weakness on exertion and began to look pale and thin .... It was observed that the eyes assumed a singular appearance, for the eyeballs were apparently enlarged. In a few months ... a tumour, of a horseshoe shape, appeared on the front of the throat and exactly in the situation of the thyroid gland.

Robert James Graves (1796–1853)

General Considerations

The appearance of the head and face, their contours and texture, often provides the first insight into the nature of illness. Sunken cheeks, wasting of the temporal muscles, and flushing of the face are important visible clues of systemic illness. Some facial appearances are pathognomonic of disease. The pale, puffy face of nephritis, the startled expression of hyperthyroidism, and the immobile stare of parkinsonism are examples of classic facies.

The appearance of the patient's face may also provide information regarding psychologic makeup: is the person happy, sad, angry, or anxious?

Thyroid disease takes many forms. The World Health Organization estimates that more than 200 million people in the world have enlarged thyroid glands, a condition known as *goiter*. Asians first described goiter around 1500 BCE. Even at that time, they recognized that seaweed in the diet tended to make goiters smaller. Iodine was not discovered until the 19th century, but it is now believed that those goiters were related to an iodine deficiency that was partially corrected by the iodine in the seaweed.

The ancient Greeks and Romans recognized that when a thin thread tied around the neck of a newly married woman broke, she was pregnant. This was caused by an increase in the size of the thyroid during pregnancy.

Thyroid cancer is the most common endocrine cancer, and its incidence has increased by about 3% per 100,000 people per year. In 2007, there were 33,550 new cases of thyroid cancer, with 1530 deaths related to it (650 men and 880 women). Of these new cases, about 8070 occurred in men and 25,480 occurred in women.

In the United States, cancer of the head and neck constitutes approximately 5% of all malignancies in men and 3% in women. Head and neck cancer includes cancers of the mouth, nose, sinuses, salivary glands, throat, and lymph nodes in the neck. Most begin in the moist tissues that line the mouth, nose, and throat. Symptoms include a lump or sore in the mouth that does not heal, a persistent sore throat, trouble swallowing, or a change or hoarseness in the voice. Using tobacco or alcohol increases the risk of developing head and neck cancer. In fact, 85% of all head and neck cancers are linked to tobacco use. If found early, these cancers may be curable. Treatment can include surgery, radiation therapy, chemotherapy, or a combination, but these treatments may affect eating, speaking, or even breathing.

In 2007, there were 34,360 (24,180 men and 10,180 women) new cases of head and neck cancer and 7550 related deaths. It has been estimated that nearly 90% of these cases are associated with poor dental hygiene, tobacco use, exposure to nickel, and alcohol use. Tobacco, whether chewed, smoked, or simply kept in the buccal pouch, predisposes an individual to tumors of the upper aerodigestive tract. Pipe smokers and tobacco chewers are at risk for tumors of the oral cavity, and the Chinese are at risk for nasopharyngeal carcinomas. On the basis of rates from 2002 to 2004, it is estimated that 1.02% of both sexes born in 2007 in the United States will receive diagnoses of cancer of the oral cavity and pharynx at some time during their lifetime.

Structure and Physiology

The Head

The skull is composed of 22 bones, 14 in the face alone. This bony structure acts as a support and protection for the softer tissues within.

The *facial skeleton* is composed of the mandible, the maxilla, and the nasal, palatine, lacrimal, and vomer bones. The unpaired *mandible* forms the lower jaw. The *maxilla* is an irregular bone and forms the upper jaw on each side. The *nasal bones* form the bridge of the nose. The other bones are not relevant to this discussion.

The main bones of the *cranial skeleton* include the frontal, temporal, parietal, and occipital bones. The *frontal bones* form the forehead. The *temporal bones* form the anterolateral walls of the brain. The *mastoid process*, which is part of the temporal bone, is particularly important in ear disease and is discussed in Chapter 11, The Ear and Nose. The *parietal bones* form the top and posterolateral portions of the skull. The *occipital bones* form the posterior portion of the skull. The bones of the face and skull are shown in Figure 9-1.

The principal muscle of the mouth is the *orbicularis oris*. This single muscle surrounds the lips, and numerous other facial muscles insert into it. The action of the orbicularis oris is to close the lips.

The *orbicularis oculi* muscle surrounds the eye. Its function is to close the eyelids. This muscle and its action are further discussed in Chapter 10, The Eye.

The *platysma* is a thin, superficial muscle of the neck, crossing the outer border of the mandible and extending over the lower anterior portion of the face. The main action of the platysma is to pull the mandible downward and backward, which results in a mournful facial expression.

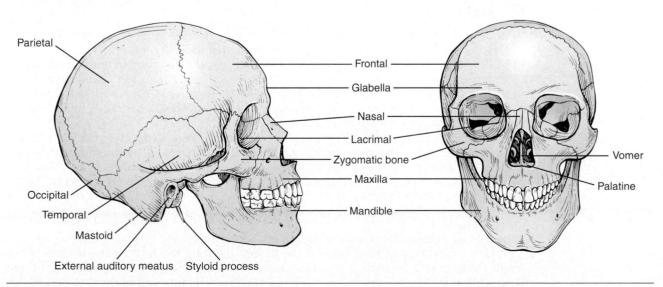

Figure 9–1 Bones of the face and skull.

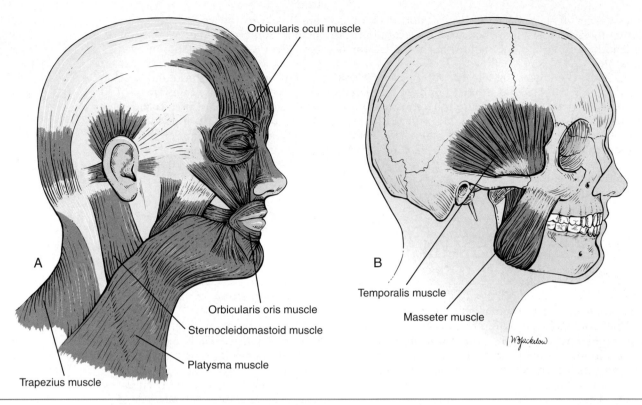

Figure 9–2 Muscles of the face and skull. *A,* The more superficial muscles. *B,* The underlying muscles.

The muscles of mastication include the masseter, pterygoid, and temporalis. These muscles insert on the mandible and effect chewing. The *masseter* is strong and thick and is one of the most powerful muscles of the face. The action of the masseter is to close the jaw by elevating and drawing the mandible backward. Tension in the masseter may be felt by clenching the jaw. Although important to jaw function, the other muscles of mastication are not clinically relevant to physical diagnosis and are not discussed here. The locations of these muscles are shown in Figure 9-2.

The *trigeminal,* or fifth cranial, nerve carries sensory fibers from the face, oral cavity, and teeth and carries efferent motor fibers to the muscles of mastication. The major divisions of this nerve are discussed in subsequent chapters.

The Neck

The neck is divided by the sternocleidomastoid muscle into the anterior, or medial, triangle and the posterior, or lateral, triangle. These are illustrated in Figure 9-3.

The *sternocleidomastoid* is a strong muscle that serves to raise the sternum during respiration. The sternocleidomastoid has two heads: The *sternal* head arises from the manubrium sterni, and the *clavicular* head originates on the sternal end of the clavicle. The two heads unite and insert on the lateral aspect of the mastoid process. The sternocleidomastoid is innervated by the *spinal accessory,* or eleventh cranial, nerve.

Anterior to the sternocleidomastoid muscle is the *anterior triangle.* The other boundaries of the anterior triangle are the clavicle inferiorly and the midline anteriorly. The anterior triangle contains the thyroid gland, larynx, pharynx, lymph nodes, submandibular salivary gland, and fat.

The *thyroid gland* envelops the upper trachea and consists of two lobes connected by an isthmus. It is the largest endocrine gland in the body. As seen from the front, the thyroid is butterfly shaped and wraps around the anterior and lateral portions of the larynx and trachea, shown in Figure 9-4.

The thyroid isthmus lies across the trachea just below the cricoid cartilage of the larynx. The lateral lobes extend along both sides of the larynx, reaching the level of the middle of the thyroid cartilage of the larynx. On occasion, the thyroid gland may extend downward and enlarge within the thorax, producing a substernal goiter. The function of the thyroid gland is to produce thyroid hormone in accordance with the needs of the body.

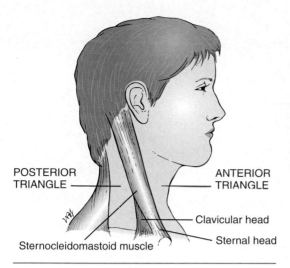

POSTERIOR
TRIANGLE

ANTERIOR
TRIANGLE

Clavicular head

Sternal head

Sternocleidomastoid muscle

Figure 9–3 Boundaries of the triangles of the neck.

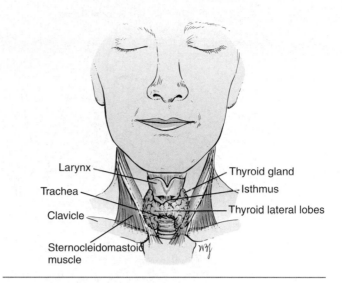

Larynx

Trachea

Clavicle

Sternocleidomastoid
muscle

Thyroid gland

Isthmus

Thyroid lateral lobes

Figure 9–4 Thyroid gland.

The pharynx and larynx are discussed in Chapter 12, The Oral Cavity and Pharynx.

The sternocleidomastoid muscle overlies the *carotid sheath*. The carotid sheath lies lateral to the larynx. This sheath contains the common carotid artery, the internal jugular vein, and the vagus nerve.

Posterior to the sternocleidomastoid is the *posterior triangle*. This is bounded by the trapezius muscle posteriorly and by the clavicle inferiorly. The posterior triangle also contains lymph nodes.

It has been estimated that the neck contains more than 75 lymph nodes on each side. The chains of these lymph nodes are named for their location. Starting posteriorly, they are the *occipital, posterior auricular, posterior cervical, superficial and deep cervical* (adjacent to the sternocleidomastoid muscle), *tonsillar, submaxillary, submental* (at the tip of the jaw in the midline), *anterior auricular,* and *supraclavicular* (above the clavicle) chains. Knowledge of the lymphatic drainage is important because the presence of an enlarged lymph node may signal disease in the area draining into it. The main groups of lymph nodes and their drainage areas are shown in Figure 9-5.

Review of Specific Symptoms

The most common symptoms related to the neck are as follows:

- Neck mass
- Neck stiffness

Neck Mass

The most common symptom is a lump or swelling in the neck. Once a patient complains of a neck lump, ask the following questions:

"When did you first notice the lump?"

"Does it hurt?"

"Does the lump change in size?"

"Have you had any ear infections? Infections in your mouth?"

"Has there been hoarseness associated with the mass?"

"Is there a family history of thyroid cancer?"

"Is there a history of prior neck or thyroid gland radiation?"

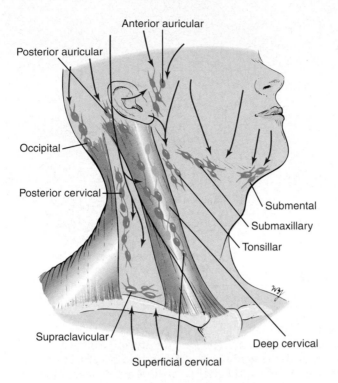

Figure 9–5 Lymph nodes of the neck and their drainage.

If there is associated pain with a mass in the neck, an acute infection is likely. Masses that have been present for only a few days are commonly inflammatory, whereas those present for months are more likely to be neoplastic. A mass that has been present for months to years without any change in size often turns out to be a benign or congenital lesion. Blockage of a salivary gland duct may produce a mass that fluctuates in size while the patient eats.

The *age of the patient* is relevant in the assessment of a neck mass. A lump in the neck of a patient younger than 20 years of age may be an enlarged tonsillar lymph node or a congenital mass. If the mass is in the midline, it is likely to be a thyroglossal cyst.*

From the ages of 20 to 40 years, thyroid disease is more common, although lymphoma must always be considered. When a patient is older than 40 years of age, a neck mass must be considered malignant until proved otherwise.

The *location* of the mass is also important. Midline masses tend to be benign or congenital lesions, such as thyroglossal cysts or dermoid cysts. Lateral masses are frequently neoplastic. Masses located in the lateral upper neck may be metastatic lesions from tumors of the head and neck, whereas masses in the lateral lower neck may be metastatic from tumors of the breast and stomach. One benign lateral neck mass is a branchial cleft cyst, which may manifest as a painless neck mass near the anterior upper third border of the sternocleidomastoid muscle.

Hoarseness associated with a thyroid nodule is suggestive of vocal cord paralysis resulting from impingement of the recurrent laryngeal nerve by tumor.

Neck Stiffness

Stiffness of the neck is usually caused by spasm of the cervical muscles and is commonly the cause of tension headache. The sudden occurrence of stiff neck, fever, and headache should raise suspicion of possible meningeal irritation. Neck pain may be associated with

---

*A thyroglossal cyst may arise anywhere along the route of the thyroid gland's descent from the foramen cecum of the tongue to its adult location in the neck. See Figure 24-41. The thyroid gland is a painless, mobile structure that moves on swallowing or with movement of the tongue.

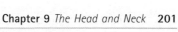

referred pain from the chest. Patients with angina or a myocardial infarction may complain of neck pain.

Impact of Head and Neck Disease on the Patient

The concept of body image is important. The head and neck are the most visible portions of the body. The shape of the eyes, mouth, face, and nose is very important to people. Many dislike their body image and want to change it by cosmetic surgery. Others require cosmetic surgery to repair alterations caused by trauma. Still others suffer from disfiguring head and neck cancer and need to undergo surgical procedures for the removal of these lesions. Many of these procedures are themselves mutilating.

Distortion of the body image, especially on the head and neck, can have a devastating effect on the patient. The most common reaction to head and neck disease is depression. Many affected patients suffer from feelings of sadness and hopelessness. They look in the mirror hoping that someday they will see themselves with a more acceptable body image. Recurrent thoughts of suicide are common. Many of these depressed patients turn to alcohol or other drugs.

On occasion, patients who have undergone cosmetic surgery are dissatisfied with the results. Many of these patients are trying to escape from feelings of inferiority and social maladjustment. They may have had only minor defects, but they viewed those defects as a major source of their interpersonal problems. Cosmetic surgery is a way to change their image in the hope of improving their social maladjustment. Some individuals may even blame their physicians for "destroying" their faces. Even after further revisions, these patients may never be satisfied. One of the keys to successful cosmetic surgery is the proper psychological evaluation of patients.

Physical Examination

No special equipment is needed for the examination of the head and neck. It is performed with the patient seated, facing the examiner. The examination consists of the following steps:

- Inspection
- Auscultation for carotid bruits (discussed in Chapter 15, The Peripheral Vascular System)
- Palpation

Inspection

Inspect the position of the head. Does the patient hold the head erect? Is there any asymmetry of the facial structure? Is the head in proportion to the rest of the body?

Inspect the scalp for lesions. Describe the hair.

Are any masses present? If so, describe their size, consistency, and symmetry. Figure 24-41 depicts a child with a midline *thyroglossal duct cyst*. This cyst results from failure of obliteration of the embryologic tract, along which the thyroid descends from the base of the tongue to the anterior neck, leaving active thyroid tissue along the path. The cyst is smooth, firm, and midline. When the patient is asked to swallow or stick out the tongue, the thyroglossal duct cyst moves upward.

Inspect the eyes for proptosis (a forward displacement, or bulging, of the eyeball). Proptosis may be caused by thyroid dysfunction or by a mass in the orbit.

Inspect the neck for areas of asymmetry. Ask the patient to extend the neck so that the neck can be inspected for scars, asymmetry, or masses. The normal thyroid is barely visible. Ask the patient to swallow while you observe any upward motion of the thyroid with swallowing. A diffusely enlarged thyroid gland often causes generalized enlargement of the neck. A patient with diffuse thyromegaly is pictured in Figure 9-6. This patient has Graves' disease with bilateral proptosis.

Is nodularity of the neck present? Nodular neck masses that are caused by a multinodular goiter are pictured in Figure 9-7.

Is superficial venous distention present? It is important to evaluate venous distention in the neck because it may be associated with a goiter.

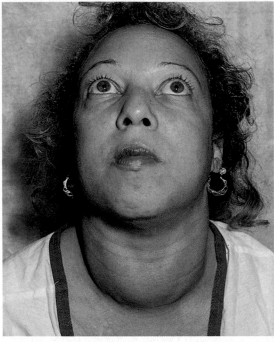

Figure 9–6 Graves' disease.

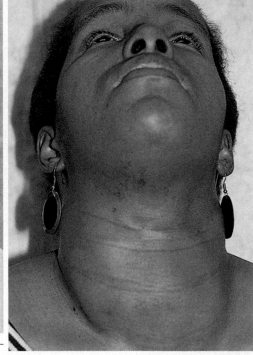

Figure 9–7 Multinodular goiter.

Palpation

Palpate the Head and Neck

Palpation confirms the information obtained by inspection. The patient's head should be slightly flexed and cradled in the examiner's hands, as demonstrated in Figure 9-8.

All areas of the cranium should be palpated for tenderness or masses. The pads of the examiner's fingers should roll the underlying skin over the cranium in circular motions to assess its contour and to feel for the presence of lymph nodes or masses. Starting from the occipital region, the examiner's hands are moved into the posterior auricular region, which is superficial to the mastoid process; down into the posterior triangle to feel for the posterior

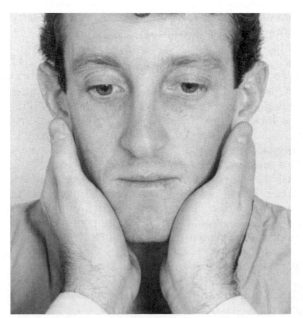

Figure 9–8 Palpation of the head and neck.

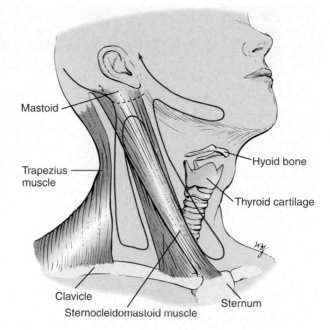

Figure 9–9 Suggested approach for palpation of the lymph nodes of the neck.

cervical chain; along the sternocleidomastoid muscle to feel for the superficial cervical chain; hooking around the sternocleidomastoid muscle to feel for the deep cervical chain deep to the muscle; into the anterior triangle region; up to the jaw margin to feel for the tonsillar group; along the jaw to feel the submaxillary chain; to the tip of the jaw for the submental nodes; and up to the anterior auricular chain in front of the ear. This sequence of examination is shown in Figure 9-9.

Enlarged posterior auricular and posterior cervical nodes are pictured in Figure 9-10.

Any nodes that are palpated should be observed for mobility, consistency, and tenderness. Tender lymph nodes are suggestive of inflammation, whereas fixed, firm nodes are consistent with a malignancy.

Palpate the Thyroid Gland

There are two approaches to palpating the thyroid gland. The anterior approach is carried out with the patient and examiner sitting face to face. By flexing the patient's neck or turning the chin slightly to the right, the examiner can relax the sternocleidomastoid muscle on that side, making the examination easier to perform. The examiner's left hand should displace the larynx to the left, and during swallowing, the displaced left thyroid lobe is palpated between the examiner's right thumb and the left sternocleidomastoid muscle. This is demonstrated in Figure 9-11.

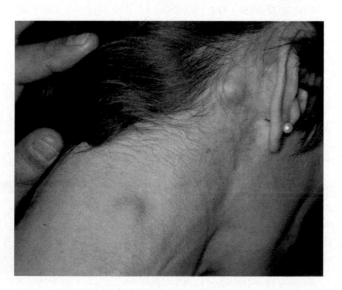

Figure 9–10 Posterior auricular and posterior cervical adenopathy.

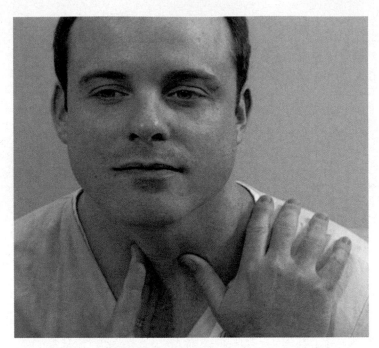

Figure 9–11 Anterior approach for palpation of the thyroid gland.

After the left lobe has been evaluated, the larynx is displaced to the right, and the right lobe is evaluated by reversing the hand positions.

At this point in the examination, the examiner should stand behind the patient to palpate the thyroid by the posterior approach. In this approach, the examiner places two hands around the patient's neck, which is slightly extended. The examiner uses the left hand to push the trachea to the right. The patient is asked to swallow while the examiner's right hand rolls over the thyroid cartilage. As the patient swallows, the examiner's right hand feels for the thyroid gland against the right sternocleidomastoid muscle. The patient is again asked to swallow as the trachea is pushed to the left, and the examiner uses his or her left hand to feel for the thyroid gland against the patient's left sternocleidomastoid muscle. The patient should be given water to drink, to facilitate swallowing. The posterior approach is shown in Figure 9-12.

Although both the anterior and the posterior approaches of palpation are usually performed, the examiner can rarely feel the thyroid gland in its normal state.

The consistency of the gland should be evaluated. The normal thyroid gland has a consistency of muscle tissue. Unusual *hardness* is associated with cancer or scarring. Softness, or sponginess, is often observed with a toxic goiter. *Tenderness* of the thyroid gland is associated with acute infections or with hemorrhage into the gland.

If the thyroid is enlarged, it should also be examined by auscultation. The bell of the stethoscope is placed over the lobes of the thyroid while the examiner listens for the presence of

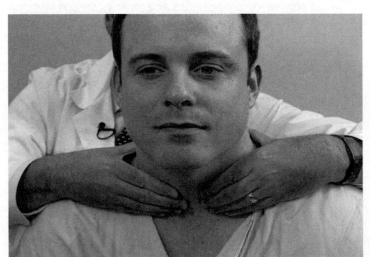

Figure 9–12 Posterior approach for palpation of the thyroid gland.

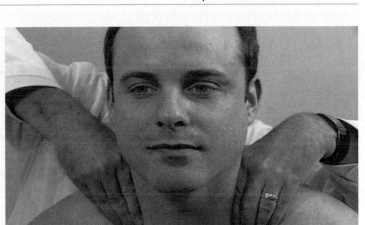

Figure 9–13 Technique for palpation of the supraclavicular lymph nodes.

a bruit (a murmur heard when there is increased turbulence in a vessel). The finding of a systolic or a to-and-fro* *thyroid bruit*, particularly if heard over the superior pole, indicates an abnormally large blood flow and is highly suggestive of a *toxic goiter*.

Palpate for Supraclavicular Nodes

Palpation for supraclavicular nodes concludes the examination of the head and neck. The examiner stands behind the patient and places the fingers into the medial supraclavicular fossae, deep to the clavicle and adjacent to the sternocleidomastoid muscles. The patient is instructed to take a deep breath while the examiner presses deeply in and behind the clavicles. Any supraclavicular nodes that are enlarged are palpated as the patient inspires. This technique is shown in Figure 9-13.

The examination of the trachea is discussed in Chapter 13, The Chest. The examination of the carotid arterial and jugular venous pulsations is discussed in Chapter 14, The Heart.

Clinicopathologic Correlations

Although iodine deficiency is still a worldwide cause of thyroid enlargement, other important causes of goiter are infection, autoimmune disease, cancer, and isolated nodules. An enlarged thyroid may be associated with *hyperthyroidism, hypothyroidism*, or a *simple* or *multinodular* goiter of normal function.

As mentioned earlier in this chapter, the thyroid may enlarge and expand into the chest cavity. If the thyroid is large enough, it may impair venous outflow from the head and neck and may even be responsible for airway or vascular compromise. Pemberton's sign is a useful maneuver for detecting latent obstruction in the thoracic inlet. To determine whether the sign is present, the patient is asked to elevate both arms until they touch the sides of the head. Facial suffusion with dilatation of the cervical veins that develops within a few seconds is Pemberton's sign, which means the test result is positive. After 1 to 2 minutes, the face may even become cyanotic. Figure 9-14 shows a patient with a positive Pemberton's sign. The patient is a 62-year-old man with an anterior neck mass, the existence of which was known for 25 years. The upper border of the thyroid was palpable on examination, but the lower pole descended below the clavicle and was not palpable.

As indicated in the quotation at the beginning of this chapter, hyperthyroidism may manifest with a variety of generalized symptoms and signs. It has been said, "To know thyroid disease is to know medicine," because there are so many generalized effects of thyroid hormone excess. Table 9-1 lists the variety of clinical symptoms related to thyroid hormone excess.

A nervous, perspiring patient with a stare and bulging eyes offers an unmistakable combination of physical signs associated with hyperthyroidism. The most common type of hyperthyroidism is the diffuse toxic goiter, known as Graves' disease. Symptomatic Graves' disease has an incidence of 1 per 1000 women in multinational studies. This disease can occur at any

---

*Refers to two separate murmurs, systolic and diastolic.

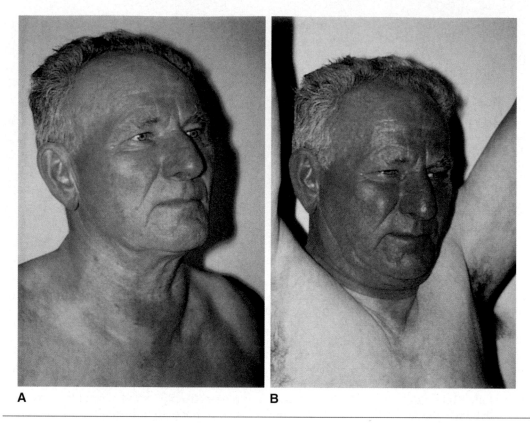

A   B

Figure 9–14 *A* and *B,* Pemberton's sign.

Table 9–1 Symptoms of Hyperthyroidism

Organ System	Symptom
General	Preference for the cold Weight loss with good appetite
Eyes	Prominence of eyeballs* Puffiness of eyelids Double vision Decreased motility
Neck	Goiter
Cardiac	Palpitations Peripheral edema[†]
Gastrointestinal	Increased numbers of bowel movements
Genitourinary	Polyuria Decreased fertility
Neuromuscular	Fatigue Weakness Tremulousness
Emotional	Nervousness Irritability
Dermatologic	Hair thinning Increased perspiration Change in skin texture Change in pigmentation

*Appears to result from mucopolysaccharide deposition behind the orbit.
[†]Appears to result from excessive mucopolysaccharide deposition under the skin, especially in the legs.

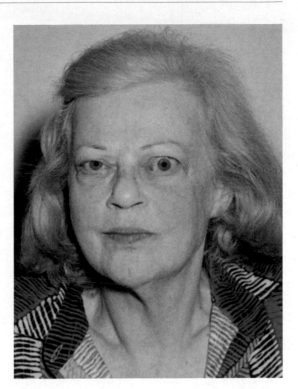

Figure 9–15 Graves' disease: unilateral proptosis.

age and in all races. Graves' disease is viewed as an autoimmune disorder provoked by the elaboration of a thyroid-stimulating immunoglobulin. The many clinical manifestations of Graves' disease are truly multisystemic and include the following:

- Warm, moist skin
- Hand tremor
- Erythema
- Easy fatigability
- Hyperhidrosis (increased sweating)
- Anxiety
- Insomnia
- Alopecia (hair loss)
- Hyperpigmentation
- Nail growth changes
- Palpitations
- Proptosis
- Lid retraction
- Gastroesophageal reflux
- Weight loss
- Increased bowel motility
- Amenorrhea
- Decreased libido
- Heat intolerance

On occasion, Graves' disease manifests with unilateral proptosis, as shown in Figure 9-15. This patient presented with proptosis and was treated for Graves' disease 20 years before this photograph was taken. As is common, the proptosis never disappeared.

Sometimes hyperthyroidism is caused by a single hot nodule.* Toxic adenomatous goiter, also known as *Plummer's disease*, accounts for fewer than 10% of all cases of hyperthyroidism.

---

*The terms hot and cold are descriptions of nodules seen on a thyroid scan and are used to indicate whether a nodule accumulates more or less radioactive iodine than the surrounding thyroid tissue. A hot nodule is functioning thyroid tissue and has a greater iodine uptake than the surrounding tissue. A cold nodule is nonfunctioning and fails to take up the radioactive tracer.

Table 9-2 Distinctive Features of Graves' Disease and Plummer's Disease

Feature	Graves' Disease (Toxic Diffuse Goiter*)	Plummer's Disease (Toxic Adenomatous Goiter†)
Age at onset	40 years	40 years
Onset	Acute	Insidious
Goiter	Diffuse	Nodular
Signs/symptoms	Clear-cut	Vague
Myopathy (muscle disease)	Present	Absent
Heart involvement	Sinus tachycardia Atrial fibrillation (occasional)	Atrial fibrillation (frequent) Congestive heart failure
Ophthalmopathy	Exophthalmos Vision changes Motility abnormalities Chemosis (conjunctival edema)‡	Eyelid lag Eyelid retraction

*See Figures 9-6 and 9-15.
†See Figure 9-7.
‡See Figure 10-40.

Hyperthyroidism may be caused by a single, autonomously functioning thyroid adenoma. The adenoma is usually papillary and is unrelated to any autoimmune process. Hyperfunction may also occur in multiple nodules. The distinctive features of hyperthyroidism caused by Graves' and Plummer's diseases are summarized in Table 9-2.

Approximately 5% of the population has a single thyroid nodule larger than 1 cm in diameter. Although most (90% to 95%) of these nodules are benign and necessitate no therapy, all should be investigated for malignancy. They develop from thyroid follicular cells and can be found in normal-sized thyroid glands and goiters. The history and physical examination can provide some clues as to the nature of the lump. Table 9-3 summarizes some of the important characteristics of benign and malignant nodules.

Many patients with thyroid cancer, especially in the early stages, do not experience any symptoms. As the cancer grows, symptoms may include a lump or nodule in the neck, hoarseness, difficulty in speaking, difficulty in swallowing, pain in the neck or throat, and swollen lymph nodes. Many symptoms and signs of thyroid disease have been evaluated for their sensitivity and specificity. Most of these findings are specific but are too insensitive to be useful. Table 9-4 summarizes the characteristics that are significant when a thyroid nodule is evaluated for malignancy. The most useful signs are a palpable, hard nodule and a fixed mass.

There are several types of thyroid cancer: papillary, follicular, medullary, and anaplastic. *Papillary* and *follicular carcinomas* are well differentiated and represent 80% to 90% of all thyroid cancers. Both types begin in the follicular cells of the thyroid. Papillary carcinomas

Table 9-3 Characteristics of Benign and Malignant Thyroid Nodules

Characteristic	Benign Nodule	Malignant Nodule
Age at onset	Adulthood	Adulthood
Predominant gender	Female	Male
Patient history	Symptoms present	Previous x-ray treatment to head or neck
Family history	Benign thyroid diseases	None
Speed of enlargement	Slow	Rapid
Change in voice	Absent	Present
Number of nodules	More than one	One
Lymph nodes	Absent	Present
Remainder of thyroid	Abnormal	Normal

Table 9–4 Characteristics of Thyroid Nodules Suspect for Cancer

Characteristic	Sensitivity (%)	Specificity (%)
Palpable, hard nodule	42	89
Fixed mass	31	94
Local symptoms	3	97
Dysphagia	10	93
Unilateral adenopathy	5	96
Nodule found on routine examination	50	56
Family history of goiter	17	79

Data from Kendall and Condon (1976) and Haff et al (1976).

are the most common (80% to 90% of all thyroid cancers). They typically grow very slowly. Usually they occur in only one lobe of the thyroid gland, but approximately 10% to 20% of the time both lobes are involved. Even though papillary thyroid cancer is slow growing, it often spreads early to the lymph nodes in the neck. Follicular cancer is much less common than papillary thyroid cancer, making up approximately 5% to 10% of all thyroid cancers. It tends to occur in older individuals, and it is more common in countries where people do not get enough iodine in their diet. If there is early detection, these cancers can be treated successfully. *Medullary thyroid carcinoma* (MTC) accounts for only 5% to 10% of all thyroid cancers. MTC is the only thyroid cancer that develops from the C cells, not the follicular cells, of the thyroid gland. There are two types of MTC: sporadic and familial. On occasion, MTC is associated with tumors of certain other organs (adrenal and parathyroid gland) and is called *multiple endocrine neoplasia type 2* (MEN 2), of which there are two subtypes: MEN 2a is associated with pheo-chromocytomas and parathyroid gland tumors; MEN 2b lacks the parathyroid gland tumors. Genetic studies should be performed on individuals with MTC. *Anaplastic thyroid carcinoma* is the least common of all thyroid cancers, accounting for 1% to 2%. It is also, however, the most aggressive type and therefore is the most difficult to control and treat.

A heavy, puffy-faced, lethargic patient with dry skin, sparse hair, and a hoarse voice provides the classic picture of hypothyroidism. Hypothyroidism develops insidiously. Often the only

Table 9–5 Symptoms and Signs of Hypothyroidism

System	Symptom	Sign
General	Weight gain with regular diet Feeling chilly while other people are warm	Obesity
Gastrointestinal	Constipation	Enlarged tongue
Cardiovascular	Fatigue	Hypotension Bradycardia
Nervous	Speech disorders Short attention span Tremor	Hyporeflexia Defective abstract reasoning Spasticity Tremor Depressed affect
Musculoskeletal	Lethargy Thickened, dry skin Hair loss Brittle nails Leg cramps Puffy eyelids Puffy cheeks	Hypotonia Puffy facies
Reproductive	Heavier menses Decreased fertility	

complaint is a tired or "run-down" feeling. The careful interviewer and examiner must be on the alert with any patient, especially one older than 60 years, who has these symptoms. Patients with hypothyroidism commonly have *hung*, or delayed, reflexes. Measurement of the relaxation time of the Achilles tendon reflex has long been used to monitor the effects of treatment in patients with hypothyroidism. However, it is useless as a screening technique because there may be many false-negative or false-positive results.

Table 9-5 lists some of the major symptoms and signs of hypothyroidism.

Useful Vocabulary

Listed here are the specific roots that are important for understanding the terminology related to diseases of the head and neck.

Root	Pertaining to	Example	Definition
capit-	head	**capit**ate	Head-shaped
cephal(o)-	head	**cephal**ometry	Measurement of the head
cleido-	clavicle	**cleido**mastoid	Pertaining to the clavicle and mastoid process
cranio-	skull	**cranio**malacia	Abnormal softening of the skull
occipito-	back portion of the skull	**occipito**parietal	Pertaining to the occipital and parietal bones
odont(o)-	tooth; teeth	**odont**orrhagia	Hemorrhage that follows tooth extraction
thyro-	thyroid gland	**thyro**megaly	Enlargement of the thyroid gland

Writing Up the Physical Examination

Listed here are examples of the write-up for the examination of the head, neck, and thyroid.

- The head is normocephalic without evidence of trauma. The neck is supple, with full range of motion. No adenopathy is present in the neck. The thyroid is nontender and is not enlarged. No thyroid nodules are felt.
- The head is normocephalic and atraumatic. There is a 2-cm, rubbery, nontender mass in the superficial cervical chain on the left side. The mass is freely mobile and is not fixed to the skin or underlying muscle. Another 4-cm, rubbery, nontender mass is felt in the right supraclavicular fossa. The thyroid is unremarkable.
- There is frontal bossing of the head with prominence of the cheek bones. There is no evidence of trauma. The neck is supple, with no adenopathy present. There is a 2-cm, soft, painless thyroid nodule felt 3 cm from the midline in the upper portion of the right lobe (at approximately the 10 o'clock position). The nodule is not fixed to the overlying skin or muscles.

Bibliography

Cancer Trends Progress Report—2007 Update. Bethesda, Md, National Cancer Institute, December 2007. Available at: *http://progressreport.cancer.gov*; accessed June 9, 2008.

Haff RC, Schecter BC, Armstrong RG, et al: Factors increasing the probability of malignancy in thyroid nodules. Am J Surg 131:707, 1976.

Jemel A, Tiwari R, Murray T, et al: Cancer Statistics, 2004. CA Cancer J Clin 54:8, 2004.

Kendall LW, Condon RE: Prediction of malignancy in solitary thyroid nodules. Lancet 1:1019, 1976.

King AD: Multimodality imaging of head and neck cancer. Cancer Imaging 7(Spec No A):S37, 2007.

Ries LAG, Melbert D, Krapcho M, et al: SEER Cancer Statistics Review, 1975–2004 [based on November 2006 Surveillance Epidemiology and End Results (SEER) data submission]. Bethesda, Md, National Cancer Institute. Available at: *http://seer.cancer.gov/csr/1975_2004/*, accessed June 9, 2007.

Wallace C, Siminoski K: The Pemberton sign. Ann Intern Med 125:568, 1996.

Werner JA: Patterns of metastasis in head and neck cancer. Cancer Treat Res 135:203, 2007.

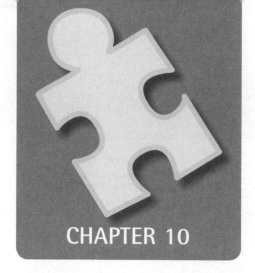

CHAPTER 10

The Eye

Who would believe that so small a space could contain the images of all the universe?
O mighty process!

Leonardo da Vinci (1452–1519)

Historical Considerations

The eyes are the human windows to the world. Most of the sensory input to the brain is through the eyes. For centuries, the eye has been considered the essence of the person, representing the "I." In mythology and the writings of ancient times, the eye is an organ associated with mystical powers.

The eye has long been associated with mythical gods. In ancient Egypt, the eye was the symbol of the Great Goddess. The Eye of Horus was believed to protect against all evil and to ensure success. The "evil eye" from the myth of Medusa was an expression of envy and greed (see Fig. 3-3).

Another interesting association is the subconscious linking of "eyeball" with genitalia. Blindness can symbolize castration because testicles and eyeballs have the same shape and are important in the development of the sense of identity. This linking goes back to the legend of Oedipus, who pierced his eyeballs when he discovered that he had been married to his mother and had killed his father. This can be thought of as an act of self-castration, as well as a means of cutting oneself off from all worldly relationships. Throughout literature, the blinding of an individual was frequently a form of punishment for lust. The age-old notion that masturbation causes blindness further reinforces this close association of organs.

Structure and Physiology

The external landmarks of the eye are shown in Figure 10-1, and the cross-sectional anatomy of the eye is shown in Figure 10-2.

The *eyelids* and *eyelashes* protect the eyes. The eyelids cover the globe and lubricate its surface. The *meibomian glands*, which are modified sebaceous glands in the eyelids, secrete an oily lubricating substance to retard evaporation. The openings of these glands are at the lid margins.

The *orbicularis oculi muscle* encircles the lids and is responsible for their closure. This muscle is supplied by the facial, or seventh cranial, nerve. The *levator palpebrae muscle* elevates the lids and is innervated by the oculomotor, or third cranial, nerve. Müller's muscle is a small part of the levator muscle that has sympathetic innervation.

The globe has six *extraocular muscles* that control its motion. There are four rectus and two oblique muscles: the medial rectus, the lateral rectus, the superior rectus, the inferior rectus,

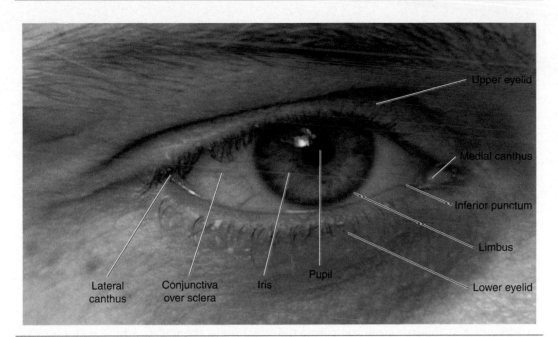

Figure 10–1 External landmarks of the eye.

the superior oblique, and the inferior oblique muscles. These six extraocular muscles are shown in Figure 10-3.

The extraocular muscles work in a parallel, conjugate manner to maintain single, binocular vision. When the head is turned to look left, for example, the *left lateral rectus* and the *right medial rectus* contract to turn the eyes to the left. The actions and innervations of the extraocular muscles are listed in Table 10-1, and the extraocular movements are illustrated in Figure 10-4.

The *lateral rectus muscle*, which is innervated by the *abducens nerve*, turns the eye laterally (*abducts* the eye), as do both oblique muscles.

The *conjunctiva* is a thin, vascular, transparent mucous membrane that lines the lids and the anterior portion of the globe continuously. The *palpebral* portion covers the inner surface of

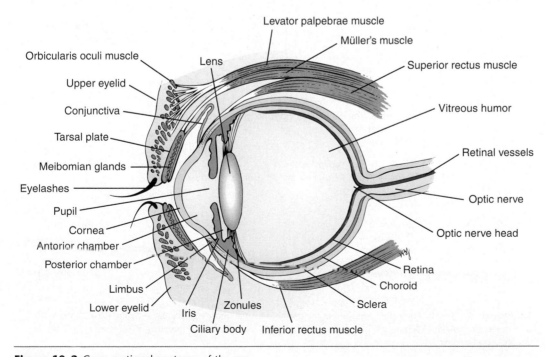

Figure 10–2 Cross-sectional anatomy of the eye.

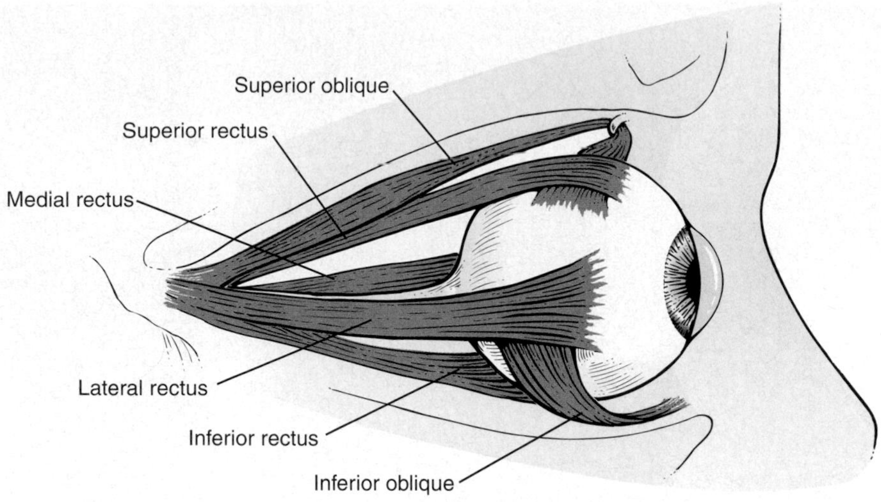

Figure 10–3 The extraocular muscles.

the lids, whereas the *bulbar* portion covers the sclera up to the *limbus*, which is the corneal-scleral junction. The conjunctiva contains many small blood vessels, which when dilated produce the appearance of a "red" eye. There is little nervous innervation to the conjunctiva.

The *lacrimal apparatus* consists of the lacrimal gland, accessory tear glands, canaliculi, tear sac, and nasolacrimal duct. These are shown in Figure 10-5.

The *lacrimal gland* produces watery tears and is located above and slightly lateral to the globe. Secretion occurs mostly as reflex tearing or crying. Tears drain through the *puncta* on the lids and into the superior and inferior *canaliculi*. These canaliculi join and enter the *tear sac*, located at the medial *canthus* of the eye. The *nasolacrimal duct* drains the sac to the nose. Of the lacrimal apparatus, only the *puncta* are visible on routine examination.

The *sclera* is the white, fibrous, outer coat of the globe visible just beneath the conjunctiva. The extraocular muscles insert into the sclera.

Table 10–1 Actions and Innervations of the Extraocular Muscles*

Muscle	Action	Cranial Nerve Innervation
Medial rectus	Adduction (eye moves nasally)	Oculomotor (III)
Lateral rectus	Abduction (eye moves temporally [away from the nose])	Abducens (VI)
Inferior rectus	Depression (eye moves down) Extorsion (the 12 o'clock position on the cornea rotates temporally) Adduction	Oculomotor (III)
Superior rectus	Elevation (eye moves up) Intorsion (the 12 o'clock position on the cornea rotates nasally) Adduction	Oculomotor (III)
Superior oblique	Intorsion Depression Abduction	Trochlear (IV)
Inferior oblique	Extorsion Elevation Abduction	Oculomotor (III)

*Remember "LR₆SO₄." This mnemonic means that the lateral rectus (LR) muscle is innervated by the sixth cranial nerve, and the superior oblique (SO) muscle is innervated by the fourth cranial nerve. All the other muscles are innervated by the third cranial nerve.

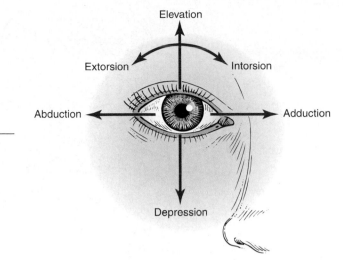

Figure 10–4 Extraocular movements.

The *cornea* is a smooth, transparent, avascular tissue that covers the iris and joins with the sclera and conjunctival reflection at the limbus. The cornea functions as a protective window, allowing light to pass into the eye. The cornea is richly innervated by the trigeminal, or fifth cranial, nerve and is therefore exquisitely sensitive to touch.

The *anterior chamber*, or space between the cornea anteriorly and the iris posteriorly, is filled with clear *aqueous humor*. Aqueous humor is produced by the *ciliary body* in the *posterior chamber*, the area behind the iris and in front of the lens. Aqueous humor circulates from the posterior chamber through the pupil into the anterior chamber and is removed through the *canal of Schlemm*, from where it eventually enters the venous system. Pressure within the eye is regulated by this filtration. The *angle* is that formed by the juncture of the cornea and the iris at the limbus. A section through the eye at this level is shown in Figure 10-6.

The *iris* is the circular, colored portion of the eye. The small, round aperture in the middle of the iris is the *pupil*. The pupil functions much like the aperture of a camera, controlling the amount of light that enters the eye.

When a light is shined on one eye, both pupils constrict consensually. This constriction is the *pupillary light reflex*. To understand this reflex, a brief review of the neuroanatomy is in order. Figure 10-7 illustrates the pathways of the pupillary light reflex.

The optic, or second cranial, nerves are composed of 80% *visual* and 20% afferent *pupillary* fibers. The optic nerves leave both retinas and travel a short course to where they join each other. This joining is the *optic chiasm*. At the optic chiasm, the nasal fibers cross and join the uncrossed fibers of the other side, forming the *optic tract*. The visual fibers continue in the optic tract to the *lateral geniculate body*, where synapses occur, the axons of which terminate

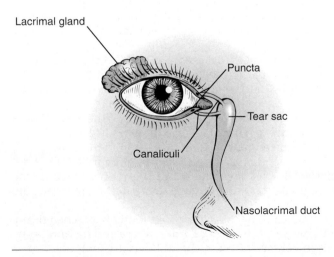

Figure 10–5 The lacrimal apparatus.

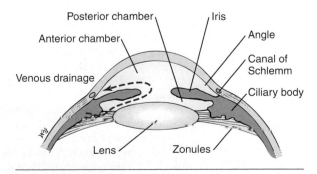

Figure 10–6 Cross section of the normal-angle structures, showing the flow of aqueous humor.

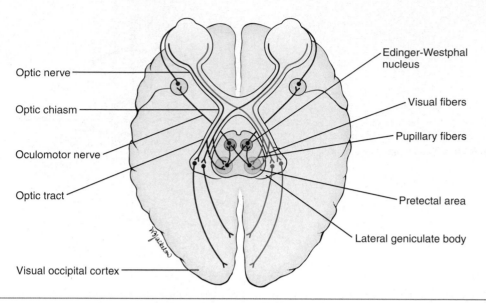

Figure 10–7 The pupillary light reflex.

in the primary visual cortex of the occipital lobe. The afferent pupillary fibers bypass the geniculate body and end in the *superior colliculus* and *pretectal* area of the midbrain.

Light impulses to the eye cause the retina to transmit nerve impulses to the optic nerve, the optic tract, the midbrain, and the visual cortex of the occipital lobes. This is the *afferent limb* of the light reflex. In the midbrain, the pupillary fibers diverge and are relayed by crossed fibers to the opposite *Edinger-Westphal* nucleus of the oculomotor, or third cranial, nerve. Some fibers remain on the same side. The third cranial nerve is the *efferent limb*, which goes via the ciliary body to the sphincter muscle of the iris to cause it to contract. The *direct effect* is the constriction of the pupil of the eye on which the light is shined (the *ipsilateral eye*). The *consensual effect* is the simultaneous constriction of the opposite pupil (the *contralateral eye*).

The *near reflex* occurs when the subject looks at a nearby target. The three parts of the near reflex are *accommodation, convergence,* and *pupillary constriction. Accommodation* is defined as the near focusing of the eye, which is effected by increasing the power of the lens by contraction of the ciliary muscle, innervated by the third cranial nerve.

There is also autonomic innervation of the eyes. The iris is supplied by sympathetic and parasympathetic fibers. When the sympathetic fibers are stimulated, the pupil dilates, and the eyelid elevates. Think of the cat stalking its prey, pupils dilated, ready to pounce in the dark. The cat needs all the light it can get. The reflex is purely sympathetic. When the parasympathetic fibers in the oculomotor nerve are stimulated, pupillary constriction occurs.

The *lens* sits directly behind the iris. It is a biconvex, avascular, colorless structure that changes its shape to focus the image on the retina. The shape is changed by the *ciliary body muscles.*

The *vitreous humor* is the transparent, avascular gel that is located behind the lens and in front of the retina. It occupies 80% of the volume of the eye. This clear matrix is made up of collagen, hyaluronic acid, and water. It is bounded by the posterior lens capsule anteriorly and the retina posteriorly.

The *choroid* is the middle, vascular layer of the globe between the sclera and the retina. It acts as a source of nourishment, as well as a heat sink, serving to remove the extreme heat produced by the light energy entering the eye. Bruch's membrane separates the choroid from the retina. Superficial to Bruch's membrane (closer to the retina) is the retinal pigment epithelium (RPE). The RPE is a monolayer of cells between Bruch's membrane and the retina. Some of the important functions of the RPE are to absorb light passing through the retina and to regenerate the visual pigments.

The *retina* is the innermost layer, or "camera film," of the eye. The retina is attached firmly to the underlying choroid at the optic nerve posteriorly and at the ora serrata anteriorly. Between these two points, the retina is in contact with the choroid, but it is not attached to it. The ora serrata is the junction of the retina and ciliary body. The retina is only 0.4 mm in

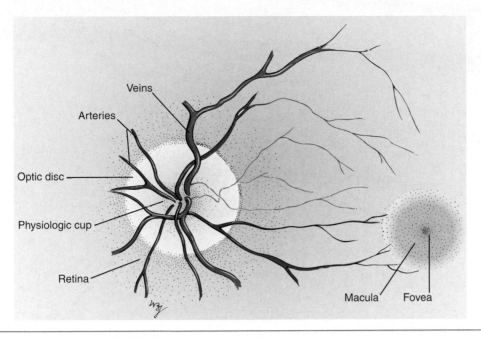

Figure 10–8 The retina of the left eye.

thickness and is thinnest in the region of the macula. Histologically, the retina is made up of 10 distinct layers. Basically, the retina senses light through the rods and cones in its outer layer (closest to the RPE), performs initial signal processing in its middle layer, and encodes and transmits the data in its inner layer, the nerve fiber layer. The nerve fiber layer is directly under the inner limiting membrane of the retina, the layer closest to the vitreous. These nerve fibers course along the inner portion of the retina and aggregate to form the optic nerve. On leaving the eye, the nerve fibers become myelinated.

Within the retina are several important structures: the optic disc, the retinal vessels, and the macula. Figure 10-8 illustrates the retina of the left eye.

The *optic disc* is located at the nasal aspect of the posterior pole of the retina. This is the head of the optic nerve, from where the nerve fibers of the retina exit the eye. The optic disc is 1.5 mm in diameter and is ovoid. It is lighter than the surrounding retina and appears yellowish-pink. The disc margins are sharp with some normal blurring of the nasal portion. African-American patients may have pigmentation at the margins. The *physiologic cup* is the center of the disc, where the retinal vessels penetrate. This small depression normally occupies about 30% of the disc diameter.

The *retinal vessels* emerge from the disc and arborize on the retinal surface. The arteries are brighter red and thinner than the veins. An artery-to-vein ratio of 2:3 is normal.

The *macula* is a small, round area, approximately the size of the disc, located 3.5 mm temporal to and 0.5 mm inferior to the disc. The macula is easily seen because it is devoid of retinal vessels. In the center of the macula is the *fovea*, a depressed area composed only of *cones*. Cones provide detailed vision and color perception.

The remaining areas of the retina contain mostly *rods*, which compose the other neurosensory element of the retina. The rods are responsible for motion detection and night vision. It should be remembered that the image on the retina is upside down and reversed left to right: The right world is projected on the left half of the retina, and the left world is projected on the right half of the retina. An image in the superior world strikes the inferior part of the retina, and an inferiorly positioned image strikes the superior part. This concept is illustrated in Figure 10-9.

At birth, there is little pigment in the iris, which is why all infants are born with blue eyes. By 6 months of age, the pigmentation is completed. The lens is more spherical at birth than in later life. Most infants are born hyperopic (farsighted). By 3 months after birth, the medullation process of the optic nerve is completed. As the child grows, hyperopia increases until the age of 8 years and then gradually decreases. After age 8, myopia (nearsightedness) appears to increase.

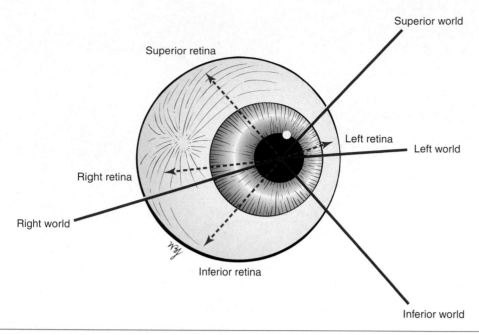

Figure 10–9 How images strike the retina.

With advancing age, there is the gradual loss of elasticity of the skin around the eyes. The cornea may show an infiltration of degenerative material around the limbus, which is known as an *arcus senilis.* The lens consistency changes from plastic to rigid, making it progressively more difficult to change its shape to focus on near objects. This condition is *presbyopia.* The lens may undergo changes resulting from metabolic disorders that cause its opacification; this condition is called a *cataract.* The vitreous humor may develop condensations, called *floaters.* The retinal arteries may develop *atherosclerosis,* with resultant retinal ischemia or infarction.

Review of Specific Symptoms

The major symptoms of eye disease are the following:

- Loss of vision
- Eye pain
- Diplopia (double vision)
- Tearing or dryness
- Discharge
- Redness

Loss of Vision

When a patient complains of loss of vision, the following two questions must be asked:

"Did the loss of vision occur suddenly?"

"Is the eye painful?"

It is extremely important to ascertain the acuteness of the loss of vision and the presence or absence of pain. Sudden, painless loss of vision may result from a retinal vascular occlusion or a retinal detachment. Sudden, painful loss of vision occurs in attacks of acute narrow-angle glaucoma. Gradual, painless loss of vision commonly occurs in chronic simple glaucoma.

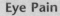

Eye Pain

Eye pain may result from a variety of causes. Ask the patient the following questions:

"Can you describe the pain?"

"Did the pain come on suddenly?"

"Does the light bother your eye?"

"Do you have pain when you blink?"

"Do you have the sensation of something in the eye?"

"Do you have headaches?"

"Do you have pain on movement of the eye?"

"Do you have pain over the brow on the same side?"

"Do you wear contact lenses?"

Pain may be experienced as "burning," "aching," "throbbing," "tenderness," or pain behind the eye. Each of these descriptions may have a range of causes. It is important to determine whether the patient has the sensation of a foreign body in the eye. Pain in the eye while blinking occurs in corneal abrasions and with foreign bodies in the eye. *Photophobia* is eye pain associated with light, as seen in inflammations of the *uveal tract* (i.e., iris, ciliary body, or choroid). Inflammations of the conjunctiva, *conjunctivitis*, produce a gritty sensation. Diseases of the cornea are associated with significant pain because the cornea is so richly innervated. Headaches and eye pain are common in acute narrow-angle glaucoma. Pain on motion of the eye occurs in optic neuritis. Eye pain associated with brow or temporal pain may be an indication of temporal arteritis (see Chapter 25, The Geriatric Patient). Contact lens wearers may have corneal irritation and may complain of eye pain.

Diplopia

Diplopia, or double vision, is a common complaint. Diplopia results from a faulty alignment of the eyes. Normally, when the eyes fixate on an object, the object is seen clearly, despite the fact that the two retinal images are not exactly superimposed. These slightly different images, however, are fused by the brain; it is this fusion that produces *binocular vision*, or the perception of depth. When the eyes are misaligned, the two images fall on different parts of the retinas, only one falling normally on the fovea. The field of vision of the deviated eye is different, so that its image is not projected on its fovea; therefore, this second image is different and not superimposable. The patient may close one eye to relieve this distressing situation. A compensatory head posture may be used by the patient to relieve the double vision (see Fig. 10-146). Elevation or depression of the patient's chin is used to overcome a vertical deviation. Tilting of the head is often used to counteract the torsional and vertical deviation. Suggested questions for the patient with diplopia are listed in Chapter 21, The Nervous System.

Tearing or Dryness

Excessive tearing or dryness of the eyes is a common complaint. Abnormal tearing may be caused either by overproduction of tears or by an obstruction of outflow. Dryness results from faulty secretion by the lacrimal or accessory tear glands. A common cause is *Sjögren's syndrome*, which is generalized failure of the secretory glands. This syndrome is associated with a variety of disease states.

Discharge

Discharge from the eye can be watery, mucoid, or purulent. A watery or mucoid discharge is often associated with allergic or viral conditions, whereas a purulent discharge occurs in association with bacterial infections.

Redness

The symptom of the red eye is very common. The interviewer should ask the following questions:

"Have you had any injury to the eye?"

"Does anyone else in the family have a red eye?"

"Have you had any recent coughing spells? vomiting?"

"Have you had any associated eye pain?"

"Does light bother your eyes?"

"Is there any associated discharge?"

"Do you wear contact lenses?"

The eye may appear bloodshot. Redness may result from trauma, infection, allergy, or increased pressure in the eye. Severe coughing spells or recurrent vomiting may cause a patient to have a conjunctival hemorrhage. A family member or friend with viral conjunctivitis may be the source of a patient's red eye. The combination of eye pain and red eye may indicate acute narrow-angle glaucoma. (Table 10-2 summarizes the differential diagnosis for the red eye.) Uveitis, inflammation of the uveal tract, which is associated with a red eye, can manifest with light sensitivity. Patients wearing contact lenses may suffer from corneal irritation and may have eye redness.

General Suggestions

It is important to determine the medications that a patient is taking, because many drugs have deleterious effects on the eye. Some antimalarial, antituberculous, antiglaucoma, and anti-inflammatory drugs can cause eye disorders. A thorough family history reveals familial disease tendencies such as glaucoma, cataracts, retinal degeneration, strabismus, or corneal dystrophies.

There are many specific symptoms related to eye disease. The common visual, nonvisual but painful, and nonvisual and painless symptoms and some possible causes are listed in Tables 10-3, 10-4, and 10-5, respectively.

Impact of Blindness on the Patient

The loss of sight is a terrifying experience. The sighted person lives mostly in a visual and auditory world illuminated by lights and colors. When blindness occurs, the person loses not only the ability to see but the perceptual center of the world. This center must now be replaced by hearing and touch. Because light is often equated with life, the inability to see light is associated with death. The newly blinded patient must take a new place in society. He or she can no longer read ordinary books, can no longer receive visual stimuli, and is unable to appreciate the world of visual communication. This can result in a reactive depression. The clinician must show genuine care for blind patients and try to understand their feelings of discouragement and despair.

The person who is blind from birth or early childhood has little or no conception of the visual world. Having never been able to see, this patient has no visual frame of reference.

On occasion, a blind individual recovers sight as a result of a surgical procedure later in life. Many difficulties may arise owing to the reorganization of the patient's perception. His or her frame of reference has been shifted from touch to sight. Surprisingly, many of these patients become depressed after attaining vision. Facial expressions mean nothing because only with experience can people understand them. The following quote from a case history by Gregory and Wallace illustrates the response of such an individual:

> *He suffered one of the greatest hardships (blindness) and yet he lived with energy and enthusiasm. When his handicap was apparently swept away, as by a miracle, he lost his peace and self-respect.*

Similarly, the patient with normal vision may develop psychosomatic eye problems as a result of anxiety. Loss of vision also can accompany panic disorders. Such individuals can have either

Table 10–2 Differential Diagnosis for Red Eye*

Manifestation	Acute Conjunctivitis†	Acute Iritis‡	Narrow-Angle Glaucoma	Corneal Abrasion
History	Sudden onset Exposure to conjunctivitis	Fairly sudden onset Often recurrent	Rapid onset Sometimes history of attack Highest incidence among Jews, Swedes, and the Inuit	Trauma Pain
Vision	Normal	Impaired if untreated	Rapidly lost if untreated§	Can be affected if central
Pain	Gritty feeling	Photophobia	Severe	Exquisite
Bilaterality	Frequent	Occasional	Occasional	Usually unilateral
Vomiting	Absent	Absent	Common	Absent
Cornea	Clear (epidemic keratoconjunctivitis has corneal deposits)	Variable	"Steamy" (like looking through a steamy window)	Irregular light reflex
Pupil	Normal, reactive	Sluggishly reactive Sometimes irregular in shape	Partially dilated, oval, nonreactive	Normal, reactive
Iris	Normal	Normal¶	Difficult to see, owing to corneal edema	Shadow of corneal defect may be projected on the iris with penlight
Ocular discharge	Mucopurulent or watery	Watery	Watery	Watery or mucopurulent
Systemic effect	None	Few	Many	None
Prognosis	Self-limited	Poor if untreated	Poor if untreated	Good if not infected

*See Figure 10-88.
†Can be viral, bacterial, or allergic.
‡See Figure 10-63.
§Seeing "rainbow" can be an early symptom during an acute attack.
¶Slit-lamp examination revealing cells in anterior chamber is diagnostic.

partial or complete vision loss in one or both eyes. Supportive care of the primary problem usually results in the return of vision.

Physical Examination

The equipment necessary for the examination of the eye is as follows: an ophthalmoscope, a penlight, a pocket visual acuity card, and a 3 × 5 inch (7.6 × 12.7 cm) card.

The physical examination of the eye includes the following:

- Visual acuity
- Visual fields
- Ocular movements
- External and internal eye structures
- Ophthalmoscopic examination

Visual Acuity

Visual acuity is expressed as a ratio, such as 20/20. The first number is the distance at which the patient reads the chart. The second number is the distance at which a person with normal

Table 10–3 Common Visual Eye Symptoms and Disease States

Visual Symptom	Possible Causes
Loss of vision	Optic neuritis Detached retina Retinal hemorrhage Central retinal vascular occlusion Central nervous system disease
Spots	No pathologic significance*
Flashes	Migraine Retinal detachment Posterior vitreous detachment
Loss of visual field or presence of shadows or curtains	Retinal detachment Retinal hemorrhage
Glare, photophobia	Iritis (inflammation of the iris) Meningitis (inflammation of the meninges)
Distortion of vision	Retinal detachment Macular edema
Difficulty seeing in dim light	Myopia Vitamin A deficiency Retinal degeneration
Colored halos around lights	Acute narrow-angle glaucoma Opacities in lens or cornea
Colored vision changes	Cataracts Drugs (digitalis increases yellow vision)
Double vision	Extraocular muscle paresis or paralysis

*May precede a retinal detachment or may be associated with ingestion of fertility drugs.

vision can read the same line of the chart. The abbreviation *OD* refers to the right eye; *OS* refers to the left eye; *OU* refers to both eyes.*

Using the Standard Snellen Chart

If a standard Snellen eye chart is available, the patient should stand 20 feet from the chart. If the patient wears glasses, he or she should wear them for the examination. The patient is asked to cover one eye with the *palm*† and read the smallest line possible. If the best he or she can see is the 20/200 line, the patient's vision in that eye is 20/200; this means that at 20 feet, the patient can see what a person with normal vision can see at 200 feet. If a patient at 20 feet cannot see the 20/200 line, he or she is moved closer until the letters are recognized. If the patient can read these letters at 5 feet, the patient's visual acuity in that eye is 5/200.

Using a Pocket Visual Acuity Card

If the standard Snellen chart is not available, a pocket visual acuity card is helpful. This is viewed at 14 inches (35.6 cm). The patient is again asked to read the smallest line possible. If neither eye chart is available, any printed material may be used. The examiner should remember that most patients older than 40 years require reading glasses. Although visual acuity cannot be quantified, the examiner can certainly determine whether the patient has any vision. In such a case, the patient is asked to cover an eye and read the smallest line possible on a given printed page.

---

*Abbreviations are Latin: OD, *oculus dexter;* OS, *oculus sinister;* OU, *oculus uterque.*
†Always ask a patient to cover the eye with the palm. When fingers are used to cover the eye, a patient may peek between the fingers.

Table 10–4 Common Nonvisual, Painful Eye Symptoms and Disease States

Nonvisual, Painful Symptom	Possible Causes
Foreign body sensation	Foreign body Corneal abrasion
Burning sensation	Uncorrected refractive error Conjunctivitis Sjögren's syndrome
Throbbing, aching	Acute iritis (inflammation of the iris) Sinusitis (inflammation of the sinuses)
Tenderness	Eyelid inflammation Conjunctivitis Iritis
Headache	Refractive errors Migraine Sinusitis
Drawing sensation	Uncorrected refractive errors

Evaluation of Patients with Poor Vision

Patients with poor vision who are unable to read any lines of print should be tested for finger-counting ability. This crude measurement of visual acuity is obtained by the examiner's holding up fingers in front of one of the patient's eyes with the other eye closed. The patient is then asked how many fingers are seen. If the patient is still unable to see, it is important to evaluate whether he or she has any light perception. This is performed by covering one eye and directing a light at the other eye. The examiner asks the patient whether he or she can see when the light is on and off. *No light perception* (NLP) is the term used when a person cannot perceive light.

Table 10–5 Common Nonvisual, Painless Eye Symptoms and Disease States

Nonvisual, Painful Symptom	Possible Causes
Itching	Dry eyes Eye fatigue Allergies
Tearing	Emotional states Hypersecretion of tears Blockage of drainage
Dryness	Sjögren's syndrome Decreased secretion as a result of aging
Sandiness, grittiness	Conjunctivitis
Fullness of eyes	Proptosis (bulging of the eyeball) Aging-related changes in the lids
Twitching	Fibrillation of orbicularis oculi
Eyelid heaviness	Fatigue Eyelid edema
Dizziness	Refractive error Cerebellar disease Vestibular disease
Excessive blinking	Local irritation Facial tic
Eyelids sticking together	Inflammatory disease of eyelids or conjunctivae

Evaluation of Patients Who Cannot Read

For individuals who cannot read, such as young children or illiterate patients, the use of the letter ''E'' in different sizes and directions is helpful. The examiner asks the patient to point in the direction of the letter: up, down, right, left.

Visual Fields

Visual field testing is useful for determining lesions of the visual pathway. Many techniques are used for this purpose. The examiner should learn to perform the technique known as *confrontation visual field testing*. In this technique, the examiner compares his or her peripheral vision with that of the patient.

Assess Fields by Confrontation Testing

The examiner stands or sits 3 feet in front of and at eye level with the patient. The patient is asked to close the right eye while the examiner closes his or her own left eye, each fixating on the other's nose. The examiner holds up fists with the palms facing him or her. The examiner then shows one or two fingers on each hand simultaneously and asks the patient how many fingers he or she sees. The hands are moved from the upper to the lower quadrants, and the examination is repeated. The examination is then repeated, with the other eye of the patient and that of examiner. The fingers should be seen by both patient and examiner simultaneously. To position the patient to better advantage, the hands are held up slightly closer to the examiner. This provides a wider field for the patient. If the examiner can see the fingers, the patient can see them unless he or she has a field deficit. This technique for examining the patient's left eye is shown in Figure 10-10.

Because lesions along the visual pathway develop insidiously, the patient may not be aware of any changes in visual fields until late in the course of the disease. Confrontation fields, performed by the internist, may provide the first objective evidence that the patient has a lesion involving the visual pathway. An area of depressed vision is called a *scotoma*.

The normal central vision extends approximately 30° in all directions of central fixation. The *blind spot* is the physiologic scotoma located about 15° to 20° temporal to central fixation, corresponding to the optic nerve head. No sensory elements such as the rods or cones are located on the nerve head.

Assess Visual Field Abnormalities

Pathologic scotomata may be appreciated on visual field testing. Scotomata may result from primary ocular disease, such as glaucoma, or from lesions in the central nervous system, such as tumors. Figure 10-11 illustrates some of the common defects.

Total loss of vision in one eye constitutes a *blind* eye, resulting from a disease of the eye or a lesion of its optic nerve.

Hemianopsia refers to absence of half of a visual field. A defect in both temporal fields is termed *bitemporal hemianopsia*. It results from a lesion involving the optic nerves at the level of the optic chiasm. Pituitary tumors are common causes.

A *homonymous hemianopsia* results from damage to the optic tract, optic radiation, or occipital cortex. The term *homonymous* indicates that the visual loss is in similar fields. A patient with a left homonymous hemianopsia is unable to see the left half of the fields of both eyes. This defect occurs with damage to the right optic tract. Homonymous hemianopsia is the most common form of field loss and occurs frequently in patients with strokes.

A *quadrantanopsia* is a field loss in one quadrant. A patient with a left upper homonymous quadrantanopsia has damage to the right lower optic radiations or the right lower occipital region.

Tunnel vision may occur in advanced glaucoma. However, the visual fields enlarge with increasing testing distance, in contrast to hysterical blindness, in which the field size typically remains the same at all times.

Assess Optokinetic Nystagmus

On occasion, a patient with psychiatric problems may feign blindness. A useful test for ruling out such malingering involves *optokinetic nystagmus* (OKN). OKN is the rapid alternating motion of the eyes that occurs when the eyes try to fixate on a moving target. For example, observe the eyes of a person riding a train as it enters the station. The eyes move rapidly back and forth as the person tries to fixate on a station sign. The presence of OKN indicates physiologic continuity of the optic pathways from the retina to the occipital cortex.

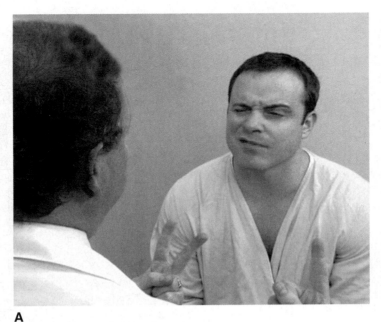

Figure 10–10 Confrontation visual field testing. *A*, View of the patient during examination of the lower fields of the patient's left eye. *B*, Position of the examiner during examination of the upper fields of the patient's left eye.

A

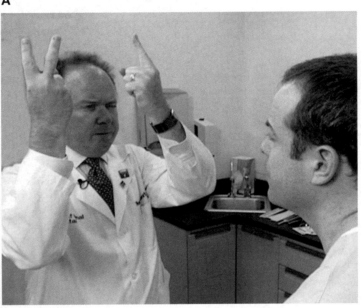

B

OKN may be elicited in the examining room by having the patient fixate on the numbers on a tape measure while you rapidly pull out the tape. Because OKN is involuntary, a positive response provides excellent verification that the patient is feigning blindness.

Ocular Movements

Ocular movements are effected by the contraction and relaxation of the extraocular muscles. This results in simultaneous movement of the eyes up or down or from side to side, as well as in convergence.

Assess Eye Alignment

Alignment of the eyes is seen by observing the location of reflected light on the cornea. The penlight should be held directly in front of the patient. If the patient is looking straight ahead into the distance, the light reflex should be in the center of each cornea. If the light falls in the corneal center of one eye but is displaced away from the corneal center in the other eye, *deviation* of the eye exists.

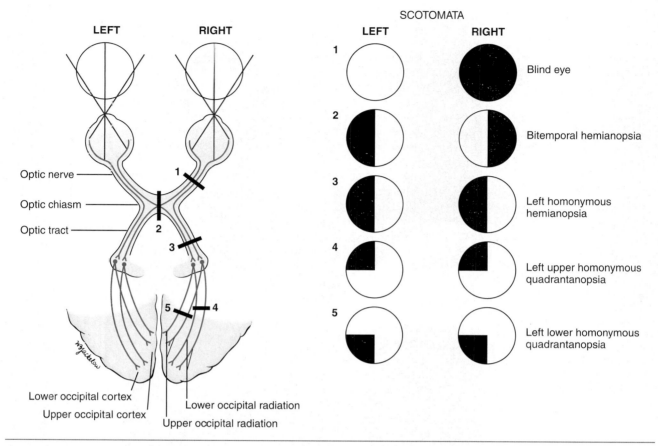

Figure 10–11 Visual field defects.

The condition of a deviated, or crossed, eye is *strabismus*, or tropia. Strabismus is the nonalignment of the eyes in such a way that the object being observed is not projected simultaneously on the fovea of each eye. *Esotropia* is deviation of an eye nasally; *exotropia* is deviation of an eye temporally; *hypertropia* is deviation upward. An *alternating tropia* is the term used to describe the condition in which either eye deviates. Figure 10-12 shows a patient with a left exotropia.

Perform the Cover Test

The cover test is useful for determining whether the eyes are straight or a deviated eye is present. The patient is instructed to look at a distant target. One eye is covered with a 3×5 inch (7.6×12.7 cm) card. The examiner should observe the uncovered eye. If the uncovered eye moves to take up fixation of the distant point, that eye was not straight before the other eye was covered. If the eye did not move, it was straight. The test is then repeated with the other eye.

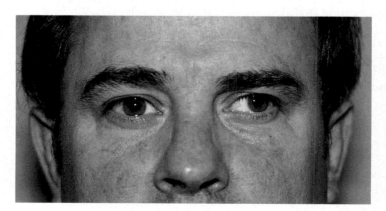

Figure 10–12 Left exotropia.

Evaluate the Six Diagnostic Positions of Gaze

An important cause of a deviated eye is *paretic* (weak), or paralyzed, extraocular muscle(s). Paralysis of these muscles is detected by examination of the *six diagnostic positions of gaze*.

Because the rotational actions of the oblique and vertical rectus muscles cannot be easily assessed, the eye must be moved into six diagnostic gaze positions that best isolate the vertical actions of these muscles to test their innervations. The oblique muscles are tested in adduction to maximize their vertical action. In contrast, the vertical rectus muscles are tested in abduction; in these positions, the superior rectus acts now as a pure elevator and the inferior rectus as a pure depressor. **These diagnostic positions of gaze are the *testing* positions for the muscles, and the abduction/adduction testing movements are different from the normal actions of the muscles as indicated in Table 10-1.**

Hold the patient's chin steady with your left hand, and ask the patient to follow your right hand as it traces a large "H" in the air. Hold your right index finger about 15 to 18 inches (38 to 46 cm) from the patient's nose. From the midline, move your finger about 12 inches (30 cm) to the patient's left and pause; then up about 8 inches (20 cm) and pause, as shown in Figure 10-13; down about 16 inches (40 cm) and pause; up about 8 inches (20 cm); and then slowly back to the midline. Switch your hands, now holding the patient's chin with your right hand. Cross the midline and repeat the finger movements on the other side. These are the six diagnostic positions of gaze. Observe the movement of both eyes, which should follow the finger smoothly. Look for the parallel movements of the eyes in all directions.

On occasion, when looking to the extreme side, the eyes develop a rhythmic motion called *end-point nystagmus*. There is a quick motion in the direction of gaze, which is followed

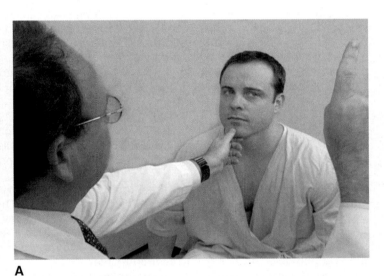

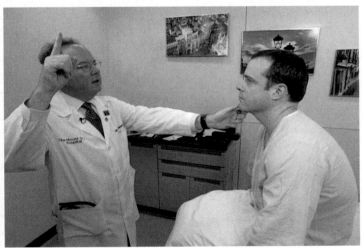

Figure 10–13 *A* and *B,* Technique for testing ocular motility.

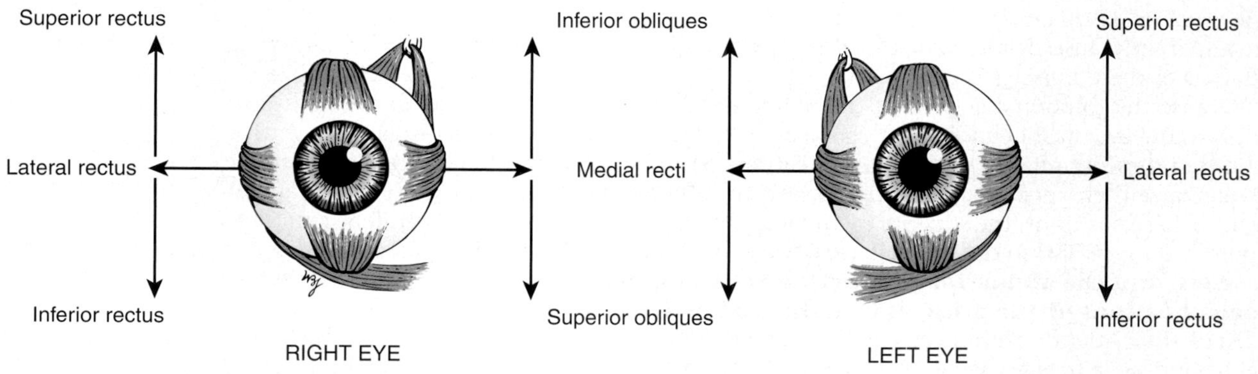

Figure 10–14 Diagnostic positions of gaze.

by a slow return. This test differentiates end-point nystagmus from pathologic nystagmus, in which the quick movement is always in the same direction, regardless of gaze.

If the eye and eyelid do not move together, *lid lag* is present.

The six diagnostic positions of gaze, with the related muscles, are illustrated in Figure 10-14, and Table 10-6 summarizes the abnormalities in ocular motility that are caused by paretic muscles.

The images projected on the retina may be interpreted by the brain in one of three ways: fusion, diplopia, or suppression. Fusion and diplopia have already been discussed. In children, strabismus leads to diplopia, which leads to confusion and then *suppression* of the image and finally to *amblyopia*. Amblyopia is the loss of visual acuity secondary to suppression. Amblyopia is reversible until the retinas are fully developed, at about the age of 7 years. Amblyopia is a phenomenon that occurs only in children. An adult who acquires strabismus secondary to a stroke, for example, cannot suppress the deviated eye's image and will have diplopia.

Evaluate the Pupillary Light Reflex

Ask the patient to look in the distance while you shine a bright light in the patient's eye. The light source should come from the side, with the patient's nose acting as a barrier to light to the other eye. Observe the direct and consensual pupillary responses. Then repeat the test on the other eye.

The *swinging light test* is a modification for testing the pupillary light reflex. This test reveals differences in the response to afferent stimuli of the two eyes. The patient fixates on a distant target while the examiner rapidly swings a light from one eye to the other, observing for constriction of the pupils. In some conditions, there is a paradoxical dilatation of the pupil on which the light is shined. This condition, called a *Marcus Gunn pupil*, is associated with an afferent limb defect in the eye being illuminated.

The most extreme example of an eye displaying the Marcus Gunn phenomenon is a blind eye. When light is shined into the blind eye, there is neither a direct nor a consensual response. When the light is moved to the other eye, there is both a direct and a consensual response because both afferent and efferent pathways are normal. When the light is swung back to the

Table 10–6 Paretic Muscles Causing Abnormal Ocular Motility

Paretic Muscle	Position to Which Eye Will Not Turn
Medial rectus	Nasal
Inferior oblique	Up and nasal
Superior oblique	Down and nasal
Lateral rectus	Temporal
Superior rectus	Up and temporal
Inferior rectus	Down and temporal

blind eye, no impulses are received by the retina (afferent), and the pupil of the blind eye no longer remains constricted; it dilates. There are different degrees of severity of Marcus Gunn pupils, depending on the involvement of the optic nerve.

Evaluate the Near Reflex

The near reflex is tested by having the patient look first at some distant target and then at a target placed about 5 inches (13 cm) away from his or her nose. When the patient focuses on the near target, the eyes should converge, and the pupils should constrict.

External and Internal Eye Structures

The examination of the external and internal eye structures includes the following:

- Orbits and eyelids
- Lacrimal apparatus
- Conjunctiva
- Sclera
- Cornea
- Pupils
- Iris
- Anterior chamber
- Lens

Inspect the Orbits and Eyelids

Are the globes present in the orbits? An *enucleation* of his left eye is pictured in Figure 10-15. The removal of the entire globe from the orbit may be caused by trauma, surgery (as in the case of a ruptured globe), or self-induced injury by a psychotic person.

Examine the eyelids for evidence of drooping, infection, erythema, swelling, crusting, masses, or other abnormalities. Have the patient open and close the eyelids. The motion should be smooth and symmetric. Do the eyes close completely?

Note the position of the eyelids. When the eye is open, the upper eyelid normally covers only the upper margin of the iris. When the eye is closed, the eyelids should approximate each other completely. The space between the upper and lower lids is the *palpebral fissure*. Drooping of the eyelid is known as *blepharoptosis*, or *ptosis*. Figure 10-16 depicts marked bilateral ptosis, causing narrowing of the palpebral fissure that resulted from a muscle-weakening disorder, myasthenia gravis.

Figure 10-17 shows a patient with *Kearns-Sayre syndrome*. In this autosomal dominant condition, there is a slowly progressive, symmetric ptosis and symmetric external ophthalmoplegia (weakness of the external eye muscles). The syndrome also is associated with retinal

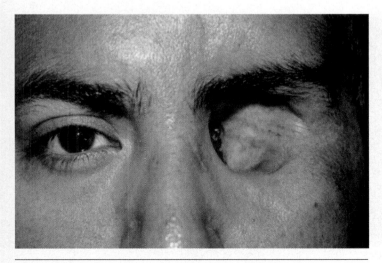

Figure 10–15 Enucleation of left eye.

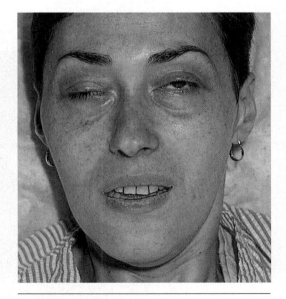

Figure 10–16 Bilateral ptosis.

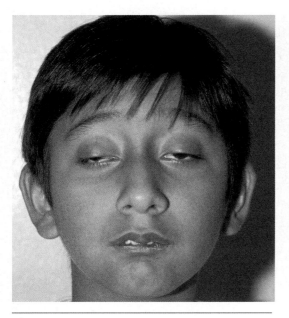

Figure 10–17 Kearns-Sayre syndrome.

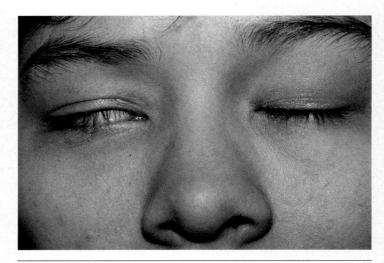

Figure 10–18 Lagophthalmos.

pigmentary degeneration and cardiac conduction defects such as complete heart block. Affected patients are frequently of short stature and may be deaf. In this patient, notice the arching of the brows in an effort to lift the eyelids to reduce the ptosis.

Lagophthalmos is a condition, pictured in Figure 10-18, in which there is an inability to close the eyelids completely. It is seen in thyroid disease secondary to orbital infiltration caused by inflammation, as a result of autonomic stimulation, or as a consequence of ocular surgery. The name comes from the Greek word *lagos*, meaning "hare," an animal believed to sleep with its eyes open.

Figure 10-19 shows a patient with an entropion. An *entropion* is a turning inward of the lid margin in such a way that the eyelashes abrade the cornea and globe. An *ectropion* is a turning outward of the eyelid margin. An ectropion is pictured in Figure 10-20. Both entropions and ectropions may be seen as involutional changes associated with aging.

A common benign lesion of the eyelid is a marginal intradermal nevus, shown in Figure 10-21. Such lesions are well differentiated, and hairs commonly grow from them. One of the associated problems is that these hairs may scratch the cornea, causing corneal abrasions like those caused by entropions.

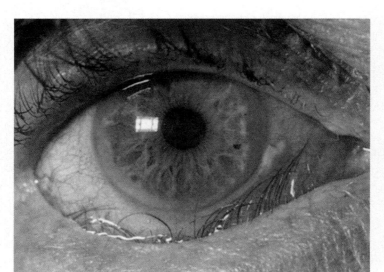

Figure 10–19 Entropion.

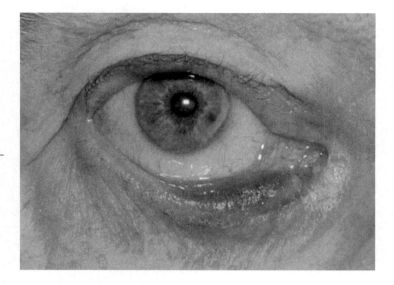

Figure 10–20 Ectropion.

A common ocular problem of aging is herniation of the orbital fat, caused by weakening of the orbital septum. Figure 10-22 shows an example of herniated orbital fat. Note the unrelated old corneal scars and the arcus senilis, discussed later in this chapter.

Figure 10-23 depicts a small hemangioma of the lower eyelid. *Sturge-Weber syndrome* is a congenital condition recognizable by a characteristic port wine stain, or *nevus flammeus*, on one side of the face that follows the distribution of one or more of the divisions of the trigeminal nerve. Hemangiomas may develop on the episclera, iris, ciliary body, and choroid. Unilateral glaucoma develops frequently on the affected side if there is extensive involvement of the eye with a uveal hemangioma. Figure 10-24 shows a patient with Sturge-Weber syndrome. Notice the sharply demarcated patch of the hemangioma with the involvement of the ophthalmic and maxillary divisions of the left trigeminal nerve. The lesion, which does not blanch on pressure, tends to darken with age from red to purple (see also Fig. 24-7).

A *chalazion* is a granulomatous reaction to inspissated secretions of the meibomian glands in the eyelid. It appears as a localized mass on the eyelid near the orifice of the gland, usually painless when chronic. Figure 10-25 shows a chalazion; Figure 10-26 shows bilateral chalazions.

In *herpes zoster ophthalmicus*, rows of vesicles, ulcers, and crusted scabs are scattered along the course of one or more of the branches of the ophthalmic division of the trigeminal nerve. The vesicles contain clear fluid. These rupture, leaving ulcers that can become infected secondarily and form crusts. The eyelids become edematous and red. Pain can be excruciating. Ophthalmoplegia secondary to involvement of the extraocular muscles may also occur. Figure 10-27 shows a patient with acquired immunodeficiency syndrome (AIDS) and herpes

Figure 10–21 Marginal nevus of upper eyelid.

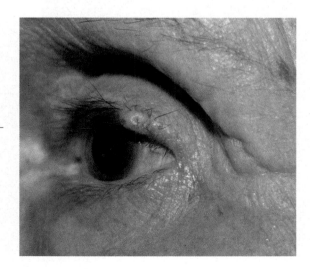

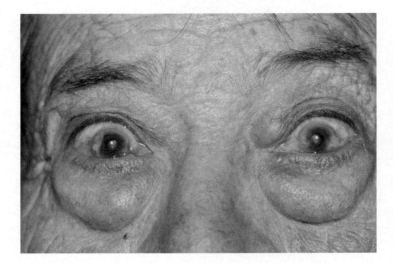

Figure 10–22 Herniated orbital fat.

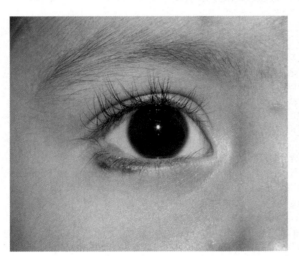

Figure 10–23 Hemangioma of lower eyelid.

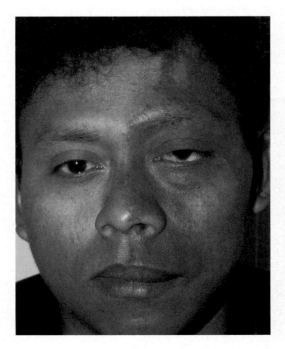

Figure 10–24 Sturge-Weber syndrome.

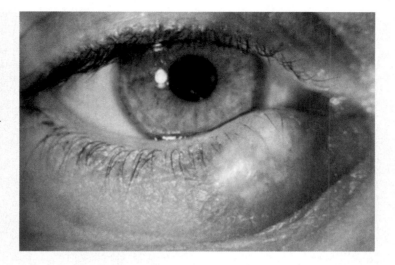

Figure 10–25 Chalazion.

zoster ophthalmicus at different stages of evolution (fresh and crusted vesicles) in the ophthalmic division of the trigeminal nerve. Treatment with antivirals can dramatically reduce the symptoms.

Is orbital pigmentation present? Orbital pigmentation, also known as *raccoon eyes*, is an important sign of a basilar skull fracture. This discoloration is caused by extravasated blood from the fracture of the base of the brain. This is an important sign to recognize, especially in an unconscious patient, when a history is not available. Figure 10-28 shows a patient with a basilar skull fracture. Notice also the subconjunctival hemorrhages on the lateral aspects.

Inspect the eyelids for *xanthelasma*. Although not specific for hypercholesterolemia, these yellowish plaques are commonly associated with lipid abnormalities and are caused by lipid deposition in the periorbital skin. Xanthelasma is shown in Figure 10-29.

A *stye*, or *acute hordeolum*, is a localized abscess in an eyelash follicle and is caused by a staphylococcal infection. It is a painful, red infection that looks like a pimple pointing on the lid margin. Figure 10-30 depicts a stye. *Blepharitis* is a chronic inflammation of the eyelid margins. The most common form is associated with small white scales around the lid margin and the eyelashes, which stick together and may fall out. There are several annoying symptoms: itching, tearing, and redness. The condition is frequently associated with seborrheic dermatitis. Figure 10-31 shows blepharitis.

Malignant tumors of the eyelids are not uncommon. Carcinoma of the eyelids has the highest incidence of any malignant ocular tumor. Men are more commonly affected than women; the average age at onset is 50 to 60 years. Ninety-five percent of eyelid carcinomas are of the

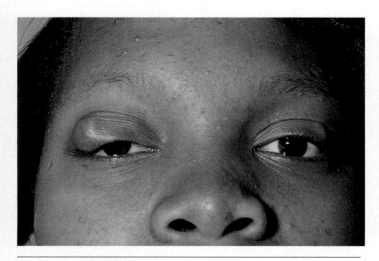

Figure 10–26 Bilateral chalazions.

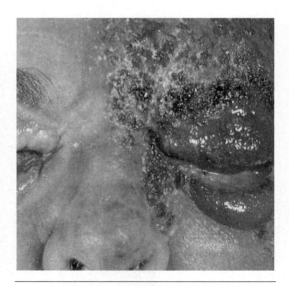

Figure 10–27 *Herpes zoster ophthalmicus.*

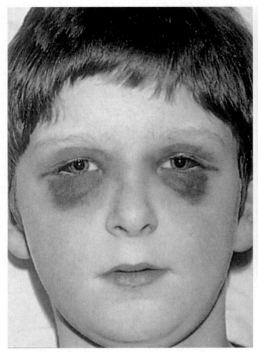

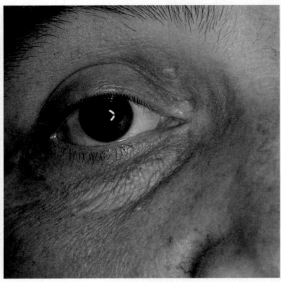

Figure 10–29 Xanthelasma.

Figure 10–28 Raccoon eyes secondary to a basilar skull fracture.

basal cell type. The remaining 5% consist of squamous cell carcinomas and meibomian gland carcinomas. Figure 10-32 shows a *basal cell carcinoma* of the lower lid, the more common location. The lesion begins growing slowly and painlessly, eventually forming the typical rodent ulcer with a raised border and an indurated base. The tumor erodes the surrounding area, forming the ulcer. Note the raised border of the lesion in Figure 10-32. *Squamous cell carcinomas*, which tend to be on the upper eyelid, grow faster than basal cell carcinomas. Early ulceration is common. A *squamous cell carcinoma* of the eyelid is shown in Figure 10-33. The base and edges of the ulcer are hard and hyperemic.

The most common ocular manifestation of AIDS affecting the eyelids is lesions of Kaposi's sarcoma. The initial manifestation may be subtle and may be mistaken for blepharitis or a chalazion. Refer to Figure 8-93C, which shows a patient with AIDS and Kaposi's sarcoma of the eyelid.

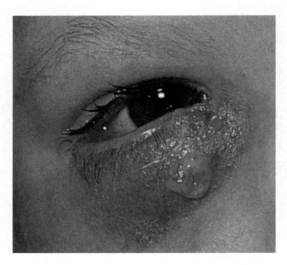

Figure 10–30 Stye.

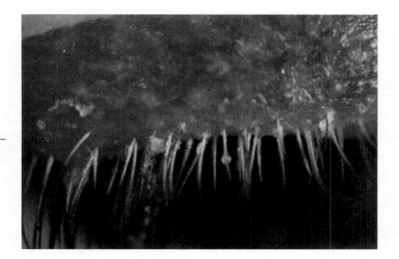

Figure 10–31 Blepharitis.

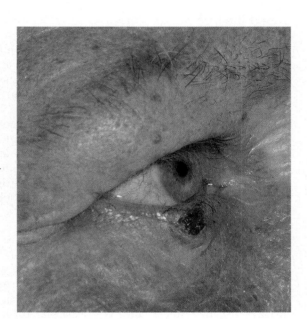

Figure 10–32 Basal cell carcinoma of the eyelid.

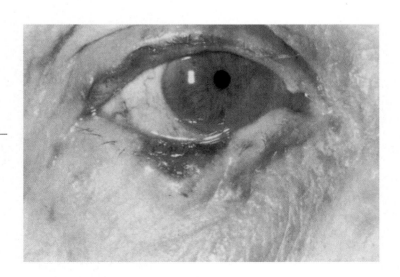

Figure 10–33 Squamous cell carcinoma of the eyelid.

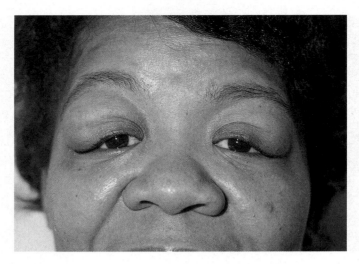

Figure 10–34 Bilateral lacrimal gland enlargement. Note the classic sigmoid shape of the eyelids.

Inspect the Lacrimal Apparatus

In general, there is little to be seen of the lacrimal apparatus, with the exception of the punctum. If tearing, also known as *epiphora*, is present, there may be some obstruction to flow through the punctum. If excessive moisture is present, check for a blockage of the nasolacrimal duct by pressing the lacrimal sac gently against the inner orbital rim. If a blockage is present, material may be expressed through the punctum. Figure 10-34 shows massive lacrimal gland enlargement as a result of sarcoidosis.

Figure 10-35 shows marked bilateral proptosis of the globe in a patient with hyperthyroidism. Note the massive lacrimal gland enlargement.

Dacryocystitis is a term describing the inflammation of the lower lacrimal passages usually seen in infants or older individuals. The causes include congenital anomalies, infection, and stenosis of the lacrimal duct. Chronic dacryocystitis, seen in Figure 10-36, is a common disorder and almost always arises secondary to ductal obstruction.

Inspect the Conjunctiva

Both conjunctivae should be examined for signs of inflammation (i.e., injection, or dilatation of its blood vessels), pallor, unusual pigmentation, swelling, masses, and hemorrhage.

The tarsal conjunctiva may be seen by everting the eyelid. Ask the patient to keep the eyes open and look downward. Grasp gently some of the eyelashes of the upper lid. Pull the eyelid away from the globe, and press the tip of an applicator stick against the upper border of the tarsal plate. Then quickly turn the tarsal plate over the applicator stick, using it as a fulcrum. Your thumb can now be used for holding the everted lid, and the applicator stick can be removed. After inspection of the tarsal conjunctiva, have the patient look up to return the lid to its normal position.

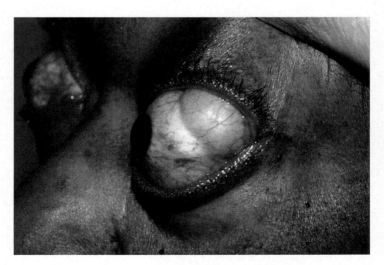

Figure 10–35 Hyperthyroidism. Note proptosis and lacrimal gland enlargement.

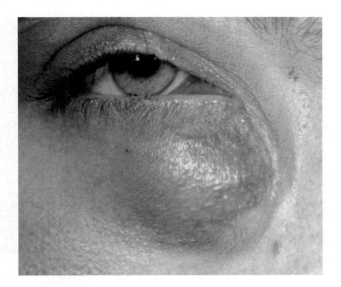

Figure 10–36 Chronic dacryocystitis.

The normal conjunctiva is transparent. Note the number of blood vessels. Normally, only a small number of vessels are seen. Ask the patient to look up, while you pull down on the lower eyelids. Compare the vascularity in the two eyes.

Conjunctivitis is the most common of all eye diseases in the Western hemisphere. The causes are numerous: bacterial, viral, chlamydial, fungal, parasitic, spirochetal, allergic, traumatic, chemical, and idiopathic. Bacterial conjunctivitis is the most frequent type and is self-limited, lasting 10 to 14 days. Figure 10-37 shows *acute hemorrhagic conjunctivitis*. This highly contagious ocular infection, often bilateral, is caused by the enteroviruses (members of the picornavirus family), *Pneumococcus* organisms, and *Haemophilus influenzae*. *Giant papillary conjunctivitis* is an ocular syndrome consisting of excessive secretion of conjunctival mucus, itching, and the development of giant papillae (1 mm or more in diameter) on the tarsal conjunctiva. This syndrome occurs mostly in patients who wear soft contact lenses, but it can occur in patients with ocular prostheses or other foreign bodies in the eye. Figure 10-38 shows a patient with giant papillary conjunctivitis.

Figure 10-39 shows a large *subconjunctival hemorrhage*. This common condition may occur spontaneously, usually in only one eye, in any age group. Because of its sudden appearance and bright red color, the patient may become alarmed. The hemorrhage is usually caused by a rupture of a small conjunctival vessel after a bout of severe coughing or sneezing. There is no treatment, and the hemorrhage resolves within 1 to 2 weeks.

The conjunctiva is attached to the episclera by loose connections. This potential space can easily be filled with fluids such as blood or serum. *Chemosis* is the presence of fluid in this space. Trauma, allergies, and chronic exposure, as seen in proptosis of hyperthyroidism and neurologic deficits, are important causes of chemosis. Figure 10-40 shows chemosis

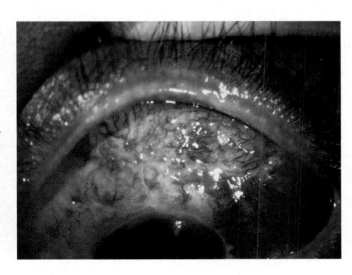

Figure 10–37 Acute hemorrhagic conjunctivitis.

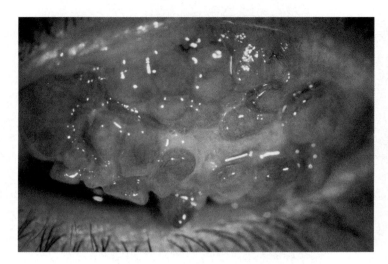

Figure 10–38 Giant papillary conjunctivitis.

secondary to hay fever. An example of hemorrhagic chemosis is pictured in Figure 10-41. The patient, a 42-year-old man, had a 10-year history of progressive proptosis secondary to a melanoma.

Two common benign growths on the conjunctiva are the pinguecula and pterygium. A *pinguecula* is a whitish-yellow, triangular, nodular growth on the bulbar conjunctiva adjacent to the corneal-scleral junction (limbus), as seen in Figure 10-42; it does not cross on to the cornea. A *pterygium* is a more vascular growth on the bulbar conjunctiva that begins at the medial canthus and extends beyond the corneal-scleral junction to the cornea. This typically triangle-shaped fibrovascular connective tissue may cause astigmatism or even decreased vision if it extends toward or occludes the pupillary margin. The cause of the pterygium is thought to be chronic dry eyes, because its frequency is higher among people living near the equator. Figure 10-43*A* shows a pterygium; Figure 10-43*B* is a close-up photograph of a pterygium in another patient. Notice the vascularity and their positions across the limbus.

Primary acquired melanosis is a unilateral condition in which melanotic pigmentation develops in the conjunctival or corneal epithelium. It starts insidiously during middle age. A biopsy is often needed to rule out a malignant melanoma. Figure 10-44 shows primary acquired melanosis. Primary acquired melanosis of the plica semilunaris in another patient is seen in Figure 10-45.

A benign pigmented tumor of the conjunctiva may be a *conjunctival nevus*. This is a solitary, well-defined, slightly elevated lesion that moves freely over the globe. Nevi have a predilection for the limbus, plica semilunaris, caruncle, and lid margin. Most nevi are tan or brown, and many have zones of clearing within known as lacunae. Figure 10-46 shows a conjunctival nevus.

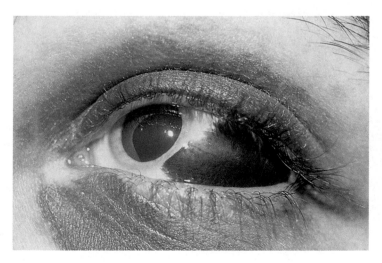

Figure 10–39 Subconjunctival hemorrhage.

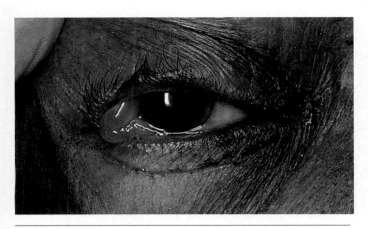

Figure 10–40 Chemosis. Note the presence of fluid in the subconjunctival space.

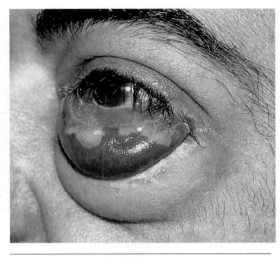

Figure 10–41 Hemorrhagic chemosis.

A *dermolipoma of the conjunctiva* is a common congenital tumor, often bilateral, that usually appears as a smoothly rounded growth in the superotemporal quadrant of the bulbar conjunctiva near the lateral canthus. Figure 10-47*A* shows bilateral dermolipomas of the conjunctiva. A close-up of the lesion in the right eye is shown in Figure 10-47*B*. The yellowish color is secondary to the increased fatty deposits in the lesion. Often, fine hairs may protrude from its surface. Treatment is usually not indicated.

Inspect the Sclera

The sclera is examined for nodules, hyperemia, and discoloration. The normal sclera is white. In dark-skinned individuals, the sclera may be slightly brownish in color due to pigment migration.

Jaundice, or *icterus*, is a yellowish discoloration of the sclera, skin, and mucous membranes and is caused by retention of bilirubin or its products of metabolism. Jaundice is more easily seen in the sclera of white individuals and may be missed in people of color or in dim light. Carotene may also cause yellowing of the skin but not of the sclera (see Fig. 17-5).

The sclera may appear bluish, normally in infants or pathologically in *osteogenesis imperfecta*. Osteogenesis imperfecta is a group of hereditary disorders with bone fragility. Individuals with these disorders may suffer bone fractures after mild trauma. The autosomal dominant form is most widely recognized. In this form, the sclerae are very thin and take on a blue hue because the uveal pigment shows through the sclera. Deafness is also seen in this form of the disorder. Figure 10-48 shows blue sclerae in a patient with osteogenesis imperfecta.

Episcleritis is a benign, usually painless, commonly recurring disorder frequently affecting both eyes of young adults, more commonly women. It is a noninfectious inflammation that is

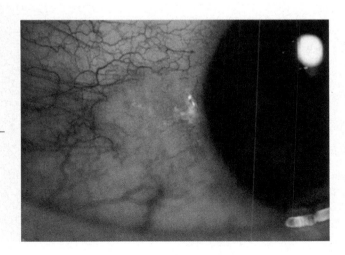

Figure 10–42 Pinguecula.

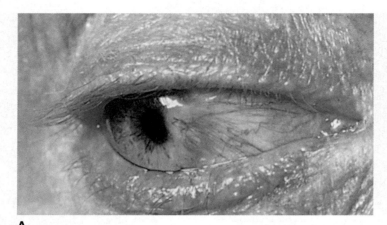

A

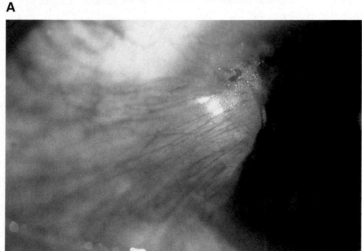

B

Figure 10–43 *A* and *B,* Pterygium. *B,* A close-up view.

subconjunctival and yet superficial to the underlying sclera. The affected area may be either flat and diffuse or localized and nodular (1 to 4 mm in diameter). Although the cause in most cases is unclear, episcleritis also occurs in patients with inflammatory bowel disease, herpes zoster, collagen vascular disease, gout, syphilis, and rheumatoid arthritis. Figure 10-49 shows the classic features of episcleritis.

Scleritis is a painful, often bilateral, recurrent disorder, less common than episcleritis, that affects older age groups and occurs in women more often than in men. There is inflammation

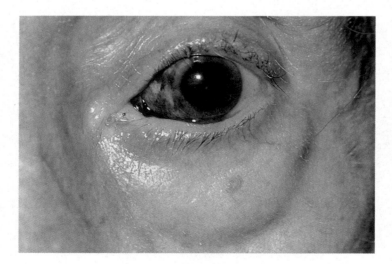

Figure 10–44 Primary acquired melanosis.

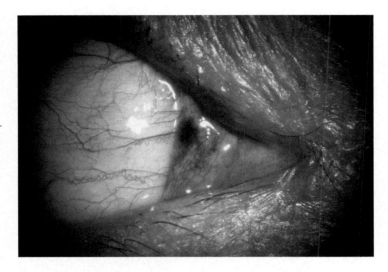

Figure 10–45 Primary acquired melanosis.

of the sclera with possible involvement of the cornea, uveal tract (i.e., iris, choroid, and ciliary body), or retina. Photophobia is common. Scleritis is usually related to a systemic disorder. It occurs much more commonly in patients with connective tissue disorders. It may be diffuse or localized and nodular. Nodular scleritis is marked by dark localized blue patches in the anterior portion of the sclera; these are seen because the choroid is visible through the translucent sclera. The condition may resolve spontaneously. Figure 10-50 shows nodular scleritis.

Scleromalacia perforans is an uncommon, painless scleral condition characterized by the appearance of one or more dehiscences in the sclera in the absence of inflammatory changes. This necrotizing scleritis without inflammation is classically seen in patients with long-standing rheumatoid arthritis. The underlying uvea is often visible, and it may bulge out, as shown in Figure 10-51. Another example of scleromalacia perforans is shown in Figure 10-52. Notice the thinning of the sclera and the underlying dark uvea, as well as the irregular border of the iris. Anterior synechiae are present, holding the iris bound down to the lens and causing the scalloped appearance of the iris. There is corneal disease as well.

Inspect the Cornea

The cornea should be clear and without cloudiness, ulceration, or opacities.

A whitish ring at the perimeter of the cornea is probably an *arcus senilis*. In patients older than 40 years, this finding is usually a normal phenomenon. Although there are many false-positive findings, patients younger than 40 years may have hypercholesterolemia. An arcus senilis is seen in Figures 10-53 and 10-54.

An abnormal greenish-yellow ring near the limbus, most evident superiorly and inferiorly, is a *Kayser-Fleischer ring*. This ring is a specific and sensitive sign of *Wilson's disease*, which is hepatolenticular degeneration as a result of an inherited disorder of copper metabolism.

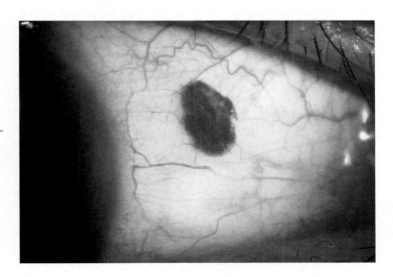

Figure 10–46 Conjunctival nevus.

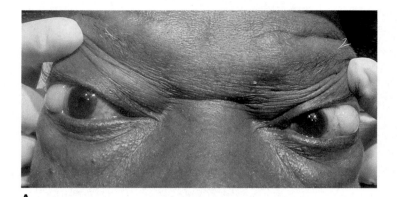

A

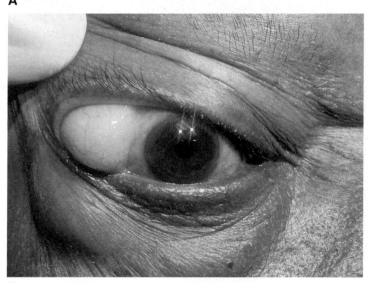

B

Figure 10–47 Dermolipoma of the conjunctiva. *A,* Bilateral view. *B,* A close-up view of the lesion in the right eye.

The Kayser-Fleischer ring is caused by deposition of copper in Descemet's membrane of the peripheral cornea. Figure 10-55 shows a Kayser-Fleischer ring. Notice that the ring is most prominent in the vertical meridian.

Corneal ulcers are extremely painful lesions caused by loss of substance from the cornea by progressive erosion and necrosis of tissue. These ulcers may be caused by a variety of agents, including bacteria, viruses, fungi, and hypersensitivity reactions. *Pneumococcus* organisms are common bacteria associated with corneal ulceration. *Pseudomonas* infection is less common but is associated with a rapid spread and corneal perforation. Herpes simplex virus (HSV) is another common cause of corneal ulceration and is the most common cause of corneal-related blindness. It is almost always unilateral and may affect any age group. The keratitis (inflammation of the cornea) is commonly accompanied by conjunctival hyperemia, tearing, and photophobia.

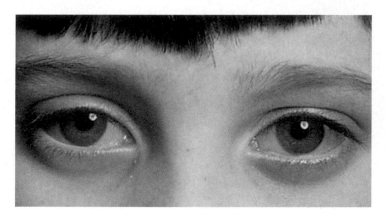

Figure 10–48 Blue sclerae secondary to osteogenesis imperfecta.

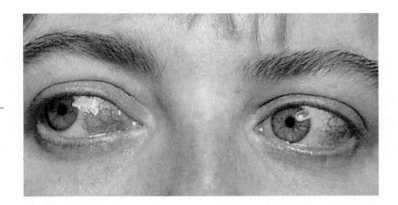

Figure 10–49 Episcleritis.

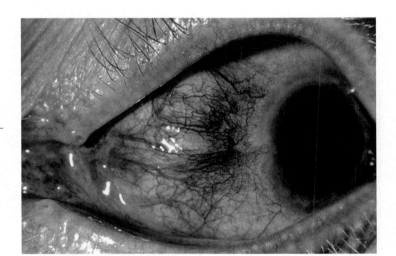

Figure 10–50 Nodular scleritis.

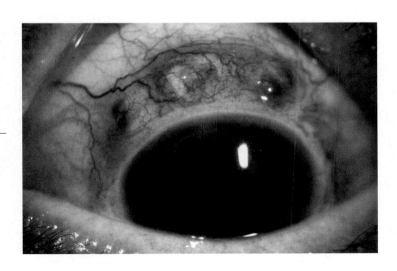

Figure 10–51 Scleromalacia perforans.

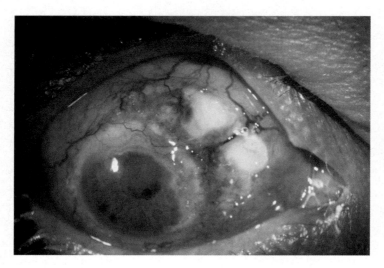

Figure 10–52 Scleromalacia perforans. Note the anterior synechiae.

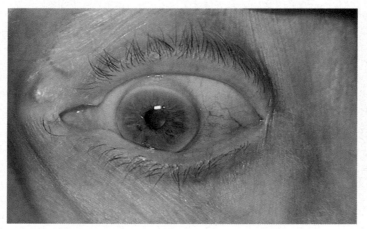

Figure 10–53 Arcus senilis.

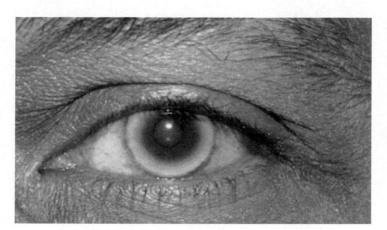

Figure 10–54 Arcus senilis.

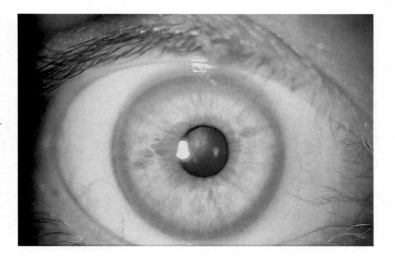

Figure 10–55 Kayser-Fleischer ring.

Recurrent attacks may be less painful to painless as generalized corneal anesthesia develops. Patients with AIDS or other immunosuppressive conditions are very susceptible to this recurring infection. Figure 10-56 shows a corneal ulceration secondary to HSV infection. Marked blepharospasm is common with corneal ulceration. The most common characteristic finding of HSV-related keratitis is the dendritic ulcer on the cornea. This ulcer is the result of active viral replication in the corneal epithelial cells. Figure 10-57 shows HSV-related keratitis. The eye has been stained with rose bengal. The devitalized, swollen cells laden with the replicating virus stain brightly with this substance. Figure 10-58 shows corneal scarring in another patient as a result of a previous herpes zoster infection. Note the discrete areas of infiltrates in the cornea, as well as the darkening of the skin on the ipsilateral side from the nose to the forehead.

Keratoconus is an acquired abnormality of the shape of the cornea. It has a gradual onset. It is usually bilateral but asymmetric. It is estimated to occur in 1 per 20,000 individuals. The cornea protrudes as a cone, with the apex becoming thin and scarred. Affected patients experience slow visual deterioration. When the patient is asked to look downward, the cone can become quite obvious, as seen in Figure 10-59. This is known as *Munson's sign*.

Patients with keratoconus or corneal scarring from other causes may require corneal transplantation. A recent corneal transplant is shown in Figure 10-60. Note the sutures and the mild edema.

Figure 10-61 shows a dermolipoma of the corneal limbus. It is a smoothly rounded, yellowish, benign growth (see also Fig. 10-47).

Inspect the Pupils

The pupils should be equal in size, round, and reactive to light and accommodation. In about 5% of normal individuals, pupillary size is not equal; this is called *anisocoria*. Anisocoria may be an indication of neurologic disease. Pupillary enlargement, or *mydriasis*, is associated with ingestion of sympathomimetic agents or with administration of dilating drops. A sluggish,

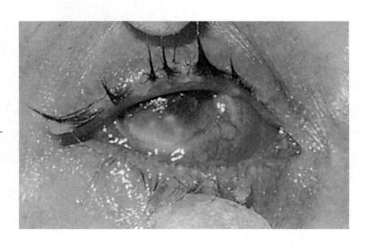

Figure 10–56 Corneal ulceration. Note the pus in the anterior chamber.

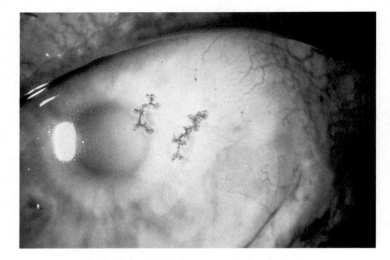

Figure 10–57 Herpes simplex virus–related keratitis. The eye has been stained with rose bengal.

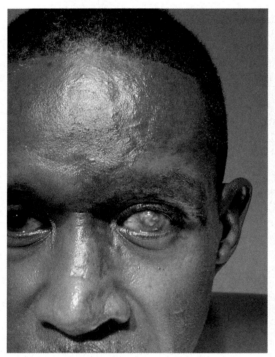

Figure 10–58 Corneal scarring secondary to previous herpes zoster infection.

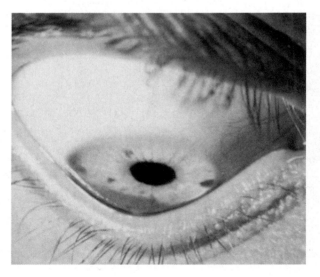

Figure 10–59 Keratoconus. Munson's sign.

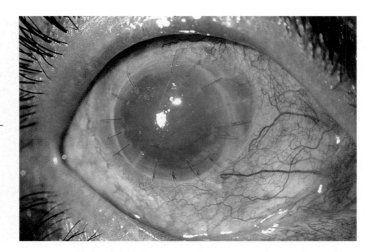

Figure 10–60 Corneal transplant.

mid-dilated pupil may be present with acute angle-closure glaucoma. Pupillary constriction, or *miosis*, occurs with ingestion of parasympathomimetic drugs, with inflammation of the iris, and with drug treatment for glaucoma. Many medications can cause anisocoria. It is therefore important to ascertain whether the patient has used any eye drops or has taken any medications.

Pupillary abnormalities are often markers of neurologic disease. A condition known as *Adie's tonic pupil* is a pupil dilated 3 to 6 mm that constricts little in response to light and accommodation. This pupil is often associated with diminished to absent deep tendon reflexes in the extremities. It occurs more commonly in women 25 to 45 years of age, and the cause is unknown. There are no serious clinical implications. The *Argyll Robertson pupil* is a pupil constricted 1 to 2 mm that reacts to accommodation but is nonreactive to light. It occurs in association with neurosyphilis. *Horner's syndrome* is sympathetic paralysis of the eye that is caused by interruption of the cervical sympathetic chain. In addition to miosis and ptosis, anhidrosis* is also present. Table 10-7 lists features of these significant pupillary abnormalities.

Inspect the Iris

The iris is evaluated for its shape, color, nodules, and vascularity. Normally, iris blood vessels cannot be seen unless the eye is observed with magnification.

An *iris coloboma* is a notch or gap in the iris. It results from failure of fusion of the embryonic tissue. The typical iris coloboma is usually part of a choroidal coloboma, which is an autosomal dominant trait. It is often bilateral, is usually located inferiorly, and involves the iris, choroid, or overlying retina (see Fig. 10-140). Visual acuity may be normal if the macula and optic nerve head are spared. Figure 10-62 shows a patient with an iris coloboma involving the ciliary body and the choroid.

Inflammation of the iris, *iritis* or *iridocyclitis*, is associated with severe pain, photophobia, lacrimation, decreased vision, and circumcorneal congestion. This congestion is caused by injection of the deep episcleral vessels (ciliary flush). The dilation of the iris vessels leads to transudation of protein into the aqueous humor and deposition of inflammatory cells on the corneal endothelium, known as keratic precipitates. As a result of this deposition, the iris becomes blurred and loses its distinctive radial appearance (a "muddy iris"). There are many causes of iritis, including exogenous infection from perforating injuries; secondary infection from the cornea, sclera, or retina; endogenous infection such as tuberculosis, gonorrhea, syphilis, and viral and mycotic infections; and systemic diseases such as rheumatoid arthritis, systemic lupus erythematosus, Reiter's disease, Behçet's syndrome, and relapsing polychondritis. Figure 10-63 shows the classic features of acute iritis.

As a result of the inflammatory reaction of the iris, the iris may adhere to the cornea, forming anterior synechiae; posterior synechiae are adhesions between the iris and lens. Glaucoma is a well-known sequela of iritis and synechiae formation.

---

*Absence of sweating in this syndrome is related to interruption of the sympathetic chain. The amount of sweating is assessed by examination of the forehead or the axilla of the affected side.

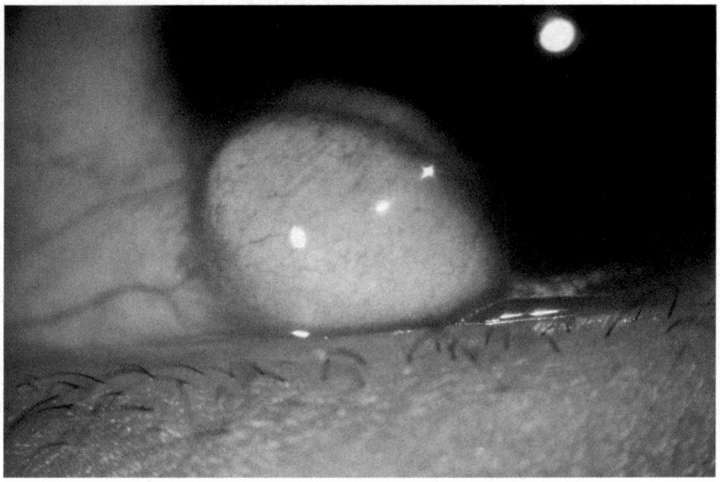

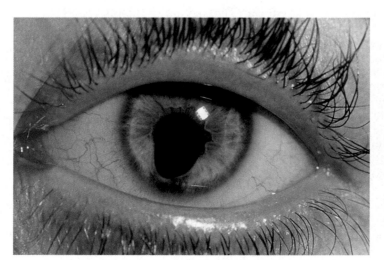

Figure 10–61 Dermolipoma of corneal limbus.

Table 10–7 Pupillary Abnormalities

Feature	Adie's Tonic Pupil	Argyll Robertson Pupil	Horner's Syndrome
Laterality	Often unilateral	Bilateral	Unilateral
Reaction to light	Minimally reactive	Nonreactive	Reactive
Accommodation	Sluggishly reactive	Reactive	Reactive
Pupillary size	Mydriatic	Miotic	Miotic
Other signs	Absent or diminished tendon reflexes	Absent knee-jerk reflexes	Slight ptosis* Anhidrosis

*The ptosis is slight owing to interruption of the sympathetic chain innervating only the Müller's muscle portion of the levator palpebrae. The rest of the levator palpebrae functions normally; thus, ptosis is not severe.

Figure 10–62 Iris coloboma.

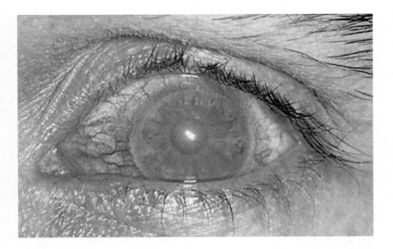

Figure 10–63 Acute iritis.

Inspect the Anterior Chamber

Is the anterior chamber clear? If not, is it filled with pus or blood? Figure 10-64*A* shows pus in the anterior chamber, known as a *hypopyon*, in a patient with HSV keratitis. Another example of hypopyon, a large hypopyon together with severe conjunctival injection, is shown in Figure 10-64*B*.

Is there blood in the anterior chamber? This condition, known as a *hyphema*, is illustrated in Figure 10-65. Note the subconjunctival hemorrhage also in the patient in Figure 10-65*A*. A hyphema always indicates that the eye has suffered significant trauma to cause bleeding. The bleeding comes from the anterior chamber angle or the iris, and, therefore, pupillary abnormalities are common. Figure 10-66 depicts an example of a "candy cane" hyphema resulting from neovascularization of the iris as a consequence of a central retinal vein occlusion. The photograph shows blood breakdown products intermingled with fresh blood.

Assess the *depth of the anterior chamber*. By shining a light obliquely across the eye, you can estimate the depth of the chamber. If a crescentic shadow on the far portion of the iris is visible, the anterior chamber may be shallow. *Shadowing of the anterior chamber* refers to the decreased space between the iris and the cornea. The technique for estimating the depth of the anterior chamber is illustrated in Figure 10-67.

The presence of a shallow anterior chamber predisposes an individual to a condition called *narrow-angle glaucoma*. The term *glaucoma* refers to a symptom complex that occurs in a variety of disease states. The characteristic finding in all types of glaucoma is an increased intraocular pressure. The *Schiotz tonometer*, which is a small, portable instrument, is used for the quantitative assessment of intraocular pressure. Palpation of the globe to determine intraocular pressure is a technique of low sensitivity. Palpation, if performed incorrectly, may be

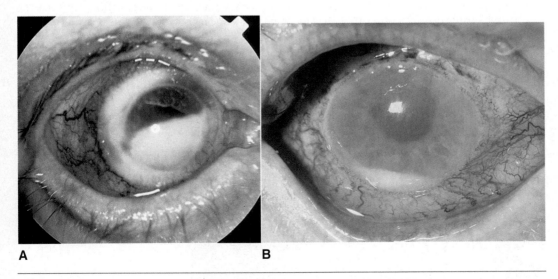

A   **B**

Figure 10–64 *A* and *B,* Two examples of hypopyon. Note the conjunctival injection.

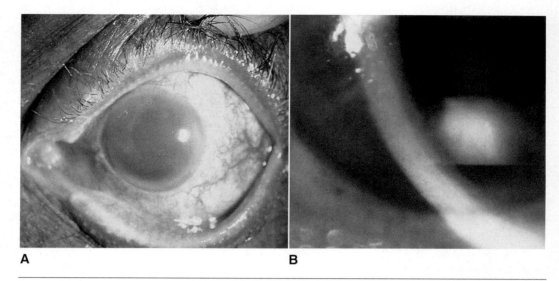

A   **B**

Figure 10–65 *A* and *B,* Two examples of hyphema.

deleterious, especially in an eye that has been subjected to recent surgery, because a retinal detachment may result. Therefore, palpation of the eye should *not* be performed.

Inspect the Lens

With oblique lighting, inspect the lens. Is the lens clear? Note any opacity that may be visible through the pupil.

The most commonly observed abnormality of the lens is opacification; the most common cause of opacification is aging. Slow, gradual vision loss is the symptom. Other causes include hereditary diseases, such as Down's syndrome and cretinism; ocular diseases, such as high myopia, iritis, and retinal dystrophy; systemic disease, such as diabetes and hypoparathyroidism; medications; and trauma, such as a penetrating eye wound.

A *cataract* is any opacification of the lens, an opacity that causes reduced visual acuity, or an opacity that interferes with the patient's everyday life. Figure 10-68*A* shows a dense cataract of the left eye. Note the leukokoria related to the cataract. Figure 10-68*B* shows a dense nuclear, or central, cataract of the left eye in another patient. Figure 10-69 is a close-up view of a dense nuclear cataract with anterior cortical spokes (opacification of the anterior cortex of the lens). The red reflex, described in the following section, Ophthalmoscopic Examination, is absent in all of these patients.

Is the lens in the normal position, or is it dislocated? The lens may be dislocated anteriorly, pressing the iris against the posterior cornea and blocking aqueous humor outflow, or it may be dislocated posteriorly. Secondary glaucoma may result. Marfan's syndrome is an autosomal

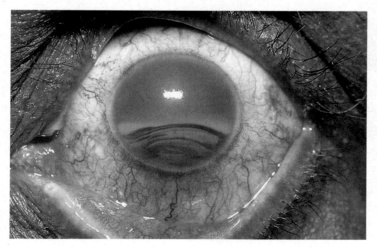

Figure 10–66 ''Candy cane'' hyphema.

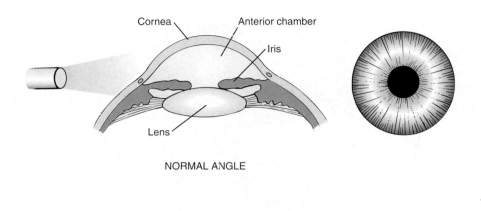

Cornea Anterior chamber

Iris

Lens

NORMAL ANGLE

NARROW ANGLE

Figure 10–67 Assessing the depth of the anterior chamber.

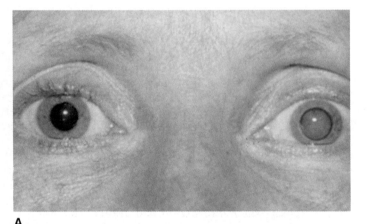

A

Figure 10–68 *A* and *B,* Cataract of the left eye.

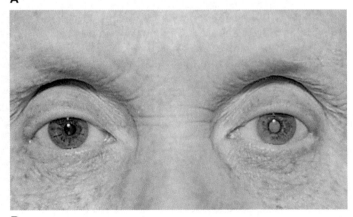

B

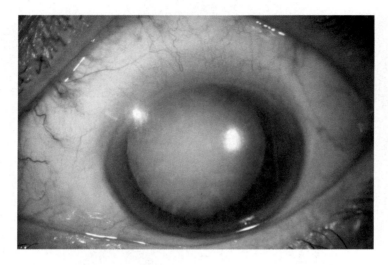

Figure 10–69 Dense nuclear cataract.

dominant condition, often with incomplete expression, in which there is increased length of the long bones; ocular complications include dislocation, or subluxation, of the lens, usually superiorly and nasally. Figure 10-70 shows a subluxated lens secondary to Marfan's syndrome. This is the pupil of the patient's left eye. Note the lower edge of the lens and the attached zonules that are apparent from the 3 o'clock to 7 o'clock positions (white lines). The red behind these lines is the red reflex of the retina in the background.

Many patients now receive intraocular lens implants after the removal of a cataractous lens. Figure 10-71 shows a dislocated intraocular lens implant. Note the dislocated wire attachment.

Ophthalmoscopic Examination

The Ophthalmoscope

Before the examination of the optic fundus is discussed, a few words about the ophthalmoscope are in order. The ophthalmoscope is an instrument with a mirror optical system for viewing the interior anatomy of the eye. There are two dials on the ophthalmoscope: one adjusts the light apertures and filters, and the other changes the lenses to correct for the refractive errors of both the examiner and the patient.

The most important apertures and filters are the *small* aperture, the *large* aperture, and the *red-free* (*green*) filter. The small aperture is for an undilated pupil; the large aperture is for a dilated pupil; and the red-free filter excludes rays of red light and is designed for visualization of blood vessels and hemorrhages. With this filter, the retina appears gray, the disc appears white, the macula appears yellow, and blood appears black.

Using the Ophthalmoscope

Hold the ophthalmoscope in your *right* hand in front of your *right* eye to examine the patient's *right* eye. Ask the patient to look straight ahead and fixate on a distant target. If you wear glasses, remove them for better visualization of the retina. The ophthalmoscope light is turned on, and the aperture is switched to the small aperture. Start with the lens diopter* dial set to 0 if you do not use glasses. The myopic examiner should start with "minus" lenses, which are indicated by red numbers; the hyperopic examiner needs "plus" lenses, which are indicated by black numbers. Your index finger remains on the dial to enable easy focusing.

Place the ophthalmoscope against your forehead while your left thumb gently elevates the patient's right upper eyelid. The ophthalmoscope and your head should function as one unit. While looking through the ophthalmoscope, approach the patient at eye level from about 15 inches (38 cm) away at an angle of about 20° lateral from center, as shown in Figure 10-72. The light should shine on the pupil. A red glow, the *red reflex*, can be seen in the pupil if the path of light is not obstructed by an opaque lens. Note any opacity in the cornea or lens.

By moving in toward the patient along the same 20° line, you begin to see the blood vessels of the retina. Move in close to the patient, bringing your hand holding the ophthalmoscope against the patient's cheek. As contact is made with the patient, the optic disc

---

*A unit of optical power of a lens to cause light rays to diverge or converge.

LEFT EYE

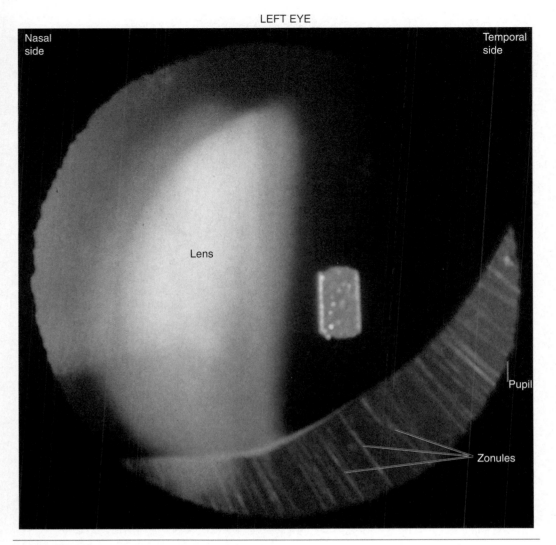

Figure 10–70 Sublaxated lens (left eye) in Marfan's syndrome.

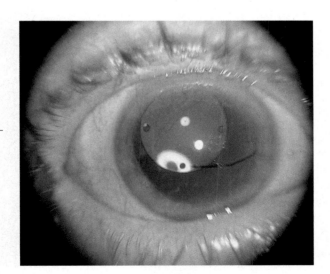

Figure 10–71 Dislocated intraocular lens implant.

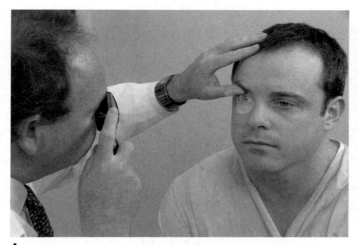

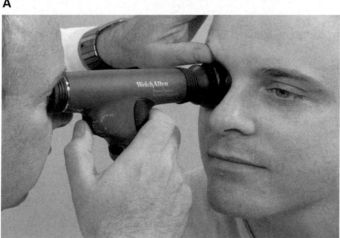

Figure 10–72 *A* and *B,* Correct positions for holding the ophthalmoscope and patient's eye. *B,* The PanOptic ophthalmoscope.

or vessels are visible. By rotating the diopter wheel with the index finger, you bring these structures into sharp focus. Figure 10-73 shows the correct position of the examiner and patient for viewing the retina; Figure 10-74*A* shows a normal optic fundus in the right eye, and Figure 10-74*B,* in the left eye. Notice that the macula is temporal to the optic disc.

After the right eye is examined, hold the ophthalmoscope in your *left* hand and use your *left* eye to examine the patient's *left* eye.

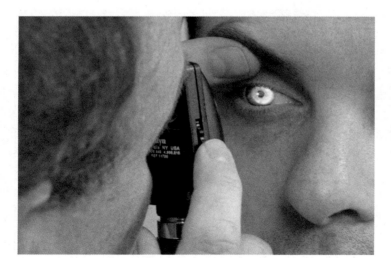

Figure 10–73 Correct position for examining the retina.

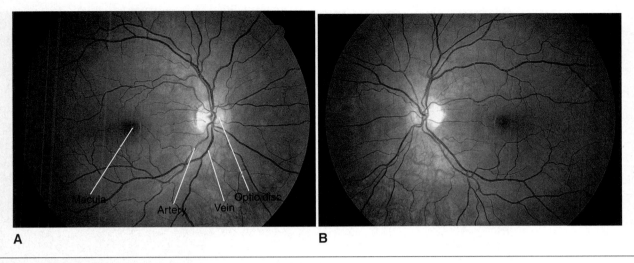

A   B

Figure 10–74 Photograph of the retinas of the right (*A*) and left (*B*) eyes.

Careful assessment of the optic fundus is important for several reasons. The optic fundus is the only area where the blood vessels can be seen in vivo; it can provide an excellent picture of the state of the vasculature of other organs. In addition, the optic fundus is frequently involved with manifestations of systemic disease such as AIDS, infective endocarditis, hypertension, and diabetes; a thorough evaluation of the fundus can provide valuable clues to their diagnosis. Finally, because the eye is an extension of the central nervous system, evaluation of the optic fundus can provide information about many neurologic disorders.

The optic fundus must be assessed methodically, starting at the optic disc, tracing the retinal vessels emerging from it, inspecting the macula, and evaluating the rest of the retina.

Inspect the Optic Disc

The most conspicuous landmark of the retina is the optic disc (Fig. 10-75). The optic disc is the intraocular portion of the optic nerve and is seen with the ophthalmoscope. Its *margins, color,* and *cup–disc ratio* should be determined. The disc should be round or slightly oval with the long axis usually vertical and with sharp borders. The nasal border is normally slightly blurred. The disc is pinkish in light-skinned individuals and yellowish-orange in darker-skinned individuals. The relative pallor of the optic disc is caused by the reflection of light from the myelin sheaths of the optic nerve. In the center of the normal optic disc, there is a funnel-shaped depression known as *physiologic cupping*. The cup is the portion of the disc that is central, lighter in color, and penetrated by the retinal vessels. The normal ratio of the cup diameter to disc diameter varies from 0.1 to 0.5. The examiner should check the cup–disc ratio in both eyes for symmetry.

The benign condition *myelinated*, or *medullated, nerve fibers* is seen in 0.3% to 0.6% of all individuals. In this condition, the nerve fiber layer continues to myelinate into the retina beyond the lamina cribrosa. The fibers appear as white patches with feathery borders that radiate from the optic disc and obscure the retinal vessels over which they pass. The condition is present at birth, does not change, and usually causes no visual impairment. Figure 10-76 shows the retina of a patient with myelinated nerve fibers. Another dramatic example of myelinated nerve fibers at the disc is shown in Figure 10-77. Figure 10-78 shows myelinated nerve fibers in the peripheral retina.

An *optic pit* is a congenital anomaly of the optic disc. It is a small depression, located temporally in 75% of cases, in the optic nerve and is usually gray or yellow. In 85% of cases, it is unilateral. Figure 10-79*A* shows an optic pit. Retinal tears and detachment can occur in 50% of patients with an optic pit, as shown in Figure 10-79*B*; that patient has an optic pit and a retinal tear involving the macula of the left eye.

Inspect the Retinal Vessels

The retinal vessels are evaluated as they arborize over the retina. The central retinal artery enters the globe through the physiologic cup. It divides within the cup and again on the surface, giving rise to four main branches that supply the superior and inferior temporal and nasal quadrants of the optic fundus. The arteries are two-thirds to four-fifths the diameter of the veins and have a prominent *light reflex*. This light reflex is a reflection of the

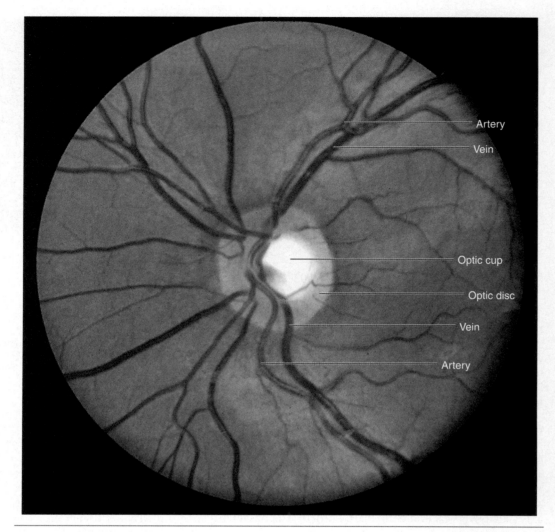

Figure 10–75 Normal optic disc, left eye.

ophthalmoscope's light on the arterial wall and is normally about one-fourth the diameter of the column of blood. The veins exhibit spontaneous pulsations in 85% of patients. This can best be demonstrated as the retinal vein enters the optic nerve, where it can be seen on end.

As all the vessels course away from the disc, they appear to narrow. The crossing of the arteries and veins occurs within two disc diameters from the disc.

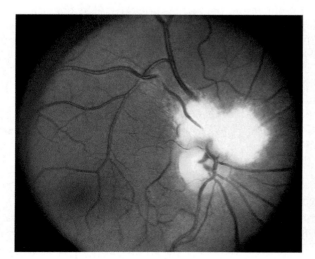

Figure 10–76 Retina with myelinated nerve fibers.

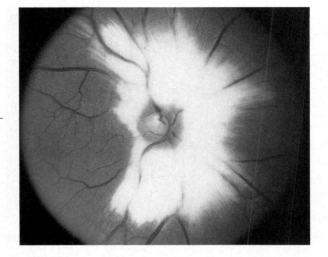

Figure 10–77 Myelinated nerve fibers at optic disc.

The normal vessel wall is invisible, with its thin light reflex. In hypertension, the vessel may have focal or generalized areas of narrowing or spasm, causing the light reflex to be narrowed. With time, the vessel wall becomes thickened and sclerotic, and there is a widening of the light reflex to greater than half of the diameter of the column of blood. The light reflex develops an orange metallic appearance called *copper wiring* (Fig. 10-80). When such an artery crosses over a vein, there appears to be a discontinuity of the venous column as a result of the widened, but invisible, arterial wall. This is termed *arteriovenous nicking*.

Follow the vessels in all four directions: superior temporal, superior nasal, inferior nasal, and inferior temporal. Remember to move your head and the ophthalmoscope as one unit.

Inspect the Macula

When the ophthalmoscope is kept level with the disc and moved temporally approximately 1.5 to 2 disc diameters, the macula is seen. This appears as an avascular area with a pinpoint reflective center, the fovea. If the examiner has difficulty in seeing the macula, the patient can be instructed to look directly into the light; the fovea is then visible. The red-free filter is also helpful in locating the macula. Figure 10-81 shows a normal macula of the right eye.

Figure 10-82 shows a patient with a macular hole of the left eye; notice the punched-out appearance at the macula. Macular holes are seen in patients with high myopia.

Describe Any Retinal Lesions

When a lesion is seen, its color and shape are important in determining its cause. Is it red, black, gray, or whitish? Red lesions are usually hemorrhages. They can be located best by using the green contrast filter of the ophthalmoscope. Linear, or *flame-shaped*, hemorrhages occur in the nerve fiber layer of the retina (Fig. 10-83), whereas round hemorrhages are located in deeper intraretinal layers. Are the borders of the lesions sharp or blurred?

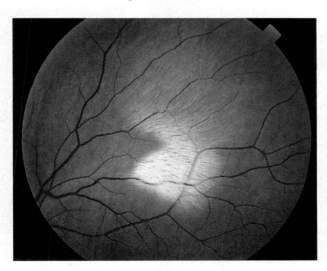

Figure 10–78 Myelinated nerve fibers at peripheral retina.

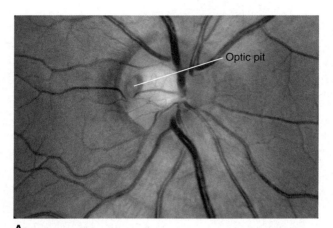

A

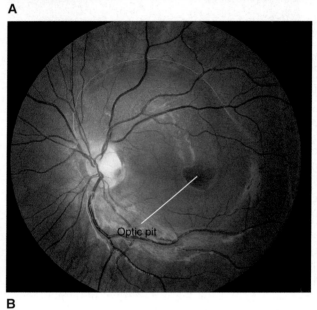

B

Figure 10–79 *A,* Optic pit, right eye. *B,* Optic pit and a retinal tear, left eye, in another patient.

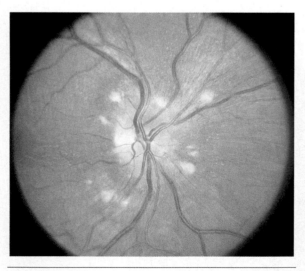

Figure 10–80 Hypertension. Note the "copper wiring" of the arteries and the numerous cotton-wool spots, which are exudates in the nerve fiber layer.

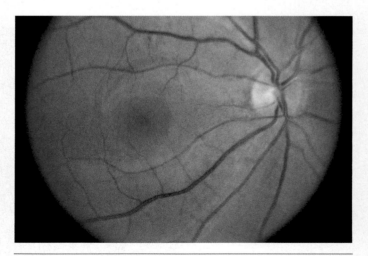

Figure 10–81 Normal macula, right eye.

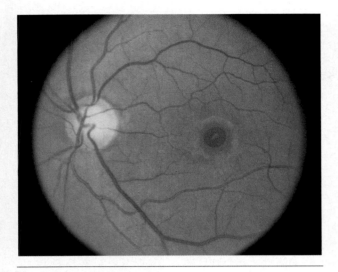

Figure 10–82 Macular hole.

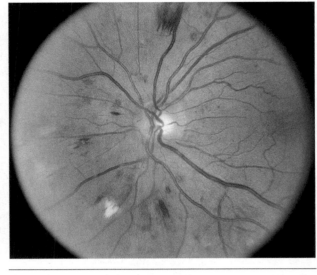

Figure 10–83 Flame-shaped hemorrhages and a cotton-wool spot in a patient with hypertension.

A common benign retinal finding is *congenital hypertrophy of the retinal pigment epithelium (RPE)*. This appears as a round, dramatically dark pigmented lesion, often one to several disc diameters in size. The surface is flat, and the edges are very sharp. Several small, punched-out holes are commonly present within. The retinal vessels appear normal. This is an asymptomatic lesion and is usually unilateral; it may occur in any position in the retina. Its recognition is important and should not be misdiagnosed as a malignant melanoma. Figure 10-84 shows a retina with congenital hypertrophy of the RPE.

Black lesions that are shaped like bone spicules are associated with retinitis pigmentosa. In this condition, melanin tends to unsheathe the retinal vessels (see Fig. 10-142 and a discussion of this condition at the end of this chapter). A doughnut-shaped lesion is often found in chronic inactive toxoplasmosis chorioretinitis (see Figs. 10-127 and 10-128). A pigmented, raised, disc-shaped lesion is suggestive of a melanoma (see Fig. 10-139). Diffuse spotting of the retina is often a degenerative state. Flat, *gray* lesions are usually benign choroidal nevi (see Fig. 10-138).

White lesions may appear as soft, cotton-wool spots or may be dense. Soft, cotton-wool spots or exudations are caused by infarctions of the nerve fiber layer of the retina (see Figs. 10-80 and 10-83). White lesions are common and are frequently associated with hypertension or diabetes. The differentiation of white lesions of the retina is summarized in Table 10-8.

Figure 10–84 Congenital hypertrophy of the retinal pigment epithelium (RPE).

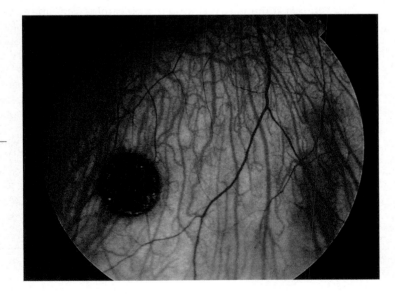

Table 10–8 Differentiation of Whitish Lesions of the Fundus

Feature	Cotton-Wool Spots*	Fatty Exudates†	Drusen‡	Chorioretinitis§
Cause¶	Hypertension Diabetic retinopathy Acquired immunodeficiency syndrome Lupus erythematosus Dermatomyositis Papilledema	Diabetes mellitus Retinal venous occlusion Hypertensive retinotherapy	Can be normal with aging Age-related macular degeneration	Toxoplasmosis Sarcoidosis Cytomegalovirus
Border	Fuzzy	Well defined	Well defined, nonpigmented	Often large with ragged edge, heavily pigmented
Shape	Irregular	Small, irregular	Round, well circumscribed	Very variable
Patterns	Variable	Often clustered in circles or stars	Variable; symmetrical in both eyes	Variable
Comments	Caused by an ischemic infarct of the nerve fiber layer of the retina; obscures retinal blood vessels; usually several in number	In deep retinal layer	Often confused with fatty exudates; deep to retinal blood vessels	Acute with white exudate; healed lesion with pigmented scar (toxoplasmosis)

*See Figures 10-80 and 10-83.
†Also known as *edema residues*. See Figures 10-104 and 10-105.
‡Also known as *colloid bodies*. See Figure 10-121.
§See Figures 10-125 to 10-135.
¶The diseases noted do not constitute a complete etiologic list. Only the most common causes are indicated.

Difficulties in Using the Ophthalmoscope

Frequently, difficulties arise in the use of the ophthalmoscope. These include the following:

- A small pupil
- Extraneous light
- Improper use of the ophthalmoscope
- Myopia in the patient
- Cataract in the patient

The use of mydriatic drops to visualize the retina better is important. Many medical students fear that these drops will precipitate an attack of narrow-angle glaucoma. It is clear from the data that more retinal findings are missed by not dilating the pupils than when the drops precipitate such an attack, which occurs in less than 0.1% of patients. If this reaction occurs, the patients are in the best possible facility for treatment.

The examiner should use one drop of tropicamide 1.0% in each eye. Care should be taken to place the drop on the inside of the lower lid and not on the cornea. The patient should be told that the drop will sting slightly and will cause photophobia in sunshine. The duration of the mydriatic action depends primarily on the patient's sensitivity to the medication: a more heavily pigmented iris requires more time to achieve mydriasis. The cycloplegic* action lasts for about 6 hours. These drops can be used in patients wearing contact lenses. Atropine should be avoided because its effect lasts for up to 2 weeks. The large aperture of the ophthalmoscope is used when the pupil is dilated. Record in the chart that the patient's pupil or pupils were dilated and which medications were used.

The room should be darkened as much as possible for the easiest evaluation of the retina. Another common problem is corneal reflection. Often, light is reflected from the cornea, which makes the examination more difficult. Use of the small aperture or a polarizing filter, which many ophthalmoscopes include, may be helpful.

Patients with myopia provide the most problems for the novice examiner. In myopic eyes, the retinal image is enlarged, making it difficult sometimes to visualize the retina adequately.

---

*Producing paralysis of accommodation.

If the patient is severely myopic, it may be necessary for the patient to wear corrective lenses while being examined.

A cataract does not allow adequate visualization of the retina, especially if the cataract is central.

Clinicopathologic Correlations

There are many ophthalmoscopic conditions with which the examiner should be familiar. An image is normally focused directly on the retina. When the image is not focused on the retina, a refractive error is present. Lenses are used to correct refractive errors. The absence of a refractive error is called *emmetropia*. Refractive errors are extremely common. Listed here are the common refractive errors and their causes:

Hyperopia (farsightedness): Light is focused posterior to the retina.

Myopia (nearsightedness): Light is focused anterior to the retina.

Astigmatism: Light is not uniformly focused in all directions. Astigmatism is commonly a result of a cornea that is not perfectly spherical.

Presbyopia: Near vision decreases progressively as a result of a decrease in the eye's ability to accommodate. Presbyopia occurs after age 40 years.

Figure 10-85 illustrates normal (emmetropic), hyperopic, myopic, and astigmatic eyes.

Cataracts (see Figs. 10-68 and 10-69) are the most common cause of blindness. A cataract is a type of degenerative eye disease. One of the first symptoms that patients with cataracts experience is a "mistiness" of vision. Affected patients typically give a history in which vision has become "like looking through a dirty window." As the lenticular opacity increases with time, there is a diminution of visual acuity in association with glare in bright light. This effect results from pupillary constriction limiting the light rays passing through the lens to the central portion of the lens, where the opacity is often most dense. These patients may wear dark glasses and hold their heads down to avoid excess light.

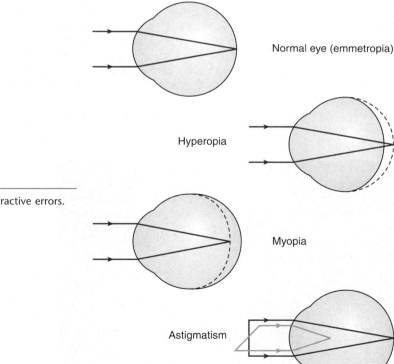

Figure 10–85 Common refractive errors.

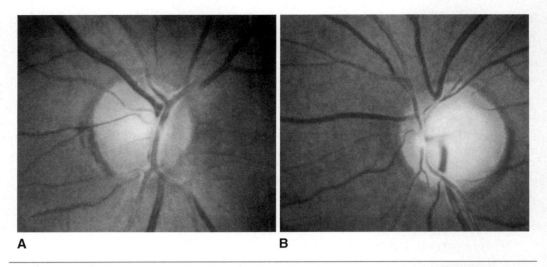

Figure 10–86 *A* and *B,* Optic cup asymmetry in glaucoma. The cup–disc ratio is approximately 30% in *A* (*right eye*) and 70% in *B* (*left eye*).

Narrow-angle glaucoma results from an obstruction to the drainage of aqueous humor at the canal of Schlemm. Patients with narrow-angle glaucoma have periodic attacks of acute elevation of intraocular pressure caused by intermittent obstruction. This is associated with pain, seeing halos, and poor vision. These attacks of glaucoma commonly occur in a darkened room, when pupillary dilatation occurs. When the pupil is fully dilated in a person with a narrow angle, the redundant iris folds at its base cause the increased obstruction and decreased drainage.

Primary open-angle, or *chronic simple, glaucoma,* in contrast, is associated with an open angle. There are many causes for simple glaucoma, which is a leading cause of slowly progressive blindness. The most important diagnostic difference from narrow-angle glaucoma is that in chronic simple glaucoma, pain is absent. Patients have reduced outflow of aqueous humor through the trabecular meshwork and into the canal of Schlemm, which results in elevated intraocular pressure. As a result, progressive cupping of the optic nerve (i.e., loss of nerve substance) occurs, accompanied by changes in the visual field. Although primary open-angle glaucoma is usually bilateral, its asymmetric onset results in a difference in optic cup size between the two eyes, one of the most characteristic early signs (Fig. 10-86). Peripheral field defects, especially in the nasal aspect, are common early in the disease. Vision is increasingly impaired as progressive atrophy of the optic nerve continues, owing to the increased intraocular pressure. Late in the disease, only a small area on the nasal aspect of the nerve head may remain. Figure 10-87 shows a close-up of the optic disc of a patient with 50% to 60% cupping of the optic nerve head. Table 10-9 lists the major characteristics of both types of glaucoma.

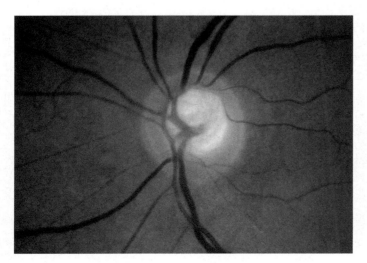

Figure 10–87 Glaucomatous cupping of the optic nerve head. The cup-to-disc ratio is approximately 50% to 60%.

Table 10–9 Characteristics of Glaucoma

Feature	Primary Open-Angle Glaucoma	Narrow-Angle Glaucoma
Occurrence	85% of all glaucoma cases	15% of all glaucoma cases
Cause	Unclear*	Closed angle prevents aqueous drainage
Age at onset	Variable	50-85 years
Anterior chamber	Usually normal	Shallow
Chamber angle	Normal	Narrow
Symptoms	Usually none Decreased vision, late	Headache Seeing halos around lights Sudden onset of severe eye pain Vomiting during attack
Cupping of disc	Progressive if not treated (see Figs. 10-86 and 10-87)	After one or more untreated attacks
Visual fields	Peripheral fields are involved early Central involvement is a very late sign	Involvement is a late sign
Ocular pressure	Progressively higher if not medically controlled Late: high	Early: detected with provocative tests only
Other signs		Fixed, partially dilated pupil Conjunctival injection "Steamy" cornea†
Treatment	Medical Laser surgery	Surgical
Prognosis	Good if recognized early Very dependent on patient compliance	Good

*Thought to be a defect in the trabecular network ultrastructure.
†Like looking through a steamy window.

Acute eye inflammations are common. They may be associated with local or systemic disease. The differential diagnosis of the red eye is important. The presence of pain, visual loss, and irregularities of the pupils are important signs signifying a serious, potentially blinding disorder. Figure 10-88 shows red eye. Table 10-2 provides an approach to the diagnosis of red eye.

Diabetic retinopathy is the leading cause of blindness in Americans aged 20 to 75 years. It is estimated that more than 12 million Americans have diabetes. Diabetic retinopathy is a highly specific vascular complication of type I and type II diabetes mellitus and is directly related to the duration of the disease. By 25 years after the onset of diabetes, nearly all patients with type I diabetes and 65% of patients with type II diabetes have some degree of retinopathy.

The retinal findings of diabetic retinopathy are the result of retinal microangiopathy, which causes increased vascular permeability that results in macular edema and decreased vision. In addition, vascular occlusive changes result in fibrovascular proliferation, hemorrhage, and scarring. The early changes of nonproliferative retinopathy are capillary microaneurysms, dilatation, tortuosity of vessels, and nonperfusion of areas of the retina. As the disease progresses to proliferative retinopathy, retinal neovascularization appears either at the optic disc (NVD) or elsewhere in the retina (NVE). Neovascularization may diminish vision still further by vitreous hemorrhage or traction detachment of the retina.

Nonproliferative, or *background, retinopathy* is the first stage of diabetic retinopathy. An early sign is the development of microaneurysms. These usually have smooth borders and sharp round shapes. In addition, intraretinal hemorrhages result from rupture of the microaneurysms, capillaries, and venules. The location of the hemorrhage within the retinal layers

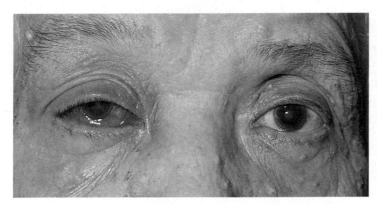

Figure 10–88 Red eye.

governs the shape of the hemorrhage: hemorrhages in the nerve fiber layer typically are flame-shaped with feathery borders, whereas hemorrhages in the deep areas of the retina have a fuzzy, blot-shaped appearance. Exudates may appear as clusters, streaks, or rings around the macula. These exudates result from leakage through the abnormally permeable capillary walls. Commonly, these microaneurysms, hemorrhages, and exudates occur near the macula. The retinal findings in a patient with nonproliferative diabetic retinopathy are shown in Figure 10-89. Note the hemorrhages and exudates. Figure 10-90 shows the marked tortuosity of the vessels in another patient with background retinopathy. Figure 10-91 shows the flame-shaped hemorrhages and exudates that are characteristic of nonproliferative diabetic retinopathy. Figure 10-92 shows circinate retinopathy in a diabetic patient.

Proliferative diabetic retinopathy is characterized by neovascularization, that is, new blood vessels that arise from the retinal and optic disc vessels. Neovascularization appears as a fine network (wisps or loops) of blood vessels that seem to bud off other vessels. Neovascularization of the disc (NVD) is shown in Figure 10-93; neovascularization elsewhere in the retina (NVE) is

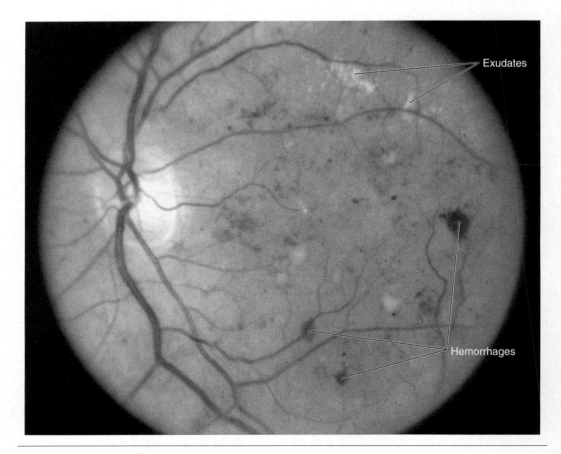

Figure 10–89 Nonproliferative diabetic retinopathy.

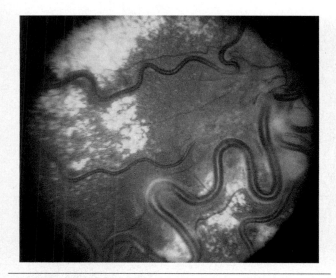

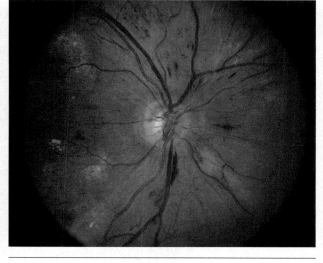

Figure 10–90 Nonproliferative diabetic retinopathy. Note the markedly tortuous vessels.

Figure 10–91 Nonproliferative diabetic retinopathy. Note the flame-shaped hemorrhages.

shown in Figure 10-94. These vessels proliferate along the retinal surface and into the vitreous humor, often with fibrous band components. The vessels are often adherent to the posterior vitreous, and preretinal hemorrhages occur as a result of vitreoretinal separation pulling on the friable vessels. The blood resulting from a preretinal hemorrhage is trapped in the potential space between the retina and the vitreous humor (under the inner limiting membrane), forming a classic boat-shaped hemorrhage (Fig. 10-95). Further pulling on the retina can progress to retinal tears and tractional retinal detachments. Figures 10-96 to 10-98 show vitreous strands in patients with proliferative diabetic retinopathy. Figure 10-98 shows vitreous traction and a macular hole. Note the light-colored area surrounding the macula.

Figure 10-99 shows a patient with proliferative diabetic retinopathy with NVE, NVD, preretinal hemorrhage, and a fatty exudative maculopathy.

The therapy for proliferative retinopathy is panretinal photocoagulation (PRP) to cause regression of the neovascularization. Figures 10-100 and 10-101 show proliferative retinopathy and the laser burns of PRP. Note the PRP-treated areas that appear as round, punched-out spots with pigmentation in the center or at the margins. The treated areas first appear white or yellow, but within several weeks, pigmentation occurs. The laser burns are brought up to the vascular arcades and up to one disc diameter from the optic disc. Vitrectomy is also indicated for tractional detachments. The final stages of diabetic retinopathy, known as *involutional* or *burned-out retinopathy*, show a tangle of new vessels, hemorrhages, traction, and fibrosis.

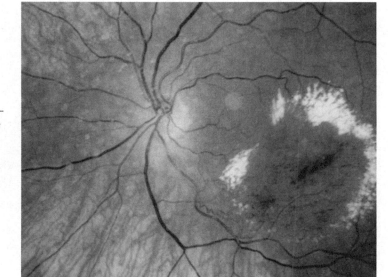

Figure 10–92 Nonproliferative retinopathy, circinate retinopathy. Note the ring of exudates around or near the macula, as well as the hemorrhages at the macula.

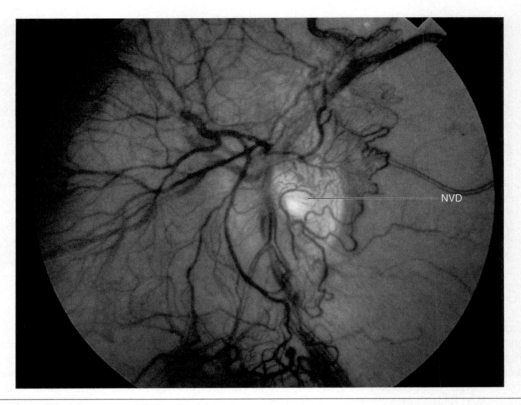

Figure 10–93 Proliferative diabetic retinopathy. Note the neovascularization of the disc (NVD).

Hypertension also produces significant characteristic retinal features. Systemic hypertension may be reflected in the retina in terms of irregularities in arteriolar size, tortuosity of the retinal arteries, retinal edema, and changes in the arteriovenous crossings. Progressive changes of hypertension include arteriolar narrowing with increasing areas of retinal ischemia, which is evident by the development of cotton-wool exudates, hemorrhages, retinal edema, and papilledema. Figure 10-102 shows the retinal changes in a patient with hypertension. Notice in Figure 10-103 the tortuosity of the retinal vessels in another patient with hypertension; a red-free (green) contrast filter is used to enhance the visualization of the vessels. Cotton-wool spots and flame-shaped retinal hemorrhages in another patient with hypertension are shown in Figure 10-83. As the arteriole walls thicken as a result of sustained hypertension, the arterioles lose their transparency, and noticeable changes are seen at the crossings of the arteries and veins. Veins appear to disappear abruptly on either side of an artery. Some of the arteries develop a burnishing of the red reflex.

Macular exudates are also common in hypertension (Fig. 10-104). These are well-defined, whitish-yellow intraretinal collections of lipids secondary to vascular leakage. A *macular star* is

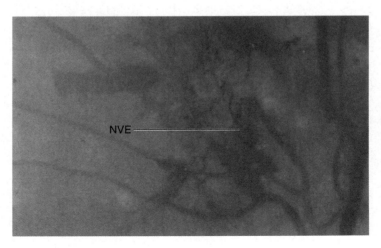

Figure 10–94 Proliferative diabetic retinopathy. Note the neovascularization elsewhere in the retina (NVE).

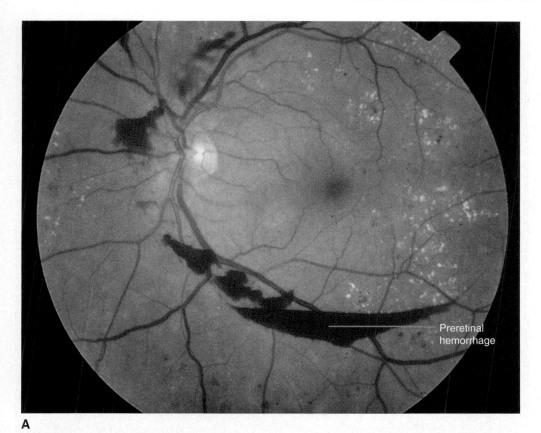

A

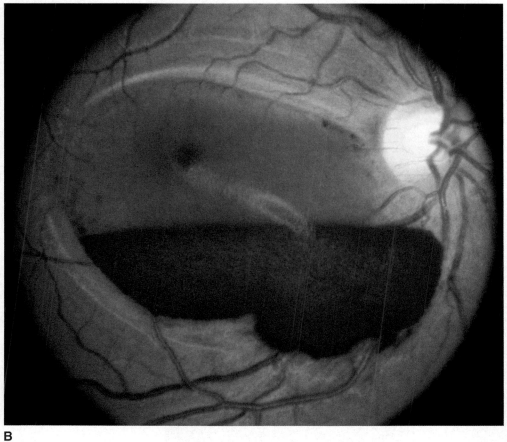

B

Figure 10–95 *A* and *B*, Proliferative diabetic retinopathy. Note the preretinal hemorrhage.

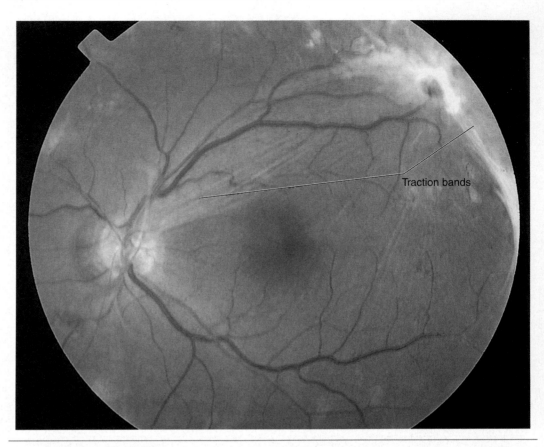

Traction bands

Figure 10–96 Proliferative diabetic retinopathy. Note the vitreoretinal fibrous bands.

an accumulation of edema residues arranged in a stellate pattern around the macula. Macular stars are commonly seen in patients with hypertension, papilledema, papillitis, and *central retinal venous occlusion* (CRVO). A macular star is shown in Figure 10-105. Arteriolar dilations may also develop. These are known as arteriolar *macroaneurysms* and are prone to leak blood and serous fluid. A hemorrhage from a macroaneurysm is shown in Figure 10-106.

Increased intracranial pressure, frequently secondary to a space-occupying intracranial lesion, produces a classic picture of *papilledema*. Papilledema is a swelling of the optic disc. It is believed that the increased pressure is transmitted to the optic nerve sheath, causing axoplasmic flow stasis in the disc. This in turn causes axonal swelling and secondary

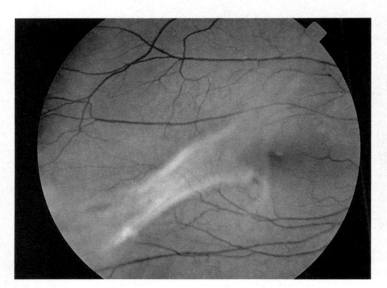

Figure 10–97 Proliferative diabetic retinopathy. Note the vitreoretinal fibrous bands.

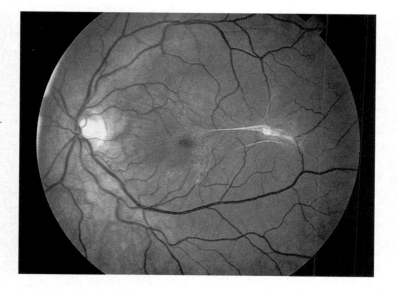

Figure 10–98 Proliferative diabetic retinopathy. Note the vitreoretinal fibrous bands and macular hole.

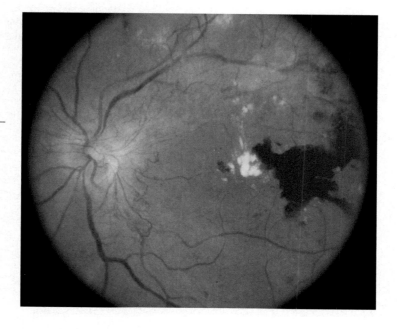

Figure 10–99 Diabetic retinopathy with neovascularization of the disc, neovascularization elsewhere in the retina, preretinal hemorrhage, and fatty macular exudates.

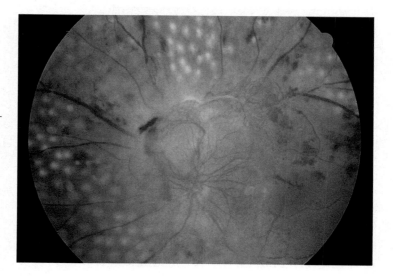

Figure 10–100 Proliferative diabetic retinopathy. Note the lesions of panretinal photocoagulation.

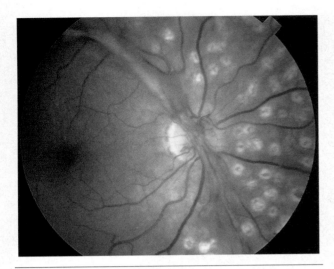

Figure 10–101 Proliferative diabetic retinopathy. Note the lesions of panretinal photocoagulation.

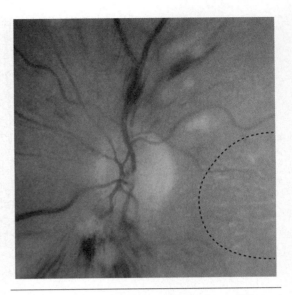

Figure 10–102 Retinal changes in a patient with long-standing hypertension. Note the cotton-wool spots and flame-shaped hemorrhages. Part of a macular star is seen on the bottom right.

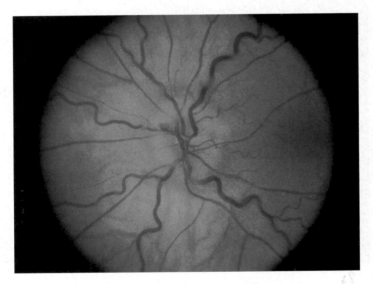

Figure 10–103 Hypertensive retinopathy. Note the markedly tortuous vessels seen through the green contrast filter.

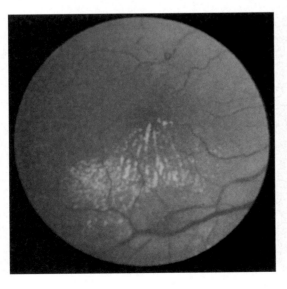

Figure 10–104 Macular exudates in a patient with hypertension.

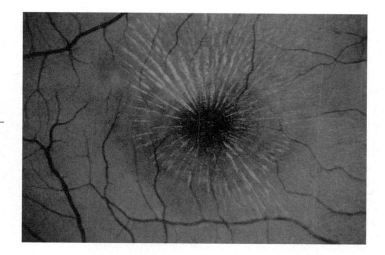

Figure 10–105 Macular star in hypertensive retinopathy.

vascular congestion. The most characteristic finding is blurring of the optic disc. This occurs in association with the loss of spontaneous retinal venous pulsation, hyperemia of the disc, hemorrhages and exudates of the disc, and dilated tortuous retinal veins. In spite of these changes, vision remains remarkably normal in the early or acute stages. Figure 10-107 is a photograph and a labeled schematic of the retinal changes in chronic papilledema. Figure 10-108 shows papilledema in another patient. Notice the blurring of the disc margins and the hyperemia of the disc. Figure 10-109 shows papilledema in yet another patient; notice the flame-shaped hemorrhages and the hyperemia of the disc. There are other causes of a blurred disc margin. Table 10-10 provides a differentiation of blurred disc margins due to different conditions.

Blood dyscrasias are frequently diagnosed from the examination of the retina. Figure 10-110 shows the retina of a patient with leukemia. Notice the multiple hemorrhages, perivascular infiltrates of the retinal arterioles, and *Roth's spots*. These spots have a clear white center and are surrounded by hemorrhage; they are believed to be areas of emboli and retinal infarcts. They are also seen in infective endocarditis and HIV retinitis.

Occlusive disorders of the retinal circulation are dramatic. A *central retinal artery occlusion* (CRAO) is usually caused by an embolus from the heart or large artery. It results in sudden, painless loss of vision in one eye. The pupillary direct light reflex is lost, and spontaneous venous pulsations are absent. Within minutes, the retina becomes pale and milky white with narrowed arteries, and a cherry-red spot appears at the macula. This cherry-red spot appears because in the foveal area, the retina is thin, allowing visibility of the underlying choroidal circulation that is obscured elsewhere by retinal edema. This is a true ocular emergency because if it is not treated within 45 minutes, the retina may not be saved. Figure 10-111 shows the left retina of a patient with a CRAO. Notice the pale retina with the cherry-red spot at the macula.

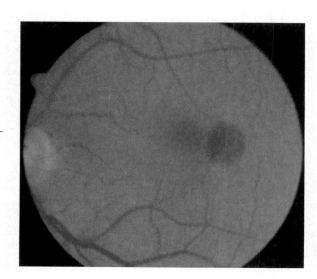

Figure 10–106 Macroaneurysms in hypertensive retinopathy. Note the hemorrhage lateral to the macula.

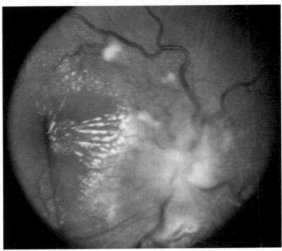

A

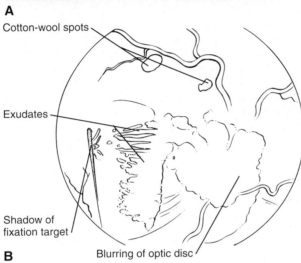

Cotton-wool spots

Exudates

Shadow of
fixation target

B

Blurring of optic disc

Figure 10–107 Photograph (*A*) and schematic (*B*) showing the retinal changes in papilledema.

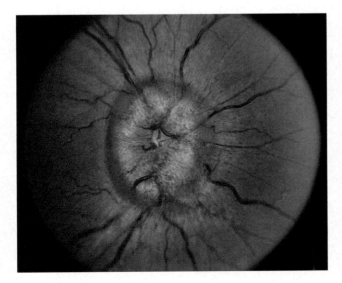

Figure 10–108 Papilledema. Note the hyperemia of the disc.

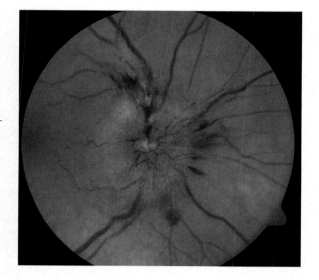

Figure 10–109 Papilledema. Note the hyperemia of the disc and the flame-shaped hemorrhages.

Figure 10-112 shows the retina of a patient with a CRAO with cilioretinal artery sparing. The cilioretinal arteries are present in 40% of normal individuals. They are derived from the posterior ciliary circulation and usually emerge from the temporal aspect of the disc to supply a small portion of the retina. Notice the area of retina that is spared as a result of perfusion by the cilioretinal artery. Figure 10-113 shows a CRAO in another patient. In this example, the retina is also pale (ischemic and edematous), but the area of the cherry-red spot at the macula is heavily pigmented. This is the finding in dark-skinned individuals with a CRAO.

Hollenhorst plaques are cholesterol emboli found at the bifurcation of the retinal arteries. The source of these emboli is usually the heart or the carotid arteries. They are usually unilateral and occur in elderly individuals with advanced atherosclerosis. Symptoms of fleeting alterations of vision may accompany these emboli. Figure 10-114 shows a classic example of a Hollenhorst plaque. Figure 10-115 shows a *branch retinal artery occlusion* (BRAO). Note the area of the ischemic retina and the cotton-wool spots and adjacent flame-shaped hemorrhage. Figure 10-116 shows a BRAO in another patient that involves the superior portion of the left retina. Note the superior pallor representing the ischemic retina.

Venous occlusion is one of the most common retinal vascular disorders. A central retinal vein occlusion (CRVO) occurs at the lamina cribrosa. The patient experiences painless loss of

Table 10–10 Differentiation of Blurred Disc Margins

Feature	Papilledema*	Papillitis†	Drusen‡	Myelinated Nerve Fibers§	Central Retinal Vein Occlusion¶
Visual acuity	Normal	Decreased	Normal	Normal	Decreased
Venous pulsations	Absent	Variable	Present	Present	Usually absent
Pain	Headache	Eye movement pain	No	No	No
Light reaction	Present	Marcus Gunn (see text)	Present	Present	Present
Hemorrhage	Present	Present	Uncommon	No	Marked
Visual fields	Enlarged blind spot	Central scotoma	Enlarged blind spot	Scotomata correspond to areas of myelination	Variable
Laterality	Bilateral	Unilateral	Bilateral	Seldom bilateral	Unilateral

*Edema of the optic disc resulting from increased intracranial pressure. See Figures 10-107 to 10-109.
†Inflammation of the optic disc.
‡See Figure 10-119.
§Myelination of the optic nerve ends at the optic disc. When it continues into the retina, white, flame-shaped areas obscure the disc margins. See Figures 10-76 to 10-78.
¶See Figure 10-117.

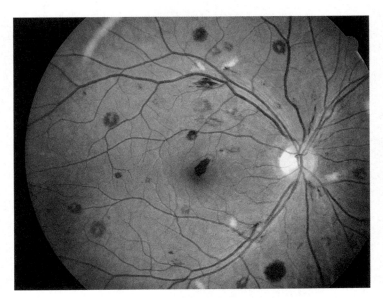

Figure 10–110 Leukemia-related retinitis. Note the multiple hemorrhages, perivascular infiltrates, and Roth's spots.

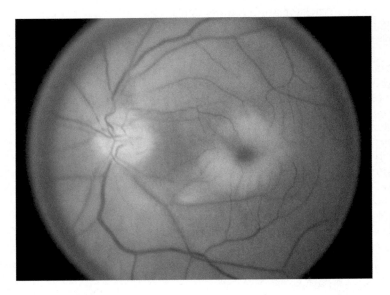

Figure 10–111 Central retinal artery occlusion.

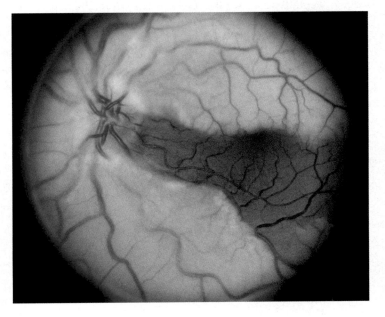

Figure 10–112 Central retinal artery occlusion with cilioretinal artery sparing.

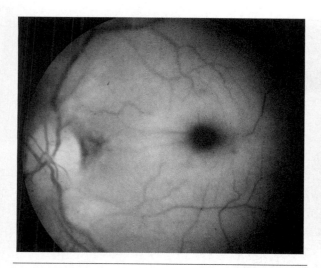

Figure 10–113 Pigmented central retinal artery occlusion in a person of color.

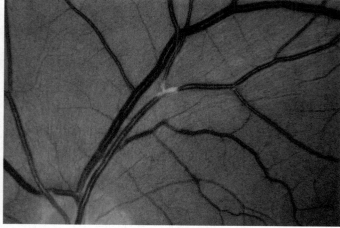

Figure 10–114 Hollenhorst plaque.

vision in one eye. The fundus exhibits venous dilatation and tortuosity, disc edema, flame-shaped hemorrhages in all quadrants, blurred optic disc, cotton-wool spots, and often a large hemorrhage at the macula. The disc is usually edematous with blurred margins. The fundus in a CRVO has been described as a "pizza thrown against a wall." The patients are usually from 70 to 80 years of age. The causes of CRVO are many: hypertension, glaucoma, atherosclerosis, diabetes, and hyperviscosity syndromes. Figure 10-117 shows the retina of a patient with a CRVO. Notice the dark, engorged, tortuous, dusky-colored retinal veins. A branch retinal vein occlusion (BRVO) occurs at a site of retinal arteriovenous crossing. BRVO is commonly

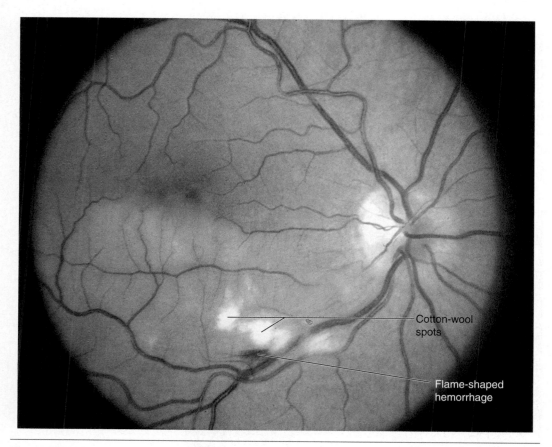

Cotton-wool spots

Flame-shaped hemorrhage

Figure 10–115 Branch retinal artery occlusion.

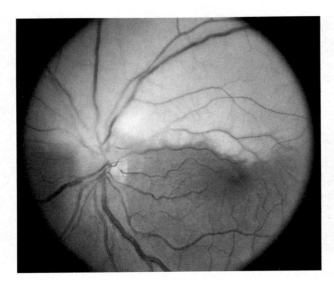

Figure 10–116 Branch retinal artery occlusion. Note the pallor of the superior left retina, resulting from occlusion of the artery supplying this area.

associated with systemic hypertension, although any systemic disease associated with hyper-coagulability may predispose to BRVO. Distal to the site of occlusion, the retinal vein becomes engorged and tortuous with associated capillary dysfunction that leads to intraretinal edema and hemorrhage. Figure 10-118 shows two examples of the retinas of patients with a BRVO.

Drusen of the optic disc are acellular, calcified hyaline deposits in the substance of the optic nerve that occur secondary to axonal degeneration. The disc margins are irregular or blurred. Drusen are found to be bilateral in 70% of affected patients, and the condition is transmitted as an irregular dominant trait with incomplete penetrance. Drusen occur almost exclusively in white individuals. Figure 10-119 shows optic disc drusen. Notice the scalloped appearance of the optic nerve border. Because of the irregular disc border, optic disc drusen sometimes can be confused with papilledema. The absence of optic disc hyperemia, exudates, and venous congestion differentiates drusen from papilledema.

Optic disc drusen should not be confused with *retinal drusen*. Diffuse retinal drusen, as shown in Figure 10-120, are not age-related phenomena and are benign. On the other hand, hard and soft retinal drusen at the level of the RPE located near the macula are part of the disorder known as *age-related macular degeneration* (AMD). AMD is the most common cause of blindness in patients older than 60 years in the United States. It is usually bilateral but may be asymmetric. Retinal drusen are yellowish-white, round lesions that may vary in size and are frequently concentrated at the posterior pole. Figure 10-121 shows the retina of a patient with AMD and subfoveal choroidal neovascularization. The neovascularization appears as the gray pigmentation around the drusen at the macula. This gray area represents new blood vessels grown in from the choroid between it and the RPE. Figure 10-122 is a close-up photograph of the macular drusen in another patient. The growing vessels leak blood, lipids, and serum under

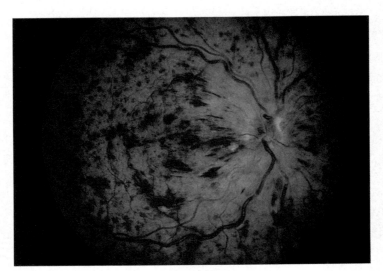

Figure 10–117 Central retinal vein occlusion.

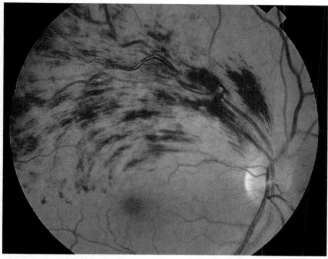

A

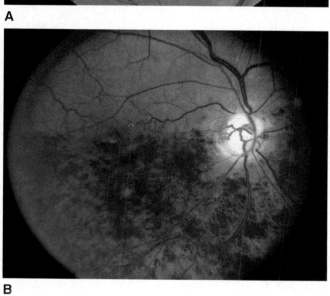

B

Figure 10–118 *A* and *B*, Two examples of branch retinal vein occlusions.

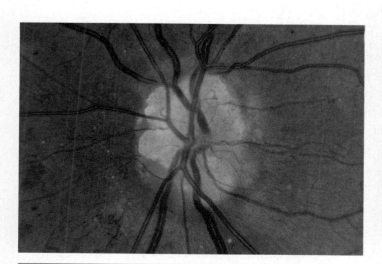

Figure 10–119 Optic disc drusen.

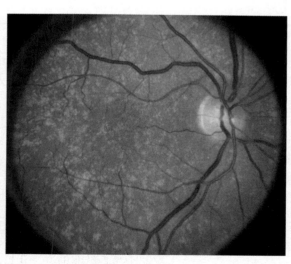

Figure 10–120 Diffuse retinal drusen, which are not age related.

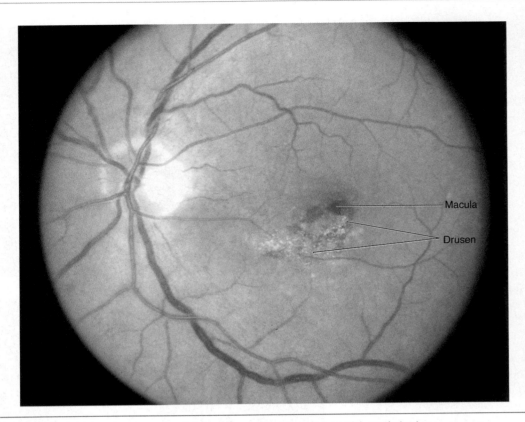

Macula

Drusen

Figure 10–121 Age-related macular degeneration and subfoveal choroidal occularization.

the sensory retinal layer that stimulate the formation of a fibrous scar, further damaging the sensory retinal layers. Studies have implicated vascular endothelial growth factor (VEGF) in the pathogenesis of AMD. This growth factor is naturally expressed in the retina, with high levels concentrated in the RPE. In the normal eye, VEGF may play a protective role in maintaining adequate blood flow to RPE and photoreceptors. Studies have indicated that a reduction of choroidal blood flow and oxidative stress may stimulate the initial overexpression of VEGF in the RPE and retina. This stimulates proliferation and permeability, promoting angiogenesis, increased vascular permeability, and the breakdown of the blood-retinal barrier, which are hallmarks of choroidal neovascularization and AMD. Figure 10-123 shows the retina of a patient with long-standing AMD; note that the macula has been destroyed and only a scar exists.

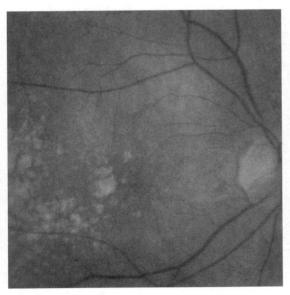

Figure 10–122 Close-up photograph of macular drusen.

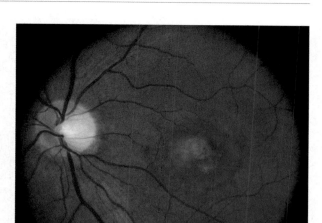

Figure 10–123 Age-related macular degeneration, late stage. Note the gray scar at the macular area.

Optic atrophy is a reduction in size and substance of the optic nerve, caused by loss of axons and myelin sheaths. Optic atrophy may result from a lesion anywhere in the anterior visual pathway between the retina and the lateral geniculate body. The ophthalmoscopic hallmark of optic atrophy is optic disc pallor. The patient may have a loss of visual acuity, narrowed visual fields, deficit in color vision, or an afferent defect. The pallor of the disc is caused by the loss of its capillary network and by glial tissue formation. There are two basic types of optic atrophy: "primary," in which disc pallor is accompanied by a clearly defined margin as a result of retrobulbar or intracranial disease; and "secondary," in which disc pallor is accompanied by a blurred disc margin as a result of optic neuritis or chronic papilledema. Figure 10-124 shows the right retina of a patient with optic atrophy. Note the pallor of the temporal aspect of the disc.

Chorioretinitis is an inflammatory process that originates in the choroidal tissues and subsequently spreads to involve the retina. Most inflammatory changes in the choroid are of endogenous origin, including tuberculosis, syphilis, Q fever, HIV, herpes zoster, cytomegalovirus (CMV), measles, sarcoidosis, histoplasmosis, *Aspergillus* infection, *Candida* infection, cryptococcosis, coccidioidomycosis, toxoplasmosis, *Toxocara* infection, onchocerciasis, and retinoblastoma. In acute chorioretinitis, there is cloudy vision resulting from vitreous haze, and the patient sees light flashes and multiple floating spots. Loss of vision may occur if the macula is involved. In chronic chorioretinitis, there is clumping of pigment around the lesions, which are whitish owing to the presence of scar tissue and the underlying sclera that is visible because the retina and choroid have been destroyed.

Toxoplasmosis, caused by the organism *Toxoplasma gondii*, is most frequently a congenital condition, transmitted to the fetus from the mother during the first trimester of pregnancy. The early lesions heal once the organisms become encysted; only retinochoroidal scarring is

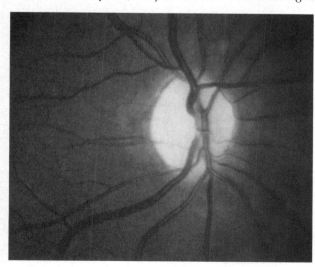

Figure 10–124 Right retina with optic atrophy. Note the marked pallor of the temporal aspect of the disc.

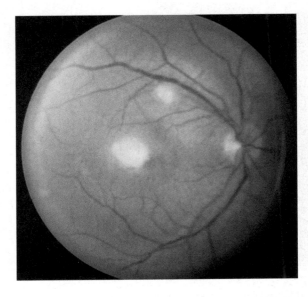

Figure 10–125 Acute toxoplasmosis chorioretinitis in a patient with acquired immunodeficiency syndrome (AIDS).

seen on routine ophthalmoscopy. The condition may recur with the liberation of the encysted organisms and further retinal damage. The visual prognosis depends on the location of the lesion. Figure 10-125 shows the retina of the right eye of a patient with AIDS and acute toxoplasmosis chorioretinitis. The acute lesions are round with an overlying yellow-white haze as a result of a vitreitis; these acute lesions have been described as looking like a ''headlight in fog.'' Notice the multifocal areas of retinal involvement. This patient had similar multifocal lesions in the left eye. The multifocal areas and bilaterality are typical of acute toxoplasmosis retinitis in patients with AIDS. Figure 10-126 shows another patient with acute toxoplasmosis; notice the dense ''fog'' caused by the active vitreitis. Figure 10-127 shows a retina of another patient with a healed, inactive lesion of toxoplasmosis chorioretinitis at the macula. Figure 10-128 shows another patient with diffuse retinal scars secondary to inactive toxoplasmosis.

The *presumed ocular histoplasmosis syndrome* (POHS) has a distinct retinal appearance characterized by small atrophic areas in the retina. Histoplasmosis is caused by a dimorphic yeast, *Histoplasma capsulatum*. It exists in humans in the yeast form and in the soil as the mold form. It is endemic in the soil along the Ohio and Mississippi River valleys and in Maryland, Florida, and Texas. Histoplasmosis enters the body through inhalation of the spores. Infection may be asymptomatic, or it may cause a mild flulike syndrome. Dissemination throughout the body may occur. Histoplasmosis infections in immuno-compromised patients may cause a fulminating, life-threatening systemic infection. In POHS, there is a ring of pigmented atrophic scarring surrounding the optic nerve. The macula may

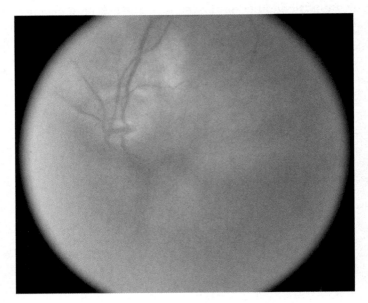

Figure 10–126 Active vitreitis secondary to acute toxoplasmosis.

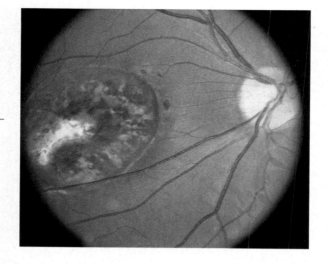

Figure 10–127 Chronic (inactive) toxoplasmosis chorioretinitis scar.

also be affected. POHS is so-named because the organism has never been isolated from the choroid of individuals who have been ill with histoplasmosis and have developed retinal lesions. Figure 10-129 shows the classic lesion of POHS.

CMV chorioretinitis is the most common ocular opportunistic infection in patients with AIDS. Autopsy studies have shown that more than 95% of viral chorioretinitis in patients with AIDS is a result of CMV infection. CMV chorioretinitis is progressive and often preterminal. It appears that the patient with AIDS is at greatest risk for CMV retinitis when the CD4$^+$ T cell count is less than 40/mm^3. Figure 10-130 depicts retinal necrosis and vasculitis in a patient with AIDS and CMV chorioretinitis. Figure 10-131 shows the retina of the left eye of a patient with CMV chorioretinitis. Notice the marked retinal necrosis extending from the optic nerve superiorly and temporally. Figure 10-132 shows the retina of the right eye of another patient with CMV retinitis. There is extensive necrotizing optic neuritis with retinal necrosis and retinal vasculitis. Notice the white sheathing of the retinal vessels (especially superiorly off the disc), which is typical of vasculitis. Figure 10-133 shows the left eye of another patient with active CMV retinitis; notice the retinal vessel sheathing and extensive necrotizing optic neuritis. Figure 10-134 shows the retina of a patient with burned-out CMV retinitis. Notice the sclerosed retinal arteries and the paucity of vessels. The patient was blind as a result of the CMV infection.

Figure 10-135*A* shows the left retina of a patient with HIV chorioretinitis. Notice the cotton-wool spots and the extremely large flame-shaped hemorrhage. Figure 10-135*B* shows another patient with HIV chorioretinitis infection. Notice the many cotton-wool spots. Roth's spots are commonly seen in patients with HIV chorioretinitis Figure 10-110 shows examples of Roth spots in a patient with leukemia.

There are several important tumors of the ocular fundus. *Retinoblastoma* is the most common malignant tumor of the sensory retina. It has been estimated to occur in 1 per

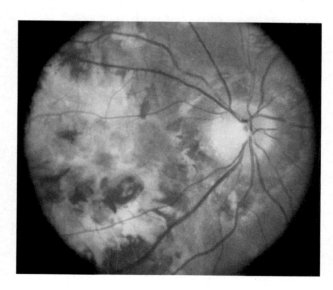

Figure 10–128 Inactive toxoplasmosis chorioretinitis. Note the diffuse retinal scars.

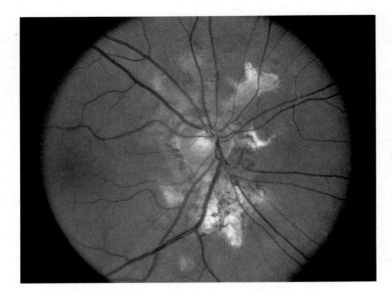

Figure 10–129 Presumed ocular histoplasmosis syndrome.

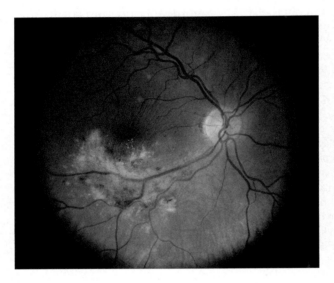

Figure 10–130 Cytomegalovirus retinitis in a patient with acquired immunodeficiency syndrome (AIDS), right retina.

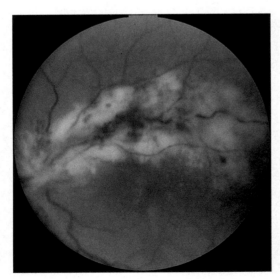

Figure 10–131 Cytomegalovirus chorioretinitis, left retina.

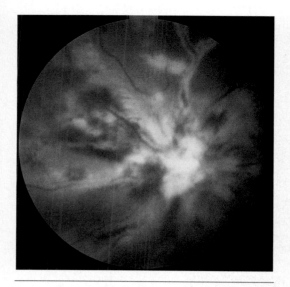

Figure 10–132 Cytomegalovirus chorioretinitis, right retina.

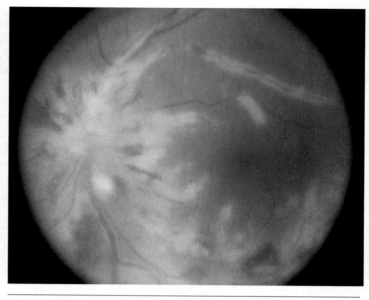

Figure 10–133 Active cytomegalovirus retinitis. Note the retinal sheathing, retinal vasculitis, and the necrotizing optic neuritis.

18,000 live births. It can be sporadic or familial with an autosomal dominant mode of inheritance. The abnormal gene has been localized to the long arm of chromosome 13. Persons who inherit the gene are more likely to have bilateral retinoblastomas than are those without the gene. Children with retinoblastomas present with leukokoria, or a white pupil. Look at Figure 10-136. Leukokoria is present because most of the globe contains the large white endophytic or exophytic tumor. Figure 10-137 shows the right and left retinas of a child with bilateral retinoblastomas. Note the large tumor mass in the left retina.

The two most important tumors of the choroid are the choroidal nevus and the choroidal melanoma. The *choroidal nevus* is the most common fundus tumor. It is commonly a flat, slate-gray lesion with a slightly ill-defined border. Figure 10-138 shows a choroidal nevus. A nevus must be differentiated from a choroidal melanoma. A *choroidal melanoma* is the most common primary intraocular malignancy. It occurs in about 6 per 1 million people per year. It has no sex predisposition and is usually nonfamilial. It is rare in African Americans and is most common in white persons. Unlike the choroidal nevus, the choroidal melanoma has depth and is frequently dome-shaped or mushroom-shaped. Figure 10-139 shows the retina of a patient with a choroidal melanoma.

Figure 10–134 Burned-out cytomegalovirus retinitis.

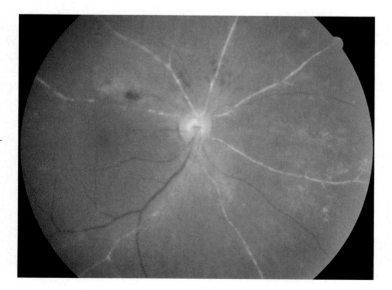

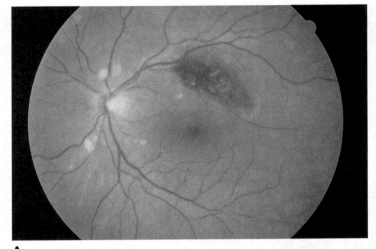

A

Figure 10–135 *A,* Human immunodeficiency virus (HIV) chorioretinitis. Note the large flame-shaped hemorrhage and the cotton-wool spots.
B, Another patient with HIV chorioretinitis. Note the many cotton-wool spots.

B

Colobomas of the retina and choroid are congenital defects in these tissues caused by failure of the embryonic fissure to fuse properly. Colobomas appear as large white areas in which the retina or choroid is absent, and thus the white sclera is seen. Retinal vessels may cross into the lesion. Typically, colobomas are seen in the inferior aspect of the fundus because the embryonic fissure is inferonasal in the developing eye. Figure 10-140 shows the classic features of a coloboma. See also Figure 10-62, which shows an iris coloboma.

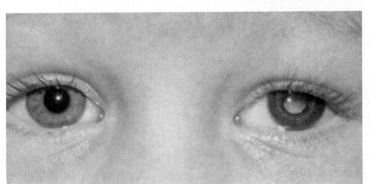

Figure 10–136 Leukokoria.

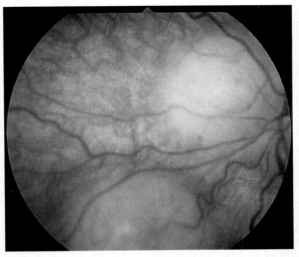

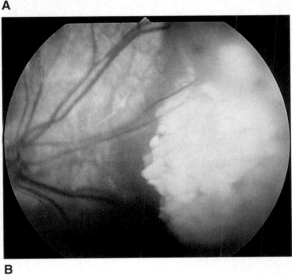

A

B

Figure 10–137 Retinoblastoma. *A,* Right retina. *B,* Left retina.

Figure 10-141 shows a giant retinal tear. A large area of bare choroid is visible through the break.

Retinitis pigmentosa is a very rare, genetically determined degenerative disease of the retina with an onset from the ages of 6 and 12 years. It is more common in boys than in girls and is almost always bilateral. Night blindness is the first symptom, followed by a gradually

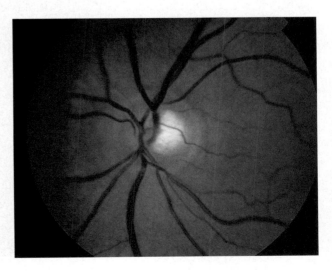

Figure 10–138 Choroidal nevus.

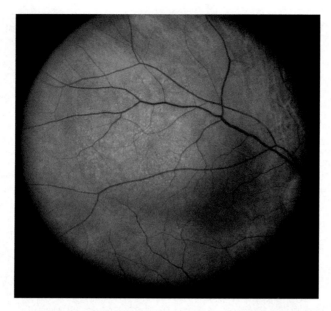

Figure 10–139 Choroidal malignant melanoma.

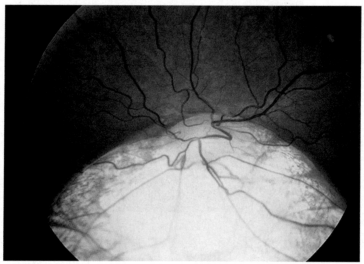

Figure 10–140 Retinal coloboma.

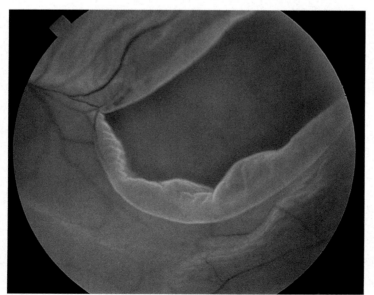

Figure 10–141 Retinal tear.

progressive constriction of the peripheral fields and eventually blurred vision. Evaluation of the retina reveals the very characteristic picture of black "bone spicule" pigmentary changes, particularly in the midperipheral retina. Macular degeneration occurs in late stages. No treatment is available. Figure 10-142*A* is the classic picture of retinitis pigmentosa. A close-up photograph of the "bone spicules" is seen in Figure 10-142*B*.

A *staphyloma* is an outward bulging of the sclera and protrusion of intraocular contents at a point where the sclera is too thin to support the ocular structure. When present in the posterior pole, as shown in Figure 10-143, it is associated with degenerative high myopia. Macular holes, retinal tears, and retinal detachment are common. Staphylomas may be congenital or may occur after trauma or chronic inflammation that has weakened the scleral wall. In most cases, no therapy is available. In severe cases, the staphyloma gradually enlarges and enucleation is eventually necessary.

Abnormalities of gaze are not uncommon. *Ophthalmoplegia* is paralysis of the eye muscles. Lesions causing this paralysis may be acute, chronic, or progressive. The abnormalities of this condition are demonstrated in Figure 10-144. When the patient is asked to look straight ahead, the right eye is abducted. Notice the ptosis of the right eyelid. When the patient is asked to look to the far right, both eyes move normally, although the right ptosis is well seen. When the patient is asked to look to the far left, the right eye cannot cross the midline. This patient has an acute oculomotor paralysis secondary to a fungal lesion near the nucleus of the third cranial nerve.

When the patient shown in Figure 10-145 is asked to look straight ahead or to the right, both eyes move smoothly in the correct motion. However, when the patient is asked to look to

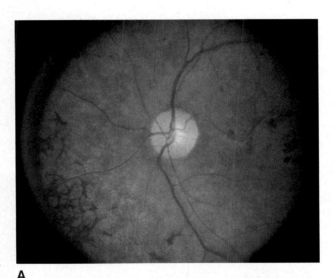

A

Figure 10–142 *A*, Retinitis pigmentosa. Note the black "bone spicules" in the midperipheral retina. *B*, Close-up photograph of the "bone spicules."

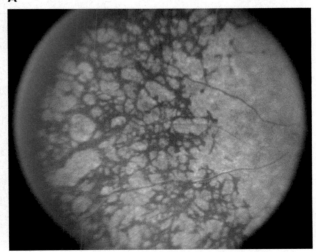

B

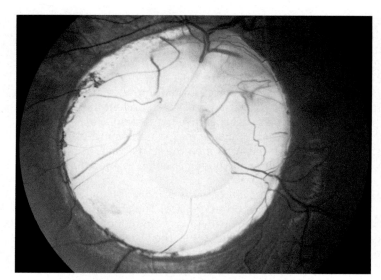

Figure 10–143 Staphyloma.

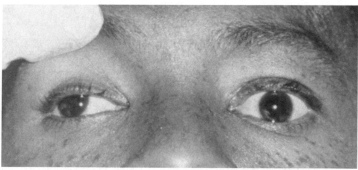

A

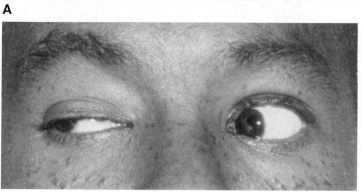

B

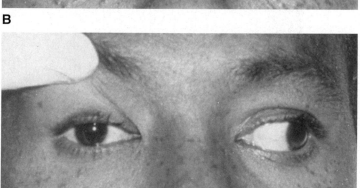

C

Figure 10–144 Acute right oculomotor nerve paralysis. *A,* When the patient is asked to look straight ahead, the right eye is turned laterally (note the position of the corneal light reflexes). The right palpebral fissure is markedly narrowed, requiring the eyelid to be elevated to visualize the position of the eye. *B,* When the patient is asked to look to the far right, both eyes are able to move in that direction. Note the marked ptosis of the right eyelid. *C,* When the patient is asked to look to the far left, the right eye cannot cross the midline.

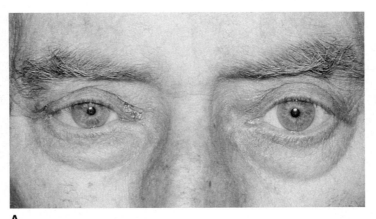

A

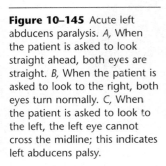

Figure 10–145 Acute left abducens paralysis. *A,* When the patient is asked to look straight ahead, both eyes are straight. *B,* When the patient is asked to look to the right, both eyes turn normally. *C,* When the patient is asked to look to the left, the left eye cannot cross the midline; this indicates left abducens palsy.

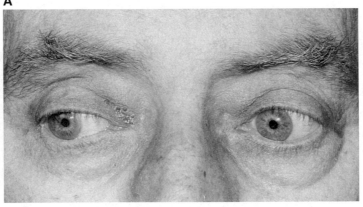

B

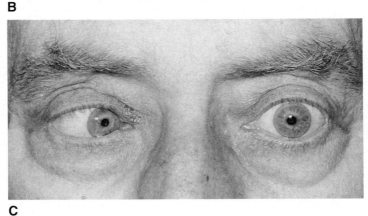

C

the left, the left eye fails to cross the midline. Diplopia occurred as a result of a left abducens palsy secondary to carcinomatous meningitis.

Head tilt may be a sign of an extraocular muscle weakness. A weakness of the superior oblique muscle, often resulting from birth trauma, may not be recognized until much later in life. Diplopia may develop associated with a characteristic head tilt. The head is habitually held in such a position as to avoid horizontal, vertical, or torsional diplopia. Figure 10-146 illustrates the classic head tilts associated with paralysis of the oblique muscles. With a *superior oblique palsy* (see Fig. 10-146A and B), the face is turned and the head is tilted to the uninvolved side; the chin is depressed. With an *inferior oblique palsy* (see Fig. 10-146C and D), the face is turned to the uninvolved side, the head is tilted to the involved side, and the chin is elevated. Head tilt also may be seen in paralysis of the vertical rectus muscles.

The retinal findings of common diseases are summarized in Table 10-11. Many common diseases display their disorders at the macula of the retina. Table 10-12 provides a differentiation of some of these lesions.

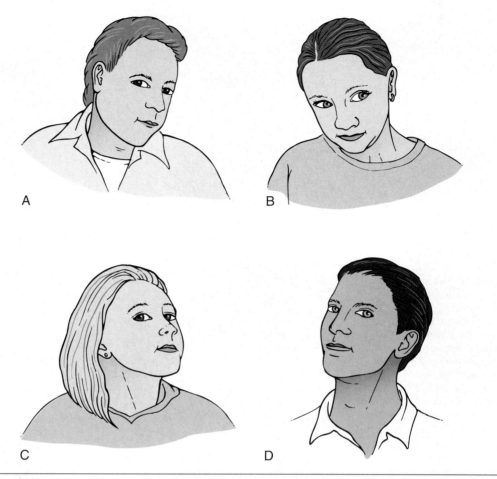

Figure 10–146 Classic head-tilt positions in patients with palsies of the oblique muscles. *A,* Right superior oblique. *B,* Left superior oblique. *C,* Right inferior oblique. *D,* Left inferior oblique.

Table 10–11 Retinal Characteristics of Common Diseases

Condition	Primary Findings	Distribution	Secondary Findings
Diabetes (see Figs. 10-89 to 10-101)	Microaneurysms Neovascularization Retinitis proliferans*	Posterior pole	Hard exudates† Deep hemorrhages Retinal venous occlusions Vitreous hemorrhages
Hypertension (see Figs. 10-80, 10-83, and 10-102 to 10-106)	Arteriolar narrowing "Copper wiring" Flame hemorrhages Arteriovenous nicking	Posterior pole	Hard exudates Deep hemorrhages Retinal venous occlusions Vitreous hemorrhages
Papilledema (see Figs. 10-107 to 10-109)	Hyperemia of the disc Venous enlargement Retinal hemorrhages Disc elevation Loss of spontaneous venous pulsations Cotton-wool spots	On or near disc	Hard exudates Optic atrophy, late
Retinal vein occlusion (see Figs. 10-117 and 10-118)	Hemorrhages Neovascularization	Confined to area drained by affected vein	Exudates
Retinal arterial occlusion (see Figs. 10-111 to 10-116)	Pallor of retina Decreased width of artery Embolus possibly visible	Confined to area supplied	Optic atrophy, late

Table 10–11 Retinal Characteristics of Common Diseases—cont'd

Condition	Primary Findings	Distribution	Secondary Findings
Arteriolar sclerosis	Widening of light reflex "Copper wiring" Arteriovenous nicking	Throughout retina	Decrease in retinal pigment
Blood dyscrasias (see Fig. 10-110)	Diffuse hemorrhages Venous dilation, common Roth's spots (hemorrhagic lesions with white centers)		
Sickle cell disease	Sharp cutoff of arterioles Arteriovenous anastomoses Neovascularization in "sea fan" formations (resembling the marine organism with a similar pattern)	Peripheral retina	Vitreous hemorrhages Retinal detachments

*A growth of a light-colored sheet of opaque connective tissue over the inner surface of the retina. Neovascularization of the tissue with tortuous vessels is seen. These vessels bleed easily.
†*Exudate* is the term used for small intraretinal lesions caused by retinal disturbances in a variety of disorders.

Table 10–12 Differentiation of Common Macular Lesions

Feature	Macular Degeneration*	Macular Star†	Circinate Retinopathy‡
Appearance	Pigmentary mottling, often with hemorrhage	Whitish exudate that radiates around macula	Broken ring-shaped whitish exudate around macula
Etiology		Hypertension Papilledema Papillitis Central retinal vein occlusion	Diabetes Central retinal vein occlusion

*Often bilateral in elderly patients. See Figures 10-121 and 10-123.
†See Figure 10-105.
‡See Figure 10-92.

Useful Vocabulary

Listed here are the specific roots that are important for understanding the terminology related to diseases of the eye.

Root	Pertaining to	Example	Definition
blepharo-	eyelid	**blepharo**plasty	Surgical repair of eyelid
choroi-	choroid	**choroi**ditis	Inflammation of the choroid
-cor- (or -kor-)	pupil	aniso**cor**ia	Unequal pupils
cyclo-	ciliary body	**cyclo**plegia	Paralysis of accommodation
dacryo-	tear	**dacryo**cystitis	Inflammation of the lacrimal sac
-duction	to lead	ab**duction**	Turning outward

Continued

Useful Vocabulary—cont'd

Root	Pertaining to	Example	Definition
irid-	iris	**irid**ectomy	Surgical excision of part of the iris
kerato-	cornea	**kerato**pathy	Disease of the cornea
lacri-	tears	**lacri**mal	Pertaining to the tears
nyct-	night	**nyct**alopia	Night blindness
-ocul-	eye	intra**ocul**ar	Within the eye
ophthalm-	eye	**ophthalm**oscope	Instrument for visualizing the retina
-opsia	vision	hemian**opsia**	Blindness in half of the visual field
-phak(os)-	lens	a**phak**ia	Without a lens
photo-	light	**photo**sensitive	Sensitive to light
presby-	old	**presby**opia	Impairment of vision as a result of increasing age
tars-	eyelid structure	**tars**orrhaphy	Surgical suturing of the lid
-trop-	turn	eso**trop**ia	Eye turning inward

Writing Up the Physical Examination

Listed here are examples of the write-up for the examination of the eye.

- Visual acuity is OD 20/20 and OS 20/30 according to the standard Snellen chart. The visual fields by confrontation field testing are normal. Examination of the external structures of the eyes is normal. The pupils are equal, round, and reactive to light and to accommodation.* The extraocular movements† are normal. On ophthalmoscopic examination, the disc margins are sharp. A normal cup–disc ratio is present. The vasculature is normal.
- Visual acuity is OD 20/60 and OS 20/20 according to the pocket visual acuity card. Examination of the eyes reveals marked conjunctival injection on the right with a dilated pupil on the same side. The pupils are round and are reactive to light. The visual fields by confrontation field testing are normal. The optic disc margins are sharp, and the vascularity of both retinas appears normal.
- The patient is able to read the newspaper without corrective lenses. The extraocular movements are normal. The left pupil is miotic and is 2 mm smaller than the right pupil. A mild ptosis of the left upper lid is present. Both pupils react to light directly and consensually. Confrontation fields are within normal limits. Funduscopic examination is within normal limits.
- The visual acuity with corrected lenses appears normal. There is a paralysis of abduction of the left eye, accompanied by diplopia on attempted left lateral gaze. The pupils are equal, round, and reactive to light. The optic disc margins are sharp. The vasculature is normal.

- There is decreased visual acuity in both eyes. The patient has difficulty reading $\frac{1}{4}$-inch [6.35-mm] print in the newspaper at about 6 inches [15 cm] with his right eye. There is OS NLP. The examination of the external eye is normal. The extraocular movements are intact. The left optic disc margin is slightly blurred on its nasal aspect. The cup–disc ratio is normal. There are multiple, soft, cotton-wool exudates seen bilaterally. A large, flame-shaped hemorrhage is seen in the right eye at the 2 o'clock position. Arteriovenous nicking is present bilaterally.
- The visual acuity is OD 20/40 and OS 20/100 according to the pocket visual acuity card. A bitemporal hemianopsia is present by confrontation field testing. EOMs are normal. Ophthalmoscopic examination reveals blurring of both optic discs with loss of spontaneous venous pulsations. A flame-shaped hemorrhage is present in the right eye one disc diameter at the 10 o'clock position.

---

*Often abbreviated as PERRLA, although accommodation cannot really be tested.
†Often abbreviated as EOMs.

Bibliography

Albert DM, Jakobiec FA: Atlas of Clinical Ophthalmology. Philadelphia, WB Saunders, 1996.

Ambati J, Ambati BK, Yoo SH, et al: Age-related macular degeneration: Etiology, pathogenesis, and therapeutic strategies. Surv Ophthalmol 48:257, 2003.

Batterbury M, Bowling B: Ophthalmology: An Illustrated Colour Text. Edinburgh, Churchill Livingstone, 1999.

Cassirer R: The Philosophy of Symbolic Forms. London, Oxford University Press, 1955.

Herbella FA, Mudo M, Delmonti C, et al: "Raccoon eyes" (periorbital haematoma) as a sign of skull base fracture. Injury 32:745, 2001.

Kanski JJ, Nischal KK: Ophthalmology: Clinical Signs and Differential Diagnosis. London, Harcourt, 2000.

Leibowitz HM: The red eye. N Engl J Med 343:345, 2005.

Michelson JB, Friedlaender MH: Color Atlas of the Eye in Clinical Medicine, Mosby-Wolfe, London, 1996.

Rowe S, MacLean CH, Shekelle PG: Preventing visual loss from chronic eye disease in primary care: Scientific review. JAMA 291:1487, 2004.

Spaide RF: Diseases of the Retina and Vitreous. Philadelphia, WB Saunders, 1999.

Steinmann WC, Millstein ME, Sinclair SH: Pupillary dilation with tropicamide 1% for funduscopic screening: A study of duration of action. Ann Intern Med 107:181, 1987.

Vafadis G: When is red eye not just conjunctivitis? Practitioner 246:469, 2002.

Witmer AN, Vrensen GFJM, Van Noorden CJF, et al: Vascular endothelial growth factors and angiogenesis in eye disease. Prog Retin Eye Res 22:1, 2003.

Zadnik K: The Ocular Examination: Measurements and Findings. Philadelphia, WB Saunders, 1997.

Zarbin MA: Current concepts in the pathogenesis of age-related macular degeneration. Arch Ophthalmol 122:598, 2004.

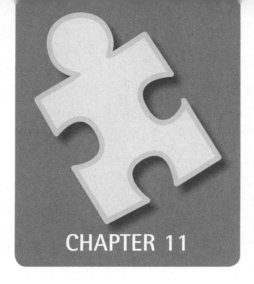

CHAPTER 11

The Ear and Nose

Yet it was not possible for me to say to people, "Speak louder, shout, for I am deaf ....
Alas! how could I declare the weakness of a sense which in me ought to be more acute
than in others—a sense which formerly I possessed in highest perfection, a perfection such
as few in my profession enjoy, or ever have enjoyed.

Ludwig van Beethoven (1770–1827)

General Considerations

Most people are fortunate to hear the sounds of music, noise, and, above all, speech. Sometimes "silence is golden," but silence can be golden only when a person can choose not to hear.

Although normal children are born with the apparatus necessary to produce speech, they are not born with speech. The ear and brain integrate and process sound, enabling the child to learn to imitate it. If sound cannot be heard, it cannot be imitated. Sounds will not become words; words will not become sentences; sentences will not become speech; speech will not become language.

Hearing is a perceptual process. To illustrate this concept, consider tinnitus as an example. *Tinnitus*, the name given to a sensation of sound in one or both ears, commonly accompanies deafness. When tinnitus is present, there is nearly always some degree of hearing loss. Conversely, when there is no appreciable hearing loss, there is rarely tinnitus. However, children who are born deaf do not complain of tinnitus.

Structure and Physiology

The Ear

The ear can be divided into the following four parts:

1. External ear
2. Middle ear
3. Inner ear
4. Nervous innervation

A cross section through the ear is illustrated in Figure 11-1.

The *external ear* consists of the *pinna* and the *external auditory canal*. The pinna is composed of elastic cartilage and skin. Figure 11-2 illustrates the parts of the pinna.

EXTERNAL
EAR

MIDDLE
EAR

INNER
EAR

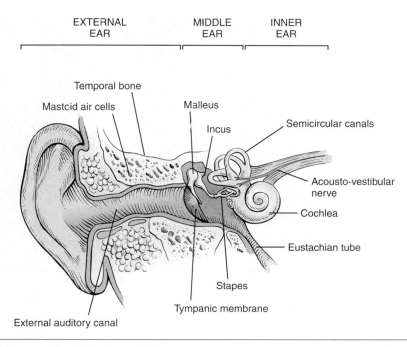

Figure 11–1 Cross-sectional view through the ear.

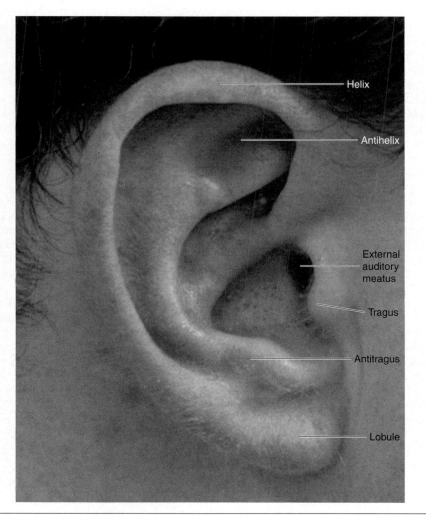

Figure 11–2 Landmarks of the pinna.

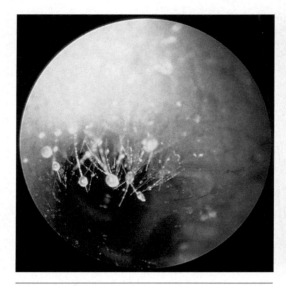

Figure 11–3 Earwax on the base of hairs.

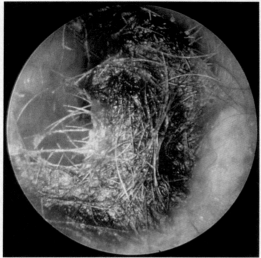

Figure 11–4 Earwax in the external ear canal.

The external auditory canal is about 1 inch in length. Its outer third is cartilaginous, and its inner two thirds are composed of bone. Within the cartilaginous portion, there are hair follicles, pilosebaceous glands, and *ceruminous*, or wax-producing, glands. Secretions of these ceruminous glands, debris, and desquamated keratin are "earwax." The glands secrete their product around the base of the hairs, as depicted in Figure 11-3. Figure 11-4 shows earwax in the external ear canal. Earwax color and consistency depend on the type of cerumen secreted, the amount of keratin present, and the presence of debris. The soft, brown form shown here is the most common type. The cartilaginous portion of the ear is continuous with the pinna. The canal curves slightly, being directed forward and downward. The innervation to most of the external canal is through the trigeminal, or fifth cranial, nerve. The innermost portion of the canal is innervated by the vagus, or tenth cranial, nerve.*

The *middle ear*, or tympanic cavity, consists of connections to the *mastoid antrum* and to its connecting air cells and, through the *eustachian tube*, to the nasopharynx. The function of the eustachian tube is to provide an air passage from the nasopharynx to the ear to equalize pressure on both sides of the tympanic membrane. The eustachian tube is normally closed but opens during swallowing and yawning.

The *tympanic membrane* forms the lateral boundary of the middle ear. The medial boundary is formed by the *cochlea*. The tympanic membrane is gray, with blood vessels at its periphery. It is composed of two parts: the *pars flaccida* and the *pars tensa*. The pars flaccida is the upper, smaller portion of the tympanic membrane. The pars tensa comprises the remainder of the membrane. The handle of the malleus is a prominent landmark and divides the pars tensa into the *anterior* and *posterior folds*. The tympanic membrane is set slightly at an angle to the external canal. The inferior portion is more medial than is the superior portion. Figure 11-5 illustrates the left tympanic membrane.

Sound is conducted from the tympanic membrane to the inner ear by three *auditory ossicles:* the *malleus*, the *incus*, and the *stapes*. The malleus is the largest ossicle. At its upper end is the *short process*, which appears as a tiny knob. The *handle* (long process) of the malleus, or *manubrium*, extends downward to its tip, called the *umbo*. The short process and the handle of the malleus attach directly to the tympanic membrane. At the other end of the malleus is its head, which articulates with the incus. The incus then articulates with the head of the stapes, the footplate of which attaches to the *oval window* of the inner ear.

The middle ear also contains two muscles: the *tensor tympani* and the *stapedius*. The tensor tympani muscle attaches to the malleus, and the stapedius muscle attaches to the neck of the stapes. The tensor tympani muscle is innervated by the trigeminal nerve, and the stapedius muscle is innervated by the facial, or seventh cranial, nerve. Both muscles contract in response to high-intensity sound.

---

*On occasion, when the distal external canal is cleaned, coughing may result. This cough reflex is mediated through the vagus nerve.

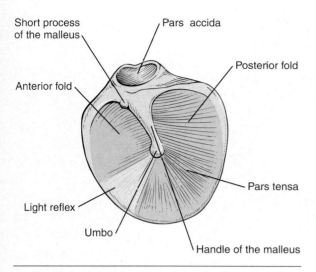

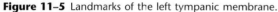

Figure 11–5 Landmarks of the left tympanic membrane.

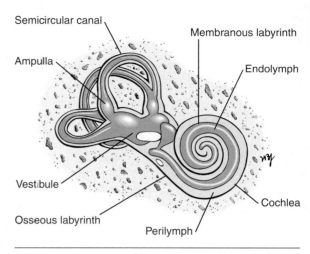

Figure 11–6 Cross-sectional view through the cochlea.

The facial nerve passes through the middle ear and provides, in addition to the nerve to the stapedius muscle, the *chorda tympani* nerve. The chorda tympani travels through the middle ear between the incus and the malleus and exits near the temporomandibular joint. It carries taste sensation from the anterior two thirds of the tongue.

The *inner ear* is the end-organ for hearing and equilibrium. It is situated in the petrous portion of the temporal bone and consists of the three *semicircular canals*, the *vestibule*, and the *cochlea*. Each of these structures is made up of three parts: the *osseous labyrinth*, the *membranous labyrinth*, and the *space between*. The osseous labyrinth is the outer bone casing. The inner membranous labyrinth is within the osseous labyrinth and contains a fluid called *endolymph* and the sensory structures. The space between these two labyrinths is filled with another fluid, called *perilymph*. A cross section through this area is illustrated in Figure 11-6.

The three semicircular canals are directed posteriorly, superiorly, and horizontally. Each canal has a dilated end, the *ampulla*, which is the sensory end-organ for balance.

The cochlea is a snail shell-shaped structure composed of $2\frac{3}{4}$ turns. Within its membranous labyrinth is the end-organ for hearing. The *acoustic*, or eighth cranial, nerve consists of two parts: the *vestibular* and *cochlear* divisions. These connect to the semicircular canals and cochlea, respectively. They join and pass through the internal auditory meatus to the brain stem.

Sound waves stimulate the afferent fibers either by *bone conduction* or by *air conduction*. Bone conduction is directly through the bones of the skull. Air conduction is through the external auditory canal, tympanic membrane, and ossicles to the oval window. Most hearing is mediated by air conduction.

Sound waves set up vibrations that enter the external canal and are transmitted to the ossicles, which vibrate. This vibration causes an inward motion of the footplate of the stapes and deforms the oval window. Waves are created in the perilymphatic fluid of the labyrinth. These fluid motion changes are transmitted in a wavelike manner to the endolymphatic fluid, which causes distortion of the *hair cells* of the *organ of Corti*. These hair cells convert the mechanical force into an electrochemical signal that is propagated down the acoustic nerve and is ultimately interpreted as sound. It has been estimated that there are more than 30,000 of these afferent hair fibers, which constitute the auditory division. After many synapses, the impulse reaches the temporal cortex, where the appreciation of the sound occurs. A cross section through the cochlear duct is shown in Figure 11-7.

The sense of *balance* is achieved by visual, vestibular, and proprioceptive* senses. The loss of one of these senses frequently goes unnoticed. The vestibular apparatus appears to be the most important. Motion within the endolymphatic fluid stimulates the hair cells in the ampulla of the semicircular canals. Electrical impulses are transmitted to the vestibular portion of the eighth cranial nerve. Synapses occur in the vestibular and oculomotor nuclei,

---

*Sensory stimulation from within the tissues of the body with regard to their movement or position.

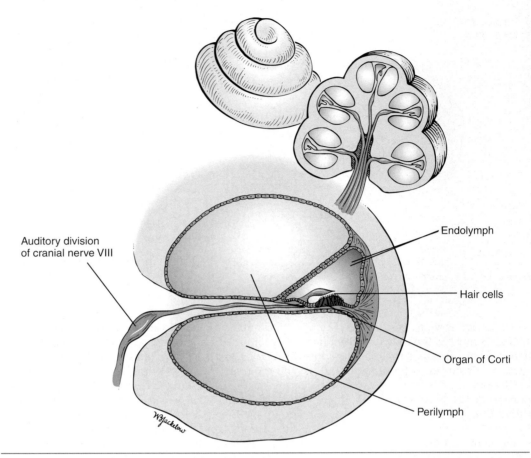

Auditory division
of cranial nerve VIII

Endolymph

Hair cells

Organ of Corti

Perilymph

Figure 11–7 Cross-sectional view through the cochlear duct.

which send efferent fibers to the extraocular and skeletal muscles. This produces a deviation of the eyes with rapid compensatory motions to maintain gaze and increased tone in the skeletal muscles.

Any alteration in the endolymphatic mechanism may affect the control of the eyes. *Nystagmus* is an involuntary, rapid back-and-forth eye motion, which can be horizontal, vertical, rotatory, or mixed. The direction of the nystagmus is determined by the direction of the quick component. Abnormalities of the labyrinth tend to produce *horizontal* nystagmus; brain-stem disorders often produce *vertical* nystagmus; and retinal lesions may produce *ocular* nystagmus, which is slow and produces an irregular, searching quality to the eyes.

The Nose

The external nasal skeleton consists of the *nasal bones*, part of the *maxilla*, and the *cartilage*. The upper third of the skeleton is composed of nasal bones, which articulate with the maxilla and frontal bones. The lower two thirds is made of cartilage.

The internal portion of the nose consists of two cavities divided by the *nasal septum*, which forms the medial wall of the nasal cavity. Projecting from the lateral wall are three *turbinates*, or *conchae*. The *inferior turbinate* is the largest and contains semierectile tissue. Inferior to each turbinate are openings to the *paranasal sinuses*; each opening is known as a *meatus*. Each meatus is named for the turbinate above it. The *nasolacrimal duct* empties into the *inferior meatus*. The *middle meatus*, below the *middle turbinate*, contains the openings of the *frontal, maxillary*, and *anterior ethmoid sinuses*. The posterior ethmoid sinus drains into the *superior meatus*. The *olfactory region* is located high in the nose between the nasal septum and the *superior turbinate*. Figure 11-8 illustrates the lateral wall of the nose.

The blood supply to the nose is derived from the internal and external carotid arteries. The turbinates are vascular and contain large vascular spaces. The blood vessels of the anterior nasal septum meet at an area about 1 inch (2.54 cm) from the mucocutaneous junction, known as *Little's area*. This is the area usually responsible for *epistaxis*, or nosebleed. The blood vessels are under autonomic nervous system control. If there is an excess of *sympathetic* stimulation, the blood vessels constrict, and the vascular spaces in the turbinates shrink. If there is an increase in *parasympathetic* tone, the blood pools in the turbinates, resulting in their swelling, obstruction to airflow, and elaboration of a watery discharge.

The nerve supply to the internal area of the nose is from branches of the trigeminal nerve. The olfactory epithelium is supplied by the *olfactory*, or first cranial, nerve. Moist air with the dissolved odorous particles acts as a stimulus. The nerve fibers from this area pierce the *cribriform plate* to the olfactory bulb in the brain. In humans, the olfactory receptors' ability to discern a stimulus diminishes rapidly with exposure to the stimulus.

The main functions of the nose are to provide the following:

- An airway
- Olfaction
- Humidification of inspired air
- Warming of inspired air
- Filtering of inspired air

The inspired air flows above and below the middle turbinate. This produces eddy currents that serve to protect the olfactory epithelium in the superior portion of the nose. The nasal mucosa produces mucus, which increases the relative humidity to nearly 100%. This prevents the epithelium from drying out and helps prevent possible infection. The air, by its circulation around the conchae, is warmed to nearly body temperature by the time it enters the nasopharynx. The mucus and the nasal hairs, or *vibrissae*, prevent particulate matter from entering the distal respiratory tract. The mucous blanket is swept posteriorly by the *cilia* and is swallowed. The mucus also contains immunoglobulins and enzymes, which serve as a line of defense.

The four *paranasal sinuses* of the head—the maxillary, the ethmoid, the frontal, and the sphenoid—are air-filled cavities lined with mucous membranes. The *maxillary sinus* is the largest and is bounded by the eye, the cheek, the nasal cavity, and the hard palate. The *ethmoid sinuses* are multiple and are present in the *ethmoid bone*, which lies medial to the orbit and extends to the pituitary fossa. The *frontal sinus* is located above the ethmoid sinuses and is bounded by the forehead, the orbit, and the anterior cranial fossa. Behind the ethmoid sinuses is the *sphenoid sinus*. The paranasal sinuses have no known functions. The maxillary, frontal, and ethmoid sinuses and their connections to the nose are illustrated in Figure 11-9.

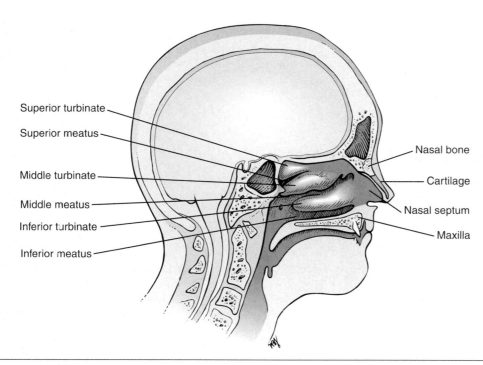

Figure 11–8 Lateral wall of the nose.

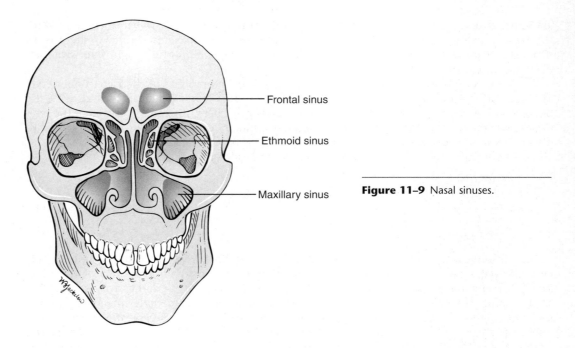

Figure 11–9 Nasal sinuses.

Review of Specific Symptoms

The Ear

The major symptoms of ear disease are the following:

- Hearing loss
- Vertigo
- Tinnitus
- Otorrhea
- Otalgia
- Itching

Hearing Loss

Hearing loss may be unilateral or bilateral and may develop slowly or occur suddenly. For any patient with a hearing loss, ask the following questions:

"Is the hearing loss in one ear?"

"For how long have you been aware of a loss of hearing?"

"Was the loss sudden?"

"Is there a family history of hearing loss?"

"What type of work do you do?" "What other work have you done?"

"What types of hobbies do you have?"

"Have you noticed that you can hear better when it is noisy?"

"What kind of medications are you currently taking?"

"Do you know if you have ever been given an antibiotic called streptomycin or gentamicin?"

Occupational history is extremely important to ascertain. Patients with otosclerosis* can often hear better in a noisy environment. Drugs are well known to cause sudden bilateral

---

*Otosclerosis is the formation of new bone in the labyrinth, causing progressive fixation of the footplate of the stapes to the oval window.

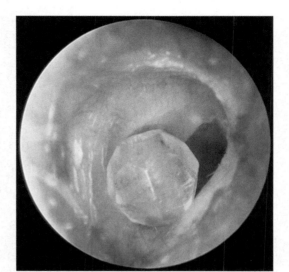

Figure 11–10 Clear plastic bead in the external ear canal.

hearing loss. Salicylates and diuretics such as furosemide and ethacrynic acid may produce transient loss of hearing when ingested in high doses. The aminoglycoside antibiotics such as streptomycin and gentamicin can destroy the hair cells of the organ of Corti and cause permanent hearing loss. An anticancer medication, cisplatin, is also linked to severe ototoxicity.

There are two main types of hearing loss: *conductive* and *sensorineural*. Any condition that interferes with or blocks the transmission of sound waves from the external ear to the inner ear may result in a conductive hearing loss. Blockage may occur as a result of cerumen (earwax), foreign bodies, infection, or congenital abnormalities. Often the position of the cerumen is more important than the amount present. Not infrequently, a small amount of cerumen lying against the tympanic membrane can produce significant hearing loss. Blockage by foreign bodies occurs primarily in 2- to 5-year-old children. Once children discover the external canal, they may experiment and place beads or other objects inside. Figure 11-10 shows a clear plastic bead in the external canal of a young child. Effusions from infections in the middle ear represent one of the most common causes of conductive deafness among children 4 to 15 years of age. The fluid impedes the transmission of sound impulses by the tympanic membrane and the ossicles. Otosclerosis is the main cause of conductive hearing loss in individuals 15 to 50 years of age. With the exception of otosclerosis, conditions causing a conductive hearing loss produce alterations in the appearance of the tympanic membrane.

Sensorineural hearing loss is caused by a disease process in the inner ear structures or auditory nerve. These conditions may be congenital or acquired, with delayed onset. Congenital deafness accounts for 50% of all deafness in children. In many cases of congenital sensorineural hearing loss, no other congenital abnormality is noted. At other times, deafness may accompany other defects, especially in the kidney. Infection with rubella during gestation accounts for most cases of sensorineural deafness that are caused by anomalous development of the fetus's cochlea. The acquired, delayed-onset types of sensorineural hearing loss may or may not be genetic in origin. There are many syndromes, too numerous to mention, as well as viral infections and ototoxic drugs that may cause acquired, delayed-onset sensorineural deafness. Systemic diseases, tumors, and noise are also associated with this type of hearing loss.

A patient's voice may provide a clue to the nature of his or her deafness. The speaking voice is regulated by the way one hears oneself. Patients with a conductive hearing loss hear their own voices better by bone conduction than by air conduction. They therefore think that their voices are loud and tend to speak softly. In contrast, patients with a sensorineural hearing defect hear less by *both* air and bone conduction; therefore, they tend to speak louder.

Vertigo

Vertigo is a sense of spinning or turning while in a resting position. It is frequently associated with a loss of vestibular function, such as unsteadiness of gait. For any patient with vertigo, ask the following questions:

"How long have you had this sensation?"

"Have you had repeated attacks?"

"How long does an attack last: seconds? minutes? hours? days?"

"Is the onset of an attack abrupt?"

"Was the sensation brought on by, or worsened by, changes in position?"

"Does the spinning sensation get worse during an attack?"

"Are there any positions that make you feel better?"

"During an attack, have you had double vision? loss of strength? decreased hearing? a disturbance of gait? nausea? vomiting? ringing in your ears?"

"What kind of medications are you currently taking?"

"Do you know if you have ever been given an antibiotic called streptomycin *or* gentamicin?*"*

Vertigo may result from otologic, neurologic, psychologic, or iatrogenic causes. *Ménière's disease* causes severe paroxysmal vertigo as a result of labyrinthine lesions. The vertigo has an abrupt onset and may last several hours. It is often associated with nausea, vomiting, headache, a ringing sensation in the ear, and decreased hearing. The auditory abnormalities frequently antedate the vertigo. Vertigo associated with an acoustic neuroma is usually mild. Some antibiotics, such as gentamicin, streptomycin, and kanamycin, are vestibulotoxic and cause vertigo. The neurologic causes of vertigo are discussed further in Chapter 21, The Nervous System.

Tinnitus

Tinnitus is the sensation of hearing sound, such as buzzing or ringing, in the absence of environmental input. It is often associated with a conductive or sensorineural hearing loss. Usually the description of the type of tinnitus (e.g., "ringing" or "buzzing") is of little help in determining its cause. The most common causes are inner ear disease such as Ménière's disease, noise trauma, ototoxic drugs, and otosclerosis. On occasion, patients describe *pulsatile tinnitus*. This type of tinnitus beats at the same rate as the heart and may be a symptom of a vascular tumor of the head or neck. See Table 11-1 for a list of common causes of tinnitus.

Otorrhea

Otorrhea, or discharge from the ear, usually indicates acute or chronic infection. For any patient complainng of an ear discharge, ask the following:

"Can you describe the discharge?"

"Have you had similar episodes?"

Table 11–1 Common Causes of Tinnitus

Location	Pulsatile/Clicking Sensation	Nonpulsatile
External ear	Otitis externa Bullous myringitis Foreign body	Cerumen Tympanic membrane perforation Foreign body
Middle ear	Otitis media Vascular anomalies Neoplasm Eustachian tube dysfunction	Otosclerosis Serous otitis media
Inner ear	Vascular anomalies	Cochlear otosclerosis Ménière's disease Labyrinthitis Noise trauma Drug toxicity Presbycusis
Central nervous system	Vascular anomalies Hypertension	Syphilis Degenerative disease Cerebral atherosclerosis

"Do you experience dizziness?"

"Do you have ear pain?"

"Have you had a recent ear or throat infection?"

"Have you had any change in your hearing?"

"Have you used ear drops?"

"Have you been swimming recently?"

"Have you had any recent head or ear injury?"

A bloody discharge may be associated with carcinoma or trauma. A clear, watery discharge may indicate a leakage of cerebrospinal fluid. Determine how long the discharge has been present, as well as its color, its smell, and its relationship to itching, pain, or trauma.

Otalgia

Otalgia, or ear pain, may be related to inflammatory conditions in or around the ear, or it may be referred* from distant anatomic sites in the head and neck. External otitis and otitis media are infections of the external and middle ear, respectively, and are common causes of locally produced pain. Pain from the teeth, pharynx, and cervical spine is commonly referred to the ear. Inflammation, trauma, and neoplasms anywhere along the course of the trigeminal, facial, glossopharyngeal, and vagus cranial nerves or cervical nerves C2 or C3 may be responsible for referred pain in the ipsilateral ear.

Itching

Pruritus (itching) of the ear may result from a primary disorder of the external ear or from a discharge from the middle ear. A systemic disease, such as diabetes, hepatitis, or lymphoma, may also be the cause.

The Nose

The specific symptoms related to the nose are the following:

- Obstruction
- Discharge
- Bleeding

Obstruction

The most common symptom of nasal disease is obstruction. If the symptom of nasal obstruction is present, ask the following questions:

"Is the obstruction on one side?"

"Have you ever had an injury to your nose?"

"How long has the obstruction been present?"

"Do you have any allergies?"

"Does the obstruction worsen with stress?"

"Is there a history of nasal polyps?"

"Is the obstruction associated with other symptoms?"

"Is there a seasonal change in your symptoms?" If so, *"Which season is the worst?"*

Rhinitis, which is inflammation of the nasal mucosa, can have allergic or nonallergic causes. *Allergic rhinitis* is congestion of the nasal mucosa triggered by an allergen such as pollen. The main symptoms include nasal obstruction, sneezing, and a clear, watery nasal discharge.

---

*Referred pain is felt in an area that is separate from the area that is actually the source of the pain. For example, pain from gallbladder disease is frequently felt in the right shoulder. Chapter 17, The Abdomen, discusses further aspects of referred pain.

It is helpful to try to determine the allergen. Weeds pollinate in the spring and fall, trees in the spring, and grasses in the summer. Nonseasonal allergic rhinitis may result from animal dander, mold, or dust. *Nonallergic rhinitis* produces the same symptoms but is nonseasonal and is not triggered by allergens. An example of nonallergic rhinitis is vasomotor rhinitis. Vasomotor rhinitis occurs at stressful times and results in venous engorgement of the conchae, causing obstruction. There are many other causes of vasomotor rhinitis, such as nasal spray abuse (also known as *rhinitis medicamentosa*), pregnancy, and hypothyroidism.

Nasal *polyps*, usually bilateral, also cause obstruction and are the most common cause of *anosmia*, or loss of smell.

Nasal obstruction may be responsible for symptoms referable to other organs. Eye tearing may result from obstruction of the nasolacrimal duct beneath the inferior turbinate. Sinus symptoms may result from obstruction to their drainage. Ear pain or a "clogged" sensation is commonly associated with eustachian tube obstruction.

Discharge

Nasal discharge can be unilateral or bilateral. It usually accompanies nasal obstruction. The discharge may be characterized as follows:

- Thin and watery
- Thick and purulent
- Bloody
- Foul smelling

A *thin and watery* discharge is usually caused by excess mucus production resulting from a viral infection or allergic condition. A *thick and purulent* nasal discharge results from bacterial infection. A *bloody* discharge can result from a neoplasm, trauma, or an opportunistic infection such as mucormycosis (fungal disease). A *foul-smelling* discharge is often associated with foreign bodies in the nose, chronic sinusitis, or malignant disease. A clear, watery discharge that is increased by bending the head forward or by coughing is suggestive of cerebrospinal fluid leakage.

Bleeding

Epistaxis, or bleeding, usually results from the traumatic or spontaneous rupture of the superficial mucosal vessels in Little's area. To exclude other causes, the clinician should determine whether the epistaxis is related to trauma or to a bleeding disorder. It may also result from chronic sinusitis or malignancy within the sinuses. The most common cause of epistaxis is nose-picking. Another prevalent causative factor is cocaine abuse.

Sinus Disease Symptoms

The symptoms of sinus disease are similar to the symptoms of nasal disease. Fever, malaise, cough, nasal congestion, maxillary toothache, purulent nasal discharge, headache, and little improvement of symptoms with decongestants increase the likelihood of sinus disease. Pain, often made worse by bending forward, is an important symptom. Pain from localized sinus disease is usually present in the area overlying the involved sinus. The only exception is sphenoid sinus disease, which is felt diffusely. Maxillary sinus pain is felt behind the eye and near the second premolar and first and second molar teeth. Frontal sinus pain is localized to above the eye. Ethmoid sinus pain is usually periorbital. Sometimes sinus pain can be referred to another area. In addition to pain, ocular abnormalities may also be present with diseases of the sinuses.

The accuracy of the symptoms and signs of sinusitis has been evaluated. Colored nasal discharge, cough, and sneezing were the symptoms with the highest sensitivities (72%, 70%, and 70%, respectively); these symptoms, however, were not very specific. Maxillary toothache was the symptom most specific for sinusitis, with a specificity of 93%; however, only 11% of patients reported this symptom. This symptom had the highest positive likelihood ratio, of 2.5. The conclusion was that the combination of maxillary toothache, poor response to decongestants, colored nasal discharge, and abnormality on sinus transillumination (discussed later in this chapter) was the strongest predictor of sinusitis in primary care populations. If all these symptoms were present in one patient, the positive likelihood ratio was 6.4, and the patient probably had sinusitis; if none were present, sinusitis was ruled out.

Table 11-2 summarizes the location of pain associated with sinus disease. Table 11-3 lists other clinical signs and symptoms associated with sinus disease.

Table 11–2 Location of Pain Associated with Sinus Disease

Sinus Involved	Local Pain	Referred Pain
Maxillary	Behind eye Cheek Nose Upper teeth Upper lip	Teeth Retrobulbar
Ethmoid	Periorbital Retronasal Retrobulbar	Occipital Upper cervical
Frontal	Supraorbital Frontal	Bitemporal and occipital headache

Impact of Deafness on the Patient

The ear is the sensory organ of hearing. Audition is one of the main avenues of communication. Any disturbance in the reception of sound waves by the external ear or the transmission of electrical impulses to the brain may result in an abnormal interpretation of language.

It is estimated that there are more than 15 million persons in the United States with some degree of hearing loss that interferes with their ability to understand speech. About half of these individuals, 7.2 million, have bilateral hearing problems. Although persons older than 70 years of age account for 30% of all deaf individuals, there are more than 250,000 deaf children younger than 3 years of age. Since the late 1970s, the overall prevalence rate has increased substantially.

To understand the impact of deafness on an individual, it is necessary to consider the *age at onset*, the *severity* of the loss, the *rapidity* of the loss, and any *residual* hearing. Persons with insidious or sudden hearing loss experience grief and depression. Consider, for example, the grief expressed in the quotation by Beethoven at the beginning of this chapter.

The psychologic effects of deafness include *paranoia, depression, withdrawal, irritability,* and *anxiety.* Although it has not been proved, it appears that deaf persons have an increased tendency toward paranoia. Most deaf individuals tend to be suspicious of others' conversations.

The most profound responses to a severe hearing deficit are depression and withdrawal. The following quotation from Beethoven dramatizes these responses:

Oh you men who think that I am malevolent, stubborn, or misanthropic, how greatly do you wrong me. You do not know the secret cause which makes me seem that way to you . . . . For me

TABLE 11-3 Clinical Signs and Symptoms in Sinus Disease

Sinus Involved	Signs and Symptoms

Maxillary	Ocular abnormalities
	   Diplopia
	   Proptosis
	   Epiphora (tearing)
	Nasal obstruction and rhinorrhea
	Epistaxis
	Loosening of teeth

Ethmoid	Orbital swelling
	Nasal obstruction and purulent rhinorrhea
	Ocular abnormalities
	   Proptosis
	   Diplopia
	Tenderness over inner canthus of eye

Frontal	Nasal obstruction and rhinorrhea Tenderness over frontal sinus Pus in middle meatus Signs of meningitis

there can be no relaxation with my fellow men, no refined conversations, no mutual exchange of ideas. I must live alone, like one who has been banished. . . . What a humiliation for me when someone standing next to me heard a flute in the distance, and I heard nothing. . . a little more of that and I would have ended my life—it was only my art that held me back.

Hearing-impaired persons have social identity problems as well. They are frequently excluded from previous associations. If they use sign language, they cannot enjoy the company of individuals who do not know sign language. Work or career may have to be altered. The stigma associated with wearing a hearing aid can reinforce the feeling of alienation from others. A patient may avoid wearing a hearing aid for fear of being stigmatized.

Deaf children experience even more severe problems. Their lack of auditory input influences character, early childhood experiences, attitudes, and interpersonal relationships. They are deprived of many of the reassuring, loving, and comforting sounds that facilitate the development of personality. They are unable to obtain verbal cues of a parent's affection. They are also unable to be alerted by auditory signs of danger.

Psychologic problems, social inadequacy, and educational retardation are common among deaf children. The worse the handicap is, the worse the psychologic and educational implications are.

A young hearing-impaired child who exhibits a delay in language development may be diagnosed as developmentally disabled. In general, children who are congenitally deaf or suffer from severe hearing impairment before 3 years of age suffer the most. As the type of lesion causing deafness progresses from the periphery inward, the deleterious effects increase.

Physical Examination

The equipment necessary for the examination of the ear and nose is as follows: otoscope, choice of specula, penlight, and 512-Hz tuning fork. A nasal illuminator attachment for the otoscope and a nasal speculum are optional.

The physical examination of the ear and the nose is performed with the examiner seated in front of the patient.

The Ear

If the patient has symptoms referable to one ear, examine the uninvolved ear first. The physical examination of the ear includes the following:

- External examination
- Auditory acuity testing
- Otoscopic examination

External Examination
Inspect the pinna and postauricular skin. Note the position, size, and shape of the pinna. The pinna should be positioned centrally and should be in proportion to the face and head. Note any obvious abnormalities or surgical scars.

Inspect the External Ear Structures
A small dimple in front of the tragus is usually a remnant of the first branchial arch.

Inspect the external ear for deformities, nodules, inflammation, or lesions. The presence of *tophi* is a highly specific but nonsensitive sign of gout. Tophi are deposits of uric acid crystals. They appear as hard nodules in the helix or antihelix. In rare cases, a white discharge may be seen in association with them. A "cauliflower ear" is a pinna that is gnarled as a result of repeated trauma. Figure 11-11 shows a squamous cell carcinoma and a malignant melanoma of one lobule.

Inspect for discharge. If discharge is present, note its characteristics, such as color, consistency, and clarity.

Palpate the External Ear Structures
Palpate the pinna for tenderness, swelling, or nodules. If pain is elicited by pulling up and down on the pinna or by pressing in on the tragus, an infection of the external canal is probably present.

Inspect the posterior auricular region for scars or swelling. Apply pressure to the mastoid tip, which should be painless. Tenderness may indicate a suppurative process of the mastoid bone.

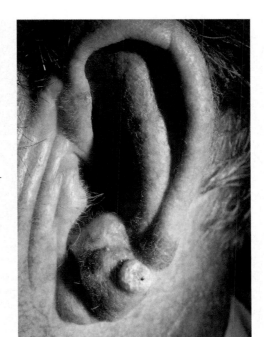

Figure 11–11 Squamous cell carcinoma (on the right) and malignant melanoma (on the left) of lobule.

Auditory Acuity Testing

Testing for auditory acuity is the next part of the physical examination. The easiest method of testing for a gross hearing loss is for the examiner to occlude one external canal by pressing inward on the tragus and to speak softly into the other ear. The examiner should hide his or her mouth to prevent lip reading by the patient. The examiner should whisper words such as "park," "dark," or "daydream" in the nonoccluded ear and determine whether the patient can hear them. This procedure is then repeated with the other ear. Asking a patient whether he or she hears a ticking watch held to the ear is generally unhelpful because the patient knows what to expect.

The use of *tuning fork testing* for hearing loss is more accurate and should be performed regardless of the results of the whisper test. Although several tuning fork frequencies are available, the best for evaluating hearing is the 512-Hz fork.* A tuning fork is held by its stem, and the tines are briskly struck against the palm of the hand. It should never be struck on a solid wooden or metal object. The two tuning fork tests to assess hearing are the Rinne test and the Weber test.

The Rinne Test

In the Rinne test, air conduction is compared with bone conduction. Each ear is tested separately. Strike a 512-Hz tuning fork and place its handle on the mastoid tip near the external auditory meatus. Ask the patient whether he or she hears the sound and to indicate when he or she no longer hears it. When the patient can no longer hear the sound, place the tines of the vibrating tuning fork in front of the external auditory meatus of the same ear, and ask the patient whether he or she can still hear the sound. The tines of the vibrating tuning fork should not touch any hair because the patient may have a hearing impairment but still feel the vibration. The Rinne test is demonstrated in Figure 11-12.

Normally, air conduction (AC) is better than bone conduction (BC), and patients are able to hear the tuning fork at the external auditory meatus after they can no longer hear it on the mastoid tip; this is a *Rinne positive* test result (AC > BC). In patients with a conductive hearing loss, however, bone conduction is better than air conduction: a *Rinne negative* test result (BC > AC). Patients with sensorineural deafness have impaired air *and* bone conduction but maintain the normal response (AC > BC). The middle ear amplifies the sound in both positions.

---

*Different examiners prefer tuning forks of different frequencies for determining auditory acuity. A tuning fork of too high a frequency yields a tone that fades too quickly.

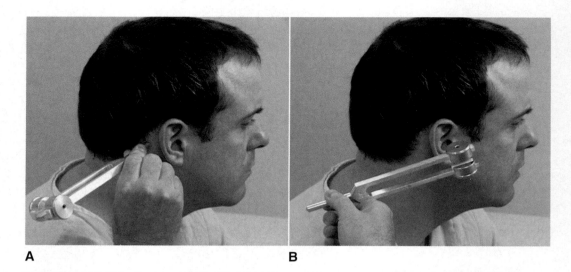

A   **B**

Figure 11–12 The Rinne test. *A,* The tuning fork is first placed on the mastoid process. *B,* When the sound can no longer be heard, the tuning fork is placed in front of the external auditory meatus. Normally, air conduction (AC) is better than bone conduction (BC); that is, AC > BC.

If there is total deafness in one ear, the patient may hear the tuning fork even when it is placed on the mastoid process of the deaf ear. This results from the transmission of vibrations by bone across the skull to the opposite side, where they are sensed by the healthy ear. This is termed a *false-negative Rinne* test result.

The Weber Test

In the Weber test, bone conduction is compared in both ears, and the examiner determines whether monaural impairment is neural or conductive in origin. Stand in front of the patient and place a vibrating 512-Hz tuning fork firmly against the center of the patient's forehead. Ask the patient to indicate whether he or she hears or feels the sound in the right ear, in the left ear, or in the middle of the forehead. Hearing the sound, or feeling the vibration, in the middle is the normal response. If the sound is not heard in the middle, the sound is said to be *lateralized,* and thus a hearing loss is present. Sound is lateralized to the *affected* side in conductive deafness. Try it on yourself. Occlude your right ear and place a vibrating tuning fork in the center of your forehead. Where do you hear it? On the *right.* You have created a conductive hearing loss on the right by blocking the right canal; the sound is lateralized to the right side. The Weber test is illustrated in Figure 11-13.

The explanation for the Weber test effect is based on the masking effect of background noise. In normal conditions, there is considerable background noise, which reaches the tympanic membrane by air conduction. This tends to mask the sound of the tuning fork heard by bone conduction. In an ear with a conductive hearing loss, the air conduction is decreased, and the masking effect is therefore diminished. Thus, the affected ear hears and feels the vibrating tuning fork better than does the normal ear.

In patients with unilateral sensorineural deafness, the sound is not heard on the affected side but is heard by, or localized to, the *unaffected* ear.

To test the reliability of the patient's responses, it is occasionally useful to strike the tuning fork against the palm of the hand and hold it briefly to silence it. The Rinne and Weber tests are then carried out as indicated, using the silent tuning fork. This serves as a good control.

In summary, consider the following two examples:

- Example 1

    Rinne: *Right ear:* AC > BC (Rinne positive); *left ear:* AC > BC (Rinne positive)

    Weber: Lateralization to the left ear

    Diagnosis: Right sensorineural deafness

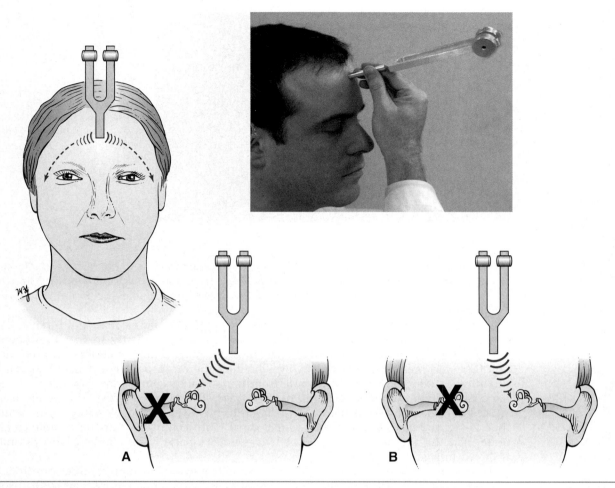

Figure 11–13 The Weber test. When a vibrating tuning fork is placed on the center of the forehead, the normal response is for the sound to be heard in the center, without lateralization to either side. *A,* In the presence of a conductive hearing loss, the sound is heard on the side of the conductive loss. *B,* In the presence of a sensorineural loss, the sound is heard better on the opposite (unaffected) side.

● Example 2

Rinne: *Right ear:* AC > BC (Rinne positive); *left ear:* BC > AC (Rinne negative)

Weber: Lateralization to the left ear

Diagnosis: Left conductive deafness

Otoscopic Examination

The remainder of the examination of the ear is performed with the otoscope. The otoscope incorporates a halogen light source and fiberoptic circumferential distribution of the light. This provides a 360° ring of light-conducting fibers within the shell of the otoscope through which the observer views the inner structures of the ear. Most otoscopes are illuminated by a bright quartz halogen bulb requiring a 3.5-V power supply. Specially designed reusable or disposable polypropylene specula slip over the tip of the instrument. Most otoscopic heads can be used with a rubber squeeze bulb for pneumatic otoscopy (described later in this chapter). Take care in the use of the otoscope. The best visualization of the structure does not require the speculum to be wedged into the canal. Be gentle, to achieve the best view of the anatomy.

Choose the correct speculum size: small enough to prevent discomfort to the patient and large enough to provide an adequate beam of light. Usually a tip 4 to 6 mm in diameter is used for adults, 3 to 4 mm in diameter for children, and 2 mm in diameter for infants.

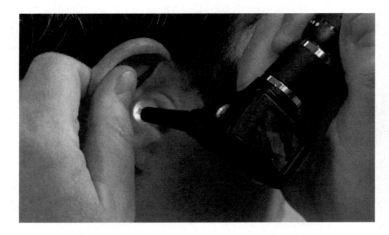

Figure 11–14 Technique for otoscopic examination. Notice that the ear is pulled up, out, and back.

The Techniques

To examine the patient's *right* ear, the examiner holds the otoscope in the *right* hand. The canal is straightened by the examiner's *left* hand pulling the pinna *up, out,* and *back.* The straighter the canal, the easier the visualization and the more comfortable the examination is for the patient.

In a child, the canal should be straightened by pulling the pinna *down* and *back.*

The patient is asked to turn his or her head to the side slightly so that the examiner can examine the ear more comfortably. The otoscope may be held in either of two positions. The first, and preferred, position involves holding the otoscope like a pencil, between the thumb and index finger, in a *downward* position with the ulnar aspect of the examiner's hand braced against the side of the patient's face. This position provides a buffer against sudden movement by the patient. By holding the end of the otoscope's handle, the examiner then angles the speculum into the external canal. This technique at first feels more cumbersome than the alternative technique, but it is safer, especially for children. This technique is shown in Figure 11-14.

The second position involves holding the otoscope *upward* as the speculum is introduced into the canal. This technique feels more comfortable, but a sudden movement by the patient can cause pain and injury to the patient. This technique is shown in Figure 11-15.

Inspect the External Canal

Gently insert the speculum and inspect the external canal. The external auditory canal is 24 mm long in the adult and is the only skin-lined, blind-ended canal in the body. The canal follows a tortuous course from the external meatus to the tympanic membrane. The techniques previously described are used to straighten the canal. There should be no evidence of redness, swelling, or tenderness, which indicates inflammation. The walls of the canal should be free of foreign bodies, scaliness, and discharge. If a foreign body is seen,

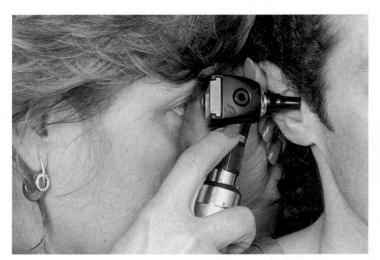

Figure 11–15 Alternative technique for otoscopic examination. The ear is pulled up, out, and back.

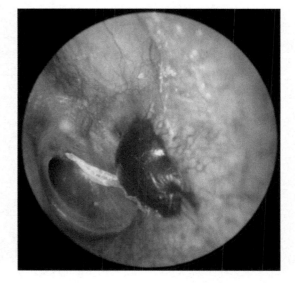

Figure 11–16 External ear canal with large hematoma.

pay particular attention when inspecting the opposite ear canal, the nose, and other accessible body orifices.

Any cerumen should be left as is, unless it interferes with the visualization of the rest of the canal and tympanic membrane. Removal of cerumen is best left to an experienced examiner because any manipulation may result in trauma or abrasions. Figure 11-16 depicts an external ear canal with a large hematoma secondary to aggressive use of a cotton-tipped applicator stick. Notice the tympanic membrane in the background.

If a discharge is present, look for the site of origin.

Inspect the Tympanic Membrane

As the speculum is introduced farther into the canal in a downward and forward direction, the tympanic membrane is visualized. The tympanic membrane should appear as an intact, ovoid, semitransparent, pearly gray membrane at the end of the canal. The lower four fifths of the tympanic membrane is called the *pars tensa;* the upper fifth, the *pars flaccida*. The handle of the malleus should be seen near the center of the pars tensa. From the lower end of the handle, there is frequently a bright triangular cone of light reflected from the pars tensa. This is called the *light reflex*, which is directed anteroinferiorly. The pars flaccida, the short process of the malleus, and the anterior and posterior folds should be identified. A normal tympanic membrane is pictured in Figure 11-17*A*, and the important landmarks are identified in Figure 11-17*B*.

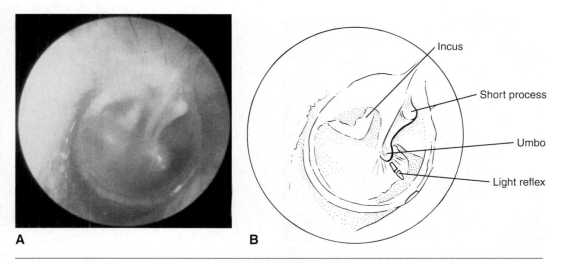

A   B

Figure 11–17 Photograph (*A*) and labeled schematic (*B*) illustrating a normal right tympanic membrane.

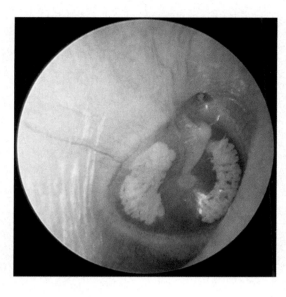

Figure 11–18 Tympanosclerosis.

The presence or absence of the light reflex should not be considered indicative of either normality or disease. The sensitivity of the light reflex for indicating disease is low. There are as many normal tympanic membranes without a light reflex as there are abnormal membranes with a light reflex.

Describe the color, integrity, transparency, position, and landmarks of the tympanic membrane.

Healthy tympanic membranes are usually pearly gray. Diseased tympanic membranes may be dull and become red or yellow. Is the eardrum injected? *Injection* refers to the dilatation of blood vessels, making them more apparent. The blood vessels should be visible only around the perimeter of the membrane. Dense, white plaques on the tympanic membrane may be caused by tympanosclerosis, which is caused by deposition of hyaline material and calcification within the layers of the tympanic membrane. This condition is commonly (in 50% to 60% of cases) secondary to the insertion of ventilation tubes. The classic horseshoe shape of tympanosclerosis is seen in the tympanic membrane shown in Figure 11-18. Despite the size of these lesions, they usually do not impair hearing and are rarely of clinical importance. If the lesion extends into the middle ear, however, conductive deafness may result.

Is the tympanic membrane bulging or retracted? Bulging of the membrane may indicate fluid or pus in the middle ear. No bubbles or fluid should be seen behind the tympanic membrane in the middle ear. A tympanic membrane becomes retracted when intratympanic cavity pressures are reduced: for example, when the eustachian tube is obstructed. Figure 11-19 depicts a "retraction pocket" just above the lateral process of the malleus, a condition known as *attic retraction*. On occasion, the entire tympanic membrane may become retracted

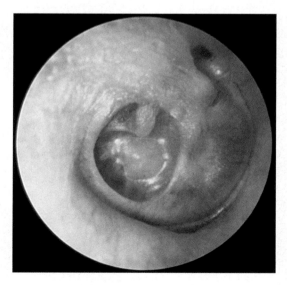

Figure 11–19 Retraction pocket.

onto the ossicles of the middle ear. The ossicles may become eroded, with the development of a conductive hearing loss.

If the tympanic membrane is perforated, describe the characteristics. Perforation of the tympanic membrane can occur after trauma or infection.

The normal position of the tympanic membrane is oblique to the external canal. The superior margin is closer to the examiner's eye. This is frequently better seen in infants than in adults.

In the normal ear, the handle of the malleus attached to the tympanic membrane is the primary landmark. Frequently, the long process of the incus may be seen posterior to the malleus. The chorda tympani nerve, which supplies innervation to the anterior two thirds of the tongue and stimulates taste there, is frequently visible in the upper posterior quadrant; it passes horizontally across the middle ear behind the tympanic membrane between the long process of the incus and the handle of the malleus. Keratin patches appear as multiple, discrete white patches on the tympanic membrane of all normal membranes; if illumination is not sufficient, however, they may not be visualized. In the presence of a retracted tympanic membrane, the malleus is seen in sharp outline.

There are many differences in the color, shape, and contour of the tympanic membrane, which can be recognized only with experience.

After examining the right ear, examine the *left* ear by holding the otoscope in the *left* hand and straightening the canal with the *right* hand.

Determine the Mobility of the Tympanic Membrane

If there is a question of middle ear infection, pneumatic otoscopy should be performed. This technique requires the use of a speculum large enough to fit snugly into the external canal to establish a closed air chamber between the canal and the interior of the otoscopic head. A rubber squeeze bulb is attached to the otoscopic head. By squeezing the bulb, the examiner can increase the air pressure in the canal. Pneumatic otoscopy must be performed gently, and the patient should be informed that he or she may experience a blowing noise during the procedure. When the pressure in the otoscopic head is increased by squeezing the bulb, the normal tympanic membrane shows a prompt inward movement. In patients with an obstructed eustachian tube, the tympanic membrane moves sluggishly inward. If fluid is present in the middle ear, a marked decrease or absence of movement is detected. The reduction of movement of the tympanic membrane increases the probability of middle ear infection by as much as 40%. This simple technique can provide invaluable assistance in the early diagnosis of many middle ear problems.

The Nose

The examination of the nose consists of the following:

- External examination
- Internal examination

External Examination

Inspect the Nose

The external examination consists of inspection of the nose for any *swelling, trauma,* or *congenital anomalies*. Is the nose straight? Does a deviation involve the upper, bony portion or the lower, cartilaginous portion?

Inspect the external nares. Are they symmetric?

Test the patency of each nostril. Occlude one nostril by gently placing a finger across the opening. Ask the patient to sniff. Do not compress the contralateral nostril by aggressive pressure.

Any swelling or deformity should be palpated for pain and firmness.

Rhinophyma is a common condition in which there is prominent hypertrophy of the sebaceous glands of the nose with overgrowth of the soft tissue. This condition is more common in men than in women. The patient pictured in Figure 11-20 also has *acne rosacea*, which is a common associated condition consisting of papules, pustules, and erythema of the face. The cause is unknown. The rash is worsened by hot drinks, highly spiced food, and alcohol.

Palpate the Sinuses

Palpation over the frontal and maxillary sinuses may reveal tenderness that is indicative of sinusitis.

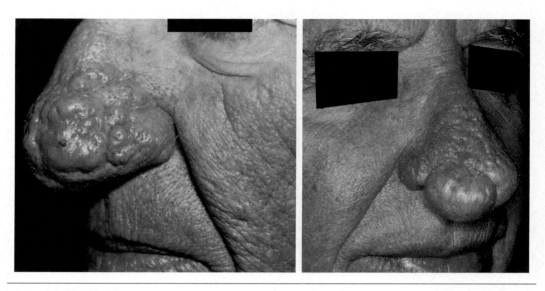

Figure 11–20 Rhinophyma.

Internal Examination

The key to the internal examination is proper positioning of the head. Ask the patient to hold his or her head back. Place your left hand firmly on top of the patient's head, and use your left thumb to elevate the tip of the patient's nose. In this manner, change the position of the patient's head to visualize the intranasal structures. Use a light source to illuminate the internal structures. This technique is shown in Figure 11-21.

Inspect the position of the septum to the lateral cartilages on each side. Examine the vestibule for inflammation and the anterior septum for deviation or perforation. Evaluate the *color* of the nasal mucous membrane. Normal nasal mucous membranes are dull red and moist and have a smooth, clean surface. Nasal mucosa is usually darker in color than oral mucosa. Inspect for exudate, swelling, bleeding, and trauma. If epistaxis has occurred, examine Little's area for vascular engorgement or crusting.

Is a discharge present? If so, describe it as purulent, watery, cloudy, or bloody. Is crusting present? Are any masses or polyps present?

Tip the patient's head farther back, and check the posterior septum for deviation or perforation. Note the size and color of the inferior turbinates. The two inferior turbinates are rarely symmetric.

Inspect the size, color, and mucosal condition of the middle turbinates. Are polyps present? Most polyps are found in the middle meatus.

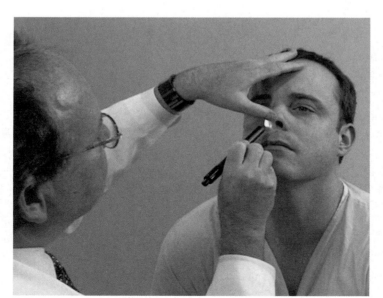

Figure 11–21 Inspection of the internal structures of the nose.

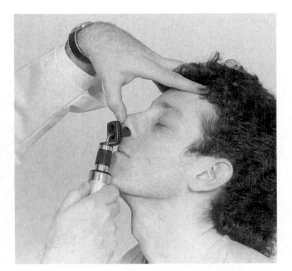

Figure 11–22 Using a nasal illuminator to inspect the internal structures of the nose.

Use a Nasal Illuminator

If a nasal illuminator is used, the examiner's left thumb is placed on the tip of the patient's nose while the palm of the examiner's hand steadies the patient's head. The patient's neck is slightly extended as the tip of the speculum of the illuminator is inserted into the nostril. After one nostril is evaluated, the illuminator is placed in the other nostril. The technique of using a nasal illuminator is shown in Figure 11-22.

Use a Nasal Speculum

If a nasal speculum is used, the instrument is held in the examiner's left hand, and the speculum is introduced into the patient's nostril in a vertical position (blades facing up and down). The speculum should not rest on the nasal septum. The blades are inserted about 1 cm into the vestibule, and the patient's neck should be slightly extended. The examiner's left index finger is placed on the ala of the patient's nose to anchor the upper blade of the speculum while the examiner's right hand steadies the patient's head. The right hand is used to change the head position for better visibility of the internal structures. After one nostril has been examined, the speculum, still being held in the examiner's left hand, is introduced into the patient's other nostril. The technique of holding the speculum is shown in Figure 11-23. Although the nasal speculum provides the best method of inspection, internists rarely use this instrument. Figure 11-24 shows a patient with nasal polyps, visible by means of the nasal speculum.

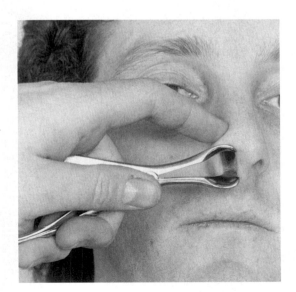

Figure 11–23 Using a nasal speculum to inspect the internal structures of the nose. Note the position of the left index finger.

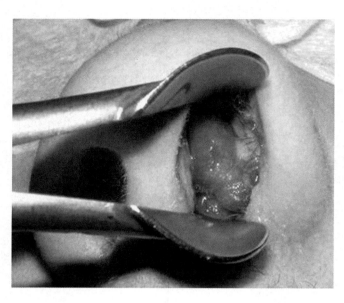

Figure 11–24 Nasal polyps.

Transilluminate the Sinuses

If a patient has symptoms referable to sinus problems, transillumination of the sinuses is performed. This examination is performed in a darkened room, and a bright light source is placed in the patient's mouth on one side of the hard palate. The light is transmitted through the maxillary sinus cavity and is seen as a crescent-shaped dull glow under the eye. The other side is then examined. Normally, the glow on each side is equal. If one sinus contains fluid, a mass, or mucosal thickening, there is a decrease in the glow, indicating loss of aeration on that side. An alternative method of examining the maxillary sinus is to direct a light downward from under the medial aspect of the eye. The patient is asked to open the mouth, and the glow is observed in the hard palate. This technique is illustrated in Figure 11-25. The frontal sinus can be examined in a similar manner by directing the light upward under the medial aspect of the eyebrow and observing the glow above the eye.

The ethmoid and sphenoid sinuses cannot be examined by transillumination.

The patient-to-patient variability of sinus transillumination is tremendous. In the absence of sinus symptoms, these differences in transillumination are nonspecific.

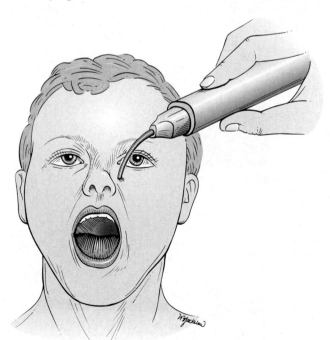

Figure 11–25 Transillumination of the maxillary sinus. Note the red glow seen on the hard palate.

Clinicopathologic Correlations

Infectious, inflammatory, traumatic, and neoplastic diseases are common in the organs of the ear and nose. Some of the more common ear infections are discussed in this section.

Acute otitis externa is a common inflammatory condition of the external ear canal, most often caused by *Pseudomonas aeruginosa*. The prominent symptom is severe ear pain (otalgia) accentuated by manipulation of the pinna and especially by pressure on the tragus. Edema of the external ear canal, erythema, and a yellowish-green discharge are prominent signs of this disease. Commonly, the canal is so tender and swollen that adequate visualization of the entire canal and tympanic membrane is impossible. "Swimmer's ear" is a form of otitis externa in which there is a loss of the protective cerumen, and chronic irritation and maceration by water and bacteria occur. Itching is a common precursor of otalgia. Figure 11-26 shows the external ear canal of a patient with acute otitis externa. Notice the follicular appearance of the canal, which resulted from epithelial swelling. As the condition progresses, the lumen may be occluded, producing conductive deafness.

Bullous myringitis is a localized form of external otitis, commonly associated with an acute viral upper respiratory infection. Severe otalgia is present, caused by bullous, often hemorrhagic, lesions on the skin in the deep external ear canal and on the tympanic membrane. A blood-tinged discharge may also occur. Fortunately, bullous myringitis is a self-limited condition. Figure 11-27 shows the tympanic membrane of a patient with bullous myringitis. Notice the blood-filled bullae on the membrane. Figure 11-28 shows the left ear of another patient with bullous myringitis. Notice the huge bulla filled with serosanguineous fluid arising from the floor of the bony external auditory canal. The bulla is so large that it obscures the tympanic membrane from view.

Acute otitis media is a bacterial infection of the middle ear, occurring most commonly in children. Up to 50% of all children experience an attack of acute otitis media before they reach 1 year of age, and 75% of children are affected before their second birthdays. After 5 years of age, the incidence declines rapidly. Affected patients suffer ear pain and have constitutional symptoms of fever and malaise, often associated with gastrointestinal problems and a conductive hearing loss. In contrast to external otitis, in which pulling on the auricle and tragus causes pain, no pain is elicited when these maneuvers are performed on a patient with acute otitis media. The tympanic membrane becomes injected, and the entire membrane is a fiery red. A mucopurulent exudate in the middle ear causes the membrane to bulge outward. In most cases, antibiotic therapy resolves the condition and restores normal hearing. Figure 11-29 shows the tympanic membrane of a young child with the classic features of acute otitis media. Notice the erythema, resulting from the acute inflammation, and the cloudiness and bulging of the tympanic membrane, resulting from the middle ear exudate.

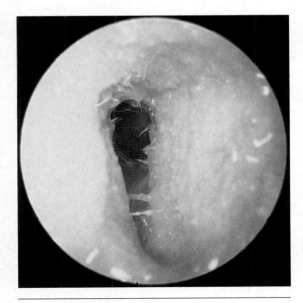

Figure 11–26 Acute otitis externa.

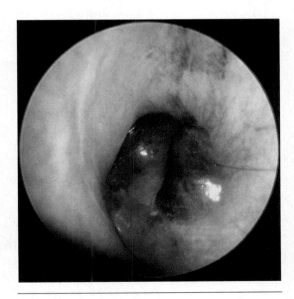

Figure 11–27 Bullous myringitis.

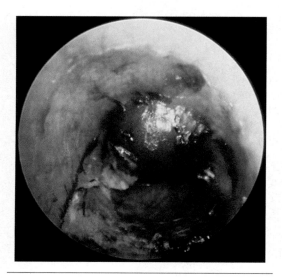

Figure 11–28 Bullous myringitis.

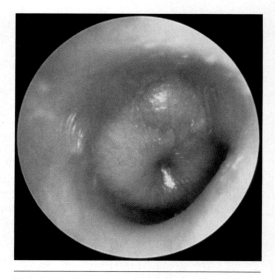

Figure 11–29 Acute otitis media.

Spontaneous rupture of the tympanic membrane may result from the increased pressure, with discharge of the mucopurulent exudate into the external ear canal. If this occurs, *advanced acute otitis media* is said to be present. Figure 11-30 illustrates perforation of a tympanic membrane as a result of otitis media.

Perforations may be *central* or *marginal* and may result from either otitis media or trauma. A central perforation does not involve the margin or annulus of the tympanic membrane; a marginal perforation involves the margin. Marginal perforations are more serious because they predispose the patient to the development of a *cholesteatoma*, which is a chronic condition of the middle ear. A marginal perforation allows squamous epithelium from the external canal to grow into the middle ear. As these cells invade, they desquamate, and debris accumulates in the middle ear, forming a cholesteatoma. Slow enlargement of the cholesteatoma leads to erosion of the ossicles and expansion into the mastoid antrum. Figure 11-31 illustrates a cholesteatoma.

A congenital cholesteatoma of the right anterior middle ear is pictured in Figure 11-32. It is smooth and white, medial to a normal tympanic membrane.

Figure 11-33 depicts chronic tympanic membrane perforation of the right ear. Notice the smooth epithelium-covered margin of chronic perforation, as well as patches of tympanosclerosis.

Serous otitis media occurs primarily in adults with viral upper respiratory infections or during sudden atmospheric pressure changes. In the presence of a blocked eustachian tube, air becomes trapped within. The tiny blood vessels in the middle ear absorb much of the air,

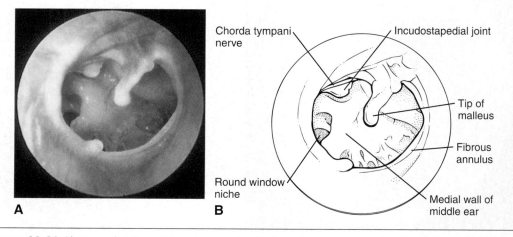

Figure 11–30 Photograph (*A*) and labeled schematic (*B*) illustrating a central perforation of the right tympanic membrane.

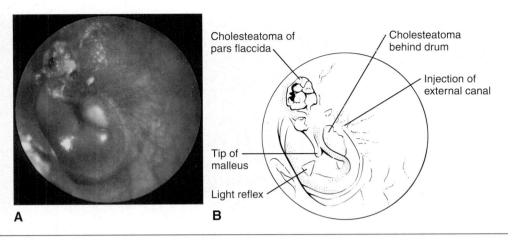

Figure 11–31 Photograph (*A*) and labeled schematic (*B*) illustrating a cholesteatoma of the left ear that resulted from a marginal perforation of the tympanic membrane. Note the injection of the distal external canal.

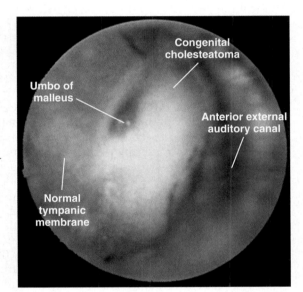

Figure 11–32 Congenital cholesteatoma.

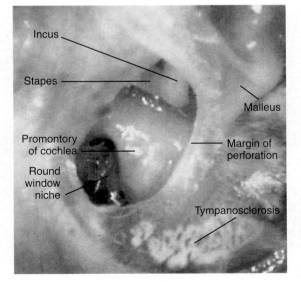

Figure 11–33 Chronic tympanic membrane perforation.

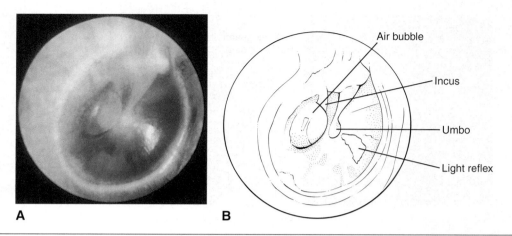

A   **B**

Figure 11–34 Photograph (*A*) and labeled schematic (*B*) illustrating serous otitis media of the right ear. Note the air bubble in the middle ear behind the tympanic membrane.

producing a vacuum that draws in or retracts the tympanic membrane. The sensation of "plugged ears" occurs. If the pressure is not relieved, this vacuum draws serous, nonpurulent fluid from the blood vessels into the middle ear. The tympanic membrane appears yellowish-orange as a result of the amber-colored fluid, and the landmarks are clearly seen as the membrane is retracted against these structures. Partial obstruction of the eustachian tube produces air bubbles or an air-fluid level in the middle ear. Figure 11-34 shows the tympanic membrane of a patient with serous otitis media.

Recurrent middle ear infections and tympanic membrane rupture may lead to *chronic otitis media*. Chronic infections may produce a foul-smelling discharge, which is the main symptom of chronic otitis media; pain is usually not present. Erosion of the ossicles with formation of scar tissue may occur, causing a conductive hearing loss.

Figure 11-35 shows the right tympanic membrane in an adult patient with chronic eustachian tube dysfunction. An early pars flaccida retraction pocket is seen. These retraction pockets result from chronic negative pressure within the middle ear and may progress to form an acquired cholesteatoma. A pressure-equalizing tube, called a *tympanostomy tube*, or T-tube, has been placed to eliminate the negative middle ear pressure. Figure 11-36 shows the right tympanic membrane in another patient with long-standing eustachian tube dysfunction whose middle ear is ventilated with a long-term T-tube. Resolving mild otitis externa is seen, with canal skin erythema and desquamation of the epithelium.

Table 11-4 summarizes the comparative features of conductive and sensorineural hearing loss. Table 11-5 enumerates the common causes of deafness. Table 11-6 differentiates acute otitis externa from acute otitis media.

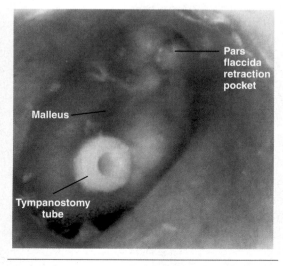

Figure 11–35 Chronic eustachian tube dysfunction.

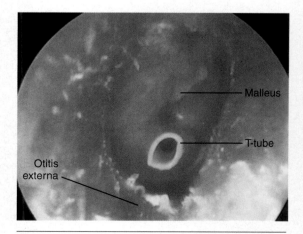

Figure 11–36 Tympanic membrane ventilated with tympanostomy tube (T-tube).

Table 11–4 Comparative Features of Conductive and Sensorineural Hearing Loss

Feature	Conductive Hearing Loss	Sensorineural Hearing Loss
Pathologic process	External canal Middle ear	Cochlea Cochlear nerve Brain stem
Loudness of speech	Softer than normal	Louder than normal
External canal	May be abnormal	Normal
Tympanic membrane	Usually abnormal	Normal
Rinne test result	Negative	Positive
Weber test result	Heard on "deaf" side	Heard on better side (only in severe unilateral loss)

Table 11–5 Common Causes of Deafness

Patient	Conductive Deafness	Sensorineural Deafness
Child	Congenital Acute otitis media Chronic otitis media Cerumen Trauma	Congenital Mumps labyrinthitis Maternal rubella during first trimester Birth trauma Congenital syphilis
Adult	Serous otitis media Chronic otitis media Otitis externa Cerumen Eustachian tube blockage Viral myringitis Cholesteatoma Otosclerosis	Delayed-onset congenital Ménière's disease Ototoxic drugs Viral labyrinthitis Acoustic neuroma Presbycusis (age-related deafness)

Table 11–6 Differentiation of Acute Otitis Externa from Acute Otitis Media

Signs and Symptoms	Acute Otitis Externa*	Acute Otitis Media†
Pressure on tragus	Painful	Painless
Lymphadenopathy	Frequent	Absent
External canal	Edematous	Normal
Season	Summer	Winter
Tympanic membrane	Normal	Fluid behind eardrum, possible perforation
Fever	Yes	Yes
Hearing	Slight loss or normal	Decreased

*See Figure 11-26.
†See Figure 11-29.

Useful Vocabulary

Listed here are the specific roots that are important to understand the terminology related to diseases of the ear and nose.

Root	Pertaining to	Example	Definition
audio-	to hear	**audio**meter	Device to measure hearing
aur-	ear	**aur**icle	Portion of the external ear not contained within the head
-cusis	hearing	presby**cusis**	Progressive decrease in hearing with age
-lalia	speech	echo**lalia**	Meaningless repetition by a patient of words addressed to him or her
myringo-	tympanic membrane	**myringo**tomy	Surgical incision of the tympanic membrane
ot(o)-	ear	**ot**itis	Inflammation of the ear
phon-	sound; the sound of a voice	**phon**asthenia	Weakness of the voice
rhino-	nose	**rhino**plasty	Plastic surgery of the nose
tympan(o)-	middle ear	**tympano**tomy	Surgical puncture of the tympanic membrane

Writing Up the Physical Examination

Listed here are examples of the write-up for the examinations of the ear and nose.

- The external ear appears normal without evidence of inflammation or lesions. The patient has no difficulty hearing the whispered word. The Weber test result is midline. Rinne test result: AC > BC. The external canals are normal, as are the tympanic membranes. There is no injection of the external canals or the tympanic membranes. No discharge is present.
- A 1-cm, round, hard, painless mass is present on the right pinna. The patient has no problem with hearing. The Weber test result shows no lateralization. The external canals and tympanic membranes are normal.
- The external structures of the ears are within normal limits. There is a hearing loss in the left ear. The Weber test result lateralizes to the left ear. The left tympanic membrane appears opaque. The ossicles are not seen on the left. The right tympanic membrane appears normal. The ossicles appear normal on the right.
- The nose is not deviated. No swellings are seen. The anterior septum appears pink without discharge or vascular engorgement. The septum is midline. No sinus tenderness is present.
- The nose appears deviated to the right. The nasal mucous membranes are bright red and moist. A whitish-yellow discharge is present on a deviated septum to the right. The sinuses are not tender.

Bibliography

Hawke M, Keene M, Alberti PW: Clinical Otoscopy, 2nd ed. Edinburgh, Churchill Livingstone, 1990.

Hawke M, Kwok P: A mini-atlas of ear-drum pathology. Can Fam Physician 33:1501, 1987.

Hawke M, McCombe A: Diseases of the Ear: A Pocket Atlas. Toronto Manticore Communication, 1995.

Orlans H (ed): Adjustment to Adult Hearing Loss. San Diego, Calif College Hill Press, 1985.

White J: Benign paroxysmal positional vertigo: How to diagnose and quickly treat it. Cleveland Clin J Med 71:722, 2004.

Williams JW, Simel DL: Does this patient have sinusitis? Diagnosing acute sinusitis by history and physical examination. JAMA 270:1242, 1993.

Williams JW, Simel DL, Roberts L, et al: Clinical evaluation for sinusitis: Making the diagnosis by history and physical examination. Ann Intern Med 117:705, 1992.

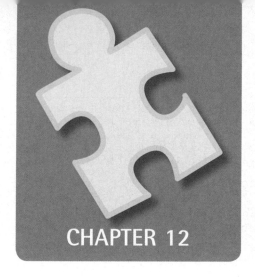

CHAPTER 12

The Oral Cavity and Pharynx

Look to thy mouth; diseases enter here.

George Herbert (1593–1632)

General Considerations

The mouth and oral cavity are used by individuals to express the entire range of emotions. As early as infancy, the mouth provides gratification and sensory pleasure.

Approximately 20% of all visits to primary care physicians are related to problems of the oral cavity and throat. Most patients with these problems present with throat pain, which may be acute and associated with fever or difficulty in swallowing. A sore throat may be the result of local disease, or it may be an early manifestation of a systemic problem.

It has been estimated that more than 90% of patients infected with human immunodeficiency virus (HIV) have at least one oral manifestation of the disease. It appears that as further immunologic impairment develops, the risk of oral lesions increases. There are several important oral manifestations that are strongly associated with early HIV infection. The presence of any of them mandates HIV testing.

Oral cancer represents about 3% of all cancers. Cancer of the oral cavity and pharynx was responsible for 7550 deaths in 2007, killing approximately 1 person per hour, 24 hours per day. The rate of death from oral cancer is higher than those from cervical cancer; Hodgkin's disease; cancer of the brain, liver, testis, kidney, or ovary; or malignant melanoma. One of the reasons for this high death rate is that the cancer is routinely discovered late in its development, with metastases to other areas or invasion deep into local structures. Oral cancer is also particularly dangerous because it has a high risk of producing second primary tumors. This means that patients who survive a first encounter with the disease have up to a 20 times higher risk for development of a second cancer. There is a 2:1 male-to-female incidence ratio and a 2:1 African-American–to–white death rate ratio. It is estimated that a man has a 1:72 lifetime risk for development of oral cancer. The American Cancer Society estimates that approximately 34,360 new cases of oral cancer were diagnosed in 2007 in the United States, with 24,180 cases occurring in men and 10,180 in women. Worldwide, the problem is much greater: More than 350,000 to 400,000 new cases are diagnosed each year. Although the exact cause of tongue cancer remains unknown, it most often occurs in people who use tobacco products (cigarettes, cigars, pipes, and smokeless tobacco), consume alcohol (especially when combined with tobacco use), or chew betel nuts. Chewing of betel nuts is not a common practice in the United States, but it is a widespread habit in many parts of the world, especially in Taiwan (see Fig. 12-51).

Many physician visits for oral problems are associated with psychiatric disturbances. Psychosomatic disease symptoms often center on the mouth. Patients with psychosomatic disease may complain of "burning" or "dryness" of the mouth or tongue. *Bruxism*, or grinding

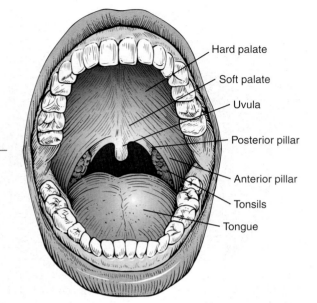

Figure 12–1 The oral cavity.

of the teeth other than for chewing, occurs especially during sleep. This overuse of the muscles of mastication has often been interpreted as a manifestation of rage or aggression that is not overtly displayed; it may also be an infantile response to reduce psychic tension. Bruxism can produce facial pain, which causes further spasm of the muscles and continued bruxism, resulting in a vicious circle. Individuals who habitually have something in their mouths, such as a pipe, a thumb, or a pencil, may cause damage to their oral cavities.

Although it is often thought that the oral cavity is examined only by dentists, other health-care professionals must have competency in evaluating this important region of the body. The health-care provider must be able to accomplish the following:

1. Appraise oral hygiene
2. Recognize dental caries and periodontal disease
3. Recognize the presence of oral lesions, as well as disorders of the regional lymph nodes, salivary glands, and bony structures
4. Recognize oral manifestations of systemic disease
5. Recognize systemic problems caused by oral disease and procedures
6. Assess physical findings concerning the range and smoothness of jaw motion
7. Identify dental appliances
8. Know when a dental consultation is required or should be postponed because of a medical problem

Structure and Physiology

The Oral Cavity

The oral cavity consists of the following structures:

- Buccal mucosa
- Lips
- Tongue
- Hard and soft palates
- Teeth
- Salivary glands

The oral cavity extends from the inner surface of the teeth to the oral pharynx. The hard and soft palates form the roof of the mouth. The soft palate terminates posteriorly at the *uvula*. The *tongue* lies at the floor of the mouth. At the most posterior aspect of the oral cavity lie the *tonsils*, between the anterior and posterior *pillars*. The oral cavity is illustrated in Figure 12-1.

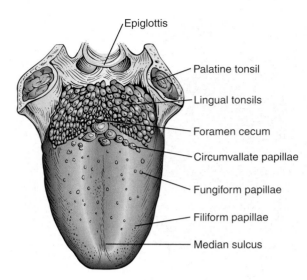

- Epiglottis
- Palatine tonsil
- Lingual tonsils
- Foramen cecum
- Circumvallate papillae
- Fungiform papillae
- Filiform papillae
- Median sulcus

Figure 12–2 The tongue viewed from above.

The *buccal mucosa* is a mucous membrane that is continuous with the gingivae and lines the insides of the cheeks. The *linea alba*, or bite line, is a pale or white line along the line of dental occlusion. It may be slightly raised and show impressions of the teeth.

Lips are red as a result of the increased number of vascular dermal papillae and the thinness of the epidermis in this area. An increase in desaturated hemoglobin, *cyanosis*, is manifested as blue lips. The common blue discoloration of the lips in a cold environment is related to the decreased blood supply and increased extraction of oxygen.

The tongue lies at the floor of the mouth and is attached to the *hyoid bone*. It is the main organ of taste, aids in speech, and serves an important function in mastication. The body of the tongue contains intrinsic and extrinsic muscles and contains the strongest muscle of the body. The tongue is supplied by the *hypoglossal*, or 12th cranial, nerve.

The dorsum of the tongue has a convex surface with a *median sulcus*. Figure 12-2 shows the tongue viewed from above. At the posterior portion of the sulcus is the *foramen cecum*, which marks the area of the origin of the *thyroid gland*. Behind the foramen cecum are mucin-secreting glands and an aggregate of lymphatic tissue called the *lingual tonsils*. The texture of the tongue is rough as a result of the presence of papillae, the largest of which are the *circumvallate papillae* (Fig. 12-3). There are approximately 10 of these round papillae, which are located just in front of the foramen cecum and divide the tongue into the anterior two thirds and the posterior one third. *Filiform papillae* are the most common papillae and are present over the surface of the anterior portion of the tongue. The *fungiform papillae* are located at the tip and sides of the tongue. These papillae can be recognized from their red color and broad surface.

The *taste buds* are located on the sides of the circumvallate and fungiform papillae. Taste is perceived from the anterior two thirds of the tongue by the *chorda tympani* nerve, a division of the facial nerve. The *glossopharyngeal*, or ninth cranial, nerve perceives taste sensation from the

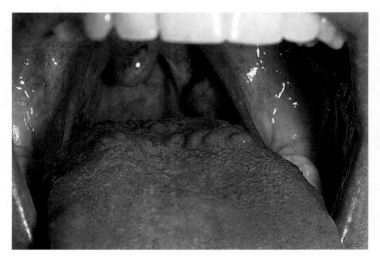

Figure 12–3 Circumvallate papillae.

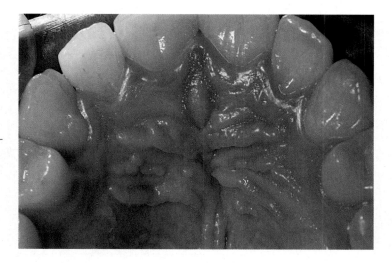

Figure 12–4 Palatal rugae.

posterior third of the tongue. There are four basic taste sensations: sweet, salty, sour, and bitter. Sweetness is detected at the tip of the tongue. Saltiness is sensed at the lateral margins of the tongue. Sourness and bitterness are perceived at the posterior aspect of the tongue and are carried by the glossopharyngeal nerve.

When the tongue is elevated, a mucosal attachment, the *frenulum*, may be seen underneath the tongue in the midline connecting the tongue to the floor of the mouth.

The *hard palate* is a concave bone structure. The anterior portion has raised folds, or *rugae*. Figure 12-4 shows the palatal rugae. The *soft palate* is a muscular, flexible area posterior to the hard palate. The posterior margin ends at the *uvula*. The uvula aids in closing off the nasopharynx during swallowing.

Teeth are composed of several tissues: enamel, dentin, pulp, and cementum. *Enamel* covers the tooth and is the most highly calcified tissue in the body. The bulk of the tooth is the *dentin*. Under the dentin is the *pulp*, which contains branches of the trigeminal, or fifth cranial, nerve and blood vessels. The *cementum* covers the root of the tooth and attaches it to the bone. Figure 12-5 shows a cross section through a molar tooth.

The *primary dentition*, or the deciduous teeth, consists of 20 teeth that erupt from the ages of 6 to 30 months. The primary dentition per quadrant of jaw consists of two incisors, one canine, and two premolars. These teeth are shed from the ages of 6 to 13 years. The *secondary dentition*, or the permanent teeth, consists of 32 teeth that erupt from the ages of 6 to 22 years. The secondary dentition per quadrant of jaw consists of two incisors, one canine, two premolars, and three molars. Figure 12-6 illustrates the primary and secondary dentition, and Table 24-5 summarizes the chronology of dentition.

Although not part of the oral cavity proper, the *salivary glands* are considered part of the mouth. There are three major salivary glands: the parotid, the submandibular, and the

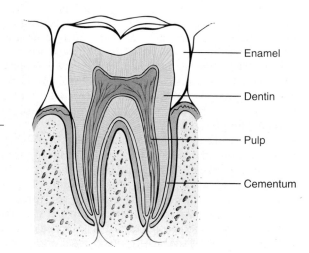

Figure 12–5 Cross-sectional view through a molar tooth.

Enamel

Dentin

Pulp

Cementum

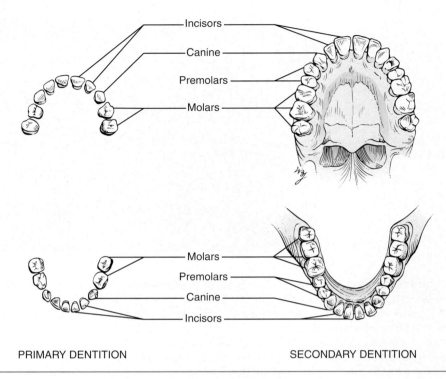

Incisors
Canine
Premolars
Molars

Molars
Premolars
Canine
Incisors

PRIMARY DENTITION

SECONDARY DENTITION

Figure 12–6 Primary dentition (*left*) and secondary dentition (*right*).

sublingual glands. The *parotid gland* is the largest of the salivary glands. It lies anterior to the ear on the side of the face. The facial, or seventh cranial, nerve courses through the gland. The duct of the parotid gland, *Stensen's duct*, enters the oral cavity through a small papilla opposite the upper first or second molar tooth. The *submandibular gland* is the second largest salivary gland. It is located below and in front of the angle of the mandible. The duct of the submandibular gland, *Wharton's duct*, terminates in a papilla on either side of the frenulum at the base of the tongue. The *sublingual gland* is the smallest of the major salivary glands. It is located in the floor of the mouth, beneath the tongue. There are numerous ducts of the sublingual gland, some of which open into Wharton's duct. In addition to these major salivary glands, there are hundreds of very small salivary glands located throughout the oral cavity.

The Pharynx

The pharynx is divided into the nasopharynx, the oropharynx, and the hypopharynx. The *nasopharynx* lies above the soft palate and is posterior to the nasal cavities. On its posterolateral wall is the opening of the *eustachian tube*. The *adenoids* are pharyngeal tonsils and hang from the posterosuperior wall near the opening of the eustachian tube. The *oropharynx* lies below the soft palate, behind the mouth, and superior to the hyoid bone. Posteriorly, it is bounded by the superior constrictor muscle and the cervical vertebrae. Below the oropharynx is the area known as the *hypopharynx* (or *laryngopharynx*). The hypopharynx is surrounded by three constrictor muscles, which are innervated by the glossopharyngeal and vagus nerves. The hypopharynx ends at the level of the cricoid cartilage, where it communicates with the esophagus through the upper esophageal sphincter. Figure 12-7 illustrates the functional parts of the pharynx.

The muscular walls of the pharynx are formed by the constrictor muscles, which function during the act of swallowing. The blood supply is derived from the external carotid artery.

Lymphatic tissue is abundant in the pharynx. The lymphoid tissue consists of the *palatine tonsils*, the *adenoids*, and the *lingual tonsils*. These tissues form *Waldeyer's ring*. The palatine tonsils lie in the tonsillar fossa, between the anterior and posterior pillars. The palatine tonsils are almond-shaped and vary considerably in size. The adenoids lie on the posterior wall of the nasopharynx, and the lingual tonsils are located at the base of the tongue. The upper portion of the pharynx drains to the retropharyngeal nodes, and the lower part drains to the deep cervical lymph nodes.

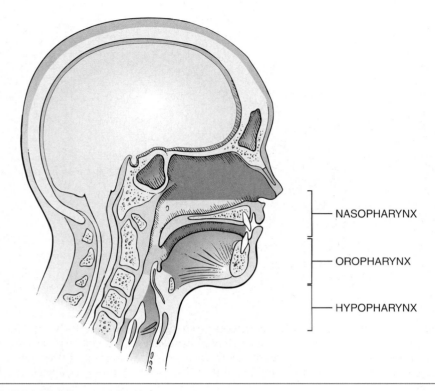

Figure 12–7 Functional parts of the pharynx.

The functions of the pharynx are as follows:

- Enable swallowing
- Enable speech
- Provide an airway

Swallowing, or *deglutition*, is divided into three stages. The voluntary stage occurs when a bolus of food is forced by the tongue past the tonsils to the posterior pharyngeal wall. The second stage is involuntary constriction by the pharyngeal muscles, propelling the bolus from the pharynx to the esophagus. The third stage is also involuntary, in which the esophageal muscles push the bolus down into the stomach. The larynx is first raised and then closed during the first two stages of swallowing. The eustachian tubes open during swallowing when the nasopharynx closes.

The pharynx also acts as a structure of resonation and articulation. *Resonation* refers to the vibration of a structure. *Articulation* is the change in shape of a structure to produce speech. Contracting the pharyngeal muscles causes a change in the acoustic quality of speech. Changes in the size and shape of the pharynx affect resonance. The soft palate affects resonance by opening and closing the partition between the oral and nasal cavities. If closure is incomplete, nasal speech results.

The Larynx

The larynx is located at the superior margin of the trachea and below the hyoid bone, which is located at the base of the tongue. The larynx is at the level of the fourth to sixth cervical vertebrae. The larynx functions as a guard against the entrance of solids and liquids into the trachea, as well as being the organ of voice production.

The *epiglottis* is attached above the larynx. The function of the epiglottis is generally believed to be protection of the airway during swallowing.

The body of the larynx consists of a series of cartilaginous structures: the thyroid, the cricoid, and the arytenoid cartilages. The *thyroid cartilage* forms the bulk of the structure of the larynx and produces the prominence in the neck known as the *Adam's apple*. Toward the top of the thyroid cartilage is the *thyroid notch*. Farther down on the thyroid cartilage, there is a space, the *cricothyroid space* and *membrane*, that separates the thyroid cartilage from the cricoid cartilage.

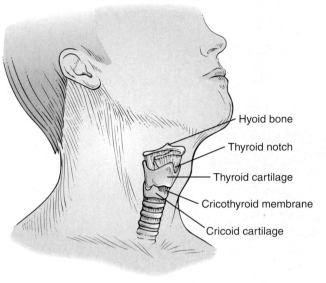

Hyoid bone

Thyroid notch

Thyroid cartilage

Cricothyroid membrane

Cricoid cartilage

Figure 12–8 Laryngeal cartilages.

The *cricoid cartilage* articulates with the cricothyroid membrane superiorly and the trachea inferiorly. It is the only complete ring of cartilage in the larynx. The paired *arytenoid cartilages* provide an important area for attachment of the vocal cords. A diagram of the thyroid and cricoid cartilages onto the neck is illustrated in Figure 12-8, and the laryngeal skeleton is illustrated in Figure 12-9.

The *vocal cords* vibrate to generate speech. Sound is produced by the rapid vibration of the vocal cords excited by the exhaled stream of air. The vocal cords are brought together, and their tension is changed, by the action of various laryngeal muscles. The nerve supply to the larynx is derived from the superior and recurrent laryngeal branches of the *vagus*, or 10th cranial, nerve. Voice produced at the larynx is modified by the pharynx and oronasal cavity.

Review of Specific Symptoms

The Oral Cavity

All patients should be asked the following:

"When did you last see a dentist?"

"What did the dentist do?"

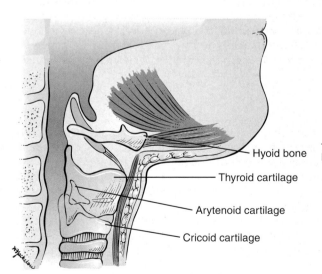

Hyoid bone

Thyroid cartilage

Arytenoid cartilage

Cricoid cartilage

Figure 12–9 Laryngeal skeleton.

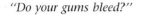

"Do your gums bleed?"

"Have you any pain, sores, or masses on your lips or in your mouth that do not heal?"

"Have you had any problems after extraction of a tooth?"

(If the patient wears dentures) *"Have you noticed any change in the way your dentures fit?"*

Cancers of the oral cavity are most often found in people who are older than 45 years of age. Cancer of the lip is more common in men than in women and is more likely to develop in people with light-colored skin who have spent extensive time in the sun. Cancer of the oral cavity is more common in people who chew tobacco or smoke pipes. A possible sign of a cancer of the mouth or gums is when dentures no longer fit well.

The most important symptoms of disease of the oral cavity are as follows:

- Pain
- Ulceration
- Bleeding
- Mass
- Halitosis (bad breath)
- Xerostomia (dry mouth)

Pain

When a patient complains of oral pain, it is important to ask the following:

"Where is the pain?"

"Describe the pain."

"Do you feel the pain anywhere else?"

"How long has the pain been present?"

"What brings the pain on?"

"What makes it better? worse?"

"When you have the pain, do you have any other symptoms?"

Tooth pain may be a symptom of underlying gingival disease. A history of dental procedures and recent dental work should be documented.

Pain in the teeth may sometimes be referred from the chest. Patients with angina may actually complain of pain in their teeth associated with exertion. Careful and thoughtful questioning is indicated.

Ulceration

Oral ulcerative lesions are common and may be manifestations of local or systemic disease of immunogenic, infectious, malignant, or traumatic origin. The patient's history is important because it indicates whether the lesions are acute or chronic, single or multiple, and primary or recurrent.

Oral pain is frequently related to ulceration of the lips or tongue. Cancer is not the most common cause of oral cavity ulceration, but it must always be considered. When a patient complains of ulceration, ask the following questions:

"Have you had a lesion like this before?"

"Are there multiple lesions?"

"How long have the lesions been present?"

"Are there lesions anywhere else on the body, such as in the vagina? In the urethra? In the anus?"

"Are the lesions painful?"

"Do you smoke?" If so, *"How much?"*

"Do you drink alcohol?"

"Do you have a history of venereal disease?"

The examiner should ask about a patient's sexual habits. These questions were discussed in Chapter 1, The Interviewer's Questions. Smoking and drinking alcohol predispose an individual to precancerous lesions of the mouth, such as leukoplakia and erythroplakia.

Bleeding

Bleeding may result from a primary hematologic disorder or from a local inflammation or neoplasm. Many medications may also cause or predispose a patient to bleeding. Always ask whether the patient is taking any medications.

Mass

If a patient complains of, or on physical examination is found to have, an intraoral mass or a mass in the region of a salivary gland, determine its duration and whether the mass is painful. A painless mass is usually a sign of a tumor.

Are there associated symptoms such as excessive salivation, known as *ptyalism,* or dryness of the mouth, known as *xerostomia?* Is dysphagia (difficulty in swallowing) present?

Halitosis

Halitosis affects about 50% of all adults. Fortunately, in only a small percentage does the problem persist the entire day. Most individuals with halitosis are told by others that they have bad breath, although they themselves may be unaware of the problem. In some cases, the odor in the mouth is so objectionable that it can compromise the patient's social and professional life.

The source of bad breath is in the oral cavity in 90% of cases; the other 10% have disorders in the nasal passages or lungs or a systemic disease. It is questionable whether the gastrointestinal tract is a source of halitosis.

It is believed that halitosis is caused by volatile sulfur and other compounds exhaled into the air during speech and respiration. These compounds are produced by putrefactive, gram-negative anaerobic bacteria colonizing on the posterior dorsum of the tongue, in periodontal pockets, and around some dental restorations and prostheses. The volatile sulfur compounds are generated by the bacterial metabolism of sulfur-containing amino acids. Xerostomia increases the level of volatile sulfur compounds.

Patients with systemic diseases such as diabetes mellitus, cirrhosis, uremia, and cancer; infections of the perioral regions; and trimethylaminuria (fish odor syndrome) can suffer from bad breath. These conditions must be considered in the absence of oral and sinonasal disease.

Treatment of halitosis should be directed toward the underlying cause. Once it has been determined that the source of the bad breath is the oral region, the patient should be instructed in procedures of good oral hygiene, including proper tooth brushing, flossing, and, most important, cleaning of the posterior dorsum of the tongue with a special scraping device or toothbrush. Appropriate mouthwash may also be used. These procedures must be performed at least twice a day to remove the bacteria and accumulated metabolic products.

Xerostomia

Xerostomia, or dry mouth, is a common symptom of reduced or absent salivary secretion. It is most common in women and in aging populations. It is frequently observed as a side effect of various medications, including antihistamines, decongestants, tricyclic antidepressants, antihypertensives, and various anticholinergic medications. It may also occur with mouth breathing, neurologic disorders, radiation therapy to the head and neck, HIV infection, and autoimmune disorders. The saliva is thick, and the oral mucosal surfaces are dry; the tongue is commonly fissured and atrophic. The dry environment predisposes to candidiasis and dental caries.

The Pharynx

The most common symptoms of disease of the pharynx include the following:

- Nasal obstruction
- Pain
- Dysphagia
- Deafness
- Snoring

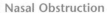

Nasal Obstruction

Nasal obstruction can result from enlarged adenoids or from tumor formation in the nasopharynx. It is important to determine whether the patient has any allergies or sinus trouble or has sustained nasal trauma.

Pain

Pain can result from inflammation of the tonsils or posterior pharynx, as well as from a tumor in this area. Acute throat pain may be caused by inflammatory processes or injury. A foreign body in the pharynx often produces severe pain that is worsened by swallowing. Often, throat pain may be referred to the ipsilateral ear. Chronic throat pain may be caused by inflammatory processes, as well as by neoplasms. Enlarged thyroid lobes or diffuse thyroid enlargement may cause throat pain associated with dysphagia. Hysteria is another cause of chronic throat pain.

Dysphagia

Dysphagia is difficulty in swallowing. Determine the site of obstruction. Does the dysphagia occur with liquids, solids, or tablets? Questions related to tonsillar infections are relevant because enlarged tonsils may interfere with swallowing. It is prudent to ask whether *regurgitation* of food occurs; this results from an abnormal pharyngeal pouch. The patient may say that the "food gets stuck." This is often associated with significant disease.

Deafness

A tumor at the distal end of the eustachian tube in the nasopharynx can produce *conductive deafness*. Benign masses such as hypertrophied adenoids may be responsible. Nasopharyngeal malignancies may also be the cause of conductive deafness. In many cases, serous effusions in the middle ear space cause eustachian tube dysfunction.

Snoring

Snoring is a common complaint. An important problem often associated with heavy snoring is obstructive sleep apnea. Many affected patients are overweight and have a history of excessive daytime sleepiness. A bed partner may describe the patient as at first sleeping quietly; then a transition occurs to louder snoring, followed by a period of cessation of snoring, during which time the patient becomes restless, has gasping motions, and appears to be struggling for breath. This period is terminated by a loud snort, and the sequence may begin again. It is common for patients with sleep apnea to have many of these episodes each night.

The Larynx

Dysphonia

The major symptom of laryngeal disease is a change in the voice, especially the development of dysphonia, or hoarseness. Ask the following questions:

> *"How long have you had the hoarseness?"*
>
> *"What seems to make it better? worse?"*
>
> *"Is there any time of day when it is worse?"*
>
> *"Have you had any surgery necessitating general anesthesia?"*
>
> *"Have you had any injury to your neck?"*

Determine whether the patient is or was a smoker. Recent onset of hoarseness may result from impingement on the recurrent laryngeal nerve as it hooks around the left bronchus. This may be caused by a tumor or by an enlarged left atrium. Voice overuse or vocal cord neoplasms are other causes of hoarseness. Procedures involving general anesthesia necessitate the use of an endotracheal tube, which could potentially damage a vocal cord and cause hoarseness.

Impact of a Voice Disorder on the Patient

Phonation is the process of sound production by the interaction of airflow through the glottis and the opening and closing of the vocal cords of the larynx. Voice loudness is proportional to the air pressure below the glottis; pitch is related to this pressure and to the length of the vocal cords. Voice quality may change when there is interference with the vocal cords or pharyngeal cavity vibration (i.e., resonance).

A voice disorder may be related to an enlarged vocal cord, a laryngeal mass, or a neurologic or psychologic problem. A voice disorder is defined as the presence of a voice that is different in pitch, quality, loudness, or flexibility in comparison with the voices of other persons of similar age, sex, and ethnic group. An abnormal voice may be a symptom or sign of illness, and its cause should be determined.

In a study of a school-aged population, voice disorders were found in up to 23% of children. Most of these disorders were related to voice abuse and not to organic problems. In another study, 7% of men and 5% of women from 18 to 82 years of age were found to have voice disorders. Most of these disorders were related to organic problems.

Many patients with organic speech disorders are rejected by other people. Their speech may be high-pitched or nasal and a cause of embarrassment. Their self-esteem is low. They are rejected by others because their voice patterns are objectionable.

Just as a voice disorder has an impact on a person, a person can use his or her voice to have an impact on others. The manner in which a person speaks—the quality, pitch, loudness, stress patterns, rate—reflects his or her personality. Psychogenic voice disorders are functional disorders that are manifestations of psychologic imbalance. Voice is a useful indicator of *affective disorders*, such as depression, manic states, and mood swings, as well as of *schizophrenia*.

Physical Examination

The equipment necessary for the examination of the oral cavity consists of a penlight, gauze pads, gloves, applicator sticks, and tongue depressors.

The Oral Cavity

The physical examination of the oral cavity includes inspection and palpation of the following structures:

- Lips
- Buccal mucosa
- Gingivae
- Teeth
- Tongue
- Floor of the mouth
- Hard and soft palates
- Salivary glands
- Twelfth cranial nerve

Sit or stand directly in front of the patient, who should be seated. The patient's face should be well illuminated. Work systematically from front to back so that no areas are omitted. Put on a pair of gloves when palpating any structure in the mouth. When any lesion is found, note its consistency and tenderness. If the patient is wearing dentures, ask him or her to remove them. Inspect the face and mouth for asymmetries and abnormalities.

Evaluate the patient's breath. Is there any distinctive odor to the patient's breath? This may suggest poor oral hygiene or systemic disease. A fetid odor may be caused by extensive caries or periodontal disease.

Have the patient open his or her mouth. If the mouth can be opened much beyond 35 mm, subluxation of the jaw may be present. Deviation of the jaw is suggestive of a neuromuscular or temporomandibular joint problem.

Inspect the Lips

Inspect the lips for localized or generalized swellings, and assess the patient's ability to open the mouth.

Assess the *color* of the lips. Is cyanosis present? Are there any lesions on the lips? If a lesion is detected, palpate it to characterize its texture and consistency. Figure 12-10 depicts the mouth of a patient with multiple herpetic ulcers, commonly known as *cold sores*, or herpes simplex labialis, on the lips and external nares. Figure 12-11 depicts multiple telangiectatic lesions on the tongue that are secondary to *Osler-Weber-Rendu syndrome*. In this syndrome,

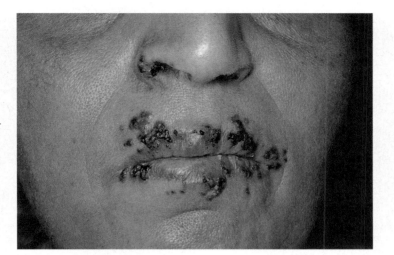

Figure 12–10 Herpes simplex labialis.

multiple telangiectases are present throughout the gastrointestinal tract. These may bleed insidiously, causing anemia. Figure 12-12 depicts the classic brown pigmentary changes on the lips of a patient with *Peutz-Jeghers syndrome*. This is an autosomal dominant disorder that is characterized by generalized gastrointestinal hamartomatous polyposis and mucocutaneous pigmentation.

A *mucocele* of the lip is a common bluish, cystic-appearing, painless, translucent, traumatically induced lesion. Mucoceles, which occur mostly on the lower lip, range in size from several millimeters to several centimeters and arise from obstruction or rupture of the minor salivary gland. When ruptured, a mucocele releases a clear, thick fluid. Figure 12-13 depicts a mucocele of the lower lip.

Inspect the Buccal Mucosa

The patient should be asked to open the mouth widely. The mouth should be illuminated with a light source. The buccal mucosa must be evaluated for any lesions or color changes, and the buccal cavity is inspected for any evidence of asymmetry or areas of injection (dilated vessels, usually indicative of inflammation). The buccal mucosa, teeth, and gingivae are easily evaluated by using a tongue depressor to retract the cheek away from the gums, as shown in Figure 12-14. The examiner should inspect for discolorations, evidence of trauma, and the condition of the parotid duct orifice.

Are there any ulcerations of the buccal mucosa? Are there *white lesions* on the buccal mucosa? A common painless white lesion in the mouth is *lichen planus*, which appears as a reticulated, or lacelike, eruption bilaterally on the buccal mucosa. An erosive, painful variant is similar in appearance except for the presence of hemorrhagic and ulcerated lesions. Nonerosive

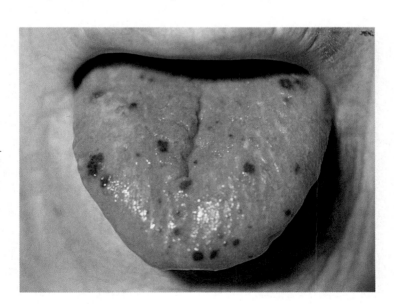

Figure 12–11 Osler-Weber-Rendu syndrome. Note the telangiectatic lesions.

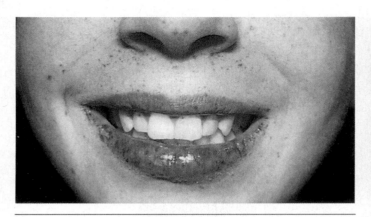

Figure 12–12 Peutz-Jeghers syndrome. Note the pigmentary changes.

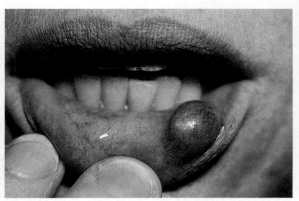

Figure 12–13 Mucocele of the lower lip.

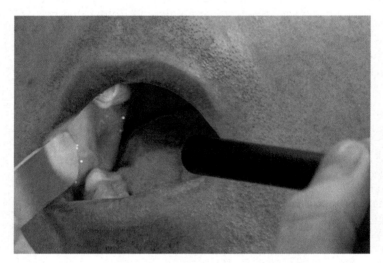

Figure 12–14 Inspection of the mouth.

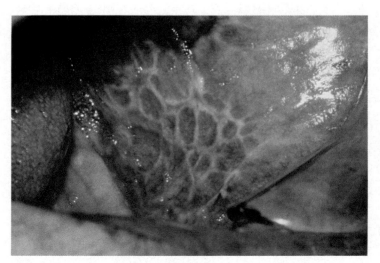

Figure 12–15 Nonerosive lichen planus of the buccal mucosa.

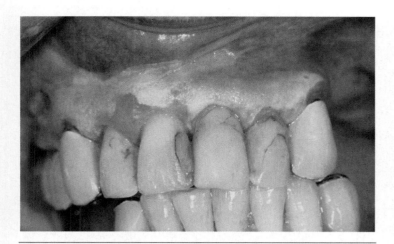

Figure 12–16 Leukoplakia of the gingiva.

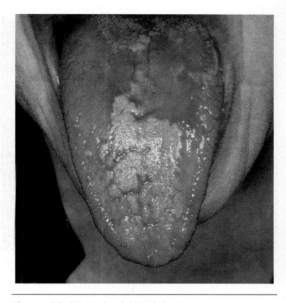

Figure 12–17 Leukoplakia of the tongue.

lichen planus is shown in Figure 12-15. Is *leukoplakia* present? In the mouth, leukoplakia can manifest as a painless, precancerous white plaque on the cheeks, gingivae, and tongue. Leukoplakia of the gingiva is pictured in Figure 12-16. Over 15 years, this lesion developed into verrucous hyperplasia, verrucous carcinoma, and finally squamous cell carcinoma. A resection of the maxilla and palate was required. Figure 12-17 depicts leukoplakia of the tongue in another patient. The thick, white, adherent patches are sharply demarcated and cannot be denuded from the tongue.

Small, pinhead-sized, yellow papules on the buccal mucous membrane are usually *Fordyce's spots* or *granules*. Fordyce's spots are normal, prominent, ectopic sebaceous glands commonly seen on the lips or buccal mucosa near the exit of the parotid duct and are probably the most common lesions in the mouth. Figure 12-18 depicts Fordyce's spots on the buccal mucosa. Ectopic sebaceous glands can also be found on the shaft of the penis (see Fig. 18-11) and on the labia (see Fig. 19-13).

Figure 12-19 shows angiokeratomas of the buccal mucosa, or *angiokeratoma corporis diffusum*, in a patient with *Fabry's disease*. Figure 18-18 depicts angiokeratomas on the scrotum of the same patient.

Inspect the Gingivae

Normal gingivae are stippled, pink, and firm. Does the gingival tissue completely occupy the interdental space? Are the roots of the teeth visible, indicating recession of the periodontal tissue? Is there pus or blood along the gingival margin? Are the gingivae swollen? Is there

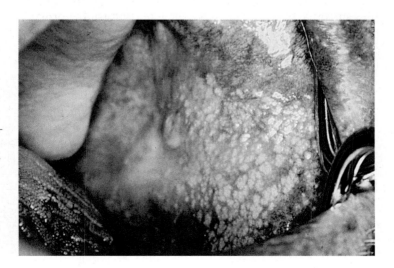

Figure 12–18 Fordyce's spots (granules) on the buccal mucosa.

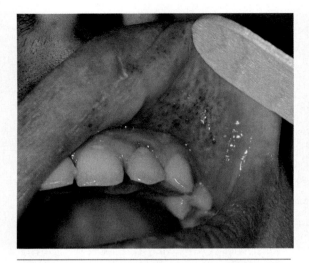

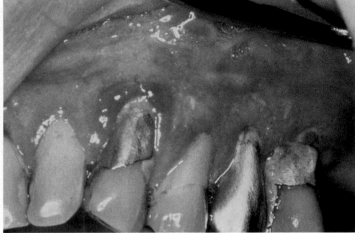

Figure 12–19 Angiokeratomas of the buccal mucosa.   **Figure 12–20** Erythroplakia of the gingiva (*right*).

evidence of bleeding? Is gingival inflammation present? Is abnormal coloration present? *Erythroplakia* is an area of mucous membrane on which there are granular, erythematous papules that bleed. Erythroplakia has a greater potential for malignancy than does leukoplakia. Figure 12-20 shows the mouth of a patient with erythroplakia of the gingiva (on the right) and inflammatory gingivitis (on the left).

There are many causes of *gingival hyperplasia*, including heredity, hormonal imbalances of puberty and pregnancy, medications, and leukemia. Gingival hyperplasia is common in patients taking phenytoin (Dilantin), an antiepilepsy medication, and in those taking nifedipine, a calcium channel blocker. It has been estimated that gingival hyperplasia develops in 30% to 50% of all patients taking phenytoin. The hyperplastic gingival changes of hormonal imbalances usually recede once the hormones have returned to their normal, lower levels. Figure 12-21 depicts marked gingival hyperplasia in a patient who was taking phenytoin. Dense leukemic infiltration of the gingiva is commonly seen in acute monocytic and acute monomyelocytic leukemia. Figure 12-22 shows gingival enlargement and bleeding caused by acute monomyelocytic leukemic infiltration.

Inspect the Teeth

There are 32 teeth in the full adult dentition. Is the dentition appropriate for the patient's age? The teeth should be inspected for caries and malocclusion. Are the teeth clean, especially around the gum line? Is there discoloration of the teeth? Is there tooth loss? Inspection of the teeth often provides insight into the patient's attitude toward general hygiene.

Are the teeth aligned properly? Ask the patient to bite normally while you retract the buccal mucosa with a tongue depressor. How many teeth bear force on mastication? Repeat this inspection on the other side. Do the maxillary teeth overlap the mandibular ones, and are they in contact with them? If so, the bite is probably normal.

If the patient is wearing dental appliances such as dentures or bridges, he or she should remove them for a complete evaluation.

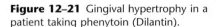

Figure 12–21 Gingival hypertrophy in a patient taking phenytoin (Dilantin).

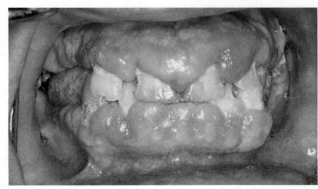

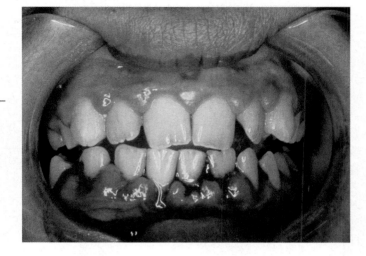

Figure 12–22 Gingival hypertrophy in a patient with acute monomyelocytic leukemia. Note the bleeding gingivae.

Inspect the Tongue

Inspect the mucosa, and note any masses or ulceration. Is the tongue moist? Ask the patient to stick out the tongue. A neuromuscular weakness may be present if the tongue cannot protrude in the midline or move rapidly in all directions. Are there any mass lesions on the sides or undersurface of the tongue? Ask the patient to lift the tongue to the roof of the mouth so that the inferior aspect of the tongue can be inspected. In older individuals, the large veins on the ventral aspect of the tongue may be tortuous. These varicosities never bleed spontaneously and have no clinical significance. Figure 12-23 shows a patient with sublingual varices. Figure 12-24 shows a patient with a benign lipoma of the tongue.

A *geographic tongue* is a benign condition in which the dorsum of the tongue has smooth, localized red areas, denuded of filiform papillae, surrounded by well-defined, raised yellowish-white margins and normal filiform papillae. These areas together give the tongue a maplike appearance. The appearance of the tongue gradually changes as the depapillated areas heal and new areas of depapillation occur. A *black hairy tongue* is another benign condition in which the filiform papillae on the dorsum of the tongue are greatly elongated; these enlarged, "hairy" papillae become pigmented with a brownish black color caused by staining from food or tobacco or proliferating chromogenic microorganisms. This condition, more commonly seen in men, may be a sequela to antibiotic therapy. A *scrotal*, or *fissured, tongue* is another normal variant; approximately 5% of the population has fissures in the tongue. The fissures first develop in late childhood and become deeper with age. The fissure pattern is quite variable. Food debris may collect in the fissures, causing inflammation, but the condition is otherwise benign. Halitosis may be a problem. Figure 12-25 shows these three normal tongue variants.

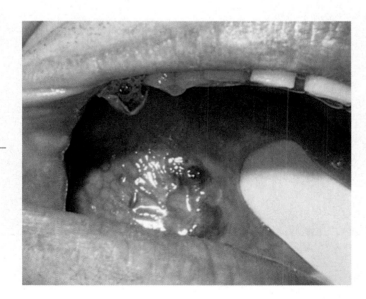

Figure 12–23 Sublingual varices of the tongue.

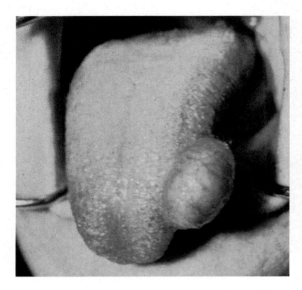

Figure 12–24 Benign lipoma of the tongue.

Is *candidiasis* present? Candidiasis, also known as *moniliasis* or *thrush*, is an opportunistic mycotic infection. It frequently involves the oral cavity, gastrointestinal tract, perineum, or vagina. The lesions appear as white, loosely adherent membranes, beneath which the mucosa is fiery red. Oral candidiasis is the most common cause of white lesions in the mouth. It is uncommon in healthy individuals who have not been receiving broad-spectrum antibiotic or steroid-based therapies. The presence of thrush in such a patient may be an initial manifestation of acquired immunodeficiency syndrome (AIDS). Candidiasis is the most common oral infection in patients with AIDS. The tongue of a patient with AIDS and oral candidiasis is pictured in Figure 12-26.

Is leukoplakia present? One form of leukoplakia, termed *oral hairy leukoplakia*, is associated with the subsequent development of AIDS. These raised white lesions appear corrugated, or "hairy," and range in size from a few millimeters to 2 to 3 cm. They are most commonly found on the lateral margins of the tongue but may also be seen on the buccal mucosa. In the absence of other causes of immunosuppression, oral hairy leukoplakia is diagnostic of HIV infection. It is seen in more than 40% of patients with HIV infection. The tongue of a patient with AIDS with oral hairy leukoplakia is pictured in Figure 12-27.

Look for indurated ulcers or masses in the middle, lateral aspect of the tongue. This is the most common site for intraoral squamous cell carcinoma. Figure 12-28 depicts squamous cell carcinoma of the tongue in the classic location.

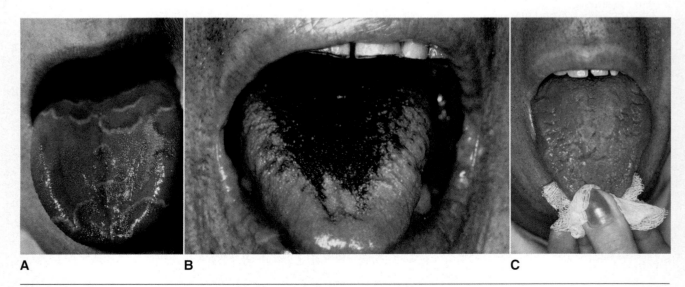

A   **B**   **C**

Figure 12–25 Three normal tongue variants. *A,* Geographic tongue. *B,* Black hairy tongue. *C,* Scrotal, or fissured, tongue.

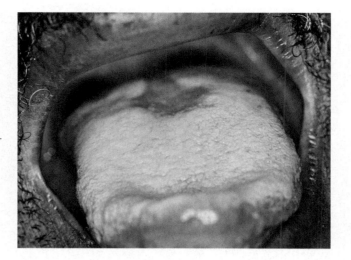

Figure 12–26 Oral candidiasis.

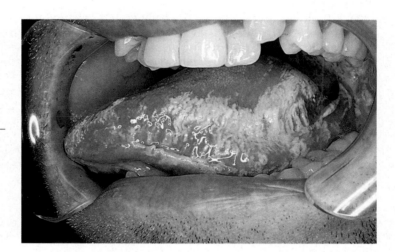

Figure 12–27 Oral hairy leukoplakia.

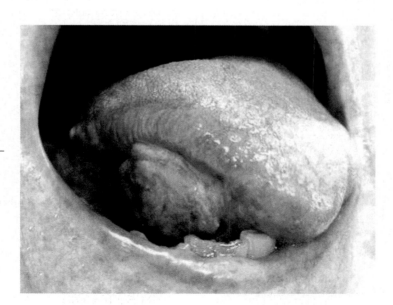

Figure 12–28 Squamous cell carcinoma of the tongue.

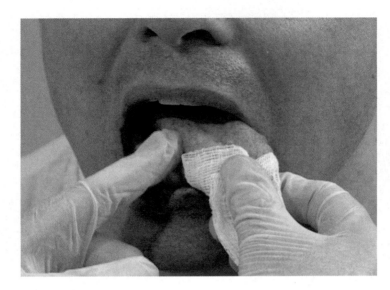

Figure 12–29 Palpation of the tongue.

Palpate the Tongue

After a thorough inspection of the tongue, the examination proceeds with palpation. The patient sticks out the tongue onto a piece of gauze. The tongue is then held by the examiner's right hand as the sides of the tongue are inspected and palpated with the left hand. This is illustrated in Figure 12-29. To examine the other side of the tongue, the examiner reverses hands.

The anterior two thirds and the lateral margins of the tongue can be evaluated without stimulating the gag reflex. The examiner should palpate the lateral margins of the tongue because more than 85% of all lingual cancers arise in this area. All white lesions should be palpated. Is there evidence of induration (hardness)? Induration or ulceration is strongly suggestive of carcinoma. After the tongue is palpated, it is unwrapped, and the gauze is discarded. Any intraoral lesion, ulcer, or mass present for more than 2 weeks should be examined through biopsy and evaluated by an oral pathologist.

Inspect the Floor of the Mouth

The patient is asked to lift the tongue to the roof of the mouth, and the examiner inspects the floor of the mouth. Is there edema on the floor of the mouth? The opening of the submandibular gland, Wharton's duct, should be observed. The examiner should look for leukoplakia, erythroplakia, or a mass.

A *ranula* is a large mucous retention cyst on the floor of the mouth in association with submandibular and sublingual glands. The lesion is unilateral, painless, and bluish. It is lateral to the frenulum and is typically larger than a mucocele. As a ranula increases in size, there may be a reduction in tongue movement and difficulty in speech and swallowing. An example of a ranula is pictured in Figure 12-30.

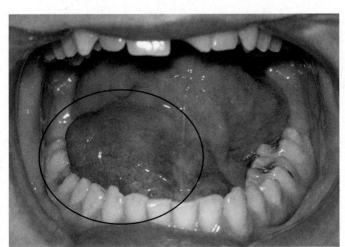

Figure 12–30 Ranula.

Palpate the Floor of the Mouth

The floor of the mouth should be examined by bimanual palpation. This is performed by placing one finger under the tongue and another finger under the chin to assess any thickening or masses. Whenever palpating in a patient's mouth, the examiner should hold the patient's cheeks, as shown in Figure 12-31. This is done as a precaution in case the patient suddenly tries to speak or bite down on the examiner's finger. The examiner's right index finger is placed under the tongue; the left thumb and third finger are pushing the patient's cheeks inward to prevent biting; and the left index finger palpates under the patient's chin.

Inspect the Hard and Soft Palates

Inspect the rugae and vault shape of the palates. Also inspect the palates for ulceration and masses. Masses are usually minor salivary gland tumors, mostly malignant. Are any white plaques present? Is the soft palate edematous? Is the uvula in the midline?

Is the palate intact? Figure 12-32 shows a severe cleft palate. Clefts of the palate and lips are distinct entities but are closely related embryologically, functionally, and genetically. The incidence of an isolated cleft palate is 1 per 1000 births. Clefts of the palate vary widely in size and shape. They can extend from the soft palate, to the hard palate, and to the incisive foramen. Recurrent otitis media, hearing loss, and speech defects are frequent complications.

In patients with impaired immunity, or in those whose microbial flora has been altered by antibiotics, *Candida albicans*, a normal commensal organism of the gastrointestinal tract, can

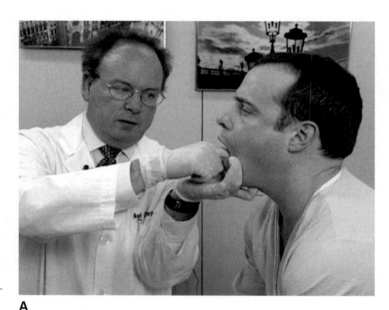

Figure 12–31 *A* and *B*, Technique for palpating the floor of the mouth.

A

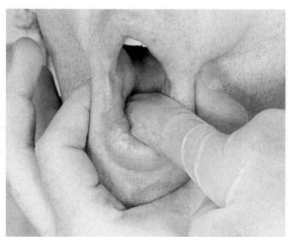

B

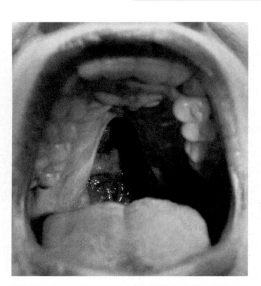

Figure 12–32 Cleft palate.

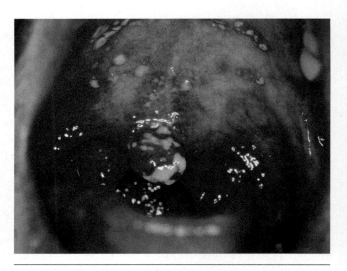

Figure 12–33 Pseudomembranous candidiasis.

become highly invasive, as seen in Figure 12-33. The patient, who has AIDS, has *pseudomembranous candidiasis* of the palate and uvula.

Are *petechiae* present? Petechiae are commonly seen in association with infective endocarditis, leukemia, oral sex, and viral infections such as infectious mononucleosis. Fellatio can result in palatal petechiae, characteristically at the junction of the hard and soft palates, as pictured in Figure 12-34.

A common finding is a *torus palatinus*, which is a discrete, hard, lobulated swelling in the midline of the posterior portion of the hard palate. This benign lesion is an overgrowth of the palatine bone. It is painless and asymptomatic and occurs twice as often in women as in men. It may remain undetected until it interferes with the fit of a denture. More than 20% of the population have at least a small torus palatinus. Figure 12-35 shows tori palatini in two patients. Not uncommonly, individuals may have multiple tori palatini; Figure 12-36 shows a patient with three tori palatini. A *torus mandibularis* is a hard, bony, often bilateral swelling that protrudes from the lingual surface of the mandible at the level of the premolar teeth. It is much less common than a torus palatinus. About 5% to 10% of the population have a torus mandibularis; however, one fifth of mandibular tori are unilateral. Figure 12-37 shows bilateral mandibular tori in two patients.

Figure 12-38 shows a patient with early invasive *erythroplakia* (red plaque) of the palate.

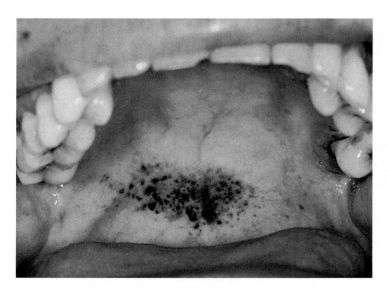

Figure 12–34 Palatal petechiae.

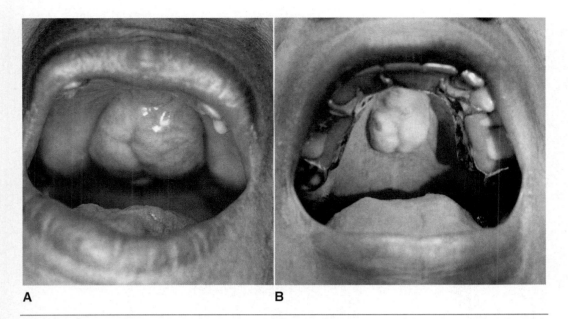

A   **B**

Figure 12–35 *A* and *B,* Torus palatinus.

Inspect the Salivary Glands

The ductal orifices of the parotid gland and the submandibular gland should be visualized. The condition of the papillae should be inspected. Is there a flow of saliva? This is best evaluated by drying the papilla with a cotton applicator and observing the flow of saliva produced by exerting external pressure on the gland itself.

The salivary glands are usually not visible. Careful observation of the face determines any asymmetry that is due to unilateral salivary gland enlargement. Obstruction to flow or infiltration of the gland results in glandular enlargement. Figure 12-39 illustrates a patient with left parotid enlargement as a result of obstruction to flow by a stone.

Palpate the parotid and submandibular glands. Determine the consistency of each gland. Is tenderness present?

Inspect the Twelfth Cranial Nerve

Ask the patient to stick out the tongue. Does the tongue deviate to one side? A *hypoglossal*, or 12th cranial, nerve palsy does not allow the lingual muscles on the affected side to contract normally. Consequently, the contralateral side "pushes" the tongue to the side of the lesion.

Figure 12–36 Multiple tori palatini.

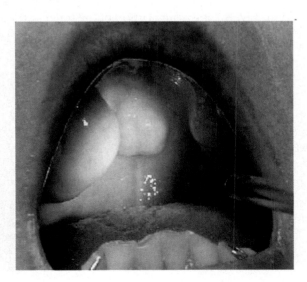

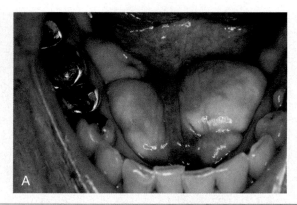

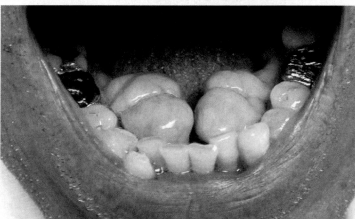

Figure 12–37 *A* and *B*, Bilateral mandibular tori.

The Pharynx

Inspect the Pharynx

Examination of the pharynx is limited to inspection. To visualize the palate and oropharynx adequately, the examiner usually must use a tongue depressor. The patient is asked to open the mouth widely, stick out the tongue, and breathe slowly through the mouth. On occasion, leaving the tongue in the floor of the mouth provides better visibility. The examiner should hold the tongue depressor in the right hand and a light source in the left. The tongue blade should be placed on the middle third of the tongue. The tongue is depressed and scooped forward behind the front teeth. The examiner should be careful not to press the patient's lower lip or tongue against the teeth with the tongue depressor. If the tongue depressor is placed too anteriorly, the posterior portion of the tongue will mound up, making inspection of the pharynx difficult; if placed too posteriorly, the gag reflex may be stimulated.

Is infection present? Is candidiasis present?

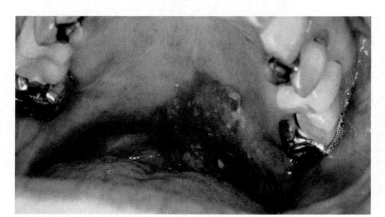

Figure 12–38 Erythroplakia of the palate.

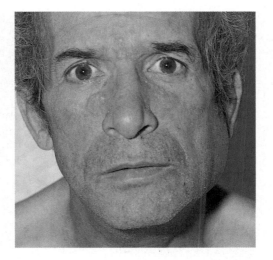

Figure 12–39 Left parotid enlargement.

An accessory for the oto-ophthalmoscope handle is a light source that holds the tongue depressor and makes the examination easier. Both techniques of holding the tongue depressor are demonstrated in Figure 12-40.

Inspect the Tonsils
Evaluate tonsillar size. Tonsillar enlargement results from infection or tumor. In chronic tonsillar infection, the deep tonsillar crypts may contain cheeselike debris. Figure 12-41 shows enormous tonsillar enlargement, known as ''kissing tonsils.'' Figure 12-42 depicts massive tonsillar enlargement in a patient with infectious mononucleosis; the cheeselike deposit in the tonsillar crypts is visible.

Is a *pseudomembranous patch* or *membrane* present over the tonsils? A membrane is associated with acute tonsillitis, infectious mononucleosis, and diphtheria. Figure 12-43 shows the oral cavity, characterized by erythema and a gray, membranous exudate, in a patient with diphtheria.

Inspect the Posterior Pharyngeal Wall
Is there a discharge, mass, ulceration, or infection present? Ask the patient to say, ''Aahhh,'' as you observe for soft palate elevation.

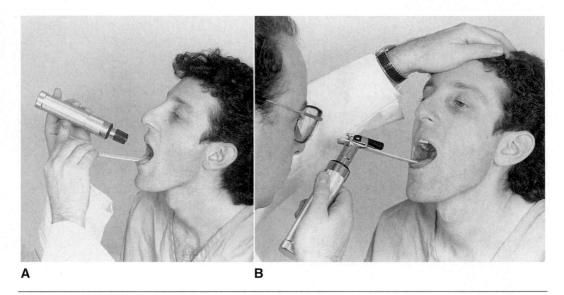

A   **B**

Figure 12–40 *A,* Use of the tongue depressor to inspect the pharynx. *B,* Use of the tongue depressor attachment to inspect the oral pharynx.

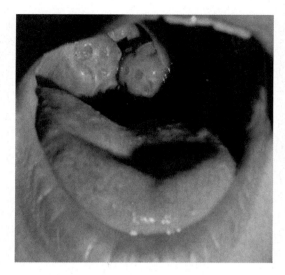

Figure 12–41 "Kissing tonsils." Notice the tonsillar crypts.

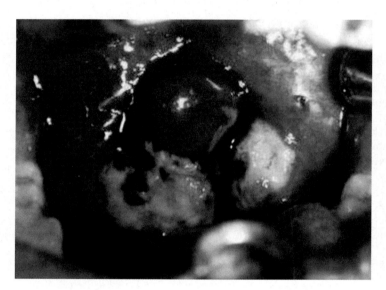

Figure 12–42 Infectious mononucleosis. Note the massive tonsillar enlargement and the cheeselike substance in the crypts.

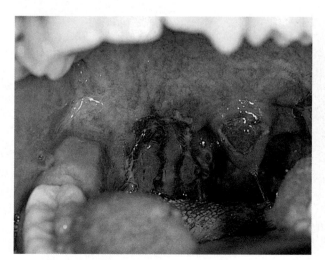

Figure 12–43 Pseudomembrane secondary to diphtheria.

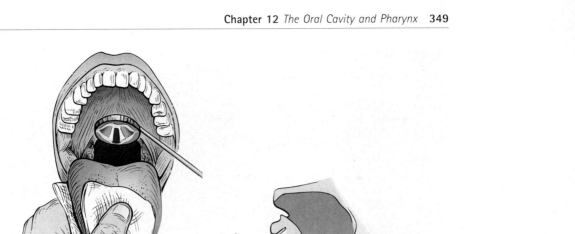

Figure 12–44 Mirror laryngoscopy. *A,* Proper technique for holding the tongue and placement of the mirror. *B,* Cross-sectional view through the pharynx, illustrating placement of the mirror. *C,* Mirror reflection of the vocal cords.

Inspect the Gag Reflex

At the end of the inspection, tell the patient that you are now going to test the gag reflex. The tip of the tongue depressor should gently touch the posterior surface of the tongue or the posterior pharyngeal wall. The gag reflex should follow rapidly.

The Larynx

Using the Laryngeal Mirror

The tongue is held while a small, slightly warmed mirror is introduced into the mouth. The mirror should not be excessively warm and should avoid contact with the tongue. The patient is asked to breathe normally through the mouth. The mirror should be pushed upward against the uvula and positioned in the oropharynx. A beam of light can then be reflected off the mirror onto the internal laryngeal structures. This technique is demonstrated in Figure 12-44.

Although the examination of the larynx is important, indirect laryngoscopy is usually performed only by specialists. Any patient exhibiting symptoms of laryngeal disease should certainly be evaluated further.

Clinicopathologic Correlations

Lesions of the oral cavity are common. The most common acute oral ulcer is the *traumatic ulcer;* the *aphthous ulcer,* or *canker sore,* is the next most common. Traumatic and aphthous lesions vary widely in size, although the latter are usually less than 1 cm in diameter. Both are relatively superficial with raised borders. Aphthous ulcers are usually located on the loose buccal or labial mucosa, whereas traumatic ulcers can occur anywhere. Despite the small size of many of these ulcers, they can be extremely painful. In addition, aphthous

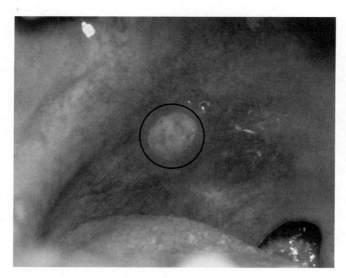

Figure 12–45 Solitary aphthous ulcer.

ulcers may recur in many patients. Both types of ulcers usually heal within 2 to 3 weeks without scarring. A *solitary*, or *giant*, aphthous ulcer of the palate is shown in Figure 12-45. The patient has *periadenitis mucosa necrotica recurrens*, also known as major aphthous ulcer. These lesions are larger than multiple aphthous ulcers and start as submucosal lesions that break down to form ulcers that may persist for many weeks before healing by secondary intention. Any part of the oropharynx may be affected, but the tonsils and soft palate are the most common sites.

Acute multiple ulcers that are preceded by or associated with vesicles may have infective or immunologic causes. Primary herpes simplex, herpes zoster, coxsackievirus, and HIV are causative infective agents. Allergic stomatitis, benign mucous membrane pemphigoid, pemphigus vulgaris, Behçet's disease, and erythema multiforme are common immunologic causes. Radiation therapy or chemotherapy may predispose an individual to the development of acute multiple ulcers.

Benign mucous membrane pemphigoid, or *cicatricial pemphigoid*, is a chronic mucocutaneous bullous disease of elderly people in which the lesions are commonly limited to the oral cavity and conjunctiva. Subepidermal bullae, up to 2 cm in size, and autoantibodies to the basement membrane are present; erosion may be present as well. Skin involvement is rare and usually not severe. Nikolsky's sign, in which the bulla or external layer of mucous membrane or skin is easily separated from the underlying tissue by slight friction, is usually positive. Figure 12-46 depictds benign mucous membrane pemphigoid. Note the denudation of the gingivae. Figure 12-47 depicts cicatricial pemphigoid. The most common oral finding is patchy, desquamative gingivitis, as seen in this figure.

Pemphigus vulgaris affects the oral cavity in 75% of cases. Autoantibodies to the epithelial intercellular substance are present. Nikolsky's sign is negative. The lesions are almost

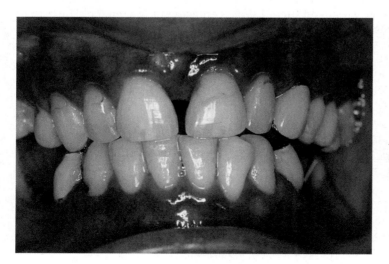

Figure 12–46 Benign mucous membrane pemphigoid.

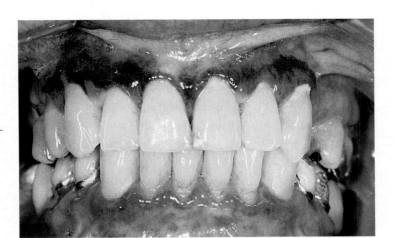

Figure 12–47 Cicatricial pemphigoid.

always painful. Figure 12-48 depicts pemphigus vulgaris; the desquamative gingivitis is visible. Another case of pemphigus vulgaris is seen in Figure 12-49. Note the large and confluent ulcerations, which were painful, on the soft palate.

Large chronic single ulcers may result from fungal infections such as aspergillosis or histoplasmosis. Infections by herpes simplex virus, cytomegalovirus, *Mycobacterium* organisms (which cause tuberculosis), and *Treponema pallidum* (which causes syphilis) are also well-known causes of this type of ulcer. Immunologic disorders such as pemphigus, systemic lupus erythematosus, bullous pemphigoid, and erosive lichen planus are often the cause of chronic multiple ulcers.

Cancer of the oral cavity is common. *Carcinoma of the lip* accounts for 30% of all cancers in this area and approximately 0.6% of all cancers. Most of these malignant tumors are squamous cell carcinomas. The lower lip is the site most frequently involved (95%). The patients are usually 50 to 70 years of age, with a strong male predominance (95%). Squamous cell carcinoma is characterized by a hard, infiltrative, usually painless ulcer. The risk factors that predispose to squamous cell carcinoma of the oral cavity are the same as for leukoplakia: smoking, spirits (alcohol), spices, syphilis, and spikes (ill-fitting dentures)—the "five Ss." Figure 12-50 depicts a squamous cell carcinoma of the lower lip.

As mentioned earlier in this chapter, risk factors for oral cancers include tobacco use, alcohol consumption, and chewing betel nuts. Betel nuts are actually seeds of the betel palm (*Areca catechu*). Betel nut chewing is a tradition that dates back thousands of years. The nuts are chewed for their mildly euphoric stimulant effect, attributed to the presence of relatively high levels of psychoactive alkaloids. Chewing betel nuts increases the capacity to work, creates a warm sensation in the body, heightens alertness, and increases sweating. Although betel nut chewing is a part of many Asian and Pacific cultures and often takes place at ceremonies and gatherings, betel nuts are often sold at roadside booths decorated with multicolored neon lights for taxi and truck drivers to keep them awake. The International Agency for Research on Cancer (IARC) regards the betel nut as a known human carcinogen. In Asian

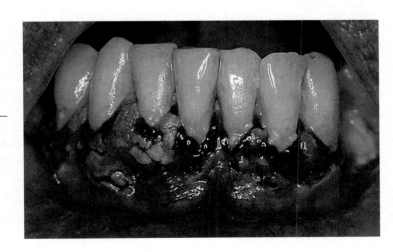

Figure 12–48 Pemphigus vulgaris.

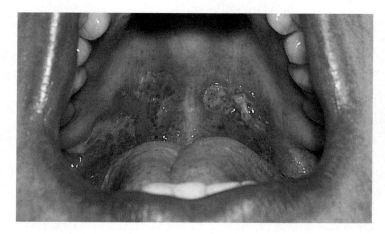

Figure 12–49 Pemphigus vulgaris.

countries and communities where betel nuts are consumed extensively, oral cancer accounts for up to 50% of all malignant cancers. Betel nut chewers in Taiwan were found to have a risk of acquiring oral cancer 28 times higher than that of nonusers, and people who chew betel nuts, smoke cigarettes, and drink alcohol are 123 times more likely to develop oral cancer. In 2006 in Taiwan, it was estimated that the government spent at least NT$5 billion (US$151 million) to cover medical expenses for betel nut–related diseases. Figure 12-51*A* shows the mouth of a patient from Taiwan with a long-standing habit of betel nut chewing; note the red stain on his teeth. Figure 12-51*B* shows a betel nut wrapped in its leaf.

In addition to these risk factors, biologic factors include viruses and fungi, which have been found in association with oral cancers. The human papillomavirus (HPV), particularly strains HPV16 and HPV18, has been implicated in some oral cancers. HPV is a common sexually transmitted virus that infects about 40 million Americans. There are more than 80 strains of HPV, most thought to be harmless. However, 1% of persons infected have the HPV16 strain, which is a causative agent in cervical cancer and now is linked to oral cancer as well. Another possible risk factor for oral cancer is lichen planus, an inflammatory disease of the oral soft tissues.

Lingual carcinoma is often easily missed because, in its early stages, it is usually painless. In 2007, it was estimated that there were 9800 new cases of lingual cancer. It occurs on the lateral aspects of the tongue or on its undersurface; there is commonly extension onto the tongue from a lesion on the floor of the mouth. Figure 12-52 depicts a carcinoma of the right lateral border of the tongue. Figure 12-53 depicts squamous cell carcinoma of the right lateral border of the tongue in another patient, with extension on the floor of the mouth.

Carcinoma of the floor of the mouth accounts for 10% to 15% of all oral cancers and is the most common site of oral cancer in African Americans. In 2007, it was estimated that there were 10,660 new cases of floor of the mouth cancer. It occurs primarily in men at an average age of 65 years. Approximately 20% of patients with carcinoma of the floor of the mouth have a

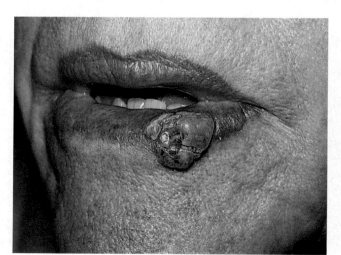

Figure 12–50 Squamous cell carcinoma of the lower lip.

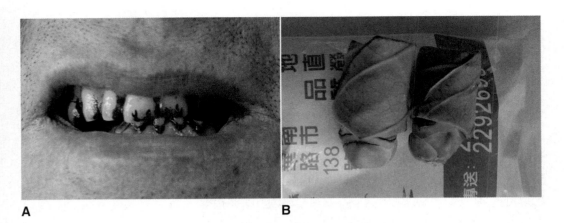

A   **B**

Figure 12–51 *A,* Red staining of teeth in a betel nut user. *B,* Betel nut wrapped in its leaf.

Figure 12–52 Squamous cell carcinoma of the tongue.

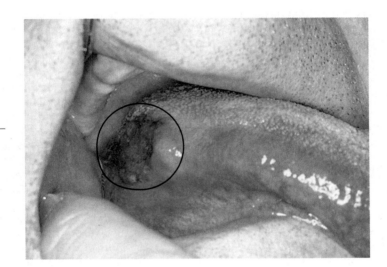

Figure 12–53 Squamous cell carcinoma of the tongue and floor of the mouth.

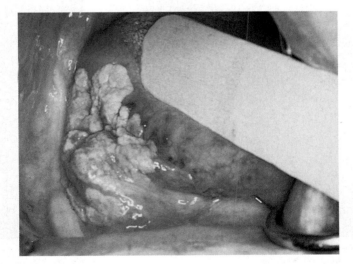

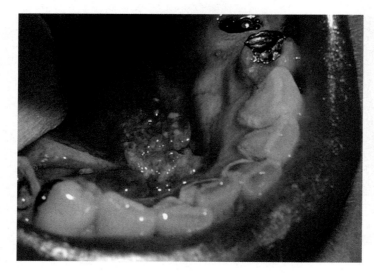

Figure 12–54 Squamous cell carcinoma of the floor of the mouth.

second primary tumor. It is particularly important to examine the area behind the last molar tooth and the associated floor of the mouth and base of the tongue. Figure 12-54 shows a squamous cell carcinoma of the floor of the mouth.

Salivary gland neoplasms are not uncommon. They occur with an annual incidence of 6 per 100,000 individuals. More than 70% occur in the parotid gland. There are more than 50 types of salivary gland tumors. The most common salivary gland tumor (65%) is the pleomorphic adenoma, and 20% of these mixed-cell tumors are malignant. Tumors of the submandibular gland are much less frequent, but 40% are malignant. Sublingual gland tumors are rare but usually malignant.

Herpetic gingivostomatitis is infection of the gums and oral mucosa by herpes simplex virus. Small vesicles form on the oral mucous membrane and rapidly break down into painful ulcers on an intensely erythematous base. Figure 12-55 depicts herpetic gingivostomatitis; the multiple erosions and marginal gingivitis are apparent. Figure 12-56 shows herpetic lesions on the palate with ulceration.

Acute necrotizing gingivostomatitis (also known as *ulcerative gingivostomatitis* or *Vincent's gingivitis*), is a severe, noncommunicable disease of young adults resulting from infection by *Fusobacterium nucleatum* or *Borrelia vincentii*. Most cases occur suddenly in the spring or autumn. The patients, commonly men with poor oral hygiene, present with gingival bleeding,

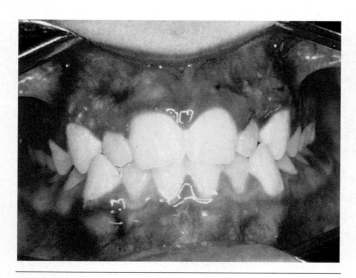

Figure 12–55 Herpetic gingivostomatitis.

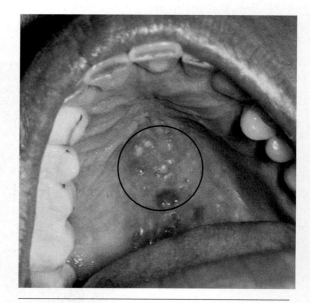

Figure 12–56 Herpetic lesions on the palate.

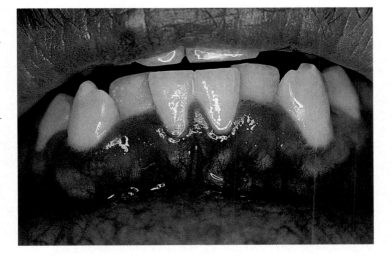

Figure 12–57 Acute necrotizing gingivostomatitis.

alteration of taste, gingival pain, malaise, fever, and halitosis. As the disease progresses, a whitish pseudomembrane develops along the gingival margins, with ulceration and blunting of the interdental papillae. Acute necrotizing gingivitis, pictured in Figure 12-57, may be an early feature of HIV infection.

On August 6, 2008, the Centers for Disease Control and Prevention (CDC) released a new estimate of the annual number of new HIV infections (HIV incidence) in the United States, revealing that the HIV epidemic is worse than previously thought. That estimate indicated that approximately 56,300 people were newly infected with HIV in the United States in 2006, which is higher than the CDC's previous estimate of 40,000. The new estimate also confirmed that gay and bisexual men of all races, African Americans, and Hispanics/Latinos were most heavily affected by HIV. Although first observed in men having sex with men, HIV is now spreading among the heterosexual population. These cases are related to the use of illegal drugs and contaminated needles, prostitution, and unprotected sex. It has been estimated that more than 90% of patients infected with HIV will have at least one oral manifestation of their disease. It appears that as further immunologic impairment develops, the risk of oral lesions increases. It has also been shown that the oral manifestations can be used as a marker of immune compromise, which is independent of the CD4$^+$ T-lymphocyte count. If left untreated, the oral lesions may interfere with chewing, swallowing, and talking. Many patients have such severe pain that they reduce their oral intake, which results in additional weight loss, malnutrition, and further wasting.

A common oral manifestation of HIV infection is *angular cheilitis*, also known as *perlèche*. This painful condition is characterized by macerated, fissured, eroded, encrusted, whitish (occasionally erythematous) lesions in the corners of the mouth. Accumulations of saliva gather in the skin folds and are subsequently colonized by yeast organisms such as *C. albicans*. Angular cheilitis may be associated with intraoral candidiasis. Angular cheilitis may also

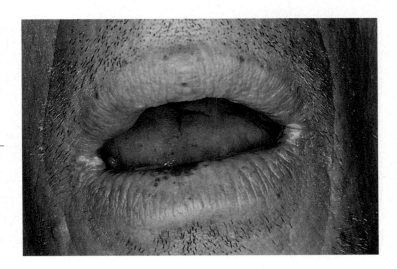

Figure 12–58 Angular cheilitis.

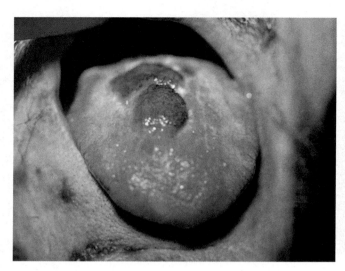

Figure 12–59 Kaposi's sarcoma of the tongue.

develop in patients with normal immunity who wear ill-fitting dentures or wear dentures during the night. An example of angular cheilitis is pictured in Figure 12-58.

Figures 12-26 and 12-33 show patients with *oral candidiasis*, another extremely common condition associated with HIV infection. Oral candidiasis is characterized by chronic severe pain in the throat that worsens on swallowing or eating. The curdlike white plaques are soft and friable and can easily be wiped off, leaving an area of intensely erythematous mucosa.

Figure 12-27 shows a patient with *oral hairy leukoplakia*. As mentioned previously, this lesion is seen most frequently either unilaterally or bilaterally on the lateral margins of the tongue. The lesion is white, does not rub off, and occasionally occurs elsewhere in the mouth and oropharynx. Although not correlated with the stage of HIV infection, oral hairy leukoplakia may be the first sign of infection. It is seen most commonly in gay and bisexual men infected with HIV. It has been suggested that the Epstein-Barr virus may be a cofactor in the development of oral hairy leukoplakia. The finding of oral hairy leukoplakia mandates HIV testing.

As discussed in Chapter 8, The Skin, the oral lesions of Kaposi's sarcoma are common. Figure 8-93 shows some of the typical oral lesions. Lesions of Kaposi's sarcoma of the tongue (Fig. 12-59) and the hard palate (Fig. 12-60) are frequently found in patients with AIDS.

Table 12-1 summarizes the important signs and symptoms of some of the more common oral lesions. Table 12-2 reviews the most common oral lesions seen during the stages of HIV infection. Table 24-5 lists the chronology of dentition.

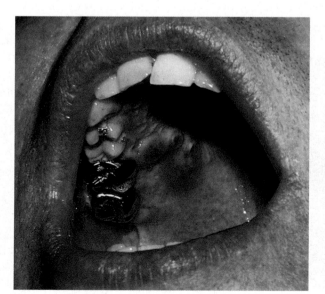

Figure 12–60 Kaposi's sarcoma of the hard palate.

Table 12–1 Symptoms and Signs of Oral Lesions

Lesion	Symptoms	Signs	Other Information
Aphthous ulcer (canker sore; see Fig. 12-45)	Painful, recurrent white sore with red border on lips, inner side of cheeks, tip and sides of tongue, or palate	Single lesion 0.5-2 cm in diameter that is first maculopapular but then ulcerates and has an area of erythema at its border; lesions usually on movable mucosal areas	Sixty percent of population have periodic canker sores lasting up to 2 weeks; cause is unknown
Herpetic ulcer (cold sore; fever blister; see Figs. 12-10, 12-55, 12-56)	Painful, recurrent sores on the lips	Multiple vesicles, papules, or ulcers on the mucocutaneous junction, hard palate, or gingivae; as the bullae break, crusting occurs	*Primary* herpetic infection in children: multiple lesions in clusters on fixed mucous membranes; small, discrete, whitish vesicles before ulceration; ulcers about 1 mm in diameter, which may coalesce; tender lymphadenopathy, fever, and malaise present *Recurrent* form, common in adults: lip lesions *Both* forms: self-limited illness, 1-2 weeks
Chancre	Painless sore on lips or tongue lasting 2 weeks to 3 months	Single ulcerated lesion with indurated border; lesion without central necrotic material; tender lymphadenitis may be present	Examiner should look for genital lesions (see Figs. 18-13 and 19-33)
Squamous cell carcinoma (see Figs. 12-28, 12-50, and 12-52 to 12-54)	Ulcerated sore of the lips, floor of mouth, or tongue (especially lateral borders); erythroplakia of floor of mouth, soft palate	Single indurated lesion with indurated and raised border; often in an area of leukoplakia or erythroplakia; absence of necrotic material in crater; base often erythematous; speech alterations may result if lesion is large; painless lymphadenopathy may be present	Frequently in alcoholic patients or smokers
Erythema multiforme	Sudden onset of multiple painful ulcers in mouth of lips	Hemorrhagic areas of ulceration with erythematous bases, often with pseudomembrane; lesions start as bullae; skin involvement common (target lesions)	Many precipitating factors include drug reactions, herpesvirus infections, endocrine changes, and an underlying malignancy; most common in winter and spring in young adults; frequently recurring
Denture hyperplasia	Painless excess tissue at border of denture	Spongy, redundant, often erythematous tissue with impression of edge of denture; frequently seen on anterior maxillary mucosa	
Candidiasis (moniliasis; thrush; see Figs. 12-26, 12-33)	Burning sensation in areas of tongue, inside of cheek, or throat	Whitish pseudomembrane, resembling milk curd, that can be peeled off, leaving a raw, erythematous area that may bleed; erythematous variant is secondary to broad-spectrum antibiotics	Often seen in individuals who are chronically debilitated, patients who are immunosuppressed, or patients receiving long-term antibiotic therapy; commonly seen in persons with AIDS

Continued

Table 12–1 Symptoms and Signs of Oral Lesions—cont'd

Lesion	Symptoms	Signs	Other Information
Erythroplakia (see Figs. 12-20, 12-38)	Painless red area on inside of cheek, tongue, or floor of mouth	Granular, erythematous papules that bleed	High potential for malignancy
Leukoplakia (see Figs. 12-16, 12-17, 12-27)	Painless white area on inside of cheek, tongue, lower lip, or floor of mouth	Hyperkeratinized, whitish lesion that cannot be scraped off; looks similar to flaking white paint; often speckled with reddish areas; associated adenopathy may indicate malignant changes of lesion	Patients are usually men over 40 years of age; linked to smoking, AIDS, alcoholism, and chewing tobacco
Lipoma (see Fig. 12-24)	Slow-growing, painless mass on inner surface of cheek or tongue	Yellowish, nontender, soft mass; freely mobile	
Lichen planus (see Fig. 12-15)	Usually no symptoms; erosive form causes painful, burning sores of inner side of cheek or tongue	White lesions on buccal mucosa bilaterally in the form of reticulated papules in lacelike pattern; erosive form appears as hemorrhagic ulcerated lesion with possible white areas or bullae; pseudomembrane may be present over lesion	Nonerosive form is a common cause of white lesions in the mouth; skin involvement in 10%-35% of affected patients and more frequently seen in patients with emotional stress
Traumatic ulcer	Pain in an area of a sore; short duration (1-2 weeks)	Single lesion with raised erythema at its border; center often with necrotic debris; occasionally purulent; mild lymphadenitis may be present	Patient frequently know the cause (e.g., biting cheek while eating)
Mucocele (see Fig. 12-13)	Intermittent, painless swelling of the lower lip or inside of cheek; slightly bluish; occasionally ruptures	Dome-shaped, 1-2 cm in diameter, freely mobile cystic lesion	Related to trauma to ductal system of minor labial salivary glands
Black hairy tongue (see Fig. 12-25B)	Gagging sensation associated with "hairy" sensation of tongue; large brown or blackish painless lesion on top of tongue	Elongation of filiform papillae on the dorsum of tongue with a change in their color to almost black or brown	History of excessive antibiotic use, excessive use of mouthwash, poor oral hygiene, smoking, or alcohol use is common
Fordyce's spots (see Fig. 12-18)	None	Clusters of small, yellowish, raised lesions best seen on the buccal mucosa opposite the molar teeth	Common in older individuals; they are normal, hyperplastic sebaceous glands

AIDS, acquired immunodeficiency syndrome.

Table 12–2 Occurrence of Oral Lesions During the Stages of HIV Infection

Oral Lesion	Occurrence During Primary HIV Infection	Occurrence During Early HIV Disease*	Advanced HIV Disease†
Candidiasis (see Figs. 12-26, 12-33)	Common	Occasional	Very common
Oral hairy leukoplakia (see Fig. 12-27)	No	Occasional	Very common
Kaposi's sarcoma (see Figs. 8-93, 12-59, 12-60)	No	Rare	Very common
Linear gingival erythema	No	Common	Very common
Acute necrotizing gingivitis (see Fig. 12-57)	No	Rare	Common
Necrotizing stomatitis	No	No	Common
Herpes simplex–related (see Figs. 12-10, 12-55, 12-56)	No	Occasional	Common
Aphthous ulcers (see Fig. 12-45)	Common	Occasional	Very common

HIV, human immunodeficiency virus.
*CD4$^+$ count > 500 cells/mm^3.
†CD4$^+$ count < 200 cells/mm^3.
Adapted from Weinert M, Grimes RM, Lynch DP: Oral manifestations of HIV infection. Ann Intern Med 125:485, 1996.

Useful Vocabulary

Listed here are the specific roots that are important to understand the terminology related to diseases of the mouth and pharynx.

Root	Pertaining to	Example	Definition
arytenoid-	pitcher-shaped structure	**arytenoid**itis	Inflammation of the arytenoid cartilage
bucco-	cheek	**bucco**pharyngeal	Pertaining to the cheek and pharynx
cheil(o)-	lip	**cheil**itis	Inflammation of the lip
dent-	tooth	**dent**al	Pertaining to the teeth
gingiv-	gingiva(e)	**gingiv**ectomy	Surgical excision of diseased gingiva(e)
gloss(o)-	tongue	**glosso**plegia	Paralysis of the tongue
-labi-	lips	naso**labi**al	Pertaining to the nose and lip
leuko-	white	**leuko**plakia	White patch on mucous membrane; often premalignant

Continued

Useful Vocabulary—cont'd

linguo-	tongue	***linguo***papillitis	Painful ulcers around the papillae of the tongue
-plakia	patch	erythro***plakia***	Red patch on mucous membrane; often premalignant
ptyal-	saliva	***ptyal***ism	Excessive salivation
stoma-	mouth; opening	***stoma***titis	Inflammation of the mouth

Writing Up the Physical Examination

Listed here are examples of the write-up for the examinations of the oral cavity and pharynx.

● The lips appear normal. The mucosa of the oral cavity is red and without masses, leukoplakia, or other lesions. There is good dentition and good dental hygiene. The tongue is midline and does not deviate to either side. The tonsils are absent. The pharynx appears normal. The palate is normal, without ulcers or masses.

● There is a 1- to 2-cm, painful vesicular lesion at the mucocutaneous junction on the right side of the mouth. There is tonsillar hypertrophy with a purulent discharge in the crypts of both tonsils. There is bilateral anterior triangle lymphadenopathy, greater on the right. The remainder of the examination of the oral cavity is unremarkable.

● There is a whitish pseudomembrane over the hard and soft palates, as well as over the tongue. When it is lifted, its erythematous base is friable and bleeds. The rest of the mouth and throat appears normal.

● The lateral border of the tongue has an ulcerated, indurated lesion, 2 × 1 cm.

● The palate has a dome-shaped 3-cm mass to the right of midline. Biopsy is recommended.

Bibliography

Aronson AE: Clinical Voice Disorders: An Interdisciplinary Approach. New York, Thieme-Stratton, 1980.

Benjamin B, Bingham B, Hawke M, et al: A Color Atlas of Otorhinolaryngology. Philadelphia, JB Lippincott, 1995.

Bingham BJG, Hawke M, Kwok P, et al: Atlas of Clinical Otolaryngology. St. Louis, Mosby–Year Book, 1992.

Cancer Facts & Figures. Atlanta, American Cancer Society, 2007.

Centers for Disease Control: Subpopulation estimates from the HIV incidence surveillance system—United States, 2006. MMWR 57(36):985, 2008.

DeBoever EH, Loesche W: Assessing the contribution of anaerobic microflora of the tongue to oral malodor. J Am Dent Assoc 126:1384, 1995.

DevCan: Probability of developing or dying of cancer software, version 5.1. Statistical Research and Applications Branch, National Cancer Institute, 2003. Available at: *http://srab.cancer.gov/devcan*; accessed June 6, 2008.

Eisen D, Lynch DP: The Mouth: Diagnosis and Treatment. St. Louis, Mosby, 1998.

Gupta PC, Warnakulasuriya S: Global epidemiology of areca nut usage. Addict Biol 7:77, 2002.

Hall HI, Ruiguang S, Rhodes P, et al: Estimation of HIV incidence in the United States. JAMA 300:520, 2008.

Jemel A, Tiwari R, Murray T, et al: Cancer Statistics, 2004. CA Cancer J Clin 54:8, 2004.

Kirby AJ, Muñoz A, Detels R, et al: Thrush and fever as measures of immunocompetence in HIV-1–infected men. J Acquir Immune Defic Syndr 7:1242, 1994.

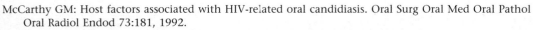

McCarthy GM: Host factors associated with HIV-related oral candidiasis. Oral Surg Oral Med Oral Pathol Oral Radiol Endod 73:181, 1992.

McIsaac WJ, Kellner JD, Aufricht P, et al: Empirical validation of guidelines for the management of pharyngitis in children and adults. JAMA 291:1587, 2004.

Moore PS, Chang Y: Detection of herpesvirus-like DNA sequences in Kaposi's sarcoma in patients with and without HIV infection. N Engl J Med 332:1181, 1995.

Nielsen H, Bentsen KD, Hojtved L, et al: Oral candidiasis and immune status of HIV-infected patients. Pathol Med 23:140, 1994.

Neuner JM, McCarthy EP, Davis RB, et al: Diagnosis and management of adults with pharyngitis: A cost-effective analysis. Ann Intern Med 139:113, 2004.

Pinkham JR, Casamassimo PS, Fields HW Jr, et al (eds): Pediatric Dentistry: Infancy Through Adolescence, 3rd ed. Philadelphia, WB Saunders, 1999.

Rosenberg M: Clinical assessment of bad breath: Current concepts. J Am Dent Assoc 127:475, 1996.

Scully C, Laskaris G, Pindborg J, et al: Oral manifestations of HIV infection and their management: I. More common lesions. Oral Surg Oral Med Oral Pathol Oral Radiol Endod 71:158, 1991.

Scully C, Laskaris G, Pindborg J, et al: Oral manifestations of HIV infection and their management: II. Less common lesions. Oral Surg Oral Med Oral Pathol Oral Radiol Endod 71:167, 1991.

Silverman S: Color Atlas of Oral Manifestations of AIDS, 2nd ed. St. Louis, Mosby–Year Book, 1996.

Speilman AL, Bivona P, Rifkin BR: Halitosis: A common oral problem. N Y State Dent J 62:36, 1996.

Tonzetich J: Production and origin of oral malodor: A review of mechanisms and methods of analysis. J Periodontol 48:13, 1977.

Vincent MT, Celestin N, Hussain AN: Pharyngitis. Am Fam Physician 69:1465, 2004.

Warnakulasuriya S, Trivedy C, Peters TJ: Areca nut use: An independent risk factor for oral cancer. BMJ 324:799, 2002.

Weinert M, Grimes RM, Lynch DP: Oral manifestations of HIV infection. Ann Intern Med 125:485, 1996.

Wu MT, Lee YC, Chen CJ, et al: Risk of betel chewing for oesophageal cancer in Taiwan. Br J Cancer 85:658, 2001.

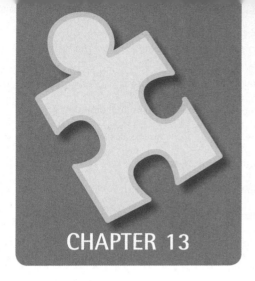

CHAPTER 13

The Chest

In the beginning the malady [tuberculosis] *is easier to cure but difficult to detect, but later it becomes easy to detect but difficult to cure.*

Niccolò Machiavelli (1469–1527)

General Considerations

Oxygen enables the breath of life; without adequate lung function, lives cannot be sustained. Patients with pulmonary disease must work harder for adequate oxygenation. These patients complain of "air hunger" or "too little air." Anyone who has traveled to areas of high altitude, where the oxygen concentration is reduced, has experienced shortness of breath.

The magnitude of pulmonary disease is enormous. In 2007, there were 115,652 deaths from chronic obstructive pulmonary disease, more than 5 million people had some degree of pulmonary disability, and more than 20 million had pulmonary symptoms. In addition, there were 91,871 deaths from pneumonia and influenza. Asthma accounted for more than 5400 deaths. In 1967, the estimated cost of morbidity and mortality from lung disease was $1.8 billion. In 2007, this figure skyrocketed to more than $65 billion.

Cancer of the lung and bronchus is the leading cause of death from cancer in the United States in both men (31% of all cancer deaths) and women (26% of all cancer deaths). In 2007, the American Cancer Society estimated that 213,380 new cases of lung and bronchus cancer were diagnosed. Cancer of the lung and bronchus is the second most common cancer in men (13%) after prostate cancer and second most common in women (12%) after breast cancer. There were 160,390 deaths, of which 89,510 were deaths in men. The highest incidence rate and death rate from cancer of the lung and bronchus are in African Americans: 73.9 per 100,000 and 60.5 per 100,000, respectively. The lifetime probability for development of cancer of the lung and bronchus is 1 per 13 in men and 1 per 17 in women.

Pulmonary diseases arise when the lungs are unable to provide adequate oxygenation or to eliminate carbon dioxide. Any derangement of these functions indicates abnormal respiratory function.

During a 24-hour period, the lungs oxygenate more than 5700 L of blood with more than 11,400 L of air. The total surface area of the alveoli of the lungs comprises an area larger than a tennis court.

Structure and Physiology

The chest forms the bony case that houses and protects the lungs, the heart, and the esophagus as it passes into the stomach. The chest skeleton consists of 12 thoracic vertebrae, 12 pairs of ribs, the clavicle, and the sternum. The bony structure is illustrated in Figure 13-1.

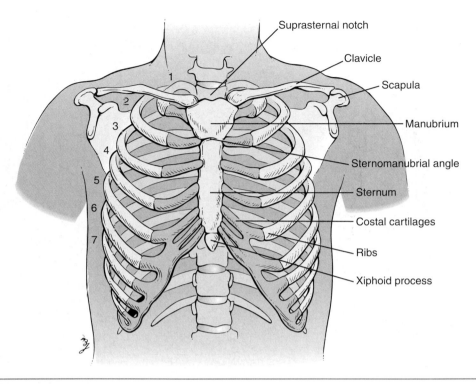

Figure 13-1 Bony chest skeleton.

The lungs continuously provide oxygen to and remove carbon dioxide from the circulatory system. The power required for breathing comes from the intercostal muscles and the diaphragm. These muscles act as a bellows to suck air into the lungs. Expiration is passive. The control of breathing is complex and is controlled by the *breathing center* in the medulla of the brain.

Inspired air is warmed, filtered, and humidified by the upper respiratory passages. After passing through the cricoid cartilage of the larynx, air travels through a system of flexible tubes, the *trachea*. At the level of the fourth or fifth thoracic vertebra, the trachea bifurcates into the *left* and *right bronchi*. The right bronchus is shorter, wider, and straighter than the left bronchus. The bronchi continue to subdivide into smaller bronchi and then into *bronchioles* within the lungs. Each respiratory bronchiole terminates in an *alveolar duct*, from which many *alveolar sacs* branch off. It is estimated that there are more than 500 million alveoli in the lungs. Each alveolar wall contains elastin fibers that allow the sac to expand with inspiration and to contract with expiration by *elastic recoil*. This system of air-conducting passages is illustrated in Figure 13-2.

The lungs are subdivided into lobes: the *upper, middle,* and *lower* on the right, and the *upper* and *lower* on the left. The lungs are enveloped in a thin sac, the *pleura*. The *visceral* pleura overlies the lung parenchyma, whereas the *parietal* pleura lines the chest wall. The two pleural surfaces glide over each other during inspiration and expiration. The space between the pleura is the pleural cavity.

To describe physical signs in the chest accurately, the examiner must understand the topographic landmarks of the chest wall. The landmarks of clinical importance are as follows:

- Sternum
- Clavicle
- Suprasternal notch
- Sternomanubrial angle
- Midsternal line
- Midclavicular lines
- Anterior axillary lines
- Midaxillary lines

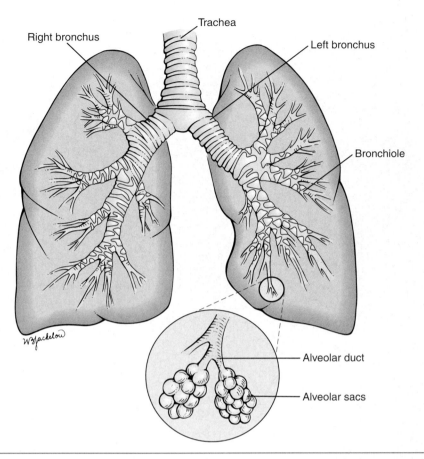

Trachea

Right bronchus

Left bronchus

Bronchiole

Alveolar duct

Alveolar sacs

Figure 13-2 System of air-conducting passages.

- Posterior axillary lines
- Scapular lines
- Midspinal line

Figure 13-3 illustrates the anterior and lateral views of the thorax, and Figure 13-4 illustrates the posterior thorax.

The *suprasternal notch* is located at the top of the sternum and can be felt as a depression at the base of the neck. The *sternomanubrial angle* is often referred to as the *angle of Louis*. This bony ridge lies approximately 5 cm below the suprasternal notch. When you move your fingers off the ridge laterally, the adjacent rib that you feel is the second rib. The interspace below the second rib is the *second intercostal space*. Using this as a reference point, you should be able to identify the ribs and interspaces anteriorly. Try it on yourself.

To identify areas, several imaginary lines can be visualized on the anterior and posterior chest in Figures 13-3 and 13-4. The *midsternal line* is drawn through the middle of the sternum. The *midclavicular lines* are drawn through the middle points of the clavicles and parallel to the midsternal line. The *anterior axillary lines* are vertical lines drawn along the anterior axillary folds parallel to the midsternal line. The *midaxillary lines* are drawn from each vertex of the axilla parallel to the midsternal line. The *posterior axillary lines* are parallel to the midsternal line and extend vertically along the posterior axillary folds. The *scapular lines* are parallel to the midspinal line and pass through the inferior angles of the scapulae. The *midspinal line* is a vertical line that passes through the posterior spinous processes of the vertebrae.

Rib counting from the posterior chest is slightly more complicated. The inferior wing of the *scapula* lies at the level of the seventh rib or interspace. Another useful landmark can be found by having the patient flex the neck; the most prominent cervical spinous process, the *vertebra prominens*, protrudes from the seventh cervical vertebra.

Only the first 7 ribs articulate with the sternum. The 8th, 9th, and 10th ribs articulate with the cartilage above. The 11th and 12th ribs are floating ribs and have a free anterior portion.

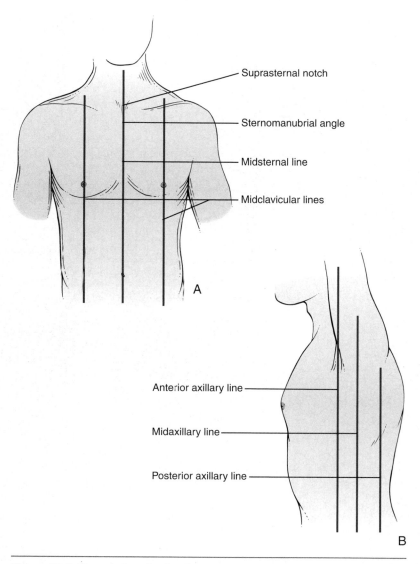

Figure 13-3 Thoracic cage landmarks. *A,* Topographic landmarks of the anterior thorax. *B,* Landmarks on the lateral view.

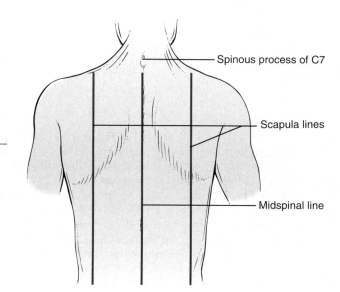

Figure 13-4 Topographic landmarks of the posterior thorax.

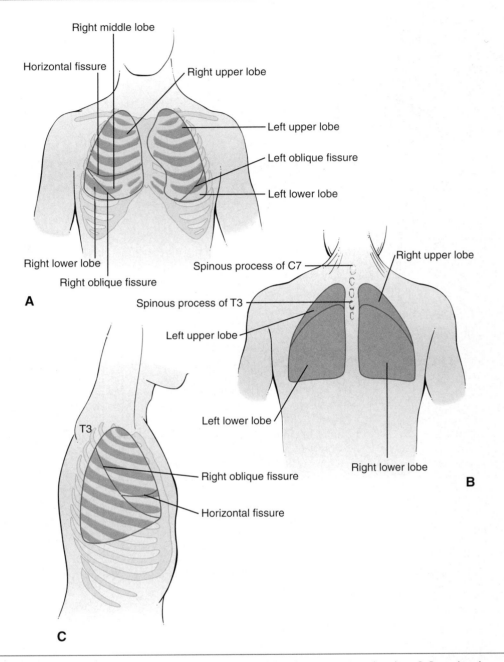

Figure 13-5 Surface topography and the underlying interlobar fissures. *A,* Anterior view. *B,* Posterior view. *C,* Lateral view.

The *interlobar fissures,* illustrated in Figure 13-5, are situated between the lobes of the lungs. Both the right and the left lungs have an *oblique fissure,* which begins on the anterior chest at the level of the sixth rib at the midclavicular line and extends laterally upward to the fifth rib in the midaxillary line, ending at the posterior chest at the spinous process of T3. The right lower lobe is below the right oblique fissure; the right upper and middle lobes are superior to the right oblique fissure. The left lower lobe is below the left oblique fissure; the left upper lobe is superior to the left oblique fissure. The *horizontal fissure* is present only on the right and divides the right upper lobe from the right middle lobe. It extends from the fourth rib at the sternal border to the fifth rib at the midaxillary line.

The lungs extend superiorly about 3 to 4 cm above the medial end of the clavicles. The inferior margins of the lungs extend to the sixth rib at the midclavicular line, to the eighth rib at the midaxillary line, and between T9 and T12 posteriorly. This variation is related to respiration. The bifurcation of the trachea, the *carina*, is located behind the angle of Louis at approximately the level of T4 on the posterior chest. The *right hemidiaphragm* at the end of expiration is located at the level of the fifth rib anteriorly and T9 posteriorly. The presence of the liver on the right side makes the right hemidiaphragm slightly higher than the left.

During quiet breathing, muscle contraction occurs only during inspiration. Expiration is passive, resulting from the elastic recoil of the lungs and chest.

Review of Specific Symptoms

The main symptoms of pulmonary disease are the following:

- Cough
- Sputum production
- Hemoptysis (coughing up blood)
- Dyspnea (shortness of breath)
- Wheezing
- Cyanosis (bluish discoloration of the skin)
- Chest pain
- Sleep apnea

Cough

The most common symptom of lung disease is the *cough*. Coughing is so common that it is frequently regarded as a trivial complaint. The cough reflex is a normal defense mechanism of the lungs that protects them from foreign bodies and excessive secretions. Infections of the upper respiratory tract are associated with coughing that usually improves in 2 to 3 weeks. A persistent cough necessitates further investigation.

Coughing is a coordinated, forced expiration, interrupted by repeated closure of the glottis. The expiratory muscles contract against the partially closed glottis, creating high pressure within the lungs. When the glottis suddenly opens, there is an explosive rush of air that clears the air passages. When a patient complains of coughing, ask these questions:

"Can you describe your cough?"

"How long have you had a cough?"

"Was there a sudden onset of coughing?"

"Do you smoke?" If so, *"What do you smoke? How much, and for how long?"*

"Does your cough produce sputum?" If so, *"Can you estimate the amount of your expectorations? What is the color of the sputum? Does the sputum have a foul odor?"*

"Does the cough occur for prolonged periods?"

"Does the cough occur after eating?"

"Is the coughing worse in any position?"

"What relieves the cough?"

"Are there any other symptoms associated with the cough? fever? headaches? night sweats? chest pain? runny nose? shortness of breath? weight loss? hoarseness? loss of consciousness?"

"Do you have any birds as pets? Do you feed pigeons?"

"Have you ever been exposed to anyone with tuberculosis?"

Coughing may be voluntary or involuntary, productive or nonproductive. In a *productive* cough, mucus or other materials are expelled. A *dry* cough does not produce any secretions.

Smoking is probably the most common cause of the chronic cough. *Smoker's cough* results from inhalation of irritants in tobacco and is most marked in the morning. Coughing is normally decreased during sleep. When the smoker awakens, productive coughing tends to clear the respiratory passages. In patients who stop smoking, the cough decreases and may disappear.

Table 13-1 Descriptors of Coughing

Description	Possible Causes
Dry, hacking	Viral infections, interstitial lung disease, tumor, allergies, anxiety
Chronic, productive	Bronchiectasis, chronic bronchitis, abscess, bacterial pneumonia, tuberculosis
Wheezing	Bronchospasm, asthma, allergies, congestive heart failure
Barking	Epiglottal disease (e.g., croup)
Stridor	Tracheal obstruction
Morning	Smoking
Nocturnal	Postnasal drip, congestive heart failure
Associated with eating or drinking	Neuromuscular disease of the upper esophagus
Inadequate	Debility, weakness

Coughing may also be *psychogenic*. This nonproductive cough occurs in individuals with emotional stress. When attention is drawn to it, the cough occurs more often. During sleep, or when the patient is distracted, the coughing stops. Psychogenic coughing is a *diagnosis of exclusion*: Only after all other causes have been eliminated can this diagnosis be made.

There are many terms used by patients and physicians to describe a cough. Table 13-1 provides a list of some of the more common descriptors and their possible causes.

Sputum Production

Sputum is the substance expelled by coughing. Approximately 75 to 100 mL of sputum is secreted daily by the bronchi. By ciliary action, it is brought up to the throat and then swallowed unconsciously with the saliva. An increase in the quantity of sputum production is the earliest manifestation of bronchitis. Sputum may contain cellular debris, mucus, blood, pus, or microorganisms.

Sputum should be described according to color, consistency, quantity, the number of times it is brought up during the day and night, and the presence or absence of blood. An adequate description may indicate a cause of the disease process. Uninfected sputum is odorless, transparent, and whitish-gray, resembling mucus; it is termed *mucoid*. Infected sputum contains pus and is termed *purulent*; the sputum may be yellow, greenish, or red. Table 13-2 lists the appearances of sputum and their possible causes.

Hemoptysis

Hemoptysis is the coughing up of blood. Few symptoms produce as much alarm in patients as does hemoptysis. Careful description of the hemoptysis is crucial because what is produced can include clots of blood, as well as blood-tinged sputum. The implications of each are very different. Coughing up clots of blood is a symptom of extreme importance because it often heralds a serious illness. Clots of blood are usually indicative of a cavitary lung lesion, a tumor of the lung, certain cardiac diseases, or pulmonary embolism. Blood-tinged sputum is usually associated with smoking or minor infections, but it can be seen with tumors and more serious diseases as well. When a patient complains of coughing up blood, the examiner should ask the following questions:

"Do you smoke?" If yes, *"What do you smoke? How much, and for how long?"*

"Did the coughing up of blood occur suddenly?"

"Have there been recurrent episodes of coughing up blood?"

"Is the sputum blood-tinged, or are there actual clots of blood?"

"How long have you noticed the blood?"

Table 13-2 Appearances of Sputum

Appearance	Possible Causes
Mucoid	Asthma, tumors, tuberculosis, emphysema, pneumonia
Mucopurulent	Asthma, tumors, tuberculosis, emphysema, pneumonia
Yellow-green, purulent	Bronchiectasis, chronic bronchitis
Rust-colored, purulent	Pneumococcal pneumonia
Red currant jelly	*Klebsiella pneumoniae* infection
Foul odor	Lung abscess
Pink, blood-tinged	Streptococcal or staphylococcal pneumonia
Gravel	Broncholithiasis
Pink, frothy	Pulmonary edema
Profuse, colorless (also known as *bronchorrhea*)	Alveolar cell carcinoma
Bloody	Pulmonary emboli, bronchiectasis, abscess, tuberculosis, tumor, cardiac causes, bleeding disorders

"What seems to bring on the coughing up of blood? vomiting? coughing? nausea?"

"Have you ever had tuberculosis?"

"Is there a family history of coughing up blood?"

"Have you had recent surgery?"

"Do you take any 'blood thinners'?"

"Are you aware of any bleeding tendency?"

"Have you had any recent travel on airplanes?"

"Have you had night sweats? shortness of breath? palpitations? irregular heartbeats? hoarseness? weight loss? swelling or pain in your legs?"

"Have you felt any unusual sensation in your chest after coughing up blood?" If so, *"Where?"*

(For a woman with hemoptysis) *"Do you use oral contraceptives?"*

Any suppurative (associated with the production of pus) process of the airways or lungs can produce hemoptysis. Bronchitis is probably the most common cause of hemoptysis. Bronchiectasis and bronchogenic carcinoma are also major causes. Hemoptysis results from mucosal invasion, tumor necrosis, and pneumonia distal to bronchial obstruction by tumor. Pneumococcal pneumonia characteristically produces rust-colored sputum. Pink and frothy sputum can result from pulmonary edema.

On occasion, patients have a warm sensation in the chest at the location from which the hemoptysis originated. Therefore, it is useful to ask patients with recent hemoptysis whether they experienced such a sensation. This information may lead to a more careful review of the physical examination and x-ray films of that area.

Patients who have undergone recent surgery or have traveled for long periods of time on airplanes are at risk for deep vein thrombophlebitis with pulmonary embolism. Women taking oral contraceptives are likewise at risk for pulmonary embolic disease. Hemoptysis occurs when pulmonary emboli result in infarction, with necrosis of the pulmonary parenchyma.

Recurrent episodes of hemoptysis may result from bronchiectasis, tuberculosis, or mitral stenosis. Atrial fibrillation is a common cause of "irregular heartbeats" and embolic phenomena.

Sometimes it is difficult to ascertain whether the patient coughed up or vomited blood. Most patients can provide a sufficiently clear history. Table 13-3 lists characteristics that help distinguish hemoptysis from hematemesis (vomiting of blood).

Table 13-3 Characteristics Distinguishing Hemoptysis from Hematemesis

Features	Hemoptysis	Hematemesis
Prodrome	Coughing	Nausea and vomiting
Past history	Possible history of cardiopulmonary disease	Possible history of gastrointestinal disease
Appearance	Frothy	Not frothy
Color	Bright red	Dark red, brown, or "coffee grounds"
Manifestation	Mixed with pus	Mixed with food
Associated symptoms	Dyspnea	Nausea

Dyspnea

The *subjective* sensation of "shortness of breath" is *dyspnea*. Dyspnea is an important manifestation of cardiopulmonary disease, although it is found in other states such as neurologic, metabolic, and psychologic conditions. It is important to differentiate dyspnea from the *objective* finding of *tachypnea*, or rapid breathing. A patient may be observed to be breathing rapidly while stating that he or she is not short of breath. The converse is also true: a patient may be breathing slowly but have dyspnea. Never assume that a patient with a rapid respiratory rate is dyspneic.

It is important for the examiner to inquire when dyspnea occurs and in which position. *Paroxysmal nocturnal dyspnea* is the sudden onset of shortness of breath occurring at night during sleep. Patients are suddenly seized with an intense strangling sensation. They frantically sit up and, classically, run to the window for "air." As soon as they assume an upright position, the dyspnea usually improves. *Orthopnea* is difficulty breathing while lying flat. Patients require two or more pillows to breathe comfortably. *Platypnea* is a rare symptom of difficulty breathing while sitting up and is relieved by a recumbent position. *Trepopnea* is a condition in which patients are more comfortable breathing while lying on one side. (Some of the more common causes of positional dyspnea are listed in Table 13-4.) For any patient complaining of dyspnea, ask the following questions:

> *"How long have you had shortness of breath?"*
>
> *"Did the shortness of breath occur suddenly?"*
>
> *"Is the shortness of breath constant?"*
>
> *"Does the shortness of breath occur with exertion? at rest? lying flat? sitting up?"*

Table 13-4 Positional Dyspnea

Type	Possible Causes
Orthopnea	Congestive heart failure Mitral valvular disease Severe asthma (rarely) Emphysema (rarely) Chronic bronchitis (rarely) Neurologic diseases (rarely)
Trepopnea	Congestive heart failure
Platypnea	Postpneumonectomy status Neurologic diseases Cirrhosis (intrapulmonary shunts) Hypovolemia

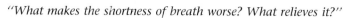

"What makes the shortness of breath worse? What relieves it?"

"How many level blocks can you walk without becoming short of breath?"

"How many level blocks could you walk 6 months ago?"

"Is the shortness of breath accompanied by wheezing? fever? cough? coughing up blood? chest pain? palpitations? hoarseness?"

"Do you smoke?" If so, *"How much? For how long?"*

"Have you had any exposure to asbestos? sandblasting? pigeon breeding?"

"Have you had any exposure to individuals with tuberculosis?"

"Have you ever lived near the San Joaquin Valley? midwestern or southeastern United States?"

It is essential to try to quantify the dyspnea. Questions such as "How many level blocks can you walk?" provide a framework for *exercise tolerance*. For example, if the patient answers, "two blocks," the patient is said to have *two-block dyspnea on exertion*. The interviewer can then ask, "How many level blocks were you able to walk 6 months ago?" and thus assess approximately the progression of the disease or the efficacy of therapy.

Careful questioning regarding *industrial exposure* is paramount for any patient with unexplained dyspnea. Examples of further questions regarding occupational and environmental history are discussed in Chapter 1, The Interviewer's Questions. Exposure to pigeons may result in psittacosis. Outbreaks of coccidioidomycosis have occurred in individuals living in the southwestern United States. Living in the midwestern and southeastern United States has been linked to outbreaks of histoplasmosis.

Wheezing

Wheezing is an abnormally high-pitched noise resulting from a partially obstructed airway. It is usually present during expiration when slight bronchoconstriction occurs. Bronchospasm, mucosal edema, loss of elastic support, and tortuosity of the airways are the usual causes. Asthma causes bronchospasm, which results in the wheezing associated with this condition. Obstruction by intraluminal material, such as aspirated foreign bodies or secretions, is another important cause of wheezing. A well-localized wheeze, unchanged by coughing, may indicate that a bronchus is partially obstructed by a foreign body or tumor. When a patient complains of wheezing, the examiner must determine the following:

"At what age did the wheezing begin?"

"How often does it occur?"

"Are there any precipitating factors, such as foods, odors, emotions, animals, and so forth?"

"What usually stops the attack?"

"Have the symptoms worsened over the years?"

"Are there any associated symptoms?"

"Is there a history of nasal polyps?"

"Do you smoke?" If so, *"What do you smoke? How much, and for how long?"*

"Is there a history of heart disease?"

An important axiom to remember is that asthma is associated with wheezing, but not all wheezing is asthma.

Do not equate wheezing with asthma. Although congestive heart failure is usually associated with abnormal breath sounds called *crackles* (discussed later in this chapter), sometimes there is such severe bronchospasm in heart failure that the main physical finding is a wheeze rather than a crackle.

A decrease in wheezing may result from either an opening of the airway or a progressive closing off of the air passage. A "silent" chest in a patient with an acute asthmatic attack is usually an ominous sign: It indicates worsening of the obstruction.

Cyanosis

Cyanosis is commonly detected by a family member or friend. The subtle bluish discoloration may go completely unnoticed by the patient. *Central* cyanosis occurs with inadequate gas exchange in the lungs that results in a significant reduction in arterial oxygenation. Primary pulmonary problems or diseases that cause mixed venous blood to bypass the lungs (e.g., intracardiac shunt) are frequently the causative factors. The bluish discoloration is best seen in the mucous membranes of the mouth (e.g., the frenulum) and lips. *Peripheral* cyanosis results from an excessive extraction of oxygen at the periphery. It is limited to the extremities (e.g., the fingers, toes, nose). Ask the following questions:

"Where is the cyanosis present?"

"How long has the cyanosis been present?"

"Are you aware of any lung problem? heart problem? blood problem?"

"What makes the cyanosis worse?"

"Is there associated shortness of breath? cough? bleeding?"

"What types of work have you performed?"

"Is there anyone else in your family who has cyanosis?"

Cyanosis from birth is associated with congenital heart lesions. The acute development of cyanosis can occur in severe respiratory disease, especially acute airway obstruction. Peripheral cyanosis results from increased oxygen extraction in states of low cardiac output and is seen in cooler areas of the body such as the nail beds and the outer surfaces of the lips. Peripheral cyanosis disappears as the area is warmed. Cyanosis of the nails and warmth in the hands suggest that the cyanosis is central. Central cyanosis occurs only after the oxygen saturation has fallen below 80%. Central cyanosis diffusely involves the skin and mucous membranes and does not disappear with warming of the area. At least 2 to 3 g of unsaturated hemoglobin per 100 mL of blood must be present for the patient to manifest central cyanosis. Exercise worsens central cyanosis because the exercising muscles require an increased extraction of oxygen from the blood. In patients with severe anemia, in whom hemoglobin levels are markedly decreased, cyanosis may not be seen. Clubbing of the nails is seen in association with central cyanosis and significant cardiopulmonary disorders. See Figure 8-12.

Some industrial workers, such as arc welders, inhale toxic levels of nitrous gases that can produce cyanosis by methemoglobinemia. Hereditary methemoglobinemia is a primary hemoglobin abnormality causing congenital cyanosis.

Chest Pain

Chest pain related to pulmonary disease usually results from involvement of the chest wall or parietal pleura. Nerve fibers are abundant in this area. *Pleuritic pain* is a common symptom of inflammation of the parietal pleura. It is described as a sharp, stabbing pain that is usually felt during inspiration. It may be localized to one side, and the patient may *splint** to avoid the pain. Chapter 14, The Heart, summarizes the important questions to ask a patient complaining of chest pain.

Acute dilatation of the main pulmonary artery may also produce a sensation of dull pressure, often indistinguishable from angina pectoris. This results from nerve endings responding to the stretch on the main pulmonary artery.

Although chest pain occurs in pulmonary disease, chest pain is the cardinal symptom of cardiac disease and is discussed more completely in Chapter 14, The Heart.

Sleep Apnea

The sleep apnea syndrome is a potentially disabling condition characterized by excessive daytime fatigue or sleepiness, disruptive snoring, episodes of upper airway obstruction during sleep, and nocturnal hypoxemia. During sleep, the pharynx repeatedly collapses. The patient

---

*Splinting means making the chest muscles rigid to avoid motion of that part of the chest.

struggles to breathe against the closed airway, which results in hypoxemia. The patient eventually awakens from sleep; the posterior pharyngeal muscles contract, opening the airway; and air rushes in, creating a loud snore or gasp. The patient falls back to sleep, only to have the events repeat. The poor sleeping pattern and the hypoxemia often lead to the symptoms of excessive daytime fatigue. The true prevalence is unknown, but it has been estimated that it is 4% among men and 2% among women from the ages of 30 to 60 years. The prevalence may be higher in individuals older than 60 years. Ask the following questions:

"Have you been told that you snore?"

"How often do you snore?"

"Does your snoring bother other people?"

"Have breathing pauses been noticed?"

"Are you tired after sleeping?"

"Are you tired during the daytime?"

"Have you ever fallen asleep while driving?"

"Do you have high blood pressure?"

The presence of snoring, sleepiness, and tiredness are suggestive of sleep apnea.

Other Symptoms

In addition to the main symptoms of pulmonary disease, there are other, less common symptoms. These include the following:

- Stridor (noisy breathing)
- Voice changes
- Swelling of the ankles (dependent edema)

Stridor is a harsh type of noisy breathing and is usually associated with obstruction of a major bronchus that occurs with aspiration. *Voice changes* can occur with inflammation of the vocal cords or interference with the recurrent laryngeal nerve. *Swelling of the ankles* is a manifestation of dependent edema, which is associated with right-sided heart failure, renal disease, liver disease, and obstruction of venous flow. As the condition worsens, abnormal accumulations of fluid produce generalized edema, known as *anasarca*.

Impact of Lung Disease on the Patient

The impact of lung disease on the patient varies greatly with the nature of the ailment, as does the subjective sensation of air hunger. Some patients with lung disease are hardly aware of the dyspnea. The decrease in exercise tolerance is so insidious that these patients may not be aware of any problem. Only when asked to try to quantify the dyspnea do these patients realize their deficiency. In other patients, dyspnea is so rapidly progressive that they experience severe depression. They recognize that little can be done to improve their lung conditions and thus markedly alter their lifestyle. Many become incapacitated and are forced to retire from work. They can no longer experience the slightest exertion without becoming dyspneic.

Often, chronic lung disease develops as a result of occupational hazards. Affected patients may become embittered and hostile. There has been much publicity about occupational exposure, but some industries still provide little protection for their employees.

Chronic obstructive pulmonary disease can be divided into two types: *emphysema* and *chronic bronchitis*. Both are characterized by a slowly progressive course, obstruction of airflow, and destruction of the lung parenchyma. Classically, patients with emphysema are the "pink puffers." They are thin and weak from severe dyspnea associated with little cough or sputum production. The classic "blue bloaters" suffer primarily from bronchitis. They are cyanotic and have a productive cough but are less troubled by dyspnea; they are usually short and stocky. These classic descriptions are interesting, but most patients with chronic obstructive pulmonary disease have characteristics of both types.

Since ancient times, clinicians have recognized that emotional factors play a role in the onset and maintenance of symptoms in bronchial asthma. Attacks of asthma can be provoked by a range of emotions: fear, anger, anxiety, depression, guilt, frustration, and joy. It is the patient's attempt to suppress the emotion, rather than the emotion itself, that precipitates the asthmatic attack.

A patient having an asthmatic attack becomes anxious and fearful, which tends to perpetuate the attack. Hyperventilation may contribute to the breathlessness of the frightened patient. Despite being given adequate medical therapy, these patients remain dyspneic. In such patients, it is the *anxiety* and its causes that require attention. They need continuing medical *and* psychologic support after an acute attack. As early as the 12th century, Maimonides recognized that "mere diet and medical treatment cannot fully cure this disorder."

Asthma in children presents a special problem. Anxiety, underachievement, peer pressure, and noncompliance with medications can exacerbate episodes of asthma. These children are absent from school more often than their nonasthmatic peers, which causes schoolwork to suffer; this creates a vicious cycle. The incidence of emotional disorders is greater than twofold higher in asthmatic school-aged children than in the general population.

Asthma can affect a person's sexual function both physiologically and psychologically. Asthmatic patients may become more dyspneic as a result of the increased physical demands of sexual intercourse. Bronchospasm may occur, owing to excitement, anxiety, or panic. Anxiety about precipitating an asthmatic attack during sexual intercourse worsens the patient's dyspnea and sexual performance; another vicious cycle is set into motion. Patients may then tend to avoid sexual intercourse.

Physical Examination

The equipment necessary for the examination of the chest is a stethoscope.

After a general assessment of the patient, the examination of the posterior chest is performed while the patient is still seated. The patient's arms should be folded in his or her lap. After the examination of the posterior chest is completed, the patient is asked to lie down, and the examination of the anterior chest is begun. During the examination, the examiner should try to imagine the underlying lung areas.

If the patient is a man, his gown should be removed to his waist. If the patient is a woman, the gown should be positioned to prevent unnecessary or embarrassing exposure of the breasts. The examiner should stand facing the patient.

The examination of the anterior and posterior aspects of the chest includes the following:

- Inspection
- Palpation
- Percussion
- Auscultation

General Assessment

Inspect the Patient's Facial Expression

Is the patient in acute distress? Is there nasal flaring or pursed lip breathing? Nasal flaring is the outward motion of the nares during inhalation. This is seen in any condition that causes an increase in the work of breathing. Are there audible signs of breathing, such as stridor and wheezing? These are related to obstruction to airflow. Is cyanosis present?

Inspect the Patient's Posture

Patients with airway obstructive disease tend to prefer a position in which they can support their arms and fix the muscles of the shoulder and neck to aid in respiration. A common technique used by patients with bronchial obstruction is to clasp the sides of the bed and use the latissimus dorsi muscle to help overcome the increased resistance to outflow during expiration. Patients with orthopnea remain seated or lie on several pillows.

Inspect the Neck

Is the patient's breathing aided by the action of the *accessory muscles?* Use of the accessory muscles is one of the earliest signs of airway obstruction. In respiratory distress, the trapezius and sternocleidomastoid muscles contract during inspiration. The accessory muscles assist in ventilation; they raise the clavicle and anterior chest to increase the lung volume and produce an increased negative intrathoracic pressure. This results in retraction of the supraclavicular fossae and intercostal muscles. An upward motion of the clavicle of more than 5 mm during respiration is associated with severe obstructive lung disease.

Inspect the Configuration of the Chest

A variety of conditions may interfere with adequate ventilation, and the configuration of the chest may indicate lung disease. An increase in the *anteroposterior diameter* is seen in advanced chronic obstructive pulmonary disease. The anteroposterior diameter tends to equal the lateral diameter, and a *barrel chest* results. The ribs lose their 45° angle and become more horizontal. A *flail chest* is a configuration in which one chest wall moves paradoxically inward during inspiration. This condition is seen with multiple rib fractures. The spinal deformity *kyphoscoliosis* results in an abnormal anteroposterior diameter and lateral curvature of the spine that severely restricts chest and lung expansion. Figure 13-6 depicts a patient with severe kyphoscoliosis. *Pectus excavatum,* or "funnel chest," is a depression of the sternum that produces a restrictive lung problem only if the depression is marked. Patients with pectus excavatum may have abnormalities of the mitral valve, especially mitral valve prolapse. Figure 13-7 depicts a patient with pectus excavatum. *Pectus carinatum,* or pigeon breast, which results from an anterior protrusion of the sternum, is a common deformity but does not compromise ventilation. Figure 13-8 depicts a patient with pectus carinatum. Notice the prominent sternal ridge and the ribs slanting steeply away on either side. Figure 13-9 illustrates the various configurations of the chest.

Assess the Respiratory Rate and Pattern

When assessing respiratory rate, never ask the patient to breathe "normally." Individuals voluntarily change their breathing patterns and rates once they are aware that respiration is being assessed. A better way is, after taking the radial pulse, to direct your eyes to the patient's chest and evaluate respirations while still holding the patient's wrist. The patient is unaware that you are no longer taking the pulse, and voluntary changes in breathing rate will not occur. Counting the number of respirations in a 30-second period and multiplying that number by two provides an accurate respiratory rate.

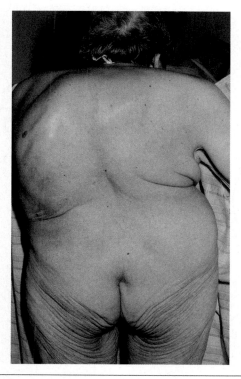

Figure 13-6 Severe kyphoscoliosis.

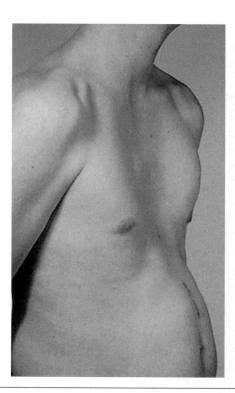

Figure 13-7 Pectus excavatum.

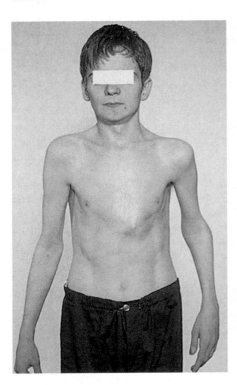

Figure 13-8 Pectus carinatum.

The normal adult takes about 10 to 14 breaths a minute. *Bradypnea* is an abnormal slowing of respiration; *tachypnea* is an abnormal increase. *Apnea* is the temporary cessation of breathing. *Hyperpnea* is an increased depth of breathing, usually associated with metabolic acidosis. It is also known as *Kussmaul's breathing*. There are many types of abnormal breathing patterns. Figure 13-10 illustrates and lists the more common types of abnormal breathing.

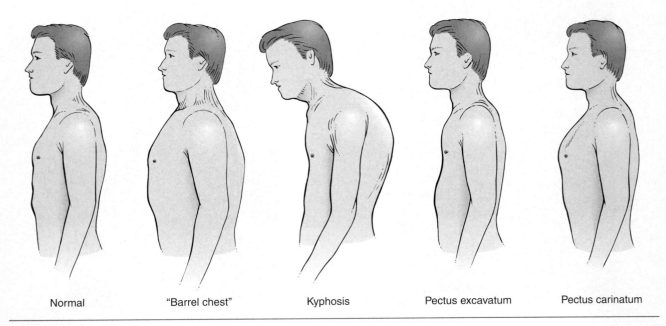

| Normal | "Barrel chest" | Kyphosis | Pectus excavatum | Pectus carinatum |

Figure 13-9 Common chest configurations.

Pattern	Characteristic	Cause
Apnea	Absence of breathing	Cardiac arrest
Biot's respiration	Irregular breathing with long periods of apnea	Increased intracranial pressure Drug-induced respiratory depression Brain damage (usually at the medullary level)
Cheyne-Stokes respiration	Irregular breathing with intermittent periods of increased and decreased rates and depths of breaths alternating with periods of apnea	Drug-induced respiratory depression Congestive heart failure Brain damage (usually at the cerebral level)
Kussmaul's respiration	Fast and deep	Metabolic acidosis

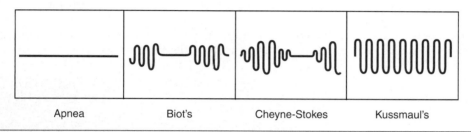

Apnea   Biot's   Cheyne-Stokes   Kussmaul's

Figure 13-10 Patterns of abnormal breathing.

Inspect the Hands

Is *clubbing* of the fingernails present? The technique for evaluating clubbing is described in Chapter 8, The Skin. The earliest finding of clubbing is loss of the angle between the nail and the terminal phalanx. Look at Figure 8-12, in which a normal index fingernail is compared with a severely clubbed index fingernail of a patient with bronchogenic carcinoma.

Clubbing has been associated with a number of clinical disorders, such as the following:

- Intrathoracic tumors
- Mixed venous-to-arterial shunts
- Chronic pulmonary disease
- Chronic hepatic fibrosis

The pathogenesis of clubbing is unclear. In many conditions, however, arterial desaturation occurs. This, in some way, may be the underlying problem. In some individuals, clubbing may be inherited without any pathologic process.

The Posterior Chest

Move behind the patient to examine the posterior chest.

Palpation

Palpation is used to assess the following:

- Areas of tenderness
- Symmetry of chest excursion
- Tactile fremitus

Palpate for Tenderness

With your fingers, firmly palpate any chest areas where tenderness is experienced by the patient. A complaint of "chest pain" may be related only to local musculoskeletal disease and not to disease of the heart or lungs. Be meticulous in assessing for areas of tenderness.

Evaluate Posterior Chest Excursion

The examiner can determine the degree of symmetry of chest excursion by placing his or her hands flat against the patient's back with the thumbs parallel to the midline at approximately the level of the 10th ribs and pulling the underlying skin slightly toward the midline. The patient is asked to inhale deeply, and the movement of the examiner's hands is noted. The hand movement should be symmetric. Localized pulmonary disease may cause one side of the chest to move less than the opposite side. The placement of the examiner's hands is shown in Figure 13-11.

Evaluate Tactile Fremitus

Speech creates vibrations that can be heard when the examiner listens to the chest and lungs. These vibrations are termed *vocal fremitus*. When the examiner palpates the patient's chest wall while the patient is speaking, these vibrations can be felt and are termed *tactile fremitus*. Sound is conducted from the larynx through the bronchial tree to the lung parenchyma and the chest wall. Tactile fremitus provides useful information about the density of the underlying lung tissue and chest cavity. Conditions that increase the density of the lung and make it more solid, such as consolidation, increase the transmission of tactile fremitus. Clinical states that decrease the transmission of these sound waves result in reduced tactile fremitus. If there is excess fat tissue on the chest, air or fluid in the chest cavity, or overexpansion of the lung, tactile fremitus is diminished.

Tactile fremitus can be evaluated in two ways. In the first technique, the examiner places the ulnar side of his or her right hand against the patient's chest wall, as demonstrated in

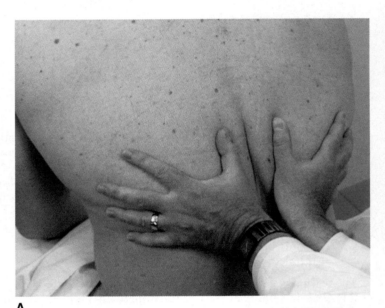

A

Figure 13-11 Technique for evaluating posterior chest excursion. *A,* Placement of the examiner's hands during normal expiration. *B,* Placement of the examiner's hands after normal inspiration.

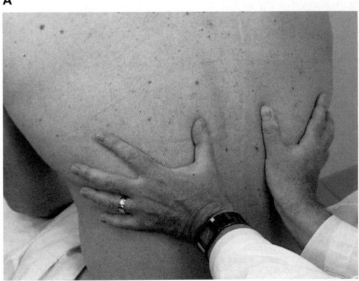

B

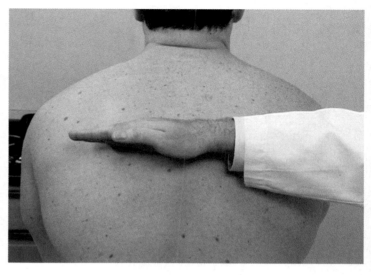

Figure 13-12 Technique for evaluating tactile fremitus.

Figure 13-12, and asks the patient to say, ''Ninety-nine.'' Tactile fremitus is evaluated, and the examiner's hand is moved to the corresponding position on the other side. Tactile fremitus on the opposite side is then evaluated and compared. By moving the hand from side to side and from top to bottom, the examiner can detect differences in the transmission of the sound to the chest wall. ''Ninety-nine'' is one of the phrases used because it causes good vibratory tones. If the patient speaks either louder or deeper, the tactile sensation is enhanced. Tactile fremitus should be evaluated in the six locations illustrated in Figure 13-13.

The other method of evaluating tactile fremitus is to use the fingertips instead of the ulnar side of the hand. The same side-to-side and top-to-bottom positions illustrated in Figure 13-13 are used. The evaluation of tactile fremitus should be performed with only one of these techniques. The examiner should try both methods initially to determine which one is preferable.

Table 13-5 lists some of the important pathologic causes of changes in tactile fremitus.

Percussion

Percussion refers to tapping on a surface to determine the underlying structure. It is similar to a radar or echo detection system. Tapping on the chest wall creates vibrations that are transmitted to the underlying tissue, reflected back, and picked up by the examiner's tactile and auditory senses. The sound heard and the tactile sensation felt depend on the air–tissue ratio. The

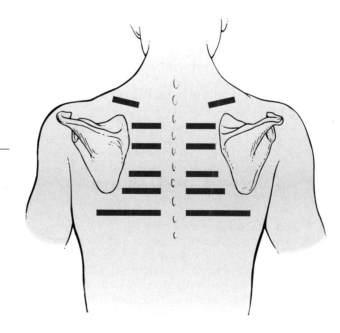

Figure 13-13 Locations on the posterior chest for evaluating tactile fremitus.

Table 13-5 Causes of Changes in Tactile Fremitus

Increased Tactile Fremitus

Pneumonia

Decreased Tactile Fremitus

Unilateral

  Pneumothorax

  Pleural effusion

  Bronchial obstruction

  Atelectasis (incomplete expansion of lung tissue)

Bilateral

  Chronic obstructive lung disease

  Chest wall thickening (muscle, fat)

vibrations initiated by percussion of the chest enable the examiner to evaluate the lung tissue to a depth of only 5 to 6 cm, but percussion is valuable because many changes in the air–tissue ratio are readily apparent.

Percussion over a solid organ, such as the liver, produces a *dull*, low-amplitude, short-duration note without resonance. Percussion over a structure containing air within a tissue, such as the lung, produces a *resonant*, higher amplitude, lower pitched note. Percussion over a hollow air-containing structure, such as the stomach, produces a *tympanic*, high-pitched, hollow-quality note. Percussion over a large muscle mass, such as the thigh, produces a *flat*, high-pitched note.

Normally, in the chest, dullness over the heart and resonance over the lung fields are heard and felt. As the lungs fill with fluid and become more dense, as in pneumonia, resonance is replaced by dullness. The term *hyperresonance* has been applied to the percussion note obtained from a lung with decreased density, such as that found in emphysema. Hyperresonance is a low-pitched, hollow-quality, sustained resonant note bordering on tympany.

In percussion of the chest, the examiner places the middle finger of one hand firmly against the patient's chest wall, parallel to the ribs in an interspace, with the palm and other fingers held off the chest. The tip of the right middle finger of the other hand strikes a quick, sharp blow to the terminal phalanx of the left finger on the chest wall. The motion of the striking finger should come from the wrist and not from the elbow. Paddleball players use this motion naturally, whereas tennis players must learn to concentrate on using this wrist motion. The technique of percussion is diagrammed in Figure 13-14 and demonstrated in Figure 13-15.

Try percussion on yourself. Percuss over your right lung (resonant), stomach (tympanic), liver (dull), and thigh (flat).

Percuss the Posterior Chest

The sites on the posterior chest for percussion are above, between, and below the scapulae in the intercostal spaces, as diagrammed in Figure 13-16. The scapulae themselves are not percussed. The examiner should start at the top and work downward, proceeding from side to side, comparing one side with the other.

Evaluate Diaphragmatic Movement

Percussion is also used to detect diaphragmatic movement. The patient is asked to take a deep breath and hold it. Percussion at the right lung base helps determine the lowest area of resonance, which represents the lowest level of the diaphragm. Below this level is dullness from the liver. The patient is then instructed to exhale as much as possible, and the percussion is repeated. With expiration, the lung contracts, the liver moves up, and the same area becomes dull; that is, the level of dullness moves upward. The difference between the inspiration and expiration levels represents diaphragmatic motion, which is normally 4 to 5 cm. In patients

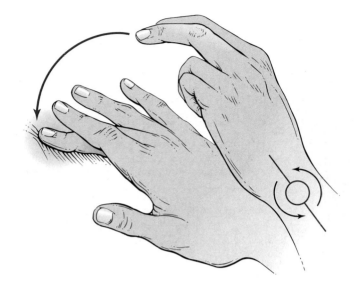

Figure 13-14 Technique of percussion.

with emphysema, the motion is reduced. In patients with a phrenic nerve palsy, diaphragmatic motion is absent. This test is illustrated in Figure 13-17.

Auscultation

Auscultation is the technique of listening for sounds produced in the body. Auscultation of the chest is used to identify lung sounds. The stethoscope usually has two heads: the bell and the diaphragm. The bell is used to detect low-pitched sounds, and the diaphragm is better at detecting higher pitched sounds. The bell must be applied loosely to the skin; if it is pressed too tightly, the skin acts as a diaphragm, and the lower pitched sounds are filtered out. In contrast, the diaphragm is applied firmly to the skin. In very cachectic individuals, the bell may be more useful because the protruding ribs in these patients make placement of the diaphragm difficult. The correct placements of the heads of the stethoscope are demonstrated in Figure 13-18.

It is *never* acceptable to listen through clothing. The bell or the diaphragm of the stethoscope must *always* be in contact with the skin.

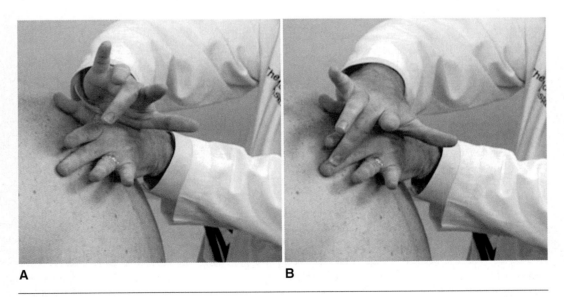

A   B

Figure 13-15 Percussion. *A,* Position of the right hand ready to percuss. *B,* Location of the fingers after striking. Notice that the motion is from the wrist.

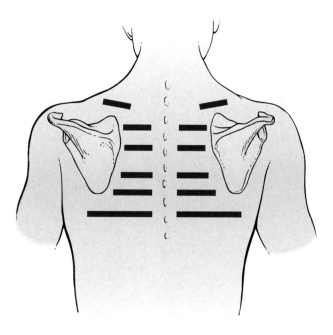

Figure 13-16 Locations on the posterior chest for percussion and auscultation.

Types of Breath Sounds

Breath sounds are heard over most of the lung fields. They consist of an inspiratory phase followed by an expiratory phase. There are four types of normal breath sounds:

- Tracheal
- Bronchial
- Bronchovesicular
- Vesicular

Tracheal breath sounds are harsh, loud, high-pitched sounds heard over the extrathoracic portion of the trachea. The inspiratory and expiratory components are approximately equal in length. Although these sounds are always heard when the examiner listens over the trachea, they are rarely evaluated because they do not represent any clinical lung problems.

Bronchial breath sounds are loud and high-pitched and sound like air rushing through a tube. The expiratory component is louder and longer than the inspiratory component.

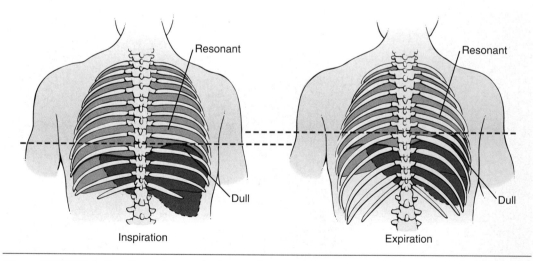

Figure 13-17 Technique for evaluating diaphragmatic motion. During inspiration (*left*), percussion in the right seventh posterior interspace at the midscapular line would be resonant as a result of the presence of the underlying lung. During expiration (*right*), the liver and diaphragm move up. Percussion in the same area would now be dull, owing to the presence of the underlying liver.

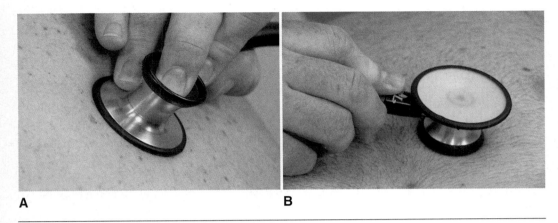

Figure 13-18 Placement of stethoscope heads. *A,* Correct placement of the diaphragm. Notice that the head is applied tightly to the skin. *B,* Placement of the bell. Notice that the bell is applied lightly to the skin.

These sounds are normally heard when the examiner listens over the manubrium. A definite pause is heard between the two phases.

Bronchovesicular breath sounds are a mixture of bronchial and vesicular sounds. The inspiratory and expiratory components are equal in length. They are normally heard only in the first and second interspaces anteriorly and between the scapulae posteriorly. This is the area overlying the carina and mainstem bronchi.

Vesicular breath sounds are the soft, low-pitched sounds heard over most of the lung fields. The inspiratory component is much longer than the expiratory component, which is also much softer and frequently inaudible.

The four types of breath sounds are illustrated and summarized in Figure 13-19.

Characteristic	Tracheal	Bronchial	Bronchovesicular	Vesicular
Intensity	Very loud	Loud	Moderate	Soft
Pitch	Very high	High	Moderate	Low
I:E ratio*	1:1	1:3	1:1	3:1
Description	Harsh	Tubular	Rustling but tubular	Gentle rustling
Normal locations	Extrathoracic trachea	Manubrium	Over mainstem bronchi	Most of peripheral lung

*Ratio of duration of inspiration to that of expiration.

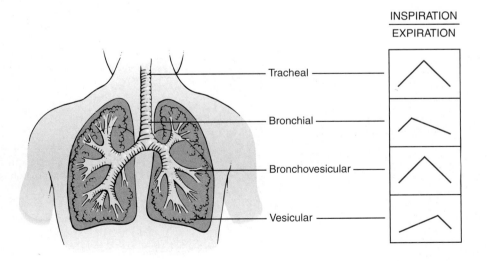

Figure 13-19 Characteristics of breath sounds.

Auscultate the Posterior Chest

Auscultation should be performed in a quiet environment. The patient is asked to breathe in and out through the mouth. The examiner should concentrate first on the length of inspiration and then on expiration. Very soft breath sounds are referred to as *distant.* Distant breath sounds are commonly found in patients with hyperinflated lungs, as in emphysema.

The examination should proceed from side to side and from top to bottom, comparing one side with the other. The positions are illustrated in Figure 13-16. Because most breath sounds are high-pitched, the diaphragm is used to evaluate lung sounds.

The Anterior Chest

The examiner should now move in front of the patient. The first part of the examination of the anterior chest is performed with the patient seated, after which the patient is asked to lie down.

Evaluate the Position of the Trachea

The examiner can determine the position of the trachea by placing his or her right index finger in the patient's suprasternal notch and moving slightly lateral to feel the location of the trachea. The examiner repeats this technique, moving the finger from the suprasternal notch to the other side. The space between the trachea and the clavicle should be equal on each side. A shift of the mediastinum can displace the trachea to one side. This technique is demonstrated in Figure 13-20.

Look at the patient pictured in Figure 13-21. Notice that the trachea is markedly displaced to the right in this very cachectic woman. The diagnosis of a mass either pushing or pulling the trachea to the right is suggested.

Now ask the patient to lie on his or her back for the rest of the examination of the anterior chest. The patient's arms are at the sides. If the patient is a woman, either have her elevate her breasts herself or displace them yourself as necessary during palpation, percussion, and auscultation. These examinations should not be performed over breast tissue.

Evaluate Tactile Fremitus

Tactile fremitus is assessed in the supraclavicular fossae and in alternate anterior interspaces, beginning at the clavicle. The techniques for evaluating tactile fremitus have already been discussed. Proceed from the supraclavicular fossae downward, comparing one side with the other.

Percuss the Anterior Chest

Percussion of the anterior chest includes the supraclavicular fossae, the axillae, and the anterior interspaces, as illustrated in Figure 13-22. The percussion note on one side is always compared with that elicited in the corresponding position on the other side. Dullness may be noted in the third to fifth intercostal spaces to the left of the sternum, which is related to the presence of the heart. Percuss high in the axilla because the upper lobes are best evaluated at these positions. Axillary percussion is sometimes easier to perform while the patient is sitting.

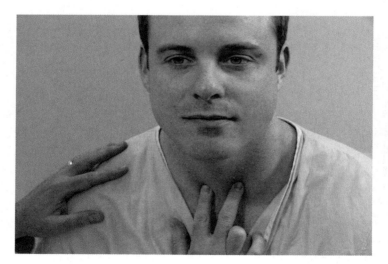

Figure 13-20 Technique for determining the position of the trachea.

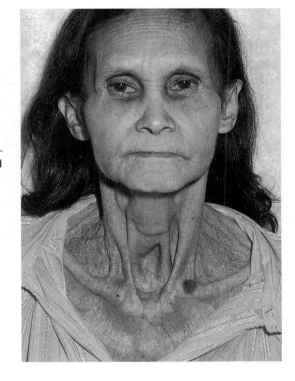

Figure 13-21 Tracheal deviation. Note the marked tracheal deviation to the patient's right.

Auscultate the Anterior Chest

Auscultation of the anterior chest is performed in the supraclavicular fossae, the axillae, and the anterior chest interspaces, as illustrated in Figure 13-22. The techniques of auscultation have already been discussed. The breath sounds of one side are compared with the breath sounds heard in the corresponding position on the other side.

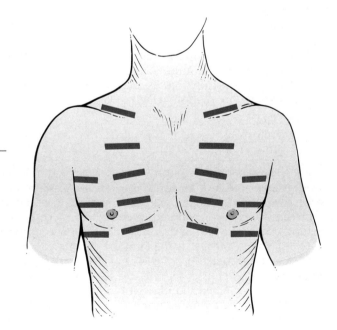

Figure 13-22 Locations on the anterior chest for percussion and auscultation.

Table 13-6 Timing of Common Inspiratory Crackles

Disease	Early Crackle	Late Crackle
Congestive heart failure	Very common	Common
Obstructive lung disease	Present	Absent
Interstitial fibrosis	Absent	Present
Pneumonia	Absent	Present

Clinicopathologic Correlations

In addition to the normal breath sounds discussed, other lung sounds may be produced in abnormal clinical states. These abnormal sounds heard during auscultation are called *adventitious* sounds. Adventitious sounds include the following:

- Crackles
- Wheezes
- Rhonchi
- Pleural rubs

Crackles are short, discontinuous, nonmusical sounds heard mostly during inspiration. Also known as *rales* or *crepitation*, crackles are caused by the opening of collapsed distal airways and alveoli. A sudden equalization of pressure seems to result in a crackle. Coarser crackles are related to larger airways. Crackles are likened to the sound made by rubbing hair next to the ear or the sound made when Velcro patches are pulled apart. They may be described as early or late, depending on when they are heard during inspiration. The timing of common inspiratory crackles is summarized in Table 13-6. The most common causes of crackles are pulmonary edema, congestive heart failure, and pulmonary fibrosis.

Wheezes are continuous, musical, high-pitched sounds heard mostly during expiration. They are produced by airflow through narrowed bronchi. This narrowing may be caused by swelling, secretions, spasm, tumor, or foreign body. Wheezes are commonly associated with the bronchospasm of asthma.

Rhonchi are lower pitched, more sonorous lung sounds. They are believed to be more common with transient mucus plugging and poor movement of airway secretions.

A *pleural rub* is a grating sound produced by motion of the pleura, which is impeded by frictional resistance. It is best heard at the end of inspiration and at the beginning of expiration. The sound of a pleural rub is like the sound of creaking leather. Pleural rubs are heard when pleural surfaces are roughened or thickened by inflammatory or neoplastic cells or by fibrin deposits.

All the adventitious sounds should be described with regard to their location, timing, and intensity.

There is much confusion regarding the terminology of adventitious sounds. Table 13-7 summarizes the adventitious sounds.

On occasion, breath sounds are transmitted abnormally. This may result in auscultatory changes known by the following terms:

- Egophony
- Whispered pectoriloquy
- Bronchophony

Egophony (egobronchophony) is said to be present when the spoken word heard through the lungs is increased in intensity and takes on a nasal or bleating quality. The patient is asked to say "eeee" while the examiner listens to an area in which consolidation is suspected. If egophony is present, the "eeee" will be heard as "aaaah" This "e-to-a" change is seen in consolidation of lung tissue. The area of compressed lung above a pleural effusion often produces egophony.

Whispered pectoriloquy is the term for the intensification of the whispered word heard in the presence of consolidation of the lung. The patient is instructed to whisper, "one-two-three" while the examiner listens to the area suspected of having consolidation. Normally, whispering produces high-pitched sounds that tend to be filtered out by the lungs. Little or nothing may be heard when the examiner listens to a normal chest. However, if consolidation is present, the transmission of the spoken words is increased, and the words are clearly heard.

Table 13-7 Adventitious Sounds

Recommended Term	Older Term	Mechanism	Causes
Crackle	Rale Crepitation	Excess airway secretions	Bronchitis, respiratory infections, pulmonary edema, atelectasis, fibrosis, congestive heart failure
Wheeze	Sibilant rale Musical rale Sonorous rale Low-pitched wheeze	Rapid airflow through obstructed airway	Asthma, pulmonary edema, bronchitis, congestive heart failure
Rhonchus		Transient airway plugging	Bronchitis
Pleural rub		Inflammation of the pleura	Pneumonia, pulmonary infarction

Bronchophony is the increased transmission of spoken words heard in the presence of consolidation of the lungs. The patient is asked to say, "ninety-nine" while the examiner listens to the chest. If bronchophony is present, the words are transmitted more loudly than normally.

One of the most important principles concerning the examination of the chest is to correlate the findings of percussion, palpation, and auscultation. Dullness, crackles, increased breath sounds, and increased tactile fremitus are suggestive of consolidation. Dullness, decreased breath sounds, and decreased tactile fremitus are suggestive of a pleural effusion.

Many physical signs are associated with obstructive lung disease. These include impaired breath sounds, barrel chest, decreased chest expansion, impaired cardiac dullness, use of accessory muscles, absent cardiac impulse, cyanosis, and diminished diaphragmatic excursion. Although all these are important physical findings, the first three have the greatest intrinsic value as diagnostic tools.

Table 13-8 lists some of the common causes of dyspnea and their associated symptoms. Table 13-9 summarizes some important manifestations of common pulmonary conditions.

Table 13-8 Common Conditions Associated with Dyspnea

Condition	Dyspnea	Other Symptoms
Asthma	Episodic; symptom free between attacks	Wheezing, chest pain, productive cough
Pulmonary edema	Abrupt	Tachypnea, cough, orthopnea, and paroxysmal nocturnal dyspnea with chronic state
Pulmonary fibrosis	Progressive	Tachypnea, dry cough
Pneumonia	Exertional, insidious onset	Productive cough, pleuritic pain
Pneumothorax	Sudden, moderate to severe	Sudden pleuritic pain
Emphysema	Insidious onset, severe	Cough as disease progresses
Chronic bronchitis	As disease progresses and with infection	Chronic, productive cough
Obesity	Exertional	

Table 13-9 Differentiation of Common Pulmonary Conditions

Condition	Vital Signs	Findings			
		Inspection	**Palpation**	**Percussion**	**Auscultation**
Asthma*	Tachypnea; tachycardia	Dyspnea; use of accessory muscles; possible cyanosis; hyperinflation	Often normal; decreased fremitus	Often normal; hyperresonant; low diaphragm	Prolonged expiration; wheezes; decreased lung sounds
Emphysema	Stable	Increased anteroposterior diameter; use of muscles; thin individual	Decreased tactile fremitus	Increased resonance; decreased excursion of diaphragm	Decreased lung sounds; decreased vocal fremitus
Chronic bronchitis	Tachycardia	Possible cyanosis; patients tend to be short and stocky	Often normal	Often normal	Early crackles; rhonchi
Pneumonia	Tachycardia; fever; tachypnea	Possible cyanosis; possible splinting on affected side	Increased tactile fremitus	Dullness	Late crackles; bronchial breath sounds[†]
Pulmonary embolism	Tachycardia; fever; tachypnea	Often normal	Usually normal	Usually normal	Usually normal
Pulmonary edema	Tachycardia; tachypnea	Possible signs of elevated right-sided heart pressures[‡]	Often normal	Often normal	Early crackles; wheezes
Pneumothorax	Tachypnea; tachycardia	Often normal; lag on affected side	Absent fremitus; trachea may be shifted to other side	Hyperresonant	Absent breath sounds
Pleural effusion	Tachypnea; tachycardia	Often normal; lag on affected side	Decreased fremitus; trachea shifted to other side	Dullness	Absent breath sounds
Atelectasis	Tachypnea	Often normal; lag on affected side	Decreased fremitus; trachea shifted to same side	Dullness	Absent breath sounds
Acute respiratory distress syndrome	Tachycardia; tachypnea	Use of accessory muscles; cyanosis	Usually normal	Often normal	Normal initially; cackles and decreased lung sounds, late

*The physical findings in asthma are often not reliable in predicting its severity.
[†]Bronchophony, whispered pectoriloquy, and egophony are also often present.
[‡]Elevated jugular venous distention, pedal edema, and hepatomegaly.

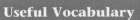

Useful Vocabulary

Listed here are the specific roots that are important for understanding the terminology related to diseases of the chest.

Root	Pertaining to	Example	Definition
bronch(o)-	bronchus	**bronch**itis	Inflammation of the bronchus
-capnia	carbon dioxide	hyper**capnia**	Excessive carbon dioxide in the blood
chondro-	cartilage	**chrondr**oma	Hyperplastic growth of cartilage
costo-	ribs	**costo**chondritis	Inflammation of the rib cartilage
muc(o)-	mucus	**muco**lytic	Agent that dissolves mucus
phren(o)-	diaphragm	**phreno**hepatic	Pertaining to the diaphragm and liver
pleur(o)-	pleura	**pleu**ritic	Pertaining to inflammation of the pleura
-pne(o)-	breath	dys**pnea**	Difficulty in breathing; shortness of breath
pneumo-	lungs	**pneumo**nectomy	Surgical removal of lung tissue
spiro-	to breathe	**spiro**gram	A tracing of respiratory movements
-stern(o)-	sternum	costo**stern**al	Pertaining to the ribs and sternum

Writing Up the Physical Examination

Listed here are examples of the write-up for the examination of the chest.

- The trachea is midline. The chest is normal in appearance. Palpation is normal. The chest is clear to percussion and auscultation.
- The trachea is midline. A mild pectus excavatum is present. There is increased tactile fremitus at the left posterior chest, up one third from the base. This area is also dull to percussion. Bronchial breath sounds and crackles are present in the area of dullness. Bronchophony and whispered pectoriloquy are also present in this area.
- The trachea is deviated to the left. The chest structure is within normal limits. There is decreased tactile fremitus on the right chest posteriorly, up three fourths from the base. The percussion note is dull in the area of decreased fremitus. There are no breath sounds heard in this area. An area of egophony is present above the area of dullness.
- The trachea is midline. Tactile fremitus is normal, as is percussion. Auscultation reveals normal breath sounds with bilateral basilar crackles.

Bibliography

Brody JS: The Lung: Molecular Basis of Disease. Philadelphia, WB Saunders, 1998.

Cancer Facts & Figures. Atlanta, American Cancer Society, 2007.

Cancer Trends Progress Report—2007 Update. Bethesda, MD, National Cancer Institute, National Institutes of Health, U.S. Department of Health and Human Services, December 2007.

Caples SM, Gami AS, Somers VK: Obstructive sleep apnea. Ann Intern Med 142:187, 2005.

DevCan: Probability of developing or dying of cancer software, version 5.1. Statistical Research and Applications Branch, National Cancer Institute, 2003. Available at: *http://srab.cancer.gov/devcan*; accessed June 6, 2008.

Espey DK, Wu XC, Swan J, et al: Annual report to the nation on the status of cancer, 1975–2004, featuring cancer in American Indians and Alaska Natives. Cancer 110:2119, 2007.

Millman RP: Do you ever take a sleep history? Ann Intern Med 131:535, 1999.

Morgan WKC, Seaton A: Occupational Lung Diseases. Philadelphia, WB Saunders, 1995.

Netzer NC, Stoohs RA, Netzer CM, et al: Using the Berlin questionnaire to identify patients at risk for the sleep apnea syndrome. Ann Intern Med 131:485, 1999.

Ries LAG, Melbert D, Krapcho M, et al: SEER Cancer Statistics Review, 1975–2004 [based on November 2006 Surveillance Epidemiology and End Results (SEER) data submission]. Bethesda, Md, National Cancer Institute. Available at: *http://seer.cancer.gov/csr/1975_2004/*; accessed June 9, 2007.

Ritz HJ: Pinning down the cause of chronic cough. JAAPA 17:27, 2004.

Sargent JD, DiFranza JR: Tobacco control for clinicians who treat adolescents. CA Cancer J Clin 53:102, 2003.

SEER Incidence 1973–1996, Surveillance, Epidemiology, and End Results Program. Bethesda, Md, Division of Cancer Control and Population Sciences, National Cancer Institute, 2000.

Stubbing DG, Mathur PN, Roberts RS: Some physical signs in patients with chronic airway obstruction. Am Rev Respir Dis 125:549, 1982.

Zackon H: Pulmonary Differential Diagnosis. Philadelphia, WB Saunders, 2000.

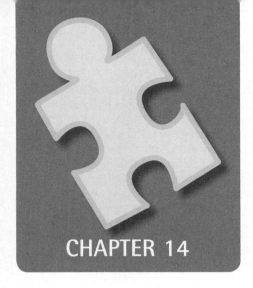

CHAPTER 14

The Heart

... For it is the heart by whose virtue and pulse the blood is moved, perfected, made apt to nourish and is preserved from corruption and coagulation. ... It is indeed the fountain of life, the source of all action.

William Harvey (1578–1657)

General Considerations

The heart does not rest for more than a fraction of a second at a time. During a lifetime, it contracts more than 4 billion times. To support this active state, the coronary arteries supply more than 10 million liters of blood to the myocardium and more than 200 million liters to the systemic circulation. Cardiac output can vary under physiologic conditions from 3 to 30 L/minute, and regional blood flow can vary by 200%. This wide range occurs without any loss of efficiency in the normal state.

Diseases of the heart are common. The major disease categories are coronary heart disease (CHD), hypertension, rheumatic heart disease, bacterial endocarditis, and congenital heart disease. The clinical consequences of these conditions are usually serious.

Nearly 65 million Americans have one or more forms of cardiovascular disease (CVD), and nearly 1 million die from such conditions each year. Although CVD death rates in the United States are declining, the illness is still the leading cause of death, by far, in the nation. It accounts for approximately 38.5% of all deaths, or 1 of every 2.6 deaths. CVD kills more Americans than the next seven causes combined, including cancer. CHD, stroke, high blood pressure, and congestive heart failure have been the leading causes of death in the United States every year since 1900, with the exception of 1918, when there was a worldwide flu pandemic. The National Center for Health Statistics reported that in 2004, there were 79,400,000 Americans with one or more forms of CVD. There are 72 million Americans with high blood pressure, 15.8 million with CHD, and 5.7 million who had suffered a stroke. There are 15.8 million people alive today who have a history of heart attack, angina pectoris, or both: about 8.5 million male patients and 7.3 million female patients. The 2004 death rates from CVD were 335.7 white male patients, 448.9 African-American male patients, 239.3 white female patients, and 331.6 African-American female patients.*

CHD is the leading cause of death in the United States. In 2004, there were 871,500 deaths from CVD (36.3% of all deaths), including 452,300 deaths related to ischemic heart disease, equivalent to 1 death every 33 seconds. By the age of 60 years, nearly one per five American

---

*Death rates are per 100,000 population. For these rates, the year 2000 standard U.S. population is used as the base for age adjustment.

men has symptomatic CHD caused by coronary atherosclerosis. The 2004 death rates from CHD were 194.4 white male patients, 222.2 black African-American male patients, 115.4 white female patients, and 148.6 African-American female patients.* Autopsy studies during the Korean War showed that 40% of all American soldiers who were killed in their early 20s had atheromatous involvement of one or more of their coronary arteries.

CHD is also the leading cause of mortality in women in the United States and is responsible for the deaths of nearly 250,000 women yearly. It claims more lives than the next 14 causes of death combined. In women, CHD is highly age dependent; one per eight or nine women from the ages of 45 to 64 years has clinical evidence of CHD, whereas one per three women older than 65 years is affected. Among women from the ages of 55 to 64 years with clinically significant CHD, 36% are disabled by its symptoms; this disability increases to 55% for women older than 75 years. Numerous studies have shown that the mortality rate from a myocardial infarction is worse for women than for men, although more men die suddenly from myocardial infarction. The lifetime risk of death from CHD in women is 31%; the lifetime risk of death from breast cancer is 2.8%.

In 2004 in the United States, 15.8 million people had suffered a myocardial infarction, angina pectoris, or both. About 325,000 people per year die of a myocardial infarction in the emergency department or without ever reaching a medical facility. In 2007, an estimated 1.2 million Americans had a new or recurrent myocardial infarction. Unlike other forms of cardiac disease, CHD may be severe and life-threatening despite normal results on physical examination, electrocardiography, and chest radiography.

The good news, however, is that from 1994 to 2004, the death rate from CHD declined 33%, perhaps because of better control of hypertension, better cholesterol management, and cigarette smoking cessation.

Systemic arterial hypertension affects approximately 20% of the American population. It is a major risk factor for coronary artery disease, as well as a prime cause of congestive heart failure and strokes. It has been well established that among patients with higher systolic or diastolic pressures, there is a greater incidence of morbidity and mortality.

Since the implementation of antibiotic therapy, the incidence of rheumatic heart disease has been decreasing in the more affluent countries. In 1998, there were 4792 deaths related to rheumatic fever and rheumatic heart disease. In areas of overcrowding and in less affluent areas, rheumatic fever and the valvular heart disease that results from it are still a major cause of cardiac morbidity and mortality.

Bacterial endocarditis remains a significant medical problem despite the wide use of antibiotics. The increasing number of cases is related to intravenous use of street drugs. The existence of endocarditis is often not suspected in a patient until serious sequelae develop. In addition to causing valvular damage, the persistent bacteremia can spread to the brain, myocardium, spleen, kidneys, and other sites in the body.

The incidence of congenital heart disease averages 5 per 1000 live births. If other commonly found congenital cardiovascular conditions, such as bicuspid aortic valve and mitral valve prolapse, are included, the incidence approaches 1 per 100 live births.

It is clear that the magnitude of cardiac disease is enormous, and the cost of the morbidity and mortality is directly proportional. In 2005, the cost of heart disease and stroke in the United States exceeded $394 billion: $242 billion for health-care expenditures and $152 billion for lost productivity resulting from death and disability. In 2005, $60 billion in health-care spending was attributed to high blood pressure alone.

Structure and Physiology

The principal function of the cardiovascular system is to deliver nutrients to and remove metabolites from every cell in the body. This metabolic exchange system is produced by a high-pressure delivery system, an area of exchange, and a low-pressure return system. The high-pressure delivery system is the *left* side of the heart and *arteries*, and the low-pressure return system includes the *veins* and the *right* side of the heart. The circulation of blood through the heart is illustrated in Figure 14-1.

---

*Death rates are per 100,000 population. For these rates, the year 2000 standard U.S. population is used as the base for age adjustment.

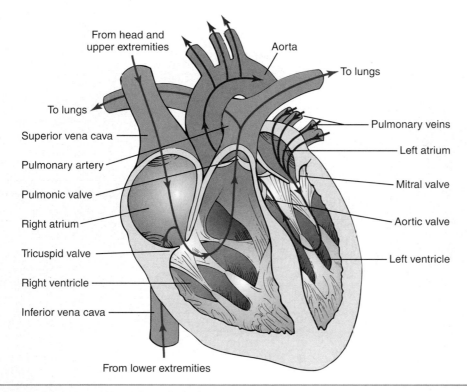

From head and
upper extremities

Aorta

To lungs

To lungs

Superior vena cava

Pulmonary artery

Pulmonic valve

Right atrium

Tricuspid valve

Right ventricle

Inferior vena cava

Pulmonary veins

Left atrium

Mitral valve

Aortic valve

Left ventricle

From lower extremities

Figure 14-1 Circulation of blood through the heart.

The heart is enveloped by a thin *pericardial sac*. The bottom of this sac is adherent to the diaphragm, and the top is loosely attached to the upper portion of the sternum. The *visceral* pericardium is the epicardial, or outermost, layer of cells of the heart. The *parietal* pericardium is the outer sac. Between these two surfaces, a small amount of pericardial fluid in the pericardial sac provides a lubricating interface for the constantly moving heart. The parietal pericardium is innervated by the phrenic nerve, which contains pain fibers. The visceral pericardium is insensitive to pain.

The synchronous contraction of the heart results from the conduction of impulses generated by the *sinoatrial (SA) node* and propagated through the *conduction system*. The SA node is located at the juncture of the superior vena cava and the right atrium. The SA impulse spreads from its point of origin concentrically. When the impulse reaches the *atrioventricular (AV) node*, in the interatrial septum near the entrance of the coronary sinus, the impulse is slowed. It is then transmitted to the specialized conducting tissue known as the *right* and *left bundle branches*, which conduct the impulse to the specialized conducting pathways in the ventricles, *Purkinje's fibers*. The impulse spreads from the endocardial to the epicardial surface of the heart. These conducting pathways are illustrated in Figure 14-2.

The heart is innervated extensively by branches of the autonomic nervous system. Both sympathetic and parasympathetic fibers are present in the SA and atrioventricular nodes. The atrial muscle is also innervated by both types of fibers. The ventricular musculature is innervated predominantly by the sympathetic nervous system.

The *parasympathetic fibers* travel along the vagus, or 10th cranial, nerve. The *sympathetic fibers* descend in the spinal cord to the level of T1 to T5, where they emerge through the ventral roots to form a synapse in the thoracic and cervical *sympathetic ganglia*. The postganglionic fibers travel through the cervical *cardiac nerves* to join the parasympathetic fibers in forming the *cardiac plexus*, which is located near the aortic arch and the tracheal bifurcation. These neural pathways are illustrated in Figure 14-3.

Sympathetic stimulation by *norepinephrine* produces marked increases in heart rate and contractility. Parasympathetic stimulation mediated by *acetylcholine* slows the heart rate and decreases contractility.

In addition, several receptor sites provide circulatory information to the *medullary cardiovascular center* in the brain. This center has cardioexcitatory and cardioinhibitory areas that regulate the neural output to the sympathetic and parasympathetic fibers. *Stretch receptors* in

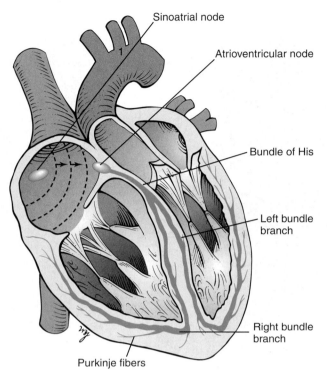

Sinoatrial node

Atrioventricular node

Bundle of His

Figure 14-2 Conducting pathways of the heart.

Left bundle branch

Right bundle branch

Purkinje fibers

the aortic arch and in the carotid sinus monitor blood pressure. These *baroreceptors* respond to a decrease in blood pressure by decreasing their impulses to the medullary center. The center senses this decreased activity and increases its sympathetic efferent activity and decreases its parasympathetic efferent activity. The net result is to increase the heart rate and contractility. An increase in blood pressure causes an increase in afferent activity to the center, and the opposite changes occur.

To describe physical signs, the examiner must be able to identify the important surface topographic landmarks. Chapter 13, The Chest, describes the major areas. These areas should be reviewed at this time.

The surface projection of the heart and great vessels is illustrated in Figure 14-4. Most of the anterior cardiac surface is the right ventricle. The right atrium forms a narrow border from the third to the fifth ribs to the right of the sternum. The left ventricle lies to the left and behind the right ventricle. The left ventricular *apex* is normally in the *fifth intercostal space* at the *midclavicular line*. This location is commonly written as *5ICS-MCL*. The *apical impulse* is called the *point of maximum impulse* (PMI). The other chambers and vessels of the heart are usually not identifiable on examination.

The four classic *auscultatory areas* correspond to points over the precordium, at which events originating at each valve are best heard. The areas are not necessarily related to the anatomic position of the valve, nor are all sounds heard in the area directly produced by the valve for which the area is named. The normal areas are as follows:

Aortic: Second intercostal space, right sternal border (2ICS-RSB)

Pulmonic: Second intercostal space, left sternal border (2ICS-LSB)

Tricuspid: Left lower sternal border (LLSB)

Mitral: Cardiac apex (5ICS-MCL)

In addition to these four areas, the third left intercostal space, known as *Erb's point*, is frequently the area at which pulmonic or aortic sounds are best heard. The five areas are illustrated in Figure 14-5. The second intercostal space to the right and left of the sternum is called the *base*.

Remember that the left atrium is the most posterior portion of the heart. When the left atrium enlarges, it extends posteriorly and to the right.

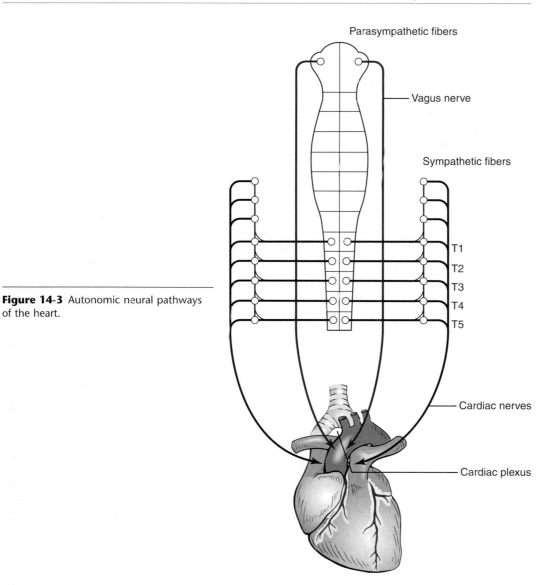

Figure 14-3 Autonomic neural pathways of the heart.

The Cardiac Cycle

To understand the cardiac cycle, the motion of the valves and the pressures within the chambers should be reviewed. The interrelationships of valve motion are critically important and must be understood. Only with the knowledge of these cycles can the clinician fully comprehend the cardiac physical examination and heart sounds. The pressure tracings and valve motions are shown in Figure 14-6.

Normally, only the closing of the heart valves can be heard. The closure of the *atrioventricular valves*, the tricuspid and the mitral, produces the *first heart sound* (S_1). The closure of the *semilunar valves*, the aortic and the pulmonic, produces the *second heart sound* (S_2).

The opening of the valves can be heard only if they are damaged. When an atrioventricular valve is narrowed, or *stenotic*, the opening of the valve may be heard and is termed an *opening snap*. If a semilunar valve is stenotic, the opening may be heard and is termed an *ejection click*. It should be noted that in Figure 14-6, the term *opening snap* refers to the opening of a pathologically damaged atrioventricular valve that occurs during *diastole*, and the term *ejection click* refers to the opening of a damaged semilunar valve that occurs during *systole*.

The sequence of the opening and closing of the four valves is as follows:

$$\mathbf{MV_c TV_c PV_o AV_o AV_c PV_c TV_o MV_o}$$

in which MV = mitral valve, TV = tricuspid valve, PV = pulmonic valve, AV = aortic valve, c = closing, and o = opening.

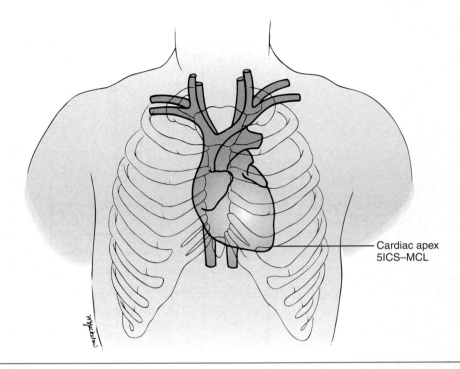

Cardiac apex
5ICS–MCL

Figure 14-4 Surface topography of the heart. 5ICS-MCL, fifth intercostal space at the midclavicular line.

The mitral component of S_1 occurs as a result of the closure of the mitral valve when the left ventricular pressure rises above the left atrial pressure; it is written M_1. The tricuspid component of S_1 occurs as a result of closure of the tricuspid valve when right ventricular pressure rises above right atrial pressure; it is written T_1.

The time between the closure of the atrioventricular valves and the opening of the semilunar valves is the period of *isovolumetric contraction*. When the pressure in the right ventricle exceeds the diastolic pressure in the pulmonary artery, the pulmonic valve opens. A pulmonic

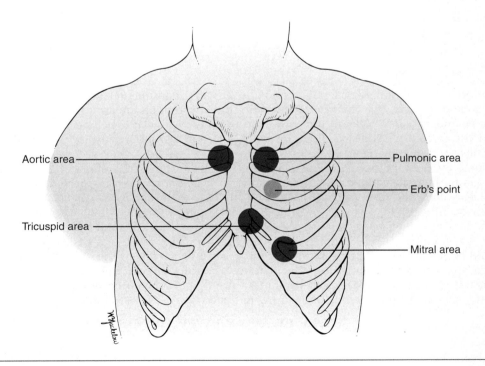

Aortic area
Tricuspid area

Pulmonic area
Erb's point
Mitral area

Figure 14-5 Auscultatory areas.

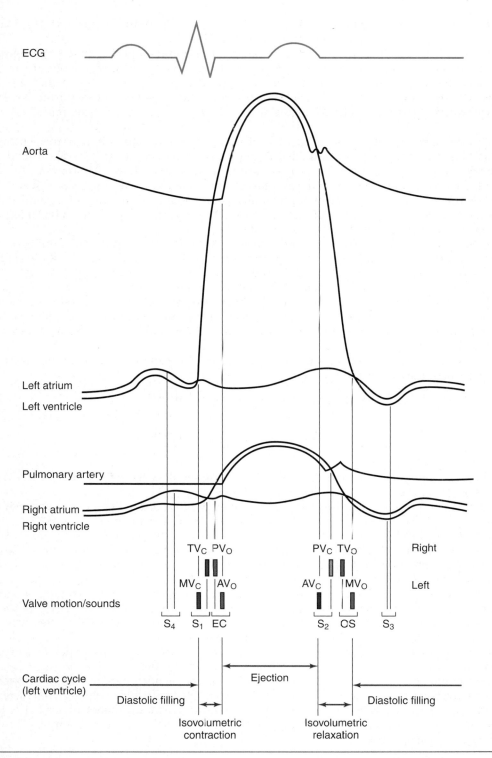

Figure 14-6 The cardiac cycle. TV_c, tricuspid valve closing; PV_o, pulmonic valve opening; MV_c, mitral valve closing; AV_o, aortic valve opening; EC, ejection click; OS, opening snap; S_1 to S_4, first to fourth heart sounds.

ejection click is heard at this time if the pulmonic valve is stenotic. When the pressure in the left ventricle exceeds the diastolic pressure in the aorta, the aortic valve opens. An aortic ejection click is heard at this time if the aortic valve is stenotic.

The time between the opening and the closing of the semilunar valves is the systolic period of *ejection*. The point at which ejection is completed and the aortic and left ventricular curves separate is called the *incisura*, or *dicrotic notch*, and is simultaneous with the aortic component of S_2, or closure of the aortic valve; this is written A_2. The pulmonic valve closes at the point when the right ventricular pressure falls below the pulmonary diastolic pressure. This is the pulmonic component of S_2 and is commonly written P_2.

The time between the closure of the semilunar valves and the opening of the atrioventricular valves is called *isovolumetric relaxation*. The tricuspid valve opens when the pressure in the right atrium exceeds right ventricular pressure. A tricuspid opening snap may be heard if the tricuspid valve is stenotic. The mitral valve opens when the pressure in the left atrium exceeds left ventricular pressure. A mitral opening snap may occur at this time if the mitral valve is stenotic.

With the opening of the atrioventricular valves, the period of rapid filling of the ventricles occurs. Approximately 80% of ventricular filling occurs at this point. At the end of the rapid filling period, a *third heart sound* (S_3) may be heard. An S_3 occurs 120 to 170 msec after S_2. This period is approximately the same time as it takes to say "me too." The "me" is the S_2, and the "too" is the S_3. An S_3 is normal in children and young adults. When present in individuals older than 30 years, it signifies a volume overload to the ventricle. Regurgitant valvular lesions and congestive heart failure may be responsible.

At the end of diastole, *atrial contraction* and the additional 20% of ventricular filling occur. A *fourth heart sound* (S_4) may be heard. The interval from the S_4 to the S_1 is approximately the time it takes to say "middle." The "mid-" is the S_4, and the "-dle" is the S_1. Note that the "mid" is much softer than the "dle," which is quite similar to the S_4-S_1 cadence. An S_4 is normal in children and young adults. When present in individuals older than 30 years, it is indicative of a *noncompliant*, or "stiff," ventricle. Pressure overload on a ventricle causes concentric hypertrophy, which produces a noncompliant ventricle. In addition, CHD is a major cause of a stiff ventricle.

Two useful mnemonics for remembering the cadence and pathophysiology of the third and fourth heart sounds are as follows:

SLOSH′-ing-in   SLOSH′-ing-in   SLOSH′-ing-in
S_1 S_2 S_3 S_1 S_2 S_3 S_1 S_2 S_3

a-STIFF′-wall   a-STIFF′-wall   a-STIFF′-wall
S_4 S_1 S_2 S_4 S_1 S_2 S_4 S_1 S_2

The presence of an S_3 or an S_4 creates a cadence resembling the gallop of a horse. These sounds are therefore called *gallop* sounds or rhythms.

The first heart sound is loudest at the cardiac apex. *Splitting* of the first heart sound may be heard in the tricuspid area. The second heart sound is loudest at the base.

The terms A_2 and P_2 indicate the aortic component and the pulmonic component of S_2, respectively. A_2 normally precedes P_2, meaning that the aortic valve closes before the pulmonic valve. With inspiration, the intrathoracic pressure lowers. This causes more blood to be drawn from the superior and inferior venae cavae into the right chambers of the heart. The right ventricle enlarges, and it takes longer for all the blood to be ejected into the pulmonary artery; thus the pulmonic valve stays open longer. P_2 occurs later in inspiration, and the split between A_2 and P_2 is widened during inspiration in comparison with expiration. This is the cause of *physiologic splitting* of S_2, which is diagrammed in Figure 14-7.

The blood in the right ventricle is then pumped into the large-capacitance bed of the lungs. Therefore, the return of blood from the lungs to the left side of the heart is decreased, and the left atrium and left ventricle become smaller. Atrial receptors trigger a reflex tachycardia that compensates for the decreased left ventricular volume. This increase in heart rate with inspiration is termed *sinus arrhythmia*. It is a misnomer because it is not really an arrhythmia but a normal physiologic response to a decreased left ventricular volume during inspiration.

The Arterial Pulse

The arterial pulse is produced by the ejection of blood into the aorta. The normal configuration of the pulse consists of a smooth and rapid upstroke that begins about 80 msec after the first component of S_1. There is sometimes a slight notch in the arterial pulsation toward the end of the rapid ejection period. This is called the *anacrotic notch*. The peak of the pulse is smooth and dome-shaped and occurs about 100 msec after the onset of the pulse. The descent from the peak is less steep. There is a gradual descent to the dicrotic notch, which represents the closure of the aortic valve. The contour and volume of the arterial pulse are determined by several factors, including the left ventricular stroke volume, the ejection velocity, the relative

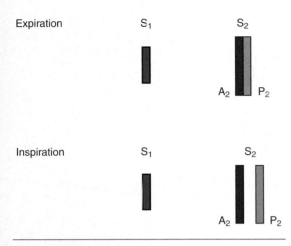

Expiration S_1 S_2

A_2 P_2

Inspiration S_1 S_2

A_2 P_2

Figure 14-7 Physiologic splitting of the second heart sound.

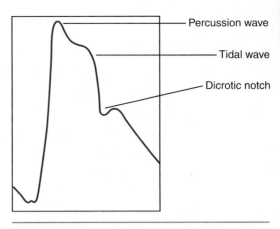

— Percussion wave

— Tidal wave

— Dicrotic notch

Figure 14-8 The arterial pulse.

compliance and capacity of the arteries, and the pressure waves that result from the antegrade flow of blood. Figure 14-8 illustrates a characteristic arterial pulse.

As the arterial pulse travels to the periphery, there are several changes. The initial upstroke becomes steeper, the systolic peak is higher, and the anacrotic notch becomes less evident. In addition, the dicrotic notch occurs later in the peripheral pulse, approximately 300 msec after the onset of the pulse. The positive wave that follows the dicrotic notch is called the *dicrotic wave*.

Commonly, two waves may be present in the arterial pulse, which precedes the dicrotic notch. The *percussion wave* is the earlier wave and is associated with the rate of flow in the artery. The percussion wave occurs during peak velocity of flow. The *tidal wave* is the second wave, is related to pressure in the vessel, and occurs during peak systolic pressure. The tidal wave is usually smaller than the percussion wave, but it may be increased in hypertensive or elderly patients.

Blood Pressure

Arterial blood pressure is the lateral pressure exerted by a column of blood against the arterial wall. It is the result of cardiac output and peripheral vascular resistance. Blood pressure depends on the volume of blood ejected, its velocity, the distensibility of the arterial wall, the viscosity of the blood, and the pressure within the vessel after the last ejection.

Systolic blood pressure is the peak pressure in the arteries. It is regulated by the stroke volume and the compliance of the blood vessels. Diastolic blood pressure is the lowest pressure in the arteries and depends on peripheral resistance. The difference in the systolic and diastolic pressures is the *pulse pressure*. Systolic blood pressure in the legs is 15 to 20 mm Hg greater than in the arms, even while the individual is lying flat. This is in part related to Poiseuille's law, according to which the total resistance of vessels connected in parallel is greater than the resistance of a single large vessel. The blood pressure in the aorta is less than the blood pressure in the branched arteries of the lower extremities.

Blood pressure varies greatly, according to the patient's degree of excitement, degree of activity, smoking habits, pain, bladder distention, and dietary pattern. There is normally an inspiratory decline of up to 10 mm Hg in systolic blood pressure during quiet respiration.

Jugular Venous Pulse

The jugular venous pulse provides direct information about the pressures in the right side of the heart because the jugular system is in direct continuity with the right atrium. During diastole, when the tricuspid valve is open, the jugular veins are continuous with the right ventricle as well. If there is no stenotic lesion at the pulmonic or mitral valves, the right ventricle indirectly monitors the pressures in the left atrium and left ventricle. The most common cause of *right*-sided heart failure is *left*-sided heart failure. Examination of the neck veins also provides information about the cardiac rhythm.

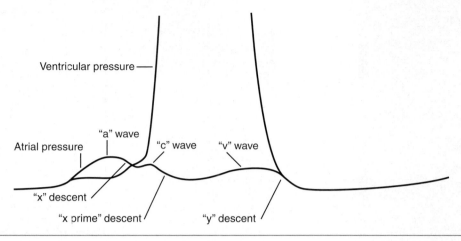

Figure 14-9 The atrial and ventricular pressure curves enlarged.

The understanding of the normal physiology is important in the consideration of the jugular venous pulsation. Figure 14-9 is an enlargement of the atrial and ventricular pressure curves in Figure 14-6.

The *"a" wave* of the jugular venous pulse is produced by right atrial contraction. When the "a" wave is timed with the electrocardiogram, it is found to occur about 90 msec after the onset of the P wave. This time delay is related to the time from electrical stimulation of the atria to atrial contraction and to the resultant wave propagated in the neck. The *"x" descent* is caused by atrial relaxation, which occurs just before ventricular contraction. This drop in right atrial pressure is terminated by the *"c" wave*. The resulting increase in right atrial pressure is caused by tricuspid valve closure secondary to right ventricular contraction. The descent of the atrioventricular valve rings, also known as the *descent of the base of the heart*, produces the next change in right atrial pressure, called the *"x prime" descent*. As the free wall of the right ventricle approaches the septum during contraction, the atrioventricular valve rings descend toward the apex as contraction progresses. This increases the size of the atrium, causing a fall in its pressure (hence the *"x prime"* descent). During ventricular systole, the right atrium begins to fill with blood returning through the venae cavae. This increase in right atrial pressure as a result of its filling produces the ascending limb of the *"v" wave*. At the end of ventricular systole, right ventricular pressure falls rapidly. When it falls below the right atrial pressure, the tricuspid valve opens. This drop in right atrial pressure produces the *"y" descent*.

Normally, only the "a" and "v" waves are visible on examination. Because the "c" wave is frequently not observed, the "x" and "x prime" descents are summated into a single "x" descent. On occasion, the later portion of the "c" wave may be enlarged by a carotid artery pulsation artifact.

Evaluation of the jugular venous pulse provides information about the level of venous pressure and the type of venous wave pattern. These are described later in the section The Jugular Venous Pulse.

Review of Specific Symptoms

The important symptoms of cardiac disease are the following:

- Chest pain
- Palpitations
- Dyspnea
- Syncope
- Fatigue
- Dependent edema
- Hemoptysis
- Cyanosis

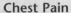

2

Chest Pain

Chest pain is probably the most important symptom of cardiac disease. It is not, however, pathognomonic for heart disease. It is well known that chest pain may result from pulmonary, intestinal, gallbladder, and musculoskeletal disorders. Ask the following questions of any patients complaining of chest pain:

"Where is the pain?"

"How long have you had the pain?"

"Do you have recurrent episodes of pain?"

"What is the duration of the pain?"

"How often do you get the pain?"

"What do you do to make it better?"

"What makes the pain worse? breathing? lying flat? moving your arms or neck?"

"How would you describe the pain: burning? pressing? crushing? dull? aching? throbbing? knifelike? sharp? constricting? sticking?"*

"Does the pain occur at rest? with exertion? after eating? when moving your arms? with emotional strain? while sleeping? during sexual intercourse?"

"Is the pain associated with shortness of breath? palpitations? nausea or vomiting? coughing? fever? coughing up blood? leg pain?"

Angina pectoris is the true symptom of CHD. Angina is commonly the consequence of hypoxia of the myocardium resulting from an imbalance of coronary supply and myocardial demand. Table 14-1 lists the characteristics that differentiate angina pectoris from the other types of chest pain.

Commonly, a patient may describe the angina by clenching the fist and placing it over the sternum. This is a pathognomonic sign of angina commonly referred to as *Levine's sign.* Figure 14-10 demonstrates this body language.

When chest pain is related to a cardiac cause, coronary atherosclerosis and aortic valvular disease are the most common ones. Table 14-2 lists some common causes of chest pain.

Palpitations

Palpitations are the uncomfortable sensations in the chest associated with a range of arrhythmias. Patients may describe palpitations as "fluttering," "skipped beats," "pounding,"

Table 14-1 Characteristics of Chest Pain*

Feature	Angina	Not Angina
Location	Retrosternal, diffuse	Left inframammary, localized
Radiation	Left arm, jaw, back	Right arm
Description	"Aching," "dull," "pressing," "squeezing," "viselike"	"Sharp," "shooting," "cutting"
Intensity	Mild to severe	Excruciating
Duration	Minutes	Seconds, hours, days
Precipitated by	Effort, emotion, eating, cold	Respiration, posture, motion
Relieved by	Rest, nitroglycerin	Nonspecific

*Angina and other chest pain may manifest in a variety of ways. The characteristics listed here are the common manifestations. This list, however, is not exhaustive and should be used only as a guide.

*In general, it is best to allow the patient to describe the character of the pain. These descriptions are provided for the interviewer to use only when the patient is unable to characterize the pain.

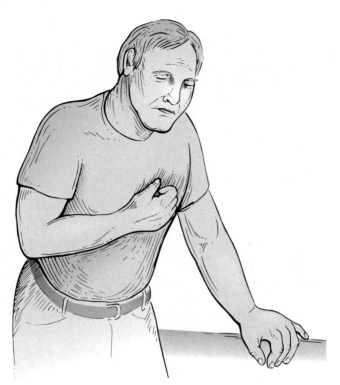

Figure 14-10 Levine's sign.

Table 14-2 Common Causes of Chest Pain

Organ System	Cause
Cardiac	Coronary artery disease
	Aortic valvular disease
	Pulmonary hypertension
	Mitral valve prolapse
	Pericarditis
	Idiopathic hypertrophic subaortic stenosis
Vascular	Dissection of the aorta
Pulmonary	Pulmonary embolism
	Pneumonia
	Pleuritis
	Pneumothorax
Musculoskeletal	Costochondritis*
	Arthritis
	Muscular spasm
	Bone tumor
Neural	Herpes zoster†
Gastrointestinal	Ulcer disease
	Bowel disease
	Hiatal hernia
	Pancreatitis
	Cholecystitis
Emotional	Anxiety
	Depression

*Tietze's syndrome, which is an inflammation of the costal cartilages.
†Shingles, which is a viral invasion of the peripheral nerves in a dermatomal distribution.

"jumping," "stopping," or "irregularity." Determine whether the patient has had similar episodes and what was done to extinguish them. Palpitations are common and do not necessarily indicate serious heart disease. Any condition in which there is an increased stroke volume, as in aortic regurgitation, may be associated with a sensation of "forceful contraction." When a patient complains of palpitations, ask the following questions:

"How long have you had palpitations?"

"Do you have recurrent attacks?" If so, *"How frequently do they occur?"*

"When did the current attack begin?"

"How long did it last?"

"What did it feel like?"

"Did any maneuvers or positions stop it?"

"Did it stop abruptly?"

"Could you count your pulse during the attack?"

"Can you tap out on the table what the rhythm was like?"

"Have you noticed palpitations after strenuous exercise? on exertion? while lying on your left side? after a meal? when tired?"

"During the palpitations, have you ever fainted? had chest pain?"

*"Was there an associated flush, headache, or sweating associated with the palpitations?"**

"Have you noticed an intolerance to heat? cold?"

"What kind of medications are you taking?"

"Do you take any medications for your lungs?"

"Are you taking any thyroid medications?"

"Have you ever been told that you had a problem with your thyroid?"

"How much tea, coffee, chocolate, or cola sodas do you consume a day?"

"Do you smoke?" If yes, *"What do you smoke?"*

"Do you drink alcoholic beverages?"

"Did you notice that after the palpitations you had to urinate?"†

In addition to primary cardiovascular causes, thyrotoxicosis, hypoglycemia, fever, anemia, pheochromocytoma, and anxiety states are commonly associated with palpitations. Hyperthyroidism is an important cause of rhythm disturbances that originate outside the cardiovascular system. Caffeine, tobacco, and drugs are also important factors in arrhythmogenicity. Sympathomimetic amines used in the treatment of bronchoconstriction are potent stimuli for arrhythmia as well. In patients with panic disorders and other anxiety states, the sensation of palpitations may occur during periods of normal rate and rhythm.

Patients who have had previous attacks of palpitations should be asked the following:

"How was your previous attack terminated?"

"How often do you get the attacks?"

"Are you able to terminate them?" If so, *"How?"*

"Have you ever been told that you have Wolff-Parkinson-White syndrome?"‡

---

*Symptoms associated with a pheochromocytoma.

†After an attack of paroxysmal atrial tachycardia, patients often have an urge to urinate. The pathophysiologic process is not well understood, but the association is present.

‡The use of this technical term is appropriate because a patient having this form of preexcitation may have been told of this condition and may recognize the name.

TABLE 14-3 Common Causes of Palpitations

Extrasystoles
Atrial premature beats*
Nodal premature beats
Ventricular premature beats[†]
Tachyarrhythmias
Paroxysmal supraventricular tachycardia
Atrial flutter
Atrial fibrillation
Multifocal atrial tachycardia
Ventricular tachycardia
Bradyarrhythmias
Heart block
Sinus arrest
Drugs
Bronchodilators
Digitalis
Antidepressants
Smoking
Caffeine
Thyrotoxicosis

*Also known as atrial premature contractions or premature atrial contractions.
[†]Also known as ventricular premature contractions or premature ventricular contractions.

Table 14-3 outlines the common causes of palpitations.

Dyspnea

The complaint of dyspnea is important. Patients report that they have "shortness of breath" or that they "can't get enough air." Dyspnea is commonly related to cardiac or pulmonary conditions. The questions relating to dyspnea are discussed in Chapter 13, The Chest. This section further delineates dyspnea as a *cardiac* symptom.

Paroxysmal nocturnal dyspnea (PND) occurs at night or when the patient is supine. This position increases the intrathoracic blood volume, and a weakened heart may be unable to handle this increased load; congestive heart failure may result. The patient is awakened about 2 hours after having fallen asleep, is markedly dyspneic, is often coughing, and may seek relief by running to a window to "get more air." Episodes of PND are relatively specific for congestive heart failure.

The symptom of PND is often associated with the symptom of *orthopnea*, the need for using more pillows on which to sleep. Inquire of all patients, "How many pillows do you need in order to sleep?" To help quantify the orthopnea, you can state, for example, "3-pillow orthopnea for the past 4 months."

Dyspnea on exertion (DOE) is usually caused by chronic congestive heart failure or severe pulmonary disease. Quantify the severity of the dyspnea by asking, "How many level blocks can you walk now?" and "How many level blocks could you walk 6 months ago?" You can now attempt to quantify the dyspnea: for example, "The patient has had 1-block DOE for the past 6 months. Before 6 months ago, the patient was able to walk 4 blocks without becoming short of breath. In addition, during the last 3 months, the patient has noted 4-pillow orthopnea."

Trepopnea is a rare form of positional dyspnea in which the dyspneic patient has less dyspnea while lying on the left or right side. The pathophysiologic process of trepopnea is not well understood.

Table 14-4 Common Causes of Dyspnea

Organ System or Condition	Cause
Cardiac	Left ventricular failure Mitral stenosis
Pulmonary	Obstructive lung disease Asthma Restrictive lung disease Pulmonary embolism Pulmonary hypertension
Emotional	Anxiety
High-altitude exposure	Decreased oxygen pressure
Anemia	Decreased oxygen-carrying capacity

Table 14-4 lists the common causes of dyspnea.

Syncope

Fainting, or syncope, is the transient loss of consciousness that results from inadequate cerebral perfusion. Ask patients what *they* mean by "fainting" or "dizziness." Syncope may have cardiac or noncardiac causes. When a patient describes fainting, ask the following questions:

"What were you doing just before you fainted?"

"Have you had recurrent fainting spells?" If so, *"How often do you have these attacks?"*

"Was the fainting sudden?"

"Did you lose consciousness?"

"In what position were you when you fainted?"

"Was the fainting preceded by any other symptom? nausea? chest pain? palpitations? confusion? numbness? hunger?"

"Did you have any warning that you were going to faint?"

"Did you have any black, tarry bowel movements after the faint?"

The activity that preceded the syncope is important because some cardiac causes are associated with syncope during exercise (e.g., valvular aortic stenosis, idiopathic hypertrophic subaortic stenosis, and primary pulmonary hypertension). If a patient describes palpitations before the syncope, an arrhythmogenic cause may be present. Cardiac output may be reduced by arrhythmias or obstructive lesions.

The position of the patient just before fainting is important because this information may help determine the cause of the syncope. For example, if a patient fainted after rising suddenly from bed in the middle of the night (e.g., to run to answer the telephone), *orthostatic hypotension* may be the cause. Orthostatic hypotension is a common form of postural syncope and is the result of a peripheral autonomic limitation. There is a sudden fall in systemic blood pressure, resulting from a failure of adaptive reflexes to compensate for an erect posture. Symptoms of orthostatic hypotension include dizziness, blurring of vision, profound weakness, and syncope. Many drugs can cause orthostatic hypotension by leading to changes in intravascular volume or tone. Older patients are most prone to orthostatic hypotension. *Micturition syncope* usually occurs in men during straining with nocturnal urination. It may occur after considerable alcohol consumption.

Vasovagal syncope is the most common type of fainting and is one of the most difficult to manage. It has been estimated that 40% of all syncopal events are vasovagal in nature. Vasovagal syncope occurs during periods of sudden, stressful, or painful experiences, such as receiving bad news, surgical manipulation, trauma, the loss of blood, or even the sight of blood. It is often preceded by pallor, nausea, weakness, blurred vision, lightheadedness, perspiring, yawning, diaphoresis, hyperventilation, epigastric discomfort, or a "sinking feeling."

Table 14-5 Common Causes of Syncope

Organic System or Condition	Cause
Cardiac	Decreased cerebral perfusion secondary to cardiac rhythm disturbance Left ventricular output obstruction
Metabolic	Hypoglycemia Hyperventilation Hypoxia
Psychiatric	Hysteria
Neurologic	Epilepsy Cerebrovascular disease
Orthostatic hypotension	Volume depletion Antidepressant medications Antihypertensive medications
Vasovagal	Vasodepression
Micturition	Visceral reflex (vasodepressor)
Cough	Chronic lung disease
Carotid sinus	Vasodepressor response to carotid sinus sensitivity

There is a sudden fall in systemic vascular resistance without a compensatory increase in cardiac output as a result of an increased vagotonia. If the patient sits or lies down promptly, frank syncope can be aborted.

Carotid sinus syncope is associated with a hypersensitive carotid sinus and is most common in the elderly population. Whenever a patient with carotid sinus syncope wears a tight shirt collar or turns the neck in a certain way, there is an increased stimulation of the carotid sinus. This causes a sudden fall in systemic pressure, and syncope results. Two types of carotid sinus hypersensitivity exist: a cardioinhibitory (bradycardia) type and a vasodepressor (hypotension without bradycardia) type. *Post-tussive syncope* usually occurs in patients with chronic obstructive lung disease. Several mechanisms have been postulated to explain its occurrence. It is generally accepted that coughing produces an increase in intrathoracic pressure, which decreases both venous return and cardiac output. There may also be a rise in cerebrospinal fluid pressure, producing a decreased perfusion to the brain.

There are other suggested questions to ask a patient with syncope that direct attention to a neurologic cause. These are summarized in Chapter 21, The Nervous System. Table 14-5 lists the common causes of syncope.

Fatigue

Fatigue is a common symptom of decreased cardiac output. Patients with congestive heart failure and mitral valvular disease frequently complain of fatigue. Fatigue, however, is not specific for cardiac problems. The most common causes of fatigue are anxiety and depression. Other conditions associated with fatigue include anemia and chronic diseases. You must attempt to differentiate organic from psychogenic fatigue. Ask the following questions:

> *"How long have you been tired?"*
>
> *"Did the fatigue start suddenly?"*
>
> *"Do you feel tired all day? in the morning? in the evening?"*
>
> *"When do you feel least tired?"*
>
> *"Do you feel more tired at home than at work?"*
>
> *"Is the fatigue relieved by rest?"*

Patients with psychogenic fatigue are tired "all the time." They are often more tired at home than at work but occasionally describe being more tired in the morning. They may feel their best at the *end* of the day, which is when most patients with organic causes feel the worst.

Dependent Edema

Swelling of the legs, a form of *dependent edema*, is a frequent complaint of patients. Ask the following questions:

"When was the swelling first noted?"

"Are both legs swollen equally?"

"Did the swelling appear suddenly?"

"Is the swelling worse at any time of the day?"

"Does it disappear after a night's sleep?"

"Does elevation of your feet reduce the swelling?"

"What kind of medications are you taking?"

"Is there a history of kidney, heart, or liver disease?"

"Do you have shortness of breath?" If so, *"Which came first, the edema or the shortness of breath?"*

"Do you have pain in the legs?"

"Do you have any ulcers on your legs?"

If the patient is a woman, ask the following questions:

"Are you taking oral contraceptives?"

"Is the edema associated with menstrual changes?"

The patient with congestive heart failure has symmetric edema of the lower extremities that worsens as the day progresses. It is least in the morning after sleeping with the legs elevated in bed. If the patient also complains of dyspnea, it is helpful to determine which symptom came first. In patients with dyspnea and edema secondary to cardiac causes, the dyspnea usually precedes the edema. Bedridden patients may have dependent edema in the sacral area.

Hemoptysis

Hemoptysis is discussed in Chapter 13, The Chest. In addition to the pulmonary causes, mitral stenosis is an important cause of hemoptysis. Rupture of the bronchial veins, which are under high back pressure in mitral stenosis, produces the hemoptysis.

Cyanosis

Cyanosis is also discussed in Chapter 13, The Chest. The important questions regarding cyanosis are indicated in that chapter.

On occasion, cyanosis is noted only in the lower extremities. This is termed *differential cyanosis*. It is related to a right-to-left shunt through a patent ductus arteriosus (PDA). In a right-to-left shunt resulting from pulmonary hypertension, blood in the pulmonary artery crosses the PDA, which is located below the level of the carotid and left subclavian arteries; deoxygenated blood is pumped only to the lower extremity, producing cyanosis in only that location. Some blood does get to the lungs for oxygenation and is ultimately pumped out through the aorta to produce normal skin color in the upper extremity.

The patient whose feet are shown in Figure 14-11 is a 30-year-old immigrant who was evaluated in the United States for cyanosis. Until the age of 20 years, he had marked "bluish discoloration" of his lower extremities and relatively normal color in his upper extremities. Over the next 10 years, there was a gradual darkening of his upper extremities. Note the marked cyanosis of the extremities and nail beds of the fingers and toes. The patient had a PDA with marked pulmonary hypertension.

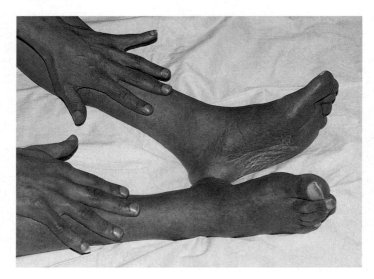

Figure 14-11 Differential cyanosis of the extremities: patent ductus arteriosus.

Impact of Cardiac Disease on the Patient

Patients with cardiac disease are intensely fearful. Once cardiac disease has been diagnosed, a series of reactions occurs. Fear, depression, and anxiety are the outcomes. The patients, who were totally asymptomatic until their episode of "sudden death" resulting from a coronary occlusion, are scared. They were resuscitated the first time; will an episode happen again? When? During recovery in the hospital, they are afraid to leave the intensive care unit for fear that "no one will be watching." At the time of discharge from the hospital, they are filled with anxiety. Although they desperately want to go home, they ask themselves, "What will happen if I have chest pain at home? Who will provide medical assistance?" They go through a period of depression, recognizing what they have gone through. After convalescence, they become fearful of daily situations that may provoke another attack. Can they go back to the daily "hassles" at work? Is it safe to have sexual intercourse? Despite appropriate reassurances from the clinician, their anxiety level may remain high.

Many patients with cardiac disease who have witnessed a fatal cardiac arrest in another patient in their room refuse to admit how stressful this event really was. The patients freely discuss the efficiency of the cardiac arrest team or complain that the noise kept them from sleeping. They refuse to identify with the deceased patient.

The patient with cardiac disease approaching surgery has the same fears as all surgical patients; these fears are discussed in Chapter 2, The Patient's Responses. However, surgical procedures for the patient with cardiac disease involve the "nucleus" of the body. The conscientious clinician takes time to explain the nature of the problem and the surgical approach. Before the procedure, the clinician should allow the patient, and especially the family, to visit the intensive care unit where the patient will be for a few days after surgery. Patients should be reassured that everything possible will be done in their behalf. *Their* courage and determination and *the clinician's* support are essential.

Physical Examination

The equipment necessary for the examination of the heart is a stethoscope, a penlight, and an applicator stick.

The physical examination of the heart includes the following:

- Inspection of the patient
- Assessment of blood pressure
- Assessment of the arterial pulse
- Assessment of the jugular venous pulse
- Percussion of the heart

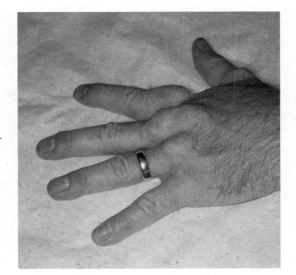

Figure 14-12 Tendon xanthomata.

- Palpation of the heart
- Auscultation of the heart
- Examination for dependent edema

The patient should be supine, and the examiner should stand on the right side of the bed. The head of the bed may be elevated slightly if the patient is more comfortable in this position.

Inspection

Evaluate General Appearance

The general inspection of the patient offers clues to cardiac diagnosis. Is the patient in acute distress? What is the patient's breathing like? Is it labored? Are accessory muscles being used?

Inspect the Skin

The skin can reveal many changes associated with cardiac disease. Inspect the skin color. Is cyanosis present? If so, does it appear central or peripheral? Is pallor present?

The *temperature* of the skin may reflect cardiac disease. Severe anemia, beriberi, and thyrotoxicosis tend to make the skin warmer; intermittent claudication is associated with coolness of the lower extremity in comparison with the upper extremity.

Are *xanthomata* present? Tendon xanthomata are stony-hard, slightly yellowish masses that are commonly found on the extensor tendons of the fingers and are pathognomonic for familial hypercholesterolemia. The Achilles tendon and plantar tendons of the soles are also common locations for tendon xanthomata. Figure 14-12 shows tendon xanthomata on the extensor surfaces of the fingers of a patient with a total serum cholesterol concentration higher than 450 mg/dL.*

Figure 14-13 shows multiple tuberous xanthomata of the hand of another patient. This patient had *primary biliary cirrhosis* and extremely elevated cholesterol levels. Primary biliary cirrhosis is a rare, progressive, and often fatal liver disease occurring mostly in women. Pruritus is a common symptom. Xanthomata develop in approximately 15% to 20% of affected patients and are typically found on the palms, soles, knees, elbows, and hands. The serum cholesterol, usually low-density lipoprotein, is often as high as 1000 to 1500 mg/dL. Antimitochondrial antibody is present in nearly 90% of patients.

Eruptive xanthomata are seen in several familial disturbances of fat metabolism, specifically hyperlipidemia types I and IV. The chest, buttocks, abdomen, back, face, and arms are most commonly affected. Figure 14-14 shows eruptive xanthomata on the abdomen of a patient with uncontrolled diabetes mellitus and hypertriglyceridemia. Eruptive xanthomata on the face of a patient are pictured in Figure 14-15. Eruptive xanthomata result from elevations

---

*The total cholesterol concentration for an adult is normally lower than 220 mg/dL.

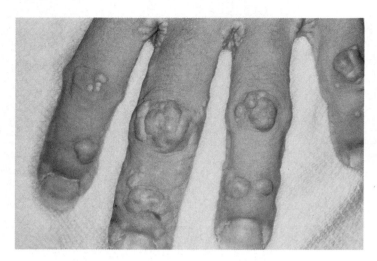

Figure 14-13 Multiple tuberous xanthomata of the hand.

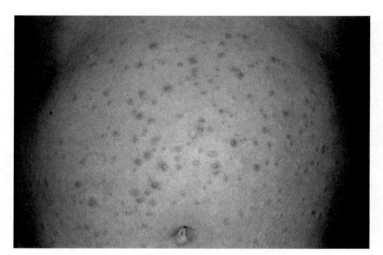

Figure 14-14 Eruptive xanthomata on the abdomen.

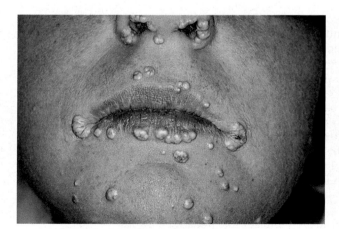

Figure 14-15 Eruptive xanthomata on the face.

in plasma triglyceride concentrations, usually to levels greater than 1500 mg/dL.* These lesions developed in this patient after excessive alcohol consumption; his serum triglyceride concentrations exceeded 2000 mg/dL. The lesions, frequently found on the abdomen, buttocks, elbows, knees, and back, are small (1 to 3 mm in diameter), yellowish papules on an erythematous base. With reduction in the level of triglycerides, the lesions may recede.

Is a rash present? The presence of *erythema marginatum* (erythema in which the reddened areas are disc-shaped with raised edges) in a febrile patient is suggestive of acute rheumatic fever.

Are any painful lesions on the fingers or toes present? *Osler's nodes* are painful lesions that occur in the tufts of the fingers and toes in patients with infective endocarditis. They are evanescent but are said to occur in 10% to 25% of patients with infective endocarditis.

Inspect the Nails

Frequently, *splinter hemorrhages* are visible as small, reddish-brown lines in the nail bed. These hemorrhages run from the free margin proximally and are classically associated with infective endocarditis. However, the finding is nonspecific because it is seen in many other conditions, even local trauma to the nail. A nail with splinter hemorrhages in a patient with endocarditis is shown in Figure 14-16.

Inspect the Facies

Abnormalities of the heart may also be associated with peculiarities of the face and head. Supravalvular aortic stenosis, a congenital problem, occurs in association with widely set eyes, strabismus, low-set ears, an upturned nose, and hypoplasia of the mandible. Moon facies and widely spaced eyes are suggestive of pulmonic stenosis. Expressionless facies with puffy eyelids and loss of the outer third of the eyebrow is seen in hypothyroidism. Affected individuals may have a cardiomyopathy. The *earlobe crease*, or Lichtstein's sign, is an oblique crease, often bilateral, seen frequently in patients older than 50 years with significant CHD. This sign is shown in Figure 14-17. Although it is a useful sign, there are too many false-positive and false-negative findings for this sign to be very reliable.

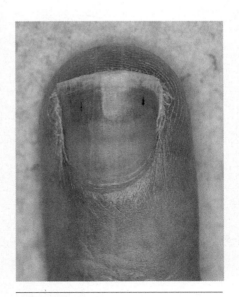

Figure 14-16 Splinter hemorrhages.

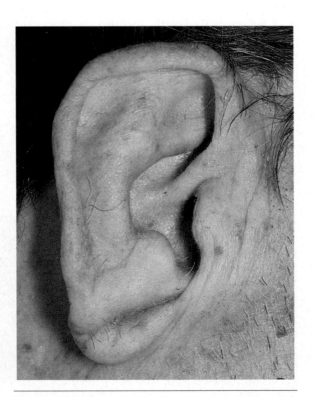

Figure 14-17 Earlobe creases.

---

*The serum triglyceride concentration for an adult is normally lower than 200 mg/dL.

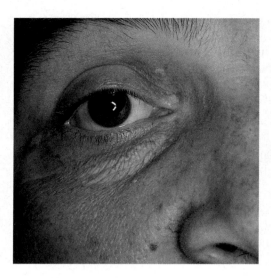

Figure 14-18 Xanthelasma.

Inspect the Eyes

The presence of yellowish plaques on the eyelids, called *xanthelasma*, should raise the suspicion of an underlying hyperlipoproteinemia, even though this lesion is less specific than the xanthoma. Xanthelasma in a patient with hypercholesterolemia is shown in Figure 14-18.

Examination of the eyes may reveal an *arcus senilis*. An arcus (see Figs. 10-53 and 10-54) seen in a patient *younger than* 40 years should raise the suspicion of *hypercholesterolemia*. Opacities in the cornea may be evidence for sarcoidosis, which may be responsible for cor pulmonale or myocardial involvement. Displacement of the lens is frequently seen in patients with *Marfan's syndrome*, an important cause of aortic regurgitation (see Fig. 10-69). Conjunctival hemorrhages are commonly seen in infective endocarditis. *Hypertelorism*, or widely set eyes, is often associated with congenital heart disease, especially pulmonic stenosis and supravalvular aortic stenosis. Retinal evaluation may furnish valuable information about diabetes (see Figs. 10-88 to 10-100), hypertension (see Figs. 10-101 to 10-105), and atherosclerosis. Roth's spots may develop in patients with infective endocarditis (see Fig. 10-109).

Inspect the Mouth

Have the patient open the mouth widely. Inspect the palate. Is the palate highly arched? A high-arched palate may be associated with congenital heart problems such as mitral valve prolapse.

Are there *petechiae* on the palate? Infective endocarditis is often associated with palatal petechiae, as seen in Figure 14-19.

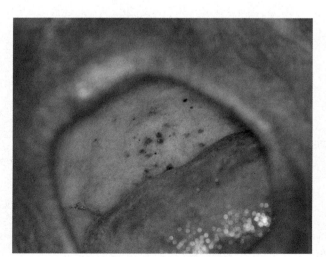

Figure 14-19 Palatal petechiae.

Inspect the Neck

Examination of the neck may reveal webbing. Webbing is seen in individuals with *Turner's syndrome,** who may have coarctation of the aorta, and in patients with *Noonan's syndrome.*[†] Pulmonic stenosis is the associated cardiac abnormality in this condition.

Inspect the Chest Configuration

Inspection of the chest often reveals information about the heart. Because the chest and the heart develop at about the same time during embryogenesis, it is not surprising that anything interfering with the development of the chest may interfere with the heart. A *pectus excavatum*, or caved-in chest, is seen in Marfan's syndrome and in mitral valve prolapse (see Fig. 13-7). *Pectus carinatum*, or pigeon breast, is also associated with Marfan's syndrome (see Fig. 13-8).

Are there any visible cardiac motions?

Inspect the Extremities

Some congenital abnormalities of the heart are associated with abnormalities of the extremities. Patients with atrial septal defects may have an extra phalanx, an extra finger, or an extra toe. Long, slender fingers may be suggestive of Marfan's syndrome and aortic regurgitation. Short stature, cubitus valgus, and medial deviation of the extended forearm are typical of patients with Turner's syndrome.

Blood Pressure Assessment

The Principles

Blood pressure can be measured directly with an intra-arterial catheter or indirectly with a *sphygmomanometer*. The sphygmomanometer consists of an inflatable rubber bladder within a cloth cover, a rubber bulb to inflate the bladder, and a manometer to measure the pressure in the bladder. Indirect measurement of blood pressure involves the auscultatory detection of the appearance and disappearance of the Korotkoff sounds over the compressed artery. *Korotkoff sounds* are low-pitched sounds originating in the vessel that are related to turbulence produced by partially occluding an artery with a blood pressure cuff. Several phases occur in sequence as the occluding pressure drops. Phase 1 occurs when the occluding pressure falls to the systolic blood pressure. The tapping sounds are clear and gradually increase in intensity as the occluding pressure falls. Phase 2 occurs at a pressure about 10 to 15 mm Hg lower than that in phase 1 and consists of tapping sounds followed by murmurs.[‡] Phase 3 occurs when the occluding pressure falls enough to allow a large amount of volume to cross the partially occluded artery. The sounds are similar to the sounds of phase 2, except that only the tapping sounds are heard. Phase 4 is the abrupt muffling and decreased intensity of the sounds as the pressure approaches the diastolic blood pressure. Phase 5 is the complete disappearance of the sounds. The vessel is no longer compressed by the occluding cuff. Turbulent flow is no longer present.

The normal blood pressure for adults is up to 140 mm Hg systolic and up to 85 mm Hg diastolic. For the diastolic blood pressure reading, the point of disappearance of the Korotkoff sounds is probably more accurate than the point of muffling. However, if the point of disappearance is more than 10 mm Hg lower than the point of muffling, the point of muffling is probably more accurate. Recording both the point of muffling and disappearance frequently helps in communication. A blood pressure might be recorded as 125/75-65: the systolic blood pressure is 125; the point of muffling is 75; the point of disappearance is 65 (the diastolic blood pressure).

Blood pressure should be recorded only to the nearest 5 mm Hg because there is a ± 3 mm Hg limit of accuracy for all sphygmomanometers. In addition, normal blood pressure changes occur from moment to moment, and measuring to less than 5 mm Hg provides a false sense of accuracy.

The size of the cuff is important for the accurate determination of blood pressure. It is recommended that the cuff be snugly applied around the arm, with its lowest edge 1 inch above the antecubital fossa. The cuff should be approximately 20% wider than the diameter of

---

*Short stature, retarded sexual development, and webbed neck in a female patient, associated with an abnormality of the sex chromosomes (45,XO).

[†]Male Turner's syndrome (46,XY).

[‡]A murmur is a blowing auscultatory sign produced by turbulence in blood flow. These vibrations can originate in the heart or in blood vessels as a result of hemodynamic changes.

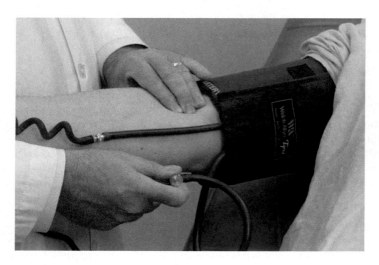

Figure 14-20 Technique for blood pressure assessment by palpation.

the extremity. The bladder should overlie the artery. The use of a cuff that is too small for a large arm results in an erroneously high reading of blood pressure.

Another cause of falsely elevated blood pressure readings is lack of support of the patient's arm. To obtain an accurate measurement, the cuff must be at heart level. If the arm is not supported, the patient is performing isometric exercise, which raises the recorded pressure. In contrast, excessive pressure on the diaphragm of the stethoscope produces a spuriously lower reading of the diastolic blood pressure without any significant alteration of systolic pressure. If the arm is held correctly, no skin indentations should occur.

The *auscultatory gap* is the silence that occurs between the disappearance of the Korotkoff sounds after the initial appearance and their reappearance at a lower pressure. The auscultatory gap is present when there is a decreased blood flow to the extremities, as is found in hypertension and in aortic stenosis. Its clinical importance lies in the fact that the systolic blood pressure may be mistaken for the lower blood pressure, the point of reappearance.

Determine Blood Pressure by Palpation

Blood pressure assessment is performed with the patient lying comfortably in the supine position. The cuff bladder is centered over the right brachial artery. If the arm is obese, a large adult or thigh cuff should be used. The arm should be slightly flexed, and it should be supported at approximately the level of the heart. To determine the systolic blood pressure adequately and to exclude an error as a result of an auscultatory gap, blood pressure is first assessed by palpation. In this procedure, the right brachial or right radial artery is palpated while the cuff is inflated above the pressure required to obliterate the pulse. The adjustable screw is opened slowly for deflation. The systolic pressure is identified by the reappearance of the brachial pulse. As soon as the pulse is felt, the adjustable screw is opened for rapid deflation. This assessment is demonstrated in Figure 14-20.

Determine Blood Pressure by Auscultation

Blood pressure by auscultation is assessed in the right arm by inflating the cuff to about 20 mm Hg above the systolic pressure that was determined by palpation. The diaphragm of the stethoscope should be placed over the artery as close to the edge of the cuff as possible, preferably just under the edge. The cuff is deflated *slowly* while the Korotkoff sounds are evaluated. The systolic blood pressure, the point of muffling, and the point of disappearance are determined. The systolic blood pressure is the point at which the initial tapping sounds are heard. The technique of determining auscultatory blood pressure is shown in Figure 14-21. If the blood pressure is high, it is useful to measure the blood pressure again at the end of the examination, when the patient may be calmer.

Rule Out Orthostatic Hypotension

After the patient has been recumbent for at least 5 minutes, measure the baseline blood pressure and pulse. Then have the patient stand, and repeat the measurements immediately.

Orthostatic hypotension is defined as a drop in systolic blood pressure of 20 mm Hg or more, in association with the development of symptoms such as dizziness or syncope, when

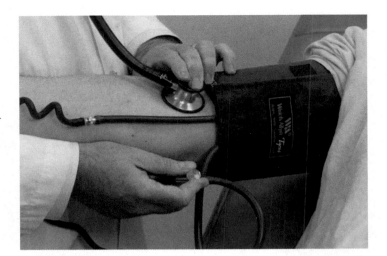

Figure 14-21 Technique for blood pressure assessment by auscultation.

the patient assumes the standing position. In most affected patients, there is also an increase in heart rate.

Rule Out Supravalvular Aortic Stenosis

If hypertension is detected in the right arm, perform the following test: Place the cuff on the patient's left arm, and determine the auscultatory pressure. It is not necessary to remeasure the palpatory pressure or reevaluate for orthostatic changes. In supravalvular aortic stenosis, there is a difference in the blood pressures in the arms; hypertension may be detected in the right arm, whereas hypotension may be present in the left arm.

Rule Out Coarctation of the Aorta

If the blood pressure is elevated in the arms, determination of the blood pressure in the lower extremities is important for ruling out coarctation of the aorta. The patient is asked to lie on the abdomen while the thigh cuff, which is 6 cm wider than the arm cuff, is placed around the posterior aspect of the midthigh. The stethoscope is placed over the artery in the popliteal fossa. The Korotkoff sounds are determined as in the upper extremity. If a thigh cuff is not available, the regular cuff can be applied to the lower leg with the distal border just at the malleoli. The stethoscope is placed over either the posterior tibial or the dorsalis pedis artery, and the auscultatory blood pressure is taken. A leg systolic blood pressure that is lower than that in the arm should raise suspicion of coarctation of the aorta.

Rule Out Cardiac Tamponade

In the presence of low arterial blood pressure and a rapid and feeble pulse, it is necessary to rule out the presence of cardiac tamponade. A valuable clinical sign suggestive of cardiac tamponade is the presence of a marked *paradoxical pulse* (also known as a *pulsus paradoxus*), which is characterized by an exaggeration of the normal inspiratory fall in systolic pressure. There is much confusion about the definition of a normal paradoxical pulse. A normal paradoxical pulse should be defined as the *normal* fall (about 5 mm Hg) in systolic arterial pressure during inspiration. It is the *magnitude* of the phenomenon that should determine whether the pulsus paradoxus is normal or abnormal.

The technique for assessing the magnitude of a paradoxical pulse is as follows: Have the patient breathe as normally as possible. Inflate the blood pressure cuff until no sounds are heard. Gradually deflate the cuff until sounds are heard in expiration only. Note this pressure. Continue to deflate the cuff slowly until sounds are heard during inspiration. Note this pressure. If the difference in these two pressures exceeds 10 mm Hg, a marked (abnormal) pulsus paradoxus is present; cardiac tamponade may be the cause. Cardiac tamponade results when there is an increase in intrapericardial pressure that interferes with normal diastolic filling. A marked paradoxical pulse is not a specific phenomenon for tamponade because it is also seen in large pericardial effusions, in constrictive pericarditis, and in conditions associated with increased ventilatory effort, such as asthma and emphysema.

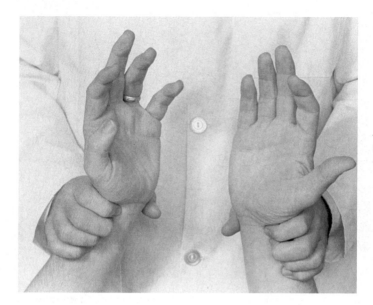

Figure 14-22 Technique for evaluating the radial artery pulses.

The Arterial Pulse

The following information is gained from palpation of the arterial pulse:

- The rate and rhythm of the heart
- The contour of the pulse
- The amplitude of the pulse

Determine the Cardiac Rate

Cardiac rate is routinely assessed by the radial pulse. The examiner should stand in front of the patient and grasp both radial arteries. The second, third, and fourth fingers should overlie the radial artery, as shown in Figure 14-22. The examiner should count the pulse for 30 seconds and multiply the number of beats by 2 to obtain the beats per minute. This method is accurate for most *regular* rhythms. If the patient has an *irregularly irregular* rhythm, as is found in atrial fibrillation, a *pulse deficit* may be present. In atrial fibrillation, many impulses bombard the atrioventricular node and ventricles. Owing to the varying lengths of diastolic filling periods, some of the contractions may be very weak and unable to produce an adequate pulse wave despite ventricular contraction. A pulse deficit, which is the difference between the apical (precordial) and radial pulses, occurs. In such cases, only auscultation of the heart, not the radial pulse, provides an accurate assessment of the cardiac rate.

Determine the Cardiac Rhythm

When palpating the pulse, carefully evaluate the regularity of the rhythm. The slower the rate, the longer you should palpate. If the rhythm is irregular, is there a pattern to the irregularity?

Cardiac rhythm may be described as *regular, regularly irregular,* or *irregularly irregular.* A regularly irregular rhythm is a pulse with an irregularity that occurs in a definite pattern. An irregularly irregular pulse has no pattern.

Electrocardiography is really the best medium for diagnosing the rhythm, but the physical examination may provide some clues. *Premature beats* may be recognized by the presence of isolated extra beats during a regular rhythm. *Bigeminy* is a coupled rhythm of beats in pairs. The first beat is the sinus beat, which is followed by a premature, usually ventricular, beat. If the premature beat is very early in the diastolic period, the pulse from this beat may be missed if the examiner evaluates the rhythm by palpation alone. A rhythm that is grossly irregular with no pattern is irregularly irregular and is the pulse in patients with *atrial fibrillation*.

Palpate the Carotid Artery

Assess the carotid artery pulse by standing at the patient's right side, with the patient lying on the back. Auscultate the patient's carotid arteries for bruits *first* (see Chapter 15, The Peripheral Vascular System). If a bruit is present, do not palpate the carotid artery. If a cholesterol plaque is present, palpation may produce an embolus.

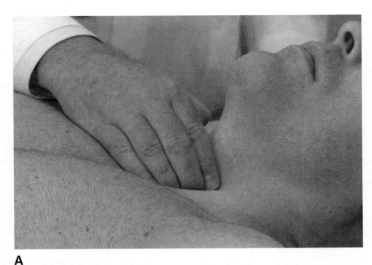

A

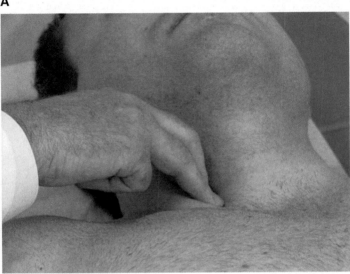

B

Figure 14-23 *A* and *B,* Technique for evaluating the carotid artery pulsations.

To palpate the carotid artery, place your index and third fingers on the patient's thyroid cartilage and slip them laterally between the trachea and the sternocleidomastoid muscle. You should be able to feel the carotid pulsations just medial to the sternocleidomastoid muscle. Palpation should be performed low in the neck to avoid pressure on the carotid sinus, which would cause a reflex drop in blood pressure and heart rate. Each carotid artery is evaluated separately. *Never* press on both carotid arteries at the same time. After the right carotid artery is evaluated, stand in the same position, and place the same fingers back on the patient's trachea and slip them laterally to the left to feel the left carotid artery. This technique is demonstrated in Figure 14-23.

Evaluate the Characteristics of the Pulse

The carotid artery is used for the assessment of the contour and amplitude of the pulse. *Contour* is the shape of the wave. It is frequently described as the speed of the upward slope, downward slope, and duration of the wave. Place a hand firmly against the carotid artery until maximal force is felt. At this moment, the wave form should be discernible. The pulse may be described as *normal, diminished, increased,* or *double-peaked.* The normal carotid pulse wave is smooth, with the upward stroke steeper and more rapid than the downward stroke. A diminished pulse is a small, weak pulse. The palpating finger feels a gentle pressure rise with a distinct peak. An increased pulse is a large, strong, hyperkinetic pulse. The palpating finger feels an increased rate of rise of the ascending limb of the pulse and a brisk tap at its peak. A double-peaked pulse has a prominent percussion and tidal wave with or without a dicrotic wave. Arterial pulse abnormalities are summarized in Figure 14-24.

Type	Description	Cause
Anacrotic*	Small, slow rising, delayed pulse with a notch or shoulder on the ascending limb	Aortic stenosis
Waterhammer (Corrigan's)	Rapid and sudden systolic expansion	Aortic regurgitation
Bisferiens	Double-peaked pulse with a midsystolic dip	Aortic regurgitation
Alternans	Alternating amplitude of pulse pressure	Congestive heart failure
Paradoxical (marked)	Detected by blood pressure assessment. An exaggerated drop in systolic blood pressure during inspiration	Tamponade Constrictive pericarditis Chronic obstructive lung disease

*Also known as plateau pulse or pulsus parvus et tardus.

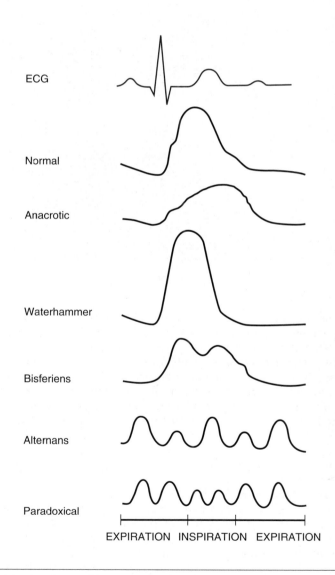

ECG

Normal

Anacrotic

Waterhammer

Bisferiens

Alternans

Paradoxical

EXPIRATION   INSPIRATION   EXPIRATION

Figure 14-24 Arterial pulse abnormalities. ECG, electrocardiogram.

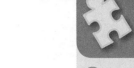

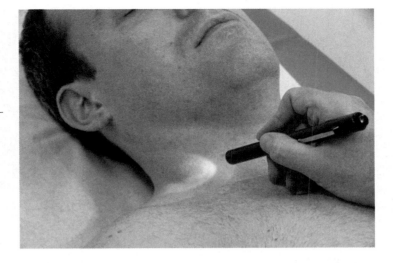

Figure 14-25 Technique for evaluating the jugular wave forms.

The Jugular Venous Pulse

The *internal jugular vein* provides information about the wave forms and right atrial pressure. The pulsations of the internal jugular vein are beneath the sternocleidomastoid muscle and are visible as they are transmitted through the surrounding tissue. The vein itself is not visible. Because the right internal jugular vein is straighter than the left, only the right internal jugular vein is evaluated. Measurements from the external jugular system, which is easier to visualize, are much less accurate and should not be used.

Determine the Jugular Wave Forms

To visualize the *jugular wave forms*, the patient should lie flat without a pillow so that his or her neck is not flexed and does not interfere with the pulsations. The patient's trunk should be at approximately 25° to the horizontal. The higher the venous pressure is, the greater the elevation that is required; the lower the pressure, the lower the elevation needed. The patient's head should be turned slightly to the right and slightly down to relax the right sternocleidomastoid muscle. Standing on the patient's right side, the examiner should place his or her right hand, holding a small pocket flashlight, on the patient's sternum and shine the light tangentially across the right side of the patient's neck. Shadows of the pulsations will be cast on the sheet behind the patient. The light and shadows magnify the wave forms. This technique is demonstrated in Figure 14-25. If no wave forms are seen, the angle of elevation of the head of the bed should be reduced. To help identify the wave forms, the examiner can time the cardiac cycle by palpating the cardiac impulse beneath his or her right hand or by feeling the left carotid impulse with his or her left hand. The descents, rather than the waves themselves, tend to be more obvious. If the neck veins are visible at the jaw margin while the patient is seated, the examiner should watch for the wave forms at the angle of the jaw with the patient seated upright.

The jugular pulse must be differentiated from the pulsation of the carotid artery. Table 14-6 lists the most important characteristic differences of these pulses.

Estimate the Jugular Venous Pressure

To assess the pressure in the right side of the heart, it is necessary to establish a reference level. The standard reference is the *manubriosternal angle*. At any degree of elevation, this position is used to measure the pressure in the internal jugular system. The examiner must first determine the height of the venous distention by noting the top of the wave forms in the internal jugular venous pulsations. An imaginary horizontal line is then drawn from this height to the sternal angle. The examiner should then measure the distance from the sternal angle to this imaginary line. The angle of elevation of the head of the bed is also estimated. It might be stated, "At 45° elevation, the jugular pulse is 7 cm above the sternal angle." At 45°, the upper limit of normal is 4 to 5 cm above the sternal angle; if the patient is at 30°, the upper limit of normal is 6 cm. When the height of the venous column is equal to or lower than the sternal angle in the supine position, venous pressure is usually normal.

There is tremendous inaccuracy in attempting to determine the pressure in the right atrium by the jugular manometer, as just indicated. It has been demonstrated numerous times that the sensitivity and specificity of this test are low, and thus it is inaccurate in

Table 14-6 Differentiation of Jugular and Carotid Pulses

Feature	Internal Jugular Pulse	Carotid Pulse
Palpation	Not palpable	Palpable
Waveforms	Multiform: two or three components	Single
Quality	Soft, undulating	Vigorous
Pressure*	Wave forms obliterated	No effect
Inspiration	Decreased height of wave forms	No effect
Sitting up	Decreased height of wave forms	No effect
Valsalva maneuver	Increased height of wave forms	No effect

*Light pressure on the vessel above the sternal end of clavicle.

predicting elevated pressures. The only accurate statement is that right atrial pressure is high when there is neck vein distention up to the jaw margin while the patient is seated at 90°. In this situation, the right atrial pressure usually exceeds 15 mm Hg. In Figure 14-26, the neck veins are distended to the angle of the jaw while the patient is seated upright. His right atrial pressure was 21 mm Hg.

Evaluate the Hepatojugular Reflux

A useful test in assessing high jugular venous pressure is that of the *hepatojugular reflux*, also known as *abdominal compression*. By applying pressure over the liver, the examiner can grossly assess right ventricular function. Patients with right ventricular failure have dilated sinusoids in the liver. Pressure on the liver pushes blood out of these sinusoids and into the inferior vena cava and right side of the heart, causing further distention of the neck veins. The procedure is performed with the patient lying in bed, mouth open, breathing normally; this prevents a Valsalva maneuver. The examiner places his or her right hand over the patient's liver in the right upper quadrant and applies a firm, progressive pressure. Compression is maintained for 10 seconds. The normal response is for the internal and external jugular veins to show a transient increase in distention during the first few cardiac cycles, which is followed by a fall to baseline levels during the later part of the compression. In patients with right ventricular failure or elevated pulmonary artery wedge pressure, the neck veins remain distended during the entire period of compression; this distention diminishes rapidly (at least 4 cm) on sudden release of the compressing hand. If the examination is incorrectly performed with the patient's mouth closed, a Valsalva maneuver results and produces inaccurate results of the hepatojugular reflux test.

Like most other clinical maneuvers, the hepatojugular reflux test must be performed in a standardized manner. If performed correctly, this test can be of considerable value in the bedside assessment of the patient. The test result correlates best with the pulmonary artery

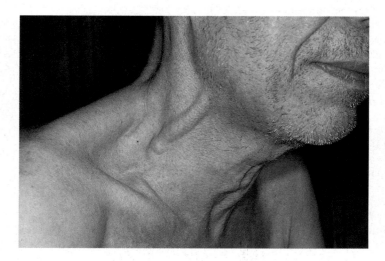

Figure 14-26 Neck vein distention.

wedge pressure and, as such, is a reflection of increased central blood volume. Ewy (1988) evaluated this test and showed that in the absence of right ventricular failure, a positive test result is suggestive of a pulmonary artery wedge pressure of 15 mm Hg or greater.

Percussion

Percuss the Heart's Borders

The technique of percussion is discussed in Chapter 13, The Chest. Percussion of the heart is performed at the third, fourth, and fifth intercostal spaces from the left anterior axillary line to the right anterior axillary line. Normally, there is a change in the percussion note from resonance to dullness about 6 cm lateral to the left of the sternum. This dullness is attributable to the presence of the heart.

A percussion dullness distance of greater than 10.5 cm in the left fifth intercostal space has a sensitivity of 91.3% and a specificity of 30.3% for detecting increased left ventricular end-diastolic volume (LVEDV) or left ventricular mass. Percussion dullness of more than 10.5 cm in the fifth intercostal space has a sensitivity of 94.4% and a specificity of 67.2% in detecting cardiomegaly. In patients with a palpable apical impulse of greater than 3 cm in the left decubitus position, the sensitivity of detecting increased LVEDV or left ventricular mass increases to 100% and the specificity is 40%.

Palpation

Palpation is performed to evaluate the apical impulse, the right ventricle, the pulmonary artery, and the left ventricular motions. The presence or absence of *thrills** is also determined by palpation. The point of maximum impulse (PMI) describes the outward motion of the cardiac apex as it rotates counterclockwise, as viewed from below, to strike the anterior chest wall during isovolumetric contraction.

Palpate the Point of Maximum Impulse

The examiner should stand on the right side of the patient, with the bed at a level comfortable for the examiner. Palpation for the PMI is most easily performed with the patient in a sitting position. Only the examiner's fingertips should be applied to the patient's chest in the fifth intercostal space, midclavicular line, because they are the most sensitive for assessing localized motion. The PMI should be noted. This technique is demonstrated in Figure 14-27. If the apical impulse is not felt, the examiner should move his or her fingertips in the area of the cardiac apex. The PMI is usually within 10 cm of the midsternal line and is no larger than 2 to 3 cm in diameter. A PMI that is laterally displaced or is felt in two interspaces during the same phase of respiration is suggestive of cardiomegaly.

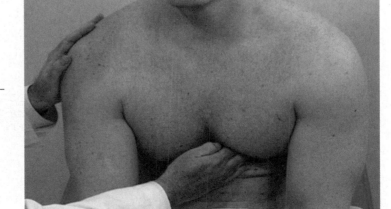

Figure 14-27 Technique for assessing point of maximum impulse.

---

*Low-frequency cutaneous vibrations associated with loud heart murmurs.

The PMI is felt in approximately 70% of normal individuals while they are sitting. If it cannot be felt in the sitting position, the patient should be reevaluated while supine and in the left lateral decubitus position. The position of the PMI in the left lateral decubitus position must be assessed with the understanding that the normal cardiac impulse is now shifted slightly to the left. If the patient is in the left lateral decubitus position and the PMI is not laterally displaced, the examiner can suspect that cardiomegaly is not present.

In a patient without conditions predisposing to left ventricular hypertrophy, a palpable apical impulse felt in the left lateral decubitus position that is greater than 3 cm is said to be a specific (91%) and sensitive (92%) indicator of left ventricular enlargement. An apical diameter greater than 3 cm is predictive (86%) of an increased LVEDV. In patients with an apical diameter of less than 3 cm and a normal LVEDV, the negative predictive value is 95%.

The PMI usually corresponds to the *left* ventricular apex, but in patients with an enlarged right ventricle, the heart is rotated clockwise, as viewed from below, and the PMI may actually be produced by the *right* ventricle. This rotation turns the left ventricle posteriorly and makes it difficult to palpate. The apical impulse by the right ventricle is diffuse, whereas that of the left ventricle tends to be more localized.

In patients with chronic obstructive lung disease, the overinflation of the lungs displaces the PMI downward and to the right. The PMI in such patients is felt in the *epigastric* area, at the lower end of the sternum. In patients with chronic obstructive lung disease, a PMI in the normal location is suggestive of cardiomegaly.

Palpate for Localized Motion

The patient should now lie down so that all four main cardiac areas can be palpated. The examiner uses his or her fingertips to assess any localized motion. This technique is demonstrated in Figure 14-28.

The presence of a systolic impulse in the second intercostal space to the left of the sternum is suspect for pulmonary hypertension. This impulse is caused by the closure of the pulmonic valve under increased pressure. The presence of this impulse is suggestive of a dilated pulmonary artery, but it may also be felt in thin individuals without pulmonary hypertension.

Palpate for Generalized Motion

After the chest has been palpated with the fingertips, the examiner uses the proximal portion of his or her hand to palpate for any large area of sustained outward motion, called a *heave* or *lift*. The examiner again palpates each of the four main cardiac areas. The technique for assessing heaves is demonstrated in Figure 14-29. The presence of a *right ventricular rock*, which is a

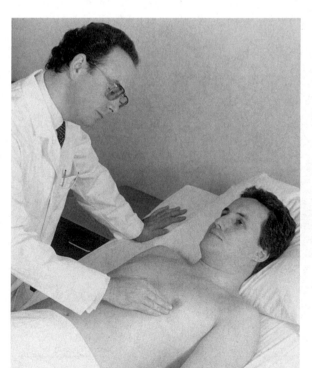

Figure 14-28 Technique for assessing localized cardiac motion.

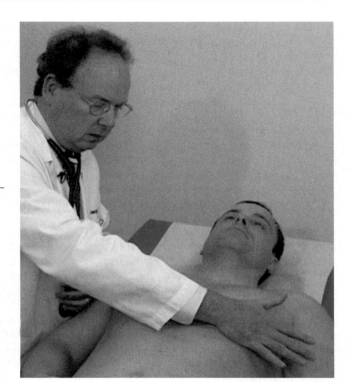

Figure 14-29 Technique for assessing generalized cardiac motion.

sustained left parasternal impulse associated with lateral retraction, is suggestive of a large right ventricle.

Any condition that increases the rate of ventricular filling during early diastole can produce a palpable impulse that occurs *after* the main left ventricular impulse. This second impulse in the area of the PMI is usually felt in association with an S$_3$. Frequently, an S$_3$ is more easily felt than heard.

The use of a tongue blade or an applicator stick can be helpful to reinforce visually what has been palpated. The tip of the stick is placed directly over the area and held in place by the examiner's finger. This acts as a fulcrum, and the motions tend to be magnified by the movement of the stick. The technique is demonstrated in Figure 14-30.

Palpate for Thrills

Thrills are the superficial vibratory sensations felt on the skin overlying an area of turbulence. The presence of a thrill indicates a loud murmur. Thrills are best felt by using the heads of your metacarpal bones rather than the fingertips and applying very gentle pressure on the skin.

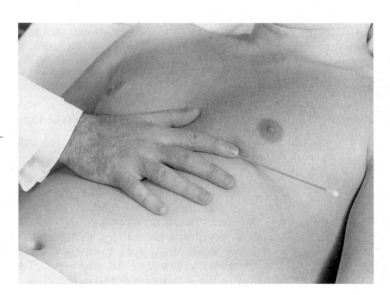

Figure 14-30 Technique for amplifying detection of cardiac movement.

If too much pressure is applied, thrills are not felt. The palpation of thrills is generally of little importance because auscultation reveals the presence of the loud murmur that has produced the thrill. Therefore, the finding of a thrill adds little to the diagnosis, but it is an interesting physical sign to alert the examiner as to what will be heard.

Auscultation

The Technique

Proper auscultation requires a quiet area. Every attempt should be made to eliminate extraneous noise from radios, televisions, and so forth. The earpieces of the stethoscope are directed anteriorly or parallel to the direction of the external auditory canal. If the earpieces are put in backward, the openings of the earpieces impinge on the wall of the external canal and lower the intensity of the sounds. The earpieces should fit properly so as to be comfortable but tight enough to exclude external noises.

It is often useful for you to close your eyes when listening to the heart. Sounds that are more difficult to hear sound louder with your eyes closed, because the brain is flooded with all types of sensory input. The input from the eyes appears to be the most important. The next important sensory input is auditory, which is followed by tactile input. If you eliminate the distraction of visual stimuli, the brain concentrates more on the auditory input, and the sounds become more evident.

As indicated in Chapter 13, The Chest, the bell of the stethoscope should be applied lightly to the skin, whereas the diaphragm should be pressed tightly against the skin. High-pitched sounds, such as valve closure, systolic events, and regurgitant murmurs, are better heard with the diaphragm. Low-pitched sounds, such as gallop rhythms or the murmur of atrioventricular stenosis, are better heard with the bell.

It is common in many countries to examine patients through their clothing or a hospital gown. In the United States, however, *never* listen through *any* type of clothing.

There are several other pitfalls in auscultation. Make sure that the stethoscope is in good shape: Cracked tubing certainly interferes with good listening. Both the examiner and the patient must be comfortable for the best hearing. An examiner who is straining over the patient and is uncomfortable will want to finish the examination quickly without a proper assessment. Always inspect and palpate *before* auscultation. Accumulate as much information as possible before listening!

Auscultate the Cardiac Areas

The examiner should be on the right side of the patient while the patient lies flat on the back. If not already at the proper height, the bed should be adjusted so that the examiner is comfortable. The examiner should listen in the aortic, pulmonic, tricuspid, and mitral areas. However, the examiner should not limit auscultation to these areas alone. The examiner should start at any area and move the stethoscope gradually over the precordium from area to area. The areas have been established to provide some degree of standardization.

While listening at the apex and left lower sternal border with the bell, the examiner should determine whether an S_3 or an S_4 is present.

Cardiac murmurs may radiate widely. The examiner should determine where the sounds are loudest or best heard. There are no acoustic walls in the chest. A murmur typically heard at the apex with radiation to the axilla may be heard in the neck, if it is loud enough. The murmur in this example is probably loudest at the apex and axilla.

The Standard Auscultation Positions

The four standard positions for auscultation are shown in Figure 14-31. They are as follows:

- Supine
- Left lateral decubitus
- Upright
- Upright, leaning forward

All precordial areas are examined while the patient is supine. Using a systematic approach, the examiner starts at either the aortic area or the apex and carefully listens to the heart sounds. After all areas are examined, the patient is then instructed to turn onto the left side. The examiner should now listen at the apex for the low-pitched diastolic murmur of *mitral stenosis*, which is best heard with the bell of the stethoscope. Then the patient sits upright, and all areas are examined with the diaphragm of the stethoscope. Finally, the patient sits up and

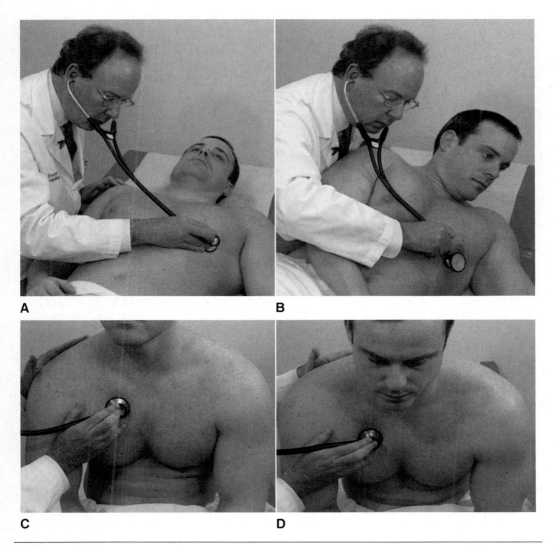

A   B

C   D

Figure 14-31 Positions for auscultation. *A,* The supine position, used for listening to all areas. *B,* The left lateral decubitus position, used for listening with the bell in the mitral area. *C,* The upright position, used for listening to all areas. *D,* The upright, leaning-forward position, used for listening with the diaphragm at the base positions.

leans forward. The patient is asked to exhale and hold his or her breath while the examiner, using the diaphragm, listens for the high-pitched diastolic murmur of *aortic regurgitation* at the right and left second and third intercostal spaces.

The Influence of Breathing
The examiner should pay special attention to the influence of breathing on the intensity of heart sounds. Most murmurs or sounds originating in the right side of the heart are accentuated with inspiration. This is related to the increased return of blood that occurs with inspiration and the resultant increased right ventricular output. In addition, an S_3 or an S_4 originating in the right side of the heart is accentuated during inspiration.

Time the Cardiac Events
To interpret heart sounds accurately, the examiner must be able to time the events of the cardiac cycle. The most reliable way of identifying S_1 and S_2 is to time the sounds by palpating the carotid artery. While the examiner's right hand is positioning the stethoscope, the left hand is placed on the patient's carotid artery. This technique is demonstrated in Figure 14-32. The sound that precedes the carotid pulse is the S_1. The S_2 follows the pulse. The carotid, *not*

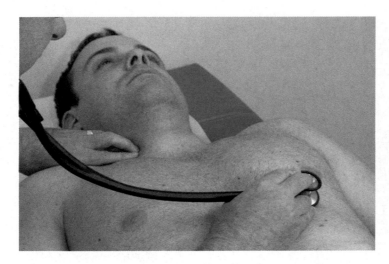

Figure 14-32 Technique for timing the heart sounds.

the radial pulse, must be used. The time delay from S_2 to the radial pulse is significant, and errors in timing will result.

Approach to Careful Auscultation

Until the examiner gains expertise in cardiac examination, heart sounds should be evaluated in the manner suggested in Table 14-7. The examiner should take time in each area before continuing on to the next area. The examiner should listen to several cardiac cycles at each position to be certain of the observations made, which include respiratory effects.

Describe Any Murmurs Present

If a murmur is present, attention should be directed to the following features:

- Timing in the cardiac cycle
- Location
- Radiation
- Duration
- Intensity
- Pitch
- Quality
- Relationship to respiration
- Relationship to body position

Timing of murmurs as to systole and diastole is paramount. Does the systolic murmur begin with, or after, S_1? Does it end before, with, or after S_2? Does the murmur occupy the entire systolic period? Murmurs occurring throughout systole are termed *holosystolic* or *pansystolic*. These murmurs begin with S_1 and end after S_2. A *systolic ejection* murmur begins after S_1 and ends before S_2. Does the murmur occur only in early systole, midsystole, or late systole? Does

Table 14-7 Approach to Cardiac Auscultation	
Position	**Evaluate**
Supine	S_1 in all areas S_2 in all areas Systolic murmurs or sounds in all areas
Left lateral decubitus	Diastolic events at apex with bell of stethoscope
Upright	S_1 in all areas S_2 in all areas Systolic murmurs or sounds in all areas Diastolic murmurs or sounds in all areas
Upright, leaning forward	Diastolic events at base with diaphragm of stethoscope

the murmur persist throughout the entire diastolic period? Such murmurs are termed *holodiastolic*.

In which area is the murmur best heard?

The *radiation* of the murmur can provide a clue as to its cause. Does it radiate to the axilla? the neck? the back?

The intensity of a murmur is graded from I to VI, based on increasing loudness. The following grading system, although antiquated, serves as a means of communicating the intensity of the murmur:

    I: Lowest intensity, often not heard by inexperienced listeners
   II: Low intensity, usually audible by inexperienced listeners
  III: Medium intensity without a thrill
  IV: Medium intensity with a thrill
   V: Loudest murmur that is audible when the stethoscope is placed on the chest; associated with a thrill
  VI: Loudest intensity: audible when stethoscope is removed from chest; associated with a thrill

Murmurs can be described, for example, as "grade II/VI," "grade IV/VI," or "grade II-III/VI." Any murmur associated with a thrill must be at least a grade IV/VI. A grade IV/VI murmur is louder than a grade II/VI murmur only because there is more turbulence; both or neither may have clinical significance. The "/VI" is used because there is another, less popular, grading system involving only four categories. An important axiom to remember is the following:

In general, the intensity of a murmur tells nothing about the severity of the clinical state.

The quality of a murmur can be described as rumbling, blowing, harsh, musical, machinery, or scratchy.

Describe Any Pericardial Rubs

Friction rubs are extracardiac sounds of short duration that have a unique quality similar to the sound of scratching on sandpaper. Rubs may result from irritation of the pleura (i.e., a pleural rub) or of the pericardium (i.e., a pericardial rub). Pericardial rubs typically have three components: one systolic and two diastolic. The systolic component occurs during ejection; the two diastolic components occur during rapid filling and atrial contraction. Pericardial rubs are best heard with the patient sitting while holding breath in expiration. Patients with pericardial rubs commonly have chest pain that is lessened by sitting forward. A rub that disappears while the patient holds the breath originates from the pleura.

The Goals of Auscultation

The goals at the end of auscultation are to be able to describe the following:

- The intensity of S_1 in all areas
- The intensity of S_2 in all areas
- The characterization of any systolic sounds
- The characterization of any diastolic sounds

With experience, the examiner is able to listen to all parts of the cardiac cycle in one area and compare the sounds and events with those of other areas. Normally, S_1 is loudest at the apex, and S_2 is loudest at the base. Splitting of S_2 into A_2 and P_2 during inspiration is best heard at the pulmonic area with the patient lying on his or her back. This increases venous return and widens the A_2-P_2 split.

Examination for Edema

When peripheral venous pressure is high, as in congestive heart failure, pressure in the veins is distributed in a retrograde manner to the smaller vessels. Transudation of fluid occurs, and edema of dependent areas results. This increase in tissue fluid produces edema that "pits."

Test for Edema

To test for pitting edema, the examiner presses his or her fingers into a dependent area, such as the patient's shin, for 2 to 3 seconds. If pitting edema is present, the fingers sink into the tissue,

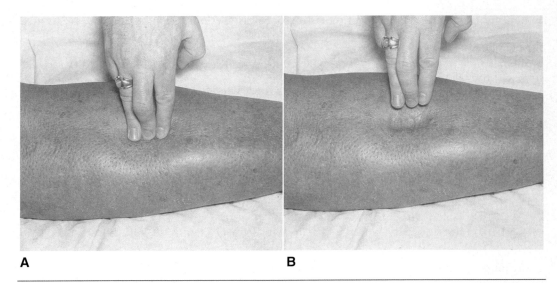

A   **B**

Figure 14-33 Technique for testing for pitting edema. *A,* The examiner presses into the patient's shin area. *B,* When pitting edema is present, indentation occurs after the fingers are lifted.

and when the fingers are removed, the impression of the fingers remains. This technique is demonstrated in Figure 14-33.

Pitting edema is usually quantified from 1+ to 4+, depending on how long the indentation persists. The most noticeable is 4+. In patients who are bedridden, the dependent area is usually the sacrum and not the shins. The examiner should evaluate for edema over the sacrum in these patients. Figure 14-34 illustrates 4+ sacral edema in a bedridden patient.

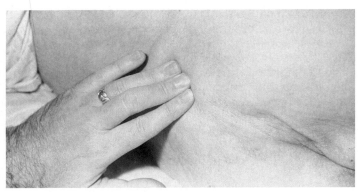

A

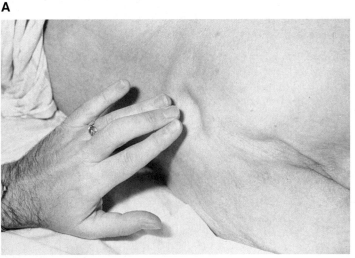

B

Figure 14-34 Technique for testing for pitting edema over the sacrum. *A,* The examiner presses into the sacrum of a bedridden patient. *B,* The pitting edema is evident.

Clinicopathologic Correlations

Discussion now focuses on the pathologic changes that result in the following:

- Abnormalities of S_1
- Abnormalities of S_2
- Systolic clicks
- Diastolic opening snaps
- Murmurs

Abnormalities of the First Heart Sound

The factors that are responsible for the intensity of S_1 are as follows:

- The rate of rise of ventricular pressure
- The condition of the valve
- The position of the valve
- The distance of the heart from the chest wall

The faster the *rate of rise* of left ventricular pressure is, the louder the mitral component of S_1 is. Increased contractility increases the intensity of S_1. Decreased contractility softens S_1.

When the atrioventricular valve stiffens as a result of fibrosis or calcification, its closure is louder. The pathologically deformed valve of mitral stenosis produces an accentuated or louder S_1. After many years, as the valve becomes increasingly calcified, it becomes unable to move, causing S_1 to soften.

The *position of the valve* at the time of ventricular contraction affects the intensity of S_1. The *arc of coaptation* is the angle through which the valve closes. If the valve is in a midposition, it travels less than when it closes from a widely opened position. The more it is opened, the wider the arc of coaptation, and the louder is S_1. This situation is directly related to the pressure in the left atrium at the moment that the left ventricular pressure exceeds it and closes the valve. This can occur in conditions in which there is a shortened PR interval on the electrocardiogram. The mitral valve is opened normally during diastole for ventricular filling. The P wave of the electrocardiogram corresponds to atrial contraction, which elevates left atrial pressure (the "a" wave of the left atrial tracing), further opening the mitral valve in late diastole. If the PR interval is short, ventricular contraction occurs so quickly after atrial contraction that the atrial pressure is still high when the left ventricular pressure exceeds it. The mitral valve stays open longer and closes later than normal, during the rapid rate of rise of pressure of the ventricle, which accentuates S_1.

In general, the longer the PR interval, the softer the S_1. Lengthening of the PR intervals, as is seen in Wenckebach's phenomenon,* produces an S_1 that softens until the dropped beat occurs.

Whenever the heart is *farther from the chest wall*, the S_1 is softer than normal. In patients who are very obese or who have chronic obstructive lung disease, the intensity of the S_1 is softer than normal. In patients with a large pericardial effusion, the S_1 is likewise soft.

Abnormalities of the Second Heart Sound

Abnormalities of the Intensity of the Second Heart Sound

The conditions that change the intensity of S_2 are the following:

- Changes in systolic pressure
- Condition of the valve

Any condition that produces an increase in the systolic pressure increases the intensity of the S_2. Conversely, conditions that lower the systolic pressure soften the S_2. Hypertension raises aortic systolic pressure and produces a loud A_2 component of S_2.

Calcification or *fibrosis* of the semilunar valves produces a softening of their closure, S_2. Because the semilunar valves are a morphologically different type of valve, fibrosis does not cause an increased intensity, as in closure of a fibrotic atrioventricular valve.

---

*Gradually increasing PR intervals until a dropped beat occurs.

Abnormalities of Splitting of the Second Heart Sound

Normal physiologic splitting of S_2 was discussed in the section The Cardiac Cycle. This section deals with abnormalities of splitting.

Any condition that delays right ventricular systole, either electrically or mechanically, delays P_2 and produces a widened splitting of S_2. Right ventricular emptying is delayed by a right bundle branch block or pulmonic stenosis. The pulmonic component of S_2 is delayed during both inspiration and expiration, and *wide splitting* of S_2 occurs.

Any condition that shortens left ventricular systole allows A_2 to occur earlier than normal, and wide splitting likewise occurs. Conditions such as mitral regurgitation, ventricular septal defect, and PDA shorten left ventricular systole, and the S_1-A_2 interval is shorter than normal. In these conditions, there is a "double outlet" to the left ventricle, and systole therefore is shorter. In a ventricular septal defect, with a left-to-right shunt, not only is left ventricular systole shorter but also right ventricular systole is prolonged. Both factors are crucial in producing the wide splitting of S_2.

Any condition, either electrical or mechanical, that delays left ventricular emptying produces *paradoxical splitting* of S_2. Left bundle branch block or aortic stenosis delays left ventricular emptying. These conditions delay the closure of the aortic valve after right ventricular systole and P_2 have occurred. The normal sequence of A_2-P_2 is reversed. During inspiration, P_2 moves normally away from S_1 toward A_2. The split is said to be *narrowed*. With expiration, P_2 moves normally and approaches S_1; the P_2-A_2 split widens. This widening during expiration is paradoxical. Other conditions, such as left ventricular failure and severe hypertension, delay left ventricular ejection and cause paradoxical splitting of S_2.

Fixed splitting of S_2 is the auscultatory hallmark of an atrial septal defect. In this situation, the split is wide and does not change with respiration. This is because inspiratory increases in venous return to the right atrium normally raise its pressure. During expiration, the right atrial pressure is lower, but the left-to-right atrial shunt keeps the volume in the right atrium constant during respiration; therefore, normal splitting does not occur.

Normal physiologic splitting of the second heart sound and abnormalities of splitting are illustrated in Figure 14-35.

Systolic Clicks

Ejection clicks are high-pitched sounds that occur early in systole at the onset of ejection and are produced by the opening of pathologically deformed semilunar valves. Pulmonic or aortic

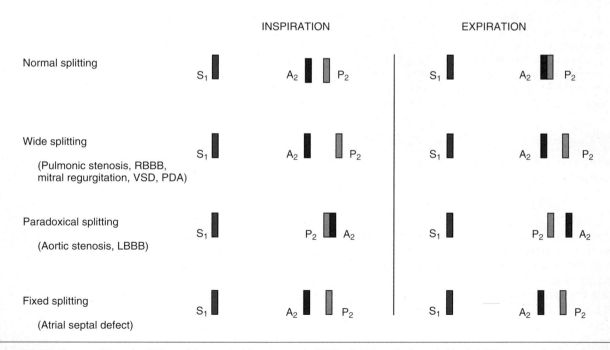

Figure 14-35 Abnormalities of splitting of the second heart sound. (RBBB, right bundle branch block; VSD, ventricular septal defect; PDA, patent ductus arteriosus; LBBB, left bundle branch block.)

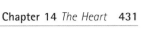

stenosis may produce ejection clicks. The sounds are short and have the quality of a "click." Pulmonic ejection clicks are best heard at the pulmonic area, and aortic ejection clicks are heard at the aortic area. As calcification progresses, the mobility of the valve decreases, and the ejection click disappears.

Midsystolic clicks are not ejection clicks. They occur in the middle of systole. They may be single or multiple, and they may change in position during the cardiac cycle with various maneuvers that change ventricular geometry. The most common condition associated with a midsystolic click is prolapse of the mitral or tricuspid valve.

Diastolic Opening Snaps

The opening of an atrioventricular valve is normally silent and occurs about 100 msec after S_2. This is about as long as it takes to say "ma-ma" quickly. An *opening snap* is a diastolic event that is the sound of the opening of a pathologically deformed atrioventricular valve. The sound is sharp and high-pitched. The mitral opening snap of mitral stenosis occurs after A_2; the tricuspid opening snap of tricuspid stenosis occurs after P_2.

The interval between S_2 and the opening snap is termed the *S_2-OS interval* and has specific significance as to the severity of the stenosis. As mitral stenosis worsens, the resistance and obstruction to flow increase. Pressure in the left atrium increases, and the gradient across the mitral valve increases. The mitral valve, therefore, opens earlier than normal when the left ventricular pressure falls below left atrial pressure. The S_2-OS time shortens as the severity increases. Try saying "ma-da" as quickly as possible. This interval is about 50 to 60 msec and approximates a very short S_2-OS interval, as heard in severe mitral stenosis.

Murmurs

Murmurs are produced when there is turbulent energy in the walls of the heart and blood vessels. Obstruction to flow or flow from a narrow vessel to a large-diameter vessel produces turbulence. Turbulence sets up eddies that strike the walls to produce vibrations that the examiner recognizes as a murmur. Murmurs can also be produced when there is a large volume of blood through a normal opening. In this circumstance, the normal opening is relatively stenotic for the increased volume. "Blowing" murmurs are produced by large gradients with variable flow volumes. "Rumbling" murmurs result from areas of small gradients that are dependent on flow. "Harsh" murmurs result from large gradients and high flow.

An ejection murmur is a murmur produced by turbulence across a semilunar valve during systole, such as in aortic stenosis or pulmonic stenosis. Ejection murmurs appear diamond-shaped and are described as "crescendo-decrescendo." They begin slightly after S_1 and end before S_2. An ejection click from stenosis of the semilunar valve may precede the murmur. These murmurs are medium-pitched and are best heard with the diaphragm of the stethoscope. Because they are based on flow, the intensity of these murmurs does not indicate the degree of severity. Increased flow across a minimally narrowed aortic valve produces a loud murmur; decreased flow across a severely stenotic aortic valve may produce a barely audible murmur. Any increase in flow or volume may produce an ejection murmur even in the presence of a normal valve. An ejection murmur as a sign of aortic stenosis is a finding of high sensitivity but low specificity. Figure 14-36 illustrates an ejection murmur.

Regurgitant systolic murmurs are produced by retrograde flow from a higher pressure area to a lower pressure area during systole, such as in mitral or tricuspid regurgitation. These murmurs are holosystolic or pansystolic. They begin with S_1 and end after S_2. They extend past S_2 because ventricular pressure is higher than atrial pressure, even after the closure of the semilunar valve. An S_3 indicative of volume overload to the ventricle is often heard. These murmurs are high-pitched and are best heard with the diaphragm of the stethoscope. The terms *regurgitation, incompetence*, and *insufficiency* are often used synonymously for this type of murmur. The preferred term is *regurgitation* because it implies the retrograde direction of flow. The holosystolic murmur of atrioventricular valve regurgitation is a finding of high sensitivity. Figure 14-37 illustrates a regurgitant murmur.

Diastolic atrioventricular murmurs begin after S_2 with the opening of the atrioventricular valve. Mitral stenosis and tricuspid stenosis are examples of this type of murmur. There is a pause between S_2 and the beginning of the murmur. Isovolumetric relaxation is occurring during this period. The murmur is decrescendo in shape, beginning with an opening snap, if

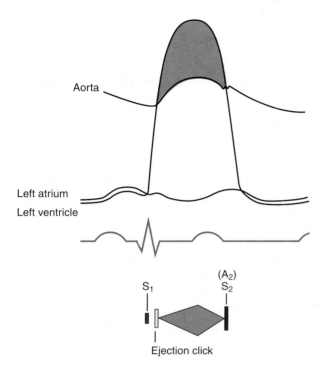

Figure 14-36 A systolic ejection murmur such as that occurring in aortic stenosis.

the valve is mobile. These murmurs are low-pitched and are best heard with the bell of the stethoscope, with the patient lying in the left lateral decubitus position. Because the atrioventricular valve is stenotic, rapid filling does not occur, and a gradient persists throughout diastole. If the patient is in normal sinus rhythm, atrial contraction increases the gradient at the end of diastole, or presystole, and there is an increase in the murmur at this time. The diastolic atrioventricular murmur is a sensitive and specific sign of atrioventricular valve stenosis.

The first heart sound is the loudest sound. The cadence and emphasis of the sounds are best heard by saying the following mnemonic:

MIT′-ral-—vaaaalve   MIT′-ral-vaaaalve
S_1 S_2 OS   DM S_1 S_2 OS DM

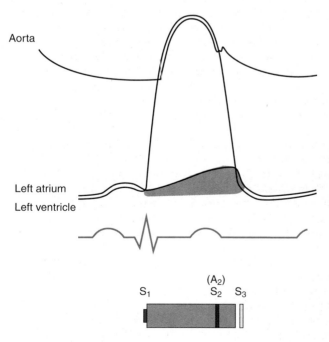

Figure 14-37 A systolic regurgitant murmur such as that occurring in mitral regurgitation.

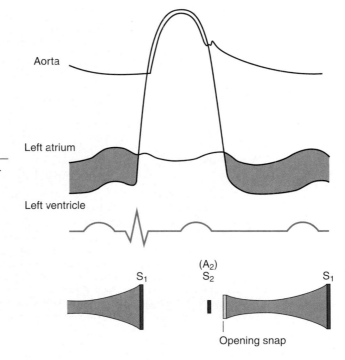

Figure 14-38 A diastolic atrioventricular murmur such as that occurring in mitral stenosis.

in which OS is the mitral opening snap, and DM is the diastolic murmur. The "aaaalve" is the presystolic accentuation heard when a patient with mitral stenosis is in normal sinus rhythm. Figure 14-38 illustrates a diastolic atrioventricular murmur.

Diastolic semilunar murmurs begin immediately after S_2, as heard in aortic or pulmonic regurgitation. In contrast to the diastolic atrioventricular murmurs, there is no delay after S_2 to the beginning of the murmur. The high-pitched murmur is decrescendo in shape and is best heard with the diaphragm of the stethoscope while the patient is sitting up and leaning forward. A diastolic semilunar murmur is a sign of low sensitivity but high specificity. Figure 14-39 illustrates the pressure curves responsible for the generation of a diastolic semilunar murmur.

Table 14-8 lists important cardiac sounds according to the cardiac cycle. Figure 14-40 lists important characteristics of the systolic murmurs of aortic stenosis and mitral regurgitation. Table 14-9 summarizes the differentiation of some additional systolic murmurs. Figure 14-41 lists important characteristics of the diastolic murmurs of mitral stenosis and aortic regurgitation.

Figure 14-39 A diastolic semilunar murmur such as that occurring in aortic regurgitation. Note the systolic ejection murmur, which is related to the increased volume and flow.

Table 14-8 Cardiac Sounds

Cardiac Cycle	Sound
Early systolic	Ejection click Aortic prosthetic valve opening sound*
Midsystolic to late systolic	Midsystolic click Rub
Early diastolic	Opening snap S_3 Mitral prosthetic valve opening sound† Tumor plop‡
Mid-diastolic	S_3 Summation gallop§
Late diastolic (sometimes called *presystolic*)	S_4 Pacemaker sound

*Opening and closure of the prosthetic aortic valve are heard with many prosthetic valves. The opening is comparable to an ejection click; the closing is a "prosthetic" S_2.
†Opening and closure of the prosthetic mitral valve are heard with many prosthetic valves. The opening is comparable to an opening snap; the closing is a "prosthetic" S_1.
‡A left atrial myxoma that is pedunculated may "plop" in and out of the mitral annulus, simulating the auscultatory signs of mitral stenosis.
§At fast heart rates, the diastolic period shortens. If an S_3 and S_4 are present, the sounds may be summated into a single sound called a *summation gallop*.

Systolic Murmurs Differentiating AS from MR

Feature	Aortic Stenosis	Mitral Regurgitation
Location	Aortic area	Apex
Radiation	Neck	Axilla
Shape	Diamond	Holosystolic
Pitch	Medium	High
Quality	Harsh	Blowing
Associated signs	Decreased A_2 Ejection click S_4 Narrow pulse pressure Slow rising and delayed pulse	Decreased S_1 S_3 Laterally displaced diffuse PMI

PMI, point of maximum impulse.

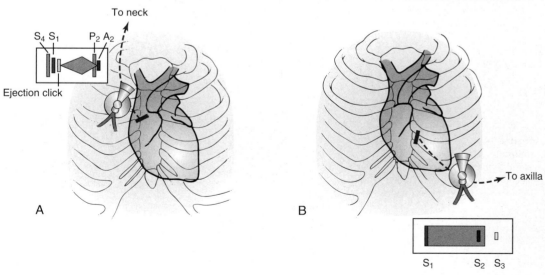

Figure 14-40 Systolic murmurs. *A,* Pathophysiology of aortic stenosis. Note the paradoxical splitting of the second heart sound (S_2), the S_4, and the ejection click. *B,* Mitral regurgitation. Note that the murmur ends after S_2, and note the presence of the S_3.

Table 14-9 Differentiation of Other Systolic Murmurs

Feature	Pulmonic Stenosis	Tricuspid Regurgitation	Ventricular Septal Defect	Venous Hum	Innocent Murmur
Location	Pulmonic area	Tricuspid area	Tricuspid area	Above clavicle	Widespread*
Radiation	Neck	Right of sternum	Right of sternum	Right neck	Minimal
Shape	Diamond	Holosystolic	Holosystolic	Continuous	Diamond
Pitch	Medium	High	High	High	Medium
Quality	Harsh	Blowing	Harsh	Roaring; humming	Twanging; vibratory

*Usually between the apex and the left lower sternal border.

Diastolic Murmurs Differentiating MS from AR

Feature	Mitral Stenosis	Aortic Regurgitation
Location	Apex	Aortic area
Radiation	No	No
Shape	Decrescendo	Decrescendo
Pitch	Low	High
Quality	Rumbling	Blowing
Associated signs	Increased S_1 Opening snap RV rock* Presystolic accentuation	S_3 Laterally displaced PMI Wide pulse pressure[†] Bounding pulses Austin Flint murmur[‡] Systolic ejection murmur[§]

PMI, point of maximum impulse; RV, right ventricular.
*Right ventricular impulse at lower left sternal border.
[†]The wide pulse pressure is the cause of the many physical signs of aortic regurgitation: Quincke's pulse, De Musset's sign, Duroziez's sign, Corrigan's pulse, and so forth.
[‡]An apical diastolic murmur heard in association with aortic regurgitation, mimicking that of mitral stenosis.
[§]A flow murmur across a valve that is relatively narrow for the increased blood volume as a result of aortic regurgitation. It is relatively stenotic and need not be anatomically stenotic, as in true aortic stenosis.

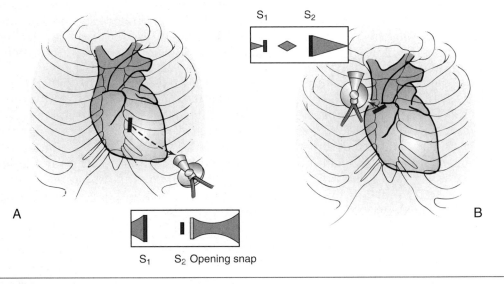

S_1 S_2 Opening snap

Figure 14-41 Diastolic murmurs. *A*, Pathophysiology of mitral stenosis. Note the intensity of S_1 and the accentuation of the diastolic murmur in late diastole. *B*, Aortic regurgitation. Note the systolic flow murmur.

Useful Vocabulary

Listed here are the specific roots that are important for understanding the terminology related to cardiac disease.

Root	Pertaining to	Example	Definition
brady-	slow	***brady***cardia	Slow heart rate
-cardio-	heart	***cardio***megaly	Enlargement of the heart
sphygmo-	pulse	***sphygmo***manometer	Instrument for measuring blood pressure
supra-	above	***supra***ventricular	Above the level of the ventricles
tachy-	fast	***tachy***cardia	Rapid heart rate

Writing Up the Physical Examination

Listed here are examples of the write-up for the examination of the heart.

- No abnormal jugular venous distention or abnormal jugular wave forms are present. The PMI is in the fifth intercostal space, midclavicular line. S_1 and S_2 are normal.* Physiologic splitting is present. No murmurs, gallops, or rubs are heard. There is no clubbing, cyanosis, or edema.
- The jugular venous pressure is elevated. There is a prominent "v" wave present in the neck. The jugular vein is distended 8 cm above the sternal angle at 45°. The PMI is in the sixth intercostal space, anterior axillary line. S_1 is soft. S_2 is widely split on inspiration and expiration. A grade III/VI, high-pitched, holo-systolic murmur is heard at the apex with radiation to the axilla. A palpable S_3 is present at the apex. There is 2+ pitting edema on the shins bilaterally. No cyanosis or clubbing is present.
- No abnormal jugular venous distention is seen. The PMI is in the fifth inter-costal space, midclavicular line. S_1 is normal. S_2 is soft. An S_4 is present at the apex. A grade IV/VI, harsh, medium-pitched, crescendo-decrescendo murmur, beginning slightly after S_1 and ending before S_2, is present at the aortic area. This murmur radiates to both carotid arteries. No clubbing, cyanosis, or edema is present.
- The jugular venous pressure is very elevated. The jugular vein is distended to the jaw margin when the patient is seated at 90°. The PMI is in the fifth inter-costal space, midclavicular line. S_1 is accentuated. S_2 is normal. An RV[†] rock is present at the left lower sternal border. There is a grade II/VI, low-pitched, diastolic rumble heard at the apex, best heard in the left lateral decubitus posi-tion. A grade III/VI, high-pitched, holosystolic murmur is heard at the left lower sternal border, which increases in intensity with inspiration. A right ventricular S_3 may be present at the left lower sternal border.[‡] There is 4+ pit-ting sacral edema. No cyanosis or clubbing is present.

---

*The descriptors for S_1 and S_2 are normal, increased, decreased, widely split, narrowly split, fixed split, or paradoxically split. Never indicate that S_1 and S_2 are present.
[†]Right ventricular.
[‡]Notice that in this example the examiner stated that a finding may be present.

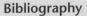

Bibliography

American Heart Association: Heart Disease and Stroke Statistics—2005 Update. Dallas, American Heart Association, 2005.

Braunwald E, Zipes DP, Libby P: Heart Disease: A Textbook of Cardiovascular Medicine, 6th ed. Philadelphia, WB Saunders, 2001.

Chandra NC, Ziegelstein RC, Rogers WJ, et al: Observations of the treatment of women in the United States with myocardial infarction: A report from the National Registry of Myocardial Infarction—I. Arch Intern Med 158:981, 1998.

Cook DJ, Simel DL: Does this patient have abnormal central venous pressure? JAMA 275:630, 1996.

Crawford MH, DiMarco JP: Cardiology. St. Louis, Mosby, 2000.

Ducas J, Magder S, McGregor M: Validity of the hepatojugular reflux as a clinical test for congestive heart failure. Am J Cardiol 52:1299, 1983.

Eilen SD, Crawford MH, O'Rourke RA: Accuracy of precordial palpation for detecting increased left ventricular volume. Ann Intern Med 99:628, 1983.

Elliott WJ: Ear lobe crease and coronary artery disease. Am J Med 75:1024, 1983.

Ewy G: The abdominojugular test: Technique and hemodynamic correlates. Ann Intern Med 109:456, 1988.

Heckerling PS, Wiener SL, Moses VK, et al: Accuracy of precordial percussion in detecting cardiomegaly. Am J Med 91:328, 1991.

Heckerling PS, Wiener SL, Wolfkiel CJ, et al: Accuracy and reproducibility of precordial percussion and palpation for detecting increased left ventricular end-diastolic volume and mass. JAMA 270:1943, 1993.

Henkind SJ, Benis AM, Teichholz LE: The paradox of pulsus paradoxus. Am Heart J 114:198, 1987.

Johnson R, Swartz MH: A Simplified Approach to Electrocardiography. Philadelphia, WB Saunders, 1986.

Julian D, Wenger NK (eds): Women and Heart Disease. London, Martin Dunitz, 1997.

Kroenke MK: Sphygmomanometry: The correct arm position. West J Med 140:459, 1984.

Maisel AS, Atwood JE, Goldberger AL: Hepatojugular reflux: Useful in the bedside diagnosis of tricuspid regurgitation. Ann Intern Med 101:781, 1984.

Marrugat J, Sala J, Masia R, et al: Mortality differences between men and women following myocardial infarction. JAMA 280:1405, 1998.

Miniño AM, Heron MP, Murphy SL, et al: Deaths: Final Data for 2004. National Vital Statistics Report, vol 55, no. 19. Hyattsville, Md, National Center for Health Statistics, 2007.

Murphy SL: Deaths: Final Data for 1998. National Vital Statistics Report, vol 48, no. 11. Hyattsville, Md, National Center for Health Statistics, 2000.

Parikh NI, Pencina MJ, Wang TJ, et al: A risk score for predicting near-term incidence of hypertension: The Framingham Heart Study. Ann Intern Med 148:102, 2008.

Pryor DB, Shaw L, McCants CB, et al: Value of the history and physical in identifying patients at increased risk for coronary artery disease. Ann Intern Med 118:81, 1993.

Rosendorff C: Essential Cardiology: Principles and Practice. Philadelphia, WB Saunders, 2000.

Schouten VW, Bohnen AM, Bosch JLHR, et al: Erectile dysfunction prospectively associated with cardiovascular disease in the Dutch general population: Results from the Krimpen Study. Int J Impotence Res 20:92, 2008.

Silverberg DS, Shemesh E, Iaina A: The unsupported arm: A cause of falsely raised blood pressure readings. BMJ 2:1331, 1977.

Thomas JE, Schirger A, Fealey RD, et al: Orthostatic hypotension. Mayo Clin Proc 56:117, 1981.

Tsang TSM, Barnes ME, Gersh BJ, et al: Risks of coronary heart disease in women: Current understanding and evolving concepts. Mayo Clin Proc 75:1289, 2000.

CHAPTER 15

The Peripheral Vascular System

Veins which by the thickening of their tunicles in the old restrict the passage of blood, and by this lack of nourishment destroy their life without any fever, the old coming to fail little by little in slow death.

Leonardo da Vinci (1452–1519)

General Considerations

Diseases of the peripheral vascular system are common and may involve the arteries, veins, or lymphatic vessels. The arterial conditions include cerebrovascular, aortoiliac, femoropopliteal, renal, aortic occlusive, and aneurysmal diseases. The two most important diseases of the peripheral arteries are atherosclerosis of the larger arteries and microvascular disease.

The most common cause of peripheral arterial occlusive disease is atherosclerosis affecting the medium-sized and large vessels of the extremities. Narrowing of the vessel causes a decreased blood supply, resulting in ischemia. In addition, atherosclerosis may become manifest by aneurysmal dilatation. The abdominal aorta is the artery most frequently involved. The aneurysm is commonly below the renal arteries and may extend as far as the external iliac arteries. Often, this aneurysm produces few, if any, symptoms. The examiner may discover a pulsatile mass as an incidental finding. Frequently, the first manifestation is the catastrophic rupture of the aneurysm. An abdominal aortic aneurysm (AAA) larger than 5 cm in diameter carries a 20% risk of rupturing within the first year of discovery and a 50% risk of rupturing within 5 years.

Vesalius described the first AAA in the 16th century. Before the development of a surgical intervention for the process, attempts at medical management failed. The initial surgical attempts at control entailed ligation of the aorta, with poor results. In 1923, Rudolph Matas performed the first successful aortic ligation on a patient. Attempts were made to induce thrombosis by inserting intraluminal wires. In 1948, C. E. Rea wrapped reactive cellophane around the aneurysm in order to induce fibrosis and limit expansion. This technique was used on Albert Einstein in 1949, and he survived 6 years before dying of rupture. However, not until 1951 was an abdominal aneurysm surgically treated by resection and grafting. In that year, C. Dubost performed the first AAA repair with a homograft. Since then, great strides have been made in understanding the natural history of vascular disease, as well as in developing new technology to help diagnose and treat it.

In autopsy studies, the frequency rate of AAA ranges from 0.5% to 3.2%. In a large U.S. Veterans Administration screening study, the prevalence rate was 1.4%. The frequency of

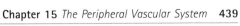

rupture is 4.4 cases per 100,000 persons. AAA is 5 times more common in men than in women and is 3.5 times more common in white men than in African-American men. The likelihood of development varies from 3 to 117 cases per 100,000 person-years.

Microvascular arterial disease occurs in patients with diabetes. Changes develop in the small arterioles that impair circulation to the skin or nerves, especially of the lower extremities, producing symptoms of ischemia. Peripheral neuropathy is a common sequela of microvascular disease. This neuropathy may be manifested as a defect in the sensory, motor, or autonomic system. Microvascular disease affects more than 15 million individuals in the United States.

Peripheral venous disease often progresses to venous stasis and thrombotic disorders. One of the dreaded complications of thrombotic disease is pulmonary embolism. In the United States, more than 175,000 deaths per year are attributed to acute pulmonary embolism.

Structure and Physiology

Diseases of the peripheral *arterial* system cause ischemia of the extremities. When the body is at rest, collateral blood vessels may be able to provide adequate circulation. During exercise, when oxygen demand increases, this circulation may not be sufficient for the actively contracting muscles, and ischemia may result.

The *venous system* consists of a series of low-pressure capacitance vessels. Nearly 70% of the blood volume is contained in this system. Although offering little resistance, the veins are controlled by a variety of neural and humoral stimuli that enhance venous return to the right side of the heart. In addition, valves aid in the return of blood.

When an individual is in the upright posture, the venous pressure in the lower extremity is the highest. Over many years, the veins dilate as a result of weakening of their walls. As the walls dilate, the veins are unable to close adequately, and reflux of blood occurs. In addition, the venous pump becomes less efficient in returning blood to the heart. Both of these factors are responsible for the venous stasis seen in patients with chronic venous insufficiency. Complications from venous stasis include pigmentation, dermatitis, cellulitis, ulceration, and thrombus formation.

The *lymphatic system* is an extensive vascular network and is responsible for returning tissue fluid (lymph) back to the venous system. The extremities are richly supplied with lymphatic tissue. Lymph nodes, many of which are located between major proximal joints, aid in filtering the lymphatic fluid before it enters the blood. The most important clinical symptoms of lymphatic obstruction are *lymphedema* and *lymphangitis*.

Review of Specific Symptoms

Many patients with peripheral vascular disease are asymptomatic. When patients are symptomatic, vascular disease causes the following:

- Pain
- Changes in skin temperature and color
- Edema
- Ulceration
- Emboli
- Stroke
- Dizziness

Pain

Pain is the principal symptom of atherosclerosis. Whenever a patient complains of pain in the calf, arch of the foot, thighs, hips, or buttocks while walking, peripheral vascular disease of the arteries must be considered. The symptom of pain in the lower extremity *during* exercise is called *intermittent claudication*. The site of the pain is always distal to the occlusive disease. As the disease progresses, pain at rest occurs. This is often severe and is aggravated by cool temperatures and elevation, especially during sleep in bed. Pain may also occur with deep vein thrombosis.

If a male patient complains of buttock or thigh pain while walking, the examiner should inquire about erectile dysfunction. *Leriche's syndrome* is chronic aortoiliac obstruction; the patient presents with intermittent claudication and erectile dysfunction. In this condition, the terminal aorta and iliac arteries are involved by severe atherosclerosis at the aortic bifurcation.

Patients occasionally complain of bilateral leg pain or numbness that occurs while walking, as well as while resting. This is called *pseudoclaudication* and is a symptom of musculoskeletal disease in the lumbar area.

Skin Changes

Skin color changes are common with vascular disease. In chronic *arterial insufficiency*, the affected extremity is cool and pale. In chronic *venous insufficiency*, the extremity is warmer than normal. The leg becomes erythematous, and erosions produced by excoriation result. With chronic insufficiency, stasis changes produce increased pigmentation, swelling, and an "aching" or "heaviness" in the legs. These changes characteristically occur in the lower third of the extremity and are more prominent medially. When venous insufficiency occurs, edema of dependent areas results.

Patients with acute deep vein thrombosis have secondary inflammation of the tissue surrounding the vein. This produces signs of inflammation: warmth, redness, and fever. Swelling is the most reliable symptom and sign associated with venous obstruction. This finding is indicative of severe deep vein obstruction because the superficial veins of the lower extremity carry only 20% of the total drainage and are not associated with swelling. The extremities should be compared, and a difference in circumference of 2 cm at the ankle or midcalf should be considered significant.

Edema

Lymphedema results from either a primary abnormality in the development of the lymphatic system or an acquired obstruction to flow. Whether the congenital or the acquired form is involved, the net result is stasis of lymph fluid in the tissues, producing a *firm, nonpitting edema*. Over several years, the skin takes on a rough consistency similar to that of pigskin. Because lymphedema is usually painless, the only symptom is "heaviness" of the extremity.

Ulceration

Persistent ischemia of a limb is associated with ischemic ulceration and gangrene. Ulceration is almost inevitable once skin has thickened and the circulation is compromised. Ulceration related to arterial insufficiency occurs as a result of trauma to the toes and heel. These ulcers are painful, have discrete edges that produce a "punched-out" appearance, and are often covered with crust. When infected, the tissue is erythematous.

In contrast to arterial insufficiency ulceration, venous insufficiency leads to stasis ulceration, which is painless and occurs in the ankle area or lower leg just above the medial malleolus. The classic manifestation is a diffusely reddened, thickened area over the medial malleolus. The skin has a cobblestone appearance resulting from fibrosis and venous stasis. Ulceration occurs with the slightest trauma. Rapidly developing ulcers are commonly caused by arterial insufficiency, whereas slowly developing ulceration is usually the result of venous insufficiency. Figures 15-1 and 15-2 show stasis dermatitis and ulcerations over the medial malleoli. Patients with leg ulcers should be asked the following:

"What did the ulcer look like when it first appeared?"

"What do you think started the ulcer?"

"How quickly did it develop?"

"How painful is the ulcer?"

"What kind of medications have you been taking?"

"Is there a history of any generalized diseases, such as anemia? rheumatoid arthritis?"

"Is there a family history of leg ulcers?"

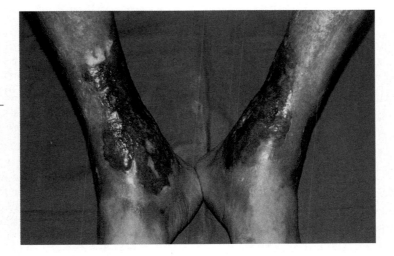

Figure 15–1 Stasis dermatitis and bilateral ulceration over the medial malleoli.

Emboli

A history of emboli is important. Thrombus formation results from stasis and hypercoagulability. It appears, however, that venous stasis is the most important cause of thrombus formation. Bed rest, congestive heart failure, obesity, pregnancy, recent extended travel on airplanes, and oral contraceptives have been linked to thrombus formation and emboli.

Symptoms secondary to emboli can include shortness of breath from pulmonary emboli; abdominal pain from splenic, intestinal, or renal artery emboli; neurologic symptoms from carotid or vertebrobasilar artery emboli; and pain and paresthesias from peripheral artery emboli.

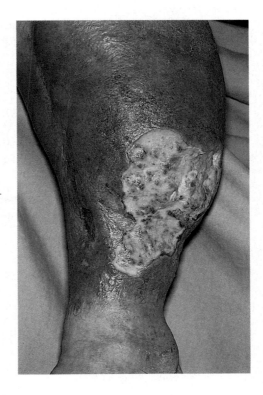

Figure 15–2 Stasis dermatitis and ulceration over the medial malleolus.

Neurologic Symptoms

Cerebrovascular occlusive disease causes many neurologic symptoms, including strokes,* dizziness, and changes in consciousness. Occlusion of the internal carotid artery produces a syndrome of contralateral hemiplegia, contralateral sensory deficits, and dysphasia. Vertebrobasilar disease is associated with diplopia, cerebellar dysfunction, changes in consciousness, and facial paresis.

Impact of Vascular Disease on the Patient

A patient with chronic arterial insufficiency has worsening pain while walking. As the condition progresses, ulceration of the toes, feet, and areas susceptible to trauma, such as the shins, develops. Pain may become excruciating. Gangrene of a toe may develop, and amputation of the toe is frequently followed by amputation of the foot and leg. In addition, the patient becomes increasingly depressed as a result of ongoing mutilation of the body.

Physical Examination

The equipment necessary for the examination of the peripheral vascular system consists of a stethoscope, a tourniquet, and a tape measure.

The physical examination of the peripheral vascular system consists of inspection, palpation of the arterial pulses, and some additional tests if disease is thought to be present. All these techniques are usually integrated with the rest of the physical examination.

The patient lies supine, with the examiner standing to the right of the bed. The evaluation of the peripheral vascular system includes the following:

- Inspection
- Examination of the arterial pulses
- Examination of the lymphatic system
- Other special techniques

Inspection

Inspect for Symmetry of the Extremities

The extremities should be compared for asymmetries in size, color, temperature, and venous patterns. Figure 15-3 depicts massive lymphedema of the right upper extremity secondary to a right total mastectomy 18 years earlier.

Inspect the Lower Extremities

The lower extremities should be inspected for pigmentary abnormalities, ulcers, edema, and venous patterns. Is cyanosis present? Is edema present? If edema is present, does it pit? Bilateral color changes and swelling of the legs of the patient are pictured in Figure 15-4. The patient had chronic venous insufficiency. She died of a massive pulmonary embolus 1 day after this photograph was taken.

Assess the Skin Temperature

Evaluate the temperature by using the back of your hand. Compare similar areas of each extremity. Coolness of an extremity is common with arterial insufficiency.

Inspect for Varicosities

Ask the patient to stand, and inspect the lower extremities for varicosities. Look at the area of the proximal femoral ring, as well as in the distal portion of the legs. Varicose veins in these locations may not have been visible when the patient was lying down.

The patient in Figure 15-5 was a 37-year-old woman with severe right-sided heart failure. Notice the marked dilated and tortuous veins in the popliteal fossa. Also notice the increased pigmentation of the skin over the lower legs.

---

*A stroke is also known as a *cerebrovascular accident*.

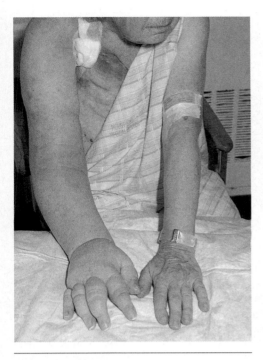

Figure 15–3 Lymphedema.

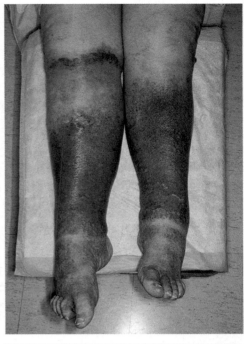

Figure 15–4 Chronic venous insufficiency.

Examination of the Arterial Pulses

The most important finding when the peripheral arterial tree is examined is a decreased or absent pulse. The radial, brachial, femoral, popliteal, dorsalis pedis, and posterior tibial pulses are routinely evaluated.

Palpate the Radial Pulse

You should stand in front of the patient. The radial pulses are evaluated by grasping both of the patient's wrists and palpating the pulses with your index, middle, and fourth fingers. Hold the patient's right wrist with your left fingers and the patient's left wrist with your right fingers, as demonstrated in Figure 14-22. The symmetry of the pulses is evaluated for timing and strength.

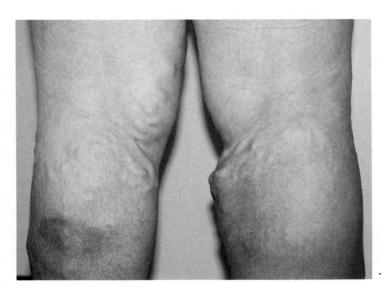

Figure 15–5 Marked varicosities of the popliteal fossa.

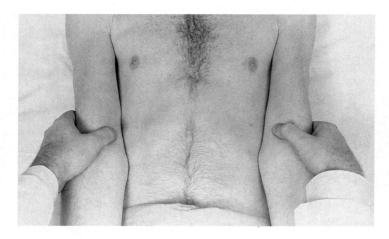

Figure 15–6 Technique for brachial artery palpation.

Palpate the Brachial Pulse

Because the brachial pulse is stronger than the digital pulses, the examiner may use his or her thumbs to palpate the patient's brachial pulses. The brachial artery can be felt medially just under the belly or tendon of the biceps muscle. With the examiner still standing in front of the patient, both brachial arteries can be palpated simultaneously. The examiner's left hand holds the patient's right arm, and the examiner's right hand holds the patient's left arm. Once the examiner's thumbs feel the brachial pulsation, the examiner should apply progressive pressure to it until the maximal systolic force is felt. This is demonstrated in Figure 15-6. The examiner should now be able to assess its wave form.

Auscultate the Carotid Artery

Auscultation for carotid bruits* is performed by placing the diaphragm of the stethoscope over the patient's carotid artery while the patient is lying supine. This is demonstrated in Figure 15-7. The patient's head should be slightly elevated on a pillow and turned slightly away from the carotid artery being evaluated. It is often helpful to ask the patient to hold his or her breath during the auscultation. Normally, either nothing or transmitted heart sounds are heard. After one carotid artery is evaluated, the other is examined. After auscultation of the carotid arteries, they are palpated (see Chapter 14, The Heart).

The presence of a murmur should be noted. This may be a bruit resulting from atherosclerotic disease of the carotid artery. On occasion, loud murmurs originating from the heart can be transmitted to the neck. With experience, the examiner is able to determine whether the disorder is local in the neck or distal in the heart.

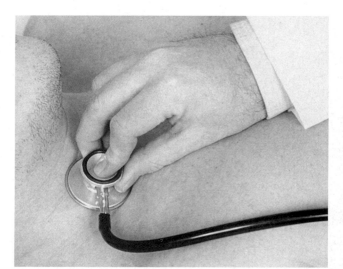

Figure 15–7 Technique for auscultation of the carotid artery.

---

*A bruit is a sound or murmur heard in a vessel as a result of increased turbulence.

Table 15–1 Characteristics of Physical Signs for Detecting an Abdominal Aortic Aneurysm

Physical Sign	Sensitivity (%)	Specificity (%)
Definite pulsatile mass	28	97
Definite or suggestive pulsatile mass	50	91
Abdominal bruit	11	95
Femoral bruit	17	87
Femoral pulse deficit	22	91

Data from Lederle FA, Walker JM, Reinke DB: Selective screening for abdominal aortic aneurysms with physical examination and ultrasound. Arch Intern Med 148:1753, 1988.

Palpate the Abdominal Aorta

AAAs kill approximately 10,000 people in the United States each year. Many of these deaths could be prevented if the patients were aware of the presence of this defect. Once the defect is recognized, the rate of operative mortality for a nonruptured aneurysm is less than 5%, and after operation, the survival rate equals that of the general population. An AAA that ruptures carries a mortality rate of nearly 90%. Even among patients who reach the operating room alive, the surgical mortality rate is 50%.

The examination is performed by palpating deeply, but gently, into the midabdomen. The presence of a mass with laterally expansive pulsation suggests an AAA. Some caution is urged in making this diagnosis in thin individuals, in whom the normal pulsatile aorta can be easily palpated. The high false-positive rate with this examination should not be a problem, however, because confirmation with abdominal ultrasonography is safe and inexpensive.

Other findings associated with an AAA include an abdominal bruit, a femoral bruit, and a femoral pulse deficit. In fewer than 10% of patients with AAAs, a bruit may be present. Acute rupture of an AAA is suggested when a bruit is associated with severe pain in the abdomen or back and when the distal pulse is absent or diminished and later returns.

Table 15-1 summarizes the physical signs useful for detecting an AAA.

Rule Out Abdominal Bruits

The patient should be supine. The examiner places the diaphragm of the stethoscope in the midline of the patient's abdomen about 2 inches (5 cm) above the umbilicus and listens carefully for the presence of an *aortic bruit*. This technique is demonstrated in Figure 15-8.

A *renal bruit* may be the only clue to renal artery stenosis. Auscultation should be performed about 2 inches (5 cm) above the umbilicus and 1 to 2 (2.5 to 5 cm) inches laterally to the right and to the left of midposition.

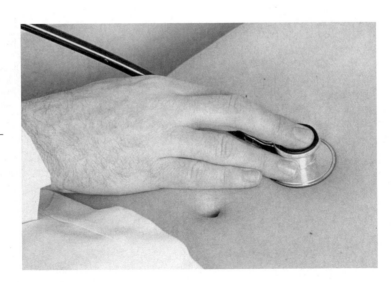

Figure 15–8 Technique for auscultation of the abdominal aorta.

Abdominal bruits that are present only during systole are frequently of little clinical value because they are found in normal individuals and in patients with essential hypertension. The presence of a systolic-diastolic abdominal bruit, however, should raise the suspicion of renovascular hypertension. Nearly 60% of all patients with renovascular hypertension have such a bruit.

The presence of a combined systolic-diastolic abdominal bruit has a sensitivity of 39% and a specificity of 99% for detecting renovascular hypertension. The presence of this type of bruit has a positive likelihood ratio (LR+) of 39 and, if absent, a negative likelihood ratio (LR−) of 0.6. In a study that evaluated the presence of any epigastric or flank bruit and its association with renovascular hypertension, the sensitivity was 63%, but the specificity dropped to 90%. The presence of any abdominal bruit confers a much lower LR+ for renovascular hypertension (i.e., 6.4).

Palpate the Femoral Pulse

The femoral pulse is evaluated with the patient lying on the back and the examiner at the patient's right side. The lateral corners of the pubic hair triangle are observed and palpated. The femoral artery should run obliquely through the corner of the pubic hair triangle inferior to the inguinal ligament at a point midway between the pubic tubercle and the anterior superior iliac spine. Both femoral pulses may be compared simultaneously. The technique is demonstrated in Figure 15-9.

If one of the femoral pulses is diminished or absent, auscultation for a bruit is necessary. The diaphragm of the stethoscope is placed over the femoral artery. The presence of a bruit may indicate obstructive aortoiliofemoral disease.

Rule Out Coarctation of the Aorta

The timing of the femoral and radial pulses is important. Normally, these pulses peak either at the same time or with the femoral pulse preceding the radial pulse. By placing one hand on the patient's femoral artery and the other on the radial artery, the examiner can determine the peaking of these pulses. This technique need be performed on one side only. Any delay in the femoral pulse should raise suspicion of coarctation of the aorta, especially in a hypertensive individual. This technique is demonstrated in Figure 15-10.

Palpate the Popliteal Pulse

The popliteal artery is often difficult to assess. Each artery is evaluated separately. While the patient is lying on the back, the examiner's thumbs are placed on the patella, and the remaining fingers of both hands are pressed in the popliteal fossa medial to the lateral biceps femoris tendon, as demonstrated in Figure 15-11. The examiner should hold the leg in a mild degree of flexion. The patient should not be asked to elevate the leg, because this tightens the muscles and makes it more difficult to feel the pulse. The examiner should squeeze both hands in the popliteal fossa. Firm pressure is usually necessary to feel the pulsation.

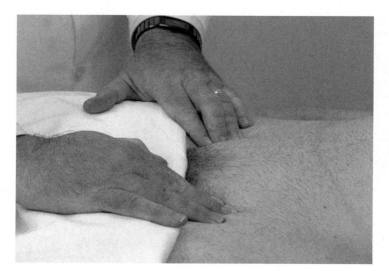

Figure 15–9 Technique for palpation of the femoral arteries.

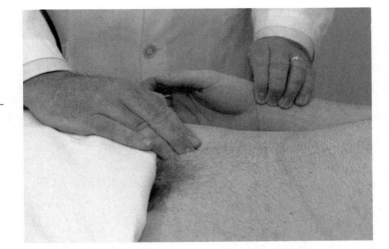

Figure 15–10 Technique for timing the femoral and radial pulses.

Palpate the Dorsalis Pedis Pulse

The dorsalis pedis pulse is best palpated when the foot is dorsiflexed. The dorsalis pedis artery passes along a line from the extensor retinaculum of the ankle to a point just lateral to the extensor tendon of the great toe. It is usually easily palpated in the groove between the extensor digitorum longus and hallucis longus tendon. The dorsalis pedis pulses may be felt simultaneously, as demonstrated in Figure 15-12.

Palpate the Posterior Tibial Pulse

The posterior tibial artery can be palpated just posterior to the medial malleoli between the tibialis posterior tendon and the flexor digitorum longus tendon. Both arteries can be evaluated simultaneously. Figure 15-13 demonstrates this procedure. Although posterior tibial pulses are absent in 15% of normal subjects, the most sensitive sign of occlusive peripheral arterial disease in patients older than 60 years of age is the absence of the posterior tibial pulse.

Grading of Pulses

The description of the amplitude of the pulse is most important. The following is the most widely accepted grading system:

0 Absent

1 Diminished

2 Normal

3 Increased

4 Bounding

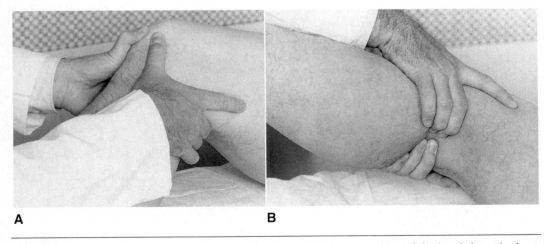

A   **B**

Figure 15–11 Technique for palpation of the popliteal artery. *A*, Correct position of the hands from the front. *B*, View from behind the popliteal fossa.

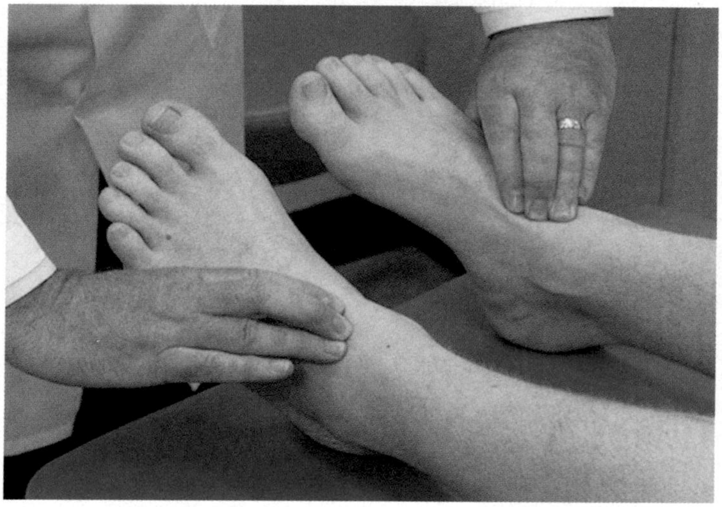

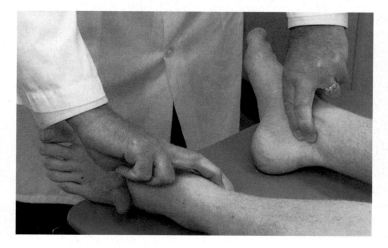

Figure 15–12 Technique for palpation of the dorsalis pedis arteries.

It is important that the patient's socks or stockings be removed when the examiner assesses the peripheral pulses of the lower extremities. If there is confusion about whether you are feeling the patient's pulse or your own pulse, you can palpate the patient's pulse with your right hand and use your left hand to palpate your own right radial pulse. If the pulses are different, you are feeling the patient's pulse with your right hand.

Examination of the Lymphatic System

Physical signs of lymphatic system disease include the following:

- Palpable lymph nodes
- Lymphangitis
- Lymphedema

Lymph nodes should be described as painless or tender and as single or matted. Generalized lymphadenopathy and localized lymphadenopathy are suggestive of different diagnoses. *Generalized* lymphadenopathy is the presence of palpable lymph nodes in three or more lymph node chains. Lymphoma, leukemia, collagen vascular disorders, and systemic bacterial, viral, and protozoal infections may be responsible. *Localized* lymphadenopathy is usually the result of localized infection or neoplasm.

Figure 15–13 Technique for palpation of the posterior tibial arteries.

Lymphangitis is lymphatic spread manifested by thin red streaks on the skin. Obstruction to lymphatic flow produces *lymphedema*, which is usually indistinguishable from other types of edema. In Figure 16-8, the patient has marked lymphedema of her left arm secondary to inflammatory breast carcinoma.

The examinations for lymphadenopathy of the head, neck, and supraclavicular areas are described in Chapter 9, The Head and Neck, and in Chapter 13, The Chest. Chapter 16, The Breast, describes the examination for palpating axillary adenopathy. Chapter 18, Male Genitalia and Hernias, describes the technique for palpating inguinal lymph nodes. The only other important lymph node chain is the epitrochlear nodes, discussed in the following section.

Palpate for Epitrochlear Nodes

To palpate epitrochlear nodes, have the patient flex the elbow approximately 90°. Feel for the nodes in the fossa about 3 cm proximal to the medial epicondyle of the humerus, in the groove between the biceps and the triceps muscles. Epitrochlear nodes are rarely palpable, but if they are present, their size, consistency, and tenderness should be described. Acute infections of the ulnar aspect of the forearm and hand may be responsible for epitrochlear adenopathy. Epitrochlear nodes are also observed in non-Hodgkin's lymphoma.

Other Special Techniques

All the special tests described here are to be used in conjunction with other forms of testing. Each of these vascular techniques is associated with many false-positive and false-negative findings. The results, therefore, must be considered as part of the total evaluation.

Evaluate Arterial Supply in the Lower Extremity

The most important sign of arterial insufficiency is a decreased pulse. In patients in whom chronic arterial insufficiency of the lower extremity is suspected, another test may be useful. The amount of pallor that develops after elevation and dependency of the ischemic extremity provides an approximate guide to the extent of decreased circulation. The patient is asked to lie on the back, and the examiner elevates the patient's legs at about 60° above the bed. The patient is asked to move the ankles to help drain the blood from the venous system, making the color changes more obvious. After about 60 seconds, the feet are inspected for pallor. Normally, no pallor is present (grade 0). Definite pallor in 60 seconds is grade 1; pallor in 30 to 60 seconds is grade 2; pallor in less than 30 seconds is grade 3; and pallor without elevation is grade 4. The patient is then asked to sit dangling the feet off the side of the bed, and the examiner assesses the time for color return. Normally it takes 10 to 15 seconds for color to return and 15 seconds for the superficial veins to fill. If it takes 15 to 25 seconds for color return, moderate occlusive disease is present; if it takes more than 40 seconds for color to return, severe ischemia is present. A dusky or cyanotic color may also develop. This test is useful only if the valves of the superficial veins are competent.

Evaluate Capillary Refill Time in the Lower Extremity

The capillary refill time is usually 3 to 5 seconds. It can be determined by compressing the toe tufts until they blanch. Prolongation of the time it takes for normal coloration to return after release is synonymous with arterial vascular insufficiency.

Evaluate Arterial Supply in the Upper Extremity

Chronic arterial insufficiency of the upper extremity is much less common than that of the lower extremity. The *Allen test*, which determines the patency of the radial and ulnar arteries, can be used to assess whether arterial insufficiency exists in the upper extremity. (The ulnar artery is normally not palpable.) This test takes advantage of the radial-ulnar loop. The examiner first occludes the radial artery by applying firm pressure over it. The patient is asked to clench the fist tightly. The patient is then asked to open the fist, and the color of the palm is observed. The test is repeated with occlusion of the ulnar artery. Pallor of the palm during compression of one artery indicates occlusion of the other.

Test for Incompetent Saphenous Veins

It is easy to demonstrate incompetent saphenous vein valves on examination. The patient is asked to stand, and the dilated varicose vein becomes obvious. The examiner compresses the proximal end of the varicose vein with one hand while placing his or her other hand about 15 to 20 cm below it at the distal end of the vein. When saphenous valves in the portion of the vein examined are incompetent, an impulse is transmitted to the examiner's distal fingers.

Test for Retrograde Filling

The *Trendelenburg maneuver* is used to assess venous valvular competency in the communicating veins, as well as in the saphenous system. A tourniquet is placed around the patient's upper thigh after it has been elevated 90° for 15 to 20 seconds. The tourniquet occludes the great saphenous vein and should not occlude the arterial pulse. The patient is then instructed to stand while the examiner watches for venous filling. The saphenous vein should fill slowly from below in about 30 seconds as the femoral artery pushes blood through the capillary bed into the venous system. Rapid filling of the superficial veins from above indicates retrograde flow through incompetent valves of the communicating veins. After 30 seconds, the tourniquet is released. Any sudden additional filling also indicates incompetent valves of the saphenous vein.

Clinicopathologic Correlations

The signs of an acute arterial occlusion are the *five Ps: p*ain, *p*allor, *p*aresthesia, *p*aralysis, and *p*ulselessness.

Chronic progressive small vessel disease is characteristic of diabetes mellitus. It is commonly observed that arterial pulses are present despite gangrene in the extremity. Figure 15-14 depicts dry gangrene of the toes in a diabetic patient.

Diabetes has been associated with many skin disorders. The cutaneous hallmark of diabetes is a waxy, yellow or reddish-brown, sharply demarcated, plaquelike lesion known as *necrobiosis lipoidica diabeticorum*. These lesions are classically found on the anterior surface of the lower legs. They are shiny and atrophic, with marked telangiectasia over their surface. The lesions have a tendency to ulcerate, and the ulcers, once present, heal very slowly. Necrobiosis lipoidica diabeticorum often predates the development of frank diabetes. The severity of the cutaneous lesion is not related to the severity of the diabetes. Figure 15-15 shows necrobiosis lipoidica diabeticorum; Figure 15-16 is a close-up photograph of the lesion in another patient with diabetes.

Deep vein thrombosis of a lower extremity is diagnosed when there is unilateral marked swelling, venous distention, erythema, pain, increased warmth, and tenderness. There is often resistance to dorsiflexion of the ankle. Calf swelling is present in most patients with femoral or popliteal venous involvement, whereas thigh swelling occurs with iliofemoral thrombosis. Figure 15-17 shows deep femoral vein thrombosis secondary to cancer. Notice the marked swelling of the left leg.

Gentle squeezing of the affected calf or slow dorsiflexion of the ankle may produce calf pain in approximately 50% of patients with femoral vein thrombosis. Pain elicited by this technique is referred to as *Homans' sign*. Unfortunately, owing to the low sensitivity of Homans' sign, this finding should not be used as a single criterion for diagnosing deep vein thrombophlebitis. A variety of unrelated conditions also may elicit a false-positive response.

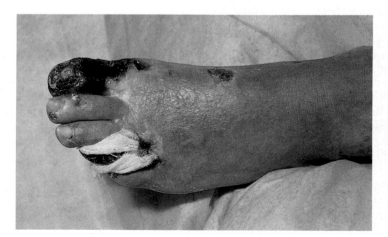

Figure 15–14 Diabetic gangrene.

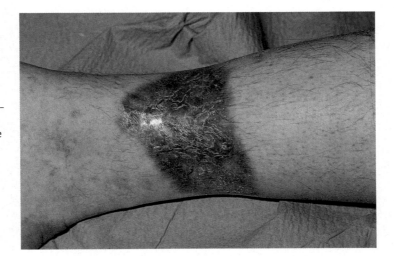

Figure 15–15 Necrobiosis lipoidica diabeticorum. Note the shiny, waxy surface.

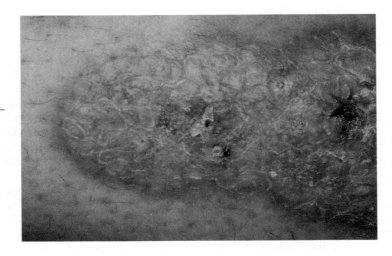

Figure 15–16 Close-up of a necrobiosis lipoidica diabeticorum lesion.

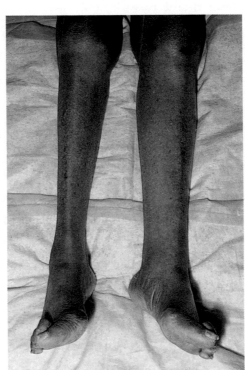

Figure 15–17 Deep vein thrombosis, left leg.

Table 15–2 Precipitating Factors in Thromboembolism

Factor	Cause
Stasis	Arrhythmia Heart failure Immobilization Obesity Varicose veins Dehydration
Blood vessel injury	Trauma Fracture
Increased coagulability	Neoplasm Oral contraceptives Pregnancy Polycythemia Previous thromboembolism

Secondary to venous thrombosis, inflammation around the vein may result. Erythema, warmth, and fever then occur, and *thrombophlebitis* is present. In many cases, the examiner can palpate this tender, indurated vein in the groin or medial thigh. This is commonly referred to as a *cord*.

Deep vein thrombophlebitis is associated with symptomatic *pulmonary embolism* in approximately 10% of patients. If the embolus is large, main pulmonary artery obstruction may occur, which can result in death. It is estimated that an additional 45% of patients with thrombophlebitis have asymptomatic pulmonary emboli.

Several factors that are important in precipitating thromboembolism are outlined in Table 15-2.

An important and common peripheral vascular condition is *Raynaud's disease* or *phenomenon*. Classically, this condition is associated with three color changes of the distal fingers or toes: white (*pallor*), blue (*cyanosis*), and red (*rubor*). These color changes are related to arteriospasm and decreased blood supply (pallor), increased peripheral extraction of oxygen (cyanosis), and return of blood supply (rubor). The patient may experience pain or numbness of the involved area as a result of the causes of pallor and cyanosis. During the hyperemic or rubor stage, the patient may complain of burning paresthesias. Between episodes, there may be no symptoms or signs of the condition.

Raynaud's disease, which is *primary* or idiopathic, must be differentiated from Raynaud's phenomenon, which is *secondary*. Table 15-3 lists some of the different characteristics of these conditions.

Gangrene is necrosis of the deep tissues resulting from a decreased blood supply. Features of the main vascular diseases causing gangrene of the lower extremities are summarized in Table 15-4.

Table 15–3 Differential Diagnosis of Raynaud's Disease and Raynaud's Phenomenon

Feature	Raynaud's Disease	Raynaud's Phenomenon
Sex	Female	Female
Bilaterality	Present (often symmetric)	± (asymmetric)
Precipitated by cold	Common	Increases symptoms
Ischemic changes	Rare	Common
Gangrene	Rare	More common
Disease association*	No	Yes

*Such as scleroderma, systemic lupus erythematosus, dermatomyositis, or rheumatoid arthritis.

Table 15–4 Differential Diagnosis of the Main Vascular Diseases Causing Gangrene

Feature	Diabetes	Atherosclerosis	Thromboangiitis Obliterans	Raynaud's Disease	Arterial Embolism
Age	Any	Older than 60 years	Younger than 40 years	Younger than 40 years	Any
Sex	Either	Either	Male	Female	Either
Onset	Gradual	Gradual	Gradual	Gradual	Sudden
Pain	Moderate	Moderate	Severe	Moderate	Often severe
Distal pulses	May be absent	May be absent	May be absent	Present	Absent*

*Affected artery does not have pulsation.

Useful Vocabulary

Listed here are the specific roots that are important for understanding the terminology related to vascular disease.

Root	Pertaining to	Example	Definition
angi(o)-	blood vessel	***angio***graphy	Radiographic visualization of blood vessels
embol(o)-	wedge; stopper	***embol***ism	Sudden blocking of a vessel by a clot
phleb(o)-	veins	***phlebo***tomy	Incision into a vein for blood removal
thrombo-	clot	***thrombo***embolism	Obstruction of a blood vessel by a clot that has broken loose from its site of formation
varico-	twisted; swollen	***varico***se	Unnaturally swollen and twisted

Writing Up the Physical Examination

Listed here are examples of the write-up for the examination of the vascular system.

- The extremities are normal in color, size, and temperature. All pulses in the upper and lower extremities are grade 2 and are equal. No bruits are present. No clubbing, cyanosis, or edema is present.
- There are yellow, waxy, sharply demarcated lesions on both anterior shins. Both legs appear slightly cool, the left greater than the right. There is a punched-out ulceration on the lateral aspect of the left ankle. The left big toe is blackened, with a sharp demarcation. The femoral pulses are grade 2 bilaterally. No distal pulses are felt. There is 1+ pretibial edema present bilaterally. No clubbing or cyanosis is present.
- The right lower extremity is 3 cm larger than the left, measured 4 cm below the inferior aspect of the patella. The right calf is tender, warm, and erythematous. A cord is palpated in the right groin. Both lower extremities are edematous

and hyperpigmented. There is 3+ pretibial edema on the right and 2+ pretibial edema on the left. A small ulceration is present above the left medial malleolus. The arterial pulses are grade 2 at the femoral arteries and grade 1 at the popliteal arteries. No pulses are palpated distal to the popliteal arteries. No clubbing or cyanosis is present.

Bibliography

Ailawadi G, Eliason JL, Upchurch GR Jr: Current concepts in the pathogenesis of abdominal aortic aneurysm. J Vasc Surg 38:584, 2003.

Bloch MJ, Basile J: Clinical insights into the diagnosis and management of renovascular disease. An evidence-based review. Minerva Med 95:357, 2004.

Grim CE, Luft FC, Myron H, et al: Sensitivity and specificity of screening tests for renal vascular hypertension. Ann Intern Med 91:617, 1979.

Hacklander T, Mertens H, Stattaus J, et al: Evaluation of renovascular hypertension: Comparison of functional MRI and contrast-enhanced MRA with a routinely performed renal scintigraphy and DSA. J Comput Assist Tomogr 28:823, 2004.

Hirsch AT, Haskal ZJ, Hertzer NR, et al: ACC/AHA 2005 Practice Guidelines for the management of patients with peripheral arterial disease (lower extremity, renal, mesenteric, and abdominal aortic): A collaborative report from the American Association for Vascular Surgery/Society for Vascular Surgery, Society for Cardiovascular Angiography and Interventions, Society for Vascular Medicine and Biology, Society of Interventional Radiology, and the ACC/AHA Task Force on Practice Guidelines (Writing Committee to Develop Guidelines for the Management of Patients with Peripheral Arterial Disease); endorsed by the American Association of Cardiovascular and Pulmonary Rehabilitation; National Heart, Lung, and Blood Institute; Society for Vascular Nursing; TransAtlantic Inter-Society Consensus; and Vascular Disease Foundation. Circulation 113(11):e463, 2006.

Lederle FA, Johnson GR, Wilson SE, et al: Prevalence and associations of abdominal aortic aneurysm detected through screening. Aneurysm Detection and Management (ADAM) Veterans Affairs Cooperative Study Group. Ann Intern Med 126:441, 1997.

Lederle FA, Walker JM, Reinke DB: Selective screening for abdominal aortic aneurysms with physical examination and ultrasound. Arch Intern Med 148:1753, 1988.

Rutherford RB, Krupski WC: Current status of open versus endovascular stent-graft repair of abdominal aortic aneurysm. J Vasc Surg 39:1129, 2004.

Tewari A, Chung K-S, Button M, et al: Differential diagnosis, investigation, and current treatment of lower limb lymphedema. Arch Surg 138:152, 2003.

Turnbull JM: Is listening for abdominal bruits useful in the evaluation of hypertension? JAMA 274:1299, 1995.

CHAPTER 16

The Breast

The shape of the breast is like a gourd. They are round for holding blood to be changed into milk. ... They have teats, that the new born child may suck therefrom.

Mondino De' Luzzi (1275–1326)

General Considerations

In the United States, the National Cancer Institute estimates that one of every eight women (approximately 12.5%) will develop breast cancer during her lifetime. Among the malignant diseases in women, breast cancer is the most common to develop and is the second most common cancer cause of death. In 2007, it accounted for 31% of new cancer cases in American women, and 15% of cancer deaths; there were 180,510 new cases of invasive breast cancer (stages I to IV) and 40,910 related deaths in the United States (40,460 women and 450 men). Breast carcinoma in situ, a very early form of the disease, was diagnosed in another 62,030 women.

The incidence of cancer of the breast is higher in the United States than in European or Asian countries. It has been well established that women in underdeveloped nations have lower rates of breast cancer than do women from more affluent societies. Among racial/ethnic groups, white and African-American women have the highest incidence rates of breast cancer (113.2 and 99.3 per 100,000 population, respectively). Asian and Pacific Islander women and Latino women have a lower risk (72.6 and 69.4 per 100,000 population, respectively). The risk is lowest among Native Americans (33.9 per 100,000 population). The rate of mortality from breast cancer is highest in African-American women (31.4 per 100,000); the mortality rate in white women is 25.7 per 100,000. The lowest rate of mortality from breast cancer is in Asian and Pacific Islander women (11.4 per 100,000). The incidence of breast cancer continues to increase, partly because of increased screening through mammography.

Once breast cancer has occurred in a family, the risk that other women in the same family will have breast cancer is significantly higher. First-degree relatives, such as sisters or daughters, have more than twice the risk for development of breast cancer if the original patient developed cancer in one breast after menopause. Women with a family history of premenopausal breast cancer in one breast have three times the risk. If the original patient had postmenopausal cancer in both breasts, the first-degree relatives have more than four times the risk. First-degree relatives of patients with cancer in both breasts before menopause have nearly nine times the risk.

The age at onset of menarche and the reproductive cycle seems to play some role in the development of breast cancer. In women with menarche before the age of 12 years, the incidence of breast cancer appears to be higher. Women who had their first child at the age of 30 years or older have three times the risk of those who had their first child at a younger age.

Most breast cancers are detected as painless masses, noticed by either the patient or the examiner during a routine physical examination. The earlier the diagnosis is made, the better the prognosis is. Screening for breast cancer is best accomplished by a thorough clinical breast examination, breast self-examination, and mammography. Mammography is the most sensitive method for the detection of breast cancer and has been demonstrated to reduce the breast cancer mortality rate.

Structure and Physiology

The *mammary glands* are the distinguishing feature of all mammals. Human breasts are conical in form and are often unequal in size. The breast extends from the level of the second or third rib to the level of the sixth or seventh rib, from the sternal edge to the anterior axillary line. The ''tail'' of the breast extends into the axilla and tends to be thicker than the other breast areas. This upper outer quadrant contains the greatest bulk of mammary tissue and is frequently the site of neoplasia. Figure 16-1 illustrates the normal breast.

The normal breast consists of glandular tissue, ducts, supporting muscular tissue, fat, blood vessels, nerves, and lymphatic vessels. The glandular tissue consists of 15 to 25 lobes, each of which drains into a separate excretory duct that terminates in the nipple. Each duct dilates as it

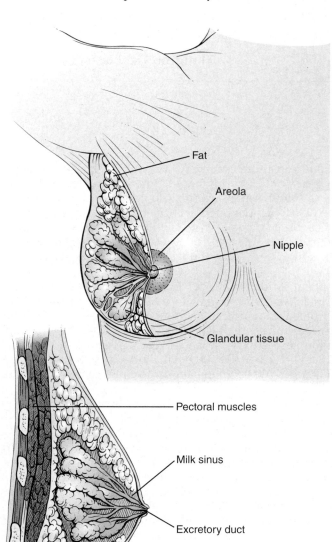

Fat

Areola

Nipple

Glandular tissue

Pectoral muscles

Milk sinus

Excretory duct

Figure 16–1 Anatomy of a normal breast.

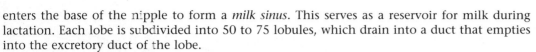

enters the base of the nipple to form a *milk sinus*. This serves as a reservoir for milk during lactation. Each lobe is subdivided into 50 to 75 lobules, which drain into a duct that empties into the excretory duct of the lobe.

Both the nipple and areola contain smooth muscle that serves to contract the areola and compress the nipple. Contraction of the smooth muscle makes the nipple erect and firm, thereby facilitating the emptying of the milk sinuses.

The skin of the nipple is deeply pigmented and hairless. The dermal papillae contain many sebaceous glands, which are grouped near the openings of the milk sinuses. The skin of the areola is also deeply pigmented but, unlike the skin of the nipple, contains occasional hair follicles. Its sebaceous glands are commonly seen as small nodules on the areolar surface and are termed *Montgomery's tubercles*.

Cooper's ligaments are projections of the breast tissue that fuse with the outer layers of the superficial fascia and serve as suspensory structures.

The blood supply to the breast is carried by the internal mammary artery. The breast has an extensive network of venous and lymphatic drainage. Most of the lymphatic drainage empties into the nodes in the axilla. Other nodes lie beneath the lateral margin of the pectoralis major muscle, along the medial side of the axilla, and in the subclavicular region. The main lymph node chains and lymphatic drainage of the breast are illustrated in Figure 16-2.

Several physiologic changes occur in the breast. These changes are a result of the following factors:

- Growth and aging
- The menstrual cycle
- Pregnancy

At birth, the breasts contain a branching system of ducts emptying into a developed nipple. There is elevation of only the nipple at this stage. Shortly after birth, there is a slight secretion of milky material. After 5 to 7 days, this secretory activity stops. Before puberty, there is elevation of the breast and nipple, called the *breast bud stage*. The areola has increased in size. At the onset of puberty, the areola enlarges further and darkens. A distinct mass of

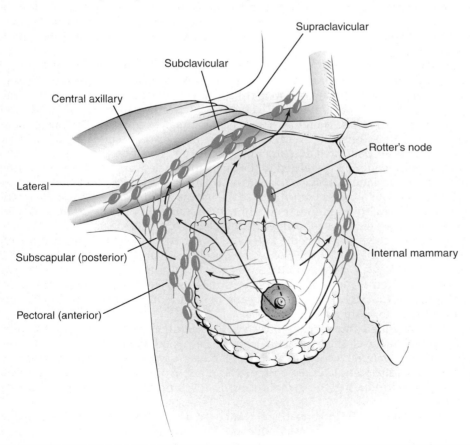

Figure 16–2 Lymphatic drainage of the breast.

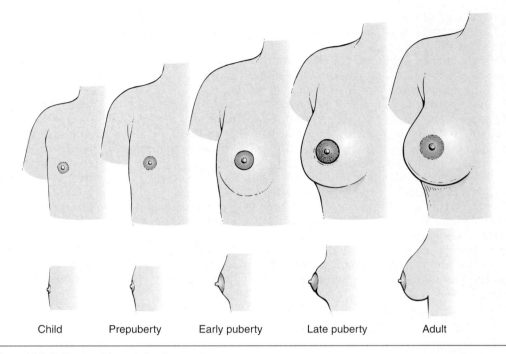

| Child | Prepuberty | Early puberty | Late puberty | Adult |

Figure 16–3 Stages of breast development.

glandular tissue begins to develop beneath the areola. By the onset of menstruation, the breasts are well developed, and there is forward projection of the areola and nipple at the apex of the breast. One to 2 years later, when the breast has reached maturity, only the nipple projects forward; the areola has receded to the general contour of the breast. The stages of breast development from birth to adulthood are illustrated in Figure 16-3. Figure 24-46 (Chapter 24, The Pediatric Patient) further illustrates and describes the breast developmental stages.

The nodularity, density, and fullness of the adult breast depend on several factors. Most important is the presence of excess adipose tissue. Because the mammary gland consists mainly of adipose tissue, women who are overweight have larger breasts. Pregnancy and nursing also alter the character of the breasts. Often, women who have nursed have softer, less nodular breasts. However, because the glandular tissue is approximately equal in all women, the size of the breast is unrelated to nursing. With menopause, the breasts decrease in size and become less dense. There is an associated decrease in elastic tissue as women age.

The major physiologic change related to the menstrual cycle is engorgement, occurring 3 to 5 days before menstruation. This is an increase in the size, density, and nodularity of the breasts. There is also an increased sensitivity of the breasts at this time. Because the nodularity of the breasts increases, the examiner should not attempt to diagnose a breast mass at this time. The patient should be reevaluated during the midperiod of the next cycle.

With pregnancy, the breasts become fuller and firmer. The areola darkens, and the nipples become erect as they enlarge. As the woman approaches the third trimester, a thin, yellowish secretion, called *colostrum*, may be noted. After the birth of the child, if the mother begins nursing within 24 hours, the secretion of colostrum stops, and the secretion of milk begins. During nursing, the breasts become markedly engorged. After the woman has stopped nursing, lactation continues for a short time.

The neuroendocrine control of the breasts can be outlined as follows. Suckling produces nerve impulses that travel to the hypothalamus. The hypothalamus stimulates the anterior pituitary to secrete *prolactin*, which acts on the glandular tissue of the breast to produce milk. The hypothalamus also stimulates the posterior pituitary to produce *oxytocin*, which stimulates the muscle cells surrounding the glandular tissue to contract and force the milk into the ductular system.

Many abnormalities of the breast are related to its embryology. An epithelial ridge, called the *milk line*, forms along each side of the body from the axilla to the inguinal region. Along this milk line are multiple rudiments for future breast development. In humans, only one rudimentary pair in the pectoral region persists and eventually develops

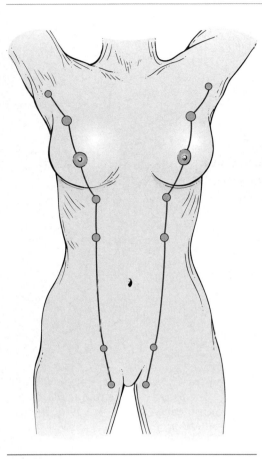

Figure 16–4 The milk line.

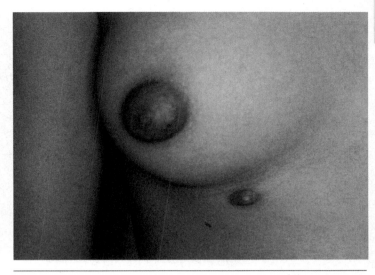

Figure 16–5 Accessory nipple.

into normal breasts. Accessory breasts or nipples are present in as many as 2% of white women. Accessory breasts may exist as glandular tissue, nipple, or only the areola. The axilla is the most common site for these anomalous structures, followed by a site just below the normal breast. In more than 50% of all patients with accessory breast tissue, the anomalies are bilateral. In general, accessory breast tissue is of little clinical significance. It usually has no physiologic function and is rarely associated with disease. Figure 16-4 illustrates the milk line. Figure 16-5 shows an accessory nipple.

Review of Specific Symptoms

The most important symptoms of breast disease are the following:

- Mass or swelling
- Pain
- Nipple discharge
- Change in skin over breast

Mass or Swelling

During self-examination, a patient may discover a breast mass. Ask the following questions:

"When did you first notice the lump?"

"Have you noticed that the mass changes in size during your menstrual periods?"

"Is the mass tender?"

"Have you ever noticed a mass in your breast before?"

"Have you noticed any skin changes on the breast?"

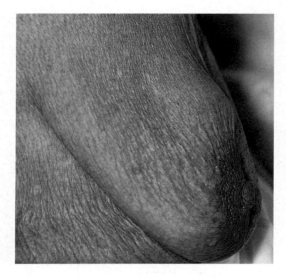

Figure 16–6 Large breast mass found on self-examination.

"Have you had any recent injury to the breast?"

"Is there any nipple discharge? nipple retraction?"

"Do you have breast implants?" If yes, *"What are they made of?"*

If the lump enlarges during the premenstrual and menstrual stages of the cycle, it is likely that the woman is detecting only physiologic nodularity. The association of nipple discharge, nipple inversion, or skin changes overlying the mass is strongly suggestive of neoplasm. Figure 16-6 shows a large breast mass found on self-examination.

Pain

Breast pain or tenderness is a common symptom. Most often, these symptoms are attributable to the normal physiologic cycle. Ask the following questions of any patient with breast pain:

"Can you describe the pain?"

"When did you first experience the pain?"

"Are there any changes in the pain with your menstrual cycle?"

"Do you have pain in both breasts?"

"Have you had any injury to the breast?"

"Is the pain associated with a mass in the breast? nipple discharge? nipple retraction?"

"Has there been a change in your bra size?"

Rapidly enlarging cysts may be painful. Cystic disease of the breasts is usually painless. Although breast pain is a relatively uncommon manifestation of breast cancer, its presence does not exclude the diagnosis. Never delay evaluation of a painful breast mass.

Nipple Discharge

Nipple discharge is not a common symptom, but it should always raise the suspicion of breast disease, especially if the discharge occurs spontaneously. Any patient who describes a nipple discharge should be asked the following questions:

"What is the color of the discharge?"

"Do you have a discharge from both breasts?"

"When did you first notice the discharge?"

"Is the discharge related to your menstrual cycle?"

"When was your last menstrual cycle?"

"Is the discharge associated with nipple retraction? a breast mass? breast tenderness?"

"Do you have headaches?"

"Are you taking any medications?"

"Are you using oral contraceptives?"

If the woman has recently delivered a child, ask

"Were there any problems during the delivery of your last child?"

The most common types of discharge are serous and bloody. A *serous* discharge is thin and watery and may appear as a yellowish stain on the patient's garments. This commonly results from an intraductal papilloma in one of the large subareolar ducts. Women taking oral contraceptives may complain of bilateral serous discharge. A serous discharge can also occur in women with breast carcinoma.

A *bloody* discharge is associated with an intraductal papilloma, which is common among pregnant and menstruating women. It may, however, be associated with a malignant intraductal papillary carcinoma. The presence of any nipple discharge is more important than its character because both types of discharge are associated with benign or malignant disease.

A milky discharge is usually milk. It is common for women to continue to secrete milk for a few months after they stop nursing. In rare instances, the secretion may continue for a year. Persistent lactation, also known as *galactorrhea*, can be a result of massive hemorrhage occurring during childbirth and producing pituitary necrosis. Abnormal lactation may also result from a pituitary tumor that interferes with the normal hypothalamic-pituitary feedback loop or from the use of certain tranquilizing medications. Mechanical stimulation or suckling may produce physiologic stimulation.

Change in Skin over Breast

A change in the color or texture of the skin of the breast or areola is an important symptom of breast carcinoma. The presence of dimpling, puckering, or scaliness warrants further investigation. The presence of unusually prominent pores, indicative of edema of the skin, is an important sign of malignancy. This clinical sign is called *peau d'orange* because of its orange-peel appearance. During the early stages of breast carcinoma, the lymphatic vessels of the breast are dilated and contain occasional emboli of carcinoma cells. Limited peau d'orange over the lower half of the areola is present. As the disease progresses, more lymphatic vessels become filled with carcinoma cells that block them, creating more generalized edema. The classic appearance of peau d'orange is pictured in Figure 16-7.

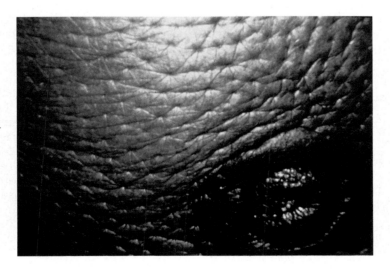

Figure 16-7 Peau d'orange.

General Suggestions

The interviewer should pay special attention to the family history of any woman presenting with symptoms of breast disease. As indicated earlier, breast cancer may be a familial disorder. The occurrence of breast disease in a close relative and the age at which it developed are relevant to the patient's disease. Ask the patient the following questions:

> *"Have you had a mammogram?"* If yes, *"When and what was the result?"*
>
> *"Have you had breast cancer?"*
>
> *"Have you had breast cancer without the removal of your breast?"*
>
> *"Do you have breast implants?"*
>
> *"Have you had any breast biopsies or breast surgery?"*
>
> *"Have you ever had radiation treatments to your breasts?"*
>
> *"Did your birth mother have breast cancer?"* If yes, *"Premenopausal or postmenopausal? At what age was her diagnosis made?"*
>
> *"Do you have a sister or daughter with breast cancer?"* If yes, *"Premenopausal or post-menopausal? "At what age was her diagnosis made?"*
>
> *"Do you use birth control pills?"*
>
> *"Do you take estrogen replacement therapy?"*

Impact of Breast Disease on the Patient

The psychosocial problems resulting from breast cancer are far-reaching. Although the loss of an extremity is more disabling in everyday life, the loss of a breast produces intense feelings of loss of the feminine identity. Many women who lose a breast become depressed because they feel their symbol of femininity has been removed. They are afraid that they will no longer be considered "whole" women because their bodies have been maimed. They fear that they can no longer be loved normally and that they can no longer experience sexual satisfaction. They fear looking at themselves in a mirror and perceive themselves as ugly. The asymmetry is often described as "mutilation" or "a bomb crater." After mastectomy, women often suffer from sexual inhibition and sexual frustration.

Once a woman has discovered a mass in her breast, she becomes intensely fearful. The fear of breast cancer is twofold: It is a cancer, often with a bad prognosis, and it is associated with disfigurement. For these reasons, the patient commonly denies the presence of the mass and delays seeking medical attention. It is not uncommon for a patient to seek medical assistance for the first time with a large tumor mass the size of an orange that has eroded through the skin and has become infected. When asked how long the mass has been present, the woman might answer that she "discovered it yesterday."

After a mastectomy, the patient will probably suffer from depression and low self-esteem. The patient should be supported, and counseled if necessary. Open communication and sharing of feelings among the patient, husband, significant other, physician, and family are important factors in the psychologic rehabilitation of the woman.

The patient pictured in Figure 16-8 had inflammatory carcinoma of her left breast, with massive lymphedema of the left arm. The patient had noticed that her arm had been swelling for the past few months, and she now needed support to raise it. She presented to the clinic complaining only about the heaviness of her arm. When examination revealed the breast lesion, she stated that she had noticed the breast changes "only a few days ago." This is another example of denial of illness (see also the patient shown in Fig. 2-1).

Most commonly, women with invasive breast cancer and axillary lymph node involvement require chemotherapy for periods up to 6 or 7 months after mastectomy. Many of the agents used to treat the patient have significant side effects, including nausea, vomiting, and alopecia. There are medicines available to help control the nausea and vomiting, but the alopecia presents another special problem. Although the woman recognizes that she will lose her hair and knows that it will grow back, she suffers further from low self-esteem. In our society, hair is a

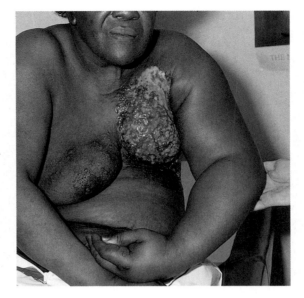

Figure 16–8 Inflammatory breast carcinoma.

woman's "persona": a bald man is acceptable; a bald woman is not. Finally, at the conclusion of chemotherapy, the woman may face further depression. While on the chemotherapeutic protocol, she feels reassured that no further cancer can develop, but what does the future hold when these medications are stopped?

Physical Examination

No special equipment is necessary for the examination of the breast.
The examination of the breast consists of the following:

- Inspection
- Axillary examination
- Palpation

The examination of the breast is in two parts. The first is performed with the patient sitting up. Inspection of the breasts and palpation of the lymph nodes are done in this position. The second is performed with the patient lying down. The examiner systematically palpates the entire breast by using firm, gentle pressure exerted by the pulp of his or her finger rather than the fingertips.

To facilitate communication, the breast is pictorially divided into four quadrants. Two imaginary lines run through the nipple at right angles to each other. By visualizing the breast as a face of a clock, one line is the "12 o'clock–6 o'clock" line, and the other is the "3 o'clock–9 o'clock" line. The resulting four quadrants are the upper outer, upper inner, lower outer, and lower inner. The "tail" is an extension of the upper outer quadrant. These regions are illustrated in Figure 16-9.

Inspection

The woman should be seated on the edge of the examination table, facing the examiner. The examiner should ask the woman to remove her gown to her waist.

Inspect the Breasts

Inspection is first accomplished with the patient's arms at her side, as shown in Figure 16-10. Tell the patient, "I am inspecting the breasts for any changes in the skin, contour, or symmetry." The breasts are inspected for size, shape, symmetry, contour, color, and edema. The nipples are inspected as to size, shape, inversion, eversion, or discharge. The nipples should be symmetric. Is any abnormal bulging present?

The skin of the breast is observed for edema. Edema of the skin of the breast that overlies a malignancy may manifest as peau d'orange.

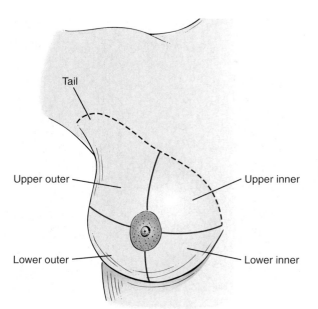

Figure 16–9 The four breast quadrants.

Tail

Upper outer

Upper inner

Lower outer

Lower inner

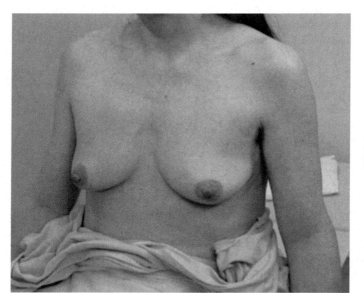

Figure 16–10 Position of patient for inspection of the breasts.

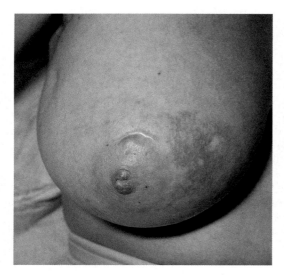

Figure 16–11 Erythema of the breast.

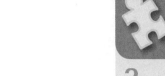

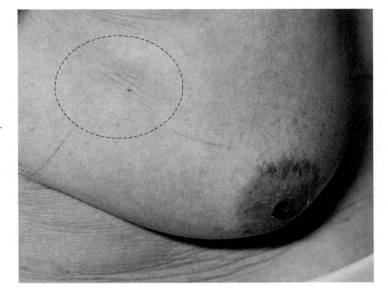

Figure 16–12 Breast carcinoma. Note dimpling of the breast and bloody nipple discharge.

Is erythema present? Erythema is associated with infection and with inflammatory carcinoma of the breast. Figure 16-11 shows marked erythema of the breast secondary to inflammatory breast carcinoma. The scar above the areola is from a previous biopsy of a benign breast mass.

Is dimpling present? The examiner must inspect the breasts for the presence of *retraction phenomena*. Dimpling is a sign of retraction phenomena that are caused by an underlying neoplasm and its fibrotic response. Skin retraction is commonly associated with malignancy that causes an abnormal traction on Cooper's ligaments. The shortening of the larger mammary ducts by cancer produces flattening or inversion of the nipple. A change in the position of the nipple is important because many women have a congenitally inverted nipple on one or both sides. The dimpling of the breast in Figure 16-12 is associated with a bloody nipple discharge; both are secondary to carcinoma.

Is there a red, scaling, crusting plaque around one nipple, areola, or surrounding skin? *Paget's disease* of the breast is a surface manifestation invariably associated with an underlying invasive or intraductal carcinoma. The lesion appears eczematous, but unlike eczema, it is unilateral. The skin may also weep and be eroded. A much less common form is extramammary Paget's disease, which is seen around the anus or genitalia and is usually associated with malignant disease of the adnexa, bowel, or genitourinary tract. Figure 16-13 shows Paget's disease of the breast; an underlying ductal adenocarcinoma was present.

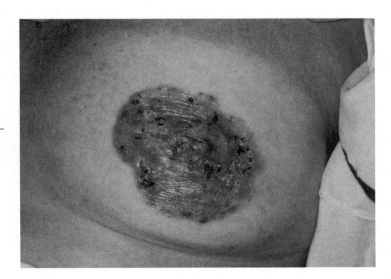

Figure 16–13 Paget's disease of the breast.

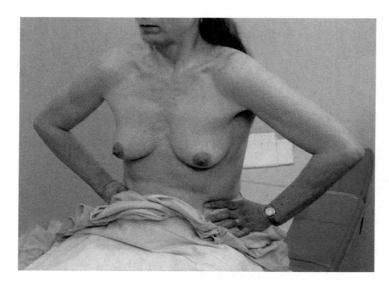

Figure 16–14 Technique for tensing the pectoralis muscles.

Inspect the Breasts in Various Postures

Inspection is next performed while the woman assumes several postures that may bring out signs of retraction that were less evident previously. Ask the woman to press her arms against her hips. This maneuver tenses the pectoralis muscles, which may bring out dimpling caused by fixation of the breast to the underlying muscles. This technique is shown in Figure 16-14. If a malignancy is present, the abnormal attachment of the tumor to the fascia and pectoralis muscle pulls on the skin and may produce skin dimpling. Any bulging may also indicate an underlying mass.

Another maneuver, which is useful for a woman with pendulous breasts, involves her bending at the waist and allowing her breasts to hang free from the chest wall. This technique is demonstrated in Figure 16-15. A carcinoma causing fibrosis in one breast produces a change in the contour of that breast.

Axillary Examination

The axillary examination is performed with the patient seated facing the examiner. Examination of the axilla is best accomplished by relaxing the pectoral muscles. To examine the right axilla, the patient's right forearm is supported by the examiner's right hand. The tips of the fingers of the examiner's left hand start low in the axilla, and, as the patient's right arm is drawn medially, the examiner advances the left hand higher into the axilla. This technique is demonstrated in Figure 16-16. The supraclavicular, subclavian, and axillary regions are palpated.

The technique of using small, circular motions of the fingers riding over the ribs is used for detecting adenopathy. Freely mobile nodes 3 to 5 mm in diameter are common and are usually

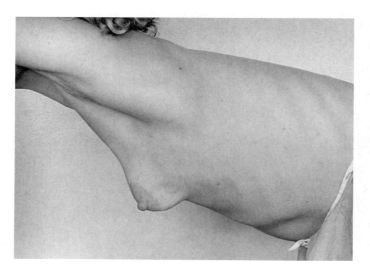

Figure 16–15 Position of patient for inspecting the breasts.

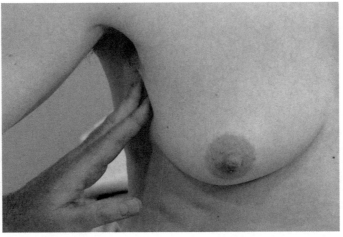

A

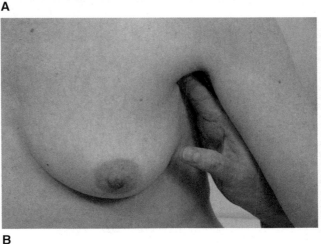

B

Figure 16–16 Technique for axillary examination. *A,* Low axilla (right side). *B,* High axilla (left side).

indicative of lymphadenitis secondary to minor trauma of the hand and arm. After one axilla is examined, the other is evaluated by the examiner's opposite hand.

Palpation

The woman is asked to lie down and is told that the breast will next be palpated. The examiner stands at the right side of the patient's bed. Although the examiner can usually palpate each breast from the patient's right side, it is often better with large-breasted women to examine the left breast from the left side.

The breast is best palpated by allowing it to lie evenly distributed over the chest wall. Small-breasted women may lie with their arms at their sides; larger breasted women should be instructed to place their hands behind their head. A pillow placed beneath the shoulder on the side being examined facilitates the examination.

Palpate the Breast

In palpation of the breast, the examiner should use both the flat of the hand and the fingertips, as demonstrated in Figure 16-17. Palpation should be performed by the "spokes of a wheel," the concentric circle, or the vertical strip method. The "spokes of a wheel" method starts at the nipple (see Fig. 16-17A). The examiner should start the palpation by moving outward from the nipple to the 12 o'clock position. The examiner then should return to the nipple and move along the 1 o'clock position and continue the palpation around the breasts. The concentric circles approach (see Fig. 16-17B) also starts at the nipple, but the examiner moves from the nipple in a continuous circular manner around the breast. Any lesion found by either technique is described as being a certain distance from the nipple in clock time: for example, "3 cm from the nipple along the 1 o'clock line." These techniques are illustrated in Figure 16-18.

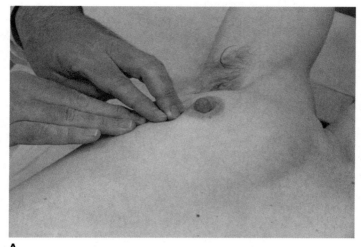

A

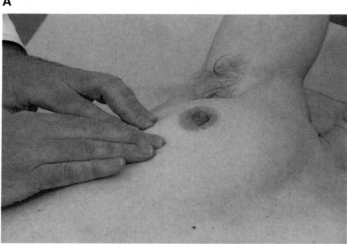

B

Figure 16–17 Technique for breast palpation. *A,* ''Spokes of a wheel.'' *B,* Concentric circles.

Another method is the vertical strip, or grid, technique. The breast is divided into eight or nine vertical strips, each approximately one finger's width. The examiner's three middle fingers are held together and slightly bowed to ensure contact with the skin. The pads, not the tips, of the fingers must be used for palpation. Using dime-sized circles, the examiner evaluates the breast at each of three different levels of pressure: light, medium, and deep. Each strip consists of 9 or 10 areas of palpation, slightly overlapping the previous area, and each vertical strip is evaluated with the three pressures. Although this method has been shown to be superior to the other traditional types of breast palpation, it is more time consuming and may be best used by women for breast self-examination.

The examiner should be careful when evaluating the *inframammary fold.* This fold is commonly observed in older women and is the area where the mammary tissue is bound tightly to the chest wall. Often, this ridge is mistaken for a breast disorder.

Describe the Findings

If a mass is palpated, the following characteristics should be described:

1. The *size* of the mass in centimeters and its position.
2. The *shape* of the mass.
3. The *delimitation*, referring to the borders of the mass. Is it well delimited, as with a cyst? Are the edges diffuse, as with a carcinoma?
4. The *consistency*, describing the ''hardness'' of the mass. A carcinoma is often stony hard. A cyst has some elastic qualities.
5. The *mobility* of the lesion. Is the lesion movable in the tissue that surrounds it? Benign tumors and cysts are freely mobile. Carcinomas are usually fixed to the skin, underlying muscle, or chest wall.

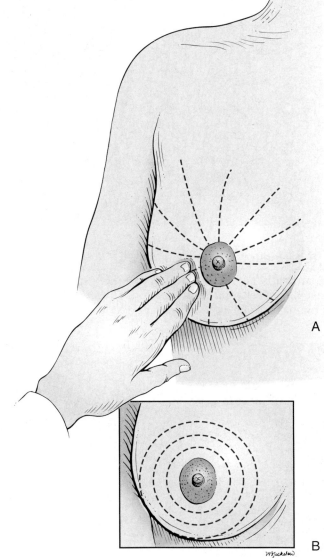

Figure 16–18 Method of breast palpation. *A,* ''Spokes of a wheel.'' *B,* Concentric circles.

Evaluate for Retraction Phenomenon

If a mass is detected, *molding* of the skin may be useful to determine whether the retraction phenomenon is present. The examiner should elevate the breast around the mass. Dimpling may occur if a carcinoma is present. Figure 16-19 demonstrates the technique of molding and its result in a patient with carcinoma of the breast. Notice the marked dimpling of the breast. This patient also had metastatic lesions of breast carcinoma on her arm, together with lymphedema. She presented to the clinic stating that she had discovered the swollen arm the day before.

Palpate the Subareolar Area

The subareolar area, the area directly under the areola, should be palpated while the patient is lying supine. In the subareolar area, the breast tissue is less dense. An abscess of Montgomery's glands in the areola may cause a tender mass in this area.

Examine the Nipple

Examination of the nipple concludes the examination of the breast. Inspect for nipple retraction, fissures, and scaling. To examine for discharge, place each hand on either side of the nipple and gently compress the nipple, noting the character of any discharge. This technique is demonstrated in Figure 16-20. Ask the woman whether she would prefer to perform this part of the examination herself.

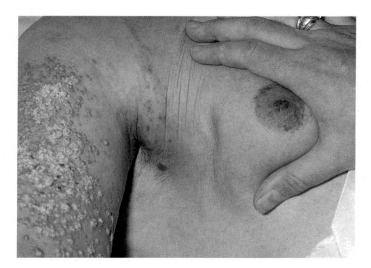

Figure 16–19 Breast dimpling. Note the satellite skin lesions of metastatic breast cancer on the upper arm.

Examination of the Male Breast

Examination of the breast should be performed on all men. The nipples should be inspected for swelling, discharge, and ulceration. The areola and the subareolar tissue should be palpated for any masses. The axillary examination is as indicated for women.

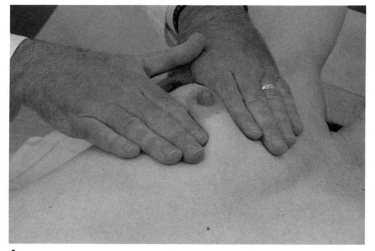

A

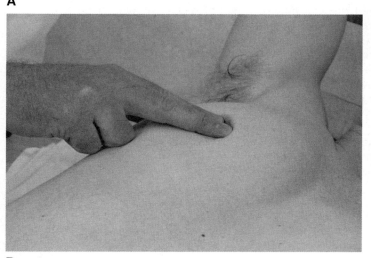

B

Figure 16–20 Technique for nipple examination. *A,* Examination for discharge. *B,* Examination for masses below the nipple.

Breast Self-Examination[*]

Women should be encouraged to perform breast self-examination monthly starting at age 20 years. It is important for a woman to learn what is normal and about the changes in her breasts that occur with her menstrual cycle. Familiarity with breast tissue makes it easier for the woman to notice any changes in the breast from month to month.

Advise the woman that the best time to perform breast self-examination is 2 to 3 days to a week after the end of her menstrual period. At this time the breasts are less tender or swollen. Women taking oral contraceptives are encouraged to do their breast self-examination each month on the day they begin their new package of pills. A woman past menopause should be advised to pick a particular day of the month and then perform the examination monthly.

Advise the patient that if she discovers anything unusual, such as a lump, discharge from the nipple, or dimpling of the skin, she should seek medical attention. Inform her that 8 of 10 breast lumps are *not* cancer.

The techniques of breast self-examination are included here for the purpose of patient education:

1. Stand with your arms at your sides in front of a mirror. Inspect both breasts for anything unusual, such as dimpling, puckering, discharge from the nipples, or scaling of the skin.
2. Raise your arms and clasp your hands behind your head. Press your hands forward. Look in the mirror for any changes in the breast tissue.
3. Put your hands down and place them on your hips. Bend slightly toward the mirror as you pull your shoulders and elbows forward.
4. Raise your right arm; using the pads of your left fingers, press into your right breast firmly, carefully, and thoroughly. Start at the upper outer edge and move in small circles, moving the circles slowly around the breast. Pay special attention to the breast tissue between the breast and the underarm. Use a massaging motion.
5. Gently squeeze your nipple and look for any discharge.
6. Repeat steps 4 and 5 while lying down with a small pillow under your right shoulder. Place your right arm over your head.
7. Repeat the examination on your left breast.

There are several errors that patients make with regard to breast self-examination. The first is failure to perform self-examination. The second is failure to examine the breasts both in the sitting (or standing) position and when lying down. The third is failure to use a pillow under the side that is being examined. The fourth is failure to raise the arm (on the side being examined) above the head and relax it.

The Male Breast

Gynecomastia is the enlargement of one or both breasts in a man. It often occurs at puberty, occurs with aging, or is drug-related. Figure 16-21 shows a 90-year-old man who was treated with diethylstilbestrol for carcinoma of the prostate and developed gynecomastia.

Carcinoma of the breast affects approximately 1000 men per year in the United States. More than 300 men per year die of metastatic breast cancer. The average age at the time of diagnosis is 59 years. The most common clinical manifestation, occurring in 75% of cases, is a painless, firm, subareolar mass or a mass in the upper outer quadrant of the breast.

The incidence of breast carcinoma in men, as well as in women, is highest in North America and in the British Isles; it is lowest in Japan and Finland. As in women, breast carcinoma in men most commonly metastasizes to the bone, lung, liver, pleura, lymph nodes, skin, and other visceral sites.

---

[*]The importance of breast self-examination has been recognized for more than 60 years. However, to date, the efficacy of this examination is not definitive. A large, randomized, controlled trial was conducted in 1997 by Thomas and associates in Shanghai and included more than 267,040 women, half of whom were given intensive training in breast self-examination; the other half were asked to attend training sessions on the prevention of low back pain. All women were observed for 5 years for the development of breast diseases. The study showed neither a significant difference in mortality rate in the two groups nor an earlier identification of breast disease in the group trained in breast self-examination. The authors' conclusion was that "there was insufficient evidence to recommend for or against the teaching of breast self-examination."

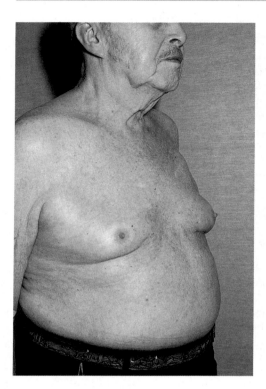

Figure 16–21 Gynecomastia.

Clinicopathologic Correlations

Cancer of the Breast

There is mounting evidence that defects in DNA repair may be significant factors for the development of breast cancer. Two genes, *BRCA1* and *BRCA2*, have been identified as *tumor suppressor genes* or *breast cancer susceptibility genes* and appear to be involved with gene repair. Tumor suppressor genes keep cellular growth in control but can cause cancer when their function is blocked. More than 2000 mutations have been described for these tumor suppressor genes. When mutations or deletions occur in these suppressor genes, the incidence of neoplastic transformation is much greater. *BRCA1* and *BRCA2* are associated with proteins, such as p53 and RAD51, which are involved with DNA repair and transcriptional activation. Carriers of germline mutations in *BRCA1*, located on chromosome 17, or *BRCA2*, located on chromosome 13, have an increased incidence of early-onset, familial breast, or ovarian cancer. Mutant *BRCA1* and *BRCA2* genes account for 50% of hereditable breast cancers. Mutations in these tumor suppressor genes have been found in only 5% to 10% of women with early-onset breast cancers. If a mutation in the *BRCA1* gene is present in a woman, however, it is estimated that her lifetime risk for development of breast cancer is approximately 60% to 80%, and she has a 33% chance for development of ovarian cancer. A man with a mutant allele of the gene has an increased incidence of prostate cancer. *BRCA2* is associated with an increased incidence of breast cancer in men and women. Researchers have discovered that 2.5% of women of Ashkenazi Jewish descent may carry one of the *BRCA* mutations—an occurrence that is about five times greater than that of the general population.

The finding of a breast mass on palpation, even in the presence of a normal mammogram, necessitates a biopsy. However, breast palpation has a much lower true-positive rate (sensitivity) than mammography. There are many false-negative findings in breast palpation. This error is related to the difficulty in palpating a small mass in large breasts, the inherent properties of breast tissue, and poor technique. The limitations of physical examination and mammography are shown in Table 16-1.

The physical examination is of great importance in determining the probability that a mass is cancerous. Any lump detected by either the patient or the examiner carries a 20% risk of cancer. As indicated in Table 16-2, benign lesions usually are freely mobile, have well-delimited borders, and feel soft or cystic. However, of all breast cancers, 60% are freely mobile, 40% have well-delimited borders, and 50% feel soft or cystic. A fixed lesion has a 50% chance of

Table 16–1 Limitations of Physical Examination and Mammography

Operating Characteristic	Physical Examination	Mammography
Sensitivity (%)	24	62
Specificity (%)	95	90

Data from Bond WH: The Treatment of Carcinoma of the Breast. In Jarrett AS (ed): Proceedings of a Symposium on the Treatment of Carcinoma of the Breast. Amsterdam, Excerpta Medica, 1968.

being malignant. If this lesion has irregular borders, the likelihood of being malignant rises to 60%. The sensitivity and specificity of certain physical findings in evaluating a breast mass for malignancy are shown in Table 16-3.

Screening Guidelines for Early Detection of Cancer of the Breast

1. The National Cancer Institute recommends that women begin receiving screening mammograms every 1 to 2 years starting at 40 years of age and every year once they reach 50 years of age, continuing for as long as a woman is in good health. Screening mammography involves taking low-dose radiographs from two views of each breast, typically from above (craniocaudal view) and from an oblique or angled position (mediolateral-oblique view). Mammography can detect approximately 85% of breast cancers. If the mammogram indicates an abnormality, the woman will most likely be urged to undergo further breast imaging (i.e., with spot-view mammography, ultrasonography, or other imaging tests). If further imaging confirms or reveals an abnormality, the woman may be referred for a biopsy to determine whether she has breast cancer. Screening mammography can miss 10% to 15% of breast cancers. These tumors can be missed (1) if the tumor is very small; (2) if the tumor is in an area not easily imaged (e.g., in the axilla); or (3) if the tumor is obscured by other shadows.
2. A clinical breast examination should be part of a periodic health examination, about every 3 years for women in their 20s and 30s and every year for women 40 years of age and older.
3. Women should know how their breasts normally feel. They should report any changes immediately to their health-care provider. Breast self-examination should be taught to women in their 20s.
4. Women at increased risk (e.g., family history, genetic tendency, past history of breast cancer) should speak to their health-care provider about the benefits and limitations of starting mammography screening earlier, having additional tests (e.g., breast ultrasonography, magnetic resonance imaging), or having more frequent examinations.

Table 16–2 Differentiation of Breast Masses

Characteristic	Cystic Disease	Benign Adenoma	Malignant Tumor
Patient age	25-60 years	10-55 years	25-85 years
Number	One or more	One	One
Shape	Round	Round	Irregular
Consistency	Elastic, soft to hard	Firm	Stony hard
Delimitation	Well delimited	Well delimited	Poorly delimited
Mobility	Mobile	Mobile	Fixed
Tenderness	Present	Absent	Absent
Skin retraction	Absent	Absent	Present

Table 16–3 Characteristics of Breast Masses Suspect for Cancer

Characteristic	Sensitivity (%)	Specificity* (%)
Fixed mass	40	90
Poorly delimited mass	60	90
Hard mass	62	90

*Based on the assumption that nonmalignant breast masses have benign characteristics.
Data from Venet L, Strax P, Venet W, et al: Adequacies and inadequacies of breast examination by physicians in mass screening. Cancer 28:1546, 1971.

Useful Vocabulary

Listed here are the specific roots that are important for understanding the terminology related to breast disease.

Root	Pertaining to	Example	Definition
gyne(co)-	woman	**gyneco**mastia	Excessive development of the male breast
lact(o)-	milk	**lact**ation	Secretion of milk
mammo-	breast	**mammo**graphy	Radiographic visualization of the breast
mast(o)-	breast	**mast**itis	Inflammation of the breast

Writing Up the Physical Examination

Listed here are examples of the write-up for the examination of the breast.

- The breasts are symmetric, with both nipples pointing outward. The overlying skin is normal. No dimpling is present. There are no masses or discharge. Axillary examination reveals no lymphadenopathy.
- The left breast is slightly larger than the right. There is a serosanguineous discharge from the left nipple. When the patient presses her arms against her hips, a dimple is seen 4 cm from the nipple at the 2 o'clock position of the left breast. Palpation reveals a 2 × 3 cm stony mass under the area of dimpling. The mass appears fixed to the underlying muscle and overlying skin. Examination of the left axilla reveals numerous hard, fixed lymph nodes.
- The right breast is larger than the left. The skin is erythematous and warm to the touch, especially around the areola. The right nipple is inverted. No masses are felt. Dimpling cannot be appreciated. No axillary adenopathy is present.
- The breasts are pendulous and symmetric. Both nipples are everted. There are multiple round, freely mobile masses in both breasts, more on the right. The masses are 2 to 3 cm in diameter, elastic in consistency, and somewhat tender. Skin retraction is absent. No discharge is present. No axillary adenopathy is present.

Bibliography

Bickell NA, Aufses AH Jr, Chassin MR: The quality of early-stage breast cancer care. Ann Surg 232:220, 2000.

Bland KI, Copeland EM III (eds): The Breast: Comprehensive Management of Benign and Malignant Diseases, 2nd ed. Philadelphia, WB Saunders, 1998.

Burnet K: Holistic Breast Care. Philadelphia, WB Saunders, 2001.

Campbell HS, Fletcher SW, Lin S: Improving physicians' and nurses' clinical breast examination: A randomized controlled trial. Am J Prev Med 7:1, 1991.

Cancer Facts & Figures. Atlanta, American Cancer Society, 2007.

Collins FS: BRCA1: Lots of mutations, lots of dilemmas. N Engl J Med 334:186, 1996.

Couch FJ, DeShano ML, Blackwood A, et al: BRCA1 mutations in women attending clinics that evaluate the risk of breast cancer. N Engl J Med 336:1409, 1997.

Dixon JM, Morrow M: Breast Disease: A Problem-Based Approach. Philadelphia, WB Saunders, 1999.

Domchek SM, Antoniou A: Cancer risk models: Translating family history into clinical management. Ann Intern Med 147:515, 2007.

Easton DF, Ford D, Bishop DT, et al: Breast and ovarian cancer incidence in BRCA1-mutation carriers. Am J Hum Genet 56:265, 1995.

Feig SA, Schwartz GF, Nerlinger R, et al: Prognostic factors of breast neoplasms detected on screening by mammography and physical examination. Radiology 133:577, 1979.

Feuer EJ, Wun LM: DEVCAN: Probability of Developing or Dying of Cancer Software, Version 4.0. Bethesda, MD, National Cancer Institute, 1999.

Fletcher SW, O'Malley MS, Earp JL, et al: How best to teach women breast self-examination: A randomized controlled trial. Ann Intern Med 112:772, 1990.

Ford D, Easton DF: The genetics of breast and ovarian cancer. Br J Cancer 72:805, 1995.

Ghafoor A, Jemal A Cokkinides V, et al: Cancer statistics for African Americans. CA Cancer J Clin 52:326, 2002.

Ghafoor A, Jemal A, Ward E, et al: Trends in breast cancer by race and ethnicity. CA Cancer J Clin 53:342, 2003.

Healy B: BRCA genes: Bookmaking, fortunetelling, and medical care. N Engl J Med 336:1448, 1997.

Hicks MJ, Davis JR, Layton JM, et al: Sensitivity of mammography and physical examination of the breast for detecting breast cancer. JAMA 242:2080, 1979.

Hughes LE, Mansel RE, Webster DJT: Benign Disorders and Diseases of the Breast, 2nd ed. Philadelphia, WB Saunders, 1999.

Jaiyesimi IA, Buzdar AU, Sahin AA, et al: Carcinoma of the male breast. Ann Intern Med 117:771, 1992.

Jemel A, Tiwari R, Murray T, et al: Cancer Statistics, 2004. CA Cancer J Clin 54:8, 2004.

Krainer M, Silva-Arrieta S, FitzGerald MG, et al: Differential contributions of BRCA1 and BRCA2 to early-onset breast cancer. N Engl J Med 336:1416, 1997.

Malumbres M, Baracid M: Timeline: RAS oncogenes: The first 30 years. Nat Rev Cancer 3:459, 2003.

Parmigiani G, Chen S, Iversen ES, et al: Validity of models for predicting BRCA1 and BRCA2 mutations. Ann Intern Med 147:441, 2007.

Pennypacker HS, Pilgrim CA: Achieving competence in clinical breast examination. Nurse Pract 4:85, 1993.

Rebbeck TR, Lynch HT, Neuhausen SL, et al: Prophylactic oophorectomy in carriers of BRCA1 and BRCA2 mutations. N Engl J Med 346:1616, 2002.

Roses DF: Breast Cancer. Philadelphia, WB Saunders, 1999.

Schulman JD, Stern HJ: Genetic predisposition testing for breast cancer. Cancer J Sci Am 2:244, 1996.

Smith IE, Dowsett M: Aromatase inhibitors in breast cancer. N Engl J Med 348:2431, 2003.

Smith RA, Cokkinides V, Eyre HJ: American Cancer Society guidelines for the early detection of cancer, 2004. CA Cancer J Clin 54:41, 2004.

Smith RA, Saslow D, Sawyer KA, et al: American Cancer Society guidelines for breast cancer screening: Update 2003. CA Cancer J Clin 53:141, 2003.

Struewing JP, Hartge P, Wacholder S, et al: The risk of developing cancer associated with specific mutations of BRCA1 and BRCA2 among Ashkenazi Jews. N Engl J Med 336:1401, 1997.

Surveillance, Epidemiology, and End Results (SEER) Program: SEER Stat Database: Incidence—SEER 9 Regs Public-Use, November 2002 Sub (1973–2000). Bethesda, Md, National Cancer Institute, Division of Cancer Control and Population Sciences, Surveillance Research Program, Cancer Statistics Branch. Released April 2003, based on the November 2002 submission. Available at *www.seer.cancer/gov*; accessed June 23, 2008.

Thomas DB, Gao DL, Self SG, et al: Randomized trial of breast self-examination in Shanghai: Methodology and preliminary results. J Natl Cancer Inst 89:355, 1997.

U.S. Mortality 1973–1996, National Center for Health Statistics, Centers for Disease Control and Prevention 1999, Surveillance, Epidemiology, and End Results Program. Bethesda, Md, National Cancer Institute, Division of Cancer Control and Population Sciences, 2000.

U.S. Preventive Services Task Force: Genetic risk assessment and BRCA mutation testing for breast and ovarian cancer susceptibility: U.S. Preventive Services Task Force recommendations (clinical guidelines). Ann Intern Med 143:355, 2005.

Venet L, Strax P, Venet W, et al: Adequacies and inadequacies of breast examination by physicians in mass screening. Cancer 28:1546, 1971.

Venkitaraman AR: Cancer susceptibility and the functions of BRCA1 and BRCA2. Cell 108:171, 2002.

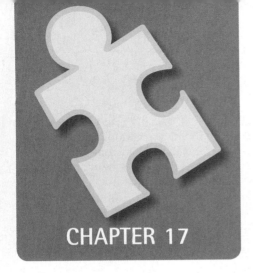

CHAPTER 17

The Abdomen

A good eater must be a good man; for a good eater must have good digestion, and good digestion depends upon a good conscience.

Benjamin Disraeli (1804–1881)

General Considerations

Diseases of the abdomen are common. In the United States, approximately 10% of the adult male population is affected by peptic ulcer disease. Five percent of the population older than 40 years has diverticular disease. Colorectal cancer is the third common malignant neoplasm (11% of all cancers) affecting American men and women. It is the second most common cause of cancer deaths in men (10%) and the third most common cause in women (11%). In 2007, approximately 158,410 new cases of cancer of the colon and rectum were diagnosed, and there were 52,870 deaths from colorectal cancer.

In the general American population, the lifetime probability for development of colorectal cancer is approximately 5.5%, or 1 per 18 people. The risk for this type of cancer differs widely among individuals. The highest incidence is in African Americans, who have a rate of 50.4 cases per 100,000 population. The incidence for the white population is second, at 43.9 per 100,000. The lowest incidence is in the Native American population, at 16.4 per 100,000. Some patients, such as those with congenital polyposis or ulcerative colitis, have a predisposition to the development of cancer of the colon, frequently at an early age. The lifetime risk of colonic cancer in patients with polyposis coli is 100%. The incidence of polyposis in the population of the United States varies from 1 per 7000 to 1 per 10,000 live births. The risk for development of colonic cancer in patients with ulcerative colitis is 20% per decade of life. Diet has been shown to have a relationship to the incidence of colonic cancer. Individuals on a low-fiber and high-fat diet are at higher risk. Earlier physical diagnosis has been clearly shown to lower the mortality rates for colorectal cancer

In 2007, in addition to deaths related to cancer of the colon and rectum, deaths from cancer of the liver and intrahepatic bile ducts accounted for 4% (12,540 patients) of all cancer deaths in men. There were also 37,170 new cases of pancreatic cancer and 33,370 deaths, which account for 6% of all cancer deaths in men and women in the United States. There were 15,560 new cases of esophageal cancer, with a 4:1 male–female ratio and 13,940 deaths, which makes esophageal cancer the seventh leading cause of cancer deaths in men (4% of all cancer deaths).

Structure and Physiology

For descriptive purposes, the abdominal cavity is usually divided visually into four quadrants. Two imaginary perpendicular lines cross at the umbilicus to divide the abdomen into the *right upper* and *right lower quadrants* and the *left upper* and *left lower quadrants*. One line extends from the sternum to the pubic bone through the umbilicus. The second line is at right angles to the first at the level of the umbilicus. The four quadrants formed and the abdominal organs within each quadrant are shown in Figure 17-1.

Another method of description divides the abdomen into nine areas: *epigastric, umbilical, suprapubic, right* and *left hypochondrium, right* and *left lumbar,* and *right* and *left inguinal.* Two imaginary lines are drawn by extending the midclavicular lines to the middle of the inguinal ligaments. These lines form the lateral extent of the rectus abdominis muscles. At right angles to these lines, two parallel lines are drawn: one at the costal margins and the other at the anterosuperior iliac spines. The nine-area system is shown in Figure 17-2.

The examiner should recognize the abdominal structures that are located in each area. Table 17-1 lists the organs present in each of the four quadrants.

Because the kidneys, duodenum, and pancreas are posterior organs, it is unlikely that abnormalities in these organs can be palpated in adults. In children, in whom the abdominal muscles are less developed, renal masses, especially on the right side, can often be palpated.

A detailed description of the pathophysiology of the gastrointestinal system is beyond the scope of this text. A brief statement regarding the basic physiology serves to integrate the signs and symptoms of abdominal disease.

As food passes into the esophagus, an obstructing lesion can produce *dysphagia*, or difficulty swallowing. Gastroesophageal reflux can lead to heartburn. Upon entry of partially digested food into the stomach, the stomach relaxes. A failure of this relaxation may lead to early satiety or pain. The stomach functions as a food reservoir, secreting gastric juice and providing peristaltic activity with its muscular wall. Between 2 and 3 L of gastric juice is produced daily by the stomach lining and affects the digestion of proteins. The semifluid, creamy material produced by gastric digestion of food is called *chyme*. Secretion of gastric juice may produce pain if a gastric ulcer is present. Intermittent emptying of the stomach occurs when intragastric pressure overcomes the resistance of the pyloric sphincter. Emptying is normally complete within 6 hours after eating. Any obstruction to gastric emptying may produce vomiting.

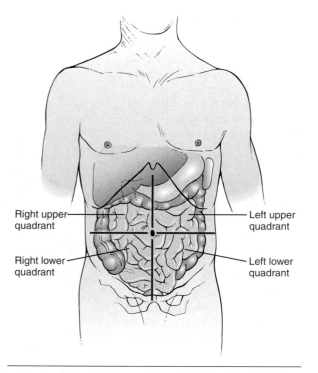

Figure 17–1 The four abdominal quadrants.

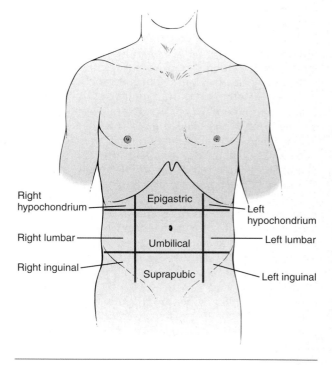

Figure 17–2 The nine abdominal areas.

Table 17–1 Abdominal Structures by Quadrants

Right	Left
Upper Quadrant	
Liver	Liver, left lobe
Gallbladder	Spleen
Pylorus	Stomach
Duodenum	Pancreas: body
Pancreas: head	Left adrenal gland
Right adrenal gland	Left kidney: upper pole
Right kidney: upper pole	Splenic flexure
Hepatic flexure	Transverse colon: portion
Ascending colon: portion	Descending colon: portion
Transverse colon: portion	
Lower Quadrant	
Right kidney: lower pole	Left kidney: lower pole
Cecum	Sigmoid colon
Appendix	Descending colon: portion
Ascending colon: portion	Left ovary
Right ovary	Left fallopian tube
Right fallopian tube	Left ureter
Right ureter	Left spermatic cord
Right spermatic cord	Uterus (if enlarged)
Uterus (if enlarged)	Bladder (if enlarged)
Bladder (if enlarged)	

The entry of chyme from the stomach into the duodenum stimulates the secretion of pancreatic enzymes and contraction of the gallbladder. The flow of pancreatic juice is maximal approximately 2 hours after a meal; the daily output is 1 to 2 L. The three enzymes of chyme—lipase, amylase, and trypsin—are responsible for the digestion of fats, starches, and proteins, respectively. In cases of pancreatic insufficiency, the stool is pale and bulky and has an odor that is more offensive than normal. The chyme and the neutralizing effect of these enzymes reduce the acidity of the duodenal contents and relieve the pain of peptic duodenal ulcer. The pain from an acutely inflamed gallbladder or from pancreatitis worsens at this phase of the digestive cycle.

The digested food continues its course through the small intestine, in which further digestion and absorption occur. Failure of bile production or its release from the gallbladder results in decreased digestion and absorption of fats, leading to diarrhea. Gallstones may form as a result of diet or hereditary predisposition.

The liver produces bile, detoxifies the byproducts of the digestion of food, and metabolizes proteins, lipids, and carbohydrates. The daily output of bile is about 1 L. In the absence of normal liver function, jaundice, ascites, and coma may result.

The jejunum and ileum further digest and absorb the nutrients. Bile acids and vitamin B_{12} are absorbed in the ileum. The dark color of stool is caused by the presence of stercobilin, a metabolite of bilirubin, that is secreted in the bile. If bile does not flow into the small intestine, the stools become pale brown to gray and are called *acholic*, or free from bile.

The colon functions to remove much of the remaining water and electrolytes from the chyme. Approximately 600 mL of fluid enters the colon daily, and only 200 mL of water is excreted in the stool daily. Abnormal colonic function leads to diarrhea or constipation. Aneurysmal pouches of colonic mucosa may cause bleeding; if they are infected, pain results. Colonic obstruction produces severe pain. Tumors may cause obstruction or bleeding.

Review of Specific Symptoms

The most common symptoms of abdominal disease are as follows:

- Pain
- Nausea and vomiting

- Change in bowel movements
- Rectal bleeding
- Jaundice
- Abdominal distention
- Mass
- Pruritus (itching)

Pain

Pain is probably the most important symptom of abdominal disease. Although abdominal neoplasia may be painless, most abdominal disease manifests itself with some amount of pain. Pain can result from mucosal irritation, smooth muscle spasm, peritoneal irritation, capsular swelling, or direct nerve stimulation. Abdominal pain necessitates speedy diagnosis and therapy. When a patient complains of abdominal pain, ask the following questions:

"Where is the pain?"

"Has the pain changed its location since it started?"

"Do you feel the pain in any other part of your body?"

"How long have you had the pain?"

"Have you had recurrent episodes of abdominal pain?"

"Did the pain start suddenly?"

"Can you describe the pain? Is it sharp? dull? burning? cramping?"

"Is the pain continuous? Does it come in waves?"

"Has there been any change in the severity or nature of the pain since it began?"

"What makes it worse?"

"What makes it better?"

"Is the pain associated with nausea? vomiting? sweating? constipation? diarrhea? bloody stools? abdominal distention? fever? chills? eating?"

"Have you ever had gallstones? kidney stones?"

If the patient is a woman, ask this question:

"When was your last period?"

Note the exact *time* at which the pain started and what the patient was doing at that time. Sudden, severe pain awakening a patient from sleep may be associated with acute perforation, inflammation, or torsion of an abdominal organ. A stone in the biliary or renal tract also causes intense pain. Note *acuteness* of the pain. Acute rupture of a fallopian tube by an ectopic pregnancy, perforation of a gastric ulcer, peritonitis, and acute pancreatitis cause such severe pain that fainting may result.

It is crucial to determine the *location* of the pain at its onset, its *localization*, its *character*, and its *radiation*. Commonly, when an abdominal organ ruptures, pain is felt "all over the belly," without localization to a specific area. Pain arising from the small intestine is commonly felt in the umbilical or epigastric regions; for example, pain from acute appendicitis begins at the umbilicus.

After time, pain may become localized to other areas. Pain from acute appendicitis travels from the umbilicus to the right lower quadrant in about 1 to 3 hours after the initial event. Pain in the chest followed by abdominal pain should raise the suspicion of a dissecting aortic aneurysm.

Note the nature of the pain. Pain caused by a perforated gastric ulcer is often described as "burning"; dissecting aneurysm as "tearing"; intestinal obstruction as "gripping"; pyelonephritis as "dull, aching"; and biliary or renal colic as "crampy, constricting."

Referred pain often provides insight as to the cause. *Referred pain* is a term used to describe pain originating in the internal organs but described by the patient as being located in

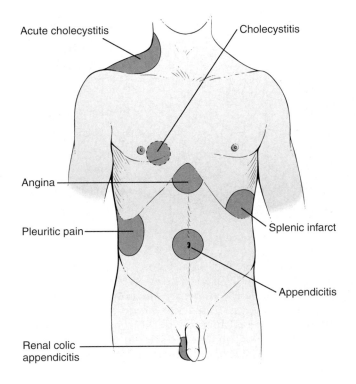

Figure 17–3 Common areas of referred pain. The dotted area is on the posterior chest.

the abdominal or chest wall, shoulder, jaw, or other areas supplied by the somatic nerves. Pain appears to originate in areas supplied by the somatic nerves entering the spinal cord at the same segment as the sensory nerves from the organ responsible for the pain. For example, right-shoulder pain may result from acute cholecystitis; testicular pain may result from renal colic or from appendicitis. The common sites for referred pain are shown in Figure 17-3. The locations of pain in abdominal disease are summarized in Table 17-2.

The time of occurrence and factors that aggravate or alleviate the symptoms (e.g., meals or defecation) are particularly important. Periodic epigastric pain occurring $\frac{1}{2}$ to 1 hour after eating is a classic symptom of gastric peptic ulcers. Patients with a duodenal peptic ulcer

Table 17–2 Location of Pain in Abdominal Disease

Area of Pain	Affected Organ	Clinical Example
Substernal	Esophagus	Esophagitis
Shoulder	Diaphragm	Subphrenic abscess
Epigastric	Stomach Duodenum Gallbladder Liver Bile ducts Pancreas	Peptic gastric ulcer Peptic duodenal ulcer Cholecystitis Hepatitis Cholangitis Pancreatitis
Right scapula	Biliary tract	Biliary colic
Midback	Aorta Pancreas	Aortic dissection Pancreatitis
Periumbilical	Small intestine	Obstruction
Hypogastrium	Colon	Ulcerative colitis Diverticulitis
Sacrum	Rectum	Proctitis Perirectal abscess

Table 17–3 Maneuvers for Ameliorating Abdominal Pain

Maneuver	Affected Organ	Clinical Example
Belching	Stomach	Gastric distention
Eating	Stomach, duodenum	Peptic ulcer
Vomiting	Stomach, duodenum	Pyloric obstruction
Leaning forward	Retroperitoneal structures	Pancreatic cancer Pancreatitis
Flexion of knees	Peritoneum	Peritonitis
Flexion of right thigh	Right psoas muscle	Appendicitis
Flexion of left thigh	Left psoas muscle	Diverticulitis

have pain 2 to 3 hours after eating or before the next meal. Food tends to lessen the pain, especially in duodenal ulcers. Perforation of a duodenal ulcer to the pancreas may produce backache, simulating an orthopedic problem. *Nocturnal pain* is a classic symptom of duodenal peptic ulcer disease. Pain after eating may also be associated with vascular disease of the abdominal viscera. Patients with this condition are older and have postprandial pain, anorexia, and weight loss. This triad is seen in *abdominal angina* resulting from obstructive vascular disease in the celiac axis or the superior mesenteric artery. Table 17-3 summarizes the important maneuvers for ameliorating abdominal pain.

Nausea and Vomiting

Vomiting may be caused by severe irritation of the peritoneum resulting from the perforation of an abdominal organ; from obstruction of the bile duct, ureter, or intestine; or from toxins. Vomiting resulting from a *perforation* is rarely massive. *Obstruction* of the bile duct or other tube produces stretching of the muscular wall, resulting in episodic vomiting that occurs at the height of the pain. Intestinal obstruction prevents the intestinal contents from passing distally; consequently, vomiting may result in the expulsion of intestinal contents. *Toxins* generally cause persistent vomiting. Not all abdominal emergencies cause vomiting. Intraperitoneal bleeding may occur in the absence of vomiting. Vomiting is frequently also caused by inflammation of intra-abdominal structures, as well as by extra-abdominal conditions, including drug toxicity, central nervous system disorders, myocardial infarction, and pregnancy. Ask the following questions if a patient complains of nausea, vomiting, or both:

> *"How long have you had nausea or vomiting?"*

> *"What is the color of the vomit?"*

> *"Is there any unusually foul odor to the vomitus?"*

> *"How often do you vomit?"*

> *"Is vomiting related to eating?"* If yes, *"How soon after eating do you vomit? Do you vomit only after eating certain foods?"*

> *"Do you have nausea without vomiting?"*

> *"Is the nausea or vomiting associated with abdominal pain? constipation? diarrhea? a loss of appetite? a change in the color of your stools? a change in the color of your urine? fever? chest pain?"*

> *"Have you noticed a change in your hearing ability?"*

> *"Have you noticed ringing in your ears?"*

If the patient is a woman, ask this question:

> *"When was your last period?"*

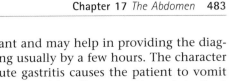

The relationship of the pain to vomiting is important and may help in providing the diagnosis. In acute appendicitis, pain precedes the vomiting usually by a few hours. The character of the vomitus may aid in determining its cause. Acute gastritis causes the patient to vomit stomach contents. Biliary colic produces bilious, or greenish-yellow, vomitus. Intestinal obstruction often causes the patient to expel bilious vomitus, followed by feculent-smelling fluid. *Feculent vomitus* is usually caused by intestinal obstruction.

Nausea without vomiting is a common symptom in patients with hepatocellular disease, pregnancy, and metastatic disease. Nausea may be associated with a hearing loss and tinnitus in patients with Ménière's disease.

Change in Bowel Movements

Take a careful history of bowel habits. A change in bowel movements necessitates further elaboration. Ask these questions of the patient with *acute* onset of diarrhea:

> *"How long have you had the diarrhea?"*
>
> *"How many bowel movements do you have a day?"*
>
> *"Did the diarrhea start suddenly?"*
>
> *"Did the diarrhea begin after a meal?"* If yes, *"What did you eat?"*
>
> *"Are the stools watery? bloody? malodorous?"*
>
> *"Is the diarrhea associated with abdominal pain? loss of appetite? nausea? vomiting?"*

The acute onset of diarrhea after a meal suggests an acute infection or toxin. Watery stools are often associated with inflammatory processes of the small bowel and colon. Shigellosis is a disease of the colon that produces bloody diarrhea. Amebiasis is also associated with bloody diarrhea.

The patient with *chronic* diarrhea should be asked the following:

> *"How long have you had diarrhea?"*
>
> *"Do you have periods of diarrhea alternating with constipation?"*
>
> *"Are the stools watery? loose? floating? malodorous?"*
>
> *"Have you noticed blood in the stools? mucus? undigested food?"*
>
> *"What is the color of the stools?"*
>
> *"How many bowel movements do you have a day?"*
>
> *"Does the diarrhea occur after eating?"*
>
> *"What happens when you fast? Do you still have diarrhea?"*
>
> *"Is the diarrhea associated with abdominal pain? abdominal distention? nausea? vomiting?"*
>
> *"Have you noticed that the diarrhea is worse at certain times of the day?"*
>
> *"How is your appetite?"*
>
> *"Has there been any change in your weight?"*

Diarrhea and constipation frequently alternate in patients with colon cancer or diverticulitis. Loose bowel movements are common in diseases of the left colon, whereas watery movements are seen in severe inflammatory bowel disease and protein-losing enteropathies. Floating stools may result from malabsorption syndromes. Patients with ulcerative colitis commonly have stool mixed with blood and mucus. Any inflammatory process of the small bowel or colon can manifest with blood mixed with stool or undigested food. Irritable bowel syndrome classically produces more diarrhea in the morning.

Patients complaining of constipation should be asked these questions:

> *"How long have you been constipated?"*
>
> *"How often do you have a bowel movement?"*

"What is the size of your stools?"

"What is the color of your stools?"

"Is the stool ever mixed with blood? mucus?"

"Have you noticed periods of constipation alternating with periods of diarrhea?"

"Have you noticed a change in the caliber of the stool?"

"Do you have much gas?"

"How's your appetite?"

"Has there been any change in your weight?"

Change in the *caliber* of the stool is significant. "Pencil"-diameter stools may result from an anal or a distal rectal carcinoma. A change in the color of stools is important. As is discussed later, pale brown to gray stools indicate an absence of bile. This can result from an obstruction to bile flow from the gallbladder or from decreased production of bile. Weight changes are important with the symptom of constipation. An increase in weight may indicate decreased metabolism seen in hypothyroidism; a decrease in weight may be associated with cancer of the colon or other hypermetabolic conditions.

Rectal Bleeding

Rectal bleeding may be manifested by bright red blood, blood mixed with stool, or black, tarry stools. Bright red blood per rectum, also known as *hematochezia*, can occur from colonic tumors, diverticular disease, or ulcerative colitis. Blood mixed with stool can be the result of ulcerative colitis, diverticular disease, tumors, or hemorrhoids. Ask the patient who describes rectal bleeding the following questions:

"How long have you noticed bright red blood in your stools?"

"Is the blood mixed with the stool?"

"Are there streaks of blood on the surface of the stool?"

"Have you noticed a change in your bowel habits?"

"Have you noticed a persistent sensation in your rectum that you have to move your bowels, but you cannot?"

Tenesmus is the painful, continued, and ineffective straining at stool. It is caused by inflammation or a space-occupying lesion such as a tumor at the distal rectum or anus. Hemorrhoidal bleeding is a common cause of hematochezia and streaking of stool with blood.

Melena is a black, tarry stool that results from bleeding above the first section of the duodenum, with partial digestion of the hemoglobin. Inquire about the presence of melena. A useful way of questioning is to show the patient the black tubing on the stethoscope and ask, "Have your bowel movements ever been this color?" If asked directly whether the bowel movements have ever been black, the patient may answer in the affirmative, equating dark (normal) stools with black stools. Ask these questions of a patient who describes melena:

"Have you passed more than one black, tarry stool?" If yes, *"When?"*

"How long have you been having black, tarry stools?"

"Have you noticed feeling lightheaded?"

"Have you had any nausea associated with these stools? any vomiting? diarrhea? abdominal pain? sweating?"

The answers to these questions can provide some information regarding the acuteness and the amount of the hemorrhage. Lightheadedness, nausea, and diaphoresis are seen with rapid gastrointestinal bleeding and hypotension.

The presence of *silver-colored stools* is rare but pathognomonic of acholic stools with melena, a condition resulting from cancer of the ampulla of Vater in the duodenum. The cancer produces biliary obstruction, and the cancerous fronds are sloughed, causing melena.

Jaundice

The presence of jaundice (*icterus*) must alert the examiner that there is either liver parenchymal disease or an obstruction to bile flow. The presence of icterus, or jaundice, results from a decreased excretion of conjugated bilirubin into the bile. This can result from intrahepatic biliary obstruction, known as *medical jaundice*, or from extrahepatic biliary obstruction, known as *surgical jaundice*. In any patient with icterus, the examiner should search for clues by asking the following questions:

"How long have you been jaundiced?"

"Did the jaundice develop rapidly?"

"Is the jaundice associated with abdominal pain? loss of appetite? nausea? vomiting? distaste for cigarettes?"

"Is the jaundice associated with chills? fever? itching? weight loss?"

"In the past year have you had any transfusions? tattooing? inoculations?"

"Do you use any recreational drugs?" If yes, *"Do you use any drugs intravenously?"*

"Do you eat raw shellfish? oysters?"

"Have you traveled abroad in the past year?" If yes, *"Where? Were you aware that you may have consumed unclean water?"*

"Have you been jaundiced before?"

"Has your urine changed color since you noticed that you were jaundiced?"

"What is the color of your stools?"

"Do you have any friends or relations who are also jaundiced?"

"What type of work do you do? What other types of work have you done?"

"What are your hobbies?"

Viral hepatitis is associated with nausea, vomiting, a loss of appetite, and an aversion to smoking. Hepatitis A has a fecal-oral route of transmission and an incubation period of 2 to 6 weeks. It may be linked to ingestion of raw shellfish. Hepatitis B is blood-borne and has an incubation period of 1 to 6 months. Health professionals are at increased risk for hepatitis. Any contact with an individual with viral hepatitis places a person at a higher risk of contracting viral hepatitis. Hepatitis C virus (HCV) is the most common chronic blood-borne infection in the United States. The Centers for Disease Control and Prevention has estimated that during the 1980s, as many as 230,000 new infections have occurred in this country. It is estimated that as many as 3.9 million Americans have antibody to HCV and are currently asymptomatic. They are, however, at risk for chronic liver disease, the 10th leading cause of death in the United States. About 40% of chronic liver disease is HCV related and results in 8000 to 10,000 deaths a year. End-stage liver disease secondary to HCV infection is the most common indication for liver transplantation. Because most of these individuals are younger than 50 years, it is anticipated that by 2020, there will be a marked increase in the number of patients with chronic liver disease.

Slowly developing jaundice that is accompanied by pale stools and cola-colored urine is *obstructive jaundice*, either intrahepatic or extrahepatic. Jaundice accompanied by fever and chills is considered *cholangitis* until proved otherwise. Cholangitis may result from stasis of bile in the bile duct that results from a gallstone or from cancer of the head of the pancreas. Determine whether chemicals are used in a patient's occupation or hobbies, because they may be related to the cause of the jaundice. Many industrial chemicals and drugs have been associated with liver disease. These agents may be responsible for a viral hepatitis-like illness, cholestasis, or for granulomas or hepatic tumors. Occupational exposure to carbon tetrachloride and vinyl chloride is well known to cause liver disease. Ask questions related to alcohol abuse. These are described in Chapter 1, The Interviewer's Questions.

Abdominal Distention

Abdominal distention may be related to increased gas in the gastrointestinal tract or to the presence of ascites. Increased gas can result from malabsorption, irritable colon, or air swallowing (*aerophagia*). *Ascites* can have a variety of causes, such as cirrhosis, congestive heart failure, portal hypertension, peritonitis, or neoplasia. To try to identify the cause of abdominal distention, ask these questions:

"How long have you noticed your abdomen to be distended?"

"Is the distention intermittent?"

"Is the distention related to eating?"

"Is the distention lessened by belching or by passing gas from below?"

"Is the distention associated with vomiting? loss of appetite? weight loss? change in your bowel habits? shortness of breath?"

Gaseous distention related to eating is intermittent and is relieved by the passage of flatus or belching. A patient with ascites has the insidious development of increased abdominal girth, noted through a progressive increase in belt size. Loss of appetite is often associated with cirrhosis and malignancy, although end-stage congestive heart failure may produce this symptom as well. Shortness of breath and ascites may be symptoms of congestive heart failure, but the shortness of breath may be the result of a decrease in pulmonary capacity owing to ascites from another cause. Questions related to alcoholic abuse are most appropriate and are outlined in Chapter 1, The Interviewer's Questions.

Mass

An abdominal mass may be a neoplasm or a hernia. An abdominal *hernia* is a protrusion from the peritoneal cavity into which peritoneal contents are extruded. The contents may be omentum, intestine, or bladder wall. An abdominal hernia may be inguinal, femoral, umbilical, or internal, depending on its location. The most common complaint is swelling, which may or may not be painful. An inguinal hernia may manifest as a mass in the groin or scrotum. The major complications of a hernia are intestinal obstruction and intestinal strangulation from interference of blood supply. A hernia is termed *reducible* when it can be emptied of its contents by pressure or a change in posture.

The sign or symptom of a pulsatile abdominal mass should alert the examiner to the possibility of an aortic aneurysm.

Pruritus

Pruritus, or itching, is a common symptom. Generalized itching may be a symptom of a diffuse skin disorder* or a manifestation of chronic renal or hepatic disease. Intense pruritus may be associated with lymphoma or Hodgkin's disease, as well as with malignancies of the gastrointestinal tract. In older individuals, pruritus may also be caused by dry skin alone. *Pruritus ani* is localized itching of the anal skin. It has many causes, including fistulas, fissures, psoriasis, parasites, poor hygiene, and diabetes.

Impact of Inflammatory Bowel Disease on the Patient

Inflammatory bowel disease constitutes a group of diseases of unknown cause. The symptoms produced depend on the location, extent, and acuteness of the inflammatory lesions. The common presenting features are fever, anorexia, weight loss, abdominal discomfort,

---

*For example, dermatitis herpetiformis, a blistering disease predominantly on the buttocks, shoulders, elbows, and knees.

diarrhea, rectal urgency, and rectal bleeding. It is a chronic, potentially disabling illness, often resulting in the need for multiple surgeries, in fistula formation, and in cancer.

Inflammatory bowel disease may lead to long absences from school or work, disruption of family life, malabsorption, malnutrition, and multiple hospitalizations. A patient can have 10 to 30 watery or bloody bowel movements each day. As a consequence, patients with inflammatory bowel disease can have many psychologic problems, particularly when they are young adults. Because of malabsorption, the prevalence of osteopenia in patients with inflammatory bowel disease ranges from 40% to 50%; osteoporosis is present in 5% to 30% of all patients. Fractures of the hip, spine, and distal radius occur. One study revealed that the incidence of fractures among persons with inflammatory bowel disease is 40% greater than in the general population.

Sexual development may be delayed as a result of malnutrition. Social development is also delayed. The necessity of constantly having to remain near a bathroom inhibits patients' abilities to develop normal dating patterns. Many of these patients are socially immature, and social introversion is common. By necessity, they remain at home. Their lives revolve around their bowel habits.

In most cases, there is a positive correlation between the severity of the physical disease and the extent of emotional disturbance. *Dependency* is the most reported characteristic of patients with inflammatory bowel disease. Repressed rage, suppression of feelings, and anxieties are also common. It is reported that many patients have a constant desire to rid themselves of events in their lives. This characteristic can be acted out through the diarrhea. Another characteristic of these patients is to be *obsessive-compulsive*. The marked obsessive character becomes even more obvious when the patient is ill. It is typical for patients to worry incessantly about what is happening in their bowels. The patients are intelligent, often having read much literature, including medical textbooks, about their disease.

Denial is usually not a prominent symptom. In contrast, these patients concentrate obsessively on the details of their bowel habits.

Sexual problems are common. Interest and participation in sexual activity tend to be at a low level. Many of these individuals prefer to be fondled like a child and largely reject any genital contact. Patients are prone to regard sexual activity in anal terms, such as "dirty," "unclean," or "soiling." They are squeamish about body contact, odors, and secretions. The loss of libido and decreased sexual drive may be related to their fear of bowel action during intercourse, of perineal pain, or that sexual intercourse may in some way further damage the bowel.

The frequent hospitalizations cause anxiety and depression, which exacerbate the disease. The fear of cancer may be the basis of depression, which is a common response to the disease. It is well established that emotional factors are important in maintaining and prolonging an existing attack. Schoolwork deteriorates as young patients are forced to miss more and more school, further increasing their anxiety.

An often unappreciated major complication of inflammatory bowel disease is substance abuse. As a result of chronic pain, as much as 5% of patients with inflammatory bowel disease are physically addicted to oral narcotics. Many more are psychologically dependent on their pain medication.

Many patients with ulcerative colitis require an ileostomy. The fear of disfigurement, the loss of self-confidence, the potential lack of cleanliness, and the dread of unexpected spillage are common.

Time for listening and an interest in a patient's problem are important in gaining the patient's confidence. Listening may reveal and help unravel the emotional problems that may be the source of the exacerbation of the bowel disease. Talking with the patient may be more efficacious than prescribing anti-inflammatory agents or tranquilizers. Careful and thoughtful discussion of the illness strengthens the doctor-patient relationship and produces immeasurable therapeutic benefits.

Physical Examination

The equipment necessary for the examination of the abdomen and rectum consists of a stethoscope, gloves, lubricant, tissues, and occult blood testing card and Hemoccult developer.

The patient should be lying flat in bed, and the abdomen should be fully exposed from the sternum to the knees. The arms should be at the sides, and the legs flat. Frequently, patients tend to place their arms behind their heads, which tightens the abdominal muscles and makes

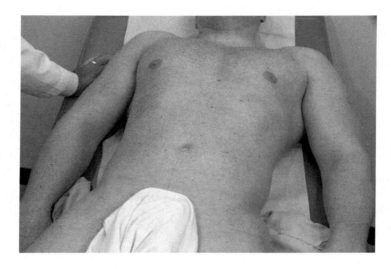

Figure 17–4 Technique for inspecting the abdomen.

the examination more difficult. Placing a pillow beneath the knees often aids in relaxation. The examiner should be standing on the patient's right side. A sheet or towel is placed over the genitalia, as shown in Figure 17-4.

If the patient has complained of abdominal pain, examine the area of pain *last*. If the examiner touches the area of maximal pain, the abdominal muscles tighten, and the examination is more difficult.

The physical examination of the abdomen includes the following:

- Inspection
- Auscultation
- Percussion
- Palpation
- Rectal examination
- Special techniques

Inspection

Evaluate General Appearance

The general appearance of the patient often furnishes valuable information as to the nature of the condition. Patients with renal or biliary *colic* writhe in bed. They squirm constantly and can find no comfortable position. In contrast, patients with *peritonitis*, who have intense pain on movement, characteristically remain still in bed because any slight motion worsens the pain. They may be lying in bed with their knees drawn up to help relax the abdominal muscles and reduce intra-abdominal pressure. Patients who are pale and sweating may be suffering from the initial *shock* of pancreatitis or a perforated gastric ulcer.

Determine Respiratory Rate

The respiratory rate is increased in patients with generalized peritonitis, intra-abdominal hemorrhage, or intestinal obstruction.

Inspect the Skin

Inspect the skin and sclera for jaundice. Whenever possible, the patient should be evaluated for jaundice in natural light because incandescent light frequently masks the existence of icterus. Jaundice becomes apparent when the serum bilirubin level exceeds 2.5 mg/dL in adults or 6 mg/dL in neonates. Figure 17-5 shows a patient with jaundice. Notice the scleral icterus as well as the yellow discoloration of the skin. Hyperbilirubinemia can also result in intense generalized pruritus.

Inspect for *spider angiomas*. Spider angiomas have a high degree of sensitivity in patients with alcoholic cirrhosis but are nonspecific because they also occur in pregnancy and collagen vascular disorders (see Fig. 8-75).

Figure 17-6 shows the leg of a patient with *pyoderma gangrenosum*. Notice the necrotic, undermined ulceration with pus. These tender ulcerations, commonly on the lower extremities, are associated with inflammatory bowel disease, especially ulcerative colitis. In general,

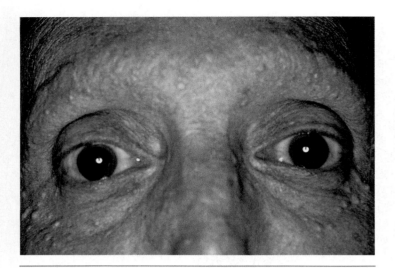

Figure 17–5 Jaundice.

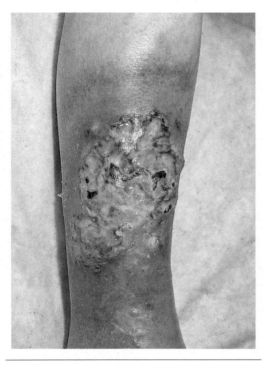

Figure 17–6 Pyoderma gangrenosum.

the clinical course of pyoderma gangrenosum follows the course of the bowel disease. This condition is also seen in patients with rheumatoid arthritis, myeloid metaplasia, and chronic myelogenous leukemia.

Inspect the Hands

Is there muscle loss in the small muscles of the hands? This is associated with wasting.

The nails are examined for changes in the nail bed, especially an increase in the size of the lunula. The fingers of a patient with cirrhosis showing "half-and-half" nails are shown in Figure 17-7 (see also Fig. 8-8).

Inspect the Facies

Are the eyes sunken? Is temporal wasting present? These signs indicate wasting and poor nutrition.

The skin around the mouth and oral mucosa may provide evidence of gastrointestinal disorders. Melanin deposition around and in the oral cavity, especially the buccal mucosa,

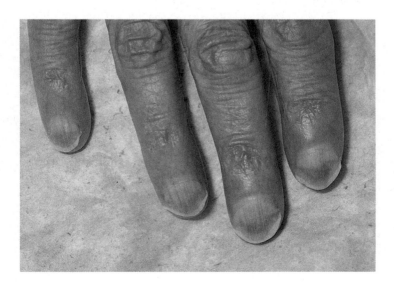

Figure 17–7 Lindsay's nails.

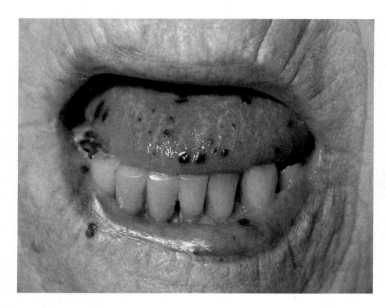

Figure 17–8 Osler-Weber-Rendu syndrome.

suggests *Peutz-Jeghers syndrome*. Figure 12-12 shows the lips of a patient with the classic brown pigmentary changes of Peutz-Jeghers syndrome. This is an autosomal dominant disorder characterized by generalized gastrointestinal, hamartomatous polyposis, and mucocutaneous pigmentation. The benign polyps are most common in the jejunum and only rarely become malignant. The polyps, however, may bleed, cause intussusception, or cause obstruction. Telangiectases of the lips and tongue are suggestive of *Osler-Weber-Rendu syndrome* (see Fig. 12-11), in which multiple telangiectases are present throughout the gastrointestinal tract. These lesions may bleed insidiously, causing anemia. The classic oral lesions of a patient with Osler-Weber-Rendu syndrome are shown in Figure 17-8.

Hypercortisolism, or *Cushing's syndrome*, has a range of clinical manifestations. The most common are obesity, facial plethora, hirsutism, and hypertension. Obesity occurs in 90% of affected patients. Most patients with hypercortisolism characteristically have round, puffy, red faces called *moon facies*. They also have prominent fat deposits in the supraclavicular and retrocervical areas (buffalo hump). Figure 17-9 shows a patient with Cushing's syndrome and the typical moon facies.

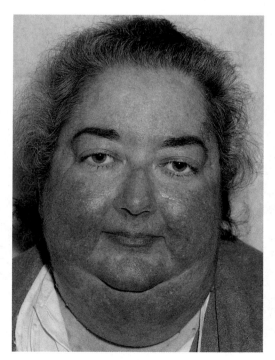

Figure 17–9 Cushing's syndrome.

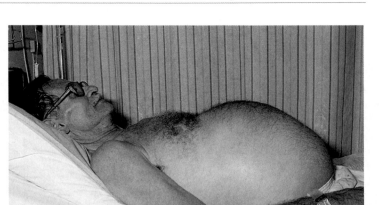

Figure 17–10 Ascites.

Inspect the Abdomen

The contour of the abdomen should be assessed. A *scaphoid*, or concave, abdomen may be associated with cachexia; a *protuberant* abdomen may result from gaseous distention of the intestines, ascites, (splenomegaly lator), or obesity. When a patient with ascites stands, the fluid sinks into the lower abdomen; when lying supine, the fluid bulges in the flanks. If a patient with ascites lies on the side, the fluid flows to the dependent lower side. A patient with a protuberant abdomen as a result of carcinomatous ascites is shown in Figure 17-10.

The examiner should focus attention on the abdomen to describe adequately the presence of any asymmetry, distention, masses, or visible peristaltic waves. The examiner should then observe the abdomen from above, looking for the same signs. Inspection of the abdomen for striae and scars may provide valuable data. Silver striae are stretch marks consistent with weight loss. Pinkish-purple striae are classic signs of adrenocortical excess. Figure 17-11 shows the characteristic purplish striae in a patient with Cushing's syndrome.

Is the umbilicus everted? An everted umbilicus is often a sign of increased abdominal pressure, usually from ascites or a large mass. An umbilical hernia may also cause an umbilicus to become everted.

Are there ecchymoses on the abdomen or on the flanks? Massive ecchymoses may occur in these areas as a result of hemorrhagic pancreatitis or strangulated bowel. This is *Grey Turner's sign*.

Cullen's sign is a bluish discoloration of the umbilicus resulting from hemoperitoneum of any cause.

Recognition of classic surgical scars may be helpful. Figure 17-12 shows the locations of some common surgical scars.

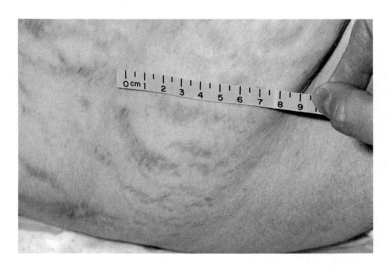

Figure 17–11 Abdominal striae.

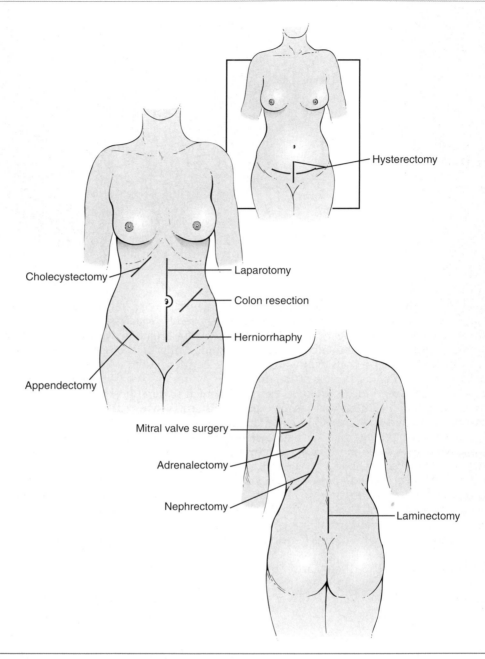

Figure 17–12 Locations of common surgical scars.

Inspect for Hernias

The patient lying in bed should be asked to cough while the examiner inspects the inguinal, umbilical, and femoral areas. This maneuver, by increasing intra-abdominal pressure, may produce a sudden bulging in these areas, which may be related to a hernia. If the patient has had surgery, coughing may reveal a bulging along the abdominal scar from the previous incision. In addition, coughing may elicit pain localized to a specific area. This technique enables the examiner to identify the area of maximal tenderness and to perform most of the abdominal examination without too much discomfort to the patient. Ascites secondary to metastatic breast carcinoma and an umbilical hernia are shown in Figure 17-13.

Inspect the Superficial Veins

The venous pattern of the abdomen is usually barely perceptible. If it is visible in the normal individual, the drainage of the lower two thirds of the abdomen is downward. In the presence of vena caval obstruction, superficial veins may dilate, and the veins drain cephalad (toward the head). In patients with portal hypertension, the dilated veins appear to radiate from the

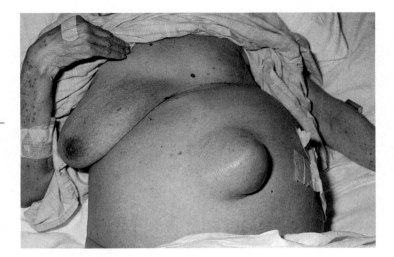

Figure 17–13 Ascites with umbilical hernia.

umbilicus. This is caused by backflow through the collateral veins within the falciform ligament, and this pattern is called *caput medusae*.

If the superficial veins are distended, evaluate the direction of drainage by the following technique: Place the tips of your index fingers on a vein that is oriented cephalad-caudad, not transverse, and compress it. Using continuous pressure, slide your index fingers apart for about 3 to 4 inches (7.5 to 10 cm). Remove one finger and observe the refilling in the direction of flow. Repeat this procedure, but this time remove your other finger and observe the direction of flow. Figure 17-14 shows the abdomen of a patient with intrahepatic portal hypertension. Notice the engorged paraumbilical veins; the flow was away from the umbilicus toward the caval system.

Auscultation

Auscultation of bowel sounds can provide information about the motion of air and liquid in the gastrointestinal tract. Many examiners perform auscultation of the abdomen before percussion or palpation, in contrast to the usual order. It is believed that percussion or palpation

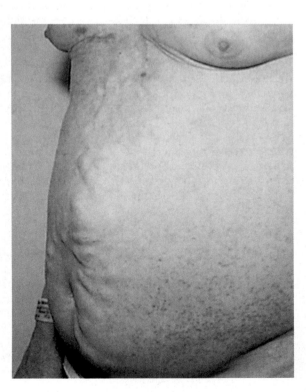

Figure 17–14 Abdominal venous pattern.

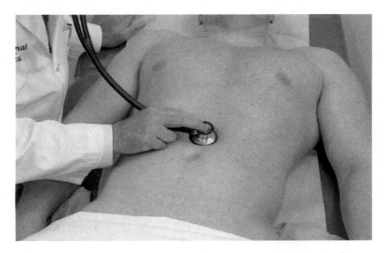

Figure 17–15 Technique for evaluating bowel sounds.

may change the intestinal motility; therefore, auscultation should be performed first to produce a more accurate assessment of the existing bowel sounds.

Evaluate Bowel Sounds

The patient is placed in a supine position. To perform auscultation of the abdomen, the examiner places the diaphragm of the stethoscope over the midabdomen and listens for bowel sounds. This technique is pictured in Figure 17-15.

Normal bowel sounds occur approximately every 5 to 10 seconds and have a high-pitched sound. If after 2 minutes no bowel sounds are heard, "absent bowel sounds" may be noted. The absence of bowel sounds suggests a paralytic ileus that results from diffuse peritoneal irritation. There may be rushes of low-pitched rumbling sounds, termed *borborygmi,* which are associated with hyperperistalsis. These sounds are similar to the sound of the word "borborygmi" itself. They are common in early acute intestinal obstruction.

Rule Out Obstructed Viscus

A *succussion splash* may be detected in a distended abdomen as a result of the presence of gas and fluid in an obstructed organ. The examiner applies the stethoscope over the patient's abdomen while shaking the patient's abdomen from side to side. The presence of a sloshing sound usually indicates distention of the stomach or colon. This technique is illustrated in Figure 17-16.

Rule Out Abdominal Bruits

Auscultation is also useful for determining the presence of bruits. Each quadrant should be evaluated for their presence. Bruits may result from stenosis of the renal artery or of the abdominal aorta. (See discussion of abdominal bruits in Chapter 15, The Peripheral Vascular System.)

Rule Out Peritoneal Rubs

A peritoneal friction rub, like a pleural or pericardial rub, is a sound that indicates inflammation. During respiratory motion, a friction rub may be heard in the right or left upper quadrants in the presence of hepatic or splenic disorder.

Percussion

Percussion is used to demonstrate the presence of gaseous distention and fluid or solid masses. In the normal examination, usually only the size and location of the liver and spleen can be determined. Some examiners prefer to palpate before percussion, especially if the patient complains of abdominal pain; either approach is correct. The technique of percussion is discussed in Chapter 13, The Chest.

Percuss the Abdomen

The patient lies supine. All four quadrants of the abdomen are evaluated by percussion. Tympany is the most common percussion note in the abdomen. It is caused by the presence

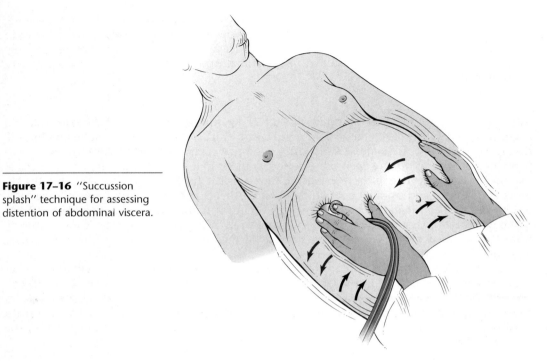

Figure 17–16 "Succussion splash" technique for assessing distention of abdominal viscera.

of gas in the stomach, small bowel, and colon. The suprapubic area, when percussed, may sound dull if the urinary bladder is distended or, in a woman, if the uterus is enlarged.

Percuss the Liver

The upper border of the liver is percussed in the right midclavicular line, starting in the mid-chest. As the chest is percussed downward, the resonant note of the chest becomes dull as the liver is reached. As percussion continues still further, this dull note becomes tympanic because the percussion is now over the colon. The upper and lower borders of the liver should be no more than 4 inches (10 cm) apart. The technique is illustrated in Figure 17-17.

There are several problems with predicting liver size by percussion. If ascites is present, the examiner can only speculate about the correct size of the liver. A more common cause of

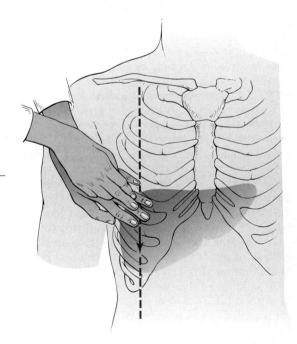

Figure 17–17 Technique for liver percussion.

overestimating liver size (false-positive measurement) is some form of chronic obstructive lung disease. This makes percussion of the upper border of the liver difficult. Obesity in a patient can cause problems in both percussion and palpation. Distention of the colon may obscure the lower liver dullness. This may result in underestimating the size of the liver (false-negative measurement).

Percuss the Spleen

Although the size of the spleen is often difficult to determine, evaluation of the spleen should begin with percussion of splenic size. In normal individuals, the spleen lies hidden within the rib cage against the posterolateral wall of the abdominal cavity in *Traube's space*. Traube's space is defined by the sixth rib superiorly, the left anterior axillary line laterally, and the costal margin inferiorly. As the spleen enlarges, it remains close to the abdominal wall, and the tip moves downward and toward the midline. Because the early enlargement is in an anteroposterior direction, considerable enlargement may occur without its becoming palpable below the costal margin. It is thought that dullness to percussion in Traube's space—the loss of tympany from the air-filled colon and stomach because of the enlarged spleen—is a useful sign for determining splenic enlargement.

Have the patient lie in the supine position. With the patient breathing normally, percuss in the lowest intercostal space in the left anterior axillary line. Normal percussion yields either a resonant or tympanic note. A positive test of splenomegaly is diagnosed when the percussion note is dull. With ultrasonography, the standard imaging technique, splenic percussion has a sensitivity of 62% and a specificity of 72%. In leaner individuals who had not eaten in the previous 2 hours, the sensitivity was 78% and the specificity was 82%.

Rule Out Ascites

On patients in whom ascites is thought to be present, a special percussion test for *shifting dullness* may be performed. While the patient is lying on the back, the examiner determines the borders of tympany and dullness. The area of tympany is present above the area of dullness and is caused by gas in the bowel that is floating on top of the ascites. The patient is then asked to turn on the side, and the examiner again determines the borders of the percussion notes. If ascites is present, dullness "shifts" to the more dependent position; the area around the umbilicus that was initially tympanic becomes dull. Shifting dullness has a sensitivity of 83% to 88% and a specificity of 56%. The test for shifting dullness is illustrated in Figure 17-18.

An additional test for ascites is the presence of a *fluid wave*. Another examiner's hand or the patient's own hand is placed in the middle of the patient's abdomen. Indenting the abdominal wall stops transmission of an impulse by the subcutaneous adipose tissue. The examiner then taps one flank while palpating the other side. The appearance of a fluid wave is suggestive of ascites. This technique is illustrated in Figure 17-19. The presence of a prominent fluid wave is the most specific of all physical diagnostic tests for ascites and has a specificity of 82% to 92%, according to several studies. A false-positive result may be obtained in obese individuals, and a false-negative result may be obtained when the ascites is small to moderate.

Another physical finding with ascites is the presence of *bulging flanks*. This change occurs when the weight of free abdominal fluid is sufficient to push the flanks outward. It has a 93% sensitivity and a 54% specificity for detecting ascites.

The most sensitive sign for ascites is the presence of shifting dullness, whereas the most specific sign is the presence of a prominent fluid wave. For an individual patient, the examiner must know the prevalence of disease or the pretest probability to apply sensitivity and specificity. Several studies have reviewed the operating characteristics of the physical examination tests for ascites. Their pooled sensitivity, specificity, and likelihood ratios for the presence of ascites are summarized in Table 17-4. The presence of a prominent fluid wave or shifting dullness is associated with the highest likelihood of the presence of ascites; the absence of bulging flanks, flank dullness, or shifting dullness decreases the likelihood.

Among the more common historical items perceived by patients, an increase in abdominal girth or recent weight gain has the highest chance of being associated with ascites. An increase in abdominal girth has a positive likelihood ratio (LR+) of 4.16; recent weight gain has an LR+ of 3.20. Conversely, the absence of the subjective increase in abdominal girth has a negative likelihood ratio (LR−) of 0.17; the absence of subjective ankle swelling carries an LR− of 0.10. With regard to the physical examination, the presence of a fluid wave or shifting dullness has the highest LR+ (9.6 or 5.76, respectively). The absence of bulging flanks or edema makes the presence of ascites least likely, with an LR− of 0.12 or 0.17, respectively.

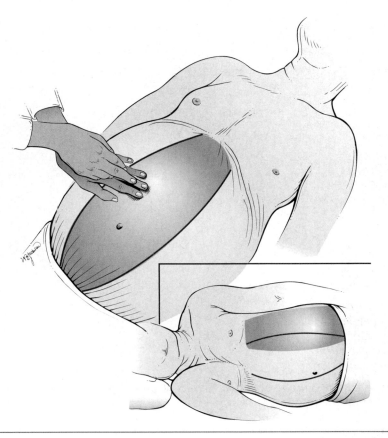

Figure 17–18 Technique for testing for shifting dullness. The *shaded areas* represent the areas of tympany.

Figure 17–19 Technique for testing a fluid wave.

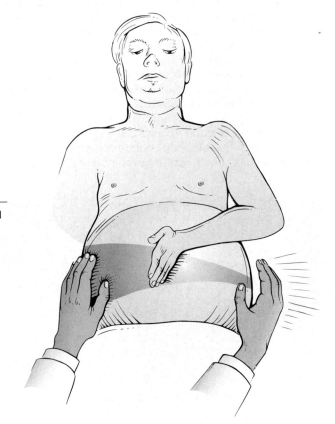

Table 17-4 Characteristics of Physical Signs (Pooled Data) for Detection of Ascites*

Physical Sign	Sensitivity %	Range	Specificity %	Range	LR+	LR−
Bulging flanks	81	69-93	59	50-68	2.0	0.3
Flank dullness	84	80-94	59	47-71	2.0	0.3
Shifting dullness	86	64-90	72	63-81	2.7	0.3
Prominent fluid wave	62	47-77	90	84-96	6.0	0.4

*95% confidence interval; data pooled from Cummings et al (1985), Simel et al (1988), Cattau et al (1982), and Williams and Simel (1992).
LR+, positive likelihood ratio; LR−, negative likelihood ratio.

Palpation

Abdominal palpation is commonly divided into the following:

- Light palpation
- Deep palpation
- Liver palpation
- Spleen palpation
- Kidney palpation

The patient is supine during palpation. Always begin palpation in an area of the abdomen that is farthest from the location of pain.

Light Palpation

Light palpation is used to detect tenderness and areas of muscular spasm or rigidity. The examiner should systematically palpate the entire abdomen by using the flat part of his or her right hand or the pads of the fingers, *not* the fingertips. The fingers should be together, and sudden jabs are to be avoided. The hand should be lifted from area to area instead of sliding over the abdominal wall. Light palpation is demonstrated in Figure 17-20.

With patients who are ticklish, it may be useful to sandwich their hand between the examiner's hands, as demonstrated in Figure 17-21.

During expiration, the rectus muscles usually relax and soften. If there is little change, rigidity is said to be present. *Rigidity* is involuntary spasm of the abdominal muscles and is indicative of peritoneal irritation. Rigidity may be *diffuse*, as in diffuse peritonitis, or *localized*, as over an inflamed appendix or gallbladder. In patients with generalized peritonitis, the abdomen is described as "boardlike."

In patients who complain of abdominal pain, palpation should be performed gently. Lightly stroking the abdomen with a pin may reveal an area of increased sensation that is caused by

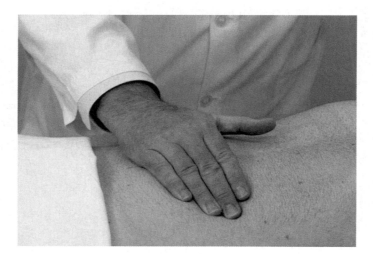

Figure 17-20 Technique for light palpation.

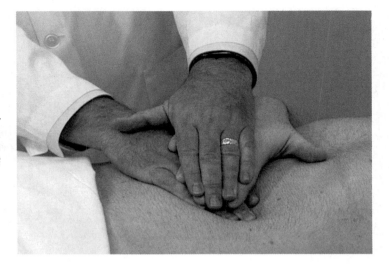

Figure 17–21 Technique used for ticklish patients. The patient's hand is sandwiched between the examiner's hands.

inflammation of the visceral or parietal peritoneum. This sensation is *hyperesthesia*. The patient is asked to determine whether the pin feels sharper on one side of the abdomen than on the corresponding area on the other side. Although useful, the presence or absence of this finding must be considered in view of all other findings.

Deep Palpation

Deep palpation is used to determine organ size, as well as the presence of abnormal abdominal masses. In deep palpation, the examiner places the flat portion of his or her right hand on the patient's abdomen, and his or her left hand is placed over the right hand. The fingertips of the left hand exert the pressure, while the right hand should appreciate any tactile stimulation. Pressure should be applied to the abdomen gently but steadily. The technique of deep palpation is demonstrated in Figure 17-22.

During deep palpation, the patient should be instructed to breathe quietly through the mouth and to keep arms at the sides. Asking the patient to open the mouth when breathing seems to aid in generalized muscular relaxation. The palpating hands should be warm, because cold hands may produce voluntary muscular spasm called *guarding*. Engaging the patient in conversation often aids in relaxing the patient's abdominal musculature. Patients with well-developed rectus muscles should be instructed to flex their knees to relax the abdominal muscles. Any tender areas must be identified.

Rule Out Rebound Tenderness

In a patient with abdominal pain, it should be determined whether rebound tenderness is present. *Rebound tenderness* is a sign of peritoneal irritation and can be elicited by palpating deeply and *slowly* in an abdominal area away from the suspected area of local inflammation.

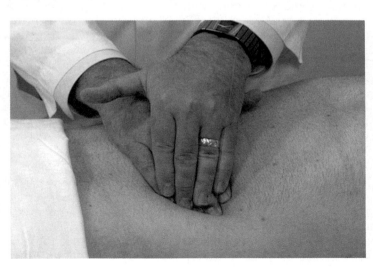

Figure 17–22 Technique for deep palpation.

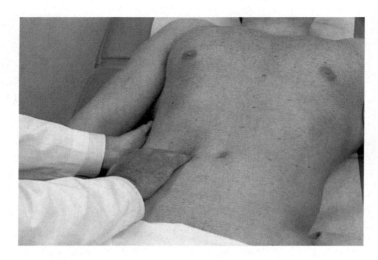

Figure 17–23 Technique for liver palpation.

The palpating hand is then quickly removed. The sensation of pain on the side of the inflammation that occurs on release of pressure is rebound tenderness. If generalized peritonitis is present, pain is felt in the area of palpation. The patient should be asked, "Which hurts more, *now* (while pressing) or *now* (during release)?" This is a useful test, but because generalized pain is elicited in the patient with peritonitis, the maneuver should be performed near the conclusion of the abdominal examination.

Liver Palpation

To perform palpation of the liver, place your left hand posteriorly between the patient's right 12th rib and the iliac crest, lateral to the paraspinal muscles. Place your right hand in the patient's right upper quadrant parallel and lateral to the rectus muscles and below the area of liver dullness. The patient is instructed to take a deep breath as you press inward and upward with your right hand and pull upward with your left hand. You may feel the liver edge slipping over the fingertips of your right hand as the patient breathes. Start as low as the pelvic brim and gradually work upward. If the examination does not start low, a markedly enlarged liver edge may be missed. The technique of liver palpation is demonstrated in Figure 17-23.

The normal liver edge has a firm, regular ridge, with a smooth surface. If the liver edge is not felt, repeat the maneuver after readjusting your right hand closer to the costal margin. Enlargement of the liver results from vascular congestion, hepatitis, neoplasm, or cirrhosis.

Another technique for liver palpation is the "hooking" method. The examiner stands near the patient's head and places both hands together below the right costal margin and the area of dullness. The examiner presses inward and upward and "hooks" around the liver edge while the patient inhales deeply. The technique of hooking the liver is shown in Figure 17-24.

On occasion, the liver appears to be enlarged, but the actual border is difficult to determine. The *scratch test* may be helpful in ascertaining the liver's edge. The examiner holds the diaphragm of the stethoscope with the left hand and places it below the patient's right costal margin over the liver. While the examiner listens through the stethoscope, his or her right index finger "scratches" the abdominal wall at points in a semicircle equidistant from the stethoscope. As the finger scratches over the liver's edge, there is a marked increase in the intensity of the sound. This technique is illustrated in Figure 17-25.

A palpable liver is not necessarily enlarged or diseased; however, its being palpable does increase the possibility of hepatomegaly. Being nonpalpable does not rule out hepatomegaly, but it does reduce the likelihood that the liver is enlarged. The LR+ for hepatomegaly, if the liver is palpable, is 2.5; if the liver is not palpable or if enlargement of the liver is detected by scintigraphic scanning, the LR− is 0.45.

Rule Out Hepatic Tenderness

To elicit hepatic tenderness, place the palm of your left hand over the patient's right upper quadrant and *gently* hit it with the ulnar surface of the fist of your right hand. Inflammatory processes involving the liver or gallbladder produce tenderness on fist palpation. Figure 17-26 demonstrates this technique.

On occasion during liver palpation, pain is elicited in the left upper quadrant during inspiration, and the patient suddenly stops inspiratory efforts. This is called *Murphy's sign* and is

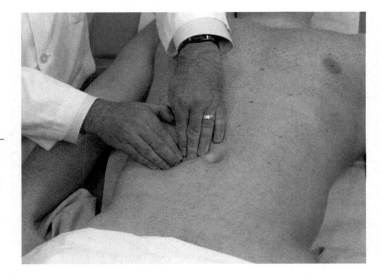

Figure 17–24 Technique for "hooking" the liver.

suggestive of acute cholecystitis. On inspiration, the lungs expand, pushing the diaphragm, liver, and inflamed gallbladder down into the abdominal cavity. As the inflamed gallbladder descends against the palpating hand, pain is produced, and there is sudden inspiratory arrest.

Spleen Palpation

Palpation of the spleen is more difficult than palpation of the liver. The patient lies on the back, with the examiner at the patient's right side. The examiner places his or her left hand over the patient's chest and elevates the patient's left rib cage. The examiner's right hand is placed flat below the patient's left costal margin and presses inward and upward toward the anterior axillary line. The left hand exerts an anterior force to displace the spleen anteriorly. Figure 17-27 illustrates the positions of the hands for splenic palpation.

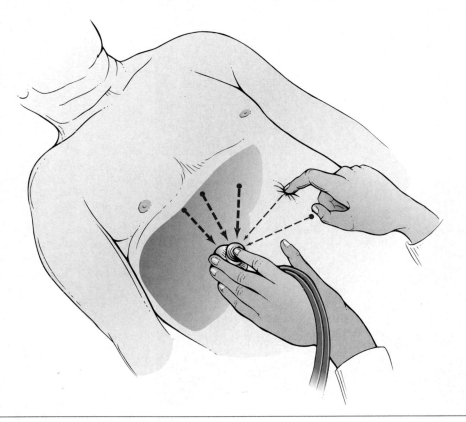

Figure 17–25 The scratch test for determining liver size.

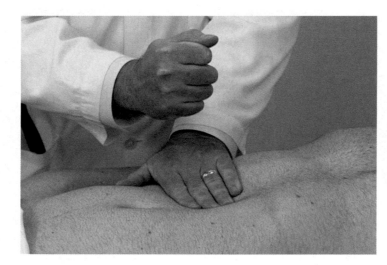

Figure 17–26 Liver tap technique for assessing liver tenderness.

The patient is instructed to take a deep breath as the examiner presses inward with the right hand. The examiner should attempt to feel the tip of the patient's spleen as it descends during inspiration. The tip of an enlarged spleen will lift the fingers of the right hand upward.

The examination of the spleen is repeated with the patient lying on the right side. This maneuver allows gravity to help bring the spleen anterior and downward into a more

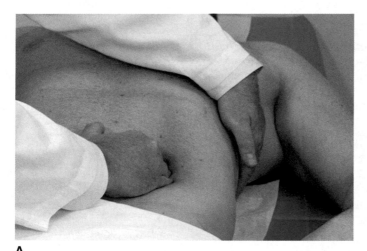

A

Figure 17–27 *A* and *B*, Technique for splenic palpation, with patient lying on the back.

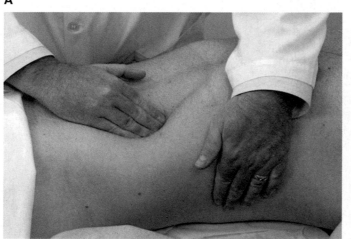

B

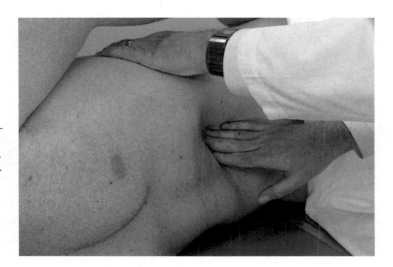

Figure 17–28 Another technique for splenic palpation, with patient lying on right side.

favorable position for palpation. The examiner places his or her left hand on the patient's left costal margin while the right hand palpates in the left upper quadrant. The technique is demonstrated in Figure 17-28.

Because the spleen enlarges diagonally in the abdomen from the left upper quadrant toward the umbilicus, the examiner's right hand should always palpate near the umbilicus and gradually move toward the left upper quadrant. This is particularly important if the spleen is massively enlarged, because starting the palpation too high may cause the examiner to miss the splenic border.

The spleen is not palpable in normal conditions, but both techniques should be used in an attempt to palpate it. Splenic enlargement may result from hyperplasia, congestion, infection, or infiltration by tumor or myeloid elements. Massive splenomegaly in a patient with chronic myelocytic leukemia is pictured in Figure 17-29.

Kidney Palpation

More often than not, neither kidney can be palpated in the adult. The technique, however, is important to know, especially in the evaluation of a newborn.

Palpation of the right kidney is performed by deep palpation below the right costal margin. The examiner stands at the patient's right side and places his or her left hand behind the patient's right flank, between the costal margin and the iliac crest. The right hand is placed just below the patient's costal margin with the tips of the fingers pointing to the examiner's left. The method of kidney palpation is demonstrated in Figure 17-30.

Very deep palpation may reveal the lower pole of the right kidney as it descends during inspiration. The lower pole may be felt as a smooth, rounded mass.

The same procedure is used for the left kidney except that the examiner is on the patient's left side. Because the left kidney is more superior than the right, the lower pole of a normal left

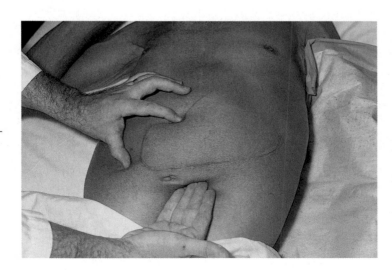

Figure 17–29 Splenomegaly. Note the splenic notch.

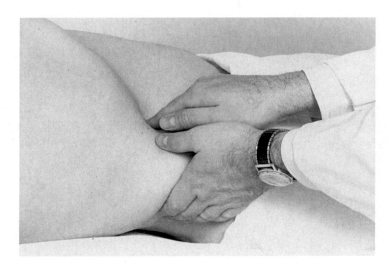

Figure 17–30 Technique for kidney palpation.

kidney is rarely palpable. On occasion, the spleen may be mistaken for an enlarged left kidney. The medial notch of the spleen is helpful in differentiating it from the kidney (see Fig. 17-29).

Rule Out Renal Tenderness

For this part of the examination, the patient should be seated. The examiner should make a fist and *gently* hit the area overlying the costovertebral angle on each side. Figure 17-31 demonstrates the technique. Patients with pyelonephritis usually have extreme pain even on slight percussion in these areas. If pyelonephritis is suspected, only digital pressure should be used. As is described in Chapter 22, Putting the Examination Together, this portion of the abdominal examination is usually performed when the posterior chest is examined.

Rectal Examination

The routine abdominal examination concludes with the digital rectal examination (DRE). Because the anterior rectum has a peritoneal surface, the DRE may reveal tenderness if peritoneal inflammation is present.

The rectal examination for the male patient is discussed here; for the female patient, it is discussed in Chapter 19, Female Genitalia.

Patient Positioning

The examination of the rectum in the male patient may be performed with the patient lying on his back, lying on the left side, or standing and bent over the examination table. The modified lithotomy position (patient on the back with knees flexed) is used when the patient has difficulty standing or when a detailed examination of the anus is not required. The examiner passes

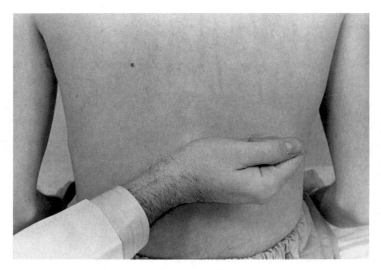

Figure 17–31 Assessing costovertebral angle tenderness (CVAT).

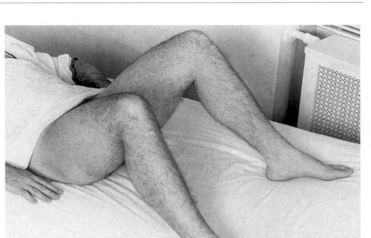

Figure 17–32 Positions for the rectal examination. *A,* Modified lithotomy position. *B,* Sims' position.

A

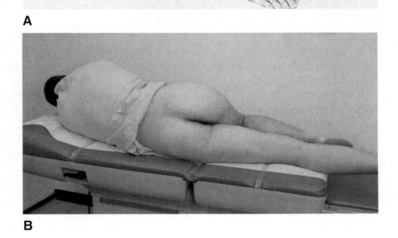

B

the right hand under the patient's right thigh. The index finger in the patient's rectum is used in conjunction with the examiner's left hand, which is placed on the patient's abdomen. This bimanual approach is useful and causes minimal disturbance of the sick patient.

The left lateral prone position, called *Sims' position,* is used commonly in patients who are weak and confined to bed. In this position, the right upper leg should be flexed while the left lower leg is semiextended. The modified lithotomy and left lateral prone positions are pictured in Figure 17-32.

The standing position is the one most commonly used for men and allows for thorough inspection of the anus and palpation of the rectum. The patient is instructed to stand bent over, with shoulders and elbows supported on the bed or examination table. The examiner's gloved right hand is used to examine the anus and the tissue surrounding it while the left hand carefully spreads the buttocks. The examiner should wear gloves on both hands. The anal skin is inspected for signs of inflammation, excoriation, fissures, nodules, fistulas, scars, tumors, and hemorrhoids. Any abnormal areas should be palpated. The patient is asked to strain while the examiner inspects the anus for hemorrhoids or fissures. Figure 17-33 shows prolapsed internal hemorrhoids.

The Technique

The patient is told that a rectal examination will now be performed. The examiner should tell the patient that a lubricant that will feel cool will be used, and this will be followed by the sensation of having to move the bowels; the patient should be assured that he will not do so.

The examiner lubricates the right gloved index finger and places the left hand on the patient's buttocks. As the left hand spreads the patient's buttocks, the examiner's right index finger is gently placed on the anal verge. The sphincter should be relaxed by gentle pressure

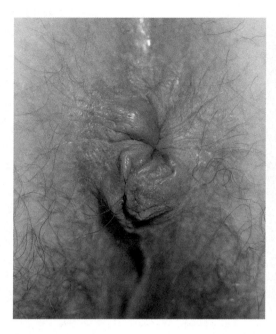

Figure 17–33 Prolapsed internal hemorrhoids.

with the palmar surface of the finger, as shown in Figure 17-34. Figure 17-35*A* illustrates the procedure.

The patient is instructed to take a deep breath, at which time the examiner's right index finger is inserted into the anal canal as the anal sphincter relaxes. The sphincter should close completely around the examining digit. The sphincter tone should be assessed. The finger should be inserted as far as possible into the rectum, although 4 inches (10 cm) is the probable limit of digital exploration. The examiner's left hand can now be moved to the patient's left buttock, while the right index finger examines the rectum. This examination is illustrated in Figure 17-35*B*.

Palpate the Rectal Walls

The lateral, posterior, and anterior walls of the rectum are palpated. To palpate the lateral walls, rotate your digit along the sides of the patient's rectum, as shown in Figure 17-36. The ischial spines, coccyx, and lower sacrum can be felt easily. Palpate the walls for polyps, which may be sessile (attached by a base) or pedunculated (attached by a stalk). Any irregularities or undue tenderness should be noted. The only way to examine the entire circumference of the rectal wall fully is to turn your back to the patient, which will allow you to hyperpronate your hand. Unless you do so, you will be unable to examine the portion of the rectal wall between the 12 o'clock and 3 o'clock positions. A small lesion in this quadrant may go undetected.

Intraperitoneal metastases may be palpated anterior to the rectum. These tumors are hard, and a shelflike structure projects into the rectum as a result of infiltration of Douglas' pouch with neoplastic cells. This is *Blumer's shelf*.

Palpate the Prostate Gland

The prostate gland lies anterior to the wall of the rectum. The size, surface, consistency, sensitivity, and shape of the prostate gland should be assessed.

The prostate is a bilobed, heart-shaped structure approximately 1.5 inches (4 cm) in diameter. It is normally smooth and firm and has the consistency of a hard rubber ball. The apex of the heart shape points toward the anus. Identify the median sulcus and the lateral lobes. Note any masses, tenderness, and nodules. Only the lower apex portion of the gland is palpable. The superior margin is usually too high to reach. The examination of the prostate is illustrated in Figure 17-37. The size of the prostate in relation to the examiner's finger is illustrated in Figure 17-38.

A hard, irregular nodule produces asymmetry of the prostate gland and is suggestive of cancer. Carcinoma of the prostate frequently involves the posterior lobe, which can easily be identified during the DRE. Carcinoma of the prostate is the third leading cause of death in men (9% of all cancer deaths) in the United States. In 2007, there were 218,890 new cases and

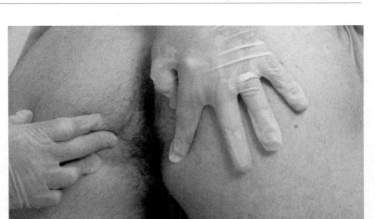

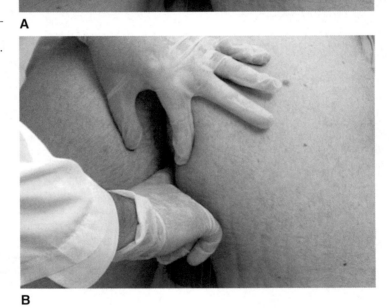

Figure 17–34 Technique of the rectal examination. *A*, Inspection. *B*, Palpation. The examiner's finger is inserted with the palm of the hand facing downward.

27,050 deaths from cancer of the prostate. Early detection is usually limited to detection of an abnormality on DRE.

Benign prostatic hypertrophy produces a symmetrically enlarged, soft gland that protrudes into the rectal lumen. This diffuse enlargement is common among men older than 60 years. A boggy, fluctuant, or tender prostate may indicate acute prostatitis. The seminal vesicles lie superior to the prostate gland and are rarely palpated, unless they are enlarged.

The rectal examination is concluded by informing the patient that you are now going to withdraw your finger. Gently remove the examining finger, and give the patient tissues to wipe himself.

Fecal Occult Blood Test

The examining digit should be inspected. The color of the fecal material should be noted. The fecal material should be placed on the fecal occult blood test (FOBT) card and examined with the Hemoccult developer.

The *guaiac* or *benzidine test* detects occult blood. If blood is present, a chemical reaction results in a blue coloration on the card. The reaction is graded by the intensity of the blue color, from light blue (trace blood) to dark blue (4+ positive).

Although the examination for inguinal hernias is part of the abdominal examination, it is discussed in Chapter 18, Male Genitalia and Hernias.

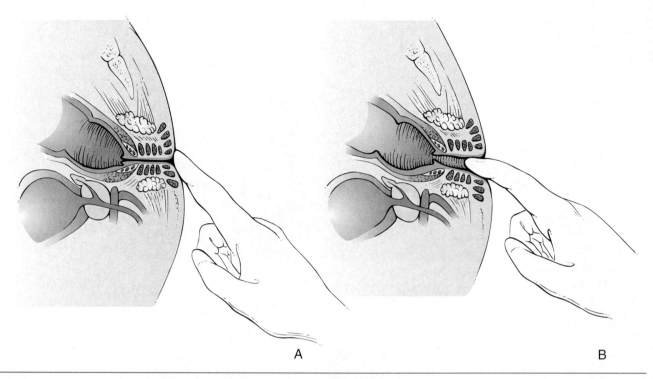

A   B

Figure 17–35 Illustration of the rectal examination. *A,* The sphincter is relaxed by gentle pressure with the palmar surface of the examiner's finger. *B,* With the examiner's left hand spreading the patient's buttocks, examination is carried out with the examiner's right index finger.

Special Techniques

Intra-abdominal inflammation may involve the psoas muscle. A special test performed when there is suspicion of intra-abdominal inflammation is the *iliopsoas test*. The patient is asked to lie on the unaffected side and extend the other leg at the hip against the resistance of the examiner's hand. A *positive psoas sign* is abdominal pain with this maneuver. Irritation of the right psoas muscle by an acutely inflamed appendix produces a right psoas sign. This test is demonstrated in Figure 17-39.

Another useful test for inflammation is the *obturator test*. While the patient is lying on the back, the examiner flexes the patient's thigh at the hip, with the patient's knees bent, and rotates the leg internally and externally at the hip. If there is an inflammatory process adjacent to the obturator muscle, pain is elicited. The obturator test is demonstrated in Figure 17-40.

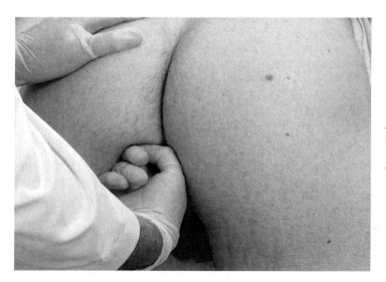

Figure 17–36 Technique for rectal examination. Note position of the examiner's left hand.

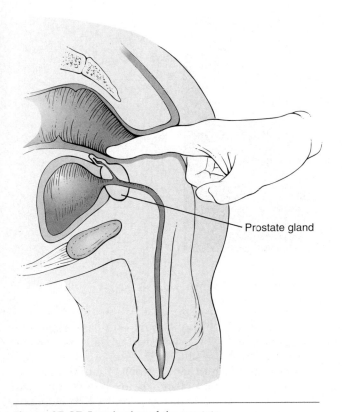

Figure 17–37 Examination of the prostate.

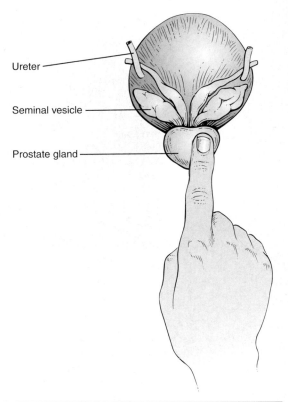

Ureter

Seminal vesicle

Prostate gland

Figure 17–38 Relationship of the size of the prostate gland to the examining finger.

Clinicopathologic Correlations

There is evidence that detecting and removing polyps reduces the incidence of colorectal cancer and that detecting early cancers lowers the mortality rate from colorectal cancer. The American Cancer Society has suggested the following guidelines for the early detection of colorectal cancer in individuals without increased risk. Beginning at age 50 years, men and women should follow one of the following examination schedules:

1. FOBT every year
2. Flexible sigmoidoscopy every 5 years
3. Annual FOBT and flexible sigmoidoscopy every 5 years

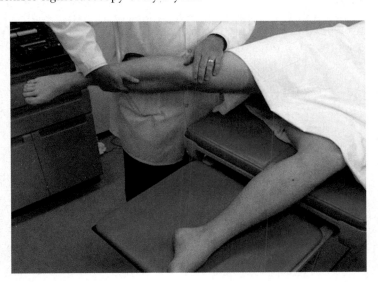

Figure 17–39 The iliopsoas test.

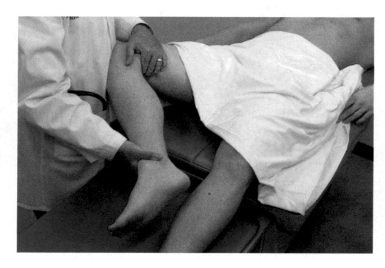

Figure 17–40 The obturator test.

4. Double-contrast barium enema testing every 5 years
5. Colonoscopy every 10 years

The colorectal cancer mortality rate can be reduced 15% to 33% by FOBT and diagnostic evaluation and treatment for positive test results. Annual FOBT screening leads to a greater reduction in the colorectal cancer mortality rate than does biennial screening. Flexible sigmoidoscopy identifies nearly all cancers and polyps greater than 0.4 inch (1 cm) in diameter and 75% to 80% of small polyps that are located in the portion of the bowel examined. Screening with flexible sigmoidoscopy has been shown to result in a 60% to 80% reduction in risk of death from colorectal cancer in the part of the colon examined. There is indirect evidence supporting the use of double-contrast barium enema testing in screening for colorectal cancer. This test can image the entire colon and detect cancers and large polyps. Screening colonoscopy offers the potential both to identify and remove cancers and premalignant lesions throughout the colon and rectum. However, no studies that show a reduction in the mortality rate associated with screening colonoscopy have been completed to date.

Anal cancer is increasing in both men and women worldwide. Men who have sex with men, HIV-positive individuals, transplant recipients, and women with cervical neoplasia have a higher risk for anal cancer than the general population. Men who have sex with men have a 44% greater risk for anal cancer than the general population (Chin-Hong, 2008). Anal cancer, like cervical cancer, is potentially preventalbe. Anal cytology has been studied and found to be a useful screening test to detect anal cancer. It has been shown that a high proportion of men who have sex with men were infected with anal human papillomavirus (HPV) (66%).

Table 17-2 lists the classic locations of pain referred from abdominal structures. Table 17-3 summarizes the maneuvers for ameliorating abdominal pain. Table 17-4 summarizes the sensitivities and specificities of the various maneuvers used to detect ascites. Table 17-5 is a comparison of the clinical manifestations of ulcerative colitis and Crohn's disease. Table 17-6 lists the clinical features of cancer of the stomach, pancreas, and colon. Table 17-7 lists the variation of symptoms in right-sided and left-sided colon cancer and in rectal cancer. Table 17-8

Table 17–5 Clinical Comparison of Ulcerative Colitis and Crohn's Disease

Feature	Ulcerative Colitis	Crohn's Disease
Diarrhea	Present	Present
Hematochezia	Common	Rare
Extraintestinal manifestations	Common	Common
Perirectal disease	Fissures	Fistulas Abscesses
Rectal disease	Present	Absent
Anal disease	Absent	Present

Table 17–6 Clinical Comparison of Cancer of the Stomach, Pancreas, and Colon

Cancer of Stomach	Cancer of Pancreas	Cancer of Colon
Major Symptoms		
Upper abdominal pain	Upper abdominal pain	Change in bowel habits
Occult bleeding	Back pain	Gastrointestinal bleeding
Weight loss	Weight loss	Lower abdominal pain
Vomiting	Jaundice	
Anorexia		
Dysphagia		
Risk Factors		
Adenomatous polyps	Smoking	Adenomatous polyps
Pernicious anemia	Alcoholism (?)	Ulcerative colitis
Family history		Familial polyposis
Immigrants from Japan		Gardner's syndrome
		Villous adenomas

compares the symptoms and signs of cirrhosis, which are numerous, as they relate to hepato-cellular failure and portal hypertension.

Prostate cancer is the leading cancer diagnosed among men in the United States, accounting for 33% of all cancers in men. However, racial/ethnic variations in the Surveillance, Epidemiology, and End Results (SEER) study data are striking: The incidence rate among African-American men (180.6 per 100,000) is more than seven times that among Koreans (24.2 per 100,000). Indeed, African Americans in the United States have the highest rates of this cancer in the world. Although the incidence among white persons is quite high, it is distinctly lower than that among African Americans. Asian and Native American men have the lowest rates. The very low rate in Korean men possibly reflects the fact that most of the Koreans in the SEER areas were recent immigrants from Asia, where rates are lower than in the United States.

Nearly 9 per 10 prostate cancers (86%) are diagnosed at a localized stage, when the 5-year survival rate is 100%. The incidence rates for prostate cancer, however, continue to increase, in part because of increased numbers of screening tests. Prostate cancer can often be found early by a DRE and by testing the amount of prostate-specific antigen (PSA) in a sample of blood. If a man has routine yearly examinations and either one of these test results becomes abnormal, any cancer that he may have has probably been found at an early, more treatable stage. Since the use of these early detection tests for prostate cancer became relatively common around 1990, the death rate from prostate cancer has dropped.

PSA is a substance made by the normal prostate gland. Although PSA is found mostly in semen, a small amount is also present in the blood. Most men have levels under 4 ng/mL of blood. When prostate cancer develops, the PSA level usually goes above 4 ng/mL. If the level is above 4 ng/mL but less than 10 ng/mL, the man has about a 25% chance of having prostate cancer. If it goes above 10 ng/mL, the chance of having prostate cancer is more than 67% and increases as the PSA level increases.

PSA occurs in two major forms in the blood. One is *bound* (attached) to blood proteins and the other circulates *free* (unattached). The *percent-free PSA test* indicates how much PSA circulates free in comparison with the total PSA level. The percentage of free PSA is lower in men

Table 17–7 Variation of Symptoms of Cancer of the Right Colon, Left Colon, and Rectum

Symptom	Cancer of Right Colon	Cancer of Left Colon	Cancer of Rectum
Pain	Ill defined	Colicky*	Steady, gnawing
Obstruction	Infrequent	Common	Infrequent
Bleeding	Brick-red	Red mixed with stool	Bright red coating stool
Weakness†	Common	Infrequent	Infrequent

*Worse with ingestion of foods.
†Secondary to anemia.

Table 17–8 Signs and Symptoms of Cirrhosis

Hepatocellular Failure	*Portal Hypertension*
Spider angiomata	Ascites
Gynecomastia	Varices: esophageal
Palmar erythema	Hemorrhoids
Ascites	Caput medusae
Jaundice	Splenomegaly
Testicular atrophy	
Erectile dysfunction	
Bleeding problems	
Changes in mental function	

who have prostate cancer than in men who do not. If the PSA results are in the borderline range (4 to 10 ng/mL), a low percent-free PSA (< 10%) means that the likelihood of having prostate cancer is about 50%, and a biopsy should be performed.

The PSA level can be affected by many factors. It is increased with noncancerous enlargement of the prostate (i.e., *benign prostatic hypertrophy*), and with *prostatitis*. PSA levels also normally rise slowly with aging. Ejaculation can cause a temporary increase in blood PSA levels, so it is often recommended that men abstain from ejaculation for 2 days before testing.

The American Cancer Society believes that health-care professionals should offer the PSA blood test and DRE yearly, beginning at age 50 years, to men who have at least a 10-year life expectancy. Men at high risk, such as African Americans and men who have a first-degree relative (father, brother, son) in whom prostate cancer was diagnosed at an early age should begin testing at age 45 years. Men at even higher risk (because they have several first-degree relatives who had prostate cancer at an early age) could begin testing at age 40 years. Depending on the results of this initial test, further testing might not be needed until age 45 years.

Useful Vocabulary

Listed here are the specific roots that are important for understanding the terminology related to abdominal disease.

Root	Pertaining to	Example	Definition
aer(o)-	air; gas	**aero**phagia	Air swallowing
celi(o)-	abdomen	**celi**ac	Pertaining to the abdomen
chol(e)-	bile	**chole**lith	Gallstone
cyst-	sac containing liquid	chole**cyst**itis	Inflammation of the gallbladder
enter(o)-	intestines	**enter**itis	Inflammation of the small intestines
gastr(o)-	stomach	**gastr**ectomy	Surgical removal of the stomach
lapar(o)-	loin; flank	**lapar**otomy	Surgical incision through the flank; generally, any abdominal incision
-phago-	eating	**phago**cyte	Any cell that ingests other cells or microorganisms
-tripsy	shock waves	litho**tripsy**	Noninvasive technique for breaking up stones by the use of shock waves

Writing Up the Physical Examination

Listed here are examples of the write-up for the examination of the abdomen.

- The abdomen is scaphoid without scars. Bowel sounds are present. The liver is felt 2 fingerbreadths below the right costal margin for a total span of 10 cm [4 inches]. Neither the spleen nor any masses are felt. The kidneys are not palpable. Rectal examination reveals normal sphincter tone. The prostate is soft, without any masses. The walls of the rectum are smooth, without masses. Results of testing of the stool for blood is negative. No costovertebral angle tenderness [CVAT] is present.

- The abdomen has a scar in the right upper quadrant. Bowel sounds are absent. Marked tympany is present throughout the abdomen. Rigidity is present throughout. Marked tenderness is present in the abdomen, especially in the left lower quadrant. Examination of the rectum reveals tenderness in the same area. Stool guaiac test result is 4+. The liver, spleen, and kidneys are not felt. No CVAT is present.

- The abdomen is obese. Bowel sounds are present. Percussion notes are normal. There is an area of significant pain in the right lower quadrant, immediately above the right midposition of the inguinal ligament. Rectal examination discloses severe pain in the same area. The obturator and straight leg raising signs are positive on the right. Stool guaiac test result is negative. Right CVAT is present. No organomegaly is felt.

- The abdomen is protuberant, with a midline well-healed scar. Bowel sounds are present. Shifting dullness and a fluid wave are present. A large mass 8 × 15 cm [3 × 6 inches] is felt in the right upper quadrant. Results of examination of the rectum are unremarkable except for a trace positive stool guaiac. There is no hepatosplenomegaly.

- The abdomen is scaphoid and soft, without guarding, rigidity, or tenderness. Bowel sounds are present. The liver measures 12 cm [4.7 inches] in span in the midclavicular line. The spleen tip is felt below the left costal margin. No masses are present. Rectal examination reveals a 2-cm [0.75-inch] hard nodule in the posterior lobe of the prostate, which is nontender. Stool guaiac test result is negative.

Bibliography

Alter MJ, Kruszon-Moran D, Nainan OV, et al: The prevalence of hepatitis C virus infection in the United States, 1988 through 1994. N Engl J Med 341:556, 1999.

Barkun AN, Camus M, Green L, et al: The bedside assessment of splenic enlargement. Am J Med 91:512, 1991.

Barkun AN, Camus M, Meagher T, et al: Splenic enlargement and Traube's space: How useful is percussion? Am J Med 87:562, 1989.

Bernstein CN, Blanchard JF, Leslie W, et al: The incidence of fracture among patients with inflammatory bowel disease: A population-based cohort study. Ann Intern Med 133:795, 2000.

Cancer Facts & Figures. Atlanta, American Cancer Society, 2007.

Cancer Trends Progress Report—2007 Update. Bethesda, Md, National Cancer Institute, National Institutes of Health, Department of Health and Human Services, December 2007. Available at: *http://progressreport.cancer.gov*; accessed June 25, 2008.

Carter HB, Ferrucci L, Kettermann A, et al: Detection of life-threatening prostate cancer with prostate-specific antigen velocity during a window of curability. J Natl Cancer Institute 98:1521, 2006.

Castell DO: The spleen percussion sign: A useful diagnostic technique. Ann Intern Med 67:1265, 1967.

Cattau EL Jr, Benjamin SB, Knoff TE, et al: The accuracy of the physical examination in the diagnosis of suspected ascites. JAMA 247:1164, 1982.

Chin-Hong PV, Berry M, Cheng SC, et al: Comparison of patient- and clinician-collected anal cytology samples to screen for human papillamovirus-associated anal intraepithelial neoplasia in men who have sex with men. Ann Intern Med 149:300, 2008.

Cotterchio M, Manno M, Klar N, et al: Colorectal screening is associated with reduced colorectal cancer risk: A case-control study within the population-based Ontario Familial Colorectal Cancer Registry. Cancer Causes Control 16:865, 2005.

Cummings S, Papadakis M, Melnick J, et al: The predictive value of physical examination for ascites. West J Med 142:633, 1985.

Espey DK, Wu XC, Swan J, et al: Annual report to the nation on the status of cancer, 1975–2004, featuring cancer in American Indians and Alaska Natives. Cancer 110:2119, 2007.

Fowler FJ Jr, Barry MJ, Walker-Corkery B, et al: The impact of a suspicious prostate biopsy on patients' psychological, socio-behavioral, and medical care outcomes. J Gen Intern Med 21:715, 2006.

Grover SA, Barkun AN, Sackett DL: Does this patient have splenomegaly? JAMA 270:2218, 1993.

Halpern S, Coel M, Ashburn W, et al: Correlation of liver and spleen size: Determinations by nuclear medicine studies and physical examination. Arch Intern Med 134:123, 1974.

Harris R, Lohr KN: Screening for prostate cancer: An update of the evidence for the U.S. Preventive Services Task Force. Ann Intern Med 137:917, 2002.

Helzer JE, Chammas S, Norland CC, et al: A study of the association between Crohn's disease and psychiatric illness. Gastroenterology 86:324, 1984.

Imperiale TF, Ransohoff DF, Itzkowitz SH, et al: Fecal DNA versus fecal occult blood for colorectal-cancer screening in an average-risk population. N Engl J Med 351:2704, 2004.

Johnson LG, Madeleine MM, Newcomer LM, et al: Anal cancer incidence and survival: the surveillance, epidemiology, and end results experience, 1973-2000. Cancer 101:281, 2004.

Leitzmann MF, Platz EA, Meir J, et al: Ejaculation frequency and subsequent risk of prostate cancer. JAMA 291:1578, 2004.

Levin B, Brooks D, Smith RA, et al: Emerging technologies in screening for colorectal cancer: CT colonography, immunochemical fecal occult blood tests, and stool screening using molecular markers. CA Cancer J Clin 53:44, 2003.

Markowitz SD, Dawson DM, Willis J, et al: Focus on colon cancer. Cancer 1:233, 2002.

Meidl EJ, Ende J: Evaluation of liver size by physical examination. J Gen Intern Med 8:635, 1993.

Naylor CD: Physical examination of the liver. JAMA 271:1859, 1994.

Ries LAG, Melbert D, Krapcho M, et al: SEER Cancer Statistics Review, 1975–2004 [based on November 2006 Surveillance Epidemiology and End Results (SEER) data submission]. Bethesda, Md: National Cancer Institute, 2007. Available at: *http://seer.cancer.gov/csr/1975_2004/*; accessed June 9, 2008.

Robertson DJ, Greenberg ER, Beach M, et al: Colorectal cancer in patients under close colonoscopic surveillance. Gastroenterology 129:34, 2005.

Schiller LR: Chronic diarrhea. Gastroenterology 127:287, 2004.

Seeff L, Shapiro J, Nadel M: Are we doing enough to screen for colorectal cancer? Findings from the 1999 Behavioral Risk Factor Surveillance System. J Fam Pract 51:761, 2003.

Simel DL, Halvorsen RA, Feussner JR: Quantitating bedside diagnosis: Clinical evaluation of ascites. J Gen Intern Med 3:423, 1988.

Smith RA, Cokkinides V, Eyre HJ: American Cancer Society guidelines for the early detection of cancer, 2004. CA Cancer J Clin 54:41, 2004.

Surveillance, Epidemiology, and End Results (SEER) Program: SEER Stat Database: Incidence—SEER 9 Regs Public-Use, November 2002 Sub (1973–2000). Bethesda, Md, National Cancer Institute, DCCPS, Surveillance Research Program, Cancer Statistics Branch. Released April 2003, based on the November 2002 submission. Available at *www.seer.cancer/gov*; accessed June 23, 2008.

Thompson IM, Pauler DK, Goodman PJ, et al: Prevalence of prostate cancer among men with a prostate-specific antigen level < or =4.0 ng per milliliter. New Engl J Med 350:2239, 2004.

Williams JW, Simel DL: Does this patient have ascites? How to divine fluid in the abdomen. JAMA 267:2645, 1992.

CHAPTER 18

Male Genitalia and Hernias

If a man's urine is like the urine of an ass, like beer yeast, like wine yeast or varnish, that man is sick ... and through a bronze tube in the penis pour oil and beer and licorice.

From the Sushruta Samhita (ca. 3000 BCE)

General Considerations

Since the beginning of recorded history, the external genitalia and the urologic system have been of special interest to people. Kidney stones and urologic surgery were well described in antiquity. One of the earliest reported kidney stones was found in a young boy who lived about 7000 BCE.

Circumcision is one of the oldest known surgical procedures in medicine. Male circumcision has been widely practiced as a religious rite since ancient times. An initiatory rite of Judaism, circumcision is also practiced by Muslims, for whom it signifies spiritual purification. Although the origin is unknown, circumcision is often depicted on the walls of temples dating from 3000 BCE. In the Egyptian Book of the Dead, it is written, "The blood falls from the phallus of the Sun God as he starts to incise himself." By the time of the Roman takeover of Egypt in 30 BCE, the practice of circumcision had a ritual significance, and only circumcised priests could perform certain religious rites. The Hindus regarded the penis and testicles as a symbol of the center of life and sacrificed the prepuce as a special offering to the gods.

The Bible has many urologic references. In Genesis 17:7, Abraham makes a covenant with God for the Jews. He is told in Genesis 17:14, "And the uncircumcised male who is not circumcised in the flesh of his foreskin, that soul shall be cut off from his people; he hath broken My covenant." In Leviticus 12:3, the Jews were told, "And in the eighth day the flesh of his foreskin shall be circumcised." Leviticus 15:2-17 deals with discharges that render a man unclean. Today, it is estimated that one in every six men worldwide is circumcised. There are more than 15 million postinfancy circumcisions a year, and thus it is one of the most common surgical procedures.

The Bible, Hindu literature, and Egyptian papyri described a disease now presumed to be gonorrhea. The Mesopotamian tablets described a variety of cures, such as this: "If a man's penis on occasions of his pleasure hurts him, boil beer and milk and anoint him from the pubis." Avicenna's *Canon of Medicine* (1000 CE) was considered the authoritative medical text for centuries and described placing a louse in the penis to counteract a penile discharge.

Gonorrhea was probably first named by Galen in the second century CE. *Gonorrhea* is the Greek translation of "a flow of offspring." Galen apparently thought that the purulent discharge was a leakage of semen. Many terms have been used to describe gonorrhea throughout the years. Perhaps the most common is *clap*, a name used for the past 400 years. It is thought that the term *clap* was derived from a specific area in Paris known for prostitution called "Le Clapier."

It is unclear when the scourge of *syphilis* began. There was much confusion between syphilis and gonorrhea. It was thought that gonorrhea was the first stage of syphilis. The cause of these diseases was also unknown. Many believed that syphilis was caused by floods, eating disguised human meat, or drinking poisoned water. It was not until 1500, when syphilis was pandemic in Europe, that the venereal origins of both diseases were understood. It is now believed that syphilis was introduced on the European continent in 1492 by the returning sailors who had been traveling with Columbus. After France's invasion of Italy and the siege of Naples in 1495, syphilis became rampant throughout Europe. The *King's pox* and the *French pox* were common terms for syphilis.

Benign prostatic hyperplasia (BPH) is the most common benign neoplasm in aging men. It has been estimated that by 60 years of age, the prevalence is greater than 50%, and by 85 years of age, the prevalence approaches 90%. In addition, by 80 years of age, one in every four men require some form of treatment for relief of symptomatic BPH. More than 300,000 surgical procedures are performed in the United States annually for BPH, most commonly a transurethral resection of the prostate (TURP).

Cancer of the genitourinary system is common. In the United States, in 2007, prostate cancer accounted for 33% of all cancer cases in men. It accounted for 9% of all cancer deaths and was the third most common cause of cancer deaths after lung/bronchus cancer (31%) and colon/rectum cancer (10%). In 2007, there were 218,890 new cases of prostate cancer and 27,050 deaths from the disease in the United States, and thus this diagnosis is the most common nondermatologic malignancy to develop in men and the third most common cause of cancer deaths in men.

The highest incidence rate for prostate cancer is in African Americans (54.8 per 100,000); for white persons, it is 23.7 per 100,000. The lowest incidence rate is in Asians and Pacific Islanders (10.7 per 100,000). The lifetime probability for development of prostate cancer is 16.7% (one per six). For a 50-year-old man with a 75-year life expectancy, the lifetime risk for development of microscopic prostate cancer is 42%; the risk for development of clinically evident prostate cancer is 10%; and the risk for development of fatal prostate cancer is 3%. Approximately 95% of all prostate cancers arise from an area of the gland where it can be readily detected by rectal examination.

Cancer of the urinary bladder accounted for an additional 6% of cancer cases but only 3% of all cancer deaths. In 2007, there were 67,160 new cases (50,040 in men, 17,120 in women) of cancer of the urinary bladder in the United States and 13,750 deaths from the disease. Cancer of the urinary bladder is the fourth most common malignancy among men and the eighth most frequent among women. Approximately 260,000 new cases of urinary bladder cancer are diagnosed worldwide every year. The highest incidence rates for bladder cancer are found in industrialized countries such as the United States, Canada, France, Denmark, Italy, and Spain. The lowest rates are in Asia and South America, where the incidence is only about 30% as high as in the United States. Cigarette smoking is an established risk factor for cancer of the urinary bladder. It is estimated that about 50% of these cancers in men and 30% in women are linked to smoking. Occupational exposures may account for up to 25% of all urinary bladder cancers. Most of the occupationally accrued risk is attributable to exposure to a group of chemicals known as *arylamines*. Occupations with high exposure to arylamines include dye workers, rubber workers, leather workers, truck drivers, painters, and aluminum workers. In recent decades, there has been a steady increase in the incidence of bladder cancer. However, health-care workers are making progress in treatment, and the survival rates are improving.

Although testicular cancer accounts for only 1% of all cancers in men, testicular carcinoma is the most common cancer in men in the 15- to 35-year-old age group. There were 7,920 new testicular cancer cases in 2007 and 380 related deaths. Testicular cancer is four times less common in African-American men than in white men. The risk for development of testicular cancer in a man's lifetime is approximately 1 per 500. Approximately 90% of all testicular tumors manifest as an asymptomatic testicular mass. Once these tumors are detected and treatment is begun, the cure rate can approach 90%, even when the tumor has spread beyond the testicle. Many patients have oligospermia or sperm abnormalities before therapy. Virtually all become oligospermic during chemotherapy with platinum-based agents. Many recover sperm production, however, and can father children, often without the use of cryo-preserved semen. In a population-based study, 70% of patients actually fathered children. Men in whom testicular cancer has been cured have approximately a 2% to 5% cumulative risk of developing a cancer in the opposite testicle during the 25 years after initial diagnosis. The most important prognostic factor has been shown to be early detection by routine physical examination and self-examination. All men should be instructed in testicular self-examination.

Erectile dysfunction (ED) is an extremely common problem. It has been estimated that more than 30 million American men have some degree of ED and that nearly a million new cases can be expected to develop annually. Studies have shown that ED affects not only a man's physical and sexual satisfaction but also his general quality of life, with especially strong links to depression. In the Massachusetts Male Aging Study, 52% of men from 40 to 70 years of age had some degree of ED. Seventeen percent reported minimal dysfunction, 25% reported moderate dysfunction, and 10% reported complete dysfunction. This study also revealed the progressive nature of ED with increasing age. At 40 years of age, 5% of the American male population has complete ED, and at 70 years of age, 15% of the population has complete ED. Sixty-seven percent of men 70 years of age have some degree of ED. As the population continues to age, clinicians will treat more and more male patients for ED in the future.

Structure and Physiology

Cross-sectional and frontal views of the male genitalia are shown in Figure 18-1.

The *penis* is composed of three elongated, distensible structures: two paired *corpora cavernosa* and a single *corpus spongiosum*. The urethra runs through the corpus spongiosum. The penis has

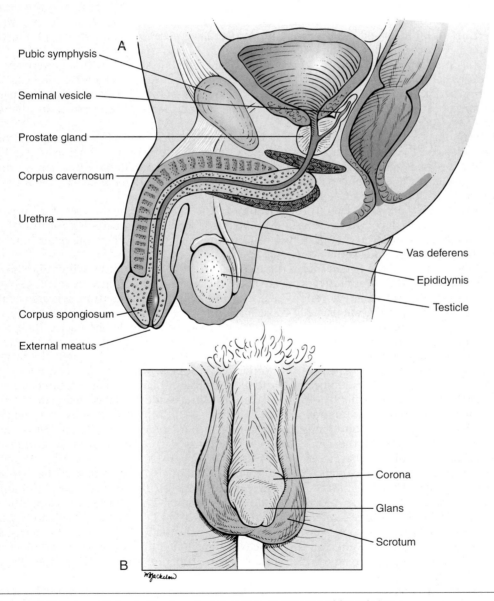

Figure 18–1 Male genitalia. *A,* Diagram of cross section. *B,* Diagram of frontal view.

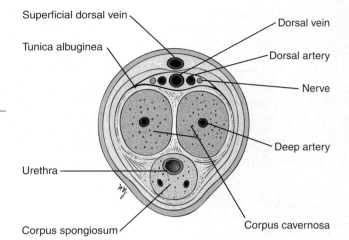

Figure 18–2 Cross-sectional view through the penis.

two surfaces, dorsal and ventral (urethral), and consists of the root, the shaft, and the head. The shaft is composed of erectile tissue that, when engorged with blood, produces a firm erection necessary for sexual intercourse. The corpora cavernosa also contain smooth muscle that contracts rhythmically during ejaculation.

On the dorsal aspect of the penis in the midline runs the dorsal vein, with an artery and a nerve on either side. The distal end of the corpus spongiosum expands to form the head, or *glans penis*. The glans penis covers the end of the corpora cavernosa. The glans has a prominent margin on its dorsal aspect, the *corona*. A slitlike opening on the tip of the glans is the *external meatus* of the urethra.

The skin of the penis is smooth, thin, and hairless. At the distal end of the penis, a free fold of skin called the *prepuce* (foreskin) covers the glans. Secreted mucus and sloughed epithelial cells called *smegma* collect between the prepuce and the glans, providing a lubricant during sexual intercourse. The prepuce can be retracted to expose the glans as far as the corona. During circumcision, the prepuce is removed.

The root of the penis lies deep to the scrotum, in the perineum. At the root, the corpora cavernosa diverge. Each corpus cavernosum is enveloped in a dense, fibroelastic covering called the *tunica albuginea*, and these tunicae fuse to form the median septum of the penis. A cross section through the penis is shown in Figure 18-2.

The blood supply to the penis is from the internal pudendal artery, from which the dorsal and deep arteries of the corpora cavernosa are derived. The veins drain into the dorsal vein of the penis. In the flaccid state, the venous channels and arteriovenous anastomoses are widely patent, whereas the arteries are partially constricted.

Erection is a complex hemodynamic and neurophysiologic event. In the flaccid state, the smooth muscles of the penile arteries and sinusoid spaces are contracted. The erectile state begins in the brain and requires relaxation of the smooth muscles of the penis. From the brain center, neural signals are sent to the corpora cavernosa, where synthesis and release of the neurotransmitter nitric oxide occur. Nitric oxide is the primary mediator responsible for endothelial and cavernous smooth muscle relaxation. Nitric oxide activates guanylate cyclase to produce cyclic guanosine monophosphate (cyclic GMP), which decreases intracellular calcium levels, allowing smooth muscle relaxation and an increase in arterial inflow and corporal veno-occlusion in the penis. Venous outflow is decreased because distention of the blood-filled sinusoidal spaces compresses the veins against the inner layer of the rigid tunica albuginea. In the erect state, the arteriovenous channels are closed, and the arteries are widely opened. Muscular pillars are present in the walls of the arteries, veins, and arteriovenous anastomoses, which aid in occluding the lumina. Phosphodiesterase, predominantly type V in penile tissue, catalyzes the conversion of cyclic GMP to GMP and results in detumescence. There are some new medications that selectively inhibit phosphodiesterase V. These agents enhance the effect of the nitric oxide–mediated increase in cyclic GMP levels and significantly improve erectile function and sexual function in men. The anatomy of erection is illustrated in Figure 18-3.

The *urethra* extends from the internal urinary meatus of the bladder to the external meatus of the penis. The urethra can be divided into three portions: the prostatic (posterior) portion,

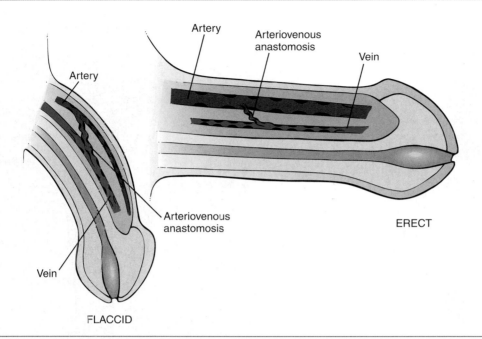

Figure 18–3 Anatomy of erection.

the membranous portion, and the cavernous (anterior) portion. The short posterior portion passes through the prostate gland. The common ejaculatory duct and several prostatic ducts enter at the distal end of this portion. The external urethral sphincter surrounds the membranous urethra, and on either side lie Cowper's bulbourethral glands. The anterior urethra is the longest portion and passes through the corpus spongiosum. The ducts of Cowper's glands enter the anterior urethra near its proximal end.

The *scrotum* is the pouch containing the testes; it is suspended externally from the perineum. The scrotum is divided into halves by the intrascrotal septum, one testis lying on each side. The wall of the scrotum contains involuntary smooth muscle and voluntary striated muscle. A major role of the scrotum is temperature regulation of the testes. The testes are maintained about 2° C lower than the temperature of the peritoneal cavity, a condition necessary for spermatogenesis. The size of the scrotum is variable according to the individual and his response to ambient temperature. During exposure to cold temperatures, the scrotum is contracted and very rugate. In a warm environment, the scrotum becomes pendulous and smoother.

The *testes*, or *testicles*, are ovoid, smooth, and approximately 1.5 to 2 inches (3.5 to 5 cm) in length. The left testicle commonly lies lower than the right. The testes are covered with a tough fibrous coat called the *tunica albuginea testis*. Each testicle has a long axis directed slightly anteriorly and upward and contains long, microscopic, convoluted seminiferous tubules that produce sperm. The tubules end in the *epididymis*, which is comma-shaped and located on the posterior border of the testis. It consists of a head that is swollen and overhangs the upper pole of the testicle. The inferior portion, or tail, of the epididymis continues into the *vas deferens*. The testicular artery enters the testicle in its posterior midportion. The veins draining the testicle form a dense network called the *pampiniform plexus*, which drains into the testicular vein. The right testicular vein drains directly into the inferior vena cava, whereas the left drains into the left renal vein. The lymphatic drainage of the testes is to the preaortic and precaval nodes, not to the inguinal nodes. This is important to recognize because the testes are embryologically intra-abdominal organs, and neoplasms and inflammations of the testis produce adenopathy of these nodal chains. In general, inguinal adenopathy is rare.

The relationship of the testicle and epididymis is illustrated in Figure 18-4.

The vas deferens is a cordlike structure, easily felt in the scrotum. The vas deferens, testicular arteries, and veins form the *spermatic cord*, which enters the inguinal canal. The vas deferens passes through the internal ring and, after a convoluted course, reaches the fundus of the bladder. It passes between the rectum and the bladder and approaches the vas deferens

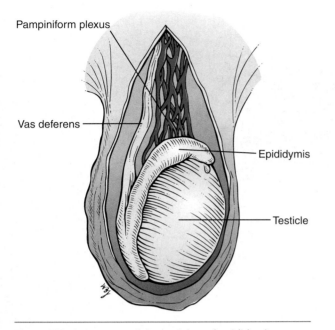

Figure 18–4 Anatomy of the testicle and epididymis.

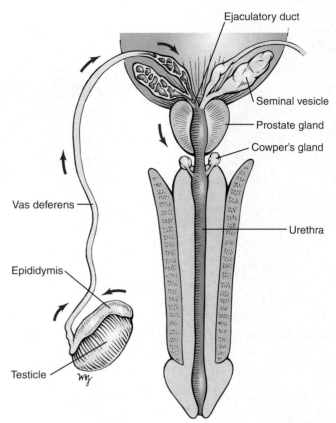

Figure 18–5 Sources and direction of seminal fluid flow.

of the opposite side near the seminal vesicles. Near the base of the prostate, the vas deferens joins with the duct of the corresponding seminal vesicle to form the *ejaculatory duct*, which passes through the prostate gland to enter the posterior urethra.

The *prostate gland* is about the size of two almonds, or approximately 1.5 inches (3.5 cm) long by 1.2 inches (3 cm) wide. Traversing the gland in the midline is the posterior urethra. On either side is an ejaculatory duct. The prostate is commonly divided into five lobes. The posterior lobe is clinically important because prostate carcinoma frequently affects this lobe. In the presence of cancer, the midline groove between the two lateral lobes may be obliterated. The middle and lateral lobes are above the ejaculatory ducts and are typically involved in benign hypertrophy. The anterior lobe is of little clinical importance.

The sources and direction of seminal fluid flow in the male genitalia are illustrated in Figure 18-5.

The descent of the testes is important to review at this time. In the normal full-term male newborn, both testes are in the scrotum at birth. The testes descend to this position just before birth. About the 12th week of gestation, the *gubernaculum* develops in the inguinal fold and grows through the body wall to an area that will ultimately lie in the scrotum. This tract marks the location of the future inguinal canal. A dimple called the *processus vaginalis* forms in the peritoneum and follows the course of the gubernaculum. By the 7th month of gestation, the processus vaginalis has reached the aponeurosis of the external oblique muscle. Each testis then begins its descent from the abdominal cavity through the internal ring to lie in the abdominal wall. During the 8th month, the testes descend along the inguinal canal; at birth, they are in the scrotum. At birth, the gubernaculum is barely distinguishable, and the processus vaginalis becomes obliterated within the spermatic cord. In about 5% of male infants, there is imperfect descent of the testis (*cryptorchidism*). The descent of the testes is illustrated in Figure 18-6.

The genital development stages for boys are illustrated in Figure 24-44 (and discussed in Chapter 24, The Pediatric Patient).

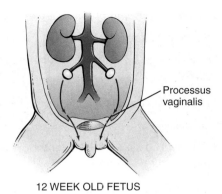

12 WEEK OLD FETUS

Figure 18–6 Descent of the testes.

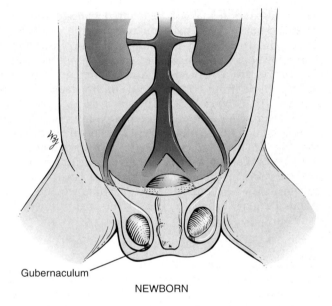

NEWBORN

Review of Specific Symptoms

The most common symptoms of male genitourinary disease are as follows:

- Pain
- Dysuria
- Changes in urine flow
- Red urine
- Penile discharge
- Penile lesions
- Genital rashes
- Scrotal enlargement
- Groin mass or swelling
- Erectile dysfunction
- Infertility

Pain

Sudden distention of the ureter, renal pelvis, or bladder may cause flank pain. Any patient with flank pain should be asked the following questions:

"When did the pain begin?"

"Where did the pain begin? Can you point to the area?"

"Do you feel the pain in any other area of your body?"

"Did the pain start suddenly?"

"Have you ever had this type of pain before?"

"Is the pain constant?"

"What seems to make the pain worse? less?"

"Has the color of your urine changed?"

"Is the pain associated with nausea? vomiting? abdominal distention? fever? chills? burning sensation on urination?"

Gradual enlargement of an organ is usually painless. An aching pain in the costovertebral angle may be related to sudden distention of the renal capsule, which results from acute pyelonephritis or obstructive hydronephrosis. The spasmodic, colicky pain from upper ureteral dilatation may cause referred pain to the testis on the same side. Lower ureteral dilatation may cause pain referred to the scrotum. The pain of ureteral distention is severe, and the patient is restless and uncomfortable in any position. Bladder distention causes lower abdominal fullness and suprapubic pain, with an intense desire to urinate. Pain in the groin may result from pathologic processes in the spermatic cord, testicle, or prostate gland; from lymphadenitis of any cause; from hernia; from herpes zoster; or from a disorder that is neurologic in origin.

Testicular pain can result from nearly any disease of the testis or epididymis. Such diseases include epididymitis, orchitis, hydrocele, spermatic cord torsion, and tumor. Referred pain from the ipsilateral ureter must always be considered. *Priapism* is a painful, persistent erection of the penis that is not a result of sexual excitation. The sustained erection results from thrombosis of veins in the corpora cavernosa. This occurs in patients with sickle cell anemia or leukemia. The exact mechanism is unknown, but it appears to result from a blockage of venous drainage from the penis while the arteries remain patent. Chronic priapism often results in organic ED.

Dysuria

Pain on urination, called *dysuria*, is frequently described as "burning." Dysuria is evidence of inflammation of the lower urinary tract. The patient may describe discomfort in the penis or in the suprapubic area. Dysuria also implies difficulty in urination. This may result from external meatal stenosis or from a urethral stricture. Painful urination is usually associated with urinary frequency and urgency. When the patient describes pain or difficulty in urination, ask the following questions:

"How long have you noticed a burning sensation on urination?"

"How often do you urinate each day?"

"How does your urination feel different?"

"Is your urine clear?"

"Does the urine smell bad?"

"Do you have a discharge from your penis?"

"Does the urine seem to have gas bubbles in it?"

"Have you noticed any solid particles in your urine?"

"Have you noticed pus in your urine?"

Pneumaturia is the passage of air in the urine, producing what the patient describes as "bubbles of gas" in the urine. The air or gas is usually emitted at the end of urination. Normally, there is no gas in the urinary tract. The symptom of pneumaturia indicates the introduction of air by instrumentation, a fistula to the bowel, or a urinary tract infection by gas-forming bacteria, such as *Escherichia coli* or clostridia.

Fecaluria is the presence of fecal material in the urine and is rare. The passage of feculent-smelling material results from either an intestinovesicular fistula or a urethrorectal fistula.

These fistulas occur as a consequence of ulceration from the bowel to the urinary tract. Diverticulitis, carcinoma, and Crohn's disease are frequent causes.

Pus in the urine, or *pyuria*, is the body's response to inflammation of the urinary tract. Bacteria are the most common cause of inflammation resulting in pyuria, although pyuria is also seen in patients with neoplasms and kidney stones. Cystitis and prostatitis are common causes of pyuria.

Changes in Urine Flow

Changes in urine flow include frequency and incontinence. Urinary frequency is the most common symptom of the genitourologic system. *Frequency* is defined as passing urine more often than normal. *Nocturia* is urinary frequency at night. There are several causes of frequency: decreased bladder size, bladder wall irritation, and increased urine volume. If an obstructed bladder cannot be completely emptied at each voiding, its effective capacity is diminished. The following questions, in addition to the ones pertaining to dysuria, should be asked to help define the problem.

"Do you find that you must wake up at night to urinate?"

"Can you estimate the amount of urine passed each time you urinate?"

"Do you have sudden urges to urinate?"

"Have you found that despite an urge to urinate, you cannot start the stream?"

"Has there been a change in the caliber of the stream?"

"Have you found that you must wait longer for the stream to start?"

"Do you have the sensation that after urination has stopped, you still have to urinate?"

"Do you have to strain at the end of urination?"

"Have you been drinking more fluids recently?"

Prostatic hyperplasia is the most common cause of reduced usable bladder capacity in men. Symptoms include frequency of urination, nocturia, urgency, weak stream, intermittent stream, and a sensation of incomplete emptying. Long-standing prostatic hypertrophy can lead to a complete inability to urinate, necessitating catheterization (a condition known as urinary retention); to urinary tract infections; or to bladder stones. Most bladder diseases, such as cystitis, cause frequency as a result of irritation of the bladder mucosa. *Polyuria*, or voiding large amounts of urine, is usually accompanied by excessive thirst, or *polydipsia*. Diabetes mellitus and diabetes insipidus are common causes of polydipsia.

Urinary *incontinence* is the inability to retain urine voluntarily. The urge to urinate may be so intense that incontinence may result. In addition to the questions regarding dysuria and frequency, ask the following:

"Do you involuntarily lose small amounts of urine?"

"Do you lose your urine constantly?"

"Do you lose your urine when lifting heavy objects? laughing? coughing? bending over?"

"Do you have to press on your abdomen to urinate?"

In patients with chronically distended bladders, as in those with prostatic hypertrophy, there is always a large amount of residual urine. The pressure within the bladder is constantly elevated. A slight increase in intra-abdominal pressure raises the intravesicular pressure sufficiently to overcome bladder neck resistance, and urine escapes. Leakage may be steady or intermittent. This type of incontinence is *overflow* incontinence. *Stress* incontinence is leakage that occurs only when the patient strains. The primary defect is a loss of muscular support in the urethrovesicular region. Residual urine is insignificant. Any increase in intra-abdominal pressure causes leakage. This type of incontinence is more common in women and is discussed in Chapter 19, Female Genitalia.

Polyuria is the production of increased amounts of urine, frequently greater than 2 to 3 L/day. The normal daily urine output varies from 1 to 2 L/day. The most important diseases to differentiate are diabetes mellitus, diabetes insipidus, and psychologic diabetes insipidus. Ask the following questions:

"How long have you been passing large amounts of urine?"

"Was the onset sudden?"

"How often do you have to urinate at night?"

"Is there any variability in the urine flow from day to day?"

"Do you have excessive thirst?"

"Do you prefer water or other fluids?"

"What happens if you don't drink? Will you still have to urinate?"

"How is your appetite?"

"Do you have any visual problems? headaches?"

"Are you aware of any emotional problems?"

Patients with diabetes mellitus have a high osmotic load and have polyuria. Increased appetite is also common. Diabetes insipidus is caused by a vasopressin deficiency related to a lesion in the hypothalamus or pituitary gland. In these patients, the urine cannot become concentrated despite a rise in plasma osmolality. Patients with psychogenic diabetes insipidus, which is more common, have polyuria related to compulsive drinking of water. It is seen in patients with psychologic problems. The onset of polyuria is abrupt in patients with psychogenic diabetes insipidus, and they have no preference for the type of fluid they drink. In contrast, patients with true diabetes insipidus prefer water. Because true diabetes insipidus is related to intracranial lesions, it is not surprising that affected individuals suffer from headaches and visual disturbances, especially visual field abnormalities.

Red Urine

Red urine is often indicative of *hematuria*, or blood in the urine. However, there are many causes of red urine, and it should not automatically be assumed that red urine indicates bleeding. Vegetable dyes, drugs such as phenazopyridine (Pyridium), and excessive ingestion of beets can cause red urine. When it is determined that the urine is red as a result of the presence of blood, the hematuria is termed *gross hematuria*. Hematuria may be the first symptom of serious disease of the urinary tract. Ask the following questions of any patient with the symptom of red urine:

"How long have you noticed red urine?"

"Have you had red urine previously?"

"Have you noticed that the urine starts red and then clears? starts clear and then turns red? is red throughout?"

"Have you noticed clots of blood in the urine?"

"Have you done any severely strenuous physical activity recently, such as prolonged hiking, running, or marching?"

"Did you have an upper respiratory infection or a sore throat a few weeks ago?"

"Is the red urine associated with flank pain? abdominal pain? burning sensation on urination? fever? weight loss?"

"Are you aware of any bleeding problems?"

"Are you taking any medications?"

"Do you eat beets often?"

Individuals who participate in strenuous activities may traumatize blood cells as these cells travel through the small vessels in the feet. A condition called *march hemoglobinuria* may result,

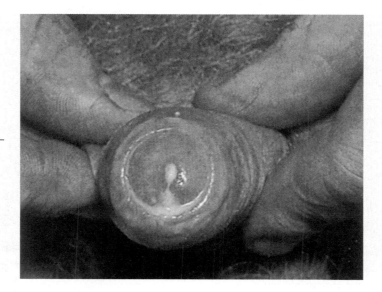

Figure 18–7 Purulent penile discharge of gonorrhea.

causing intravascular hemolysis and hemoglobinuria. The temporal relationship of blood in the urine is an important factor. Blood only at the beginning, or *initial* hematuria, usually has a source in the urethra. Blood only at the end of urination, or *terminal* hematuria, indicates a disorder at the bladder neck or the posterior urethra. Blood evenly distributed throughout urination is *total* hematuria and implies disease above the prostate gland or a massive hemorrhage at any level. Blood staining of undergarments without blood in the urine indicates pathologic processes in the external urethral meatus. Weight loss and hematuria are seen in renal cell carcinoma. Red urine that occurs 10 to 14 days after an upper respiratory infection may indicate acute glomerulonephritis.

Penile Discharge

Discharge from the penis is a continuous or intermittent flow of fluid from the urethra. Ask the patient whether he has ever had a discharge and, if he has, whether it was bloody or purulent. Bloody penile discharges are associated with ulcerations, neoplasms, or urethritis. Purulent discharges are thick and yellowish-green and may be associated with gonococcal urethritis or chronic prostatitis. Determine when the discharge was first noted. Figure 18-7 shows a purulent penile discharge in a man with gonococcal urethritis. Gonorrhea is caused by *Neisseria gonorrhoeae*. After exposure, approximately 25% of men and more than 50% of women contract the disease. In men, the acute symptoms of dysuria and a purulent urethral discharge begin 2 to 10 days after exposure. In women, a vaginal discharge and dysuria develop days to weeks after exposure; however, in up to 50% of women, the infection may be asymptomatic.

Tactful direct questioning about any history of or exposure to sexually transmitted diseases is essential. The interviewer should determine the patient's sexual orientation and the type of sexual exposure—oral, vaginal, or anal—because this information can help determine the types of bacteriologic cultures necessary. It is appropriate to ask whether the patient has more than one sexual partner and whether the partner or partners have any known illnesses. The sexual history questions suggested in Chapter 1, The Interviewer's Questions, may be helpful.

Penile Lesions

A history of lesions on the penis should alert the examiner to the possibility of venereal disease. Ask the patient whether he has had gonorrhea, syphilis, herpes, trichomoniasis, venereal warts, or other sexually transmitted diseases.

Genital Rashes

Male genital rashes are very common. They may be confusing to identify and are often difficult to treat. Some rashes may occur exclusively on the genitalia; others, which are typically found on other parts of the body, have an atypical appearance when present on the genitalia. The skin over the genitalia is thin and moist, so typical dry scaliness may not be present.

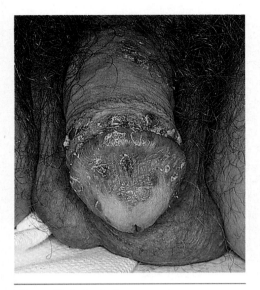

Figure 18–8 Psoriasis.

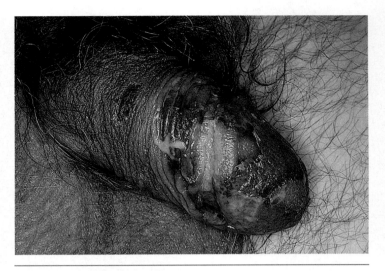

Figure 18–9 Fixed drug reaction.

The most common inflammatory reaction affecting the male genitalia is *psoriasis*. The patient develops bright red, well-defined, scaling plaques. Often the entire scrotum, inguinal folds, and penis are involved. Figure 18-8 shows psoriasis of the penis.

Another form of genital rash is *contact dermatitis*. It may develop from soaps or disinfectants. Irritants used for facial actinic keratoses may inadvertently be transferred to the genitalia. Itching is a major symptom.

Fixed drug eruptions are unique reactions that appear in the same area of the body each time the responsible drug is given. Fixed drug reactions manifest as a sudden onset of multiple, well-defined, macular, eczematous, bullous patches. When the genitalia are involved, these eruptions typically occur on the distal penis and glans and may be very painful. Antibiotics and laxatives containing phenolphthalein may cause such rashes. Figure 18-9 shows a fixed drug reaction. More than 500 medications have been implicated in fixed drug reactions; therefore, the examiner should take a careful medication history.

Lichen planus is an inflammatory disorder characterized by violaceous, flat, shiny papules ranging from 0.75 to 3 inches (2 to 8 mm) in diameter. The glans penis is frequently involved. An oral examination may reveal the classic serpiginous white streaks on the buccal mucosa (see Fig. 12-15). Figure 18-10 shows lichen planus of the penis (see also Fig. 8-99).

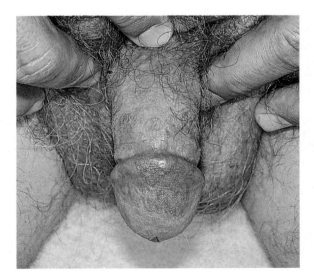

Figure 18–10 Lichen planus.

Scrotal Enlargement

It is not uncommon for a man to complain of enlargement of his scrotum, but it is often difficult for him to determine which anatomic structures in the scrotum are enlarged. Ask these questions:

"When did you first notice the enlargement?"

"Is the enlargement painful?"

"Have you sustained any injury to your groin?"

"Does the enlargement change in size?"

"Have you ever had the enlargement before?"

"Have you ever had a hernia?"

"Have you had any problems with fertility?"

Swellings in the scrotum can be related to testicular or epididymal enlargement, a hernia, a varicocele, a spermatocele, or a hydrocele. Testicular enlargement can result from inflammation or tumor. Most of the time, enlargement is unilateral. Painful scrotal enlargement can result from acute inflammation of the epididymis or testis, torsion of the spermatic cord, or a strangulated hernia. Varicoceles are often a cause of decreased fertility.

Groin Mass or Swelling

If a patient describes a mass in the groin, ask the following questions:

"When did you first notice the mass?"

"Is the mass painful?"

"Does the mass change in size with different positions?"

"Have you had any venereal diseases?"

The most common cause of swelling in the groin is a hernia. Hernias are reduced in size after the patient has been lying down. Adenopathy from any infection of the external genitalia may produce inguinal swelling. Carcinoma of the testis produces inguinal node enlargement only if the scrotal skin is involved.

Erectile Dysfunction

Erectile dysfunction (ED), or impotence, is defined as the persistent inability to achieve or maintain a penile erection sufficient for satisfactory sexual performance. The typical patient is at least 50 years old, is usually married or in a long-term monogamous relationship, and has had a year or more of gradually progressive ED. Often he is otherwise in good mental and physical health. Because penile erection is a neurovascular phenomenon, however, there are a number of neurologic and vascular conditions that can lead to ED. Vascular disease such as atherosclerotic stenosis or occlusion of the cavernosal arteries, or vascular problems secondary to smoking, can cause ED. Antihypertensives, antidepressants, antiandrogens, histamine type 2 (H_2) receptor blockers, and recreational drugs are commonly associated with ED. Diabetes, hypertension, hyperlipidemia, and alcohol use are risk factors in ED. ED frequently provides insight into the patient's emotional problems.

A delicate approach must be taken. It is necessary to use tact and appropriate language that will be understood by the patient. Explaining that ED is a common problem often sets the tone. Deep-seated problems necessitate careful questioning. The interviewer may discover latent homosexuality; guilt and taboos experienced early in life may have left a lasting impression, affecting sexual performance. It is most important to classify the origin of the ED, because there are specific therapies for different causes.

Start by asking some of the following questions:

"If you were to spend the rest of your life with your sexual function just the way it is now, how would you feel about that?"

"Are you satisfied with your sexual function?" If not, *"What are the reasons?"*

"What is your relationship status? Is it a happy one?"

"Is your partner satisfied with your sexual function?" If not, *"What are the reasons?"*

"When was the last time you had a satisfactory erection?"

"Over the last 4 weeks, how would you rate your confidence that you could get and keep an erection?"

"When you had erections with sexual stimulation, how often were your erections hard enough for penetration (entering your partner)?"

"During sexual intercourse, how often were you able to maintain your erection after you had penetrated (entered) your partner?"

"During sexual intercourse, how difficult was it to maintain your erection to completion of intercourse?"

A careful history is the most essential component in the evaluation of ED. Key and direct questions are important:

"How much do/did you enjoy sexual intercourse?"

"When you have sexual stimulation or intercourse, how often do you ejaculate?"

"How easily can you reach an orgasm (climax)?"

"How strong is your sex drive?"

"How easily are you sexually aroused?"

"Are your orgasms satisfying?"

Some other questions may help determine the cause of ED. Psychogenic causes for ED should be suspected in men who have a history of unusual anxiety, stress, or sexual abuse or in those with ethnic, cultural, sexual, or religious inhibitions. ED is often psychogenic in men younger than 40 years. Ask the following questions:

"Do you have early morning erections or nighttime emissions?"

"Do any individuals other than your partner arouse you?"

"Are you able to masturbate to an erection or climax?"

An affirmative answer to any of these questions reassures the interviewer that the ED is probably psychologic in origin. Letting the patient discuss his problems may allow him to vent some of his anxieties, but the patient's confidence must first be secured by guaranteeing confidentiality. The interviewer must also resolve his or her own sexual anxieties in order to have a confident and straightforward discussion. An open dialogue about the anxieties surrounding sexual intercourse may be productive. The interviewer must be careful not to impose his or her own moral standards on the patient, however. Improving communication between partners is also helpful.

Infertility

Infertility is the inability to conceive or to cause pregnancy. Infertility is a common problem found in as many as 10% of all marriages. A couple is said to be infertile when after 1 year of normal intercourse without the use of contraceptives, pregnancy does not occur. It has been estimated that almost 30% of all infertility is attributable to a male factor. Any patient with a history of infertility should be questioned regarding a history of mumps, testicular injury, venereal disease, history of diabetes, history of a varicocele (see Fig. 18-27), exposure to radiation, or any urologic surgical procedure. Diabetic men may be infertile because of retrograde ejaculation, or ejaculation into the urinary bladder. Determine the frequency of sexual intercourse and any difficulty in achieving or maintaining an erection. Document a careful history of general work habits, medications taken, alcohol consumption, and sleeping habits.

Impact of Erectile Dysfunction on the Patient

ED is the inability of a man to achieve or maintain an erection sufficient to accomplish coitus. ED may be either erectile or ejaculatory. This inability may also be partial or complete. Men may complain of difficulty in achieving or maintaining an erection or of premature ejaculation. The prevalence of some degree of ED ranges from 20% to 30% of the married population. As a man ages, there is a natural loss of both libido and potency. In general, this does not occur before 50 years of age. Some men remain sexually vigorous well into old age. If a patient suffering from ED has occasional erections or can achieve orgasm during masturbation, he may have a primarily emotional problem. In almost 90% of patients complaining of ED, the inadequacy is found to be caused by emotional rather than anatomic factors.

Hearing about a friend's sexual activities, especially if they are exaggerated, can deflate a patient's ego and heighten his sense of inadequacy. The cultural environment of the patient must set the standard for adequacy. It is almost impossible to compare Western and Eastern cultural patterns. In 1948, Alfred Kinsey and his colleagues obtained factual data on Anglo-American sexual patterns. The frequency of sexual intercourse varied from one to four times per week. The period of maximum sexual activity was from 20 to 30 years of age. It was shown that there were marked variations among individuals as well as among socioeconomic groups. The lower the socioeconomic group was, the more frequent were the sexual encounters.

Boredom, anxiety, peer pressure, aging, deterioration of the stereotypical male role, and female "aggressiveness" are factors contributing to psychogenic ED. Diabetes mellitus is one of the more common causes of organic ED. Patients with multiple sclerosis, spinal cord tumors, degenerative diseases of the spinal cord, and local injuries suffer from a gradual loss of potency. Certain medications can cause ED: beta blockers, carbonic anhydrase inhibitors, and antihypertensive agents, for example.

Guilt, anxiety, and hypochondriasis are common in men with psychogenic ED. Sexual indifference in a woman may make the man feel more insecure in his own marital adjustment, worsening his ED. The man's self-image may be poor. It is common for a man with marginal difficulties to worry incessantly about his next attempt at coitus. His fear of failure generates enormous anxiety, which reinforces his inadequacy, and a vicious circle is begun. Each failure worsens the next attempt. If the act of coitus is not satisfactory to the patient or his partner, embarrassment and guilt develop.

Some men may be able to maintain erections but have difficulty in ejaculation. They may become physically exhausted and have to stop intercourse before ejaculating. The ejaculatory ducts may become so inflamed or even ulcerated that if ejaculation does occur, blood is present in the semen. This produces further anxiety and emotional upset that aggravate the situation.

Regardless of the cause, ED has vast implications. The man may feel emasculated and develop an inferiority complex. Anger and depression are common. If the patient's ED is associated with an anatomic defect, there may be additional changes in his self-image related to the physical disease. If sexual problems are not resolved, personality changes may develop in the patient. Fear of losing his sexual partner can interfere with his work. Sleep and rest may be disturbed. If sexual maladjustment continues, neurotic complaints may ensue. Without proper guidance, the man may experience complete ED, and suicidal tendencies may develop.

Severe psychiatric disturbances must be treated by a trained psychiatrist or sexual therapist. To a large extent, success depends on the ability of the clinician and the patient's sexual partner to inspire confidence in the patient.

Physical Examination

The only equipment necessary for the examination of the male genitalia is disposable latex gloves. Although the wearing of protective gloves may decrease the examiner's sensitivity, disposable latex gloves should always be worn.

Many students are concerned about the possibility that a patient will have an erection during the examination. Although this is possible, it is rare for a man to become sexually excited because he is usually somewhat uncomfortable under these circumstances. If the examination is performed in an objective manner, it should not be a source of stimulation to the patient.

Examination of the male genitalia is performed with the patient first lying down and then standing. This postural change is important, because hernias or scrotal masses may not be apparent in the lying-down position.

The examination of the male genitalia consists of the following:

- Inspection and palpation with the patient lying down
- Inspection and palpation with the patient standing
- Hernia examination

Inspection and Palpation with the Patient Lying Down

Inspect the Skin and Hair

While the patient is lying down, the skin in the groin should be inspected for the presence of a superficial fungal infection, excoriations, and other rashes. Excoriations may indicate a scabies infection.

Observe the distribution of hair. Inspect the pubic hair for the presence of crab lice or nits (egg cases) attached to the hair. Are any burrows of scabies present?

Inspect the Penis and Scrotum

In the examination of the penis and scrotum, note the following:

- Whether the patient is circumcised
- The size of the penis and scrotum
- Any lesions on the penis and penile edema

Figure 18-11 shows ectopic sebaceous glands on the shaft of the penis. The glands appear as pinhead-sized, whitish-yellow papules. These are commonly seen in normal men on the corona, the inner foreskin, and the shaft of the penis. Their appearance is very similar to Fordyce's spots of the oral mucosa (see Fig. 12-18). Ectopic sebaceous glands also may be found in normal women on the labia minora and labia majora (see Fig. 19-13).

Pearly penile papules are very common around the coronal sulcus and have no racial predilection. They are thought to be embryonic remnants of a copulative prehensile organ. These fine papules are small, asymptomatic lesions that develop after puberty in 10% to 15% of men. They are skin colored, filiform in shape, and arranged in rows at the junction of the glans penis and sulcus coronarius; they are more common in uncircumcised men. They should not be confused with condylomata acuminata. Figure 18-12 shows pearly penile papules.

Figure 18-13 shows the penis of a patient with the chancre of *primary syphilis*. Although the typical syphilitic chancre is described as nontender, approximately 30% of patients with primary syphilis describe some pain or tenderness. Usually only a single lesion is present. The edge of the chancre is usually indurated. Moderate nontender inguinal adenopathy was present in this patient.

Figure 18-14 shows *chancroid* in two patients. In contrast to the chancre of syphilis, the ulceration of chancroid is extremely painful. The ulceration has a purulent, grayish surface that becomes granulating. Characteristically, the base of the ulcer and its vicinity are not infiltrated.

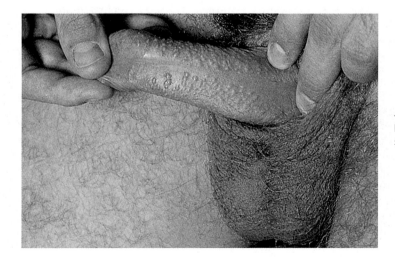

Figure 18–11 Ectopic sebaceous glands on the penis.

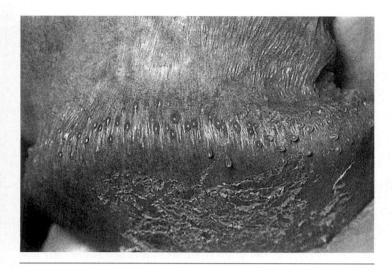

Figure 18–12 Pearly penile papules.

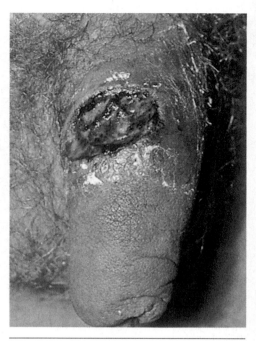

Figure 18–13 Chancre of primary syphilis.

There is usually moderate tender adenopathy associated with the genital lesions. Another important difference between the ulceration of chancroid and the chancre of syphilis is the frequent presence of multiple lesions in the former, as shown in Figure 18-14*A*. The patient in Figure 18-14*B* had a similar lesion on the other side of his penis.

Venereal warts, or *condylomata acuminata*, may be found near the meatus, on the glans, in the perineum, at the anus, and on the shaft of the penis. Condylomata acuminata are the characteristic lesions of human papillomavirus (HPV) infection. Typically, these papules have a verrucous surface resembling cauliflower. They are highly contagious, with transmission occurring in 30% to 60% of patients after a single exposure. Figure 18-15 shows a patient with condylomata acuminata on the shaft of his penis (see also Fig. 18-40).

Are there any papules on the penis or scrotum? Figure 18-16 shows the classic genital papular lesions in a patient with *scabies*.

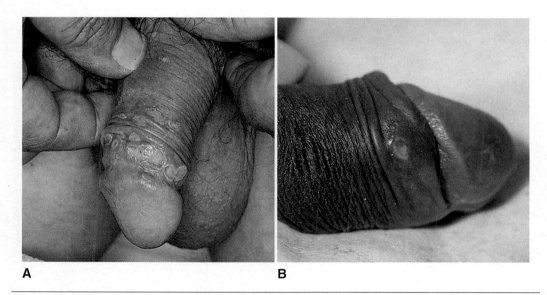

A   **B**

Figure 18–14 Chancroid. *A,* Note the multiple lesions. *B,* The patient had another lesion on the other side of his penis.

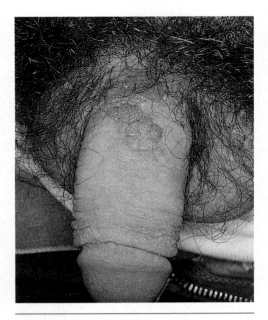

Figure 18–15 Condylomata acuminata of the shaft of the penis.

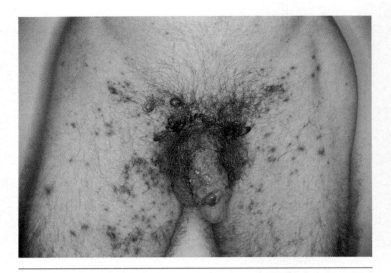

Figure 18–16 Scabies in the groin and on the penis.

Balanitis is inflammation of the glans penis. It is most often caused by *Candida* infection and is found mostly in uncircumcised men. The warmth and moisture in this area facilitate the growth of the yeast organisms. The infection begins as flat erythema on the inner side of the foreskin and glans. Pustules develop that break open and leave a moist, bright red, eroded surface. If the infection involves the glans and foreskin, the term *balanoposthitis* is used. Figure 18-17 shows *Candida* balanitis. Notice the erosions on the distal shaft and glans penis. The foreskin has been retracted.

The scrotum is inspected for any sores or rashes. Pinpoint, dark red, slightly raised, telangiectatic lesions on the scrotum are common in individuals older than 50 years. They are *angiokeratomas* and are benign. *Fabry's disease*, which is a rare, sex-linked inborn error of glycosphingolipid metabolism, is characterized by pain, fever, and diffuse angiokeratomas in a "bathing suit" distribution, especially around the umbilicus and scrotum. The scrotum of an 18-year-old patient with Fabry's disease and multiple angiokeratomas is shown in Figure 18-18.

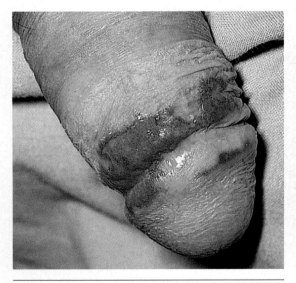

Figure 18–17 *Candida* balanitis.

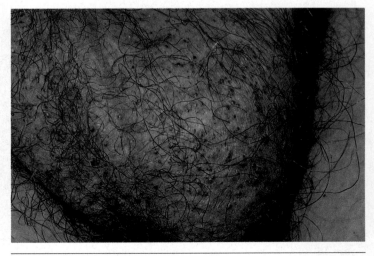

Figure 18–18 Angiokeratomas in a patient with Fabry's disease.

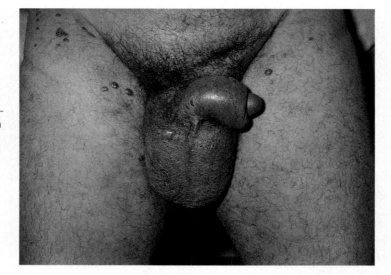

Figure 18–19 Kaposi's sarcoma and acquired immunodeficiency syndrome (AIDS)–related scrotal edema.

The patient in Figure 18-19 has acquired immunodeficiency syndrome (AIDS) and Kaposi's sarcoma. Notice the marked penile and scrotal edema, as well as the lesions of Kaposi's sarcoma on his thighs and scrotum.

The examiner elevates the patient's scrotum to inspect the perineum carefully for any inflammation, ulceration, warts, abscesses, or other lesions.

Palpate the Inguinal Nodes

By rolling the fingers along the inguinal ligament, the examiner can assess the presence of inguinal adenopathy. Commonly, small (0.2-inch [0.5-cm]), freely mobile lymph nodes are present in this area. Because the lymphatic vessels from the perineum, legs, and feet drain into this area, it is not surprising that small lymph nodes are frequently encountered.

Inspect for Groin Masses

Ask the patient to cough or strain while you inspect the groin. A sudden bulge may indicate an inguinal or femoral hernia.

Inspection and Palpation with the Patient Standing

Ask the patient to stand while you sit in front of him.

Inspect the Penis

If the patient is not circumcised, the foreskin should be retracted. Some examiners ask the patient to retract it himself; others prefer to determine the tightness of the foreskin. The cheesy, white material under the foreskin is smegma and is normal.

Phimosis is the condition in which the foreskin cannot be retracted, and it prevents adequate examination of the glans. Because the glans also cannot be cleaned, smegma builds up, leading to possible inflammation of the glans and prepuce (*balanoposthitis*). This chronic irritation may be a causative factor in cancer of the penis.

The glans is inspected for ulcers, warts, nodules, scars, and signs of inflammation.

Inspect the External Meatus

The examiner should note the position of the external urethral meatus. It should be central on the glans. To inspect the meatus, the examiner places his or her hands on either side of the glans penis and opens the meatus. The technique for examining the meatus is demonstrated in Figure 18-20.

The meatus should be observed for any discharge, warts, and stenosis. Figure 18-21 shows a patient with meatal condylomata acuminata.

On occasion, the urethral meatus opens on the ventral surface of the penis; this condition is called *hypospadias*. A less common condition is *epispadias*, in which the meatus is located on the dorsal surface of the penis.

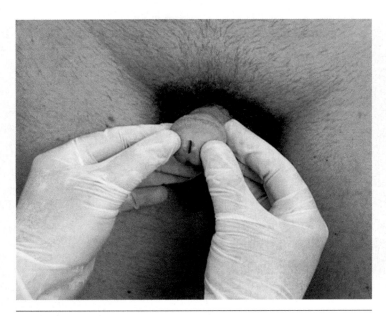

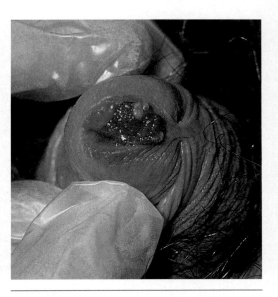

Figure 18–21 Condylomata acuminata of the urethral meatus.

Figure 18–20 Technique for inspecting the external urethral meatus.

Palpate the Penis

Palpate the shaft from the glans to the base of the penis. The presence of scars, ulcers, nodules, induration, and signs of inflammation must be noted. To palpate the corpora cavernosa, hold the penis between the fingers of both your hands and use your index fingers to note any induration. Figure 18-22 illustrates the method of palpation of the shaft of the penis.

The presence of nontender induration or fibrotic areas under the skin of the shaft is suggestive of *Peyronie's disease*. Patients with this condition may also complain of penile deviation during erection. The erect penis has a deviation in the long axis, making sexual intercourse difficult or impossible. The patient or his partner may also complain of pain during intercourse. The site of predilection is the dorsal aspect of the penis, especially in the middle or proximal third. Figure 18-23 shows the penis of a patient with Peyronie's disease.

Palpate the Urethra

The urethra should be palpated from the external meatus through the corpus spongiosum to its base. To palpate the base of the urethra, the examiner elevates the penis with the left hand while the right index finger invaginates the scrotum in the midline and palpates deep to the

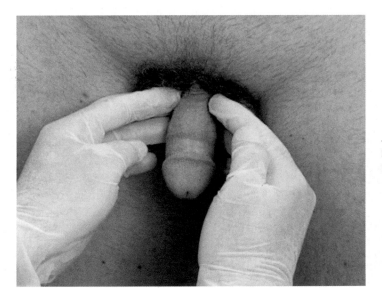

Figure 18–22 Technique for palpation of the penis.

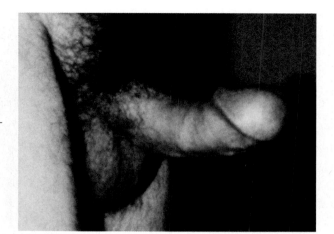

Figure 18–23 Peyronie's disease.

base of the corpus spongiosum. The pad of the examiner's right index finger should palpate the entire corpus spongiosum from the meatus to its base. This technique is demonstrated in Figure 18-24. If a discharge is present, "milking the urethra" may allow a drop to be placed on a glass slide for microscopic evaluation.

The foreskin, if retracted, should be replaced. *Paraphimosis* is a condition in which the foreskin can be retracted but cannot be replaced and becomes caught behind the corona.

Inspect the Scrotum

The scrotum is now reevaluated while the patient is standing. Observe the contour and contents of the scrotum. Two testicles should be present. Normally the left testicle is lower than the right. The presence of any fullness not seen while the patient was lying down should be noted.

Palpate the Testes

Each testis is palpated separately. Use both hands to grasp the patient's testicle gently. While your left hand holds the superior and inferior poles of the testicle, your right hand palpates the anterior and posterior surfaces. The technique for palpation of the testicle is demonstrated in Figure 18-25.

Note the size, shape, and consistency of each testicle. No tenderness or nodularity should be present. Normal testicles have a firm, rubbery consistency. The size and consistency of one

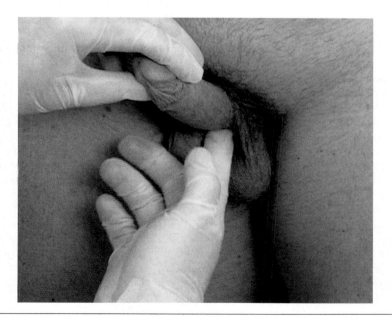

Figure 18–24 Technique for palpation of the base of the urethra.

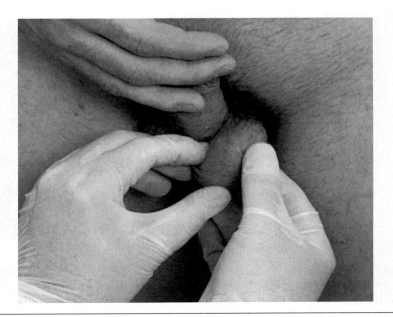

Figure 18–25 Technique for palpation of the testicle.

testicle are compared with those of the other. Does one testicle feel heavier than the other? If a mass is present, can the examining finger palpate above the mass within the scrotum? Because inguinal hernias arise from the abdominal cavity, the examining finger is unable to get above such a mass. In contrast, the examining finger can frequently get above a mass that arises from within the scrotum.

Palpate the Epididymis and Vas Deferens

Next, locate and palpate the epididymis on the posterior aspect of the testicle. The head and tail should be carefully palpated for tenderness, nodularity, and masses.

The spermatic cord is palpated from the epididymis up to the external abdominal ring. The patient is asked to elevate his penis gently. If the penis is elevated too much, the scrotal skin is reduced, and the examination is more difficult. Hold the scrotum in the midline by placing both your thumbs in front of and both your index fingers on the perineal side of the patient's scrotum. Using both hands, simultaneously palpate both spermatic cords between your thumbs and index fingers as you pull your fingers laterally over the scrotal surface. The most prominent structures in the spermatic cord are the vasa deferens. The vasa are firm cords about 0.08 to 0.15 inches (2 to 4 mm) in diameter and feel like partially cooked spaghetti. The sizes are compared, and tenderness or beading is noted. Absence of the vas deferens on one side is often associated with absence of the kidney on the same side. The technique of spermatic cord palpation is demonstrated in Figure 18-26.

A common enlargement of the spermatic cord resulting from dilatation of the pampiniform plexus is a *varicocele*. These varicosities are usually on the left side, and the impression on palpation has been likened to feeling a bag of worms. Because the varicocele is gravity dependent, it is usually visible only while the patient is standing or straining. The patient is asked to turn his head and cough while the spermatic cords are held between the examiner's fingers, as indicated previously. A sudden pulsation, especially on the left side, confirms the diagnosis of a varicocele. Although the diagnosis is usually made from palpation, large varicoceles may be discovered on mere inspection, as can be seen in the patient in Figure 18-27.

Transilluminate Scrotal Masses

If a scrotal mass is detected, transillumination is necessary. In a darkened room, a light source is applied to the side of scrotal enlargement. Vascular structures, tumors, blood, hernias, and normal testicles appear opaque on transillumination. Transmission of the light as a red glow indicates a serous fluid-containing cavity, such as a *hydrocele* or a *spermatocele*. A hydrocele is an abnormal collection of clear fluid in the tunica vaginalis. The testicle is contained within this cystic mass, preventing actual palpation of the testis itself. By transillumination, it may be possible to view the orientation of the normal-sized testicle within the hydrocele. A spermatocele

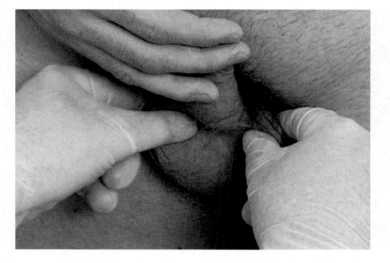

Figure 18–26 Technique for palpation of the spermatic cord.

is a pea-sized, nontender mass that contains spermatozoa and is usually attached to the upper pole of the epididymis. A hydrocele, seen only as massive scrotal enlargement, is shown in Figure 18-28. Transillumination of a hydrocele in another patient is shown in Figure 18-29. A cross section of a hydrocele is illustrated in Figure 18-30.

Hernia Examination

Inspect Inguinal and Femoral Areas

Although hernias may be defined as any protrusion of a viscus, or part of it, through a normal or abnormal opening, 90% of all hernias are located in the inguinal area. Commonly, a hernial impulse is better seen than felt.

Instruct the patient to turn his head to the side and to cough or strain. Inspect the inguinal and femoral areas for any sudden swelling during coughing, which may indicate a hernia. If a sudden bulge is seen, ask the patient to cough again, and compare the impulse with that of the other side. If the patient complains of pain while coughing, determine the location of the pain, and reevaluate the area.

Palpate for Inguinal Hernias

To palpate for inguinal hernias, the examiner places his or her right index finger in the patient's scrotum above the left testis and invaginates the scrotal skin. There should be

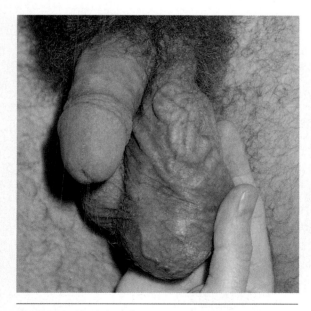

Figure 18–27 Varicocele.

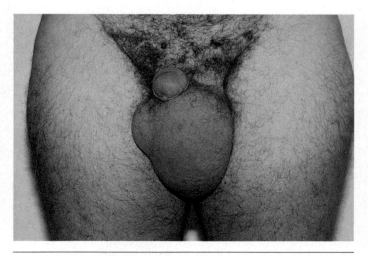

Figure 18–28 Hydrocele.

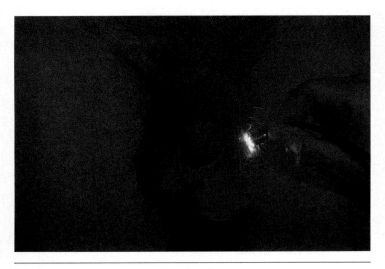

Figure 18–29 Transilluminated hydrocele.

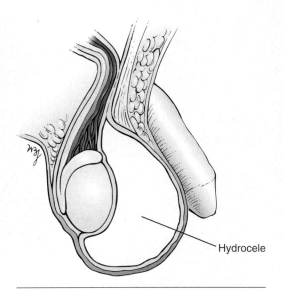

Figure 18–30 Cross section of a hydrocele, illustrating its anatomy.

sufficient scrotal skin to reach the external inguinal ring. The finger should be placed with the nail facing outward and the pad of the finger inward. This is demonstrated in Figure 18-31. The examiner's left hand may be placed on the patient's right hip for better support.

The examiner's right index finger should follow the spermatic cord laterally through the external inguinal ring, into the inguinal canal parallel to the inguinal ligament, and upward toward the internal inguinal ring, which is superior and lateral to the pubic tubercle. The external ring may be dilated and allow the finger to enter easily. The correct position of the right hand is shown in Figure 18-32 and is illustrated in Figure 18-33.

With your index finger placed either against the external ring or in the inguinal canal, ask the patient to turn his head to the side and to cough or strain down. If a hernia is present, a sudden impulse against either the tip or the pad of the examining finger is felt. If a hernia is detected, have the patient lie down, and observe whether the hernia can be reduced by gentle, sustained pressure on the mass. If the hernia examination is performed with adequate scrotal skin and is done *slowly*, it is painless. The characteristics of hernias are discussed in the next section.

After the left side is evaluated, repeat the procedure by using your right index finger to examine the patient's right side. Some examiners prefer to use the right index finger to

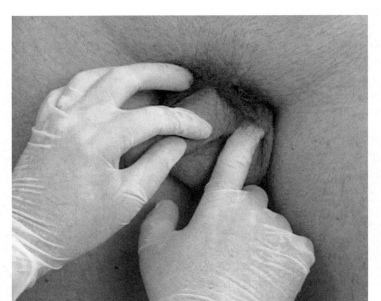

Figure 18–31 Technique for examination for inguinal hernias.

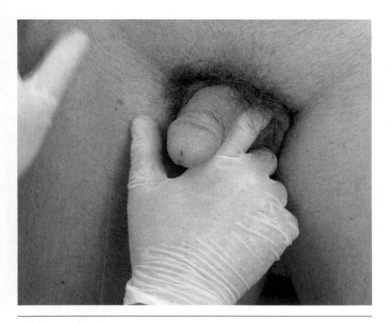

Figure 18–32 Technique for palpation of inguinal hernias.

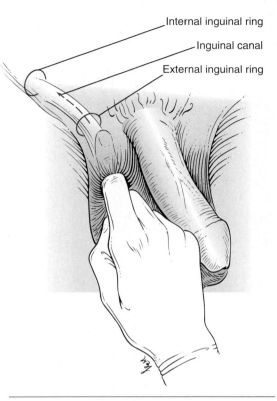

Internal inguinal ring
Inguinal canal
External inguinal ring

Figure 18–33 Position of the examining finger in the inguinal canal.

examine the patient's right side and the left index finger for the patient's left side. Try both techniques to see which one is more comfortable for you.

If there is a large scrotal mass that appears opaque on transillumination, an indirect inguinal hernia may be present in the scrotum. Auscultation of the mass can be performed to determine whether bowel sounds are present in the scrotum, a useful sign in diagnosing an indirect inguinal hernia.

Examination of the prostate is discussed in Chapter 17, The Abdomen. If the rectal examination has not yet been performed, this is the appropriate time to examine the rectum and prostate.

Clinicopathologic Correlations

Gross hematuria that is usually painless is often the first indication of a urinary tract tumor, commonly located in the bladder. Table 18-1 lists the common causes of gross hematuria in different age groups and by sex.

Scrotal disorders are relatively common. In a man with scrotal swelling, a careful history and a thorough physical examination often provide enough information for a correct diagnosis. Intrascrotal masses are common findings on physical examination. Although most masses are benign, testicular cancer is the leading solid malignancy in men younger than 35 years of age.

Some of the important considerations in the history include the patient's age, time of onset of symptoms (if any), associated problems (e.g., fever, weight loss, dysuria), past medical history, and sexual history.

Intrascrotal masses can be categorized as acute or nonacute, intratesticular or extratesticular, and neoplastic or non-neoplastic.

The most common pathologic disorders in the category of *acute, non-neoplastic lesions* include testicular torsion, epididymitis, and trauma. Testicular torsion is a surgical emergency in which a twisting of the testis leads to venous obstruction, edema, and eventual arterial obstruction. Prompt recognition (within 10 to 12 hours) of this condition enables physicians to salvage the testis in 70% to 90% of cases. Torsion is most commonly seen in adolescents from 12 to 18 years of age. Patients complain of acute, unilateral testicular pain that is often

Table 18–1 Causes of Hematuria by Age and Sex

Age (Years)	Male	Female
Younger than 20	Congenital urinary tract anomaly Acute glomerulonephritis Acute urinary tract infection	—
20-40	Acute urinary tract infection Kidney stone Bladder tumor	—
40-60	Bladder tumor Kidney stone Acute urinary tract infection	Acute urinary tract infection Kidney stone Bladder tumor
Older than 60	Prostatic disorder Bladder tumor Acute urinary tract infection	Bladder tumor Acute urinary tract infection

accompanied by nausea and vomiting. On physical examination, the testis is enlarged and extremely sensitive. It may be retracted and is often lying in a horizontal position.

Epididymitis is the most common cause of acute scrotal swelling. It accounts for more than 600,000 visits to physicians annually in the United States. It occurs in young, sexually active men and in older men with associated genitourinary problems. Patients usually complain of recent onset of testicular pain that is associated with fever, dysuria, and scrotal swelling. On examination, the epididymis is tender and indurated. The testis may also be enlarged and tender; this variant is called *epididymo-orchitis*.

Trauma is the third major cause of acute scrotal swelling. Trauma may produce a scrotal or testicular hematoma. An important fact to keep in mind is that 10% to 15% of patients with testicular tumors seek medical attention after trauma.

The most common types of intrascrotal pathologic conditions are the *nonacute, non-neoplastic lesions*. These include hydrocele, spermatocele, and varicocele. A hydrocele (see Fig. 18-28) is a collection of fluid within layers of the tunica vaginalis. It manifests as a painless swelling of the scrotum. A hydrocele may be congenital, acquired, or idiopathic. Acquired hydroceles may result from trauma, infection, renal transplantation, and neoplasm. Idiopathic hydroceles are the most common; patients may have no symptoms or may complain of a dull ache or scrotal heaviness. In general, hydroceles are anterior to the testis. They are smooth walled and can be transilluminated. Figure 18-29 depicts a transilluminated hydrocele.

Spermatoceles are cystic collections of fluid in the epididymis. They are frequently found on routine physical examination because they usually produce no symptoms. Because they are fluid filled, they can often be transilluminated.

A varicocele is a common intrascrotal mass resulting from abnormal dilatation of the veins of the pampiniform plexus. A man with a varicocele is usually asymptomatic but may have a history of infertility or a sensation of heaviness in the scrotum. The varicocele can best be visualized by observing the patient in a standing position. A mass resembling a bag of worms may be seen and palpated superior to the testis. These varicosities typically enlarge during a Valsalva maneuver and are reduced when the patient lies down. Varicoceles are found predominantly on the left side. A right-sided varicocele suggests some obstruction of the inferior vena cava, whereas an acute left-sided varicocele may indicate a left-sided hypernephroma or other left renal tumor. Figure 18-27 shows a patient with a varicocele. Notice the markedly dilated veins in the scrotum.

Most *testicular neoplasms* are asymptomatic, but some patients may seek medical attention because of acute pain related to trauma, hemorrhage, hydrocele, and epididymitis. Other men may present with weight loss, fever, abdominal pain, lower extremity edema, or bone pain resulting from advanced metastatic disease. A history of cryptorchidism is important because of a high association between this condition and testicular malignancies. The most common finding on physical examination is a nodule or a painless swelling of one testicle. About 1% to 3% of testicular neoplasms are bilateral. If found early, testicular carcinoma is almost always curable. Extratesticular tumors are uncommon and are usually benign. Pure seminomas constitute approximately 40% of all testicular cancer cases. Forty percent of testicular cancers have mixed histologic characteristics.

Table 18–2 Differential Diagnosis of Common Scrotal Swellings

Diagnosis	Usual Age (Years)	Able to Be Transilluminated	Scrotal Erythema	Pain
Epididymitis	Any	No	Yes	Severe, increasing severity
Torsion of testes	<20	No	Yes	Severe, sudden
Testis tumor	15-35	No	No	Minimal or absent
Hydrocele (see Fig. 18-28)	Any	Yes (see Fig. 18-29)	No	None
Spermatocele	Any	Yes	No	None
Hernia (see Figs. 18-42 and 18-43)	Any	No	No	None to moderate*
Varicocele (see Fig. 18-27)	>15	No	No	None

*Unless the hernia is incarcerated, in which case pain may be severe.

Table 18-2 provides a differential diagnosis of common scrotal swellings.

Sexually transmitted diseases are common. Of every 100 outpatient visits to a venereal disease clinic, 25% of men have gonorrhea, 25% have nongonococcal urethritis, 4% have venereal warts, 3.5% have herpes, 1.7% have syphilis, and 0.1% have chancroid. The incidence of both gonococcal and nongonococcal urethritis has increased dramatically since the early 1980s. On college campuses, 85% of urethritis is nongonococcal in origin.

Genital lesions of venereal diseases may be ulcerative or nonulcerative. The incidence of genital lesions has changed greatly since the 1950s. At one time, chancroid was common, and herpes was rare; today, herpes simplex virus type 2 (HSV-2) infection is common, and chancroid is rare. Figure 18-34 shows the vesicular stage of a herpetic infection. Another example of HSV-2 infection is shown in Figure 18-35. Anal ulcerative lesions are becoming more common, particularly among gay men.

Molluscum contagiosum is a common, usually self-limited, cutaneous eruption affecting the skin and mucous membranes. It is often seen in the pediatric population and is caused by a

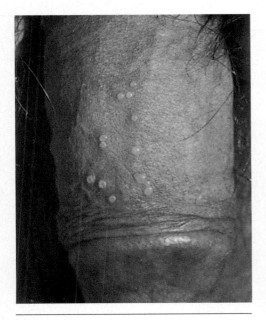

Figure 18–34 Herpes simplex virus type 2 infection.

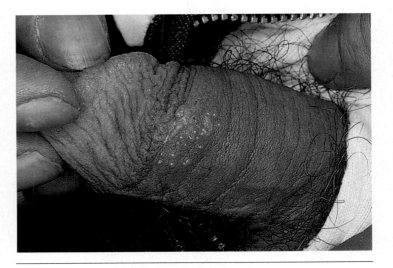

Figure 18–35 Herpes simplex virus type 2 infection.

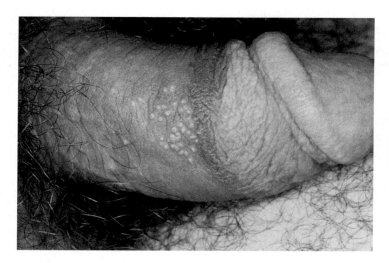

Figure 18–36 Lesions of molluscum contagiosum of the penis.

large DNA poxvirus. Adults can acquire the infection through sexual contact with infected adults. The characteristic lesions are flesh-colored papules that range in size from pinpoint to 0.4 inch (1 cm) in diameter. The central depression is the most important diagnostic sign. The painful lesions may occur anywhere on the body: on the face and trunk in children and around the genitals of adults. Any adult with this disease must be screened for other sexually transmitted diseases. The lesions, as the name indicates, are highly contagious. As the lesions develop, there may be a surrounding patch of eczema. In patients with AIDS, the lesions become widespread, attaining sizes up to 0.8 inch (2 cm) in diameter. Figure 18-36 shows lesions of molluscum contagiosum of the penis. Figure 18-37 is a close-up photograph of the classic, umbilicated lesions of molluscum contagiosum. Table 18-3 lists a differential diagnosis of genital papular lesions.

The primary lesion of *syphilis* is the chancre (see Fig. 18-13), which occurs from 10 days to 3 weeks after infection at the site of the inoculation. The chancre is a painless ulcer with an indurated edge. It usually heals spontaneously within a month. If the patient is not treated for syphilis, the disease may evolve to the secondary stage. This occurs about 2 months after the appearance of the chancre. The patient may present with a widespread, nonpruritic, maculopapular rash over the genitalia, trunk, palms, and soles. There is a tendency for cropping of the lesions. The healed chancre may still be evident. There is also generalized lymphadenopathy. In the genital and perianal areas, the papules may coalesce and erode. These large, moist, painful papules, which look as if they were "pasted" on the skin, are called *condylomata lata*. They are covered with an exudate and are teeming with active spirochetes. If untreated, the patient may recover but may have a relapse of the eruption within 2 years. After this period, there is a long latent period during which the disease may progress to cardiovascular syphilis or neurosyphilis, a condition known as tertiary syphilis.

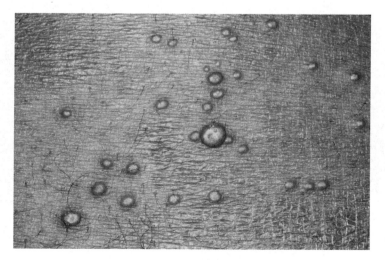

Figure 18–37 Close-up photograph of the umbilicated lesions of molluscum contagiosum.

Table 18–3 Differential Diagnosis of Genital Papules

Condition	Appearance	Pain	Lymphadenopathy
Herpes (see Figs. 18-34 and 18-35)	Multiple, ulcers, vesicles	Painful	Present
Condylomata lata (see Fig. 18-39)	Multiple, moist, flat, round	Painful	Present
Condylomata acuminata (see Figs. 18-15, 18-21, and 18-40)	Multiple, verrucous	Absent	Absent
Molluscum contagiosum (see Figs. 18-36 and 18-37)	0.04- to 0.2-inch (1- to 5-mm) umbilicated papules, often in clusters; caseous material expressible from center	Painful	Rarely

The skin lesions of syphilis are important to recognize. Figure 18-38 shows the typical skin lesions of secondary syphilis on the feet. Figure 18-39 shows condylomata lata in the perineum of the same patient. The healing chancre of primary syphilis is also seen on the penis of this patient.

Human papillomavirus (HPV) infection of the genital tract is one of the most common sexually transmitted diseases among young adults and is the cause of venereal warts. In the United States, it is estimated that 20 million people have genital HPV infections at any one time, with 5.5 million acquiring it annually. Risk factors associated with HPV infection include younger age, belonging to an ethnic minority, alcohol consumption, and a high frequency of anal or vaginal sexual encounters. The annual cost burden in the United States of genital HPV infection is $6 billion, which makes it the second most costly sexually transmitted disease after human immunodeficiency virus (HIV) infection. Condylomata acuminata are typically caused by HPV type 6 or HPV type 11, which are considered low-risk HPV types because these strains are rarely found in association with genital dysplasias or invasive cancer. Patients with immunodeficiencies are at higher risk for persistent HPV infection and progressive disease. Figure 18-40 shows the classic cauliflower lesions of condylomata acuminata on the penis of a renal transplant recipient (see also Figs. 18-15 and 18-21).

Reiter's syndrome is defined as the classic triad of nongonococcal urethritis, arthritis, and conjunctivitis. It most often affects men (20:1) during the third decade of life, and there is a high prevalence of human leukocyte antigen (HLA)–B27. It is one of the most common causes of acute inflammatory arthritis in men. Approximately one third of patients with Reiter's syndrome have a prodromal enteric or urethral inflammation. The most common enteric pathogens are *Shigella*, *Salmonella*, *Yersinia*, and *Campylobacter*; the most common urogenital

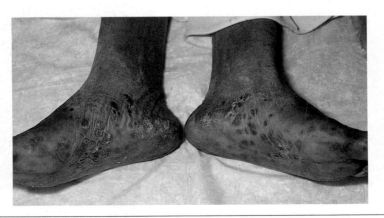

Figure 18–38 Secondary syphilis lesions on the feet.

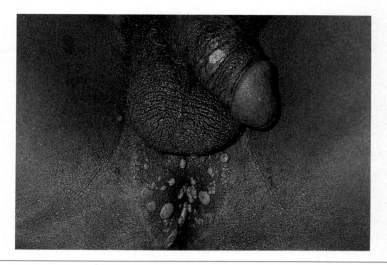

Figure 18–39 Condylomata lata. Note the healing primary chancre on the penis.

pathogens are *Chlamydia* and *Ureaplasma*. Reiter's syndrome is often associated with a psoriasis-like dermatitis on the palms and soles known as *keratoderma blennorrhagicum*. This painless, papulosquamous, "barnacle-like" eruption is pictured in Figure 18-41.

Hernias are common. The major types of external hernias are indirect and direct inguinal hernias and femoral hernias. Figure 18-42 shows a patient with a left indirect inguinal hernia. Figure 18-43 shows a patient with a small right direct inguinal hernia. Figure 18-44 illustrates and lists the major differences in the types of hernias.

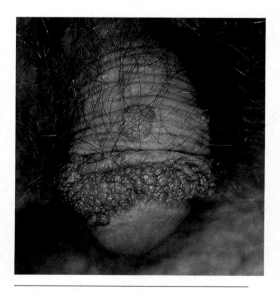

Figure 18–40 Condylomata acuminata of the penis.

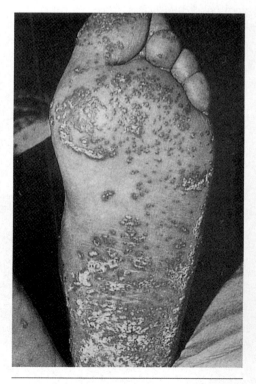

Figure 18–41 Keratoderma blennorrhagicum in a patient with Reiter's syndrome.

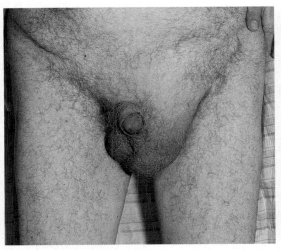

Figure 18–42 Left indirect inguinal hernia.

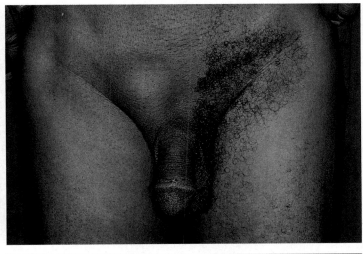

Figure 18–43 Right direct inguinal hernia.

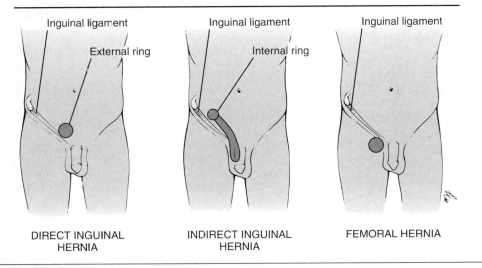

DIRECT INGUINAL
HERNIA

INDIRECT INGUINAL
HERNIA

FEMORAL HERNIA

Figure 18–44 Differential diagnosis of hernias.

Feature	Direct Inguinal*	Indirect Inguinal†	Femoral
Occurrence	Middle-aged and elderly men	All ages	Least common: more frequently found in women
Bilaterality	55%	30%	Rarely
Origin of swelling	Above inguinal ligament; directly behind and through external ring	Above inguinal ligament; hernial sac enters inguinal canal at internal ring and exits at external ring	Below inguinal ligament
Scrotal involvement	Rare	Common	None
Impulse location	At side of examining finger in inguinal canal	At tip of examining finger in inguinal canal	Not felt by examining finger in inguinal canal; mass below canal

*See Figure 18-43.
†See Figure 18-42.

Useful Vocabulary

Listed here are the specific roots that are important for understanding the terminology related to urologic disease.

Root	Pertaining to	Example	Definition
andr-	man	**andr**ogen	Substance possessing masculinizing properties
cyst(o)-	urinary bladder	**cysto**tomy	Incision of the urinary bladder
litho-	stone	**litho**tomy	Incision of an organ for the removal of a stone
nephro-	kidney	**nephro**pathy	Disease of the kidneys
orchi(o)-	testes	**orchi**tis	Inflammation of the testis
pyel(o)-	pelvis of kidney	**pyelo**gram	X-ray film of the kidney and ureter
ureter(o)-	ureter	**uretero**lith	A stone lodged or formed in the ureter
urethr(o)-	urethra	**urethro**plasty	Plastic surgery of the urethra
vas(o)-	vas deferens	**vas**ectomy	Excision of the vas deferens

Writing Up the Physical Examination

Listed here are examples of the write-up for the examination of the male genitalia.

- The penis is circumcised. Both testes are in the scrotum and are within normal limits. There are no abnormal scrotal masses. No inguinal hernias are present. No inguinal adenopathy is present.
- The penis is uncircumcised. The foreskin is easily retracted. The left hemiscrotum is markedly enlarged by a painless mass that can be transilluminated. The left testicle cannot be palpated. The right testicle is within normal limits. No inguinal hernias are present. A small, 2 × 2 cm [0.75 × 0.75 inch], soft, nonfixed, nontender lymph node is present in the right inguinal area.
- The penis is circumcised. There is a 1- to 2-cm [0.40- to 0.75-inch] verrucous mass at the external meatus. A thick, yellow, purulent urethral discharge, which can be milked from the urethra, is seen at the meatus. The scrotal contents are within normal limits. No inguinal hernias are present.
- The penis is uncircumcised. The foreskin is tight, although it can be retracted by the patient. A large amount of smegma is present behind the corona.

There is a large mass of nontender, dilated veins present in the left hemiscrotum that can be seen and felt when the patient stands. An impulse is felt in the left spermatic cord upon coughing. No inguinal hernias are present.

- The penis is circumcised. The left testicle is soft and measures 2×3 cm [0.75 × 1.20 inch]. The right testicle appears normal. The scrotal contents are within normal limits. The hernia examination on the left side reveals a prominent impulse when the patient coughs. This impulse is felt at the tip of the examiner's finger.

- The penis is circumcised. There is a 1-cm [0.4-inch] painless ulcer with a clean, nonpurulent base at the corona. The ulcer is indurated and has a smooth, regular, sharply defined border. Painless, firm, movable inguinal lymphadenopathy is present bilaterally. The testes are normal, as are the other scrotal contents. No inguinal hernias are present.

Bibliography

American Cancer Society: Cancer Facts and Figures 2007. Atlanta, Ga: American Cancer Society, 2007.

Baldwin K, Ginsberg P, Harkaway RC: Under-reporting of erectile dysfunction among men with unrelated urologic conditions. Int J Impot Res 15(2):87, 2003.

Bosl GJ, Bajorin DF, Sheinfeld J, et al: Cancer of the testis. In DeVita VT Jr, Hellman S, Rosenberg SA (eds): Cancer: Principles and Practice of Oncology, 7th ed. Philadelphia, Lippincott Williams & Wilkins, 2005.

Brown JS, Bradley CS, Subak LL, et al: The sensitivity and specificity of a simple text to distinguish between urge and stress urinary incontinence. Ann Intern Med 144:715, 2006.

Brydøy M, Fosså SD, Klepp O, et al: Paternity following treatment for testicular cancer. J Natl Cancer Inst 97:1580, 2005.

Centers for Disease Control and Prevention, Division of Sexually Transmitted Disease Prevention: Prevention of Genital HPV Infection and Sequelae: Report of an External Consultants' Meeting. Atlanta, Centers for Disease Control and Prevention, U.S. Department of Health and Human Services, 1999.

Del Mistro A, Chieco Bianchi L: HPV-related neoplasias in HIV-infected individuals. Eur J Cancer 37:1227, 2001.

English JC, Laws RA, Keough GC, et al: Dermatoses of the glans penis and prepuce. J Am Acad Dermatol 37:1, 1997.

Espey DK, Wu X, Swan J, et al: Annual report to the nation on the status of cancer, 1975–2004, featuring cancer in American Indians and Alaska Natives. Cancer 110:2119, 2007.

Feldman HA, Goldstein I, Hatzichristou DG, et al: Impotence and its medical and psychological correlates: Results of the Massachusetts Male Aging Study. J Urol 151:54, 1994.

Fosså SD, Chen J, Schonfeld SJ, et al: Risk of contralateral testicular cancer: A population-based study of 29,515 U.S. men. J Natl Cancer Inst 97:1056, 2005.

Glass C: Sexual problems of disabled patients. BMJ 318:518, 1999.

Hodges FM: The ideal prepuce in ancient Greece and Rome: Male genital aesthetics and their relation to *lipodermos*, circumcision, foreskin restoration, and the *kynodesme*. Bull Hist Med 75:375, 2001.

Johannes CB, Araujo AB, Feldman HA, et al: Incidence of erectile dysfunction in men 40 to 69 years old: *Longitudinal* results from the Massachusetts Male Aging Study. J Urol 163:460, 2000.

Kuthe A: Phosphodiesterase 5 inhibitors in male sexual dysfunction. Curr Opin Urol 13:405, 2003.

Laumann EO, Paik A, Rosen RC: Sexual dysfunction in the United States: Prevalence and predictors. JAMA 281:537, 1999.

Leitzmann MF, Platz EA, Meir J, et al: Ejaculation frequency and subsequent risk of prostate cancer. JAMA 291:1578 2004.

Montorsi F, Salonia A, Deho' F, et al: Pharmacological management of erectile dysfunction. BJU Int 91:446, 2003.

Rosen RC, Cappelleri JC, Smith MD, et al: Development and evaluation of an abridged, 5-item version of the International Index of Erectile Function (IIEF) as a diagnostic tool for erectile dysfunction. Int J Impot Res 11:319, 1997.

Rosen RC, Riley A, Wagner G, et al: The International Index of Erectile Function (IIEF): A multidimensional scale for assessment of erectile dysfunction. Urology 49:822, 1997.

Schouten VW, Bohnen AM, Bosch JLHR, et al: Erectile dysfunction prospectively associated with cardiovascular disease in the Dutch general population: Results from the Krimpen Study. Int J Impot Res 20:92, 2008.

Shabsigh R, Klein LT, Seidman S, et al: Increased incidence of depressive symptoms in men with erectile dysfunction. Urology 52:848, 1998.

U.S. Mortality 1973–1996, National Center for Health Statistics, Centers for Disease Control and Prevention 1999: SEER Incidence 1973–1996 Surveillance, Epidemiology, and End Results Program. Bethesda, Md, Division of Cancer Control and Population Sciences, National Cancer Institute, 2000.

van den Belt-Dusebout AW, Nuver J, de Wit R, et al: Long-term risk of cardiovascular disease in 5-year survivors of testicular cancer. J Clin Oncol 24:467, 2006.

Walsh PC, Retik AB, Vaughan ED Jr, et al: Campbell's Urology. Philadelphia, WB Saunders, 1997.

Waugh MA: Balanitis. Dermatol Clin 16:757, 1998.

CHAPTER 19

Female Genitalia

In young girls, as I said, and in women past childbearing, it [the uterus] is without blood, and about the size of a bean. In a marriageable virgin it has the magnitude and form of a pear. In women who have borne children, and are still fruitful, it equals in bulk a small gourd or a goose's egg; at the same time, together with the breasts, it swells and softens, becomes more fleshy, and is heat increased.

William Harvey (1578–1657)

General Considerations

Records of obstetrics and gynecology date back to the time of Hippocrates in 400 BCE. He was probably the first physician to describe midwifery, menstruation, sterility, symptoms of pregnancy, and puerperal (the period after labor) infections. Most of the early gynecologic history stems from Soranus in the second century CE. His works included chapters on anatomy, menstruation, fertility, signs of pregnancy, labor, care of the infant, dysmenorrhea (painful menstruation), uterine hemorrhage, and even the use of vaginal specula.

William Harvey, who devised the theory of blood circulation, was also responsible for a monumental treatise on obstetrics. This work, published in 1651, included a detailed assessment of uterine changes throughout life.

The 18th century was a period of a further understanding of pregnancy, labor, and fertility. However, it was not until the 19th century that diseases of the female genitalia were better understood. As recently as 1872, Emil Noeggerath published his investigations on gonorrhea, which ultimately changed the opinion of the medical world about the significance of this disorder. He was the first to suggest that "latent gonorrhea" was associated with sterility in women. Although the first cesarean section was described in 1596 by Scipione Mercurio, the development of the current technique of Max Sänger was described as recently as 1882.

In 2007, cancer of the uterine corpus, also known as *endometrial cancer*, the most common cancer of the female reproductive organs, accounted for 6% of all cancers and 3% of all cancer deaths in women in the United States. It is the fourth most common cancer found in women, after breast cancer, lung cancer, and colorectal cancer. In 2007, there were 39,080 new cases and 7400 deaths from cancer of the uterus. The lifetime risk for development of cancer of the uterus is 1 per 38. For all cases of cancer of the uterus, the 5-year relative survival rate is 84%. Although the mortality rate has declined slightly since the 1980s among white women, it has remained stable among other racial and ethnic groups. Although the incidence rate of uterine cancer is lower for African-American women than for white women, the mortality rate among African-American women is nearly twice as high.

Between the mid-1950s and 1992, deaths from invasive cancer of the cervix in the United States dropped by 74%. The decline in mortality from cervical cancer is largely attributed to early detection by physical examination. It has been estimated that noninvasive cervical cancer (carcinoma in situ) is about four times more common than invasive cervical cancer. In the United States, the widespread use of the Papanicolaou (Pap) test has decreased the incidence and mortality rate by 40% since the mid-1970s. Most invasive cervical carcinomas are found in women who have not had regular Pap tests. In 2007, there were 11,150 new cases of invasive cervical cancer diagnosed, and 3670 women died from this disease. The death rate continues to decline by about 2% per year. An American woman has a 0.78% lifetime risk (1 per 128) for development of cervical cancer and a 0.27% risk of dying from the disease. The 5-year relative survival rate for the earliest stage of invasive cervical cancer is 92%, and the overall (all cases considered together) 5-year survival rate is 71%.

Of the many risk factors that have been evaluated, young age at first sexual intercourse, multiple sexual partners, infection with the human papillomavirus (HPV), infection with herpes simplex virus, infection with human immunodeficiency virus (HIV), immunosuppression, and a history of cervical dysplasia are most often associated with an increased risk of cervical cancer. The most important risk factor for cervical cancer is infection by the HPV. Because the course of dysplasia development takes several years from the time of initial HPV infection, the guidelines indicate that a woman should be screened after being sexually active for 3 years. HPVs are a group of more than 100 types of viruses, some of which can cause warts, or papillomas; these are noncancerous (benign) tumors. Certain other types of HPV can cause cancer of the cervix. These are called *high-risk* or *carcinogenic* types of HPV, and about 70% of all cervical cancers are caused by HPV types 16 and 18. In women older than 30, an HPV test may be conducted at the same time as a Pap test.

Vaccines have been developed that may protect against infection with some types of HPV, which may reduce cervical cancer rates in the future. One of these, Gardasil, protects against types 6, 11, 16 and 18 and is now available for girls and women aged 9 to 26 years. Another vaccine, Cervarix, protects against types 16 and 18. The Gardasil vaccine entails a series of three injections over a 6-month period. To be most effective, the vaccine should be given before a person becomes sexually active. At the time of this writing, the American Cancer Society recommends that the vaccine be routinely given to girls aged 11 to 12 and as early as age 9 years at the discretion of clinicians.

Although ovarian carcinoma accounts for only 3% of all cancers in women, it is the cause of 6% of all cancer deaths in women. It is the fourth leading cause of cancer death and the leading gynecologic malignancy in women in the United States. Cancer of the ovary accounts for nearly 50% of all deaths from gynecologic malignancies. In 2007, there were 22,430 new cases of ovarian cancer and 15,280 deaths from it. The lifetime risk for development of ovarian cancer is 1 per 59; the incidence is 1.4 per 100,000 women younger than 40 years, but it increases to 45 per 100,000 women older than 60 years. The carefully performed pelvic examination has been shown to be the cornerstone of diagnosis of ovarian cancer.

Structure and Physiology

The external female genitalia are shown in Figure 19-1. The *vulva* consists of the mons veneris, the labia majora, the labia minora, the clitoris, the vestibule and its glands, the urethral meatus, and the vaginal introitus. The *mons veneris* is a rounded prominence of fat tissue overlying the pubic symphysis. The *labia majora* are two wide skinfolds that form the lateral boundaries of the vulva. They meet anteriorly at the mons veneris to form the anterior commissure. The labia majora and the mons veneris have hair follicles and sebaceous glands. The labia majora correspond to the scrotum in the man. The *labia minora* are two narrow, pigmented skinfolds that lie between the labia majora and enclose the *vestibule*, which is the area lying between the labia minora. Anteriorly, the two labia minora form the prepuce of the *clitoris*. The clitoris, analogous to the penis, consists of erectile tissue and a rich supply of nerve endings. It has a glans and two corpora cavernosa. The external *urethral meatus* is located in the anterior portion of the vestibule below the clitoris. Paraurethral glands, or *Skene's glands*, are small glands that open lateral to the urethra. Secretion of sebaceous glands in this area protects the vulnerable tissues against urine.

The major vestibular glands are known as *Bartholin's glands*, or vulvovaginal glands. These pea-sized glands correspond to the male Cowper's glands. Each Bartholin's gland lies posterolaterally to the vaginal orifice. During sexual intercourse, a watery fluid is secreted that serves as a vaginal lubricant.

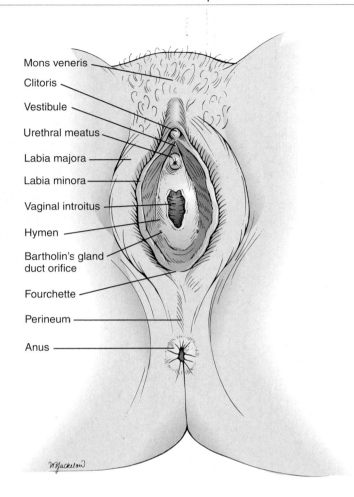

Mons veneris

Clitoris

Vestibule

Urethral meatus

Labia majora

Labia minora

Vaginal introitus

Hymen

Bartholin's gland
duct orifice

Fourchette

Perineum

Anus

Figure 19–1 The external female genitalia.

Inferiorly, the labia minora unite at the posterior commissure to form the *fourchette*. The *perineum* is the area between the fourchette and the anus.

The *hymen* is a circular fold of tissue that partially occludes the *vaginal introitus*. There are marked variations in its size, as well as in the number of openings in it. The vaginal introitus is the border between the external and internal genitalia and is located in the lower portion of the vestibule.

The blood supply to the external genitalia and perineum is predominantly from the internal pudendal arteries. The lymphatic drainage is into the superficial and deep inguinal nodes.

The internal genitalia are shown in Figure 19-2. The *vagina* is a muscularly walled, hollow canal that passes upward and slightly backward, at a right angle to the uterus. The vagina lies between the urinary bladder anteriorly and the rectum posteriorly. The vaginal walls are lined by transverse rugae, or folds. The lower portion of the cervix projects into the upper portion of the vagina and divides it into four fornices. The anterior fornix is shallow and is just posterior to the bladder. The posterior fornix is deep and is just anterior to the rectovaginal pouch, known as the *cul-de-sac (pouch) of Douglas*, and the pelvic viscera lie immediately above this pouch. The lateral fornices contain the broad ligaments. The fallopian tubes and ovaries may be palpated in the lateral fornices. The superficial cells of the vagina contain glycogen, which is acted on by the normal vaginal flora to produce lactic acid. This is in part responsible for the resistance of the vagina to infection.

The arterial supply to the vagina is derived from the internal iliac, uterine, and middle hemorrhoidal arteries. The lymphatic channels of the lower third of the vagina drain into the inguinal nodes. The lymphatic channels of the upper two thirds enter the hypogastric and sacral nodes.

The *uterus* is a hollow muscular organ with a small central cavity. The lower end is the *cervix*, and the upper portion is the *fundus*. The size of the uterus is different during various stages of life. At birth, the uterus is only 3 to 4 cm long. The adult uterus is 7 to 8 cm long and 3.5 cm wide, with an average wall thickness of 2 to 3 cm. The growth of the uterus and the relationship of the size of the fundus to the size of the cervix are shown in Figure 19-3.

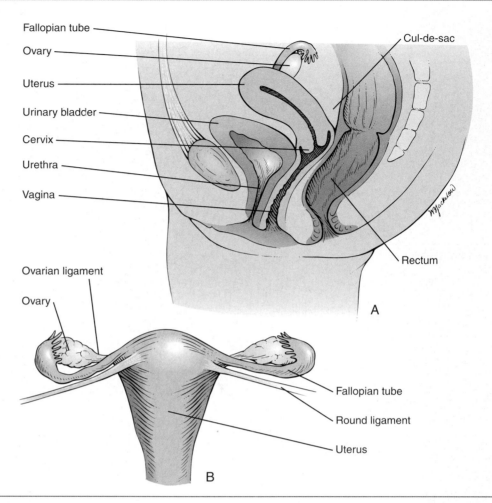

Figure 19–2 *A,* Cross-sectional view of the internal female genitalia. *B,* Frontal view of the uterus, fallopian tubes, and ovaries.

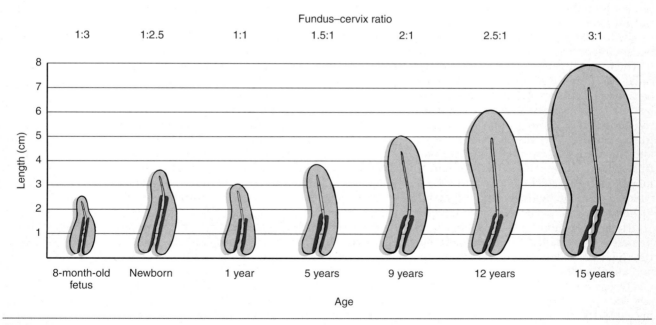

Figure 19–3 Growth of the uterus and changes in the fundus–cervix ratio with development. The darker red area represents the length of the cervix.

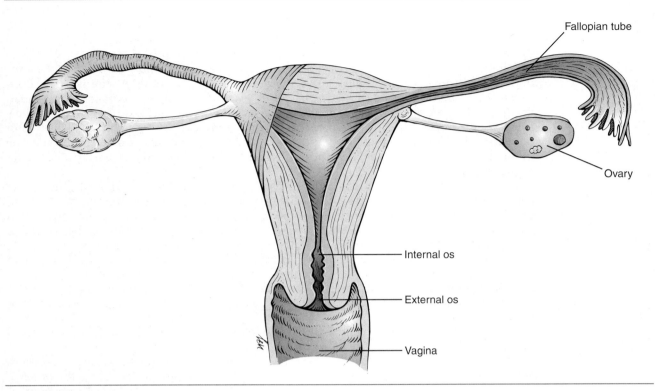

Figure 19–4 Anatomy of the uterus.

The triangular uterine cavity is 6 to 7 cm in length and is bounded by the *internal cervical os* inferiorly and the entrances of the fallopian tubes superiorly. Normally, the long axis of the uterus is bent forward on the long axis of the vagina. This is *anteversion*. The fundus is also bent slightly forward on the cervix. This is *anteflexion*.

The uterus is freely mobile and is located centrally in the pelvic cavity. It is supported by the broad and uterosacral ligaments, as well as by the pelvic floor. The peritoneum covers the fundus anteriorly down to the level of the internal cervical os. Posteriorly, the peritoneum covers the uterus down to the pouch of Douglas. The function of the uterus is childbearing. Figure 19-4 is a detailed anatomic representation of the uterus.

The cervix is the vaginal portion of the uterus. The greater portion of the cervix has no peritoneal covering. The cervical canal extends from the *external cervical os* to the internal cervical os, where it continues into the cavity of the fundus. The external cervical os in women who have not given birth vaginally is small and circular. In women who have had vaginal deliveries, the external cervical os is linear or oval.

With increasing levels of estrogens, the external cervical os begins to dilate, and cervical mucus secretion becomes clear and watery. With high levels of estrogens, cervical mucus, when placed between two glass slides that are then pulled apart, can be stretched 15 to 20 cm before breaking. This property of cervical mucus—the ability to be drawn into a fine thread—is termed *spinnbarkeit*. When cervical mucus is allowed to dry on a glass slide and is examined under low power by light microscopy, a *fern pattern* made up of salt crystals may be seen. Spinnbarkeit and ferning reach a maximum at the midpoint of the menstrual cycle. Sperm can more easily penetrate mucus with these characteristics.

The blood supply to the uterus comes from the uterine and ovarian arteries. The lymphatic vessels of the fundus enter into the lumbar nodes.

The *fallopian tubes*, or *oviducts*, enter the fundus at its superior aspect. They are small muscular tubes that extend outward into the broad ligament toward the pelvic wall. The other end of the oviduct opens into the peritoneal cavity near the ovary. These endings are surrounded by fringe-shaped projections called *fimbriae*. The primary function of the fallopian tube is to provide a conduit for and convey the egg from the corresponding ovary to the uterus, a trip that takes several days. Sperm traverse the oviduct in the opposite direction, and it is usually in the oviduct that fertilization takes place.

The *ovaries* are almond-shaped structures about 3 to 4 cm long and are attached to the broad ligament. The primary functions of the ovary are oogenesis and hormone production.

The ovaries, fallopian tubes, and supporting ligaments are termed the *adnexa*.

The female reproductive system is under the influence of the hypothalamus, whose releasing factors control the secretion of the anterior pituitary gonadotropic hormones: *follicle-stimulating hormone* and *luteinizing hormone*. In response to these hormones, the ovarian graafian follicle secretes estrogens and discharges its ovum. After ovulation, the ovarian follicle is termed the *corpus luteum*, which secretes estrogens and progesterone. With the secretion of progesterone, the basal body temperature rises. This is a reliable sign of ovulation. Under the influence of the ovarian hormones, the uterus and breasts undergo the characteristic changes of the menstrual cycle.

If pregnancy does not occur, the corpus luteum regresses, and the level of ovarian hormones begins to fall. At this time, before menstruation, many women have symptoms of weakness, depression, and irritability. Breast tenderness is also common. These symptoms are termed *premenstrual syndrome*. About 5 days after the fall in the level of hormones, the menstrual period begins. Menstrual fluid throughout the 5-day period measures about 50 to 150 mL, only half of which is blood; the remainder is mucus. Because menstrual blood does not contain fibrin, it does not clot. When the menstrual flow is heavy, as it is on days 1 to 2, "clots" may be described. These clots are not fibrin clots but are combinations of red blood cells, glycoproteins, and mucoid substances that are believed to form in the vagina rather than in the uterine cavity.

Some of the hormone-dependent changes related to the menstrual cycle are shown in Figure 19-5.

About 1.5 years before puberty, gonadotropins are measurable in the urine. The ovaries enter a period of rapid growth at, on average, 8 to 9 years of age, which marks the onset of puberty. Secretion of estrogens begins to increase rapidly at about 11 years of age. Concomitant with estrogen production, the sexual organs begin to mature. During puberty, the secondary sex characteristics begin to develop. The breasts enlarge, hair develops on the pubis, the vulva enlarges, the labia minora become pigmented, and the body contour changes. Puberty lasts for approximately 4 to 5 years. The first menstrual cycle, called *menarche*, occurs at the end of puberty at about 12.5 years of age. There is, however, a wide variation in the age at menarche. The cycles continue approximately every 28 days, with a flow lasting 3 to 5 days. The first day of the period is designated the first day of the cycle. It is rare for a woman to be absolutely regular, and cycles of 25 to 34 days are considered normal.

At the time of menarche, the menstrual cycle is usually anovulatory* and irregular. After 1 to 2 years, ovulation begins. After stabilization of the menses, ovulation occurs about midcycle in a woman with a regular cycle.

Menopause marks the ends of menstruation. *Menopause* is defined as the last uterine bleeding induced by ovarian function. It usually occurs between 45 and 55 years of age. Ovulation and corpus luteum formation no longer occur, and the ovaries decrease in size. The period after menopause is termed *postmenopausal*.

Review of Specific Symptoms

The most common symptoms of female genitourinary disease are as follows:

- Abnormal vaginal bleeding
- Dysmenorrhea
- Masses or lesions
- Vaginal discharge
- Vaginal itching
- Abdominal pain
- Dyspareunia
- Changes in hair distribution
- Changes in urinary pattern
- Infertility

---

*Not accompanied by the release of an ovum from the ovaries.

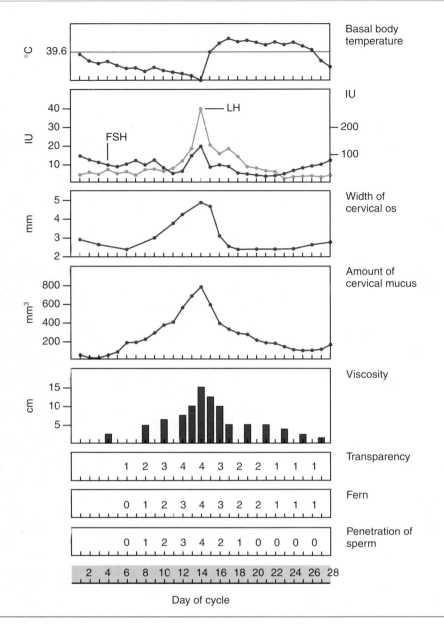

Figure 19–5 Physiologic changes associated with the menstrual cycle. The numbers 0 to 4 indicate an increasing characteristic of cervical mucus. Notice that ferning, transparency, and penetration of sperm are maximal at midcycle. FSH, follicle-stimulating hormone; LH, luteinizing hormone.

Abnormal Vaginal Bleeding

Ask these questions of any woman with abnormal vaginal bleeding:

"How long have you noticed the vaginal bleeding?"

"What types of contraceptives do you use?"

"How often are your periods?"

"What is the duration of your menstrual flow?"

"How many tampons or napkins do you use on each day of your flow?"

"Are there any clots of blood?"

"When was your last period?"

"Have you noticed bleeding between your periods?"

"Do you have abdominal pain during your periods?"

"Do you have hot flashes? cold sweats?"

"Do you have children?" If yes, *"When was your last one born?"*

"Do you think you might be pregnant?"

"Are you under any unusual emotional stress?"

"Have you noticed an intolerance to cold? heat?"

"Have you noticed a change in your vision?"

"Have you had any headaches? nausea? change in hair pattern? milk discharge from your nipples?"

"What is your diet like?"

Abnormal uterine bleeding, also known as *dysfunctional uterine bleeding*, includes amenorrhea, menorrhagia, metrorrhagia, and postmenopausal bleeding. *Amenorrhea* is the cessation or nonappearance of menstruation. Before puberty, amenorrhea is physiologic, as it is during pregnancy and after menopause. In primary amenorrhea, menstruation has never occurred; in secondary amenorrhea, menstruation has occurred but has ceased, as in pregnancy. Long-distance joggers, patients with anorexia, or any woman with abnormally low body fat may have secondary amenorrhea. Diseases of the hypothalamus, pituitary gland, ovary, uterus, and thyroid gland are associated with amenorrhea. Galactorrhea, or milk discharge from the nipples, occurs in many individuals with pituitary tumors. Chronic disease is also frequently associated with secondary amenorrhea.

Menorrhagia is excessive bleeding at the time of the menstrual period. The flow may be increased, the duration may be increased, or both may occur. The number of pads or tampons a patient uses each day of the cycle helps quantify the flow. Menorrhagia in some cases may be associated with blood disorders such as leukemia, inherited clotting abnormalities, and decreased platelet states. Uterine fibroids are a leading cause of menorrhagia. Menorrhagia secondary to fibroids is related to the large surface area of the endometrium from which bleeding occurs.

Metrorrhagia is uterine bleeding of normal amount at irregular, noncyclic intervals. Foreign bodies such as intrauterine devices, as well as ovarian and uterine tumors, can cause metrorrhagia. Often there is increased bleeding between cycles as well as heavier periods; this is termed *menometrorrhagia*.

Bleeding that occurs more than 6 to 8 months after menopause is termed *postmenopausal bleeding*. Any postmenopausal bleeding must be investigated. Uterine fibroids or tumors of the cervix, uterus, or ovary may be responsible.

Dysmenorrhea

Dysmenorrhea, or painful menstruation, is a common symptom. It is often difficult to define as abnormal, because many healthy women have some degree of menstrual discomfort. In most women, these cramps subside soon after the commencement of the menstrual flow. There are two types of dysmenorrhea: primary and secondary. Primary dysmenorrhea is far more common. It begins shortly after menarche, is associated with colicky uterine contractions, and occurs with every period. Childbirth frequently alleviates this state permanently. Secondary dysmenorrhea is caused by acquired disorders within the uterine cavity (e.g., intrauterine devices, polyps, or fibroids), obstruction to flow (e.g., cervical stenosis), or disorders of the pelvic peritoneum (e.g., endometriosis or pelvic inflammatory disease*). It usually occurs after several years of painless periods. Regardless of its cause, dysmenorrhea is described as intermittent, crampy pain accompanying the menstrual flow. The pain is felt in the lower abdomen and back, sometimes radiating down the legs. In severe cases, fainting, nausea, or vomiting may occur.

---

*Endometriosis is the presence of endometrial tissue outside the uterus and is a cause of chronic pelvic pain.

Masses or Lesions

Masses or lesions of the external genitalia are common. They may be related to venereal diseases, tumors, or infections. Ask these questions of any woman with a lesion on the genitalia:

"When did you first notice the mass (lesion)?"

"Is it painful?"

"Has it changed since you first noticed it?"

"Have you ever had it before?"

"Have you been exposed to anyone with venereal disease?"

Syphilis may result in a chancre on the labia. Often unnoticed, it is a small, painless nodule or ulcer with a sharply demarcated border. Small, acutely painful ulcers may be chancroid or genital herpes. A patient with an abscess of Bartholin's gland may present with an extremely tender mass in the vulva. Benign tumors, such as venereal warts (condylomata acuminata), and malignant conditions manifest as a mass on the external genitalia.

Some affected patients complain of a sensation of fullness or mass in the pelvis as a result of pelvic relaxation. *Pelvic relaxation* refers to the descent or protrusion of the vaginal walls or uterus through the vaginal introitus. This is caused by a weakening of the pelvic supports. The anterior vaginal wall can descend, producing a *cystocele* that triggers urinary symptoms such as frequency and stress incontinence. The posterior vaginal wall can descend, producing a *rectocele*, which triggers bowel symptoms such as constipation, tenesmus, or incontinence. The uterus can also descend, which results in uterine prolapse. In the most severe state, the uterus may lie outside the vulva with complete vaginal inversion, a condition known as *procidentia*. The consequences of pelvic relaxation are discussed further in the Clinicopathologic Correlations section of this chapter.

Vaginal Discharge

Vaginal discharges, also known as *leukorrhea*, are common. Is there an associated foul odor? Although a whitish discharge is often normally present, a fetid discharge often indicates a pathologic problem. The most common pathologic odor is a foul, fishy odor related to the volatilization of amines that are produced by anaerobic metabolism. Is itching also present? Women with moniliasis (candidiasis) complain of intense pruritus and a white, dry discharge that looks like cottage cheese. Has the woman recently taken any medications, such as antibiotics? Antibiotics change the normal vaginal flora, and an overgrowth of *Candida* may result. Table 19-1 summarizes the important characteristics of vaginal discharge.

Table 19–1 Characteristics of Common Vaginal Discharges

Feature	Physiologic Discharge	Nonspecific Vaginitis	*Trichomonas*	*Candida*	Gonococcal
Color	White	Gray	Grayish-yellow	White	Greenish-yellow
Fishy odor	Absent	Present	Present	Absent	Absent
Consistency	Nonhomogeneous	Homogeneous	Purulent, often with bubbles	Cottage cheese–like	Mucopurulent
Location	Dependent	Adherent to walls	Often pooled in fornix	Adherent to walls	Adherent to walls
Discharge at introitus	Rare	Common	Common	Common	Common
Vulva	Normal	Normal	Usually normal	Erythematous	Erythematous
Vaginal mucosa	Normal	Normal	Usually normal	Erythematous	Normal
Cervix	Normal	Normal	May have red spots	Has patches of discharge	Has pus in os

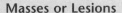

Vaginal Itching

Vaginal itching is associated with monilial infections, glycosuria,* vulvar leukoplakia, and any condition that predisposes a woman to vulvar irritation. Pruritus may also be a symptom of psychosomatic disease.

Abdominal Pain

Ask the following questions, in addition to those listed in Chapter 17, The Abdomen, of any woman with abdominal pain:

> *"When was your last period?"*
>
> *"Have you ever had any type of venereal disease?"*
>
> *"Is the pain related to your menstrual cycle?"* If yes, *"At what time in your cycle does it occur?"*
>
> *"Do you experience a burning sensation when you urinate?"*

Abdominal pain may be acute or chronic. Is the patient pregnant? Acute abdominal pain may be a complication of pregnancy. Spontaneous abortion, uterine perforation, and ectopic tubal pregnancy all are life-threatening situations. Acute inflammation by gonococci of the fallopian tubes and ovary, *salpingo-oophoritis*, can produce intense lower abdominal pain. Acute lower abdominal pain localized to one side that occurs at the time of ovulation is termed *mittelschmerz*. This pain is related to a small amount of intraperitoneal bleeding at the time of ovum release. Urinary tract infection may also cause acute pain. Patients with urinary tract infections usually have associated urinary symptoms of burning sensation or frequency.

Chronic abdominal pain may result from ectopic endometrial tissue, chronic pelvic inflammatory disease of the fallopian tubes and ovaries, and pelvic muscle relaxation with protrusion of the bladder, rectum, or uterus.

Dyspareunia

Dyspareunia is pain during or after sexual intercourse. Dyspareunia may be physiologic or psychogenic. Infections of the vulva, introitus, vagina, cervix, uterus, fallopian tubes, and ovaries have been associated with dyspareunia. Tumors of the rectovaginal septum, uterus, and ovaries have been described in patients who experienced painful sexual intercourse. Dyspareunia is often present in the absence of a physiologic disorder. A history of painful pelvic examinations and a fear of pregnancy are common in these patients. Women may have "penetration anxiety" until they are assured that the vagina can be penetrated by a penis. In these individuals, such anxiety may lead to *vaginismus*, a condition of severe pelvic pain and spasm when the labia are merely touched. In other women, dyspareunia may develop during times of stress or emotional conflict. The examiner can obtain valuable information by asking, "What else is going on in your life now?" Dryness of the vagina and labia may cause irritation that can result in dyspareunia.

Changes in Hair Distribution

Hair loss or change in hair distribution may occur during certain states of hormonal imbalance. *Hirsutism* is an excessive growth of hair on the upper lip, face, earlobes, upper pubic triangle, trunk, or limbs. *Virilization* is extensive hirsutism associated with receding temporal hair, a deepening of the voice, and clitoral enlargement. Increased androgen production by the adrenal glands or ovaries may be responsible for these phenomena. Tumors of the ovary are commonly associated with amenorrhea, rapidly developing hirsutism, and virilization. Polycystic ovarian disease is the most common ovarian cause of hirsutism, dysfunctional uterine bleeding, infertility, acne, and obesity. Figure 19-6 shows the increased hair growth

---

*High levels of glucose in the urine, as in diabetes.

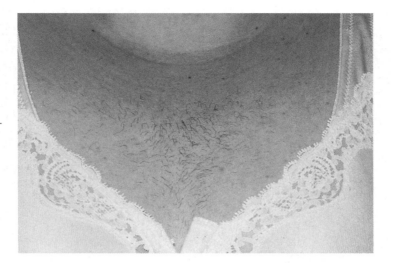

Figure 19–6 Increased hair growth in a patient with polycystic ovary syndrome.

on the chest of a 34-year-old woman with polycystic ovary syndrome. She also presented with amenorrhea and obesity. Figure 19-7 shows the face of a 68-year-old woman with an androgen-secreting ovarian tumor. Note the male-pattern baldness and the facial hair. This patient also had clitoral enlargement.

It is important to determine whether the patient is taking any medications. Several drugs such as cyclosporine, minoxidil, diazoxide, penicillamine, and glucocorticoids have the unexpected side effect of causing diffuse hair growth on the face. Figure 19-8 shows such growth in a 42-year-old woman who was taking minoxidil for hypertension. This drug is now used as a topical treatment for androgenetic alopecia. The pathophysiologic process behind the increased hair growth is unknown.

Hair loss, or *alopecia*, is a distressing problem. Many drugs may have a profound effect on hair growth. The interviewer must inquire whether the patient has taken any chemotherapeutic agents or has been exposed to radiation. Different areas of the head seem to respond differently to androgens. The top and front of the scalp respond to increased androgen production by hair loss, whereas the face responds with increased hair growth. Has the patient been dieting? Because hair has a high metabolic rate, crash diets and

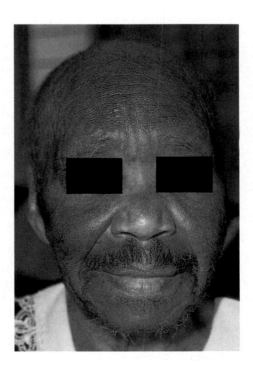

Figure 19–7 Increased hair growth in a patient with an androgen-secreting ovarian tumor.

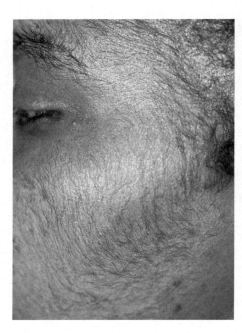

Figure 19–8 Increased hair growth caused by minoxidil antihypertensive therapy.

infectious diseases reduce the nutrients available for hair growth, and secondary alopecia may result.

Changes in Urinary Pattern

Changes in the patterns of urination are common. Chapter 18, Male Genitalia and Hernias, reviews many of the symptoms associated with changes in the urinary pattern. These symptoms may occur in women as well.

Stress incontinence is urinary incontinence that occurs with straining or coughing. Stress incontinence is more common among women than among men. The female urinary bladder and urethra are maintained in position by several muscular and fascial supports. It has been postulated that estrogens may be responsible, at least in part, for a weakening of the pelvic support. With aging, the support of the bladder neck, the length of the urethra, and the competence of the pelvic floor are decreased. Repeated vaginal deliveries, strenuous exercise, and chronic coughing increase the chance for stress incontinence. Ask an affected patient these questions:

> *"Do you lose your urine on straining? coughing? lifting? laughing?"*
>
> *"Do you lose your urine constantly?"*
>
> *"Do you lose small amounts of urine?"*
>
> *"Are you aware of a full bladder?"*
>
> *"Do you have to press on your abdomen to void?"*
>
> *"Are you aware of any weakness in your limbs?"*
>
> *"Have you ever had a loss of vision?"*
>
> *"Do you have diabetes?"*

Patients with pure stress incontinence describe urine loss without urgency that occurs during any activity that momentarily increases intra-abdominal pressure. Although stress incontinence is common among women, it is important to rule out other types of incontinence, such as neurologic, overflow, and psychogenic. *Neurologic incontinence* may result from cerebral dysfunction, spinal cord disease, and peripheral nerve lesions. Multiple sclerosis is a chronic relapsing neurologic disorder causing urinary incontinence. Most affected individuals suffer from an episode of temporary loss of vision as an early symptom. *Overflow incontinence* occurs when the pressure in the bladder exceeds the urethral pressure in the absence of bladder contraction. This may occur in patients with diabetes and an atonic bladder. In *psychogenic incontinence*, individuals have been known to urinate in bed at night to "warm" themselves or during the daytime in group settings to draw attention to themselves.

Infertility

Infertility may result from failure to ovulate, called *anovulation*, or from inadequate function of the corpus luteum. Both these conditions can occur in women with cyclic menstrual bleeding. Therefore, having a period does not indicate fertility. A woman with the symptom of infertility should be asked these questions:

> *"Do you have regular menstrual periods?"*
>
> *"Have you kept a chart of your basal body temperature?"*
>
> *"Have you ever had venereal disease?"*
>
> *"Have you been tested for thyroid disease?"*
>
> *"Have you taken any medications to promote fertility?"*

Charting basal body temperature is a reliable method for detecting ovulation. Gonococcal disease in a woman may lead to salpingo-oophoritis, with scarring of the fallopian tubes and infertility. Hypothyroidism is a well-known cause of infertility.

General Suggestions

Even in the absence of specific symptoms, all women, regardless of age, should be asked several important questions. The answers to the following questions provide a complete gynecologic, obstetric, and reproductive history. The first group of questions is related to the *gynecologic history* and menstrual cycle:

> *"At what age did you start to menstruate?"*
>
> *"How often do your periods occur?"*
>
> *"Are they regular?"*
>
> *"For how many days do you have menstrual flow?"*
>
> *"How many pads or tampons do you use each day of your flow?"*
>
> *"During your menstrual cycle, do you experience any breast tenderness or breast pain? bloating? swelling? headache? edema?"*
>
> *"When was your last menstrual period?"*

The *catamenia* refers to the menstrual history and summarizes the age at menarche, the cycle length, and the duration of flow. If a woman reached menarche at age 12 years and has had regular periods every 29 days lasting for 5 days, the catamenia can be summarized as "CAT 12 × 29 × 5." The date of the last menstrual period can be abbreviated as, for example, "LMP: August 10, 2008."

Any recurrent, midcyclic symptom associated with the menstrual period, such as breast tenderness, bloating, and so forth, is termed *molimen*. The presence of molimen is correlated with ovulation, although not all women experience molimen when ovulation occurs. Therefore, molimen is a specific but nonsensitive sign of ovulation.

The next group of questions is related to the *obstetric history:*

> *"Have you ever been pregnant?"*

If the woman has been pregnant, ask the following questions:

> *"What was the outcome of your pregnancy?"*
>
> *"How many full-term pregnancies have you had?"*

"Have you had any children born prematurely?"

"How many living children do you have?"

"How were your children delivered (vaginally, cesarean)?"

"What were the birth weights of your children?"

The obstetric history includes the number of pregnancies, known as *gravidity*, and the number of deliveries, known as *parity*. If a woman has had three full-term infants (born at 37 weeks or more of gestation), two premature infants (born at less than 37 weeks of gestation), one miscarriage (or abortion), and four living children, her obstetric history can be summarized as "para 3-2-1-4." An easy way to remember this four-digit parity code is with the mnemonic *"Florida Power And Light,"* which stands for *f*ull term, *p*remature, *a*bortions (miscarriages), *l*iving. The woman in this example is *gravida 6*.

In the United States, *never* ask a woman whether she has had an abortion. This word is charged with many religious, political, and cultural feelings. In many other parts of the world, however, the term *abortion* is often acceptable because it means the loss of a pregnancy, not the voluntary termination of a pregnancy.

When asking a woman about the date of her last menstrual period, never assume that menopause has occurred. Women of any age should be asked when their last menstrual period occurred. Allow the patient to say that she has not had a period in, for example, 12 years.

A careful sexual history is important. Chapter 1, The Interviewer's Questions, provides several ways of broaching the topic. The interviewer might start by asking, "Are you satisfied with your sex life?" It is important for the examiner to determine the marital status of the patient. Is the patient married? How many times? For how long? Are there other sexual partners? If the patient is not married, is she currently having sexual relationships? What type of birth control is being used? It is important to ask all sexually active women the following:

"How easily can you reach an orgasm or climax?"

"How strong is your sex drive?"

"How easily are you sexually aroused?"

"How easily does your vagina become moist during sex?"

"Are your orgasms satisfying?"

Always determine whether the patient's mother was given diethylstilbestrol (DES)* during her pregnancy.

Use words that the patient will understand. It may be necessary to use such terms as "lips" to refer to the labia or "privates" to refer to the genitalia.

Impact of Infertility on the Patient

The problem of infertility is not new. From ancient times, cultures have practiced fertility rites to ensure the continuation of their people. Many societies considered a woman's worth in terms of her ability to have children. The "barren woman" was frequently banished.

The average time it takes for a woman to conceive is 4 to 5 months. The American Fertility Society defines infertility as the inability to conceive "after one year of regular coitus without contraception." During this time, more than 80% of women conceive. After 3 years of regular sexual intercourse, 98% of women become pregnant.

It has been estimated that approximately one of every six couples in the United States has some problem with fertility. Infertility should be considered a problem of both men and

---

*DES was given to many pregnant women from 1940 to 1975 for a variety of reasons, such as threatened abortion and premature labor. Vaginal involvement by adenosis often developed in exposed daughters. Carcinoma of the vagina or cervix, as well as cervical incompetence, has also occasionally been reported in the offspring.

women. It was previously thought that infertility was *functional* (no demonstrable organ disorder) in 30% to 50% of all cases, but it is now recognized that more than 90% of infertile couples have a pathologic cause. However, only about 50% of these couples achieve pregnancy. Fifty percent of infertility is related to a female problem,* 30% to a male problem,† and 20% to a combined problem.

Infertility is one of several important developmental crises of adult life. The impact of infertility on a woman can be severe. The influence of the higher nervous system on ovulation is well known but only partially understood. When a woman is told that she is infertile, she may be shocked and distressed about the loss of an important function of her body. This psychologic injury lasts for variable amounts of time. Often the woman feels defective or inadequate. This extends to her interactions with others, in addition to her sexual function. Her attitude toward her job may change; her work productivity may decline. There is a significant decrease in sexual desire. Depression, loss of libido, and concern over whether conception will ever occur combine to make sex a less pleasurable activity and decrease the possibility of normal ovulation. A period of mourning and frustration usually occurs.

Often the woman becomes preoccupied with her menstrual periods. When will the next one come? Is she pregnant? Did she have any symptoms of ovulation? When the next menstrual cycle occurs, the woman suffers further grief.

The infertile woman may fear that her partner will resent her, and she may feel alienated from him. She may experience jealousy and resentment toward friends or relations who have children. Her infertility lowers her self-esteem and may make her feel that she is unfit to be a parent.

Regardless of the cause of infertility, the treatment must work to lessen the psychologic side effects. Both partners must be encouraged to communicate. Education regarding the physical problem is important throughout the medical work-up. Communication between the partners and the physician is paramount. The patient needs to be protected from her own insecurities and treated with empathy and compassion.

In some women, psychogenic factors may be the sole cause of infertility. Such factors may act at various phases in the reproductive process. These women may have immature personalities and fear the responsibilities of motherhood. They use their infertility as a defense mechanism. In other cases, emotional conflicts may lead to somatic symptoms and signs. Vaginismus is the most common psychosomatic disorder causing infertility. In this condition, the introitus may become so constricted that it inhibits the penis from entering. Vaginismus protects the patient from conception. Many of these women view sexual intercourse as exploitative and degrading. Intercourse is feared because it is painful. These patients do well with psychotherapy that allows them to express their fears about intercourse, genitalia, and childbearing.

Physical Examination

The equipment necessary for the examination of the female genitalia and rectum consists of a vaginal speculum, lubricant, cervical scrapers, cotton-tipped applicators, gloves, glass slides, occult blood testing card and Hemoccult developer, culture media (as appropriate), fixative, tissues, and a light source.

General Considerations

Unlike most other parts of the physical examination, the pelvic examination is often viewed with apprehension by the patient. This is frequently related to a previous bad experience. An examination performed slowly and gently with adequate explanations goes a long way in developing a good doctor-patient relationship. Communication is the key to a successful pelvic examination. The examiner should talk to the patient and tell her exactly what is going to be done. Eye contact is also necessary to decrease the patient's anxiety. The patient's ability to relax enables a more accurate and less traumatic examination.

---

*In general, fallopian tubal patency or ovulation problems.
†Vas deferens obstruction, varicocele, chromosomal defects, testicular infection, autoimmune states, and decreased sperm count are the most important.

If the examiner is a man, he should examine the patient's genitalia in the presence of a female attendant. Although not required by law, the presence of a female attendant is important for assistance, as well as for medicolegal considerations, especially when the patient appears overly upset or seductive. At times, the patient may request that a family member be present. The examiner should grant such a request if no other attendant is available.

Throughout the world, various patient positions are preferred to facilitate the pelvic examination. These include the woman's lying on her back on an examining table, lying in bed on her left side, lying on her back in bed with her legs abducted, and sitting upright in a chair with her legs abducted. In the United States, the woman usually lies on her back on an examination table with her feet in heel rests. This position can be uncomfortable and demeaning.

Preparation for the Examination

The patient should be instructed to empty her bladder and bowels before the examination. The patient is assisted onto an examination table with her buttocks placed near its edge. The heel rests of the table are extended, and the patient is instructed to place her heels in them. If possible, some cloth should be placed over the rests. Alternatively, the patient can be given plastic foam booties to protect her feet from cold metal heel rests. Shortening the heel rest brackets helps the woman bend her knees to lower the position of the cervix. An older patient with osteoarthritis may need the heel rests to be longer because she may have limited hip and knee motion. Offer the patient a mirror that she can use to observe the examination.

The head of the examination table should be elevated so that eye contact between the physician and the patient can occur. A sheet is usually draped over the lower abdomen and knees of the patient. Some patients prefer not to have the sheet used. The patient should be asked her preference.

The knees are drawn up sufficiently to relax the abdominal muscles as the thighs are abducted. Ask the patient to let her legs relax to the sides or to drop her knees to each side. Never tell a patient to "spread her legs."

Gloves should be worn for the examination of the female genitalia. The examiner should be seated on a stool between the legs of the patient. Good lighting, including a light source directed into the vagina, is essential.

The examination of the female genitalia consists of the following:

- Inspection and palpation of external genitalia
- Examination with speculum
- Bimanual palpation
- Rectovaginal palpation

Inspection and Palpation of External Genitalia

Inspect the External Genitalia and Hair

To make the woman more comfortable during inspection of the external genitalia, it is often useful to touch the patient. Tell the patient that you are going to touch her leg. Use the *back* of your hand.

The external genitalia should be inspected carefully. The mons veneris is inspected for lesions and swelling. The hair is inspected for its pattern and for pubic lice and nits. The skin of the vulva is inspected for redness, excoriation, masses, leukoplakia, and changes in pigmentation. Lesions should be palpated for tenderness.

Lichen sclerosus, previously known as *kraurosis vulvae*, is a relatively common condition in which the genital skin shows a uniform reddened, smooth, shiny, almost transparent appearance. It is a destructive inflammatory condition with a predilection for genital skin. It is much more common in women, although it can be seen in men with involvement of the glans penis and foreskin. Whitish atrophic patches of thin skin are typical, as is fine crinkling of the skin. Pruritus is a common symptom, and the fragile skin is susceptible to secondary infection. Although most common in white and Latino postmenopausal women, lichen sclerosus may be seen in patients of all ages. It is rare in African-American women. Lichen sclerosus should be thought of as a premalignant lesion because one complication is the development of squamous cell carcinoma. Figure 19-9 shows an early stage of lichen sclerosus in a female patient. Notice the resorption of the labia minora; the clitoris is preserved. Figure 19-10 shows a later stage in

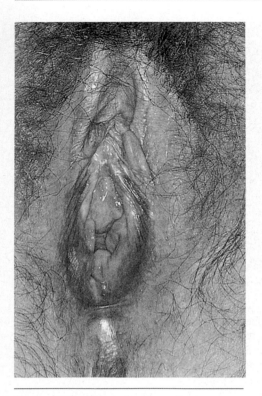

Figure 19–9 Lichen sclerosus, early stage.

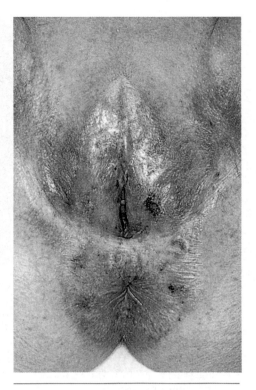

Figure 19–10 Lichen sclerosus, later stage. Note the classic whitish crinkling of the skin and resorption of the labia and clitoris.

another patient. Notice the classic whitish crinkling of the skin and the resorption of the labia and clitoris. Figure 19-11 shows vulvar squamous cell carcinoma with the background of lichen sclerosus in another patient.

Inspect the Labia

Tell the patient that you are now going to touch and spread the labia, as demonstrated in Figure 19-12. Inspect the vaginal introitus.

Figure 19–11 Squamous cell carcinoma with background of lichen sclerosus.

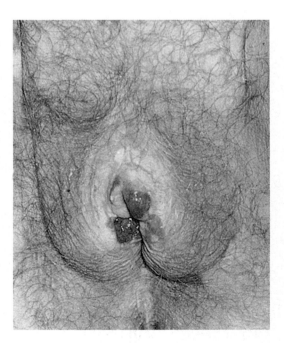

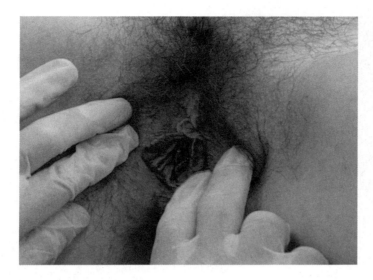

Figure 19–12 Technique for inspecting the labia.

The labia minora may show wide variation in size and shape; they may be asymmetric. On occasion, yellowish-white, asymptomatic papules may be seen over the inner labia minora. These are called *Fordyce's spots* and are normal; they represent ectopic sebaceous glands. Figure 19-13 shows Fordyce's spots. Ectopic sebaceous glands are also common in the mouth (see Fig. 12-18) and on the shaft of the penis (see Fig. 18-11).

Inflammatory lesions, ulceration, discharge, scarring, warts, trauma, swelling, atrophic changes, and masses are noted. Figures 19-14 and 19-15 show condylomata acuminata of the labia.

Inspect the Clitoris

Inspect the clitoris for size and lesions. The clitoris is normally 3 to 4 mm in size.

Inspect the Urethral Meatus

Is pus or inflammation present? If pus is present, determine its source. Dip a cotton-tipped applicator into the discharge, and spread the sample on a microscope slide for later evaluation. Are any masses present?

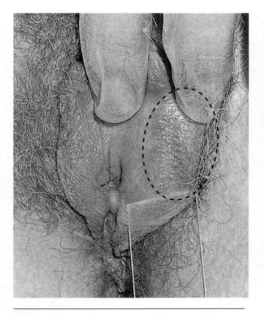

Figure 19–13 Fordyce's spots of the labia.

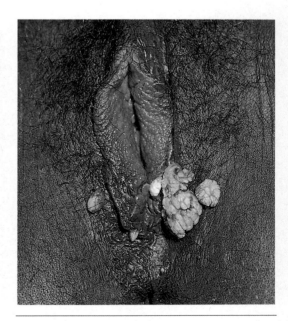

Figure 19–14 Condylomata acuminata.

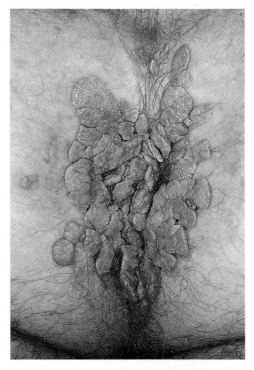

Figure 19–15 Condylomata acuminata.

A *urethral caruncle* is a small benign tumor at the urethral orifice and is relatively common in postmenopausal women. It appears as a bright red or flesh-colored mass extending through the urethral orifice. It may be asymptomatic or may cause pain or bleeding. Urethral caruncles must be differentiated from other tumors by biopsy.

Inspect the Area of Bartholin's Glands

Tell the patient that you are going to palpate the glands of the labia. With a moistened glove, palpate the area of the right gland (at the 7 to 8 o'clock position) by grasping the posterior portion of the right labia between your right index finger in the vagina and your right thumb on the outside, as demonstrated in Figure 19-16. Is any tenderness, swelling, or pus present? Normally, Bartholin's glands can be neither seen nor felt. Use your left hand to examine the area of the left gland (at the 4 to 5 o'clock position).

Figure 19-17 shows an abscess in the left Bartholin's gland.

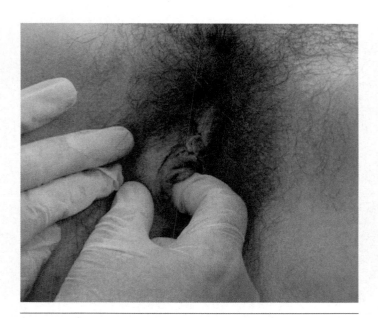

Figure 19–16 Technique for palpation of Bartholin's glands.

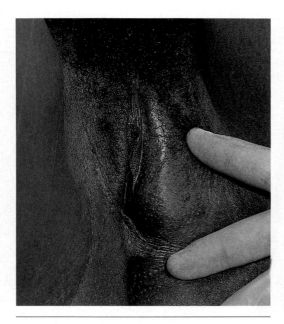

Figure 19–17 Bartholin's gland abscess.

Inspect the Perineum

The perineum and anus are inspected for masses, scars, fissures, and fistulas. Is the perineal skin reddened? The anus should be inspected for hemorrhoids, irritation, and fissures.

Test for Pelvic Relaxation

While you gently separate the labia widely and depress the perineum, ask the patient to bear down or cough. If vaginal relaxation is present, ballooning of the anterior or posterior walls may be seen. Bulging of the anterior wall is associated with a cystocele; bulging of the posterior wall is indicative of a rectocele. If stress incontinence is present, the coughing or bearing down may trigger a spurt of urine from the urethral orifice.

Examination with Speculum

Preparation

The speculum examination entails inspecting the vagina and cervix. There are several types of specula. The metal *Cusco*, or *bivalve*, speculum is the most popular. This speculum consists of two blades or bills that are introduced closed into the vagina and are then opened by squeezing the handle mechanism. The vaginal walls are held apart by the bills, and adequate visualization of the vagina and cervix is achieved. There are basically two types of bivalve specula: Graves' and Pedersen's. *Graves'* speculum is more common and is used for most adult women. The bills are wider and are curved on the sides. *Pedersen's* speculum has narrower, flat bills and is used for women with a small introitus. The plastic, disposable bivalve speculum is becoming more common. A disadvantage to its use is the loud click made as the lower bill is disengaged during removal from the vagina. If a plastic speculum is used, the patient should be informed that this sound will occur. Check the bills to make sure that there are no rough edges.

Before using the speculum in a patient, practice opening and closing it. If the patient has never had a speculum examination, show the speculum to her. You should warm the speculum with warm water and then touch it to the dorsum of your hand to ensure that the temperature is suitable. Jelly lubricant should not be used because it may interfere with cervical cytologic determination and gonococcal cultures. Tell the patient that you are now going to perform the speculum part of the internal examination.

Technique

While the examiner's left index and middle fingers separate the labia and firmly depress the perineum, the closed speculum, held in the examiner's right hand, is introduced *slowly* into the introitus at an oblique angle of 45° from the vertical over the examiner's left fingers. This procedure is demonstrated in Figures 19-18 and 19-19 and is diagrammed in Figure 19-20. Do not introduce the speculum vertically, because injury to the urethra or meatus may occur.

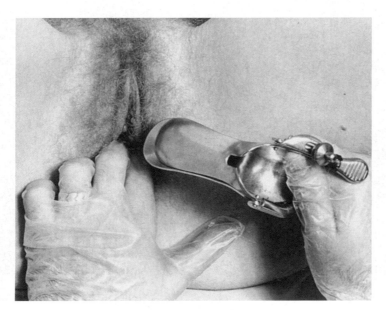

Figure 19–18 Technique for insertion of the vaginal speculum. Note the examiner's fingers pressing downward on the perineum.

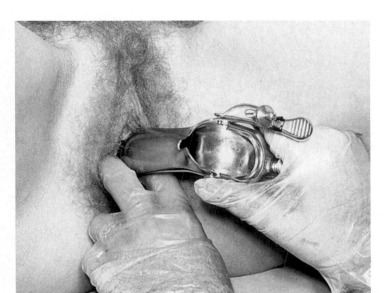

Figure 19–19 Technique for insertion of the vaginal speculum. Note that the speculum rides over the examiner's fingers, avoiding contact with the external urethral meatus and clitoris.

Inspect the Cervix

The speculum is introduced to full depth. When it is inserted completely, the speculum is rotated to the horizontal position, with the handle now pointing downward, and is opened *slowly*. With the bills open, the vaginal walls and cervix can be visualized. The cervix should rest within the bills of the speculum. This is demonstrated in Figure 19-21 and diagrammed in Figure 19-22. To keep the speculum open, the set screw can be tightened. If the cervix is not immediately seen, gently turn the bills in various directions to expose the cervix. The most common reason for not visualizing the cervix is failure to insert the speculum far enough before opening it.

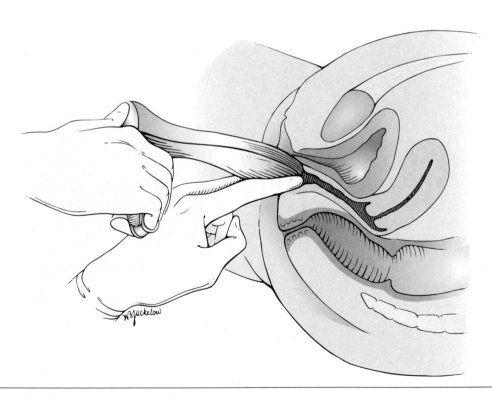

Figure 19–20 Cross-sectional view of the speculum examination.

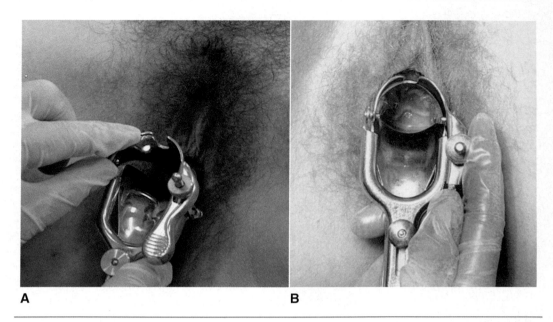

A   B

Figure 19–21 Technique for inspecting the cervix. *A,* Opening of the speculum bills after the speculum has been fully inserted and rotated to the transverse position. *B,* Internal view of the cervix when the speculum is correctly inserted.

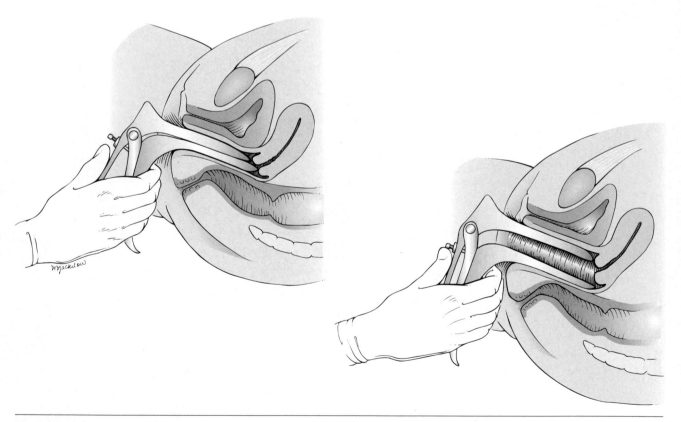

Figure 19–22 Cross-sectional view illustrating the position of the speculum during inspection of the cervix.

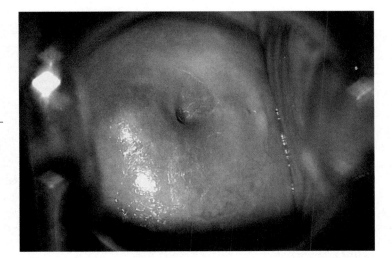

Figure 19–23 A normal cervix. Note the round external cervical os in a nulliparous woman.

If a discharge is obscuring any part of the vaginal walls or cervix, the discharge should be removed with a cotton-tipped applicator and spread onto a glass microscope slide.

Inspect the cervix for color, discharge, erythema, erosion, ulceration, leukoplakia, scars, and masses. What is the shape of the external cervical os? A bluish discoloration of the cervix may be an indication of pregnancy or a large tumor.

A normal cervix is seen in Figure 19-23. Notice that the external cervical os is round, which is characteristic of the cervix of a woman who has never had a vaginal delivery.

Pap Smear

A Pap* smear is obtained with a wooden Ayres' cervical scraper inserted through the speculum, as demonstrated in Figure 19-24. The longer end of the scraper is inserted into the external cervical os (Fig. 19-25). The scraper is then rotated 360° while it scrapes off cells from the external cervical os. Other specimens are taken with a cotton-tipped applicator from the posterior and lateral vaginal fornices and from the endocervix.

Traditionally, the sample is smeared directly onto a glass microscope slide, fixed, and then sent to the laboratory. The average conventional slide contains 50,000 to 300,000 cells to review. For more than 50 years, all cervical cytology samples were handled this way. This method works quite well and is relatively inexpensive. However, cells smeared onto the slide are sometimes mounded up on each other, so cells at the bottom of the pile cannot be clearly seen. Excessive blood, bacteria, mucus, inflammatory cells, or yeast cells may hide the cervical cells, making review more difficult. A newer method, the *liquid-based cytology*, or *liquid-based Pap, test*, can remove most of the blood, mucus, bacteria, yeast, and pus cells in a sample and can spread the cervical cells more evenly on the slide. The cervical/endocervical sample is collected in the same conventional manner with a broom-type or Cytobrush/plastic spatula cervical sampling device. Instead of being directly placed on a slide, the sample is placed into a vial with a special preservative solution. This new method, performed with the *ThinPrep* or *SurePath* system, also prevents cells from drying out and becoming distorted.

Studies have revealed that liquid-based testing can slightly improve detection of cancers, greatly improve detection of precancerous conditions, and reduce the number of tests that need to be repeated. This method is, however, more expensive than a usual Pap smear. The liquid-based Pap test has a higher sensitivity and lower specificity than conventional Pap tests; more false-positive results are obtained with this type of Pap test. Women with positive test results must receive a full diagnostic work-up to distinguish the true-positive results from the false-positive results. According to the National Cervical Cancer Coalition, in the United States today, approximately 90% of all Pap tests are performed with the liquid-based technology. Although liquid-based Pap smears demonstrate distinct advantages in slide quality and

---

*Named for George N. Papanicolaou, the physician who developed this screening technique. When properly performed, the Pap test can accurately diagnose cervical carcinoma in 98% of cases and can detect 80% of cases of endometrial carcinoma.

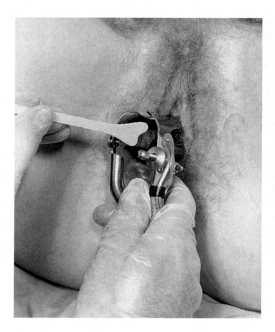

Figure 19–24 Technique for obtaining a smear for the Papanicolaou (Pap) test.

adjunctive HPV testing, there is no consensus recommendation in favor of abandoning conventional Pap smears.

Because the Pap smear may cause the cervix to bleed slightly, advise the patient that she may have a little spotting, which is normal. Any significant bleeding, however, should be evaluated. The results of the Pap smear are usually available in 2 to 3 weeks.

Inspect the Vaginal Walls

The patient is told that the speculum will now be removed. The set screw is released with the examiner's right index finger, and the speculum is rotated back to the original oblique

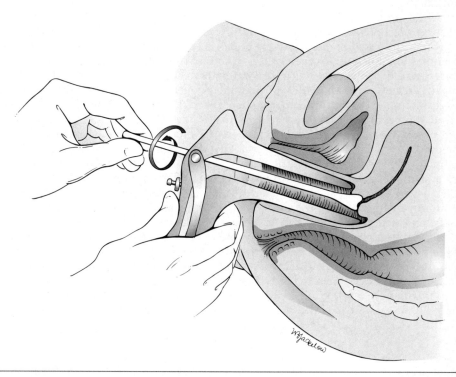

Figure 19–25 Technique for obtaining a smear for the Papanicolaou (Pap) test. Note that the longer end of the wooden spatula is placed in the cervical os.

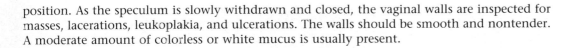

position. As the speculum is slowly withdrawn and closed, the vaginal walls are inspected for masses, lacerations, leukoplakia, and ulcerations. The walls should be smooth and nontender. A moderate amount of colorless or white mucus is usually present.

Bimanual Palpation

The bimanual examination is used to palpate the uterus and adnexa. Lower the head of the examination table to a 15° angle or flat, depending on the patient's preference. In this examination, the examiner's fingers are placed in the patient's vagina and on the abdomen, and the pelvic structures are palpated between the hands. In general, the right hand is inserted into the vagina and the left hand palpates the abdomen, but this is a matter of personal preference.

Technique

The examiner should be positioned between the patient's legs. If the examiner's right hand is to be used vaginally, the examiner places his or her right foot on a small footrest or stool. A suitable jelly lubricant is held in the left hand, and a small amount is dropped from the tube onto the examiner's gloved right index and middle fingers. The examiner should not touch the tube of lubricant to the gloves, because such touching will contaminate the lubricant. The patient is told that the internal examination will now begin.

As the bimanual examination is being performed, the examiner should observe the patient's face. Her expression will quickly reveal whether the examination is painful. The labia are spread, and the examiner's lubricated right index and middle fingers are introduced vertically into the vagina. A downward pressure toward the perineum is applied. The right fourth and fifth fingers are flexed into the palm of the hand. The right thumb is extended. The area around the clitoris should not be touched. The examiner may now rest the right elbow on his or her right knee so that undue pressure is not placed on the patient. There is no need to palpate deeply with the "abdominal hand" if the uterus is sufficiently elevated with the "vaginal hand."

The correct positions of the examiner, assistant, and patient are demonstrated in Figure 19-26.

The vaginal walls are palpated for nodules, scarring, and induration.

Once inserted into the vagina, the examiner's right (vaginal) hand is rotated 90° clockwise so that the palm is facing upward. Some clinicians prefer not to rotate the vaginal hand because this may decrease the depth of penetration. The left hand is now placed on the abdomen approximately one third of the way to the umbilicus from the pubic symphysis. The wrist of the abdominal hand should not be flexed or supinated. The vaginal hand pushes the pelvic organs up out of the pelvis and stabilizes them while they are palpated by the abdominal hand. It is the abdominal, not the vaginal, hand that performs the palpation. The technique for the bimanual examination is shown in Figure 19-27 and diagrammed in Figure 19-28.

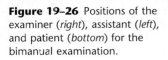

Figure 19–26 Positions of the examiner (*right*), assistant (*left*), and patient (*bottom*) for the bimanual examination.

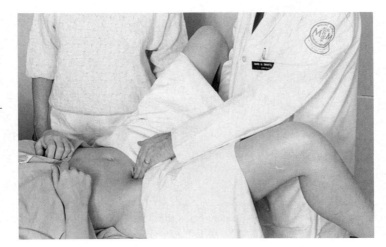

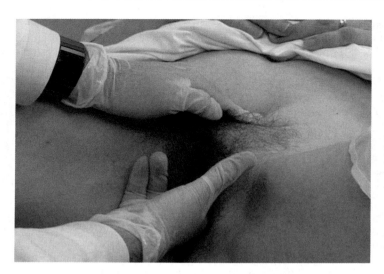

Figure 19–27 Technique for the bimanual examination.

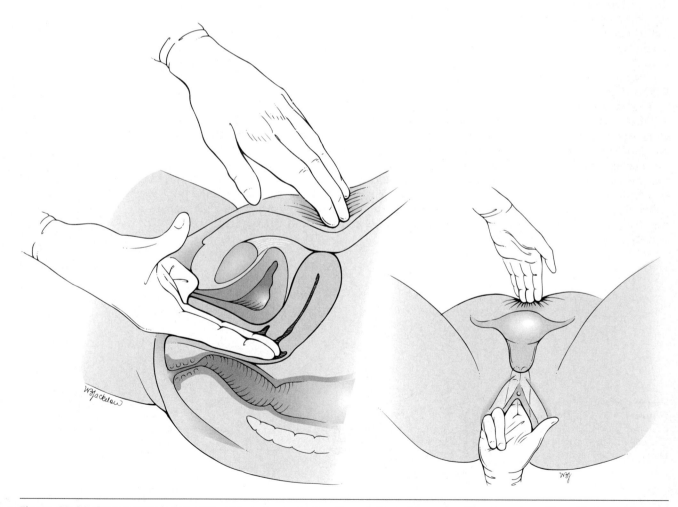

Figure 19–28 Cross-sectional view of the bimanual examination through the pelvic organs. The uterus is positioned between the examining hands. Note the position of the right thumb, held away from the clitoris.

Palpate the Cervix and Uterine Body

The cervix is palpated. What is its consistency (soft, firm, nodular, friable)?

Tell the patient that she will now feel you move her cervix and uterus, but this should not be painful. The cervix can usually be moved 2 to 4 cm in any direction. The cervix is pushed backward and upward toward the abdominal hand as the abdominal hand pushes downward. Any restriction of motion or the development of pain on movement should be noted. Pushing the cervix up and back tends to tip an anteverted, anteflexed uterus forward into a position where it is more easily palpated. The uterus should then be felt between the two hands. Describe its *position, size, shape, consistency, mobility*, and *tenderness*. Determine whether the uterus is anteverted or retroverted. Is it enlarged, firm, or mobile? Are any irregularities felt? Is there any tenderness when the uterus is moved?

Palpation by the bimanual technique is possible only if the uterus is anteverted and anteflexed, which is the most common uterine position. A retroverted uterus is directed toward the spine and is not easily felt by bimanual palpation.

Palpate the Adnexa

After the uterus has been evaluated, the right and left adnexa are palpated. If the patient has complained of pain on one side, start the examination on the other side. The right hand should move to the left lateral fornix while the left (abdominal) hand moves to the patient's left lower quadrant. The vaginal fingers lift the adnexa toward the abdominal hand, which attempts to palpate the adnexal structures. This is illustrated in Figure 19-29.

The adnexa should be explored for masses. Describe the *size, shape, consistency*, and *mobility*, as well as any *tenderness*, of the structures in the adnexa. The normal ovary is sensitive to pressure when squeezed. After the left side is examined, the right adnexa are palpated by moving the right (vaginal) hand to the right lateral fornix and the left (abdominal) hand to the patient's right lower quadrant.

In many women, the adnexal structures cannot be palpated. In thin women, the ovaries are frequently palpable. Adnexal tenderness or enlargement is relatively specific for a pathologic state.

After completion of the examination of the adnexa, the examining vaginal fingers move to the posterior fornix to palpate the uterosacral ligaments and the pouch of Douglas. Marked tenderness and nodularity are suggestive of endometriosis.

If the patient has borne children, the examiner should have no difficulty using the right index and middle fingers in the vagina for bimanual palpation. If the introitus is small, the examiner should introduce the right middle finger first and gently push downward toward the anus. By stretching the introitus, the right index finger can be introduced with little discomfort. If the patient is a virgin, only the right middle finger should be used.

Rectovaginal Palpation

Palpate the Rectovaginal Septum

Tell the patient that you will now examine the vagina and rectum. The rectovaginal examination allows for better evaluation of the posterior portion of the pelvis and the cul-de-sac than does the bimanual examination alone. You can often reach 1 to 2 cm higher into the pelvis with the rectovaginal examination. Remove your fingers from the vagina, and change your glove. Explain to the patient that the examination will make her feel as if she were going to have a bowel movement but that she will not do so. Lubricate the gloved index and middle fingers. Inspect the anus for hemorrhoids, fissures, polyps, prolapse, or other growths. Insert the index finger back into the vagina while the middle finger is introduced into the anus. The examining right index finger is positioned as far up the posterior surface of the vagina as possible. This technique is shown in Figure 19-30 and diagrammed in Figure 19-31.

The rectovaginal septum is palpated. Is it thickened or tender? Are nodules or masses present? The right middle finger should feel for tenderness, masses, or irregularities in the rectum.

The patient is told that the internal examination is completed and that you are about to remove your fingers. When you withdraw your fingers, inspect them for discharge or blood. Offer the patient tissues to wipe off any excess lubricant.

Test Stool for Occult Blood

Any fecal material on the middle (rectal) finger should be tested with the occult blood testing card and Hemoccult developer.

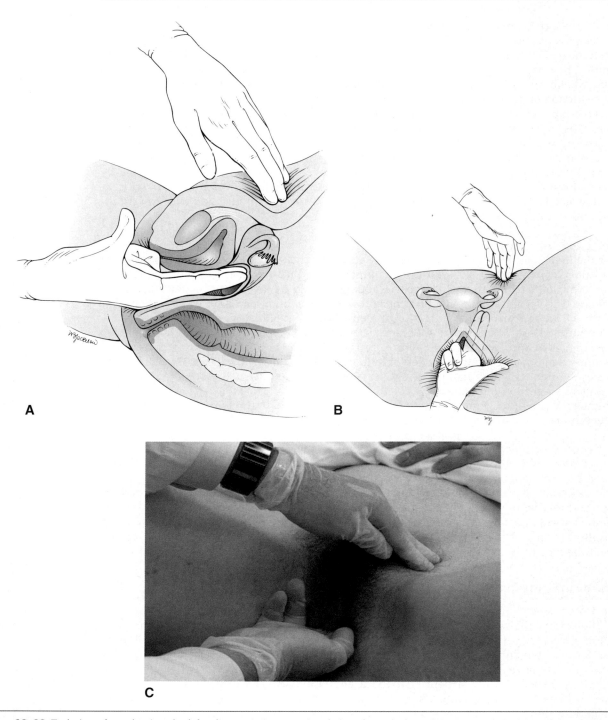

Figure 19–29 Technique for palpating the left adnexa. *A,* Cross-sectional view through the pelvic organs. *B,* Position of the ovary and fallopian tube between the examining hands. *C,* Position of examiner's hands.

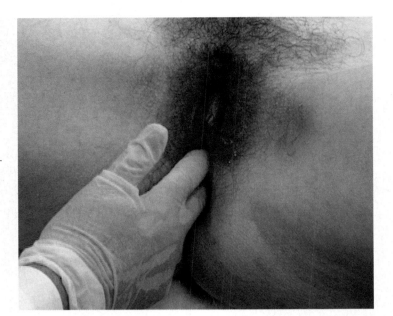

Figure 19–30 Technique for performing the rectovaginal examination.

Completion of the Examination

Ask the woman to move back on the examination table, remove her legs from the heel rests, and then sit up slowly. Remove your gloves and wash your hands. This concludes the examination of the female genitalia.

Clinicopathologic Correlations

Vaginitis is an inflammation of the vagina and vulva that is marked by pain, itching, and vaginal discharge. Normal vaginal discharge consists of mucous secretions from the cervix and vagina, as well as exfoliated vaginal cells. A normal vaginal discharge is thin and transparent and has little odor. When the normal bacterial flora in the vagina is disturbed, one or more organisms can multiply out of their normal proportions. This change in the normal flora may also make the vagina more susceptible to other invading organisms. The rapid growth of organisms produces an excess of waste products that irritate tissues, cause a burning sensation and itching, and produce a discharge with an unpleasant odor. The discharges caused by different organisms have different appearances.

Lesions of the vulva are very common. Figure 19-32 shows the vesicular stage of herpes simplex infection. Figure 19-33 shows a chancre in a woman with primary syphilis. Chancroid is a disease in which 5 to 15 days after exposure small papules or vesicles appear that break down to form tender, nonindurated ulcers. Lymphadenopathy develops. Figure 19-34 shows the classic ulceration of vulvar chancroid.

Figure 19-35 shows several of the common uterine positions.

Pelvic relaxation is a common problem. The consequences include cystocele, rectocele, and uterine prolapse. Figure 19-36 illustrates these sequelae of relaxation of the pelvic floor.

A summary of dysfunctional uterine bleeding is illustrated in Figure 19-37.

Table 19-1 lists the characteristics of common vaginal discharges. Table 19-2 summarizes the clinical features of genital ulcerations.

Although the pelvic examination can reveal many cancers of the female reproductive system, including advanced uterine cancers, it is not very effective in detecting early uterine cancer. The Pap test can reveal some early endometrial cancers, but most cases are not detected

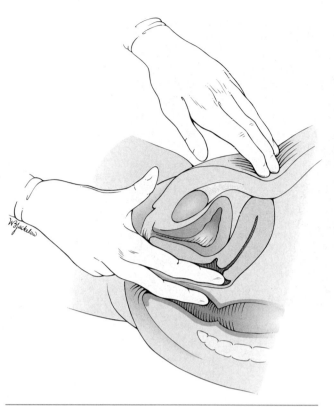

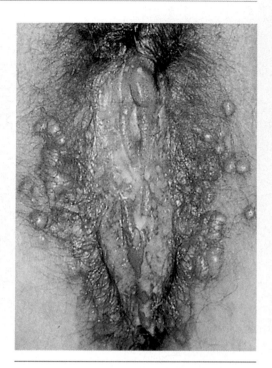

Figure 19–32 Herpes simplex infection.

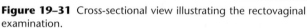

Figure 19–31 Cross-sectional view illustrating the rectovaginal examination.

by this test. In contrast, the Pap test is very effective in revealing early cancers of the cervix. For this reason, the American Cancer Society recommends the following:

1. All women should begin screening for cervical cancer about 3 years after they begin having vaginal intercourse or at age 21 years, whichever occurs first. Screening should be performed every year with the regular Pap test or every 2 years with the newer liquid-based Pap test.
2. Beginning at age 30 years, women who have had three normal Pap test results in a row may undergo screening every 2 to 3 years with either the conventional or liquid-based Pap test. Women who have certain risk factors such as DES exposure before birth, HIV infection, or a weakened immune system as a result of organ transplantation, chemotherapy, or chronic steroid use should continue to undergo screening annually.
3. Another option for women older than 30 years is to undergo screening every 3 years (but not more frequently) with either the conventional or liquid-based Pap test and with the HPV DNA test. As mentioned earlier in this chapter, an important risk factor for the development of cervical cancer is infection with HPV. It is now possible to test for the types of HPV that are most likely to cause cervical carcinoma by looking for pieces of their DNA in the cervical cells. The cells are collected in the same manner as with the Pap test.
4. Women 70 years of age or older who have had three or more normal Pap test results in a row and no abnormal Pap test results in the previous 10 years may choose to stop having cervical cancer screening. Women with a history of cervical cancer, DES exposure before birth, HIV infection, or a weakened immune system should continue to undergo screening as long as they are in good health.
5. Women who have had a total hysterectomy may also choose to stop having cervical cancer screening, unless the surgery was performed as a treatment for cervical cancer. Women who have had a hysterectomy without removal of the cervix should continue to follow the guidelines outlined previously.

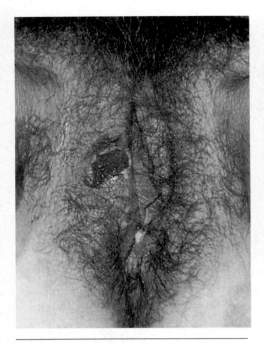

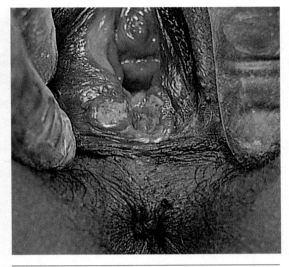

Figure 19–34 Chancroid.

Figure 19–33 Chancre of primary syphilis.

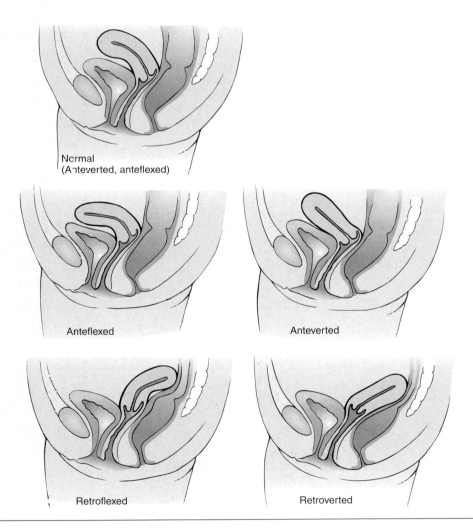

Normal
(Anteverted, anteflexed)

Anteflexed

Anteverted

Retroflexed

Retroverted

Figure 19–35 Common uterine positions.

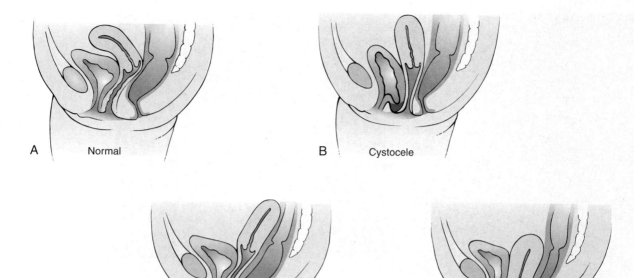

Figure 19–36 Sequelae of pelvic floor relaxation. *A,* Normal anatomy. *B,* Cystocele, which is a protrusion of the wall of the urinary bladder through the vagina. *C,* Rectocele, which is a protrusion of the rectal wall through the vagina. *D,* Uterine descent, which is a protrusion of the uterus through the vagina.

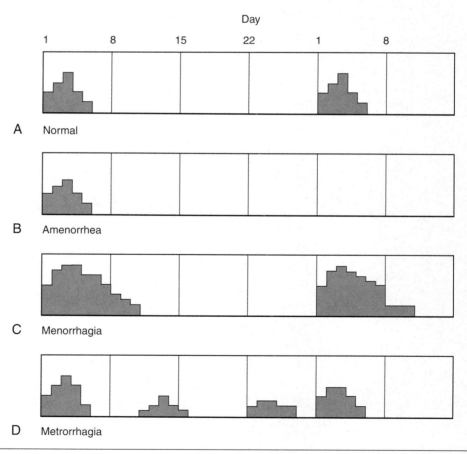

Figure 19–37 Types of uterine bleeding. *A,* Normal 28-day cycle. Note that menstrual flow occurs on day 1 and lasts for approximately 5 days. *B,* Amenorrhea. After a menstrual flow of 5 days, the period does not recur. *C,* Menorrhagia. Note that the flow occurs at 28-day intervals, but the amount of flow is heavier, and its duration is longer than normal. *D,* Metrorrhagia. In this condition, flow is regular, but there is bleeding between the normal menstrual flow cycles.

Table 19–2 Clinical Features of Genital Ulcerations

Feature	Genital Herpes*	Primary Syphilis†	Chancroid‡
Incubation period	3-5 Days	9-90 Days	1-5 Days
Number of ulcers	Multiple	Single	Multiple
Appearance at onset	Vesicle	Papule	Papule/pustule
Later appearance	Small, grouped	Round, indurated	Irregular, ragged
Ulcer pain	Present	Absent	Present
Inguinal adenopathy	Present, tender	Present, painless	Present, painful
Healing	Within 2 weeks	Slowly for weeks	Slowly for weeks
Recurrence (even if not infected)	Common	Rare	Common

*See Figure 19-32.
†See Figure 19-33.
‡See Figure 19-34.

Useful Vocabulary

Listed here are the specific roots that are important for understanding the terminology related to diseases of the female genitalia.

Root	Pertaining to	Example	Definition
amni(o)-	amnion	**amnio**rrhexis	Rupture of the amnion
colp(o)-	vagina	**colpo**scopy	Examination of vagina (and cervix)
-cyesis	pregnancy	pseudo**cyesis**	False pregnancy
gyn(e)-	woman	**gyne**cology	Branch of medicine that deals with treating diseases of the genital tract in women
hyster(o)-	uterus	**hyster**ectomy	Surgical removal of the uterus
metro-	uterus	**metro**rrhagia	Uterine bleeding
oophor(o)-	ovary	**oophoro**tomy	Incision of an ovary
ov-	egg	**ov**ulation	Discharge of an egg from the ovary
salping(o)-	fallopian tube	**salping**itis	Inflammation of the fallopian tube

Writing Up the Physical Examination

Listed here are examples of the write-up for the examination of the female genitalia.

- Examination of the vulva is within normal limits. No lesions are present. The cervix appears pink, smooth, and nulliparous. There is no discharge from the external cervical os. The vaginal walls appear normal. Bimanual palpation reveals an anteverted, anteflexed uterus without masses or tenderness. The adnexa are unremarkable. Rectovaginal examination reveals a thin rectovaginal membrane without tenderness. Stool guaiac result is negative.
- Examination of the vulva reveals groups of tense vesicles and scattered erosions that are covered with exudate. The cervix is pink and multiparous. No cervical lesions are present. No discharge is present. The vagina is within normal limits. The uterus is anteverted and anteflexed. A 6 × 6 cm mass is felt within the uterus. The ovaries and tubes are unremarkable. Rectovaginal examination findings are within normal limits.
- The vulva appears within normal limits without masses or lesions. The cervix has an erosion, and there is a thick, white, cottage cheese–like discharge in the vagina. The discharge is adherent to the vaginal walls. The uterus is retroverted and cannot be adequately examined. A walnut-sized mass is felt in the left adnexa. It appears rubbery and is freely mobile. The rectovaginal examination findings are normal. Stool guaiac result is negative.
- The vulva is normal. On straining, a rectocele becomes apparent. The vagina is normal. The cervix is smooth, pink, and multiparous. The uterus is anteverted and anteflexed and is not enlarged. The adnexa are difficult to assess because of obesity of the patient. No tenderness is present.

Bibliography

Arbyn M, Bergeron C, Klinkhamer P, et al: Liquid compared with conventional cervical cytology: A systematic review and meta-analysis. Obstet Gynecol 111:167, 2008.
Brown JS, Bradley CS, Subak LL, et al: The sensitivity and specificity of a simple text to distinguish between urge and stress urinary incontinence. Ann Intern Med 144:715, 2006.
Carnes M, Mahoney JE: Update in women's health. Ann Intern Med 140:538, 2004.
Denton KJ: Liquid based cytology in cervical cancer screening. BMJ 335:1, 2007.
Drife J: Clinical Obstetrics and Gynecology. Philadelphia, WB Saunders, 2001.
Dwyer PL: Differentiating stress incontinence from urge urinary incontinence. Int J Gynecol Obstet 86(Suppl 1):S17, 2004.
Eifel PJ, Berek JS, Markman M: Cancer of the cervix, vagina, and vulva. In DeVita VT, Hellman S, Rosenberg SA (eds): Cancer: Principles and Practice of Oncology, 7th ed. Philadelphia, Lippincott Williams & Wilkins, 2005.
French L: Dysmenorrhea. Am Fam Physician 71:285, 2005.
Hacker NF, Moore JG: Essentials of Obstetrics and Gynecology, 3rd ed. Philadelphia, WB Saunders, 1998.
Hathaway JK, Pathak PK, Maney R: Is liquid-based Pap testing affected by water-based lubricant? Obstet Gynecol 107:66, 2006.
Jemel A, Tiwari R, Murray T, et al: Cancer statistics, 2004. CA Cancer J Clin 54:8, 2004.
Magee J: The pelvic examination: A view from the other end of the table. Ann Intern Med 83:563, 1975.
Magowan BA: Churchill's Pocketbook of Obstetrics and Gynaecology, 2nd ed. Philadelphia, Churchill Livingstone, 2000.
Practice Committee of the American Society for Reproductive Medicine: Current evaluation of amenorrhea. Fertil Steril 82:266, 2004.
Ries LAG, Melbert D, Krapcho M, et al: SEER Cancer Statistics Review, 1975–2004 [based on November 2006 Surveillance Epidemiology and End Results (SEER) data submission]. Bethesda, Md, National Cancer Institute. Available at: *http://seer.cancer.gov/csr/1975_2004/*; accessed June 9, 2008.
Rollins G: Developments in cervical and ovarian cancer screening: Implications for current practice. Ann Intern Med 133:1021, 2000.
Ronco G, Cuzick J, Pierotti P, et al: Accuracy of liquid based versus conventional cytology: Overall results of new technologies for cervical cancer screening randomised controlled trial. BMJ 335:28, 2007.

Saslow D, Castle PE, Cox JT, et al: American Cancer Society guideline for human papillomavirus (HPV) vaccine use to prevent cervical cancer and its precursors. CA Cancer J Clin 57:7, 2007.

Sawaya GF, Sox HC: Trials that matter: Liquid-based cervical cytology: Disadvantages seem to outweigh advantages. Ann Intern Med 147:668, 2007.

Smith RA, Cokkinides V, Eyre HJ: American Cancer Society guidelines for the early detection of cancer, 2004. CA Cancer J Clin 54:41, 2004.

Surveillance, Epidemiology, and End Results (SEER) Program: SEER Stat Database: Incidence—SEER 9 Regs Public-Use, November 2002 Sub (1973–2000) [released April 2003, based on the November 2002 submission]. Bethesda, Md, National Cancer Institute, Division of Cancer Control and Population Sciences, Surveillance Research Program, Cancer Statistics Branch. Available at *www.seer.cancer.gov*; accessed June 25, 2008.

Welch B, Howard A, Cook K: Vaginal itch. Australian Fam Physician 33:505, 2004.

Wilbur DC, Cibas ES, Merritt S, et al: ThinPrep® Processor: Clinical trials demonstrate an increased detection rate of abnormal cervical cytologic specimens. Am J Clin Pathol 101:209, 1994.

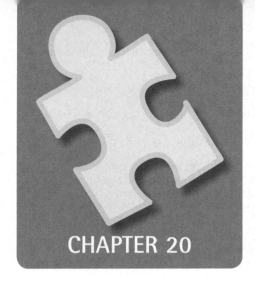

CHAPTER 20

The Musculoskeletal System

The hand of the Lord was upon me ... and set me down in the midst of the valley which was full of bones ... behold, there were very many in the open valley; and, lo, they were very dry. ... Thus saith the Lord God unto these bones: Behold, I will cause breath to enter into you, and ye shall live. And I will lay sinews upon you, and will bring up flesh upon you, and cover with skin, and put breath in you, and ye shall live ... there was a noise, and behold a commotion, and the bones came together, bone to bone ... and skin covered them ... and the breath came into them, and they lived, and stood up upon their feet.

Ezekiel 37:1–10

General Considerations

Diseases of the musculoskeletal system rank first among disease conditions that alter the quality of life. This is related to limitation of activity, disability, and impairment. In the United States, one of every seven persons suffers from some sort of musculoskeletal disorder, the cost of which exceeds $60 billion annually. This includes lost earnings and medical expenses.

Diseases of the musculoskeletal system are divided into two categories: *systemic* and *local*. Patients with systemic disease, such as rheumatoid arthritis, systemic lupus erythematosus, or polymyositis, may appear chronically ill, with generalized weakness, pain, and episodic stiffness of the joints. Patients with local disease are basically healthy individuals who suffer restriction of motion and pain from a single area. Included in this group are patients suffering from back pain, tennis elbow, arthritis, or bursitis. Although these patients may have only local symptoms, their disability can greatly limit their work capacity, and the disease can have a severe impact on the quality of their life.

Diseases of the musculoskeletal system rank first in cost to workers' compensation insurance carriers. Nearly 100,000 workers receive disability payments annually, with a total cost to the carriers of more than $200 billion annually.

It has been estimated that musculoskeletal problems rank second (after cardiovascular disorders) in accounting for visits to internists and third for surgical procedures in hospitals (after gynecologic and abdominal surgery). According to a Gallup poll, nearly 75% of individuals older than 18 years complained of foot pain at some time. More than $300 million is spent annually on insoles, corn remedies, bunion removers, other foot care products, and over-the-counter medications for foot care. Despite this widespread problem, fewer than 50% of clinicians know how to examine a foot correctly!

Although not usually fatal disorders, musculoskeletal conditions affect the quality of life. Studies indicate that backache is experienced by more than 80% of all Americans at some time in their lives. Patients with backache for longer than 6 months constitute a large portion of permanently disabled individuals. More than 50% of these patients never return to work.

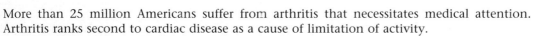

More than 25 million Americans suffer from arthritis that necessitates medical attention. Arthritis ranks second to cardiac disease as a cause of limitation of activity.

In the United States at least 10% of the population experiences a bone fracture, dislocation, or sprain annually. Each year more than 1.2 million fractures are sustained by women older than 50 years. There are more than 200,000 hip fractures annually, and these are associated with prolonged disability. Osteoporosis* is the most common musculoskeletal disorder in the world and is second only to arthritis as a leading cause of morbidity in the geriatric population. Postmenopausal osteoporosis and age-related osteoporosis increase the risk of fractures in the older population. There are more than 40 million women in the United States older than 50 years, and more than 50% of them have evidence of spinal osteoporosis. Almost 90% of women older than 75 years have significant radiographic evidence of osteoporosis.

The high prevalence of musculoskeletal disease in elderly patients who require assistance has a significant impact on the American economy. The annual cost of nursing home care for patients with musculoskeletal disease is almost $75 billion. More than 10 million individuals in the United States have some form of inflammatory arthritis, the most prevalent being rheumatoid arthritis. It is estimated that more than 7 million patients have this form of arthritis.

Musculoskeletal problems have the most significant financial impact on the aged population. More than $1 billion is spent annually by Medicare for hospitalization of patients with these conditions. This represents 20% of all Medicare payments.

Structure and Physiology

The principal functions of the musculoskeletal system are to support and protect the body and to bring about movement of the extremities for locomotion and the performance of tasks.

The parts of the musculoskeletal system are composed of variable forms of dense connective tissue, which include the following:

- Bone
- Skeletal muscle
- Ligaments and tendons
- Cartilage

Bone is composed of an organic matrix that consists of collagen fibers embedded in a cementing gel made up of calcium and phosphate. Bone is an actively changing tissue constantly undergoing *remodeling* while reappropriating its mineral stores and matrix according to mechanical stresses. Normal bone is composed of collagen fibers aligned parallel to the tension stresses to which the bone is exposed. The long bones in adults are composed of tubes of *cortical*, or compact, bone surrounding a medullary cavity of *cancellous*, or spongy, bone. Cortical bone exists in areas where support is necessary, whereas cancellous bone is found in areas where hematopoiesis and bone formation occur. In cortical bone, the bone cells, or *osteocytes*, are enclosed in lacunae, which are spaces in the sheets of bone tissue called *lamellae*. Several lamellae are arranged concentrically around a vascular channel and are termed a *haversian canal*. In cancellous bone, the lamellae are not arranged in haversian systems but are organized into a spongy network called *trabeculae*. These trabeculae align along lines of stress.

The ends of the long bones, called *epiphyses*, are expanded near the articular surfaces and are composed of spongy bone. The shaft of the long bone, the *diaphysis*, is covered with a layer of *periosteum*. The inner cavity of the long bone is lined with *endosteum* and is filled with marrow.

For a period of time, a layer of cartilage exists between the diaphysis and the epiphysis. This cartilage is known as the *growth plate* or *epiphyseal plate*. The purpose of the growth plate is to determine the longitudinal growth of the bone. The parts of a long bone are illustrated in Figure 20-1.

Cells in the periosteum can develop into *osteoblasts*, which lay down new bone, or into *osteoclasts*, which resorb bone. Trauma, infection, and tumors stimulate the development of osteoblasts. Osteoblasts secrete the matrix that is refashioned into lamellae and arranged to endure the mechanical stresses to which the bone is subjected.

---

*Osteoporosis is a state of decreased density of normal mineralized bone.

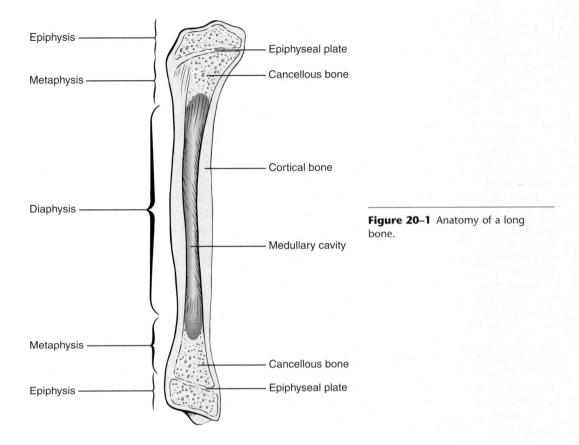

Epiphysis

Metaphysis

Diaphysis

Metaphysis

Epiphysis

Epiphyseal plate

Cancellous bone

Cortical bone

Medullary cavity

Cancellous bone

Epiphyseal plate

Figure 20–1 Anatomy of a long bone.

A pathologic process that interferes with the normal architecture of bone tends to weaken it. Paget's disease is a disease of bone in which there is a disruption of the normal architecture. Patients with this condition are extremely susceptible to pathologic fractures.

Skeletal muscle is an organ, the contraction of which produces movement.

Ligaments attach bone to bone, and *tendons* attach muscle to bone. Both are dense connective tissues that offer great resistance to pulling forces.

Cartilage is a type of connective tissue with great resilience. It plays an important role in joint function and in determining bone length.

The basic functional unit of the musculoskeletal system is the *joint*. A joint is a union of two or more bones. There are several types of joints in the body:

- Immovable
- Slightly movable
- Movable

Immovable joints are fixed as a result of fibrous tissue banding. Examples of this type of joint are the sutures of the skull. *Slightly movable joints* are termed *symphyses*. In this type of joint, fibrocartilage joins the articulating bones. The pubic symphysis is an example of a slightly movable joint. The most common type of joint is the *movable joint*. The body has many different types of movable joints, also known as *synovial joints*. In synovial joints, the bone structures come in contact with each other and are covered with hyaline articular cartilage. A capsule surrounds the joint by attaching to the bones on either side of the joint. Within the capsule is a small amount of synovial fluid, which plays a role in joint lubrication and nourishment of the articular cartilage. Synovial joints are classified according to the type of movement their structure permits. The classifications are as follows:

- Hinge joint
- Pivot joint
- Condyloid joint
- Saddle joint
- Ball-and-socket joint
- Plane joint

A *hinge joint* permits movement in only one axis: namely, flexion or extension. The axis is transverse. An example of a hinge joint is the elbow. A *pivot joint* permits rotation in one axis. The axis is longitudinal along the shaft of the bone. One bone moves around a central axis without any displacement from that axis. An example of a pivot joint is the proximal radio-ulnar joint. A *condyloid joint* permits movement in two axes. The articular surfaces are oval; thus these joints have been described as "egg-in-spoon" joints. One axis is the long diameter of the oval, and the other axis is the short diameter of the oval. The wrist joint is an example of a condyloid joint. A *saddle joint* is also a biaxial joint. The articular surfaces are saddle-shaped, with movements similar to those of a condyloid joint. The carpometacarpal joint of the thumb is an example of a saddle joint. The *ball-and-socket joint* is an example of a polyaxial joint; motion is possible in many axes. In a ball-and-socket joint, the articular surfaces are reciprocal segments of a sphere. The hip and shoulder joints are examples of ball-and-socket joints. A *plane joint* is also a polyaxial joint. In the plane joint, the articular surfaces are flat, and one bone merely rides over the other in many directions. The patellofemoral joint is an example of a plane joint. These different types of movable joints are shown in Figure 20-2.

The stability of a joint depends on the following:

- Shape of the articular surfaces
- Ligaments
- Associated muscles

It is necessary to be familiar with certain anatomic terms that refer to position (Table 20-1). The *median plane* bisects the body into right and left halves. A plane parallel to the median plane is a *sagittal plane*. The terms *medial* and *lateral* are used in reference to the sagittal plane. A position closer to the median plane is medial; farther from the median plane, it is lateral. In the upper limb, the term *ulnar* is often used to denote medial, and *radial* to denote lateral. In the lower limb, *tibial* is used to denote medial, and *peroneal* or *fibular* denotes lateral. These anatomic terms are illustrated in Figure 20-3.

The front of the body is the *anterior*, or *ventral*, surface, and the back of the body is the *posterior*, or *dorsal*, side. The *palmar*, or *volar*, aspect of the hand is the anterior surface. The *dorsal aspect* of the foot faces upward, and the *plantar aspect* is the sole. *Proximal* refers to the part of an extremity that is closest to its root; *distal* refers to the part farthest from the root.

The most important terms relating to deformities of the bone structure are *valgus* and *varus*. In a valgus deformity, the distal portion of the bone is displaced away from the midline, and angulation is toward the midline. In a varus deformity, the distal portion of the extremity is displaced toward the midline, and angulation is away from the midline. The name of the deformity is determined by the joint involved. A valgus deformity of the knees, knock-knee, is termed *genu valgum*. A varus deformity of the knee, bowleg, is termed *genu varum*.

In the evaluation of a joint, assess the *range of motion*. Each joint has a characteristic range of motion that can be measured passively and actively. *Passive* range of motion is the motion elicited when the examiner moves the patient's body. *Active* range of motion is the motion the patient performs as a result of moving the musculature. The passive range of motion usually equals the active range of motion except in cases of paralyzed muscles or ruptured tendons. The range of motion of individual joints is discussed later in this chapter. Joint motion is measured in degrees of a circle, with the joint at the center. If a limb is extended with the bones in a straight line, the joint is at *zero position*. The zero position is the neutral position of the joint. As the joint is flexed, the angle increases. The concept of range of motion is illustrated in Figure 20-4.

The six basic types of joint motion are as follows:

- Flexion and extension
- Dorsiflexion and plantar flexion
- Adduction and abduction
- Inversion and eversion
- Internal and external rotation
- Pronation and supination

The definitions of these motions and the joints at which they occur are summarized in Table 20-2.

The anatomy of the *shoulder joint* is illustrated in Figure 20-5. The joint movements at the shoulder are abduction and adduction, flexion and extension, and internal and external rotation. These motions are illustrated in Figure 20-6.

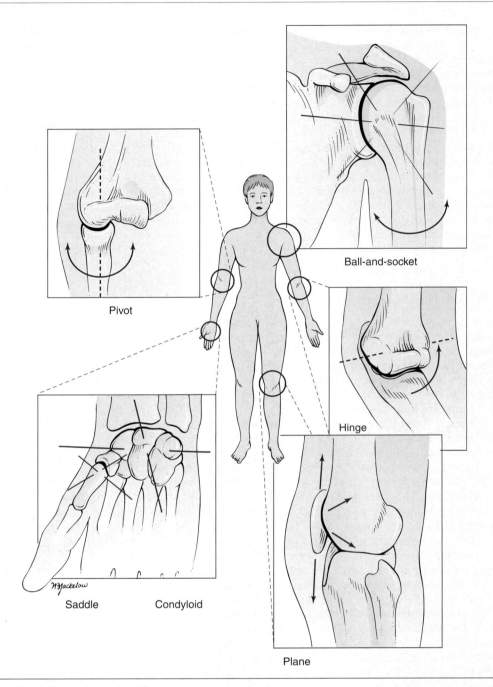

Pivot

Ball-and-socket

Hinge

Saddle   Condyloid

Plane

Figure 20–2 Types of movable joints.

Table 20–1 Anatomic Terms for the Upper and Lower Limb

Limb	Medial	Lateral
Upper	Ulnar	Radial
Lower	Tibial	Peroneal fibular

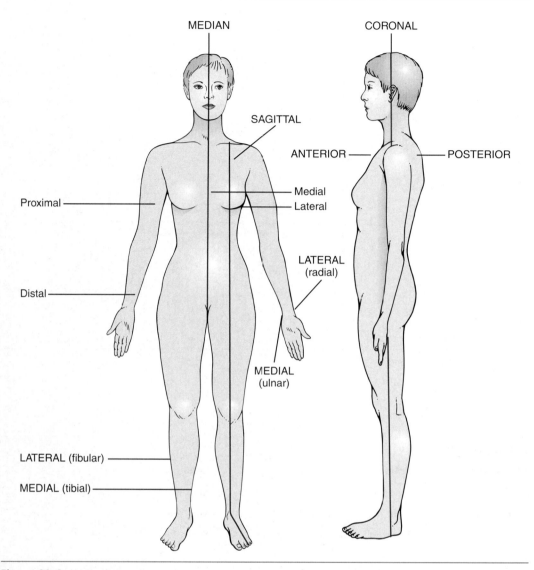

Figure 20–3 Anatomic terms.

The anatomy of the *elbow joint* is shown in Figure 20-7. The joint movements at the elbow are flexion and extension and supination and pronation. These motions are illustrated in Figure 20-8.

The anatomy of the *wrist* and *fingers* is illustrated in Figure 20-9. The joint movements at the wrist are dorsiflexion (or extension) and palmar flexion and supination and pronation. These motions are illustrated in Figure 20-10. The joint movements at the fingers are abduction and adduction and flexion. These motions are illustrated in Figure 20-11. The joint movements of the *thumb* are flexion and extension and opposition. These motions are illustrated in Figure 20-12.

The anatomy of the *hip* is illustrated in Figure 20-13. The joint movements at the hip are flexion and extension, abduction and adduction, and internal and external rotation. These motions are illustrated in Figure 20-14.

The anatomy of the *knee* is shown in Figure 20-15. The joint movements at the knee are flexion and hyperextension. These motions are illustrated in Figure 20-16.

The anatomy of the *ankle* and *foot* is illustrated in Figure 20-17. There are 26 bones and 55 articulations in the foot. The bones can be divided into three regions: forefoot, midfoot, and rear foot. The *forefoot* is represented by the 14 bones of the toes and 5 metatarsals. The big toe (hallux) has two phalanges, two joints (interphalangeal joints), and two tiny, round *sesamoid bones* that enable it to move up and down. The sesamoid bones are about the size of a kernel of corn. These bones are embedded in the flexor hallucis brevis tendon, one of several tendons that exert pressure from the big toe against the ground and help initiate the act of walking: the

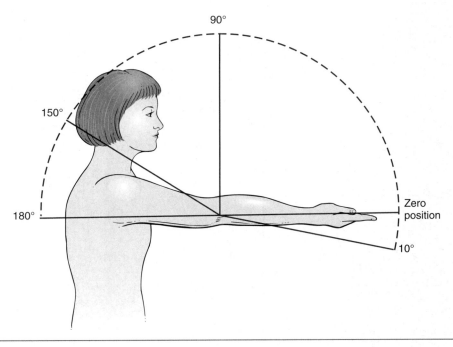

Figure 20–4 Range of motion.

Table 20–2 Joint Motion

Motion	Definition	Example
Flexion	Motion away from the zero position	Most joints
Extension	Return motion to the position*	Most joints
Dorsiflexion	Movement in the direction of the dorsal surface	Ankle, toes, wrist, fingers
Plantar (or palmar) flexion	Movement in the direction of the plantar (or palmar) surface	Ankle, toes, wrist, fingers
Adduction	Movement toward the midline†	Shoulder, hip, metacarpophalangeal, metatarsophalangeal joints
Abduction	Movement away from the midline	Shoulder, hip, metacarpophalangeal, metatarsophalangeal joints
Inversion	Turning of the plantar surface of the foot inward	Subtalar and midtarsal joints of the foot
Eversion	Turning of the plantar surface of the foot outward	Subtalar and midtarsal joints of the foot
Internal rotation	Turning of the anterior surface of a limb inward	Shoulder, hip
External rotation	Turning of the anterior surface of a limb outward	Shoulder, hip
Pronation	Rotation so that the palmar surface of the hand is directed downward	Elbow, wrist
Supination	Rotation so that the palmar surface of the hand is directed upward	Elbow, wrist

*Extension that goes beyond the zero position is called *hyperextension*.
†In the hand or foot, the midline is an imaginary line through the middle finger or middle toe, respectively.

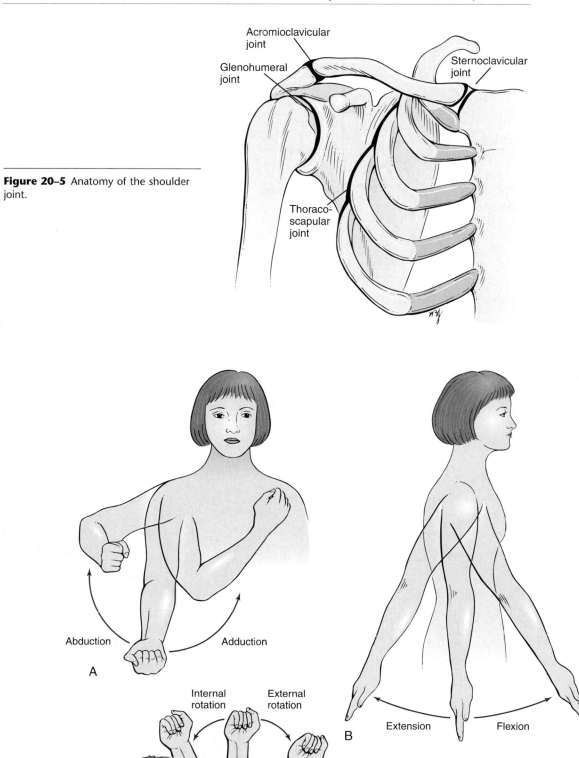

Figure 20–5 Anatomy of the shoulder joint.

Figure 20–6 Range of motion at the shoulder. *A,* Abduction and adduction. *B,* Flexion and extension. *C,* Internal and external rotation.

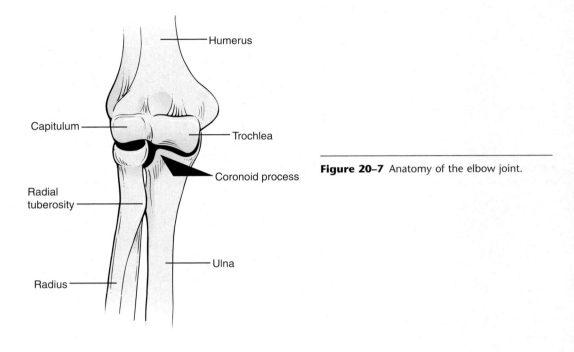

Figure 20–7 Anatomy of the elbow joint.

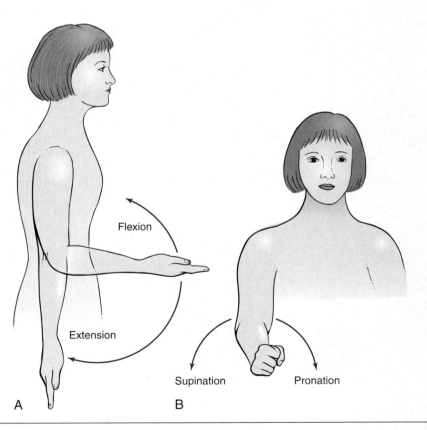

Figure 20–8 Range of motion at the elbow joint. *A,* Flexion and extension. *B,* Supination and pronation.

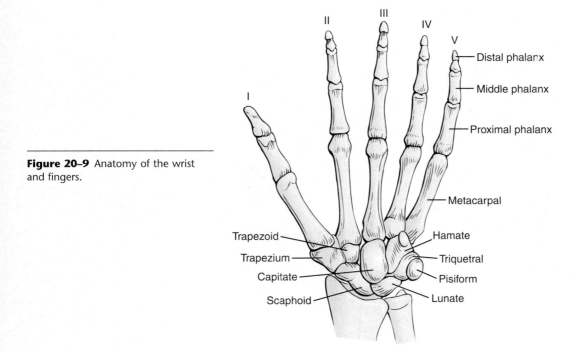

Figure 20–9 Anatomy of the wrist and fingers.

propulsive phase of the gait cycle. The other four toes each have three bones and two joints. The phalanges are connected to the metatarsals by five metatarsophalangeal joints at the ball of the foot. The forefoot bears half the body's weight and balances pressure on the ball of the foot.

The *midfoot* consists of the three cuneiform bones, the cuboid, and the navicular. The midfoot has five irregularly shaped tarsal bones, forms the foot's arch, and serves as a shock absorber. The bones of the midfoot are connected to the forefoot and the hindfoot by muscles and the plantar fascia (arch ligament).

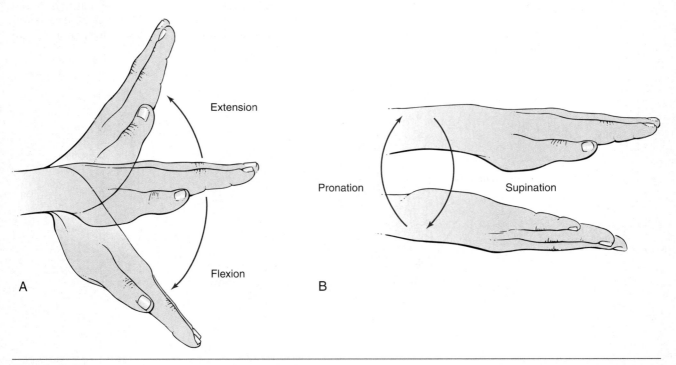

Figure 20–10 Range of motion at the wrist joint. *A,* Dorsiflexion (extension) and palmar flexion. *B,* Supination and pronation.

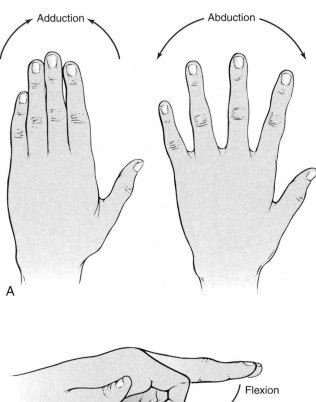

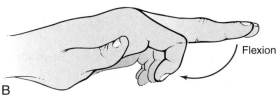

Figure 20–11 Range of motion at the finger joints. *A,* Abduction and adduction. *B,* Flexion.

The *rear foot* is composed of the talus and the calcaneus. The foot contains two arches: the longitudinal in the midpart and the transverse in the forepart. The midtarsal joint is formed by the articulations of the navicular to the talus and the calcaneus to the cuboid. The largest tarsal bone is the calcaneus, the bottom of which is cushioned by a layer of fat. The attachment of the foot to the leg occurs through the talus. The joint movements at the ankle are dorsiflexion and plantar flexion. The motion of the subtalar joint is inversion and eversion. These motions are illustrated in Figure 20-18.

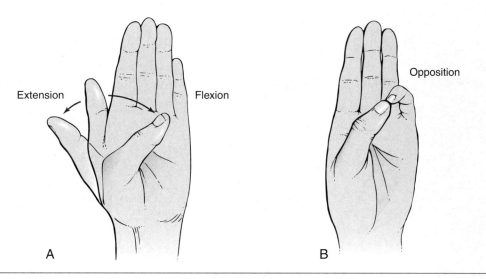

Figure 20–12 Range of motion of the thumb. *A,* Flexion and extension. *B,* Opposition.

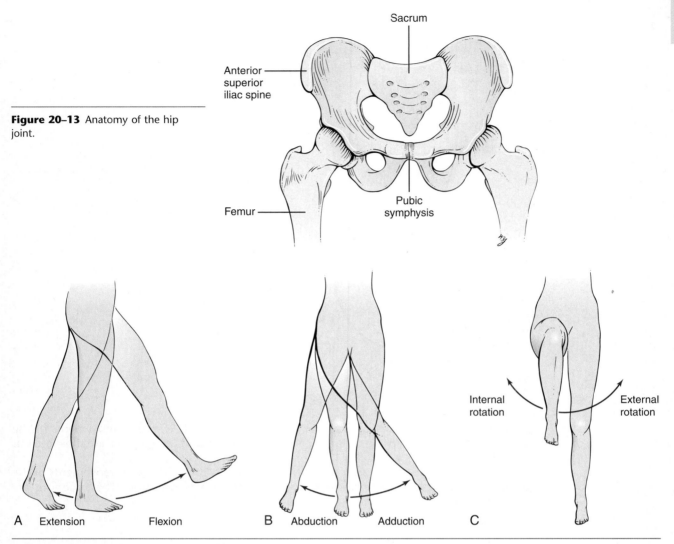

Figure 20–13 Anatomy of the hip joint.

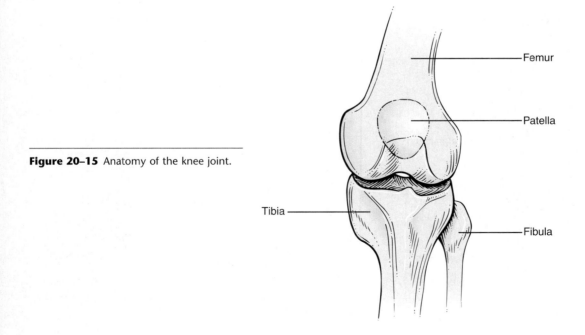

Figure 20–14 Range of motion at the hip joint. *A,* Flexion and extension. *B,* Abduction and adduction. *C,* Internal and external rotation.

Figure 20–15 Anatomy of the knee joint.

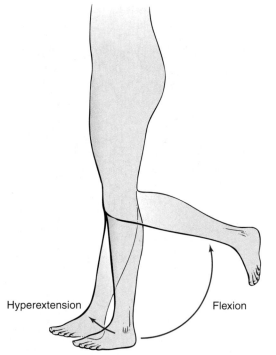

Figure 20–16 Range of motion at the knee joint: flexion and hyperextension.

The anatomy of the *cervical spine* is shown in Figure 20-19. The joint movements of the neck are flexion and extension, rotation, and lateral flexion. These motions are illustrated in Figure 20-20.

The anatomy of the *lumbar spine* is illustrated in Figure 20-21. The joint movements of the lumbar spine are flexion and extension, rotation, and lateral extension. These motions are illustrated in Figure 20-22.

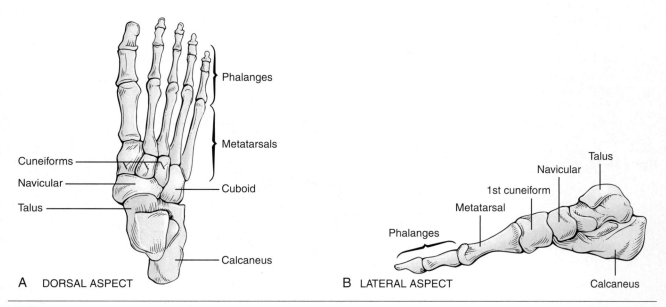

Figure 20–17 Anatomy of the ankle and foot joints. *A,* View from above. *B,* Medial view.

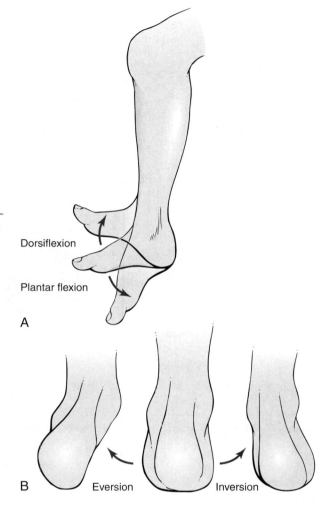

Figure 20–18 Range of motion at the ankle and foot joints. *A*, Dorsiflexion and plantar flexion. *B*, Eversion and inversion.

Dorsiflexion

Plantar flexion

A

B   Eversion   Inversion

Review of Specific Symptoms

The most common symptoms of musculoskeletal disease are as follows:

- Pain
- Weakness
- Deformity
- Limitation of motion
- Stiffness
- Joint clicking

The location, character, and onset of each of these symptoms must be ascertained. It is important for the interviewer to determine the time course of any of these symptoms.

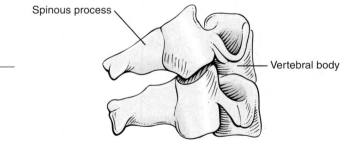

Spinous process

Vertebral body

Figure 20–19 Anatomy of the cervical spine.

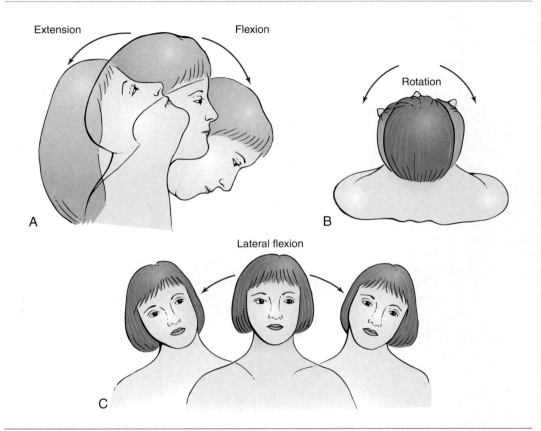

Figure 20–20 Range of motion at the cervical spine. *A,* Flexion and extension. *B,* Rotation. *C,* Lateral flexion.

Pain

Pain can result from disorders of the bone, muscle, or joint. Ask the following questions:

> *"When did you first become aware of the pain?"*
>
> *"Where do you feel the pain? Point to the most painful spot with one finger."*
>
> *"Did the pain occur suddenly?"*
>
> *"Does the pain occur daily?"*
>
> *"During which part of the 24-hour day is your pain worse: morning? afternoon? evening?"*
>
> *"Did a recent illness precede the pain?"*
>
> *"What makes the pain worse?"*
>
> *"What do you do to relieve the pain?"*

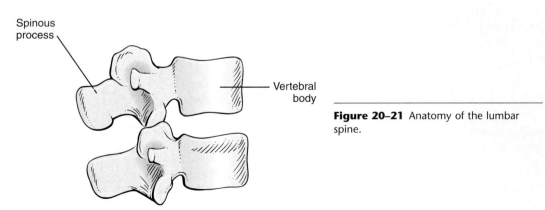

Figure 20–21 Anatomy of the lumbar spine.

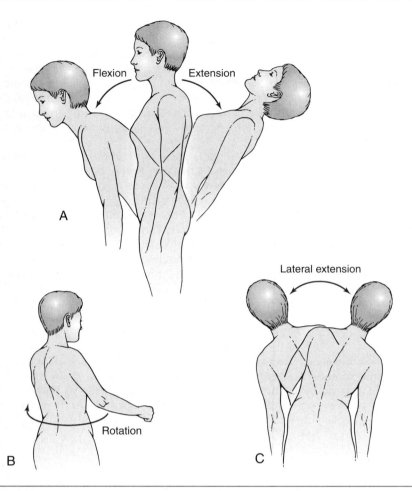

Figure 20–22 Range of motion at the lumbar spine. *A,* Flexion and extension. *B,* Rotation. *C,* Lateral extension.

"Is the pain relieved by rest?"

"What kinds of medications have you taken to relieve the pain?"

"Have you noticed that the pain changes according to the weather?"

"Do you have any difficulty putting on your shoes or coat?"

"Does the pain ever awaken you from sleep?"

"Does the pain shoot to another part of your body?"

"Have you noticed that the pain moves from one joint to another?"

"Has there been any injury, overuse, or strain?"

"Have you noticed any swelling?"

"Are other bones, muscles, or joints involved?"

"Have you had a recent sore throat?"

Bone pain may occur with or without trauma. It is typically described as "deep," "dull," "boring," or "intense." The pain may be so intense that the patient is unable to sleep. Typically, bone pain is not related to movement unless a fracture is present. Pain from a fractured bone is often described as "sharp." Muscle pain is frequently described as "crampy." It may last only briefly or for longer periods. Muscle pain in the lower extremity on walking, described in Chapter 15, The Peripheral Vascular System, is suggestive of ischemia of the calf or hip muscles. Muscle pain associated with weakness is suspect for a primary muscular disorder. Joint pain is felt around or in the joint. In some conditions, the joint may be exquisitely tender. Movement usually worsens the pain, except with rheumatoid arthritis, in which movement often reduces the pain. Pain of several years' duration rules out an acute septic process and usually malignancy. Chronic infection with tuberculosis or fungal infections may smolder for years before pain is present. The severity of the pain can often be assessed by determining the interval between the pain's onset and the patient's seeking medical attention.

The time of day when the pain is worse may be helpful in diagnosing the disorder. The pain of many rheumatic disorders tends to be accentuated in the morning, particularly on rising. Tendinitis worsens during the early morning hours and eases by midday. Osteoarthritis worsens as the day progresses.

Sudden onset of pain in a metatarsophalangeal joint should raise suspicion of gout. Entrapment syndromes are apt to radiate pain distally. Severe pain may awaken the patient from sleep. Rheumatoid arthritis and tendinitis often cause early awakening because of pain, particularly when the patient is lying on the affected limb.

Acute rheumatic fever, leukemia, gonococcal arthritis, sarcoidosis, and juvenile rheumatoid arthritis are commonly associated with *migratory polyarthritis*, in which one joint is affected, the disease subsides, and then another joint becomes involved.

Viral illnesses are commonly associated with muscle aches and pains. A recent history of a sore throat, with joint pain occurring 10 to 14 days later, is suspect for rheumatic fever. If rest does not relieve the pain, serious musculoskeletal disease may be present. The interviewer should keep in mind the possibility of *referred pain*. Pain from a hip disorder is frequently referred to the knee, especially in a child.

Weakness

Muscular weakness should always be differentiated from fatigue. Ascertain which functions the patient is unable to perform as a result of "weakness." Is the weakness related to proximal or distal muscle groups? *Proximal weakness* is usually a myopathy; *distal weakness* is usually a neuropathy. A patient with the symptom of muscular weakness should be asked these questions:

"Do you have difficulty combing your hair?"

"Do you have difficulty lifting objects?"

"Have you noticed any problem with holding a pen or pencil?"

"Do you have difficulty turning doorknobs?"

"Do you have trouble standing up after sitting in a chair?"

"Do you find that, as the day goes on, there is a change in the weakness?" If yes, *"Does the weakness worsen or improve?"*

"Have you noticed any decrease in your muscle size?"

"Are the weak muscles stiff?"

"Do you have trouble with double vision? swallowing? chewing?"

A patient with proximal weakness of the lower extremity has difficulty walking and crossing the knees. A proximal weakness of the upper extremity is manifested by difficulty brushing the hair or lifting objects. Patients with polymyalgia rheumatica have proximal muscle weakness. This condition is discussed in Chapter 25, The Geriatric Patient. A distal weakness of the upper extremity is manifested by difficulty turning doorknobs or buttoning a shirt or blouse. Patients with myasthenia gravis have generalized weakness, diplopia, and difficulty swallowing and chewing.

Deformity

Deformity may be the result of a congenital malformation or an acquired condition. In any patient with a deformity, it is important to determine the following:

"When was the deformity first noticed?"

"Did the deformity occur suddenly?"

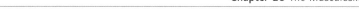

"Did the deformity occur as a result of trauma?"

"Has there been any change in the deformity with time?"

Limitation of Motion

Limitation of motion may result from changes in the articular cartilage, scarring of the joint capsule, or muscle contractures. Determine the types of motion the patient can no longer perform easily, such as combing the hair, putting on shoes, or buttoning a shirt or blouse.

Stiffness

Stiffness is a common symptom of musculoskeletal disease. For example, a patient with arthritis of the hip may have difficulty crossing his or her legs to tie shoes. Ask the patient whether the stiffness is worse at any particular time of day. Patients with rheumatoid arthritis tend to experience stiffness after periods of joint rest. These patients typically describe morning stiffness, which may take several hours to subside.

Joint Clicking

Joint clicking is commonly associated with specific movements in the presence of dislocation of the humerus, displacement of the biceps tendon from its groove, degenerative joint disease, damaged knee meniscus, and temporomandibular joint problems.

Impact of Musculoskeletal Disease on the Patient

Musculoskeletal diseases have an enormous impact on the lives of patients and their families. The perturbation of a patient's personal life and restriction of activities as a result of disability are frequently more catastrophic than the muscle or joint pain itself.

Diseases of the musculoskeletal system range from minor aches and pains to severe crippling disorders, often associated with premature death. Rheumatoid arthritis is a crippling disorder that strikes many patients in the prime of life. In addition to having joint pain and reduced activity, patients with rheumatoid arthritis fear the possibility of being crippled. They become more dependent on others as the disease progresses. The disability alters patients' self-image and self-esteem. The altered body image may be devastating; patients often become withdrawn.

The physical limitations of musculoskeletal disease, especially when accompanied by joint or muscle pain, threaten patients' integrity in their social world. Marital and familial ties may suffer as patients become more debilitated and withdrawn. Because of their disability, patients may have to change occupations, which causes further anxiety and depression. The loss of status and financial adjustments may jeopardize the marital situation. The fear of losing independence is extremely common. Patients are forced to make more demands on others but recognize that this may only worsen their relationships.

Rehabilitation is important for the physical and psychologic improvement of the patient. The patient is the key contributor to this rehabilitative process. Initially, motivation may be provided by people caring for the patient, but it is the patient's own attitude that determines whether the rehabilitation will be successful. The patient's motivation to tackle the disability depends on many factors, including self-image, as well as psychologic, social, and financial resources. It is important for the clinician to gain the patient's confidence to help him or her overcome the disability.

Physical Examination

No special equipment is necessary for the examination of the musculoskeletal system.

The purpose of the internist's musculoskeletal examination is as a screening examination to indicate or exclude functional impairment of the musculoskeletal system. The examination should take only a few minutes and should be part of the routine examination of all patients. If an abnormality is noted or if the patient has specific symptoms referable to a particular joint, a more detailed examination of that area is indicated. Detailed descriptions of the examination of specific joints follow the discussion of the screening examination.

Screening Examination

In the screening examination, the clinician should pay particular attention to the following:

- Inspection
- Palpation
- Passive and active range of motion
- Muscle strength
- Integrated function

General Principles

During inspection, asymmetry should be assessed. Nodules, wasting, masses, or deformities may be responsible for the absence of symmetry. Are there any signs of inflammation? *Swelling, warmth, redness,* and *tenderness* are suggestive of inflammation. To determine a difference in temperature, use the back of your hand to compare one side with the other.

Palpation may reveal areas of tenderness or discontinuity of a bone. Is *crepitus* present? Crepitus is a palpable crunching sensation often felt in the presence of roughened articular cartilages.

The *assessment of range of motion* of specific joints is next. Keep in mind that inflamed or arthritic joints may be painful. Move these joints *slowly.*

Muscle strength and *integrated function* are usually evaluated during the neurologic examination, and these topics are discussed in Chapter 21, The Nervous System.

Evaluate Gait

The first part of the screening examination consists of inspection of gait and posture. To determine any eccentricity of gait, ask the patient to disrobe down to underwear and walk barefoot. Have the patient walk away from you, then back to you on tiptoes, away from you on the heels, and finally back to you in tandem gait. If there is any gait difficulty, these maneuvers must be modified. The positions of the foot during the normal gait cycle are shown in Figure 20-23.

Observe the rate, rhythm, and arm motion used in walking. Does the patient have a staggering gait? Are the feet lifted high and slapped downward firmly? Does the patient walk with an extended leg that is swung laterally during walking? Are the steps short and shuffling? A complete discussion of gait abnormalities can be found in Chapter 21, The Nervous System. Figure 21-59 illustrates common gait abnormalities.

Evaluate the Spine

Attention should then focus on the spine to detect any abnormal spinal curvatures. Have the patient stand erect, and stand at the patient's side to inspect the profile of the patient's spine. Are the cervical, thoracic, and lumbar curves normal?

Move to inspect the patient's back. What is the level of the iliac crests? A difference may result from a leg length inequality, scoliosis, or flexion deformity of the hip. An imaginary line extending from the posterior occipital tuberosity should run over the intergluteal cleft. Any lateral curvature is abnormal. Figure 20-24 illustrates this point. Figure 20-25*A* shows severe kyphoscoliosis. See also Figure 13-6.

Ask the patient to bend forward, flexing at the trunk as far as possible with the knees extended. Note the smoothness of this action. This position is best for determining whether scoliosis is present. As the patient bends forward, the lumbar concavity should flatten. Figure 20-25*B* shows the patient in Figure 20-25*A* when bending forward. A persistence of the concavity may indicate an arthritic condition of the spine called *ankylosing spondylitis.*

Ask the patient to bend to each side from the waist and then bend backward from the waist to test *extension of the spine,* as shown in Figure 20-26*A*.

To test *rotation of the lumbar spine,* sit on a stool behind the patient and stabilize the patient's hips by placing your hands on them. Ask the patient to rotate the shoulders one way and then reverse, as shown in Figure 20-26*B*.

Evaluate Strength of the Lower Extremities

To assess the function of all major joints of the lower extremities, stand in front of the patient. Have the patient squat, with knees and hips fully flexed. Assist the patient by holding his or her hands to secure balance. This is shown in Figure 20-27. Ask the patient to stand. Observing the

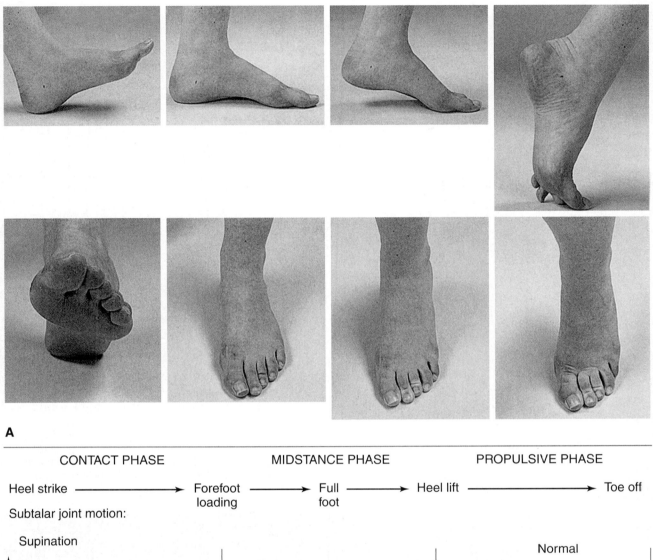

A

CONTACT PHASE	MIDSTANCE PHASE	PROPULSIVE PHASE

Heel strike ⟶ Forefoot loading ⟶ Full foot ⟶ Heel lift ⟶ Toe off

Subtalar joint motion:

Supination

Normal

Neutral

Rigid foot
for propulsion

Abnormal

Pronation

Flexible foot for
propulsion
→ pathology

B

Figure 20–23 *A* and *B*, Positions of the foot in the normal gait cycle.

manner in which the patient squats and then stands provides an excellent impression of the muscle strength and joint action of the lower extremities.

In addition, assessment of specific muscle groups can be performed and integrated into the arthrometric examination. Muscle strength can be graded according to the scale described in Chapter 21, The Nervous System.

Measure the dorsiflexors and plantar flexors. With the patient seated, have the patient dorsiflex and plantarflex the foot against resistance. This can also be accomplished by asking the patient to walk toward and away from you on the heels and then on the toes. Injury to the common peroneal nerve causes weakness of the anterior muscle group, with a diminished

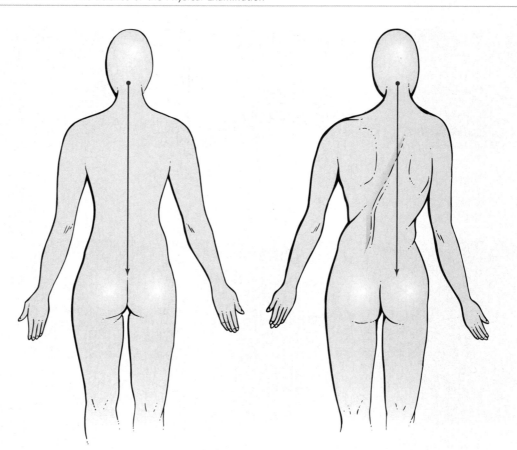

Figure 20–24 Technique for evaluating ''straightness'' of the spine. Lateral deviation of the spine may be related to a herniated disc or to spasm of the paravertebral muscles. This functional deviation is often termed a *list*. True scoliosis may result from an actual deformity of the spine. In many cases, the spine twists in the opposite direction, so that a plumb line may actually be in the center.

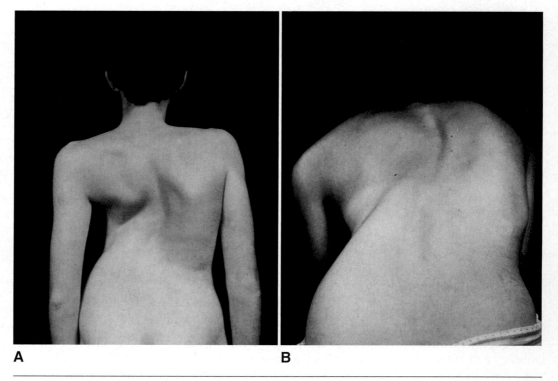

Figure 20–25 *A,* Severe kyphoscoliosis. *B,* Patient asked to bend forward.

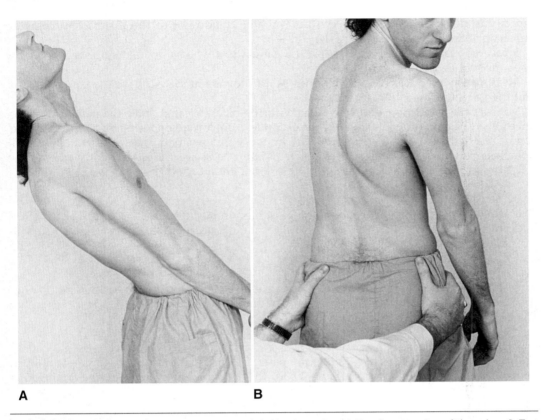

A   B

Figure 20–26 Technique for evaluating motion of the lumbar spine. *A,* Test for extension of the spine. *B,* Test for rotation of the spine.

Figure 20–27 Technique for evaluating strength of the lower extremities.

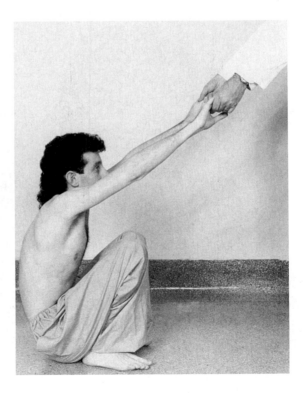

capacity to dorsiflex the foot. Injury to the Achilles tendon or to the gastrosoleus complex impairs plantar flexion.

Measure invertors and evertors. With the patient seated, have the patient invert and then evert the foot against resistance.

Measure the quadriceps and hamstrings. With the patient seated, have the patient extend and then flex the knee against resistance.

Measure the hip flexors and extensors. With the patient seated, have the patient raise the knee off the examination table against the examiner's downward opposing force. Hip extensors can be assessed by asking the patient to rise from a seated position unassisted. Human immunodeficiency virus–related myopathy affects proximal muscle groups first, and patients may initially complain of difficulty rising from a chair or climbing stairs.

Evaluate Neck Flexion

The patient is instructed to sit, and the range of motion of the neck is assessed. The patient is asked to put his or her chin on the chest, with the mouth closed, as shown in Figure 20-28. This tests full flexion of the neck.

Evaluate Neck Extension

To test full extension of the neck, place your hand between the patient's occiput and spinous processes of C7. Instruct the patient to trap your hand by extending the neck. This is shown in Figure 20-29.

Evaluate Neck Rotation

Evaluate rotation of the neck by asking the patient to rotate the neck to one side and touch chin to shoulder. This is shown in Figure 20-30. The examination is then repeated on the other side.

Evaluate Intrinsic Muscles of the Hand

The patient is instructed to stretch out the arms, with the fingers spread. The examiner attempts to compress the fingers together against resistance, as shown in Figure 20-31. This tests the intrinsic muscles of the hands.

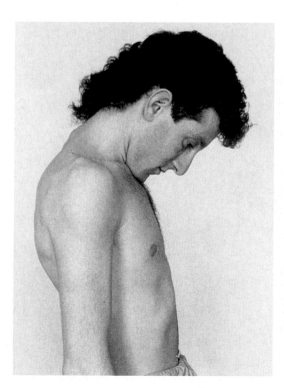

Figure 20–28 Technique for testing flexion of the neck.

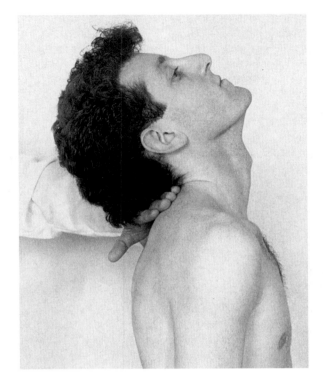

Figure 20–29 Technique for testing extension of the neck.

Evaluate External Rotation of the Arm

To test the functional range of rotation of the humerus and the *shoulder, acromioclavicular*, and *sternoclavicular joints*, instruct the patient to abduct the arms fully and place the palms together above the head. The arms should touch the patient's ears with the head and cervical spine in the vertical position. This is shown in Figure 20-32.

Evaluate Internal Rotation of the Arm

The patient is then asked to place his or her hands on the back between the scapulae. The hands should normally reach the level of the inferior angle of the scapulae. This is shown

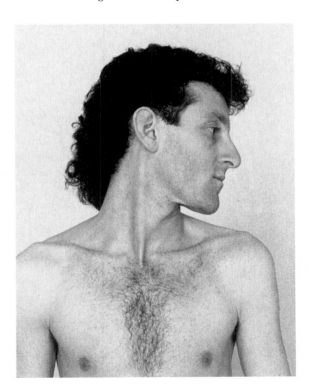

Figure 20–30 Technique for testing rotation of the neck.

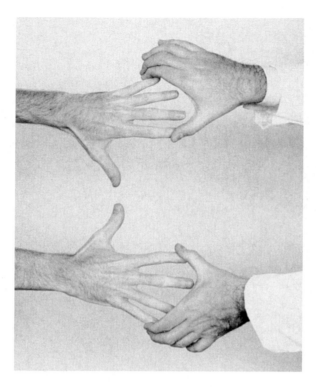

Figure 20–31 Technique for testing the intrinsic muscles of the hand.

in Figure 20-33. This maneuver tests internal rotation of the humerus and range of motion at the elbow.

Evaluate Strength of the Upper Extremities

The final test of the screening examination assesses the power of the major groups of muscles in the upper extremities. The patient is asked to grasp the examiner's index and middle fingers in each hand. The patient is instructed to resist upward, downward, lateral, and medial movement by the examiner. This position is shown in Figure 20-34.

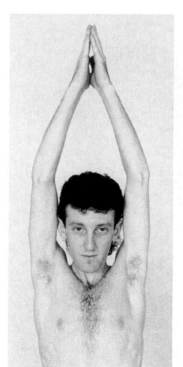

Figure 20–32 Technique for testing external rotation of the arm.

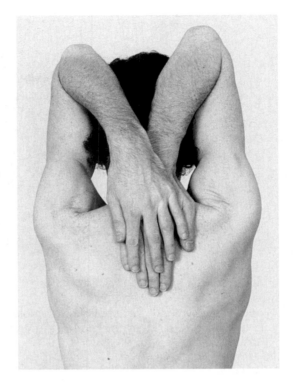

Figure 20–33 Technique for testing internal rotation of the arm.

This completes the basic musculoskeletal screening examination. The remainder of this section describes the symptoms and examination of specific joints.

Examination of Specific Joints

Any area must be inspected for evidence of swelling, atrophy, redness, and deformity, as well as palpated for swelling, muscle spasm, and local painful areas. The range of motion is assessed both actively and passively.

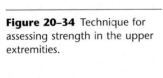

Figure 20–34 Technique for assessing strength in the upper extremities.

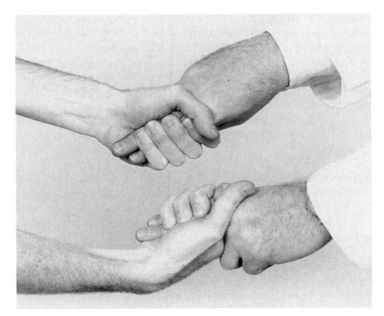

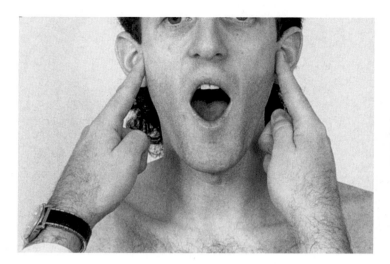

Figure 20–35 Technique for evaluating the temporomandibular joint.

Temporomandibular Joint

Symptoms

A patient with temporomandibular joint problems may complain of unilateral or bilateral jaw pain. The pain is worse in the morning and after chewing or eating. The patient may also complain of "clicking" of the jaw.

Examination

To examine this joint, the examiner places his or her index fingers in front of the tragus and instructs the patient to open and close the jaw slowly. The examiner observes the smoothness of the range of motion and notes any tenderness. This is illustrated in Figure 20-35.

Shoulder

Symptoms

Although shoulder pain may be related to a primary shoulder disorder, *always* consider the possibility that shoulder pain is referred from either the chest or the abdomen. Coronary artery disease, pulmonary tumors, and gallbladder disease are commonly associated with pain referred to the shoulder.

Pain is the main symptom of shoulder disorders. Inflammation of the *supraspinatus muscle* causes pain that is usually worse at night or when the patient lies on the affected shoulder. The pain often radiates down the arm as far as the elbow. The pain is commonly referred to the lower part of the deltoid area and is characteristically aggravated by combing the hair, putting on a coat, or reaching into the back pocket. Diffuse tenderness of the shoulder associated with pain on moving the humerus posteriorly is associated with disorders of the teres minor, infraspinatus, and subscapularis muscles. In this case, the pain usually does not radiate into the arm and is usually absent when the arm is dependent.

The movements of the shoulder occur at the *glenohumeral, thoracoscapular, acromioclavicular,* and *sternoclavicular joints.* The glenohumeral joint is a ball-and-socket joint. In contrast to the hip joint, which is also a ball-and-socket joint, in the glenohumeral joint the humerus sits in the very shallow glenoid socket. Therefore, the function of the joint depends on the muscles surrounding the socket for stability. These muscles and their tendons form the *rotator cuff* of the shoulder. For this reason, many shoulder problems are muscular, not bone or joint related, in origin.

Examination

Inspect the shoulder for deformity, wasting, and asymmetry. The shoulder should be palpated for local areas of tenderness. The range of motion for abduction, adduction, external and internal rotation, and flexion is evaluated and compared with that of the other side. Any pain is noted.

Special tests are necessary to determine specific diagnoses. The impingement syndrome, tears of the rotator cuff, and bicipital tendinitis are common. The examinations for these conditions are described in this section.

The *impingement syndrome*, also known as *rotator cuff tendinitis*, is usually secondary to sports trauma. Irritation of the avascular portion of the supraspinatus tendon progresses to an inflammatory response termed *tendinitis*. This inflammatory response later involves the biceps tendon, subacromial bursa, and acromioclavicular joint. With continued trauma, rotator cuff tears and calcification may occur. The most reliable test for the impingement syndrome is the reproduction of pain when the examiner forcibly flexes the patient's arm with the elbow extended against resistance.

Sudden onset of shoulder pain in the deltoid area 6 to 10 hours after trauma suggests a *rotator cuff tear* or *rupture*. Extreme tenderness over the greater tuberosity of the humerus and pain and restricted motion at the glenohumeral joint are usually present. Active abduction of the glenohumeral joint is markedly reduced. When the examiner attempts to abduct the arm, pain and a characteristic *shoulder shrug* result.

Generalized tenderness anteriorly over the long head of the biceps that is associated with pain, especially at night, should raise suspicion of *bicipital tendinitis*. In this condition, there is normal abduction and forward flexion. The hallmark of bicipital tendinitis is the reproduction of anterior shoulder pain during resistance to forearm supination. The patient is asked to place the arm at the side with the elbow flexed 90°. The patient is instructed to supinate the arm against the examiner's resistance. If there is pain in the triceps area with resisted extension of the elbow, *tricipital tendinitis* may be present.

Elbow

Symptoms

The most common symptom of elbow disorders is well-localized elbow pain.

Although it is a simple hinge joint, the elbow is the most complicated joint of the upper extremity. The distal end of the humerus articulates with the proximal ulna and radius. Flexion and extension of the elbow are effected through the humeroulnar portion of the joint. The radius plays little role in this action; its role is primarily in pronation and supination of the forearm. The ulnar nerve lies in a vulnerable position as it passes around the medial epicondyle of the humerus.

Examination

Palpate the elbow for swelling, masses, tenderness, and nodules. Test flexion and extension.

To test for pronation and supination, the elbows should be flexed at 90° and placed firmly on a table. The patient is asked to rotate the forearm with wrist down (pronation), as shown in Figure 20-36*A*, and wrist up (supination), as shown in Figure 20-36*B*. Any limitation of motion or pain is noted.

Tennis elbow, also known as *lateral epicondylitis*, is a common condition characterized by pain in the region of the lateral epicondyle of the humerus. The pain radiates down the extensor surface of the forearm. Patients with tennis elbow often experience pain when attempting to

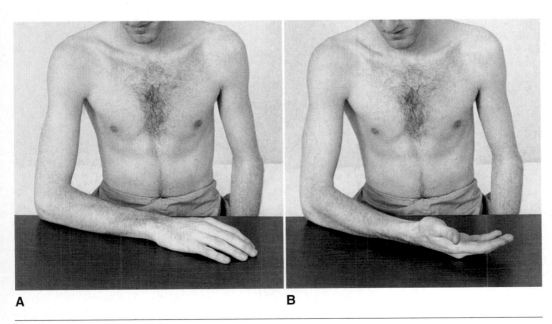

A   **B**

Figure 20–36 Technique for evaluating pronation and supination at the elbow. *A,* Pronation. *B,* Supination.

open a door or when lifting a glass. To test for tennis elbow, the examiner should flex the patient's elbow and fully pronate the hand. Pain over the lateral epicondyle while the elbow is extended is diagnostic of tennis elbow. Another test involves having the patient clench the fist, dorsiflex the wrist, and extend the elbow. Pain is elicited by trying to force the dorsiflexed hand into palmar flexion.

Wrist

Symptoms

The symptoms of wrist disorders include pain in the wrist or hand, numbness or tingling in the wrist or fingers, loss of movement and stiffness, and deformities. Pain in the hand may be referred from the neck or elbow.

The wrist is composed of the articulation of the distal end of the radius with the proximal row of the carpal bones. The stability of the wrist is caused by the banding together of these bones by strong ligaments. The distal ulna does not articulate with any of the carpal bones. On the volar aspect of the wrist, the carpal bones are connected by the carpal ligament. The passage under this ligament is the *carpal tunnel*, through which the median nerve and all the flexors of the wrist pass. Entrapment of the nerve, known as *carpal tunnel syndrome*, produces symptoms of numbness and tingling.

Examination

Palpate the patient's wrist joint between your thumbs and index fingers, noting tenderness, swelling, or redness (Fig. 20-37).

The range of motion of dorsiflexion and palmar flexion is noted. With the forearms fixed, the degree of supination and pronation is evaluated. Is ulnar or radial deviation present?

When the diagnosis of carpal tunnel syndrome is suspected, a sharp tap or pressure directly over the median nerve may reproduce the paresthesias of carpal tunnel syndrome, called *Tinel's sign*. Another useful test is for the examiner to stretch the median nerve by extending the patient's elbow and dorsiflexing the wrist. The development of pain or paresthesias is suggestive of the diagnosis. A third test entails the patient's holding both wrists in a fully palmar-fixed position for 2 minutes. The development or exacerbation of paresthesias is suggestive of carpal tunnel syndrome.

Hand

Symptoms

Pain and swelling of joints are the most important symptoms of disorders of the hand.

Examination

Palpate the patient's metacarpophalangeal joints and note swelling, redness, or tenderness, as demonstrated in Figure 20-38. Palpate the medial and lateral aspects of the proximal and distal interphalangeal joints between your thumb and index finger, as shown in Figure 20-39. Again, note swelling, redness, or tenderness.

Figure 20–37 Technique for palpation of the wrist joint.

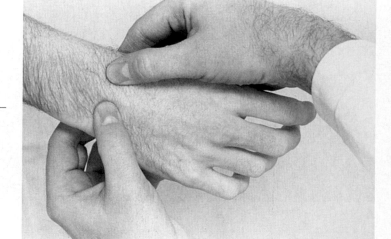

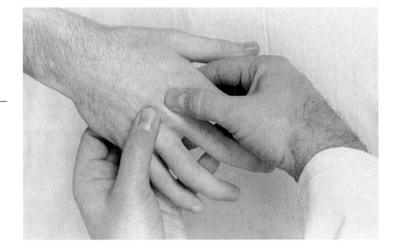

Figure 20–38 Technique for palpation of the metacarpophalangeal joints.

The range of motion of the fingers includes movements at the distal interphalangeal joint, the proximal interphalangeal joint, and the metacarpophalangeal joints of the fingers and the thumb.

Ask the patient to make a fist with the thumb across the knuckles and then extend and spread the fingers. Normally, the fingers should flex to the distal palmar crease. The thumb should oppose to the distal metacarpal head. Each finger should extend to the zero position in relation to its metacarpal.

Tenosynovitis of the thumb abductors and extensors is known as *de Quervain's disease*. The patient complains of weakness of grip and pain at the base of the thumb that is aggravated by certain movements of the wrist. To confirm the diagnosis, ask the patient to flex the thumb and close the fingers over it. You should now attempt to move the hand into ulnar deviation. Excruciating pain will accompany this maneuver if de Quervain's tenosynovitis is present.

Spine

Symptoms

The most common symptom of disorders of the spine is pain. Pain from the thoracic spine often radiates around the trunk along the lines of the intercostal nerves. Pain from the upper lumbar spine may be felt in the front of the thighs and knees. Pain originating in the lower lumbar spine can be felt in the coccyx, hips, and buttocks, as well as shooting down the back of the legs to the heels and feet. The pain is often intensified by movement. Patients with herniated vertebral discs may complain of pain that is exacerbated by sneezing or coughing. Determine whether there is associated numbness or tingling in the lower extremity, which is related to nerve root lesions.

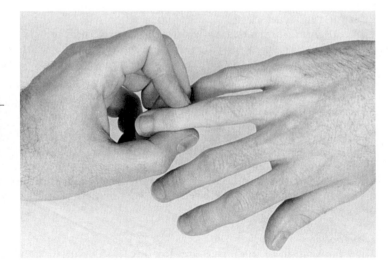

Figure 20–39 Technique for palpation of the interphalangeal joints.

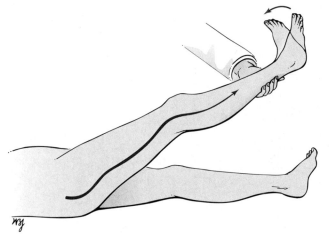

Figure 20–40 Straight leg raising test.

Examination

The cervical spine can be examined with the patient seated. You should inspect the cervical spine from the front, back, and sides for deformity and unusual posture. Test range of motion of the cervical spine. Palpate the paravertebral muscles for tenderness and spasm.

The thoracolumbar spine is examined with the patient standing in front of you. Inspect the spine for deformity or swelling. Inspect the spine from the side for abnormal curvature. Test ranges of motion. Palpate the paravertebral muscles for tenderness. Percuss each spinous process for tenderness.

The ranges of motion tested in the spine are forward flexion, extension, lateral flexion, and rotation.

The presence of a *cervical rib* may cause coldness, discoloration, and trophic changes as a result of ischemia to an upper extremity. To test for a cervical rib, palpate the radial pulse. Move the arm through its range of motion. Obliteration of the pulse by this maneuver is suggestive of the presence of a cervical rib. Ask the patient to turn the head toward the affected side and take a deep breath while you are palpating the radial pulse on the same side. Obliteration of the pulse by this maneuver is also suggestive of a cervical rib. Often, auscultation over the subclavian artery reveals a bruit suggestive of mechanical obstruction by a cervical rib. Repeat any of these tests on the opposite side. Cervical ribs are rarely bilateral.

Pain from entrapment of the sciatic nerve is called *sciatica*. Patients with sciatica describe pain, burning sensation, or aching in the buttocks radiating down the posterior thigh to the posterolateral aspect of the calf. Pain is worsened by sneezing, laughing, or straining at stool. One of the tests for sciatica is the straight leg raising test. The patient is asked to lie supine while the examiner flexes the extended leg to the trunk at the hip. The presence of pain is a positive test result. The patient is asked to plantarflex and dorsiflex the foot. This stretches the sciatic nerve even more. If sciatica is present, this test reproduces pain in the leg. The test is illustrated in Figure 20-40.

Another test for sciatica is the sitting knee extension test. The patient sits off the side of the bed and flexes the neck, placing the chin on the chest. The examiner fixes the thigh on the bed with one hand while the other hand extends the leg. If sciatica is present, pain is reproduced as the leg is extended. This test is demonstrated in Figure 20-41.

Hip

Symptoms

The main symptoms of hip disease are pain, stiffness, deformity, and a limp. Hip pain may be localized to the groin or may radiate down the medial aspect of the thigh. Stiffness may be related to periods of immobility. An early symptom of hip disease is difficulty putting on shoes. This requires external rotation of the hip, which is the first motion to be lost with degenerative disease of the hip. This is followed by loss of abduction and adduction; hip flexion is the last movement lost.

Examination

The examination of the hip is performed with the patient standing and lying on the back.

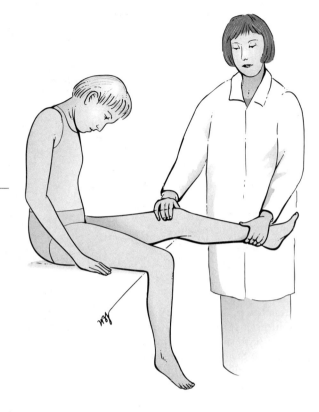

Figure 20–41 Sitting knee extension test.

Inspection of the hips and gait has already been described. The *Trendelenburg test* is used to detect a disorder between the pelvis and the femur. The patient is asked to stand on the "good" leg, as illustrated in Figure 20-42A. The examiner should note that the pelvis on the opposite side elevates, demonstrating that the gluteus medius is working efficiently. When the patient is asked to stand on the "bad" leg, as shown in Figure 20-42B, the pelvis on the opposite side falls. This is a positive Trendelenburg test result.

Figure 20–42 Trendelenburg test. *A,* Position of the hips when standing on the normal left leg. Note that the hip elevates as a result of contraction of the left hip musculature. *B,* Position of the hips when standing on the abnormal right leg. Note that the left hip falls as a result of lack of adequate contraction of the right hip muscles.

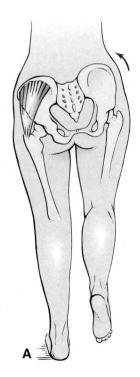

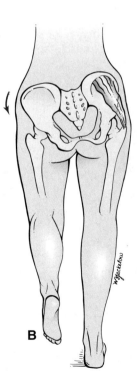

A

B

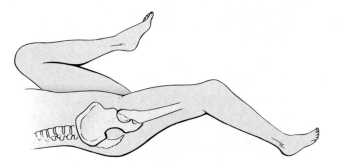

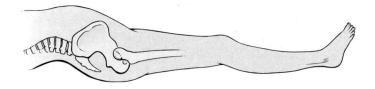

Figure 20–43 Evaluation for flexion deformity of the hip.

Ask the patient to lie on his or her back. The hip is acutely flexed on the abdomen to flatten the lumbar spine. Flexion of the opposite thigh is suggestive of a flexion deformity of that hip. Figure 20-43 illustrates the technique.

Leg length measurements are useful in evaluating hip disorders. The distance between the anterosuperior iliac spine and the tip of the medial malleolus is measured on each side, and the two measurements are compared. A difference in leg length may be caused by hip joint disorders.

As indicated, loss of rotation of the hip is an early finding in hip disease. To test this movement, ask the patient to lie on his or her back. Flex the patient's hip and knee to 90°, and rotate the ankle inward for external rotation, as illustrated in Figure 20-44*A*, and outward for internal rotation, as shown in Figure 20-44*B*. Restriction of this motion is a sensitive sign of degenerative hip disease.

Knee

Symptoms

Although the knee is the largest joint in the body, it is not the strongest. The knee is a hinge joint between the femur and the tibia and enables flexion and extension. When it is flexed, a small degree of lateral motion is also normal. As with the shoulder, the knee depends on the strong muscles and ligaments around the joint for its stability.

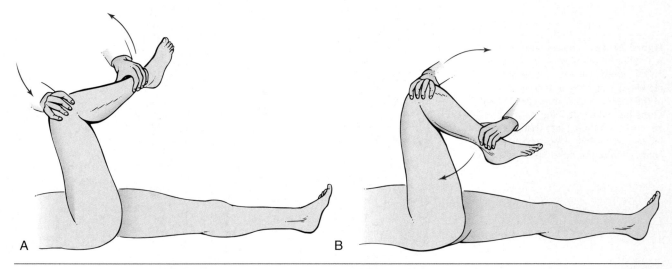

A   B

Figure 20–44 Testing the range of motion at the hip. The examiner flexes the patient's hip and knee to 90° and rotates the ankle inward for external rotation (*A*) and outward for internal rotation (*B*).

Pain, swelling, joint instability, and limited movement are the main symptoms of knee disorders. Knee pain is exacerbated by movement and may be referred to the calf or thigh. Swelling of the knee indicates a synovial effusion or bleeding into the joint, also known as *hemarthrosis*. Knee trauma may result in hemarthrosis and limitation of joint motion. *Locking* of the knee results from small pieces of broken cartilage lodged between the femur and the tibia, blocking full extension of the joint.

Examination

The examination of the knee is performed with the patient standing and lying on the back.

While the patient is standing, any varus or valgus deformity should be noted. Is there wasting of the quadriceps muscle? Is there swelling of the knee? An early sign of knee joint swelling is loss of the slight depressions on the lateral sides of the patella. Inspect for swelling in the popliteal fossa. A *Baker's cyst* in the popliteal fossa may be responsible for swelling in the popliteal fossa, causing calf pain.

The patient is then asked to lie on the back. The contours of the knee are evaluated. The patella is palpated in extension for tenderness. By stressing the patella against the femoral condyles, pain may be elicited. This occurs in osteoarthritis.

Testing for *knee joint effusion* is performed by pressing the fluid out of the suprapatellar pouch down behind the patella. Start about 15 cm above the superior margin of the patient's patella and slide your index finger and thumb firmly downward along the sides of the femur, milking the fluid into the space between the patella and the femur. While you maintain pressure on the lateral margins of the patella, tap on the patella with the other hand. This technique is termed *ballottement*. In the presence of an effusion, a distinct bump is felt in response to your tap, and the transmitted impulse is felt by the fingers on either side of the patella. This technique is shown in Figure 20-45.

To palpate the *collateral ligaments*, the patient's foot should be resting on the bed, with the knee flexed at 90°. Grasp the patient's leg and, using your thumbs, try to elicit tenderness over the patellar tendon beneath the femoral epicondyles. This technique and a *medial collateral ligament* rupture are illustrated in Figure 20-46.

Another test for collateral ligament rupture is performed by placing the examiner's left hand on the lateral aspect of the patient's knee at the level of the joint. The knee is flexed about 25°, and the lower leg is pushed outward by the examiner's right hand, with the left hand acting as a fulcrum. This maneuver is an attempt to "open up" the medial side of the knee joint. The result should be compared with that on the other side. Abnormal lateral motion is seen in rupture of the medial collateral ligament, as illustrated in Figure 20-47. The maneuver can be used to test for rupture of the lateral collateral ligament by reversing the positions.

The drawer test is used to test for rupture of the *cruciate ligaments*. The patient is instructed to flex the knee to 90°. The examiner should sit close to the foot to steady it. The examiner then grasps the leg just below the knee with both hands and jerks the tibia forward, as illustrated in Figure 20-48. Abnormal forward mobility of 2 cm or more is suggestive of rupture of the anterior cruciate ligament. This maneuver can be used to test the posterior cruciate ligament by flexing the knee to 90°, steadying the foot, and attempting to jerk the leg backward. Abnormal backward motion of 2 cm or more indicates rupture of the posterior cruciate ligament.

Ankle and Foot

Symptoms

The ankle is a hinge joint between the lower end of the tibia and the talus.

Although symptoms in the ankle and foot usually have a local cause, they can also be secondary to systemic disorders. Symptoms may include pain, swelling, and deformities.

The patient's only complaint may be uneven shoe wear. Patients with flatfoot wear down their soles on the medial side extending to the tip of the shoe. The outer portion of the heel is also worn out early. Scuff marks are usually present on the medial sides of the heels. Excessive wear under the toes may indicate an equinus foot type or a tight Achilles tendon. Asymmetric shoe wear may result from a difference in limb length. Isolated areas of wear under the ball of the foot may result from a plantar-flexed metatarsal and indicate areas of potential ulceration in a patient with diabetes and neuropathy.

Examination

The examination of the ankle and foot is performed with the patient standing, walking, and then sitting.

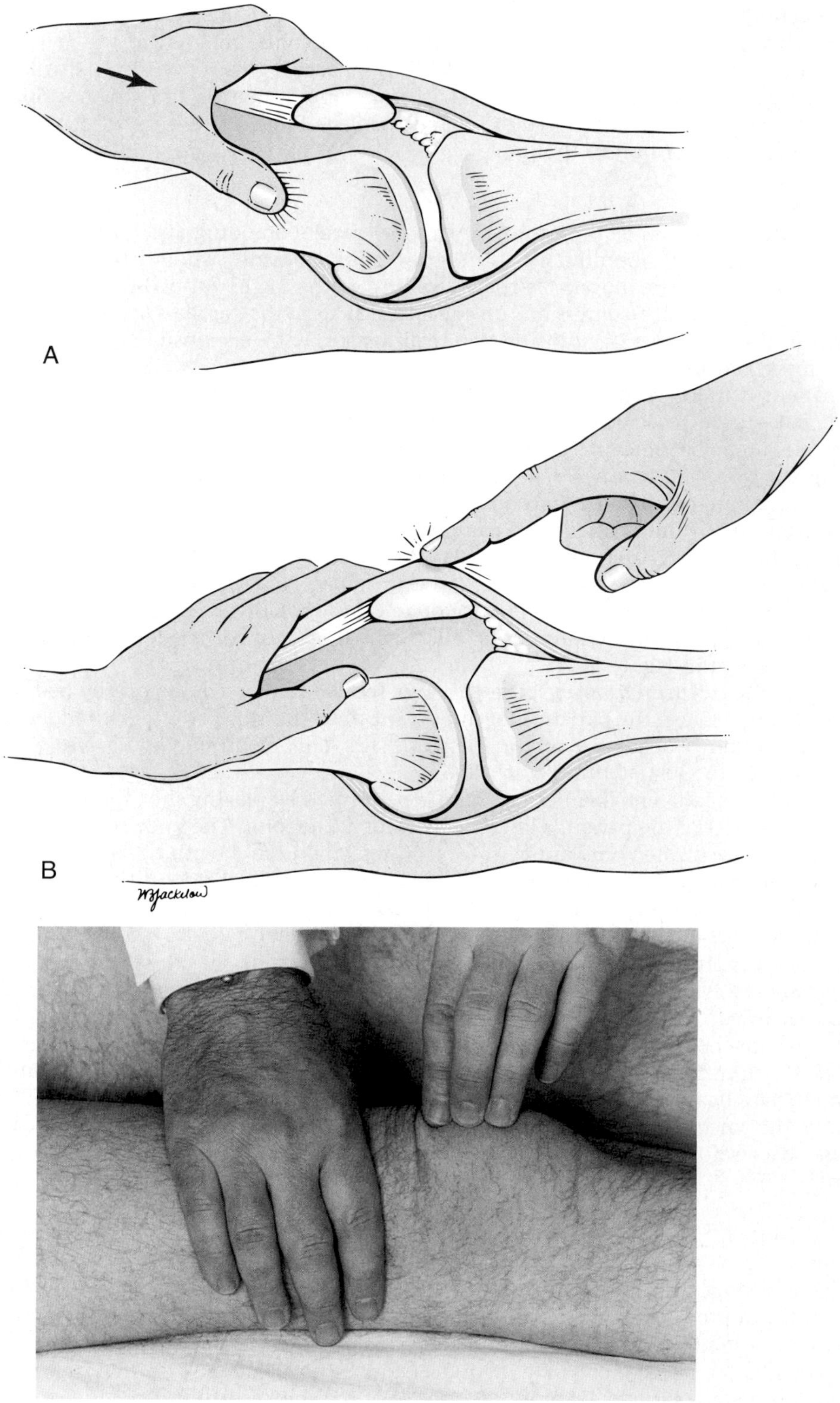

Figure 20–45 Technique for testing for knee joint effusion. *A,* Position of the hand when pushing fluid out of the bursae. *B* and *C,* Position for tapping the patella.

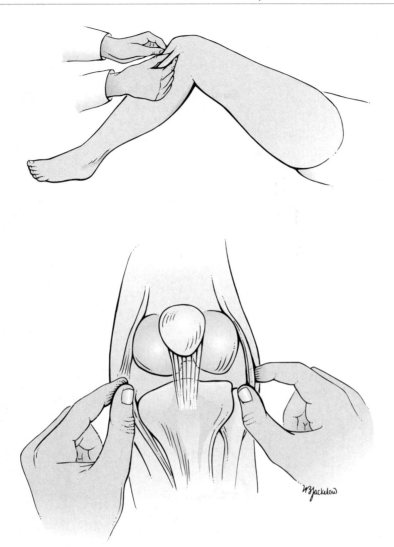

Figure 20–46 *Top,* Technique for testing the collateral ligaments. *Bottom,* Rupture of the medial collateral ligament.

Ask the patient to stand. Inspect the ankles and feet for swelling and deformities. The number and position of toes should be noted. The toes should be straight, flat, and proportional to one another in comparison with the other foot. Compare one foot with the other with regard to symmetry. Are any toes overlapping? Describe abnormalities of the longitudinal arch. A *cavus foot* has an abnormally high arch. In *flatfoot,* the longitudinal arch is flatter than normal. Common foot abnormalities are illustrated in Figure 20-49.

Ask the patient to walk without shoes and socks, and observe the gait. The patient should be able to walk normally, on heels, on toes, and one foot in front of the other (tandem walking). Note any deformities such as the width or length of the feet, heel varus or valgus, calf atrophy, varicose veins, and in-toeing or out-toeing. Take note of the patient's posture and any shuffling or other abnormality.

Ask the patient to sit with the feet dangling off the side of the bed. Normally, there is mild plantar flexion and inversion of the feet. Palpate the medial and lateral malleoli. The distal portion of the fibula constitutes the lateral malleolus. It extends more distally than the medial malleolus. Palpate the Achilles tendon. Are any nodules present? Is tenderness present?

Test the range of motion at the ankle, which includes dorsiflexion and plantar flexion. The range of motion necessary for normal gait is 10° dorsiflexion and 20° plantar flexion. Ankle joint dorsiflexion with the knee flexed should approach 15°.

If dorsiflexion at the ankle joint is less than 10°, measurement should be taken again with the knee flexed. If dorsiflexion is less than 10° in both positions, limitation of motion is usually caused by an osseous block at the ankle. If dorsiflexion increases with knee flexion, a tight gastrosoleus complex is probably responsible.

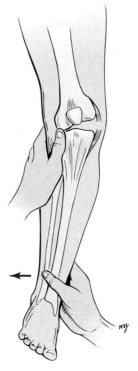

Figure 20–47 Another technique for testing the collateral ligaments.

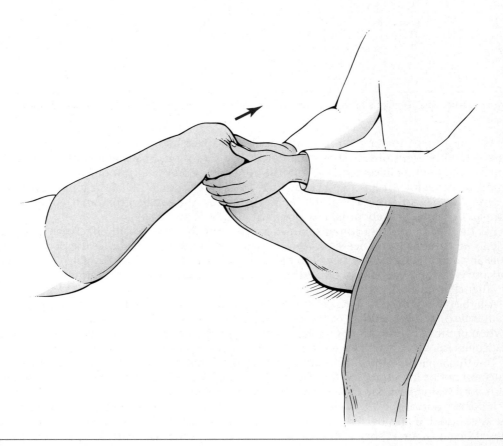

Figure 20–48 Technique for testing the cruciate ligaments: the drawer test.

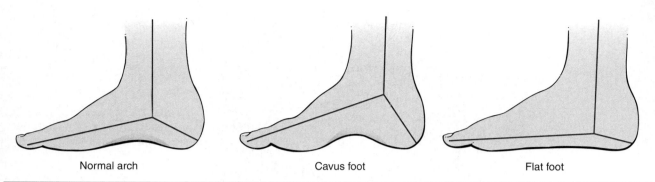

| Normal arch | Cavus foot | Flat foot |

Figure 20–49 Common foot abnormalities.

Test the range of motion at the subtalar joint, which includes eversion and inversion. With the patient lying prone on the examination table, hold the patient's leg in one of your hands, and move the heel with your other hand into inversion and eversion. Measure the excursion of the heel with regard to the bisection of the lower one third of the leg. This technique is illustrated in Figure 20-50. The average range of motion of the subtalar joint is 20° of inversion and 10° of eversion.

Test the range of motion at the midtarsal joint, which includes eversion and inversion. With the patient in the prone position, stabilize the heel with one of your hands, and rotate the forefoot into inversion and eversion. Measure excursion of the plane of the metatarsal heads with regard to the bisection of the heel. This technique is illustrated in Figure 20-51.

The movements of the metatarsophalangeal joints are tested individually. Palpate the head of each metatarsal and the base of each proximal phalanx, as well as the groove between them. Is tenderness or joint effusion present?

The Achilles tendon, which is the combined tendon of the gastrocnemius and soleus muscles, may rupture. You can test for its integrity by direct observation and having the patient jump up and down on the balls of the feet or walk on the toes. Another test for its integrity is known as the *Thompson-Doherty squeeze test*. This test is performed by squeezing the calf while you observe the motion of the foot. Normally, squeezing produces plantar flexion; a ruptured tendon produces little or no motion. When examining the tendon for continuity, remember that the most common place for rupture is approximately 1 to 2 inches (2.5 to 5.0 cm)

Figure 20–50 Evaluating the range of motion at the subtalar joint.

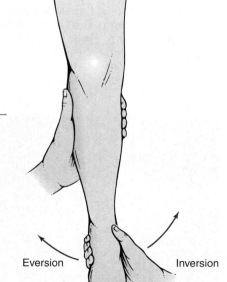

Eversion   Inversion

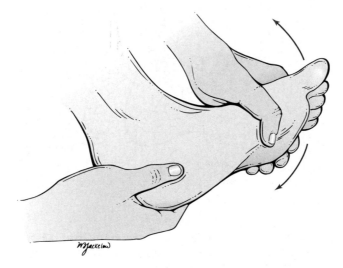

Figure 20–51 Evaluating the range of motion at the midtarsal joint.

proximal to its insertion on the calcaneus. This lies within a region of poorest blood supply that is often referred to as the "watershed area."

Describe abnormalities of the joints, including hallux abductovalgus (*bunion*), and deformities and flexion contractures of the lower digits (*hammer toes*). Figure 20-52 shows hallux abductovalgus deformity, flexion contractures of the interphalangeal joints, and bowstringing of the extensor tendons. This is a typical presentation in the geriatric age group. Note the hyperkeratotic lesion over the right bunion from shoe pressure.

Palpate the soft tissue over the first metatarsophalangeal joint. Is bursal inflammation caused by pressure, friction, or urate deposition? Measure the range of motion of the joint. Dorsiflexion of the hallux is measured against the bisection of the first metatarsal. The normal dorsal range of motion is 65° to 75°. Limitation of motion of this joint is termed *hallux limitus* and is most commonly caused by osteoarthritis.

Bunion deformities can be a source of undue pressure in diabetic patients, leading to ulceration and infection. A large pressure ulceration over the medial eminence of the first metatarsophalangeal joint resulting from shoe irritation in a diabetic patient is shown in Figure 20-53.

Figure 20-54 depicts ulceration over the distal interphalangeal joint of the fourth toe of a patient with chronic tophaceous gout. Note the bunion deformity and underlapping hallux. An acute attack of gout commonly manifests with severe pain, swelling, and inflammation in the first metatarsophalangeal joint, a condition termed *podagra*. Podagra in a patient with acute gout is pictured in Figure 20-55. Notice the erythema of the left hallux and the generalized swelling of the left foot.

Examine the lesser metatarsophalangeal joints. Grasp the metatarsophalangeal joints between your thumb and index finger, and attempt to compress the forefoot. Pain elicited by this maneuver is often an early sign of *rheumatoid arthritis*. This test is demonstrated in Figure 20-56.

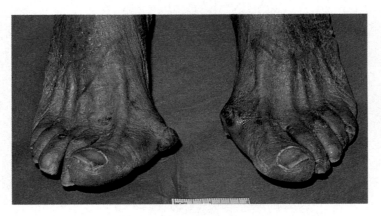

Figure 20–52 Bunion deformity and hammer toes. Notice bowstringing of the extensor tendons.

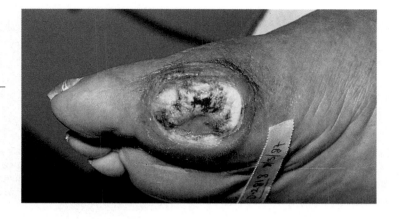

Figure 20–53 Hallux abductovalgus deformity and ulceration.

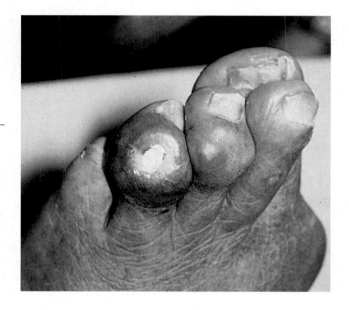

Figure 20–54 Gout of the lesser metatarsophalangeal joints.

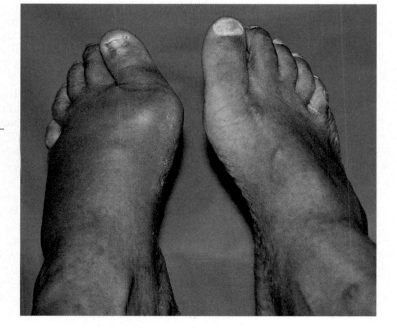

Figure 20–55 Acute gout and podagra, left big toe.

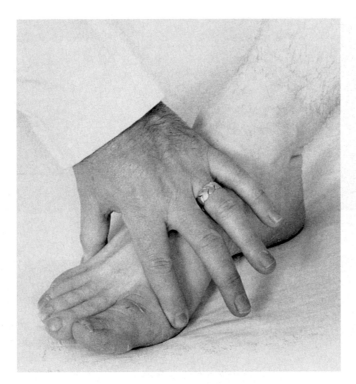

Figure 20–56 Technique for evaluating the metatarsophalangeal joints.

Clinicopathologic Correlations

Rheumatoid arthritis is a common musculoskeletal disorder and is the most destructive and disabling of the principal joint diseases. It is an autoimmune disease that causes chronic inflammation of the joints and of many other organs such as the skin, heart, kidneys, lungs, digestive tract, blood vessels, nervous system, and eyes. However, the joints display the most marked destructive changes. Rheumatoid arthritis is a progressive illness that can cause significant functional disability as a result of pain, swelling, and stiffness of the involved joints. More than 2 million Americans suffer from rheumatoid arthritis, which is two to three times more common in women than in men. Although rheumatoid arthritis generally occurs between the ages of 40 and 60 years, it can also affect young children and older adults.

The most characteristic changes are in the hands. In the early stages of the disease, there is swelling of the proximal interphalangeal, the metacarpophalangeal, and the wrist joints. As the disease progresses, there is bone erosion, which produces the classic signs of the disease. The most characteristic deformity of the fingers is ulnar deviation at the metacarpophalangeal joints. The two main deformities of the interphalangeal joints are the swan-neck deformity and the boutonnière deformity.

The *swan-neck deformity*, which results from shortening of the interosseous muscles, produces flexion of the metacarpophalangeal joints, hyperextension of the proximal interphalangeal joints, and flexion of the distal interphalangeal joints. The *boutonnière deformity* is a flexion deformity of the proximal interphalangeal joints with hyperextension of the distal interphalangeal joints. Figure 20-57 shows the hands of a woman with rheumatoid arthritis. Note the marked ulnar deviation of the metacarpophalangeal joints. Figure 20-58 depicts the characteristic swan-neck deformity.

Osteoarthritis, or degenerative joint disease, is very common, affecting more than 20 million people in the United States. Osteoarthritis is related mostly to aging. Before age 45 years, osteoarthritis occurs more frequently in men; after age 55 years, it occurs more frequently in women. In the United States, all races appear to be affected in equal proportions. A higher incidence of osteoarthritis exists in the Japanese population, whereas black people from South Africa, people from the East Indies, and people from southern China have lower rates.

Osteoarthritis is a type of arthritis that is caused by the breakdown and eventual loss of the cartilage of one or more joints. In most cases, the inflammatory response is minimal in comparison with that of rheumatoid arthritis. Osteoarthritis causes pain, swelling and reduced

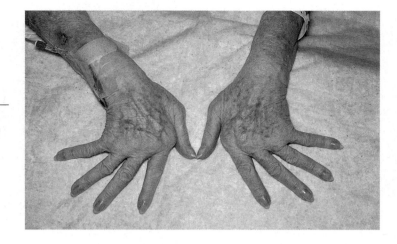

Figure 20–57 Rheumatoid arthritis. Note the marked ulnar deviation of the wrists.

motion in the joints. The form of osteoarthritis depends on the joints involved. Osteoarthritis commonly affects the hands, feet, spine, and large weight-bearing joints, such as the hips and knees. One of the joints that are frequently involved is the distal interphalangeal joint of the hands. Progressive enlargement of these joints is termed *Heberden's nodes*. As the disease progresses, the proximal interphalangeal joints may become involved, resulting in *Bouchard's nodes*. Figure 20-59 shows the hands of a woman with osteoarthritis.

Gout is a metabolic disease characterized by high levels of uric acid, recurrent attacks of acute arthritis, and deposition of urate crystals in and around the joints. The initial manifestation is frequently acute pain in the first metatarsophalangeal joint, often waking the patient from sleep. Even at rest, the pain is severe, but the slightest movement of the joint is agonizing. Within a few hours, the joint becomes swollen, shiny, and red. The higher the level of uric acid, the more likely the patient is to develop *tophi*, which are subcutaneous and periarticular deposits of urate crystals. The commonly involved sites are over the first metatarsophalangeal joint, the finger, the ear, the elbow, and the Achilles tendon. Figure 20-60 shows a gouty deposit on the big toe. Figure 20-61 shows the arms of a patient with chronic tophaceous gout who has large tophi on her elbows, as well as smaller tophi on her hands. Tophi frequently develop over the distal interphalangeal joints of the fingers and in the olecranon and prepatellar bursae. Figure 20-62 shows the hands of a patient with tophi on her fingers.

As discussed in Chapter 8, The Skin, psoriasis is one of the most common skin diseases in the United States. The pustular variant is characterized by pustules localized to the palms and soles. The patient may be quite ill, with fever and leukocytosis. Figure 20-63 shows pustular psoriasis of the soles. Note the hyperkeratosis on an erythematous base.

Joint disease develops in approximately 7% of patients with psoriasis. The most common form of *psoriatic arthritis* (70%) is asymmetric arthritis involving only two or three joints at a time. *Arthritis mutilans* is the most deforming type of psoriatic arthritis. In the most severe cases, there is osteolysis of the phalangeal and metacarpal joints, resulting in "telescoping of

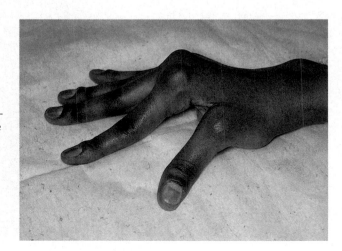

Figure 20–58 Rheumatoid arthritis. Note the swan-neck deformity.

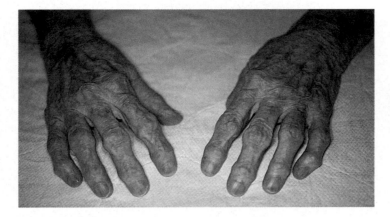

Figure 20–59 Osteoarthritis. Note Heberden's and Bouchard's nodes.

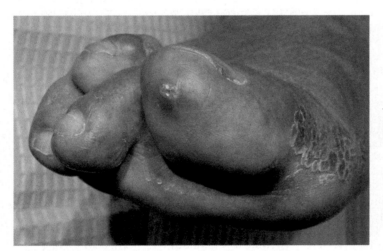

Figure 20–60 Gout affecting big toe.

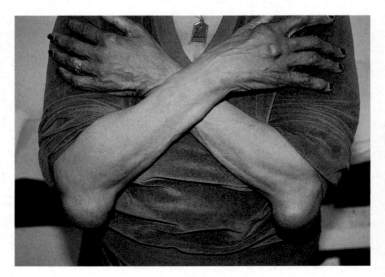

Figure 20–61 Gout. Note tophi on the elbows and hands.

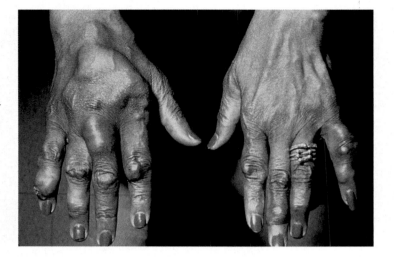

Figure 20–62 Gout. Note tophi on the fingers.

the digits," also known as the *opera-glass deformity*. The hands of a patient with this deforming type of psoriatic arthritis are shown in Figure 20-64.

Tuberous sclerosis is a dominantly inherited hamartomatous disorder characterized by mental retardation, seizures, eye lesions, and skin lesions. The classic triad of symptoms is mental retardation, seizures, and adenoma sebaceum. *Adenoma sebaceum* occurs near the nasolabial folds and over the cheeks. These lesions are facial angiofibromas. Other common skin lesions are periungual and subungual fibromas. Figure 20-65*A* shows the foot of a patient with tuberous sclerosis and periungual fibromas. Figure 20-65*B* shows the foot of another patient with tuberous sclerosis and subungual fibromas.

Lesions of Kaposi's sarcoma are frequently seen on the feet. Figure 20-66 shows the foot of a patient who presented with this lesion between his fourth and fifth toes. A biopsy of the lesion confirmed the diagnosis of Kaposi's sarcoma. This was the patient's first manifestation of acquired immunodeficiency syndrome. Figure 20-67 shows the plantar arch of another patient who presented with painful nodules. A biopsy confirmed the diagnosis of Kaposi's sarcoma. Kaposi's sarcoma of the heel is pictured in another patient in Figure 20-68.

Figure 20–63 Pustular psoriasis.

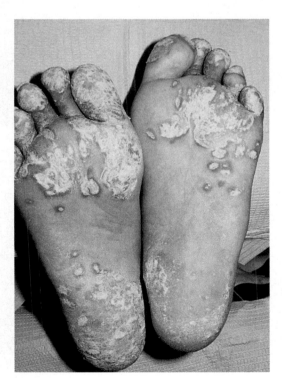

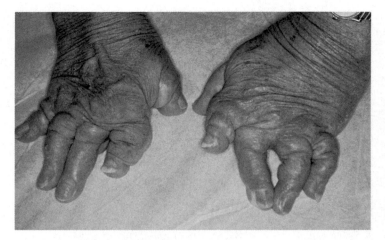

Figure 20–64 Psoriatic arthritis.

Another common podiatric complaint is an exostosis at the metatarsocuneiform joint, which produces a painful dorsal lesion. Figure 20-69A depicts this type of problem; Figure 20-69B is an x-ray film of the foot showing the bony abnormality.

Figure 20-70 shows severe paronychia with exuberant granulation tissue. Such lesions must be differentiated from amelanotic melanomas.

Although *squamous cell carcinomas* are usually found in sun-exposed areas, the lesion pictured in Figure 20-71 is on the plantar aspect of the foot. A callus is also present under the head of the first metatarsal.

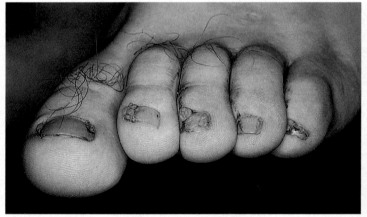

A

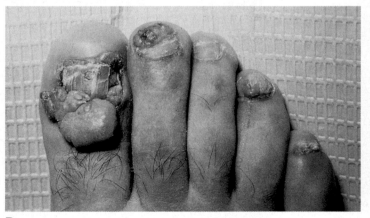

B

Figure 20–65 *A* and *B,* The feet of two patients with tuberous sclerosis and periungual fibromas.

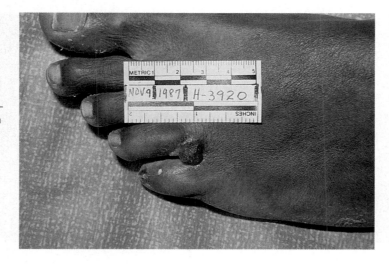

Figure 20–66 Kaposi's sarcoma between the toes.

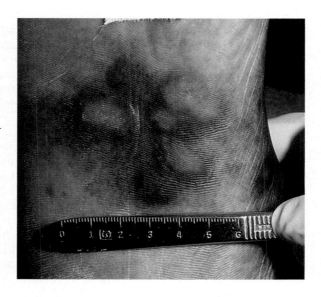

Figure 20–67 Kaposi's sarcoma on the plantar arch.

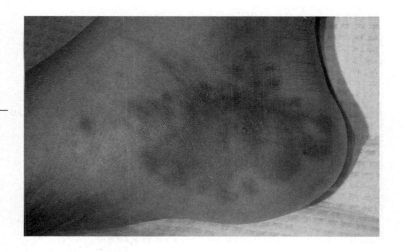

Figure 20–68 Kaposi's sarcoma on the heel.

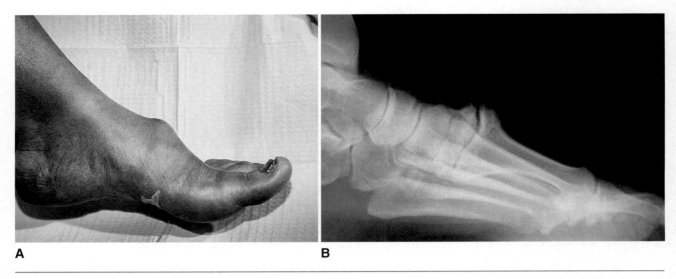

A   B

Figure 20–69 *A,* Exostosis at the metatarsocuneiform joint. *B,* X-ray film of the affected metatarsocuneiform joint.

Approximately 30% of patients with diabetes mellitus have disease-related dermatologic problems. Neurotrophic foot ulcers are very common in diabetic patients. Figure 20-72 shows bilateral neurotrophic ulcers. Painless plantar ulcers heal slowly after apparently insignificant trauma. The "diabetic foot" is characterized by chronic sensorimotor neuropathy, autonomic neuropathy, and poor peripheral circulation. The sensorimotor neuropathy results in a loss of normal sensation, which prevents the detection of traumatic events. See also Figure 15-14, which depicts diabetic dry gangrene of the big and fourth toes; Figure 15-15, which depicts a patient with the classic lesion of necrobiosis lipoidica diabeticorum; and Figure 15-16, which is a close-up photograph of the same skin lesion in another patient. It is common for diabetic patients, owing to the decreased sensitivity in their feet, to present with foreign bodies in their toes or feet. Figure 20-73 shows a foreign body protruding from the tip of the right third toe of a diabetic patient. This patient had dropped a needle on the carpet and later stepped on the needle, which penetrated the toe. Only after noticing it visually did the patient seek medical attention.

Bullosis diabeticorum (Fig. 20-74) is a relatively uncommon, noninflammatory, blistering condition of unknown origin that occurs in patients with long-standing diabetes. The tense bullae develop on normal-appearing skin in acral areas (feet, lower legs, hands). It has been associated with insulin-dependent diabetes mellitus, as well as non–insulin-dependent (type 2) diabetes. Intraepidermal and subepidermal blisters occur spontaneously, usually without trauma, and heal within 2 to 6 weeks. Treatment consists of aspiration of the bullae and topical antibiotics.

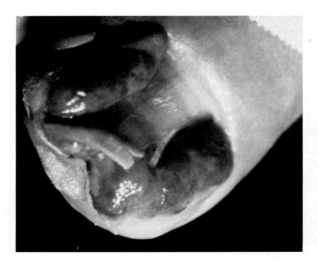

Figure 20–70 Paronychia with extensive granulation.

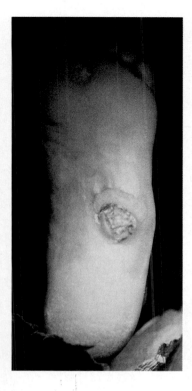

Figure 20–71 Squamous cell carcinoma on the plantar surface.

Bacterial and fungal infections are common in diabetic patients. Figure 20-75 depicts bacterial cellulitis and *tinea pedis* in a diabetic patient. Tinea pedis produces macerated, scaling, fissured toe webs; inflammatory epidermis; and thick, hypertrophic, discolored nails. *Necrotizing fasciitis* is a very severe form of cellulitis that can develop in diabetic patients. It involves the deep fascial structures underlying the skin and is caused by a mixture of aerobic and anaerobic gram-negative organisms. Figure 20-76 shows necrotizing fasciitis. Notice the sharply demarcated painful area of the infection. Surgical débridement and broad-spectrum antibiotics are necessary to treat the infection.

Scleroderma, or progressive systemic sclerosis, is a chronic multisystem disease manifested by thickening of the skin and varying degrees of organ involvement. There is a broad spectrum of disease manifestations of scleroderma, ranging from limited skin lesions associated with calcinosis, *R*aynaud's phenomenon, *e*sophageal motility problems, *s*clerodactyly, and *t*elangiectasia (CREST variant) to full encasement of the body by diffuse sclerosis. Calcification of the soft tissues can produce a stony-hard tissue and can range from a small area of involvement to

Figure 20–72 Diabetic neurotrophic foot ulcers.

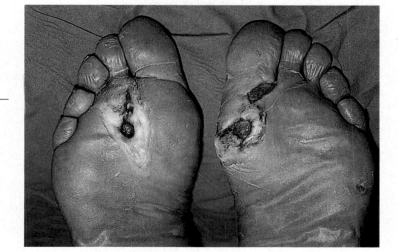

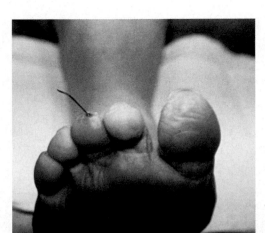

Figure 20–73 Foreign body in the toe of a diabetic patient.

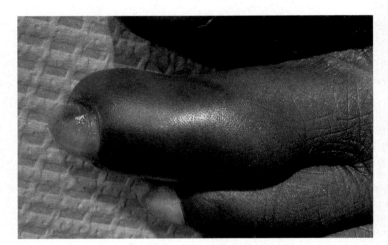

Figure 20–74 Bullous diabeticorum.

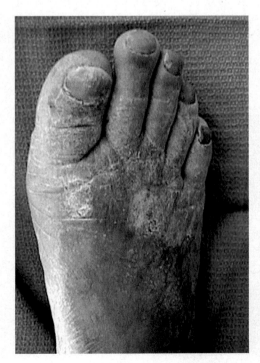

Figure 20–75 Tinea pedis and bacterial cellulitis in a diabetic patient.

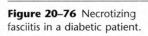
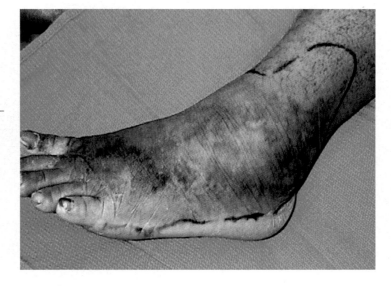

Figure 20–76 Necrotizing fasciitis in a diabetic patient.

massive calcium deposits. Figure 20-77*A* shows Raynaud's phenomenon and calcinosis cutis in a patient with the CREST syndrome. Note the telangiectases of the fingertips. Figure 20-77*B* shows calcinosis cutis of the heel in the same patient. Commonly, the distal finger pad assumes a tapered appearance, with a tuft of scarred tissue between the fingertip and the nail bed. Ulceration can also occur, which can lead to osteomyelitis. Figure 20-78 shows the plantar view of the hallux in the same patient with CREST syndrome; note the characteristic tapering of the digit and pterygium inversus (growth of soft tissue along the ventral aspect of the nail plate).

Figure 20-79 shows a subungual presentation of *malignant melanoma* of the hallux. Determine the cause of all subungual pigmented lesions. Unusual pigmentation under the nail, especially if of long duration, should always be regarded with suspicion. Subungual melanomas represent approximately 20% of melanomas in dark-skinned and Asian populations, in comparison with about 2% of cutaneous melanomas in white populations. Ultraviolet radiation exposure seems to be an important risk factor for cutaneous melanoma; however, because ultraviolet radiation is unlikely to penetrate the nail plate, it does not appear to be a risk factor for subungual melanomas. There is a considerable predominance of subungual melanoma localized on the thumb (58% of all affected fingers) and the hallux (86% of all affected toes).

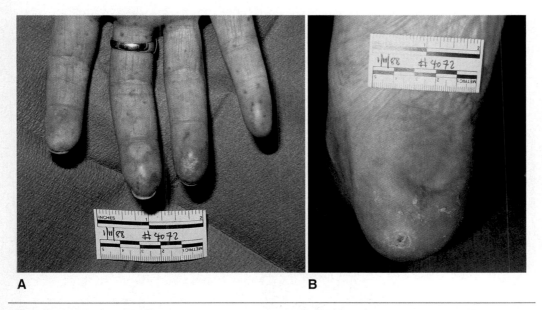

A   B

Figure 20–77 Calcinosis, Raynaud's phenomenon, esophageal motility problems, sclerodactyly, and telangiectasia (CREST) syndrome. *A,* Telangiectases of the fingertips. *B,* Calcinosis cutis of the heel.

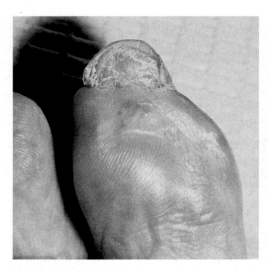

Figure 20–78 Calcinosis, Raynaud's phenomenon, esophageal motility problems, sclerodactyly, and telangiectasia (CREST) syndrome with tapered digit and pterygium inversus.

Cutaneous larva migrans is caused by animal hookworms, commonly the dog parasites *Ancylostoma braziliense* or *Ancylostoma caninum.* The creeping eruption occurs when the skin comes in direct and prolonged contact with the hookworm larva contained in the feces of dogs, cats, or humans. Moist areas visited by the infected animals, such as beaches or exposed soil covered by porches, are common sites for acquiring infection. The clinical appearance is that of a raised, serpiginous, erythematous, pruritic eruption, and it represents the paths of migration within the epidermis. Because the organism lacks collagenase and cannot disrupt the basement membrane, the parasite is unable to invade the dermis. The lesions migrate about 1 to 2 cm per day and may evolve into bullae. Topical application of thiabendazole is the treatment, although the infection is usually self-limited. Figure 20-80 shows the sole of a foot of an infected 31-year-old man after a beach vacation in Jamaica.

Pain in the heel and pain in the first metatarsophalangeal joints are common complaints, most often caused by mechanical factors. *Plantar fasciitis* is an inflammation caused by excessive stretching of the plantar fascia. The plantar fascia is a broad band of fibrous tissue that runs along the bottom surface of the foot, attaching at the bottom of the calcaneus and extending to the forefoot. When the plantar fascia is excessively stretched, plantar fasciitis can occur, leading to heel pain, arch pain, and heel spurs. Tight calf muscles or a tight Achilles tendon may cause the foot to flatten, which can lead to a painful "bowstringing" of the fascia. The most common causes of excessive stretching of the plantar fascia are as follows:

- Overpronation (flatfoot), which results in the arch's collapsing with weight bearing
- A foot with an unusually high arch
- A sudden increase in physical activity
- Excessive weight on the foot, usually attributed to obesity or pregnancy
- Improperly fitting footwear

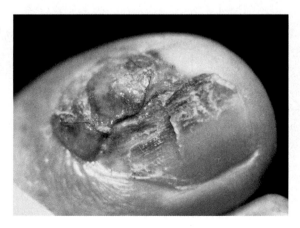

Figure 20–79 Subungual manifestation of malignant melanoma.

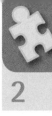

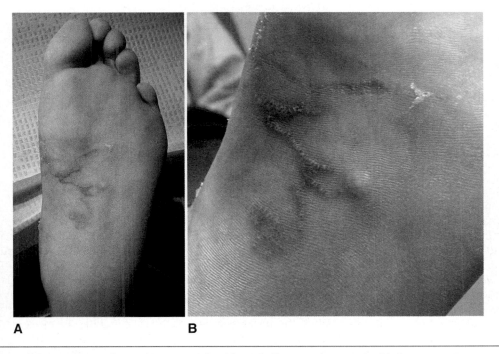

A   **B**

Figure 20–80 Cutaneous larva migrans. *A,* Sole of foot. *B,* Close-up photograph of lesion.

Overpronation is the leading cause of plantar fasciitis. Overpronation occurs in the walking process, when a person's arch collapses with weight bearing, causing the plantar fascia to be stretched away from the calcaneus. With plantar fasciitis, the patient experiences pain on the inside of the foot where the heel and arch meet. The pain is often acute upon arising in the morning or after a long rest, because while resting, the plantar fascia contracts back to its original shape. As the day progresses and the plantar fascia continues to be stretched, the pain often subsides. However, heel pain can be secondary to several other causes. Table 20-3 lists the most common disorders associated with heel pain.

Table 20-4 lists disorders associated with first metatarsophalangeal joint pain. *Sesamoiditis* is a common ailment that affects the forefoot, typically in young people who engage in physical activity such as dancing or jogging. This is a common problem among ballet dancers and people who play the position of catcher in baseball. Any activity that places constant force on the ball of the foot—even walking—can cause sesamoiditis. Its most common symptom is pain in the ball of the foot, especially on the medial or inner side. Sesamoiditis is a general description for any irritation of the sesamoid bones, which are tiny bones within the tendons that run to the big toe. The sesamoids function as a pulley, increasing the leverage of the tendons controlling the toe. With walking and pushing off against the toe, the sesamoids

Table 20–3 Disorders Causing Heel Pain

Plantar calcaneal spur (enthesopathy)
Plantar fasciitis
Inferior calcaneal bursitis
Atrophy of plantar fat pad
Rheumatoid arthritis
Ankylosing spondylitis
Reiter's syndrome
Gout
Fracture
Neoplasm
Foreign body
Nerve entrapment

Table 20–4 Disorders Causing Pain in the First Metatarsophalangeal Joint

Osteoarthritis
Bursitis/capsulitis
Fracture
Sesamoiditis
Gout
Rheumatoid arthritis
Reiter's syndrome
Septic arthritis

are involved; eventually they can become irritated and even fractured. Because the bones are actually within the tendons, sesamoiditis is a form of tendinitis. Sesamoiditis typically can be distinguished from other forefoot conditions by its gradual onset. The pain usually begins as a mild ache and increases gradually as the aggravating activity is continued; the pain may build to an intense throbbing.

Morton's neuroma is a common foot problem associated with pain, swelling, or an inflammation of an interdigital nerve, usually at the ball of the foot between the third and fourth toes. The digital nerve traveling between the toes becomes entrapped or pinched during the push-off phase of walking just before the nerve separates into two separate nerves to supply sensation to the toes. Neuroma formation is attributable to compression of the interdigital nerve against the intermetatarsophalangeal bursa. Symptoms of this condition include sharp pain, burning, and even a lack of feeling in the affected area. Morton's neuroma may also cause numbness, tingling, or cramping in the forefoot. A patient may also complain that it feels as if a marble or pebble were inside the ball of the foot. Neuromas or neural swellings usually develop in only one foot and are more common in women than in men. Symptoms of Morton's neuroma often occur during or after application of significant pressure on the forefoot area, while walking, standing, jumping, or sprinting. It can also be caused by footwear selection; footwear with pointed toes or high heels can often lead to this condition. Constricting shoes can also pinch the nerve between the toes, causing discomfort and extreme pain.

In the evaluation of a patient with foot pain and a possible Morton's neuroma, palpate the area to try to elicit pain by squeezing the toes from the side. Next, try to feel the neuroma by

Table 20–5 Clinical Features Differentiating Rheumatoid Arthritis from Osteoarthritis

Clinical Feature	Rheumatoid Arthritis*	Osteoarthritis[†]
Patient's age (years)	3-80	Older than 45
Morning stiffness	More than 1 hour	Less than 1 hour
Disability	Often great	Variable
Joint distribution		
Distal interphalangeal joint	Rare	Very common
Proximal interphalangeal joint	Very common	Common
Metacarpophalangeal joint	Very common	Absent
Wrist	Very common	Absent
Soft tissue swelling	Very common	Rare
Interosseous muscle wasting	Very common	Rare
Swan-neck deformity	Common	Rare
Ulnar deviation	Common	Absent

*See Figures 20-57 and 20-58.
[†]See Figure 20-59.

Table 20–6 Clinical Features Differentiating Diseases Affecting the Hands and Wrists

Clinical Feature	Rheumatoid Arthritis	Psoriatic Arthritis*	Acute Gout**	Osteoarthritis	Carpal Tunnel Syndrome
Age (years)	3-80	10-60	30-80	50-80	40-80
Sex	Female	Male	Male	Female	Male, female
Pain onset	Gradual	Gradual	Abrupt	Gradual	Gradual
Stiffness	Very common	Common	Absent	Common	Absent
Swelling	Common	Common	Common	Common	Common
Redness	Absent	Uncommon	Common	Uncommon	Absent
Deformity	Flexion of PIP and MCP; swan-neck,[†] boutonnière deformities; ulnar deviation[‡]	Frequent DIP, PIP, and MCP involvement; "sausage-shaped" digits[§]	None in acute stage; resembles rheumatoid arthritis if deposits occur in tendon sheaths in chronic gout	Flexion and lateral deviation of DIP and PIP[¶]	Thenar muscle atrophy

DIP, distal interphalangeal joint; MCP, metacarpophalangeal joint; PIP, proximal interphalangeal joint.
*Needlepoint pitting of the nails is often associated with psoriatic arthritis. See Figures 8-14 and 8-15.
**See Figure 20-55.
[†]See Figure 20-58.
[‡]See Figure 20-57.
[§]See Figure 20-64.
[¶]See Figure 20-59.

pressing your thumb into the third interspace. Hold the patient's first, second, and third metatarsal heads with one of your hands and the fourth and fifth metatarsal heads in the other, and push half the foot up and half the foot down slightly. In many cases of Morton's neuroma, this maneuver causes an audible click, known as *Mulder's sign*.

Table 20-5 summarizes the clinical features that differentiate rheumatoid arthritis from osteoarthritis. Table 20-6 summarizes some of the features of diseases affecting the hands and wrists. Table 20-7 outlines the clinical features that differentiate common musculoskeletal disorders affecting the elbow. Table 20-8 lists the clinical features that differentiate significant diseases affecting the knee. Table 20-9 lists the clinical features differentiating diseases of the foot. Table 20-10 summarizes the normal joint ranges of motion.

Table 20–7 Clinical Features Differentiating Diseases Affecting the Elbow

Clinical Feature	Rheumatoid Arthritis	Psoriatic Arthritis	Acute Gout*	Osteoarthritis	Tennis Elbow
Age (years)	3-80	10-60	30-80	50-80	20-60
Sex	Female	Male	Male	Female	Male, female
Pain onset	Gradual	Gradual	Abrupt	Gradual	Gradual
Stiffness	Very common	Common	Absent	Common	Occasional
Swelling	Common	Common	Common	Common	Absent
Redness	Absent	Uncommon	Common	Absent	Absent
Deformity	Flexion contractures, usually bilateral	Flexion contractures, usually bilateral	Flexion contractures only in chronic state	Flexion contractures	None

*See Figure 20-61, which shows a patient with chronic tophaceous gout and painless tophi on the elbows.

Table 20–8 Clinical Features Differentiating Diseases Affecting the Knee

Clinical Feature	Rheumatoid Arthritis	Psoriatic Arthritis	Acute Gout	Osteoarthritis	Torn Meniscus
Age (years)	3-80	10-60	30-80	50-80	20-60
Sex	Female	Male	Male	Female	Male
Pain onset	Gradual	Gradual	Abrupt	Gradual	Abrupt
Stiffness	Very common	Common	Absent	Common	Occasional
Swelling	Common	Common	Common	Common	Common
Redness	Absent	Uncommon	Common	Absent	Absent
Deformity	Flexion contractures	Flexion contractures	Flexion contractures only in chronic state	Flexion contractures	None

Table 20–9 Clinical Features Differentiating Diseases Affecting the Foot

Clinical Feature	Rheumatoid Arthritis	Psoriatic Arthritis	Acute Gout	Osteoarthritis	Reiter's Syndrome
Age (years)	3-80	10-60	30-80	50-80	10-80 (peak, 30s)
Sex	Female	Male	Male	Female	Male
Pain onset	Gradual	Gradual	Abrupt	Gradual	Gradual
Stiffness	Very common	Common	Common	Common	Common
Swelling	Common	Common	Very common	Uncommon	Common
Redness	Uncommon	Uncommon	Very common	Uncommon	Common
Joint predilection and deformity	Abductovalgus deformity of MTP	Fusiform swelling of DIP	First MTP (may also have hallux abductovalgus deformity)	Hallux abductovalgus deformity	Ankle, heel, toes ("sausage" swelling of digits)

DIP, distal interphalangeal joint; MTP, metatarsophalangeal joint.

Table 20–10 Normal Joint Ranges of Motion

Joint	Flexion	Extension	Lateral Bending	Rotation
Cervical spine	45°	55°	40°	70°
Thoracic and lumbar spine	75°	30°	35°	30°
Shoulder	180°	50°	Abduction; 180°	Adduction; 50°
Elbow	150°	180°	Pronation; 80°	Supination; 80°
Wrist	80°	70°	Radial motion; 20°	Ulnar motion; 55°
Metacarpophalangeal joint	90°	20°	—	—
Hip	90° with knee extended	30° with knee extended	40°	45°
	120° with knee flexed	—	Abduction; 45°	Adduction; 30°
Knee	135°	0-10°	—	—
Ankle	50°	15°	—	—
Subtalar	—	—	Inversion; 20°	Eversion; 10°
First metatarsophalangeal joint	40°	65-75°	—	—

Useful Vocabulary

Listed here are the specific roots that are important for understanding the terminology related to musculoskeletal diseases.

Root	Pertaining to	Example	Definition
ankyl(o)-	stiff	**ankylo**sis	Immobility or stiffness of a joint
arthr(o)-	joint	**arthro**gram	Radiograph of a joint
chir(o)-	hand	**chiro**spasm	Writer's cramp
dactyl(o)-	finger or toe	**dactylo**spasm	Cramping of a digit
myo-	muscle	**myo**pathy	Disease of muscle
oste(o)-	bone	**osteo**malacia	A condition marked by softening of the bones
pod-	foot	**pod**iatrist	Specialist in conditions of the foot
scolio-	twisted	**scolio**sis	Lateral deviation of the spine
spondyl(o)-	vertebrae	**spondy**litis	Inflammation of vertebrae
teno-	tendon	**teno**tomy	Surgical cutting of a tendon

Writing Up the Physical Examination

Listed here are examples of the write-up for the examination of the musculoskeletal system.

- All the joints have full range of motion. No deformities, tenderness, or abnormalities are detected.
- There is marked ulnar deviation of both hands in association with a flexion deformity of all the proximal interphalangeal joints and hyperextension of all the distal interphalangeal joints. Marked tenderness of both wrists is present.
- There is abnormal forward mobility of the knee. There is 3 to 4 cm of motion detected.
- The left first metatarsophalangeal joint is markedly erythematous and painful. The joint is shiny and edematous.
- No joint deformities are noted. There is marked reduction of hip internal and external rotation. No pain is produced by these movements. Pain is produced by abduction of the right shoulder against resistance. The range of right shoulder abduction is reduced. The range of motion of the hands, wrists, spine, knees, and ankles is normal.

Bibliography

Aldrige T: Diagnosing heel pain in adults. Am Fam Physician 70:332, 2004.

Balint GP, Korda J, Hangody L, et al: Foot and ankle disorders. Best Prac Res Clin Rheumatol 17:887, 2003.

Benjamin M, McGonagle D: Histopathologic changes at "synovio-entheseal complexes" suggesting a novel mechanism for synovitis in osteoarthritis and spondylarthritis. Arthritis Rheum 56:3601, 2007.

Birrer RB, DellaCorte MP, Grisafi PJ: Common Foot Problems in Primary Care. St. Louis, Mosby–Year Book, 1992.

Buchbinder R: Plantar fasciitis. N Engl J Med 350:2159, 2004.

Busija L, Hollingsworth B, Buchbinder R, et al: Role of age, sex, and obesity in the higher prevalence of arthritis among lower socioeconomic groups: A population-based survey. Arthritis Rheum 57:553, 2007.

Chou R, Qaseem A, Snow V, et al: Diagnosis and treatment of low back pain: A joint clinical practice guideline from the American College of Physicians and the American Pain Society. Ann Intern Med 147:478, 2007.

Ciccotti MC, Schwartz MS, Ciccotti MG: Diagnosis and treatment of medial epicondylitis of the elbow. Clin Sports Med 23:693, 2004.

Helmick CG, Felson DT, Lawrence RC, et al: Estimates of the prevalence of arthritis and other rheumatic conditions in the United States: Part I. Arthritis Rheum 58:15, 2008.

Jackson JL, O'Malley PG, Kroenke K: Evaluation of knee pain in primary care. Ann Intern Med 139:575, 2003.

Jellinek NJ: Primary malignant tumors of the nail unit. Adv Dermatol 21:33, 2005.

Kosinski MA, Stewart D: Nail changes associated with systemic disease and vascular insufficiency. Clin Podiatr Med Surg 6:295, 1989.

Lawrence RC, Felson DT, Helmick CG, et al: Estimates of the prevalence of arthritis and other rheumatic conditions in the United States: Part II. Arthritis Rheum 58:26, 2008.

Lee DM: Cadherin-11 in synovial lining formation and pathology in arthritis. Science 315:1006, 2007.

Lichota DK: Anterior knee pain: Symptom or syndrome? Curr Womens Health Rep 3:81, 2003.

Stevenson JH, Trojian T: Evaluation of shoulder pain. J Fam Pract 51:605, 2002.

Swartz MH: Essentials of a complete physical examination. Clin Podiatr Med Surg 15:619, 1998.

West SG, Woodburn J: Pain in the foot. BMJ 310:860, 1995.

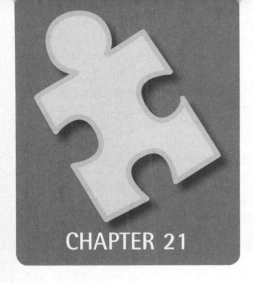

CHAPTER 21

The Nervous System

As the debility increases and the influence of the will over the muscles fades, the tremulous agitation becomes more vehement. It now seldom leaves him for a moment; but even when exhausted nature seizes a small portion of sleep, the motion becomes so violent as not only to shake the bed-hangings, but even the floor and sashes of the room. The chin is now almost immovably bent down upon the sternum. The slops with which he is attempted to be fed, with the saliva, are continually trickling from the mouth. The power of articulation is lost. The urine and faeces are passed involuntarily; and at the last, constant sleepiness, with slight delirium, and other marks of extreme exhaustion, announce the wished-for release.

James Parkinson   (1755–1824)

General Considerations

By the second century CE, Galen had already described the cerebral ventricles, 7 of the 12 cranial nerves, and the cerebral convolutions. There was, however, little further interest in the anatomy and physiology of the neurologic system until the 16th century. In 1543, Andreas Vesalius illustrated the basal ganglia, and in 1552, Bartolommeo Eustachius described the cerebellar peduncles and the pons.

In the 17th century, Thomas Willis published descriptions and illustrations of the cerebral circulation, the "striate body," and the internal capsule. Caspar Bartholin and others thought that the function of the cerebral cortex was to protect the blood vessels, whereas other investigators believed that the cerebrum possessed higher functions. François Pourfour du Petit stressed that the cortex was responsible for motor activity. This concept lay dormant until the end of the 19th century.

Careful anatomic descriptions of the tracts, nuclei, and gyri were contained in the writings of scientists of the 18th and early 19th centuries. Johann Christian Reil and Karl Friedrich Burdach provided names for the many gross anatomic structures that had been illustrated by others in previous centuries. Reil has been credited with the naming of the insula, capsule, uncinate and cingulate fasciculi, and tapetum. The uncus, lenticular nucleus, pulvinar, and gyrus cinguli were named by Burdach. During this same period, Samuel von Soemmering, Felix Vicq d'Azyr, Franz Josef Gall, Louis Gratiolet, and Luigi Rolando made many detailed illustrations of the cerebral convolutional patterns.

In the early 19th century, the first descriptions of several disease states were published. In 1817 James Parkinson wrote an essay describing the "shaking palsy" that bears his name. In 1829 Charles Bell wrote:

> *The next instance was in a man wounded by the horn of an ox. The point entered under the angle of the jaw and came out before the ear. . . . He remains now a singular proof of the*

effects of the loss of function in the muscles of the face by this nerve being divided. The forehead of the corresponding side is without motion, the eyelids remain open, the nostril has no motion in breathing, and the mouth is drawn to the opposite side.

This is the classic description of facial nerve (seventh cranial nerve) palsy, also known as Bell's palsy.

In the mid-19th century, an interest in microscopic neuroanatomy developed. Jan Purkinje, Theodor Schwann, and Hermann von Helmholtz were a few of the many neuroanatomists who contributed valuable information about the intricacies of the nervous system. However, not until the late 19th century were specific staining techniques developed by Camillo Golgi, Vittorio Marchi, and Franz Nissl, which led to the current understanding of neuronal disease. The nerve cell had finally been discovered.

The 20th century was a period of further progress in the description of the cerebral cortex, anterior commissure, thalamus, and hypothalamus. A major advance came from the work of Santiago Ramón y Cajal in 1904. His histologic exploration clarified the complexities of the neuron. Not until 1925 were the hypophysial-hypothalamic connections described, and even today, the function of the hypothalamus is not fully understood.

It has been suggested that more than 40% of patients who present to internists have symptoms referable to neurologic disease. The internist must be able to identify the early signs and symptoms of neurologic disease and initiate the appropriate therapy. All too often, subtle signs and symptoms may be ignored, and a diagnosis is not made until advanced disability is apparent.

Cerebrovascular disease is one of the most devastating diseases of our time. It remains the third leading cause of death in the United States. More than 700,000 Americans suffer a stroke yearly, and it is the number one cause of disability; more than 3 million Americans currently live with permanent brain damage caused by such an event. On average, someone in the United States suffers a stroke every 53 seconds, and every 3.3 minutes, someone dies of one. In 2007, there were 151,147 deaths from cerebrovascular disease, and 5.2 million noninstitutionalized adult Americans have had a stroke. In addition, 8.1% of all hospital inpatient deaths are related to stroke and cerebrovascular disease. The debilitating consequences of stroke and the economic impact on society are enormous.

The generalist or internist holds an important position because a patient with a neurologic problem usually seeks help from that physician first. A thorough knowledge of basic neuroanatomy and physiology is the cornerstone of neurologic diagnosis.

Structure and Physiology

The brain, which is enclosed in the cranium and surrounded by the meninges, is the center of the nervous system. The brain can be divided into paired cerebral hemispheres, basal ganglia, diencephalon (thalamus and hypothalamus), brain stem, and cerebellum.

The two *cerebral hemispheres* make up the largest portion of the brain. Each hemisphere can be subdivided into four major lobes named for the cranial bones that overlie them: frontal, parietal, occipital, and temporal. The fissures and sulci divide the cerebral surface. A deep midline, longitudinal fissure separates the two hemispheres. The convolutions, or *gyri*, lie between the sulci. A lateral view of the left cerebral hemisphere is pictured in Figure 21-1. Figure 21-2 is a medial view of the right cerebral hemisphere. A basal view of the cerebral hemispheres is pictured in Figure 21-3.

The *cerebrum* is responsible for motor, sensory, associative, and higher mental functions. The primary *motor cortex* is located in the precentral gyrus. Neurons in this area control voluntary movements of the skeletal muscles on the opposite side of the body. An irritative lesion in this area may cause seizures or changes in consciousness. Destructive lesions in this area can produce contralateral flaccid paresis or paralysis.

The primary *sensory cortex* is located in the postcentral gyrus. Irritative lesions in this area may produce paresthesias ("numbness" or a "pins-and-needles" sensation) on the opposite side. Destructive lesions produce an impairment in cutaneous sensation on the opposite side.

The primary *visual cortex* is located in the occipital lobe along the calcarine fissure, which divides the cuneus from the lingual gyri. Irritative lesions in this area produce visual symptoms

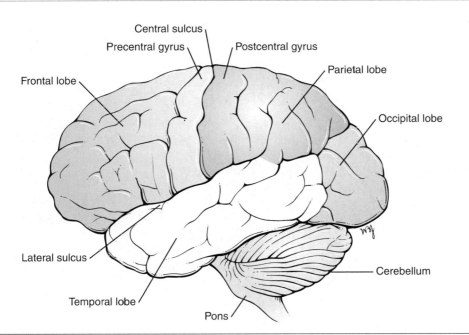

Figure 21–1 Lateral view of the left cerebral hemisphere.

such as flashes of light or rainbows. Destructive lesions cause homonymous hemianopsia on the contralateral side. Central macular vision is spared.

The primary *auditory cortex* is located in the temporal lobe along the transverse temporal gyrus. Irritative lesions in this area produce a buzzing or ringing in the ears. Destructive lesions almost never produce deafness.

The *basal ganglia* are situated deep within the cerebral hemispheres. The structures constituting the basal ganglia include the caudate and lenticular nuclei, as well as the amygdala. The amygdala is part of the limbic system and is concerned with emotion. All other components are important structures in the extrapyramidal system, which is concerned with

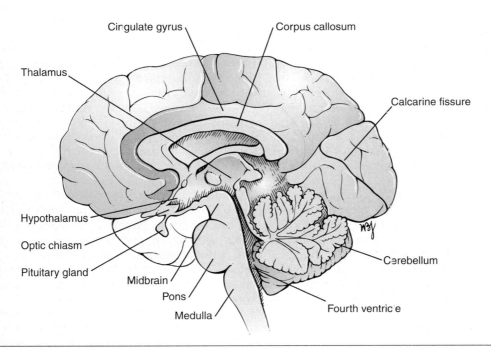

Figure 21–2 Medial view of the right cerebral hemisphere.

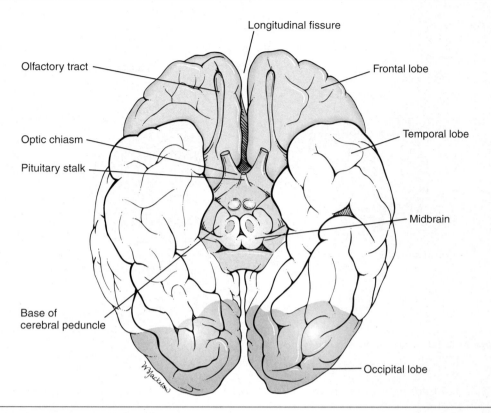

Figure 21–3 Basal view of the cerebral hemispheres.

modulating voluntary body movements, postural changes, and autonomic integration. The basal ganglia are especially involved with fine movements of the extremities. Disturbances of the basal ganglia can result in tremors and rigid movements.

The *thalamus* is a large nuclear mass located on each side of the third ventricle. The thalamus is the chief sensory and motor integrating mechanism of the neuraxis. All sensory impulses, except olfactory ones, and the major output from systems that modulate and modify motor function (i.e., the cerebellum and corpus striatum) terminate in the thalamus, from which they are projected to specific areas of the cerebral cortex. The thalamus is involved in certain emotional connotations that accompany most sensory experiences. Through its connections with the hypothalamus and striatum, the thalamus can influence visceral and somatic effectors serving primarily affective reactions. Through its control of the electrical excitability of the cerebral cortex, the thalamus plays a dominant role in the maintenance and regulation of the state of consciousness, alertness, and attention. The thalamus may be the critical structure for pain perception and thermal sense, which remain after complete destruction of the primary sensory cortex. Thermal sense endows sensation with discriminative faculties and is not concerned with the recognition of crude sensory modalities.

The *hypothalamus* is located below the thalamus. It includes the optic chiasm and the neurohypophysis. The hypothalamus is responsible for many regulatory mechanisms, such as temperature regulation; neuroendocrine control of catecholamines, thyroid-stimulating hormone, adrenocorticotropic hormone, follicle-stimulating and luteinizing hormones, prolactin, and growth hormones; thirst; appetite; water balance; and sexual behavior.

The *brain stem* consists of the midbrain, pons, and medulla. Figure 21-4 shows the external anatomy of the brain stem. The brain stem is responsible for relaying all messages between the upper and lower levels of the central nervous system. Cranial nerves III to XII also arise from the brain stem. The brain stem contains the reticular formation, a network that provides for constant muscle stimulation to counteract the force of gravity. In addition to its antigravity effects, this area of the brain is essential for the control of consciousness. The neurons in the reticular activating system are capable of waking and arousing the entire brain.

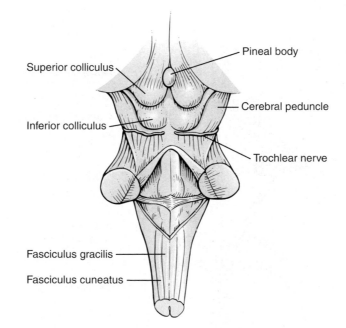

Figure 21–4 Anatomy of the brain stem.

The *midbrain* contains the superior and inferior colliculi, the cerebral peduncles, and the motor nuclei of the trochlear (CN IV) and oculomotor (CN III) nerves. The superior colliculi are associated with the visual system, and the inferior colliculi are associated with the auditory system. The cerebral peduncles converge from the inferior aspect of the cerebral hemispheres and enter the pons. A destructive lesion of the superior colliculi causes paralysis of upward gaze. Destructive lesions of the cranial nerve nuclei produce paralysis of the affected nerve. A destructive lesion of the cerebral peduncle gives rise to spastic paralysis on the other side of the body. Destruction of other tracts in the midbrain results in rigidity and involuntary movements.

The *pons* lies ventral to the cerebellum and rostral to the medulla. The abducens, facial, and acoustic (and vestibular) nuclei are found in the pons, and their nerves exit through a groove that divides the pons from the medulla. The motor and sensory nuclei of the trigeminal nerve are also located in the pons. At this level, the corticospinal tracts (also known as the pyramidal tracts) have not yet crossed, and a lesion at this level produces loss of voluntary movement on the opposite side. Destructive lesions of the pons may produce a variety of clinical syndromes, such as the following:

- Contralateral hemiplegia with ipsilateral trigeminal hemiplegia (paralysis of the jaw muscles and loss of sensation over the same side of the face)
- Contralateral hemiplegia with ipsilateral facial palsy (Bell's palsy)
- Contralateral hemiplegia with ipsilateral facial palsy and ipsilateral abducens palsy (paralysis of the lateral rectus muscle on the same side of the face)
- Contralateral hemiplegia with ipsilateral abducens palsy
- Quadriplegia and nystagmus

The *medulla* is the portion of the brain stem between the pons and the spinal cord. The nuclei of the hypoglossal, vagus, glossopharyngeal, and spinal accessory nerves are located in the medulla. It is within the medulla that the majority of fibers in the corticospinal tracts cross to the opposite side. Destructive lesions in the medulla produce symptoms that are referable to the tracts interrupted by the lesion. Some clinical syndromes are as follows:

- Contralateral hemiplegia with ipsilateral hypoglossal palsy*
- Ipsilateral vagal palsy† with contralateral loss of pain and temperature sense
- Ipsilateral vagal palsy with ipsilateral spinal accessory palsy‡

---

*Paralysis of the tongue muscles on the same side as the lesion. The tongue deviates to the side of the lesion when the patient is asked to stick out the tongue.
†Paralysis of the soft palate and difficulty speaking, termed *dysarthria*.
‡Paralysis of the sternocleidomastoid or trapezius muscle, or both. This results in the inability to turn the head to the side opposite the lesion and to shrug the shoulder.

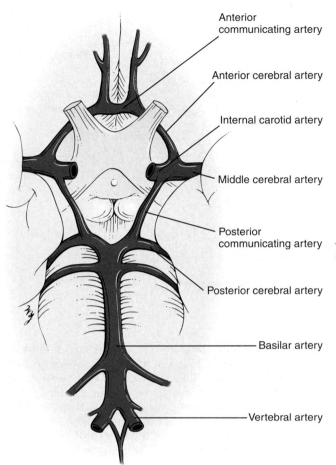

Anterior
communicating artery

Anterior cerebral artery

Internal carotid artery

Middle cerebral artery

Posterior
communicating artery

Posterior cerebral artery

Basilar artery

Vertebral artery

Figure 21–5 Circle of Willis.

- Ipsilateral vagal palsy with ipsilateral hypoglossal palsy
- Ipsilateral vagal palsy, ipsilateral spinal accessory palsy, and ipsilateral hypoglossal palsy

There are many more clinical syndromes that are beyond the scope of this text. The reader is advised to review the neuroanatomy further to understand the complexities of these neurologic syndromes.

The *cerebellum* is located in the posterior fossa of the skull and is composed of a small midline vermis and two large lateral hemispheres. The cerebellum acts to keep the individual oriented in space and to halt or check motions. The cerebellum is also responsible for the fine movements of the hands. Essentially, the cerebellum coordinates and refines the action of muscle groups to produce steady and precise movements. Destructive lesions of the cerebellum cause swaying, staggering, intention tremors,* and inability to change movements rapidly.

Of the blood supply to the brain, 80% is through the internal carotid arteries and 20% is through the vertebral basilar arteries. Each internal carotid artery terminates at the anterior cerebral and middle cerebral arteries. The posterior cerebral artery arises from the basilar artery, which joins with the posterior communicating artery, a branch of the internal carotid artery. The two anterior cerebral arteries are joined by the anterior communicating artery. This vascular network forms the circle of Willis, located at the base of the brain. This is illustrated in Figure 21-5.

Continuous with the medulla is the *spinal cord*, a cylindric mass of neuronal tissue measuring 40 to 50 cm in length in adults. Its distal end attaches to the first segment of the coccyx. The spinal cord is divided into two symmetric halves by the anterior median fissure and the

---

*Tremors that result when the individual moves the hands to do something but that may not be present at rest.

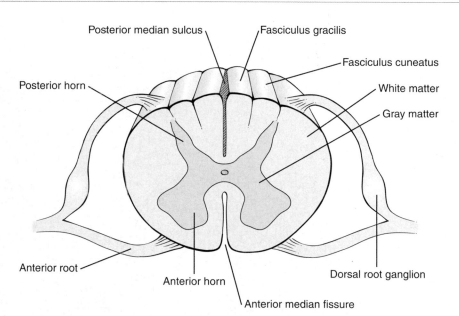

Posterior median sulcus

Fasciculus gracilis

Fasciculus cuneatus

Posterior horn

White matter

Gray matter

Anterior root

Anterior horn

Dorsal root ganglion

Anterior median fissure

Figure 21–6 Cross-sectional view through the spinal cord.

posterior median sulcus. Each half contains white and gray matter, which can be further subdivided. This is illustrated in Figure 21-6.

In the center of the spinal cord is the *gray matter*. The anterior gray matter, or the *anterior horn*, is the motor portion of the spinal cord and contains multipolar cells of origin of the *anterior roots* of the peripheral nerves. The *lateral horn* (sympathetic preganglionic neurons) is found at the T1 to L2 spinal levels. The posterior gray matter, or the *posterior horn*, is the receptor portion of the spinal cord.

The *white matter* of the spinal cord consists of tracts that link segments of the spinal cord and connect it to the brain. There are three main columns (funiculi). Between the anterior median fissure and the anterolateral sulcus is the *anterior white column*, which contains the descending fibers of the *ventral corticospinal tract* and the ascending fibers of the *ventral spinothalamic tract*. The ventral corticospinal tract is involved with voluntary motion, and the ventral spinothalamic tract carries impulses related to light touch.

The *lateral white column* is located between the anterolateral and posterolateral sulci and contains the descending fibers of the *lateral corticospinal tract* and the ascending *spinocerebellar* and *lateral spinothalamic tracts*. The lateral corticospinal tract is responsible for voluntary movement; the spinocerebellar tracts, for reflex proprioception; and the lateral spinothalamic tract, for pain and temperature sensation.

The *posterior white column* is located between the posterolateral and posterior median sulci. The most important fibers in this column are the ascending fibers of the *fasciculus gracilis* and *fasciculus cuneatus*. These tracts are involved with vibration sense, passive motion, joint position, and two-point discrimination.

There are 31 pairs of spinal nerves, each with a ventral (motor) and dorsal (sensory) root. The ventral root consists of *efferent* nerve fibers, which originate in the anterior and lateral gray matter (T1 to T2 only) and travel to the peripheral nerve and muscle, which constitute the motor root. The dorsal root consists of *afferent* nerve fibers whose cell bodies are in the *dorsal root ganglion*, which is the sensory root.

The spinal nerves are grouped into 8 cervical (C1 to C8), 12 thoracic (T1 to T12), 5 lumbar (L1 to L5), 5 sacral (S1 to S5), and 1 coccygeal nerve. These nerves are illustrated in Figure 21-7.

A *spinal reflex* involves an afferent neuron and an efferent neuron at the same level in the spinal cord. The basis for this reflex arc is an intact sensory limb, functional synapses in the spinal cord, an intact motor limb, and a muscle capable of responding. The afferent and efferent limbs travel together in the same spinal nerve. When a stretched muscle is suddenly stretched further, the afferent sensory limb sends impulses through its spinal nerve that travel to the dorsal root of that nerve. After reaching a synapse in the gray matter of the spinal cord, the impulse is transmitted to the ventral nerve root. These impulses are then conducted through the ventral root to the neuromuscular junction, where a brisk contraction of the muscle completes the reflex arc. Figure 21-8 illustrates a reflex spinal arc.

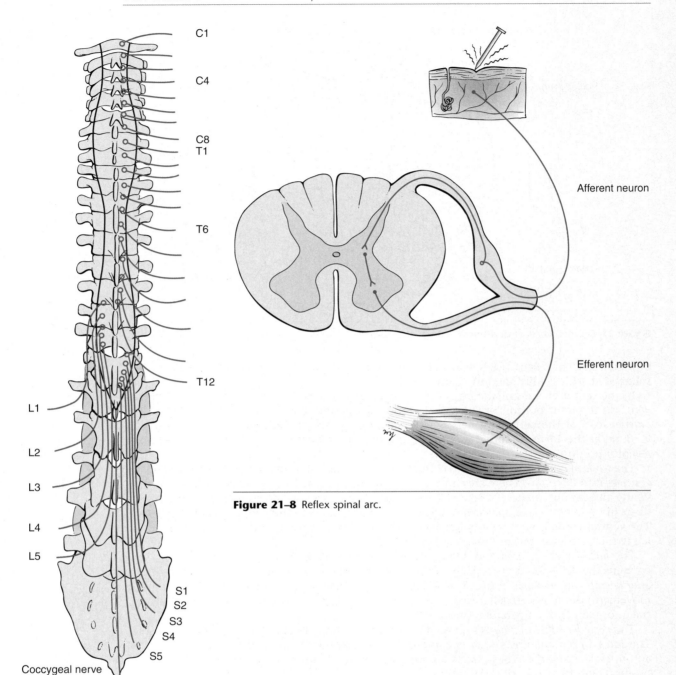

Figure 21–8 Reflex spinal arc.

Figure 21–7 Spinal nerves.

The afferent sensory limb is important not only in the reflex arc but also in the conscious appreciation of sensation. Nerve fibers carrying pain and temperature sensation enter the spinal cord and cross to the other side within one or two spinal segments. They ascend in the contralateral *lateral spinothalamic tract*, travel through the brain stem and the thalamus, and end in the postcentral gyrus of the parietal lobe, as illustrated in Figure 21-9A. Fibers carrying *proprioceptive* sensation from muscles, joints, and tendons enter the dorsal root and participate in the reflex arc. Other fibers carrying proprioceptive sensation pass directly into the *posterior columns* and ascend in the fasciculi gracilis and cuneatus to their ipsilateral nuclei, cross in the medial lemniscus, reach a synapse in the thalamus, and end in the postcentral gyrus of the parietal lobe. Still other proprioceptive fibers ascend crossed and uncrossed in the spinocerebellar tracts to the cerebellum. These additional pathways are illustrated in Figure 21-9B.

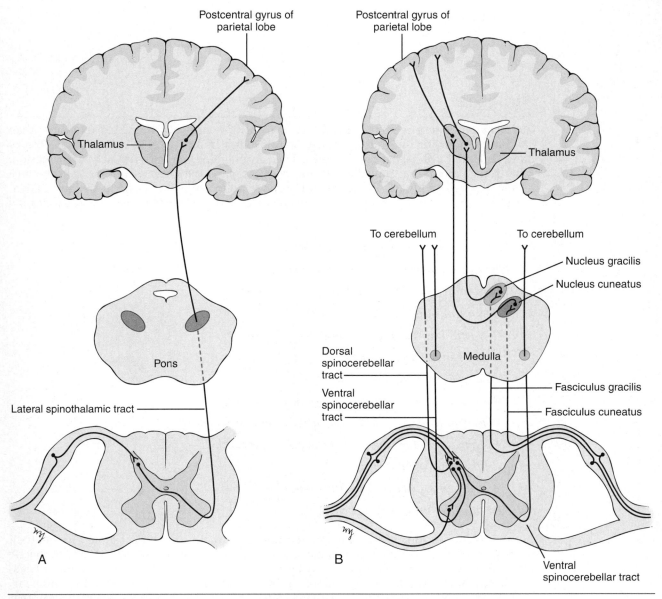

Figure 21–9 Conscious appreciation of sensation. *A,* Nerve pathways for pain and temperature sensation through the lateral spinothalamic tracts. *B,* Pathways of the fibers carrying proprioceptive sensation through the posterior columns and in the spinocerebellar tracts.

Review of Specific Symptoms

The most common symptoms of neurologic disease are as follows:

- Headache
- Loss of consciousness
- "Dizziness"
- Ataxia
- Changes in consciousness
- Visual disturbance
- Dysphasia
- Dementia
- Cerebrovascular accident
- Gait disturbance

- Tremor
- "Numbness"
- "Weakness"
- Pain

Headache

Headache is the most common neurologic symptom. It has been estimated that more than 35 million individuals in the United States suffer from recurrent headaches. Most of these patients have headaches that are related to migraine, muscle contraction, or tension. A headache pattern that is unchanged and has been present for several years is unlikely to be related to present illness of the patient. Several points must be clarified for any patient complaining of a recent change in the frequency or severity of headaches. Ask the following questions:

"How long have you been having headaches?"

"When did you notice a change in the pattern or severity of your headaches?"

"How has the pattern of your headaches changed?"

"How often do your headaches occur?"

"How long does each headache last?"

"Which part of your head aches?"

"What does the headache feel like?"

"How quickly does the headache reach its maximum?"

"When you get headaches, do you have any other symptoms?"

"Are you aware of anything that produces the headaches?"

"Are there any warning signs?"

"Does anything make the headaches worse?"

"What makes the headaches better?"

Patients complaining of a *sudden* onset of headache usually have more serious illnesses than patients with headaches of chronic duration. A continuous headache can be related to muscle spasm, whereas a *recurrent* headache may be a migraine or cluster headache. A *throbbing* headache often has a vascular cause. Certain headaches are associated with visual phenomena, nausea, or vomiting. In patients with increased intracranial pressure, any maneuver that increases the pressure, such as coughing or bending, may worsen the headache. In any patient who experiences a severe, sudden headache, stroke should be suspected.

Migraine is a biphasic type of headache associated with a prodromal phase, called the *aura*, followed by the headache phase. During the aura, one or more physiologic events may occur. These include transient experiences of autonomic, visual, motor, or sensory phenomena. Common visual symptoms are photophobia, blurred vision, and scotomata. As the aura fades, the headache begins. It is usually unilateral and is often described as pulsating; it can last for hours to days. Migraine headaches are often triggered by stress, anxiety, the use of birth control pills, and hormonal changes. Many patients experience migraine headaches after a period of excitement. Other important triggers are hunger and the ingestion of certain foods such as chocolate, cheese, cured meats, and highly spiced foods. There is often a family history of migraine.

Cluster headaches are associated with oculosympathetic disturbances. The typical patient is a middle-aged man complaining of recurrent episodes of pain around the eye that last for up to 1 hour. Classically, cluster headaches awaken the patient from sleep on successive nights for 2 to 4 weeks. There is ipsilateral miosis, ptosis, conjunctival edema, tearing, and nasal stuffiness during the headache. It is thought that alcohol may precipitate such attacks.

Headache may be the result of referred pain from sinus infections, ocular disease, or dental disease. Systemic conditions such as viral infections, chronic obstructive pulmonary disease, and poisoning may produce headaches. Determine whether the patient is taking any medications that may be producing the head pain. (See Table 21-2, which provides an approach to patients with the symptom of headache.)

Loss of Consciousness

Loss of consciousness—syncope—may result from cardiovascular or neurologic causes. The cardiovascular causes are discussed in Chapter 14, The Heart, and Chapter 15, The Peripheral Vascular System. The term *blackout* is commonly used, but it may mean different conditions to the patient and the interviewer. Any patient who uses this term should be asked to clarify its meaning. The patient may be referring to an actual loss of consciousness, a dimming of vision, or a decreased awareness of the environment without an actual loss of consciousness.

A useful way to clarify the symptom of loss of consciousness is to ask the patient, "Have you ever lost consciousness, fainted, or felt that you were not aware of your surroundings?" If the patient answers in the affirmative, identify the cause of the loss of consciousness. Ask the following questions:

"Can you describe the attack to me—every event as it occurred until you lost consciousness?"

*"Did anyone witness the attack?"**

"Were there any symptoms that preceded the attack?"

"Were you told that there were body movements?"

"Can you describe everything you remember after the attack until you felt completely normal?"

"Was there a period of sleepiness that followed?" If yes, *"For how long did this period last?"*

"How did you feel after the attack? Were you confused?"

"Did you notice afterward that you had urinated or had a bowel movement during the attack?"

Epileptic seizures may produce a loss of consciousness and are caused by the sudden, excessive, disorderly discharge of neurons. The first step in approaching the symptom of seizure is to identify its type. If the discharge is *focal*, the clinical seizure reflects the effect of the excessive discharge in that area of the body. For example, if the discharge is located in the inferior precentral gyrus, involved with hand and arm motion, the seizure is characterized by involuntary motion of the hand and arm. A *generalized* seizure results from a discharge in the subcortical structures, such as the thalamocortical radiations. These have widespread bilateral cortical connections. There are three main types of generalized seizures:

- Petit mal (absence seizure)
- Grand mal (generalized tonic-clonic)
- Myoclonic

A *petit mal* seizure is characterized by a sudden attack of unconsciousness lasting only about 10 seconds, usually without any warning. During the petit mal seizure, the patient appears to be staring or daydreaming. There is no associated falling or involuntary limb motion. The patient rapidly returns to normal activity without being aware of the attack. These seizures are most common in children 5 to 15 years of age. On occasion, they may persist into adulthood.

A *grand mal* seizure is a generalized major motor convulsion. Affected patients lose consciousness, and many fall down rigidly. In 50% of patients with grand mal seizures, there is an aura of giddiness, involuntary twitching, change in mood, confusion, or epigastric discomfort as the seizure begins. Some patients may cry out initially. During this *tonic* phase, there is an increase in muscle tone, resulting in a rigid, flexed posture and then a rigid, extended posture. The patient may become apneic and cyanotic. The eyes may open and stare or may be deviated to one side. The *clonic* phase follows, with involuntary movements of the body. These are often associated with salivation, eye rolling, and incontinence. Biting the tongue is common.

---

*Document a history with an observer, if possible.

After the clonic phase, the individual passes into a phase resembling sleep from which she or he cannot be easily awakened. *Postictally*, or after the seizure, the patient may be confused and often falls into a deep sleep that lasts for hours. Accompanying muscle pain and headache are common.

A *myoclonic* seizure is a minor motor seizure characterized by sudden muscle contractions of the face and upper extremities. The eyelids and forearms are commonly affected. There is no detectable loss of consciousness.

Febrile convulsions are common in children from 6 months to 6 years of age and are similar to grand mal seizures. When a child has a high fever, a seizure lasting less than 10 minutes may occur. The younger the child is at the time of the first febrile seizure, the greater is the likelihood that seizures will recur.

"Dizziness"

Dizziness is a term used frequently by patients and should be avoided by the interviewer. "Dizziness" may be the patient's description of vertigo, ataxia, or lightheadedness. Any time the patient uses this term, it must be clarified by additional questioning, because different pathophysiologic mechanisms may be responsible. The interviewer needs to differentiate vertigo from ataxia. If the patient complains of "dizziness," it is important to ask these questions:

> *"Would you describe the dizziness as a strange spinning sensation in your head?"*
>
> *"Did the room spin, or did it feel as if you were spinning?"*
>
> *"Were you unsteady while walking?"*

Vertigo is partially discussed in Chapter 11, The Ear and Nose. Vertigo is the hallucination of movement. Acute vertigo may be associated with nausea, vomiting, perspiration, and a sense of anxiety. Ask patients whether they have the sensation that objects are moving around them or that they are spinning or moving. In addition to the questions in Chapter 11, ask the following:

> *"During the attack, did you experience any nausea or vomiting?"*
>
> *"Have you noticed any problem with your hearing or ringing in your ears?"*
>
> *"Have you ever been given an antibiotic called gentamicin?"*

Ménière's disease can result in protracted attacks of severe vertigo associated with vomiting. Many patients with Ménière's disease also have the symptoms of tinnitus and hearing loss. During the attack, the patient is unsteady, with horizontal nystagmus directed away from the affected ear. Certain drugs (such as gentamicin) are associated with changes in the labyrinth of the ear and can cause vertigo and deafness.

Dizziness and stumbling are commonly associated with a stroke.

Ataxia

Disruption of the vestibular-ocular-cerebellar control mechanism produces ataxia. Ataxia is persistent unsteadiness in the upright position. Any patient complaining of dizziness must be evaluated for abnormal function of the vestibular, visual, proprioceptive, and cerebellar systems. Equilibrium requires the integration of sensory input and motor output, acting primarily at a reflex level for the maintenance of balance. The ears and eyes and their central connections in the brain stem and the cerebellum are intimately involved in balance. Any patient with ataxia should be asked the following questions:

> *"Are you unsteady when you walk?"*
>
> *"Have you noticed that the dizziness is worse when your eyes are open or closed?"*
>
> *"What does your diet consist of? What did you eat yesterday?"*
>
> *"Have you ever had syphilis?"*

Abnormal proprioceptive input from the lower extremities can cause ataxia. Severe posterior column damage from syphilis, vitamin B_{12} deficiency, or multiple sclerosis may produce a "sensory" ataxia, resulting in a wide-based, high-stepping gait. The gait is worsened by having the patient close the eyes and is improved by having the patient observe the feet. Vitamin B_{12} deficiency may result from pernicious anemia or from inadequate intake, although poor nutrition is a rare cause. "Motor" ataxia results from an abnormality in the cerebellum and central vestibular pathways. It is characterized by wide-based, irregular placement of the feet and poor placement of the center of gravity, with a lurching to either side.

Changes in Consciousness

Changes in consciousness may be related to changes in attention span, perception, arousal, or a combination. In *confusional states*, the patient has the ability to receive information normally, but the processing is disturbed. In *delirium*, the individual perceives the information abnormally. Any patient, or member of the patient's family, who indicates that a change in consciousness has occurred should be asked the following:

"Did the change occur suddenly?"

"Have there been other symptoms associated with the change in consciousness?"

"Do you use any medications? depressants? insulin? alcohol? recreational drugs?"

"Is there a history of psychiatric illness?"

"Is there a history of kidney disease? liver disease? thyroid disease?"

"Have you ever had an injury to your head?"

Many factors can produce changes in consciousness. The acuteness of the change in consciousness is often helpful in making a diagnosis. Hemiparesis, paresthesia, hemianopsia, garbled speech, and arm and leg weakness are common associated symptoms of supratentorial lesions. Brain-stem lesions are often associated with changes in consciousness and with nystagmus, vomiting, double vision, nausea, and excessive yawning. Drugs of any type can produce acute changes in consciousness. A history of earlier psychiatric illness is important. Toxic and metabolic changes are frequently associated with changes in consciousness. Liver or kidney failure, myxedema, and diabetic ketoacidosis are common causes of metabolic abnormalities. A history of head trauma may result in a subdural hematoma and produce a gradual change in consciousness.

Visual Disturbance

Visual disturbances are common neurologic presenting symptoms. The most important symptoms are acute visual loss, chronic visual loss, and double vision. Ask any patient complaining of visual disturbances the following questions:

"How long have you noticed these visual changes?"

"Is the visual loss associated with pain?"

"Did it occur suddenly?"

"Do you have a history of glaucoma?"

"Have you ever been told that you had a thyroid problem?"

"Do you have diabetes?"

Acute painless visual loss is caused by either a vascular accident or a retinal detachment. Painless loss of vision over a longer period occurs with compression of the optic nerve or tract or radiation. Glaucoma is often the cause of chronic, insidious, painless loss of vision. Acute narrow-angle glaucoma, however, may be responsible for transient loss of vision in association with intense ocular pain. Episodes of migraine may produce transient episodes of visual loss before the development of the headache. *Amaurosis fugax* is transient visual loss lasting up to 3 minutes and is a feature of internal carotid artery disease.

Double vision, or *diplopia*, is discussed in Chapter 10, The Eye. Ocular motor palsies, thyroid abnormalities, myasthenia gravis, and brain-stem lesions are well-known causes of diplopia. Ocular motor palsies can occur in trauma, multiple sclerosis, myasthenia gravis, aneurysms of the circle of Willis, diabetes, and tumors. Ask the following questions of any patient complaining of diplopia:

> *"Are you diabetic?"*
>
> *"In which field of gaze do you have double vision?"*
>
> *"Did the double vision occur suddenly?"*
>
> *"Was there any pain associated with the double vision?"*
>
> *"Has there been any injury to your head or eye?"*
>
> *"Have you ever been told that your blood pressure was elevated?"*
>
> *"Does the double vision get worse when you are tired?"*
>
> *"Have you been exposed to the AIDS [acquired immunodeficiency syndrome] virus?"*

When a cranial nerve is affected, resulting in an extraocular muscle palsy, the patient may complain of diplopia in one field of gaze when the affected eye is unable to move conjugately with the other. Ocular palsies involve the third, fourth, and sixth cranial nerves. A complete third (oculomotor) nerve palsy causes ptosis, mydriasis, and loss of all extraocular movements except abduction. Trauma, multiple sclerosis, tumors, and aneurysms are the most frequent causes. Aneurysms of the posterior communicating artery can involve the third nerve, which passes near the artery on its way to the cavernous sinus. Cavernous sinus thrombosis, not infrequently seen in patients with AIDS, may also produce a complete third nerve palsy. Pupil-sparing third nerve, fourth (trochlear) nerve, and sixth (abducens) nerve palsies are seen in diabetic patients and in patients with long-standing hypertension. Patients with myasthenia gravis often have diplopia in the later part of the day as the muscles tire and weaken.

Visual disturbances, including blocked vision or loss of vision in one eye, blurry vision, or "graying out" are seen frequently in patients suffering a stroke.

Dysphasia

Speech abnormalities, or dysphasia, may be either nonfluent (expressive) or fluent (receptive). In *expressive aphasia*, the speech pattern is hesitant and labored, with poor articulation. The patient has no problem with comprehension. When asked to say, "no ifs, ands, or buts," the patient has great difficulty. In *receptive aphasia*, the speech is rapid and appears fluent but is full of syntax errors, with the omission of many words. Handwriting changes are nonspecific but indicate an impairment of neuromuscular control. Ask the following questions:

> *"Have you noticed any recent change in your speech pattern, such as slurring of your words?"*
>
> *"Do you have trouble understanding things that are said to you?"*
>
> *"Have you had any difficulty finding the right word in conversation?"*
>
> *"Has your handwriting changed recently?"*

Language problems, as well as slurred speech, are found commonly in patients suffering a stroke.

Dementia

An important symptom of neurologic disease is failing memory. Dementia can be defined as the progressive impairment of orientation, memory, judgment, and other aspects of intellectual function. Dementia is a symptom rather than a specific disease entity. The most common cause of dementia is *Alzheimer's disease*. Other causes include Parkinson's disease, vascular

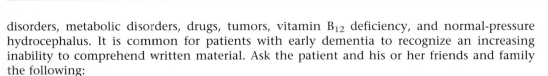

disorders, metabolic disorders, drugs, tumors, vitamin B_{12} deficiency, and normal-pressure hydrocephalus. It is common for patients with early dementia to recognize an increasing inability to comprehend written material. Ask the patient and his or her friends and family the following:

"Have you noticed any change in your memory lately?"

"Do you have difficulty reading or understanding what you have read?"

"What was the patient's personality like a few years ago?"

"When was the last time the patient seemed normal?"

"What does the patient's diet consist of? Does he or she eat well?"

"Can the patient live alone?"

Cerebrovascular Accident

Strokes, or cerebrovascular accidents, are common. Most are thromboembolic (80%), but some are hemorrhagic (20%). Thirty percent of patients who sustain a stroke die within the first month. Most patients with strokes have paresis of at least one limb. *Transient ischemic attacks (TIAs)* are short episodes manifested by focal neurologic dysfunction. They usually last only a few minutes, after which complete recovery occurs. The importance of TIAs is that, in 30% of affected patients, a stroke occurs within 4 to 5 years.

Gait Disturbance

Gait disturbances may occur for a variety of reasons. Gait may be changed by local pain in the foot, pain in a joint, claudication of the hip or leg, bone disease, vestibular problems, and extrapyramidal disorders. Interruption of the corticospinal tracts in the cerebrum after a stroke produces a spastic weakness in the contralateral leg. The foot is dragged, and the whole leg appears stiff and extended. Lesions in the spinal cord may produce a spastic paralysis affecting both legs. The gait is slow and stiff, with small steps. Patients with Parkinson's disease walk stooped over, with short, quick, shuffling steps. Any patient with a gait disturbance should be asked the following:

"Do you have pain in your leg or hip when you walk?"

"Do you have diabetes?"

"Have you ever had syphilis?"

"What do you eat? Tell me everything you ate yesterday."

Patients with vascular occlusive disease of the hip or leg may experience pain while walking and may alter their gait. Diabetes, syphilis, and pernicious anemia may produce a sensory loss, and each condition can result in gait abnormalities.

Tremor

A tremor is a rhythmic motion of the distal parts of the limbs or head. A physiologic tremor has an oscillation of 10 to 12 cycles per second and is more obvious after exercise. A pathologic tremor is slower. *Parkinson's disease* is the most frequently encountered extrapyramidal movement disorder. In this condition, the tremor is present at rest and is decreased with action. It has a frequency of three to six cycles per second and is worsened by anxiety. An intention, or *ataxic*, tremor is slow (two to four cycles per second) and worsens on attempted movement. Multiple sclerosis is one of the many causes of intention tremor. Metabolic problems from liver or kidney failure are frequently responsible. Withdrawal from alcohol or caffeine is often a precipitating factor. Any patient with the symptom of tremor should be asked these questions:

"Does the tremor worsen when you try to do something?"

"Is there a history of thyroid disease?"

"Have you ever been told about any problems with your liver or kidneys?"

"What is your daily consumption of alcoholic beverages?"

"How much coffee or tea do you drink?"

"How much chocolate do you eat?"

Chorea is involuntary jerky motions of the face and limbs. A common cause is *Huntington's disease*, in which chorea is accompanied by personality changes and progressive mental deterioration terminating in dementia.

"Numbness"

Numbness is another term used by patients to indicate a variety of problems. "Numbness" can be used by patients to describe a "pins-and-needles" sensation, coolness, pain, or clumsiness. The interviewer should be sure to clarify the meaning. The examiner must be careful during the physical examination to palpate the distal pulses in any patient complaining of numbness, because arterial insufficiency is a possible cause.

"Weakness"

Weakness may be a symptom of the motor system. A patient with a *proximal arm* motor weakness complains of difficulty brushing hair, shaving, or reaching up to shelves. A patient with *distal arm* motor weakness complains of difficulty putting a button through a buttonhole, using keys, or writing with a pen or pencil. *Proximal leg* motor weakness is characterized by difficulty climbing stairs or getting into bed or the bathtub. Footdrop is a classic sign of *distal leg* motor weakness. Chapter 20, The Musculoskeletal System, reviews some of the important questions related to weakness.

Face droop and weakness are common signs of a stroke, as is the presence of numbness or clumsiness in one arm or hand.

Pain

Pain is an infrequent symptom of neurologic disease, but it merits mention. *Trigeminal neuralgia*, also known as *tic douloureux*, is the occurrence of severe, jabbing pain lasting only seconds in the distribution of the maxillary or mandibular divisions of the trigeminal nerve (Fig. 21-10). It is frequently provoked by motion, touch, eating, or exposure to cold temperatures. Another cause of facial pain is the cluster headache, already discussed. *Herpes zoster* infection of a sensory nerve root, also known as *shingles*, manifests with intense pain

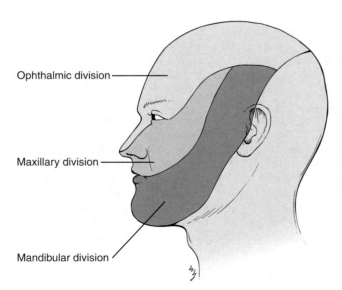

Ophthalmic division

Maxillary division

Mandibular division

Figure 21–10 Areas innervated by divisions of the trigeminal nerve.

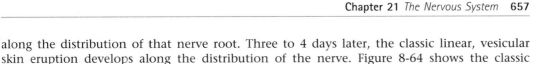

along the distribution of that nerve root. Three to 4 days later, the classic linear, vesicular skin eruption develops along the distribution of the nerve. Figure 8-64 shows the classic dermatologic manifestations of herpes zoster infection of spinal nerve T3.

Sciatica is intense pain shooting down the leg in the distribution of the sciatic nerve. In this condition, there is impingement of portions of the sciatic nerve by the vertebrae. Arthritis of the lumbosacral spine is frequently the cause.

Sometimes the paresthesias associated with demyelinating diseases are so intense that the patient may describe them as pain.

Patients with *inflammation of the meninges* often complain of pain in the neck and a resistance to flexion of the neck. If *meningitis* is suspected, have the patient lie on his or her back. Place your hand behind the patient's neck and flex it until the chin touches the sternum. In patients with meningitis, there is neck pain and resistance to motion. This is called *Brudzinski's sign*. There may also be flexion of the patient's hips and knees. Jósef Brudzinski described at least five different physical signs indicative of meningeal irritation. This sign is the best known and most reliable sign. Another sign of meningeal irritation can be elicited while the patient lies on the back and you flex one of the patient's legs at the hip and knee. If pain or resistance is elicited as the knee is extended, a positive *Kernig's sign* is present.

Impact of Chronic Neurologic Disease on the Patient

The ramifications of chronic neurologic disease on the patient and his or her family are enormous. All family members experience emotional pain while observing the progressive clinical changes. The family bears an immense personal burden in assisting the patient to cope with disability.

One example of a progressive neurologic condition is Alzheimer's disease. A devastating chronic disorder of unknown cause, Alzheimer's disease is the most common diffuse brain degeneration causing brain failure. This condition is characterized by progressive and widespread brain degeneration with a hopeless prognosis.

Memory problems and impairment of intellectual function are the main symptoms of Alzheimer's disease. Depression is common. Patients may have significant cognitive impairment, which ruins their ability to negotiate their environment. They may forget where they live. They may forget to turn off a gas burner on the stove or to put out a cigarette. They may wander aimlessly outdoors.

Manifestations of Alzheimer's disease span a clinical spectrum from awareness of the disability to a vegetative state. Many patients lose touch with reality. During an interview with such a patient, it may become clear that even the ability to describe the patient's own medical history has been lost.

Early in the course of the disease, affected patients may use a number of circumlocutions, such as substituting words when they cannot find more appropriate ones. Another early change is disorientation with regard to time and place. Visual hallucinations are common. Lack of interest in sex is almost universal. Motor behavior diminishes progressively as impairment of consciousness increases. An important characteristic is the development of bizarre thoughts and fantasies that come to dominate consciousness. Delusions, especially delusions of persecution, are common.

In the early stages of the disease—when patients are still aware of their environment but have experienced the symptom of memory loss—mild depression, anxiety, and irritability are common. As the disease progresses, apathy is the dominant feature. Patients may actually appear indifferent and emotionally withdrawn. In others in whom there is increased motor activity, anxiety and fear are common. In these individuals, terror and panic attacks are not uncommon. Hostility and paranoia develop rapidly. Regression and sudden displays of highly charged emotion are the responses to their frequent hallucinations.

In milder cases, depression, hypochondriasis, and phobic features abound. Hysterical conversion reactions, such as hysterical blindness, may occur. Social interaction is lost, and the patient may suddenly explode with anger, anxiety, or tears. As the disease progresses, suicide attempts are common. Emotional lability is often extreme, with periods of laughter followed by crying. With progressive disease, dullness of affect and lack of an emotional response occur as gross neurologic disability develops. In the terminal stages, patients with Alzheimer's disease may show severe body wasting with profound brain failure.

Physical Examination

The equipment necessary for the neurologic examination consists of safety pins, cotton-tipped applicators, a 128-Hz tuning fork, gauze pads, familiar objects (coins, keys), and a reflex hammer.

The neurologic examination consists of assessment of the following:

- Mental status
- Cranial nerves
- Motor function
- Reflexes
- Sensory function
- Cerebellar function

Mental Status

During the interview, the examiner has already gained much insight into the mental status of the patient. The interviewer may have already been able to assess the patient's remote memory, affect, and judgment. The formal mental status portion of the neurologic examination is introduced by saying to the patient, "I would like to ask you a few routine questions. Some of them you will find very easy. Others will be more difficult. Do the best you can."

The mental status examination consists of evaluation of the following:

- Level of consciousness
- Speech
- Orientation
- Knowledge of current events
- Judgment
- Abstraction
- Vocabulary
- Emotional responses
- Memory
- Calculation ability
- Object recognition
- Praxis

Assess Level of Consciousness

The level of consciousness can be assessed as soon as you introduce yourself to the patient. Is the patient awake? Alert? Is the patient's sensorium clouded by exogenous or endogenous insults? Does the patient appear confused? If the patient does not respond to your introduction, hold the patient's hand and softly say, "Hello, Mr./Ms. ____, can you hear me? If you hear me, squeeze my hand." If there is no response, try gently shaking the patient. If there is still no response and the patient appears obtunded, squeezing the nipple or applying pressure with your thumb to the bony ridge under the eyebrow is a painful maneuver that may rouse the patient. If these maneuvers fail to awaken the patient, the patient is in *coma*. Patients who are in coma are completely unconscious and cannot be roused even by painful stimuli. If either painful stimulus is used, be careful not to pinch the skin or bruise the patient. If friends or relatives are present, make sure to explain to them what you are doing.

Evaluate Speech

If the patient is awake and alert, you have already observed his or her speech. The patient should now be asked to recite short phrases such as "no ifs, ands, or buts." Is dysarthria, dysphonia, dysphasia, or aphasia present? *Dysarthria* is difficulty in articulation. In general, lesions of the tongue and palate are responsible for dysarthria. *Dysphonia* is difficulty in phonation. The result is an alteration in the volume and tone of the voice. Lesions of the palate and vocal cords are often responsible. *Dysphasia* is difficulty comprehending or speaking as a result of cerebral dysfunction. Patients with a total loss of speech have *aphasia*. Different areas of the brain are responsible for the different types of aphasia. A motor, expressive, nonfluent aphasia is present when patients know what they want to say but have motor impairment and cannot articulate properly. They understand written and verbal commands but cannot repeat them. A frontal lobe lesion is often the cause. A sensory, receptive, fluent aphasia is present when the patient articulates spontaneously but uses words inappropriately. The patient has difficulty understanding written and verbal commands and cannot repeat them. A temporoparietal lesion is frequently the cause.

Evaluate Orientation

The patient's orientation to person, place, and time must be established. *Orientation* refers to the person's awareness of self in relation to other persons, places, and time. Disorientation occurs in association with impairment of memory and attention span. The patient should be asked these questions:

> *"What is today's date?"*
>
> *"What is the day of the week?"*
>
> *"What is the name of this hospital (or building)?"*

Evaluate Knowledge of Current Events

A knowledge of current events can be assessed by asking the patient to name the last four presidents of the United States. Asking the patient the name of the local mayor or governor is also useful. If the patient is not American or is unfamiliar with American affairs, asking the patient about more general current events may be more useful. The ability to name current events requires an intact orientation, intact recent memory, and the ability to think abstractly.

Assess Judgment

Evaluation of judgment is performed by asking the patient to interpret a simple problem. Ask the patient the following:

> *"What would you do if you noticed an addressed envelope with an uncanceled stamp on it on the street near a mailbox?"*
>
> *"What would you do if you were in a crowded movie theater and a fire started?"*

A correct response to the first question would be to pick up the letter and mail it. An example of an incorrect response might be, "I'd throw it in the trash." Judgment requires higher cerebral function.

Assess Abstraction

Abstraction is a higher cerebral function that requires comprehension and judgment. Proverbs are commonly used to test abstract reasoning. The patient should be asked to interpret the following:

> *"People who live in glass houses shouldn't throw stones."*
>
> *"A rolling stone gathers no moss."*

A patient with an abnormality in abstract reasoning might respond to the first quotation with a *concrete* interpretation, such as, "The glass will break if you throw a stone through it." A concrete interpretation of the second proverb might be "Moss grows only under rocks that don't move and not under a rolling stone." Concrete responses are common in patients with mental retardation or brain failure. Schizophrenic patients often answer with concrete interpretations, but bizarre assessments are also common. Be careful when assessing abstraction in patients who are not fluent in English.

Another method of testing abstract reasoning is to ask the patient how two items are similar or dissimilar. You might ask, "What is similar about a dog and a cat?" "What is similar about a church and a synagogue?" or "What is dissimilar about an apple and a chicken?"

Assess Vocabulary

Vocabulary is often difficult to assess. It is based on many factors, which include the patient's education, background, work, environment, and cerebral function. It is, however, an important parameter in assessing intellectual capacity. Patients who are mentally retarded have a limited vocabulary, whereas those with mild brain failure have a well-preserved vocabulary. Patients should be asked to define words or use them in sentences. Any words can be used, but they should be asked in order of increasing level of difficulty. The following list is an example:

Car

Ability

Dominant

Voluntary

Telescope

Reticent

Enigma

Assess Emotional Responses

Although emotional response has probably been informally observed already, inquire specifically whether the patient has noticed any sudden mood changes. It is appropriate to ask, "How are your spirits?" During the interview, the interviewer has already noticed the patient's *affect*, which is the emotional response to an event. The response may be *appropriate*, *abnormal*, or *flat*. An appropriate response to a loved one's death may be to cry. An inappropriate response is to laugh. A flat response shows little emotion. Patients with bilateral cerebral damage lose control of their emotions.

Assess Memory

To test memory, have the patient recall the recent and the remote past. *Recent* memory is easily tested by presenting three words to the patient and asking for them to be repeated 5 minutes later. For example, tell the patient, "Repeat these words after me and remember them. I will ask for them later: necklace, thirty-two, barn." Continue with the mental status examination. Five minutes later, ask the patient, "What were those words I asked you to remember?"

A simpler test of memory is to have the patient recall as many elements in a category as possible. Request that the patient do one of the following:

"Name as many flowers as you can."

"Name as many occupations as you can."

"Name as many tools as you can."

An abnormality in recent memory may be related to a lesion in the temporal lobe.

To test the *remote past* memory, ask the patient about well-known events in the past. Do not ask about events that you cannot verify.

Assess Calculation Ability

The ability to calculate depends on the integrity of the dominant cerebral hemisphere, as well as on the patient's intelligence. Ask the patient to perform simple arithmetic problems, such as subtracting 7 from 100, then 7 from the result, then 7 from the result, and so forth. This is the *serial sevens* test. If there is difficulty with serial sevens, ask the patient to add or subtract several numbers, such as "How much is 5 plus 7? How much is 12 plus 9? How much is 27 minus 9?"

Assess Object Recognition

Object recognition is termed *gnosia*. *Agnosia* is the failure to recognize a sensory stimulus despite normal primary sensation. Show the patient a series of well-known objects, such as coins, pens, eyeglasses, or pieces of clothing, and ask the patient to name them. If the patient has normal vision and fails to recognize the object, *visual agnosia* is present. *Tactile agnosia* is the inability to recognize an object by palpation in the absence of a sensory deficit. This occurs with a lesion in the nondominant parietal lobe. *Autotopagnosia* is the term used to describe a patient's inability to recognize his or her own body part, such as the hand or leg.

Assess Praxis

Praxis is the ability to perform a motor activity. *Apraxia* is the inability to perform a voluntary movement in the absence of deficits in motor strength, sensation, or coordination. *Dyspraxia* is the decreased ability to perform the activity. The patient hears and understands the command but cannot integrate the motor activities that will complete the action. Ask a patient to pour water from the bedside pitcher into a glass and drink the water. A patient with dyspraxia may either drink the water from the pitcher or try to drink from the empty glass. A deep frontal lobe lesion is frequently responsible for this disorder.

Another type of apraxia is *constructional apraxia*. In this condition, the patient is unable to construct or draw simple designs. The examiner draws a shape and asks the patient to copy it. Alternatively, the patient can be asked to draw the face of a clock. Patients with constructional apraxia often have a lesion in the posterior portion of the parietal lobe.

Cranial Nerves

The examination of the cranial nerves should be carried out in an orderly manner. Several of the cranial nerves have already been evaluated. Table 21-1 lists the cranial nerves, their functions, and the clinical findings when a lesion exists.

Cranial Nerve I: Olfactory

The olfactory nerve supplies nerve endings to the superior nasal concha and upper one third of the nasal septum. The olfactory nerve is not routinely tested. However, in any patient with a suspected frontal lobe disorder, the olfactory nerve should be evaluated.

Table 21–1 Cranial Nerves

Cranial Nerve	Function	Clinical Findings with Lesion
I: Olfactory	Smell	Anosmia
II: Optic	Vision	Amaurosis
III: Oculomotor	Eye movements; papillary constriction; accommodation	Diplopia; ptosis; mydriasis; loss of accommodation
IV: Trochlear	Eye movements	Diplopia
V: Trigeminal	General sensation of face, scalp, and teeth; chewing movements	"Numbness" of face; weakness of jaw muscles
VI: Abducens	Eye movements	Diplopia
VII: Facial	Taste; general sensation of palate and external ear; lacrimal gland and submandibular and sublingual gland secretion; facial expression	Loss of taste on anterior two thirds of tongue; dry mouth; loss of lacrimation; paralysis of facial muscles
VIII: Vestibulocochlear	Hearing; equilibrium	Deafness; tinnitus; vertigo; nystagmus
IX: Glossopharyngeal	Taste; general sensation of pharynx and ear; elevation of palate; parotid gland secretion	Loss of taste on posterior one third of tongue; anesthesia of pharynx; partially dry mouth
X: Vagus	Taste; general sensation of pharynx, larynx, and ear; swallowing; phonation; parasympathetic innervation to heart and abdominal viscera	Dysphagia; hoarseness; palatal paralysis
XI: Spinal accessory	Phonation; head, neck, and shoulder movements	Hoarseness; weakness of head, neck, and shoulder muscles
XII: Hypoglossal	Tongue movements	Weakness and wasting of tongue

Test Olfaction

The patient is asked to close the eyes and one nostril as the examiner brings a test substance close to the patient's other nostril. The patient is instructed to sniff the test substance. The substance must be volatile and nonirritating, such as cloves, vanilla beans, freshly ground coffee, or lavender. The use of an irritating agent such as alcohol would involve cranial nerve V, as well as cranial nerve I, and the test results would be inaccurate.

Each nostril is tested separately. The examiner asks the patient to identify the test material. A unilateral loss of smell, known as unilateral *anosmia*, is more important than a bilateral loss, because it indicates a lesion affecting the olfactory nerve or tract on that side.

Cranial Nerve II: Optic

The optic nerve ends in the retina. The examinations for visual acuity and the ophthalmoscopic examination are discussed in Chapter 10, The Eye.

Cranial Nerve III: Oculomotor

The oculomotor nerve supplies the medial, superior, and inferior rectus muscles and the inferior oblique muscle, which control most eye movements. The third nerve also innervates the intrinsic muscles, controlling pupillary constriction and accommodation.

Extraocular muscle movements are discussed in Chapter 10. A patient with an oculomotor palsy is shown in Figure 10-144. The pupillary light reflex depends on the function of cranial nerves II and III (see Chapter 10). Visual fields are part of both the eye examination and the neurologic examination. The technique for visual field testing is discussed in Chapter 10.

Cranial Nerve IV: Trochlear

The trochlear nerve is responsible for movement of the superior oblique muscle. Extraocular muscle movements are discussed in Chapter 10.

Cranial Nerve V: Trigeminal

The trigeminal nerve is responsible for supplying sensation to the face, the nasal and buccal mucosa, and the teeth. The motor division supplies the muscles of mastication. The three major subdivisions of the trigeminal nerve are the ophthalmic, the maxillary, and the mandibular. These divisions are illustrated in Figure 21-10.

The *ophthalmic division* supplies sensation to the frontal sinuses, the conjunctiva, the cornea, the upper eyelid, the bridge of the nose, the forehead, and the scalp as far as the vertex of the skull. The *maxillary division* supplies sensation to the cheek, the maxillary sinus, the lateral aspects of the nose, the upper teeth, the nasal pharynx, the hard palate, and the uvula. The *mandibular division* supplies sensation to the chin, the lower jaw, the anterior two thirds of the tongue, the lower teeth, the gums and floor of the mouth, and the buccal mucosa of the cheek. The motor division innervates the muscles of mastication and the tensor tympani.

The examination of the trigeminal nerve consists of the following:

- Testing the corneal reflex
- Testing the sensory function
- Testing the motor function

Test Corneal Reflex

The corneal reflex depends on the function of cranial nerves V and VII. To evaluate the corneal reflex, the examiner uses a cotton-tipped applicator, the tip of which has been pulled into a thin strand about 1.3 cm in length. The examiner stabilizes the patient's head by placing a hand on the patient's eyebrow and head. The patient is asked to look to the left side as the cotton tip is brought in from the right side to touch the right cornea gently. This is demonstrated in Figure 21-11. A prompt bilateral reflex closure of the eyelids is the normal response. The examination is repeated on the other side by reversing the directions.

The responses on the two sides are compared. The sensory limb of the corneal reflex is the ophthalmic division of the trigeminal nerve; the motor limb is conducted through the facial nerve.

In performing the corneal reflex test, touch the cornea and not the eyelashes or conjunctiva, which will elicit an inaccurate result.

2

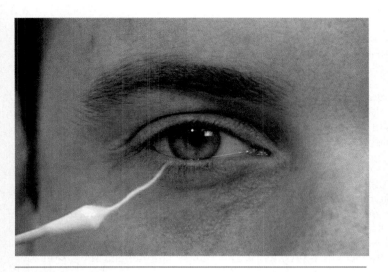

Figure 21–11 Technique for evaluating the corneal reflex.

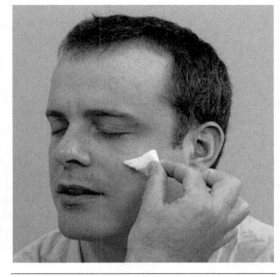

Figure 21–12 Technique for testing the sensory function of the trigeminal nerve, maxillary division.

Test Sensory Function

The sensory function of the trigeminal nerve is tested by asking the patient to close the eyes and to respond when a touch is felt. A piece of gauze is brushed against one side of the forehead and then the corresponding position on the other side. This test is then performed on the cheeks and the jaw, so that all three subdivisions of the nerve are tested. The patient is also asked whether one side feels the same as or different from the other side. The examination is demonstrated in Figure 21-12.

Test Motor Function

The motor function of the trigeminal nerve is tested by having the patient bite down or clench the teeth while the masseter and temporalis muscles are palpated bilaterally. This is demonstrated in Figure 21-13. Unilateral weakness causes the jaw to deviate toward the side of the lesion.

Figure 21–13 Technique for testing the motor function of the trigeminal nerve.

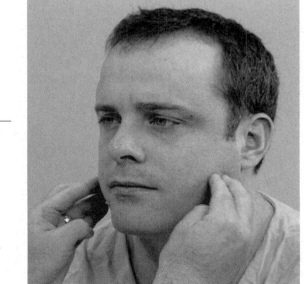

Cranial Nerve VI: Abducens

The abducens nerve is responsible for movement of the lateral rectus muscle. Extraocular muscle movements are discussed in Chapter 10, The Eye.

Cranial Nerve VII: Facial

The facial nerve innervates the facial muscles and enables taste on the anterior two thirds of the tongue. A small component also supplies general sensation to the external ear. The facial nerve carries parasympathetic motor fibers to the salivary glands and chorda tympani. Testing for abnormalities of taste is usually not performed by an internist.

Test Motor Function

The patient is asked to bare the teeth while the examiner observes for asymmetry. The patient is asked to puff out the cheeks against resistance and then to wrinkle the forehead. It is helpful if the examiner actually demonstrates these maneuvers for the patient. These maneuvers are demonstrated in Figure 21-14.

The patient is then asked to close the eyes tightly while the examiner tries to open them. The patient is told to close the eyes as tightly as possible. The examiner can say, "Don't let me open them." This procedure is demonstrated in Figure 21-15A. Each eye is examined separately, and the strengths are compared. Normally the examiner should not be able to open the patient's eyes. The patient in Figure 21-15B had marked weakness of the left orbicularis oculi muscle as a result of a stroke involving the facial nucleus.

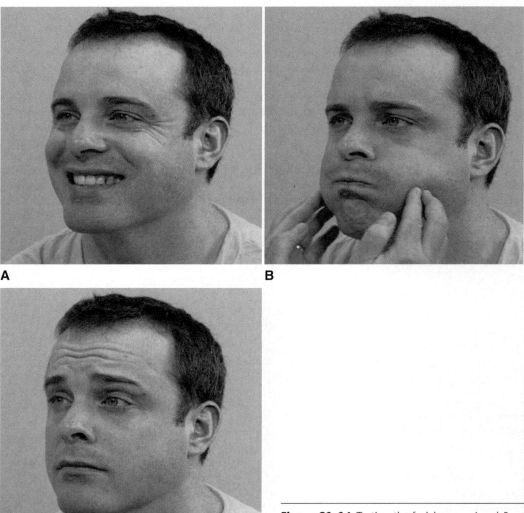

A

B

C

Figure 21–14 Testing the facial nerve. *A* and *B*, Tests for the lower division. *C*, Test for the upper division.

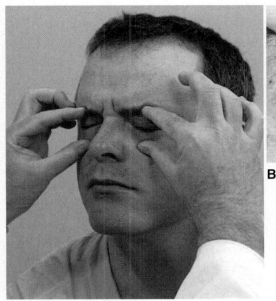
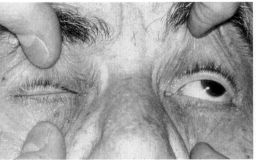

Figure 21–15 Testing the strength of eyelid closure. *A,* Normal response. Note that the eyelids cannot be opened by the examiner. *B,* Test in a patient with a stroke that involved the facial nerve nucleus. Note the loss in strength of the muscle around the left eye.

The innervations of the facial nerve are illustrated in Figure 21-16. There are two types of facial weakness. Upper motor neuron lesions such as a stroke involving the corticobulbar pathways produce contralateral weakness of the lower face, with normal function of the upper face. The patient is still able to wrinkle the forehead. This is related to the bilateral innervation of the upper face by the corticobulbar fibers. The lower face has only unilateral innervation from contralateral cortical centers. This type of upper motor neuron lesion is illustrated by lesion A in Figure 21-16. The second type of facial weakness produces total involvement of the ipsilateral facial muscles, with no area being spared. This may result from lesions of the nerve as it exits from the skull or from involvement of the facial nucleus in the pons, as illustrated by lesion B in Figure 21-16.

When the patient in Figure 21-17 was asked to smile, the right side of his face was drawn to the left. This patient has right facial palsy, also known as *right Bell's palsy*. Further maneuvers revealed that the entire right side of his face was involved as a result of a lesion affecting the right facial nucleus.

Cranial Nerve VIII: Vestibulocochlear
The vestibulocochlear nerve is responsible for hearing, balance, and awareness of position. Auditory testing is discussed in Chapter 11, The Ear and Nose. Tests for the vestibular function of cranial nerve VIII usually are not performed.

Cranial Nerve IX: Glossopharyngeal
The glossopharyngeal nerve supplies sensation to the pharynx, posterior one third of the tongue, and tympanic membrane, as well as secretory fibers to the parotid gland.

Test Sensory Function
Examination of the glossopharyngeal nerve involves the gag reflex. The examiner may use either a tongue blade or an applicator stick. By touching the posterior third of the tongue, the soft palate, or the posterior pharyngeal wall, the examiner should elicit a gag reflex. The sensory portion of the loop is through the glossopharyngeal nerve; the motor portion is mediated through the vagus nerve.

Another way to test the nerve is to ask the patient to open the mouth widely and to say, "Ah ... ah." Symmetric elevation of the soft palate demonstrates normal function of cranial nerves IX and X. The uvula should remain in the midline.

Taste sensation of the posterior third of the tongue is not routinely tested.

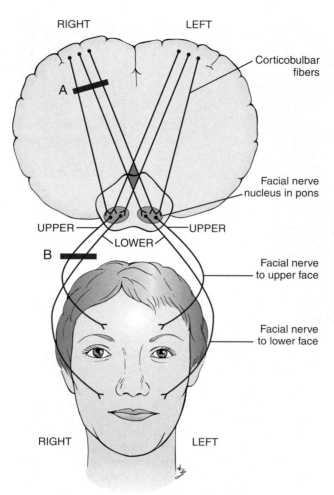

Figure 21–16 Innervations of the facial nerve and types of facial weakness. Lesion *A* produces an upper motor nerve palsy that causes contralateral weakness of the lower face but spares the contralateral forehead. Lesion *B* produces a lower motor nerve palsy that causes total paralysis of the ipsilateral face.

Cranial Nerve X: Vagus

The vagus nerve supplies parasympathetic fibers to the viscera of the chest and abdomen; motor fibers to the pharynx and larynx; and sensory fibers to the external ear canal, the meninges of the posterior cranial fossa, the pharynx, the larynx, and the viscera of the body cavities above the pelvis.

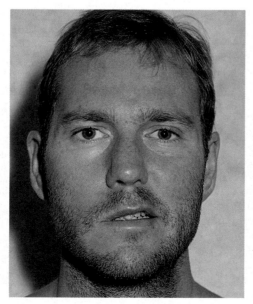

Figure 21–17 Right facial palsy.

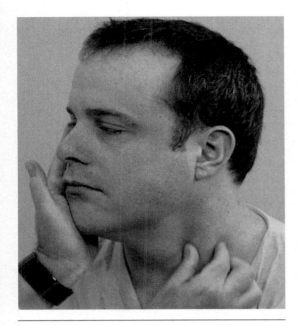

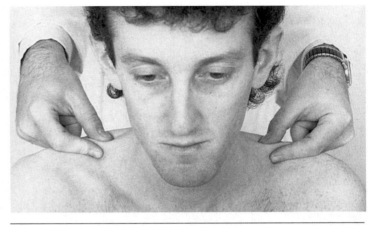

Figure 21–19 Alternative technique for evaluating the spinal accessory nerve.

Figure 21–18 Technique for evaluating the spinal accessory nerve.

Examination of the vagus nerve was performed during evaluation of the glossopharyngeal nerve.

Dysphonia or dysarthria may result from paralysis of the vagus nerve.

Cranial Nerve XI: Spinal Accessory

The spinal accessory nerve is a motor nerve that supplies the sternocleidomastoid and trapezius muscles.

Test Motor Function

The left spinal accessory nerve is examined by asking the patient to turn the head to the right against the resistance of the examiner's hand. This is demonstrated in Figure 21-18. The right spinal accessory nerve is examined by reversing the directions.

An alternative test is to evaluate the trapezius muscles. The examiner places both hands on the patient's trapezius muscles. Both muscles are palpated between the examiner's thumbs and index fingers. The patient is then asked to shrug the shoulders against the resistance of the examiner's hands. Both sides should move equally. This technique is demonstrated in Figure 21-19.

Cranial Nerve XII: Hypoglossal

The hypoglossal nerve supplies motor fibers to the muscles of the tongue. The examination of the hypoglossal nerve is performed by asking the patient to open the mouth, with the tongue resting quietly on the floor of the mouth. Inspection for *fasciculations** is performed. Fasciculations are indicative of a hypoglossal lower motor neuron lesion.

Test Motor Function

Ask the patient to open the mouth and stick out the tongue. Normally, the tongue is protruded and lies in the midline. This is demonstrated in Figure 21-20. Deviation of the tongue to either side is abnormal. Because the tongue muscles push rather than pull, weakness of one side results in the tongue's being pushed by the normal side to the side of the lesion.

In Figure 21-21, notice the marked scalloping of the tongue's surface. The patient has a chronic neurologic disease known as *amyotrophic lateral sclerosis*,[†] characterized by progressive

---

*Spontaneous contractions of groups of muscles that are visible on inspection.
[†]This disease is also called *Lou Gehrig's disease*, after the famous baseball player who was one of its victims.

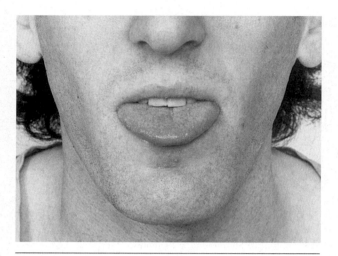

Figure 21–20 Technique for evaluating the hypoglossal nerve.

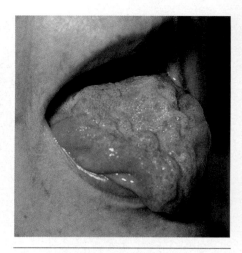

Figure 21–21 Amyotrophic lateral sclerosis. Note the scalloping of the tongue.

degeneration of motor neurons. The patient has the typical features of a lower motor neuron bulbar palsy affecting the hypoglossal nucleus: wasting of the tongue with fasciculations.

Motor Function

Basic Principles

The motor system is evaluated for the following:

- Muscle bulk
- Muscle strength
- Muscle tone

The motor examination begins with inspection of each area being tested. The contours of symmetric *muscle masses* in both the upper and lower extremities are compared. Inspection is used to detect muscle atrophy and the presence of fasciculations.

Test *muscle strength* by having the patient move actively against your resistance. Compare one side with the other. The following is an arbitrary scale that is commonly used for the grading of muscle strength:

0, Absent: No contraction detected

1, Trace: Slight contraction detected

2, Weak: Movement with gravity eliminated (sideways)

3, Fair: Movement against gravity (upward)

4, Good: Movement against gravity with some resistance

5, Normal: Movement against gravity with full resistance

If muscle weakness is found, compare the proximal and distal strengths. In general, proximal weakness is related to muscle disease; distal weakness is related to neurologic disease.

Tone can be defined as the slight residual tension in a voluntarily relaxed muscle. Tone is assessed by resistance to passive movement. Ask the patient to relax. Perform passive motion of the muscle. Compare one side with the other. Upper motor neuron lesions produce spasticity,* hyperreflexia, clonus,† and Babinski's sign.‡ Lower motor neuron lesions produce atrophy,

---

*An increase in muscle tone that results in continuous resistance to stretching. Spasticity is usually worse at extremes of range.

†Spasm in which rigidity and relaxation alternate in rapid succession.

‡Dorsiflexion of the big toe on stimulation of the sole of the foot.

fasciculations, decreased tone, and hyporeflexia. Both types of lesions result in weakness. Fasciculations may become more apparent by gently tapping the muscle with a reflex hammer.

It is impractical to test all muscles during the neurologic examination. By testing key muscle groups, the examiner can determine whether a gross deficit exists. Further testing of specific muscles and nerve roots may then be necessary. The student is referred to the many textbooks on neurology for these detailed examinations.

Examine Upper Extremities

In the assessment of motor function, the upper extremities are examined first.

Inspect the Upper Extremities for Symmetry

Ask the patient to sit on the side of the bed facing you. Inspect both arms and hands for size differences, paying special attention to the size of the thumbs and the small muscles of the hands. Is muscle wasting present?

Test Flexion and Extension of the Arm

Test flexion and extension strength of the upper extremity by having the patient pull and push against your resistance. You might say, "Push down... relax," "Push up... relax," "Push back... relax," and "Push forward... relax." Say "relax" after each direction so that the patient does not continue to push or pull after you have removed your hands. After one side is tested, the other is tested, and the results of the two sides are compared.

Test Arm Abduction

Ask the patient to extend the arms, with palms facing down. Place your hands at the lateral aspect of the patient's arms. Instruct the patient to abduct the arms against resistance. This is a test of abduction of the arm by the *axillary nerve* from roots C5 to C6. This test is demonstrated in Figure 21-22.

Test Forearm Flexion

Have the patient make a fist and flex the forearm. Hold the patient's fist or wrist. Ask the patient to pull the arm in against your resistance. This is a test of flexion of the forearm by the *musculocutaneous nerve* from roots C5 to C6. This test is demonstrated in Figure 21-23.

Test Forearm Extension

Ask the patient to abduct the arm and hold it midway between flexion and extension. Support the patient's arm by holding the wrist. Instruct the patient to extend the arm

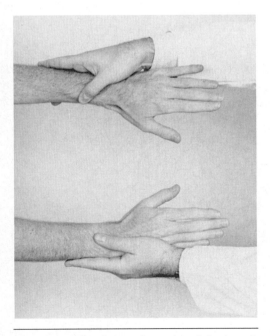

Figure 21–22 Technique for testing abduction of the arm.

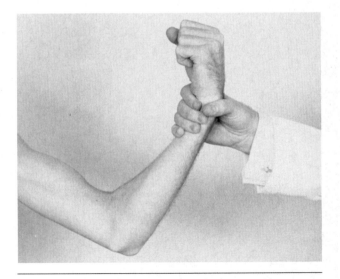

Figure 21–23 Technique for testing flexion of the forearm.

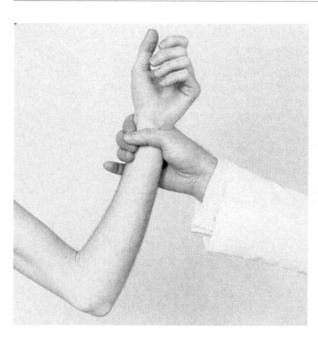

Figure 21–24 Technique for testing extension of the forearm.

against your resistance. This is a test of extension of the forearm by the *radial nerve* from roots C6 to C8. This test is demonstrated in Figure 21-24.

Test Wrist Extension
Instruct the patient to make a fist and extend the wrist while you attempt to push it up. This is a test of extension of the wrist by the *radial nerve* from roots C6 to C8. This test is demonstrated in Figure 21-25.

Test Wrist Flexion
Ask the patient to make a fist and flex the wrist while you attempt to pull it down. This is a test of flexion of the wrist by the *median nerve* from roots C6 to C7. This test is demonstrated in Figure 21-26.

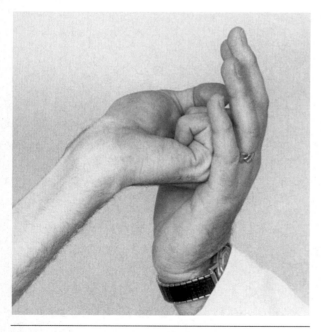

Figure 21–25 Technique for testing extension of the wrist.

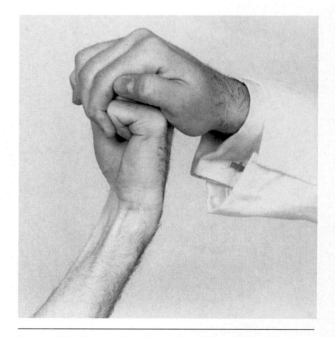

Figure 21–26 Technique for testing flexion of the wrist.

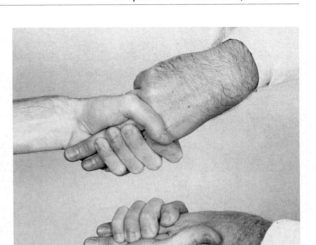

Figure 21–27 Technique for testing finger adduction.

Test Finger Adduction

Ask the patient to grasp your extended index and middle fingers and to squeeze them as hard as possible. Compare the strengths of both hands. (It is important for you to remove any rings, which may produce discomfort.) This is a test of adduction of the fingers by the *median nerve* from roots C7 to T1. This test is demonstrated in Figure 21-27.

Test Finger Abduction

Ask the patient to extend the hand with the palm down and to spread the fingers as widely as possible. Tell the patient to resist your attempt to bring the fingers together. This is a test of abduction of the fingers by the *ulnar nerve* from roots C8 to T1. This test is demonstrated in Figure 21-28.

Test Thumb Adduction

Instruct the patient to touch the base of the little finger with the tip of the thumb against resistance while the thumbnail remains parallel to the palm. This is a test of adduction of the thumb by the *median nerve* from roots C8 to T1. This test is demonstrated in Figure 21-29.

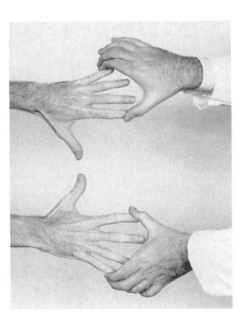

Figure 21–28 Technique for testing finger abduction.

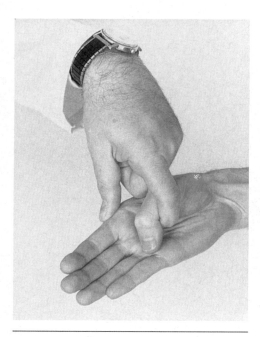

Figure 21–29 Technique for testing thumb adduction.

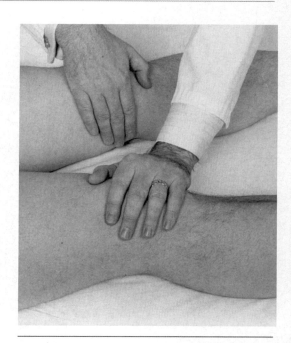

Figure 21–30 Technique for testing hip adduction.

Assess Upper Extremity Tone

Tone is assessed in the patient's upper limbs by passively flexing and extending the limbs to determine the amount of resistance to the examiner's movements. Increased resistance, such as that in muscle rigidity or spasticity, means increased muscle tone. Decreased resistance, such as that in limpness or flaccidity, means decreased muscle tone. Normal tone has a smooth sensation. In extrapyramidal disease, palpation of a proximal muscle during passive movement detects the presence of *cogwheeling*, which is a ratchety jerkiness to the motion.

Examine Lower Extremities

Inspect the Lower Extremities for Symmetry

The lower extremities are now examined for muscle bulk and muscle wasting. This examination is performed with the patient lying on his or her back in bed. As with the upper extremities, proximal and distal muscle strengths are compared, as are the legs with regard to symmetry.

Test Hip Adduction

Ask the patient to move the legs apart. Place your hands on the medial aspect of the patient's knees. Instruct the patient to close the legs against your resistance. This is a test of adduction of the hips by the *obturator nerve* from roots L2 to L4. This test is demonstrated in Figure 21-30.

Test Hip Abduction

Place your hands on the lateral margins of the patient's knees. Ask the patient to open the legs against your resistance. This is a test of abduction of the hips by the *superior gluteal nerve* from roots L4 to S1. This test is demonstrated in Figure 21-31.

Test Knee Flexion

Ask the patient to elevate a knee, with the foot resting on the bed. Instruct the patient to hold the foot down as you try to extend the leg. This is a test of flexion of the knee by the *sciatic nerve* from roots L4 to S1. This test is illustrated in Figure 21-32.

Test Knee Extension

Instruct the patient to elevate the knee, with the foot resting on the bed. Place your left hand under the knee. Ask the patient to straighten the leg against the resistance of your right hand, which is placed on the patient's shin. This procedure tests extension of the knee by the *femoral nerve* from roots L2 to L4. This test is illustrated in Figure 21-33.

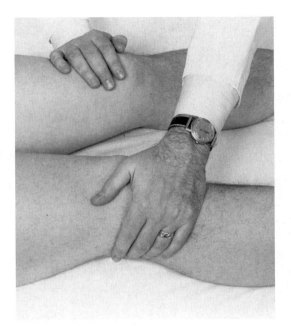

Figure 21–31 Technique for testing hip abduction.

Test Ankle Dorsiflexion

Place your hands on the dorsum of the foot, and ask the patient to dorsiflex the foot at the ankle against your resistance. This is a test of dorsiflexion of the ankle by the *deep peroneal nerve* from roots L4 to L5. This maneuver is demonstrated in Figure 21-34.

Test Ankle Plantar Flexion

Place your hand on the sole, and ask the patient to plantarflex the foot at the ankle against your resistance. This is a test of plantar flexion of the ankle by the *tibial nerve* from roots L5 to S2. This test is demonstrated in Figure 21-35.

Test Great Toe Dorsiflexion

Place your hand on the dorsal aspect of the patient's big toe. Ask the patient to dorsiflex the big toe against your resistance. This is a test of dorsiflexion of the big toe by the *deep peroneal nerve* from roots L4 to S1. This test is demonstrated in Figure 21-36.

Test Great Toe Plantar Flexion

Place your hand on the plantar surface of the patient's big toe. Ask the patient to plantarflex the great toe against your resistance. This is a test of plantar flexion of the great toe by the *posterior tibial nerve* from roots L5 to S2. This test is demonstrated in Figure 21-37.

Assess Lower Extremity Tone

Tone in the lower extremities is assessed in the same way as in the upper extremities.

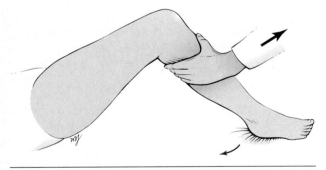

Figure 21–32 Technique for testing knee flexion.

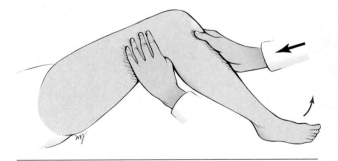

Figure 21–33 Technique for testing knee extension.

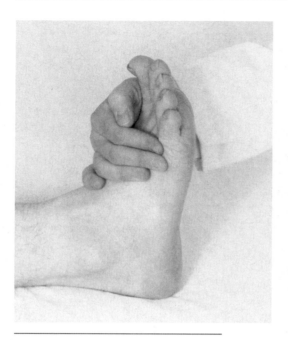

Figure 21–34 Technique for testing ankle dorsiflexion.

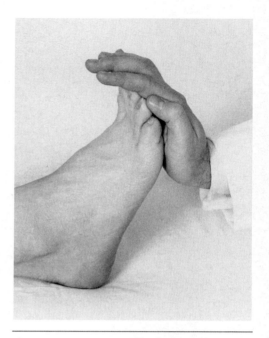

Figure 21–35 Technique for testing plantar flexion.

Grasp the foot and passively dorsiflex and plantarflex it several times, ending with dorsiflexion of the foot. If a sudden rhythmic involuntary dorsiflexion and plantar flexion occur, *ankle clonus* is present. This frequently occurs in conditions of increased tone.

If any abnormality is noted in the motor strength of the upper or lower extremity, a more detailed examination should be performed. See Table 21-7 for a list of the muscle innervations and their actions.

Reflexes

Basic Principles

Two main types of reflexes are tested. They are the *stretch*, or deep tendon, reflexes and the *superficial* reflexes.

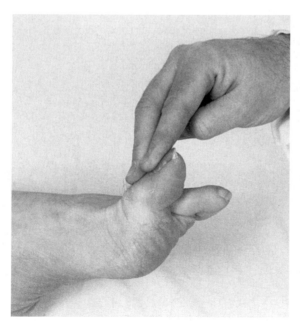

Figure 21–36 Technique for testing great toe dorsiflexion.

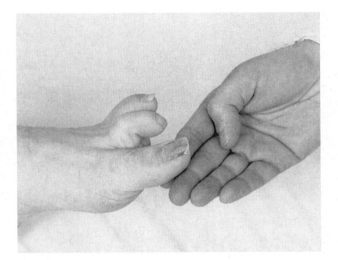

Figure 21–37 Technique for testing great toe plantar flexion.

To elicit a stretch reflex, support the joint being tested so that the muscle is relaxed. Hold the reflex hammer between your thumb and index finger, and swing it by motion at the wrist, not the elbow. In general, the pointed end of a triangular reflex hammer is used. A gentle tap over the tendon being tested should produce muscle contraction. To assess muscle contraction, it is often necessary both to palpate and to observe the muscle. Test each reflex, and compare it with the other side. Reflexes should be symmetrically equal.

There is individual variation in the reflex response. Only with experience is the examiner able to make an adequate assessment of normal reflexes. Reflexes are commonly graded on a scale from 0 to 4+ as follows:

0: No response
1+: Diminished
2+: Normal
3+: Increased
4+: Hyperactive

Hyperactive reflexes are characteristic of pyramidal tract disease. Electrolyte abnormalities, hyperthyroidism, and other metabolic abnormalities may be the cause of hyperactive reflexes. *Diminished* reflexes are characteristic of anterior horn cell disorders and myopathies. The examiner should always consider the strength of the reflex in relation to the bulk of the muscle mass. A patient may have diminished reflexes as a result of a decrease in muscle bulk. Patients with hypothyroidism have decreased relaxation after a deep tendon reflex, which is termed a *hung* reflex.

In a patient with a diminished reflex, the technique of *reinforcement* may be useful. If the patient performs isometric contraction of other muscles, the generalized reflex activity may be increased. When testing reflexes in the upper extremities, have the patient clench the teeth or push down on the bed with the thighs. When testing reflexes in the lower extremities, have the patient lock fingers and try to pull them apart at the time of testing. This procedure, sometimes called *Jendrassik's maneuver*, is demonstrated in Figure 21-38.

Test the Deep Tendon Reflexes
The deep tendon reflexes that are routinely tested are as follows:

- Biceps
- Brachioradialis
- Triceps
- Patellar
- Achilles

Test the Biceps Tendon Reflex
The *biceps tendon* reflex is assessed by having the patient relax the arm and pronate the forearm midway between flexion and extension. The examiner should place a thumb firmly on the biceps tendon. The hammer is then struck on the examiner's thumb. This is demonstrated in Figure 21-39. The examiner should observe for contraction of the biceps tendon, followed by

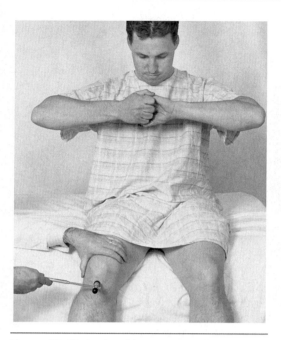

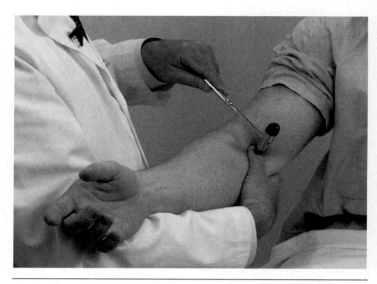

Figure 21–39 Technique for testing the biceps tendon reflex.

Figure 21–38 Jendrassik's maneuver.

flexion at the elbow. The examiner may also palpate the contraction of the muscle. This procedure is a test of the nerves at roots C5 to C6.

Test the Brachioradialis Tendon Reflex

The *brachioradialis tendon reflex* is performed by having the patient's forearm in semiflexion and semipronation. The arm should be rested on the patient's knee. If a triangular reflex hammer is used, the wide end should strike the styloid process of the radius about 2.5 to 5 cm above the wrist. The examiner should observe for flexion at the elbow and simultaneous supination of the forearm. The position is demonstrated in Figure 21-40. This procedure is a test of the nerves at roots C5 to C6.

Test the Triceps Tendon Reflex

The *triceps tendon reflex* is tested by flexing the patient's forearm at the elbow and pulling the arm toward the chest. The elbow should be midway between flexion and extension. Tap the triceps tendon above the insertion of the ulna's olecranon process about 2.5 to 5 cm above the elbow. There should be a prompt contraction of the triceps tendon with extension at

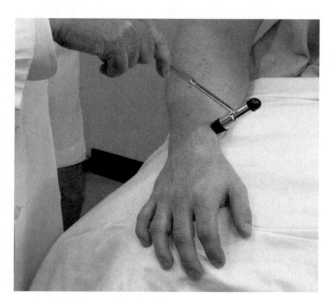

Figure 21–40 Technique for testing the brachioradialis tendon reflex.

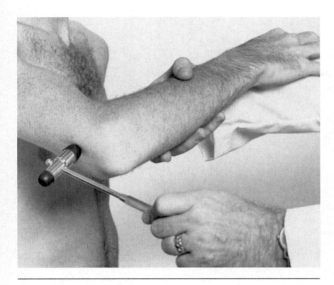

Figure 21–41 Technique for testing the triceps tendon reflex.

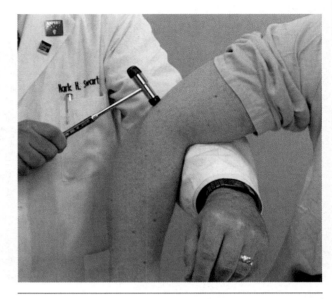

Figure 21–42 Another test of the triceps tendon reflex.

the elbow. This technique is demonstrated in Figure 21-41. This procedure is a test of the nerves at roots C6 to C8.

If the triceps tendon reflex cannot be elicited by this maneuver, try to hang the patient's arm over your arm, as demonstrated in Figure 21-42. Tapping the triceps tendon in this position often elicits the reflex.

Test the Patellar Tendon Reflex

Perform the *patellar tendon reflex*, also known as the *knee jerk*, by having the patient sit with his or her legs dangling off the side of the bed. Place your hand on the patient's quadriceps muscle. Strike the patellar tendon firmly with the base of the reflex hammer. A contraction of the quadriceps should be felt, and extension at the knee should be observed. This technique is demonstrated in Figure 21-43. It is a test of the nerves at roots L2 to L4.

Test the Achilles Tendon Reflex

The *Achilles tendon reflex*, also known as the *ankle jerk*, is elicited by having the patient sit with his or her feet dangling off the side of the bed. The leg should be flexed at the hip and the knee. The examiner places a hand under the patient's foot to dorsiflex the ankle. The Achilles tendon is struck just above its insertion on the posterior aspect of the calcaneus with the wide end of the reflex hammer. The result is plantar flexion at the ankle. This technique is demonstrated in Figure 21-44. It is a test of the nerves at roots S1 to S2.

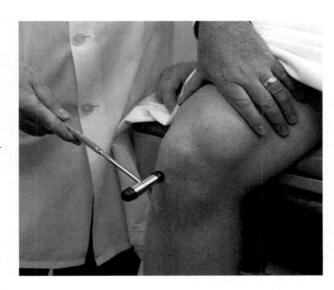

Figure 21–43 Technique for testing the patellar tendon reflex.

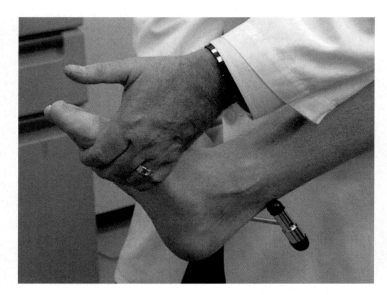

Figure 21–44 Technique for testing the Achilles tendon reflex.

Another method of testing for the Achilles reflex is to have the patient lie in bed. Flex one of the patient's legs at the hip and knee, and rotate the leg externally so that it lies on the opposite shin. Dorsiflex the ankle as the tendon is struck. This test is demonstrated in Figure 21-45*A*.

A patient with a depressed Achilles reflex should be asked to kneel, if possible, on the bed with the feet hanging off the side, as shown in Figure 21-45*B*. Tap the Achilles tendon, and observe the reflex response in this position.

Test the Superficial Reflexes

The most commonly tested superficial reflexes are the abdominal and the cremasteric. The *abdominal* superficial reflex is elicited by having the patient lie on his or her back. An applicator stick or tongue blade is quickly stroked horizontally laterally to medially toward the umbilicus. The result is a contraction of the abdominal muscles, with the umbilicus deviating toward the stimulus. The abdominal reflex is frequently not seen in obese individuals. The *cremasteric* superficial reflex in men is elicited by lightly stroking the inner aspect of the thigh with an applicator stick or tongue depressor. The result is a rapid elevation of the testicle on the same side. Although the superficial reflexes are absent on the side of a corticospinal tract lesion, there is little clinical significance to their presence or absence. They are described here for completeness only.

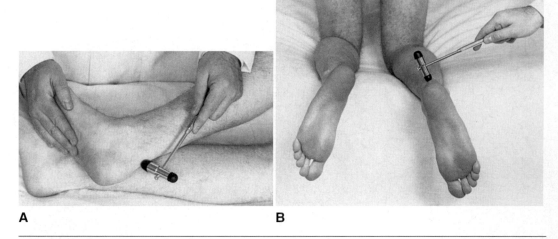

A   **B**

Figure 21–45 *A,* Alternative technique for evaluating the Achilles tendon reflex. *B,* Technique for assessing the Achilles tendon reflex when the reflex appears to be depressed.

Test for Abnormal Reflexes

Babinski's sign or *reflex* is a pathologic reflex. Normally, when the lateral aspect of the sole is stroked from the heel to the ball of the foot and curved medially across the heads of the metatarsal bones, there is plantar flexion of the big toe. This is a test of the nerve roots at L5 to S2. The foot should be stroked with a stimulus such as a key. A pin should *never* be used. In the presence of pyramidal tract disease, when the described movement is performed, there is *dorsiflexion* of the big toe, with fanning of the other toes. This is Babinski's reflex. Because Babinski's sign is an abnormal reflex, the clinician should note it only when it is present. It is correct to describe the plantar reflex as either plantar flexion (normal) or dorsiflexion (abnormal, Babinski's). The technique for evaluating the plantar reflex is shown in Figure 21-46.

Pyramidal tract disease is also suggested when the big toe dorsiflexes on stroking the lateral aspect of the foot. This is *Chaddock's sign*. In the presence of pyramidal tract disease, downward

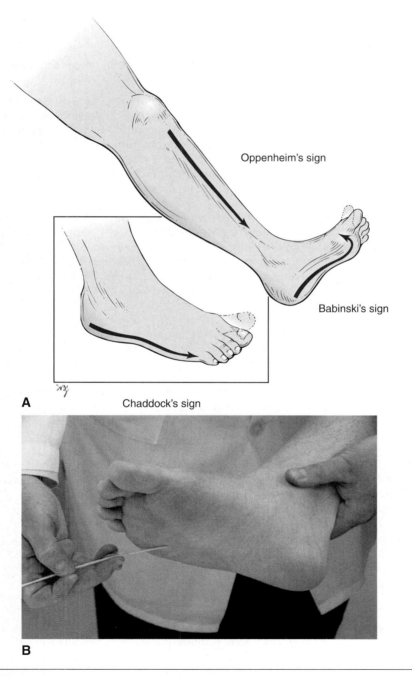

Oppenheim's sign

Babinski's sign

A   Chaddock's sign

B

Figure 21–46 *A* and *B,* Techniques for evaluating the plantar reflex.

pressure along the shin also causes the big toe to dorsiflex. This is *Oppenheim's sign*. The elicitation of these signs is less sensitive than stroking the plantar surface.

Another abnormal reflex associated with pyramidal tract disease is *Hoffmann's sign*. To elicit this sign, the patient's hand is pronated, and the examiner grasps the terminal phalanx of the middle finger between the index finger and thumb. With a sharp jerk, the phalanx is passively flexed and suddenly released. A positive response consists of adduction and flexion of the thumb as well as flexion of the other fingers.

Sensory Function

Basic Principles
The sensory examination consists of testing for the following:

- Light touch
- Pain sensation
- Vibration sense
- Proprioception
- Tactile localization
- Discriminative sensations (two-point discrimination, stereognosis, graphesthesia, and point localization)

In a patient without any symptoms or signs of neurologic disease, the examination for sensory function can be performed by quickly assessing the presence of normal sensation on the distal fingers and toes. The examiner can choose to test for light touch, pain, and vibration sense. If these are normal, the rest of the sensory examination is not required. If symptoms or signs are referable to a neurologic disorder, complete testing is indicated.

As with the motor examination, the examiner compares side with side and proximal with distal aspect. Neurologic disorders usually result in a sensory loss that is first seen more distally than proximally.

The hand is supplied by the median, ulnar, and radial nerves. The median nerve is the chief nerve of sensation because it supplies the palmar surfaces of the digits, the parts of the hand most commonly used for feeling. The ulnar nerve supplies sensation only to the ulnar one and a half fingers. The radial nerve has its sensory distribution to the dorsum of the hand. There is considerable overlap in innervation. The most reliable cutaneous areas for testing these nerves are illustrated in Figure 21-47. These areas have the least likelihood of overlapping innervation.

Test Light Touch
Light touch is evaluated by lightly touching the patient with a small piece of gauze. Ask the patient to close his or her eyes and to tell you when the touch is felt. Try touching the patient on the toes and fingers. This is demonstrated in Figure 21-48. If sensation is normal, continue with the next test. If sensation is abnormal, work proximally until a *sensory level* can be determined. A sensory level is a spinal cord level below which there is a marked decrease in sensation. Figure 21-49 illustrates the segmental distribution of the spinal nerves that transmit sensation to the spinal cord.

Test Pain Sensation
Pain sensation is tested by using a safety pin and asking the patient if it is felt. Ask the patient to close his or her eyes. Open the safety pin and touch the patient with its tip. Tell the patient, "This is sharp." Now touch the patient with the blunt end of the pin and say, "This is dull." This is demonstrated in Figure 21-50. Start testing pain sensation on the toes and fingers and say, "What is this, sharp or dull?" If the patient has no loss of sensation, proceed with the next examination. If there is a sensory loss to pain, continue proximally to determine the sensory level. **A new pin should be used for each patient**. Instead of using a pin, you can use a wooden applicator stick that has been broken. Use the broken end for sharp testing and the cotton tip for dull testing.

Test Vibration Sense
Vibration sense is tested using a 128-Hz tuning fork. Tap the tuning fork on the heel of your hand and place it on the patient on a bony prominence distally. Instruct the patient to inform you when the vibration is no longer felt. Ask the patient to close his or her eyes. Place the vibrating tuning fork over the distal phalanx of the patient's finger with your own finger under the patient's finger, as demonstrated in Figure 21-51*A*. In this manner, you will be able to feel

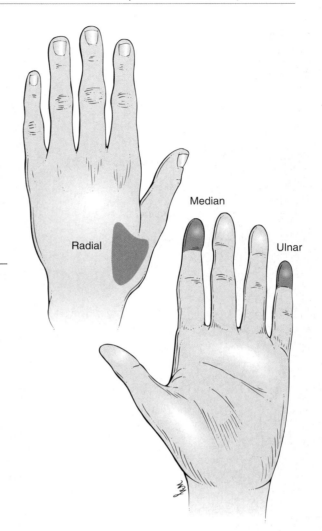

Figure 21–47 Most reliable cutaneous areas for testing hand sensation.

the vibration through the patient's finger to determine the accuracy of the patient's response. After the fingers are tested, test the big toes, as demonstrated in Figure 21-51*B*. If there is no loss of vibration sense, proceed with the next examination. If a loss is present, determine the level.

Test Proprioception

Position sense, or proprioception, is tested by moving the distal phalanx. Hold the distal phalanx at its *lateral* aspects, and move the digit up while telling the patient, "This is up." Move the distal phalanx down and tell the patient, "This is down." With the patient's eyes closed,

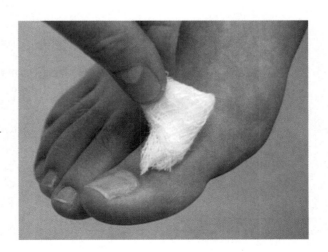

Figure 21–48 Technique for testing light touch.

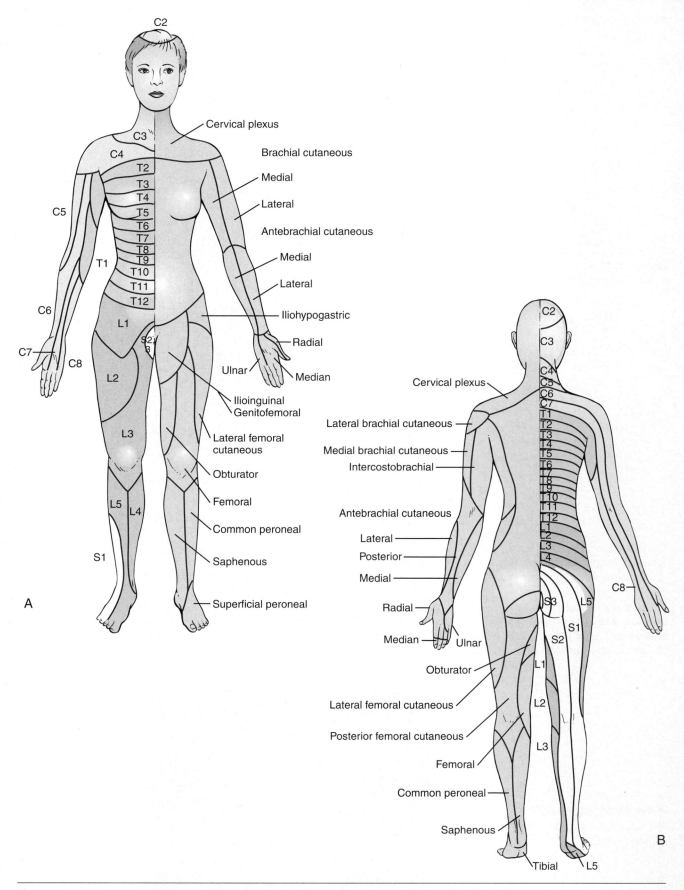

Figure 21–49 Segmental distribution of the spinal nerves. *A,* Distribution in the front. *B,* Distribution in the back.

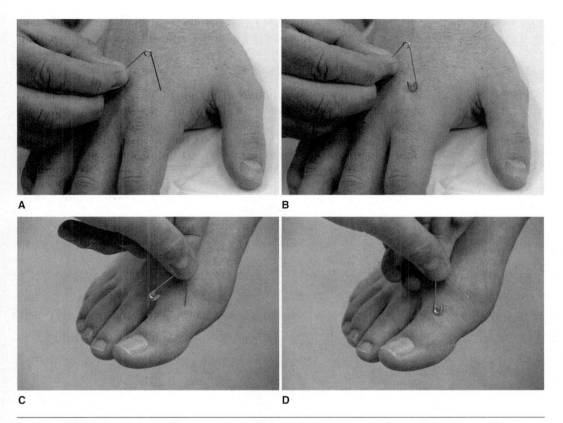

A   B

C   D

Figure 21–50 Technique for testing pain sensation. *A* and *C,* The examiner should hold the pin as demonstrated and say, "This is sharp." *B* and in *D,* The examiner should hold the other end of the pin and say "This is dull."

move the distal phalanx up and down and finally stop and ask, "What is this, up or down?" This is demonstrated in Figure 21-52*A*. Grasp only the *sides* of the digit so that the patient cannot be clued by the pressure exerted on the digit. It is routine to test the terminal phalanx of a finger on each hand and the terminal phalanx of the toes (see Fig. 21-52*B*). If no loss of position sense is detected, continue with the rest of the examination. A loss of proprioception necessitates further evaluation to determine the level of loss.

Test Tactile Localization

Tactile localization, also known as *double simultaneous stimulation,* is assessed by having the patient close his or her eyes and identify where your touch was felt. Touch the patient on the right cheek and the left arm. The patient is then asked, "Where did I touch you?" This is demonstrated in Figure 21-53. Normally, patients have no problem identifying both areas. A patient with a lesion in the parietal lobe may feel the individual touches but may "extinguish" the sensation on the side contralateral to the side of the lesion. This is the phenomenon termed *extinction.*

Test Two-Point Discrimination

Two-point discrimination tests the patient's ability to differentiate one stimulus from two. Gently hold two pins 2 to 3 mm apart, and touch the patient's fingertip. Ask the patient to state the number of pins felt. This is demonstrated in Figure 21-54. Compare this finding with that from the corresponding area on a fingertip of the other hand. Because different areas of the body have different sensitivities, you must know these differences. At the fingertips, two-point discrimination is 2 mm apart. The tongue can discriminate two objects 1 mm apart; the toes, 3 to 8 mm apart; the palms, 8 to 12 mm apart; and the back, 40 to 60 mm apart. A lesion in the parietal lobe impairs two-point discrimination.

Test Stereognosis

Stereognosis is the integrative function of the parietal and occipital lobes. It is tested by having the patient attempt to identify an object placed in the hands. Have the patient

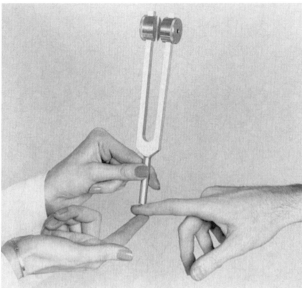

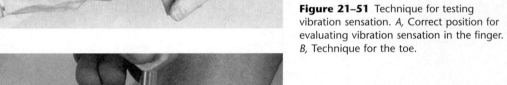

A

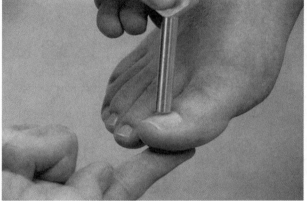

B

Figure 21–51 Technique for testing vibration sensation. *A,* Correct position for evaluating vibration sensation in the finger. *B,* Technique for the toe.

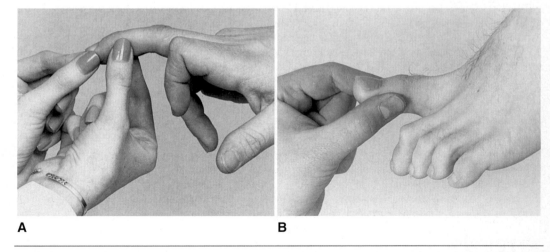

A   **B**

Figure 21–52 Technique for testing proprioception. *A,* Correct manner of holding the finger. *B,* Technique for holding the toe.

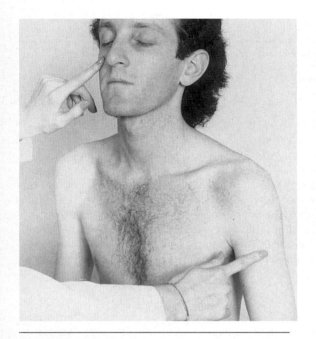

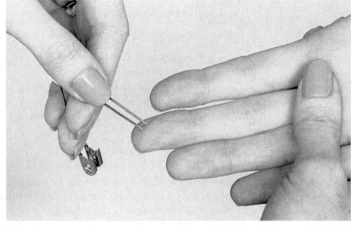

Figure 21–54 Technique for testing two-point discrimination.

Figure 21–53 Technique for testing tactile localization.

close his or her eyes. Place a key, pencil, paper clip, or coin in the palm of the patient's hand, and ask what it is. Test the other hand and compare the findings.

Test Graphesthesia

Graphesthesia is the ability to identify a number "written" in the palm of one's hand. Ask the patient to close his or her eyes and extend the hand. Use the blunt end of a pencil to "write" numbers from 0 to 9 in the palm. The numbers should be oriented facing the patient. This is demonstrated in Figure 21-55. Normally, the patient should be able to identify the numbers. Compare one hand with the other. The inability to identify the numbers is a sensitive sign of parietal lobe disease.

Test Point Localization

Point localization is the ability of a person to point to an area where he or she was touched. Have the patient close his or her eyes. Touch the patient. Ask the patient to open the eyes and point to the area touched. Abnormalities of the sensory cortex impair the ability to localize the area touched.

Figure 21–55 Technique for testing graphesthesia.

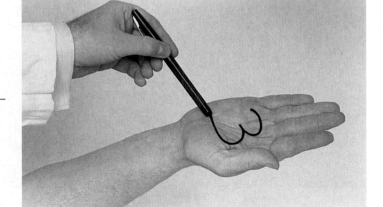

Cerebellar Function

Cerebellar function is tested by the following:

- Finger-to-nose test
- Heel-to-knee test
- Rapid alternating movement
- Romberg test
- Gait assessment

Perform the Finger-to-Nose Test

The finger-to-nose test is performed by asking the patient to touch his or her own nose and the examiner's finger alternately as quickly, accurately, and smoothly as possible. The examiner holds a finger at arm's length from the patient. The patient is instructed to touch the finger and then the nose. This is repeated several times, after which the patient is asked to perform the test with eyes closed. This is demonstrated in Figure 21-56. Patients with cerebellar disease persistently overshoot the target, a condition known as *past pointing*. They may also have a tremor as the finger approaches the target.

Perform the Heel-to-Knee Test

The heel-to-knee test is performed by having the patient lie on his or her back. The patient is instructed to slide the heel of one lower extremity down the shin of the other, starting at

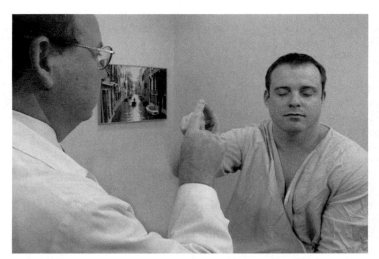

A

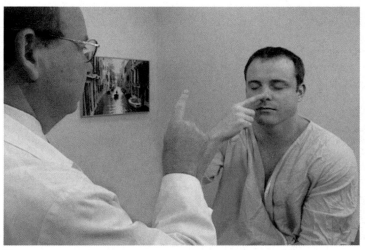

B

Figure 21–56 *A* and *B,* Finger-to-nose test.

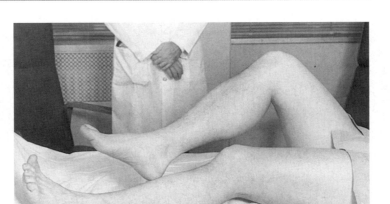

Figure 21–57 Heel-to-knee test.

the knee. This is demonstrated in Figure 21-57. A smooth movement should be seen, with the heel staying on the shin. In patients with cerebellar disease, the heel wobbles from side to side.

Assess Rapid Alternating Movements
The ability to perform rapid alternating movements is called *diadochokinesia*. These motions may be tested in the upper extremity or the lower extremity. The patient can be asked to pronate and supinate one hand on the other hand rapidly. Another technique involves having the patient touch the thumb to each finger as quickly as possible. The patient may also be asked to slap the thigh, raise the hand, turn it over, and slap the thigh again rapidly. This pattern is repeated over and over as quickly as possible. These techniques are illustrated in Figure 21-58. An abnormality in performing rapid alternating movements is called *adiadochokinesia*.

Perform Romberg Test
The Romberg test is performed by having the patient stand in front of the examiner with feet together so that the heels and toes are touching. The examiner instructs the patient to extend the arms with palms facing upward and to close the eyes. If the patient can maintain this posture without moving, the test result is negative. The result is positive if the patient begins to sway and has to move the feet for balance. Another common finding is for one of the arms to drift downward, with flexion of the fingers. This is called *pronator drift* and is seen in patients with mild hemiparesis. The Romberg test is used to examine the posterior columns rather than actual cerebellar function. The examiner should be at the patient's side during this test because an occasional patient may suddenly sway and fall if assistance is not provided.

Assess Gait
Foremost in the examination of cerebellar function is the observation of gait. The patient is asked to walk straight ahead while the examiner observes the gait. The patient is then instructed to return on tiptoes; to walk away again on the heels; and to return to the examiner by walking in tandem gait: one foot placed in front of the other, the heel of one foot touching the toes of the other on each step. The examiner may need to demonstrate this gait for the patient. The patient should have normal posture, and there should be normal associated movements of the arms. The examiner should pay special attention to the way in which the patient turns around. These maneuvers often accentuate cerebellar ataxia, as well as indicate weakness in the lower extremities (see Figure 20-23).

Many neurologic disorders produce striking and characteristic gaits. A patient with *hemiplegia* tends to drag or circumduct a weak and spastic leg. The arm is frequently flexed at the elbow across the abdomen as the patient walks. A patient with *Parkinson's disease* shuffles, with short, hurried steps. The head is bowed, with the back bent over. A patient with *cerebellar ataxia* walks with a wide-based gait. The feet are very far apart as the patient staggers from side to side. A patient with *footdrop* has a characteristic slapping gait resulting from weakness of the dorsiflexors of the ankle. A patient with *sensory ataxia* has a high-stepping gait in which the feet are slapped down firmly, as if the person is unsure of their location. Figure 21-59 illustrates these gaits.

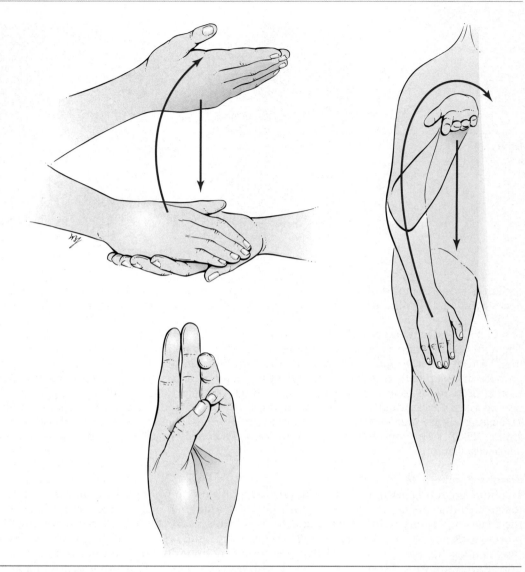

Figure 21-58 Techniques for testing rapid alternating movements.

Clinicopathologic Correlations

The Comatose Patient

Coma is the state in which the patient is unable to respond to any stimuli. The causes of coma include the following:

- Meningeal infection
- Increased intracranial pressure of any cause
- Subarachnoid hemorrhage
- Focal cerebral lesion
- Brain-stem lesion affecting the reticular system
- Metabolic encephalopathy*
- Status post seizure activity

*Common causes include electrolyte abnormalities, endocrine disorders, liver or kidney failure, vitamin deficiencies, poisoning, intoxications, and marked changes in body temperature.

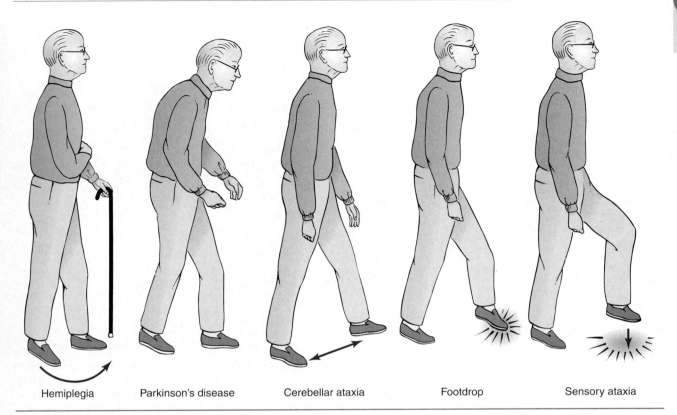

| Hemiplegia | Parkinson's disease | Cerebellar ataxia | Footdrop | Sensory ataxia |

Figure 21–59 Common types of gait abnormalities.

If the patient's friends or family members are available, speak with them. They can help in the evaluation of the patient by giving valuable information. Is there a history of hypertension, diabetes, epilepsy, substance abuse, or recent head trauma?

If there is any evidence of head trauma, radiographs of the cervical spine must be taken before the examiner moves the patient's neck.

The physical examination of the comatose patient should start with inspection. The clothing, age, and evidence of chronic illness provide valuable clues as to the cause of the coma. Does the patient have gingival enlargement consistent with antiepileptic medical therapy?* Is there a characteristic odor to the breath? The sweet smell of ketones may be present in diabetic ketoacidosis. An odor of alcohol may be present. Are there stigmata of chronic liver disease?

What is the *posture* of the patient? Patients with cerebral hemispheric dysfunction or a destructive lesion of the pyramidal tracts maintain a *decorticate* posture, whereas those patients with a midbrain or pons lesion maintain a *decerebrate* posture. In decorticate rigidity, the arms are adducted and the elbows, wrists, and fingers are flexed. The legs are internally rotated. In decerebrate rigidity, the arms are also adducted but they are rigidly extended at the elbows, and the forearms are pronated. The wrists and fingers are flexed. In both postures, the feet are plantarflexed. The positions of the arms and hands are shown in Figure 21-60.

The head should be evaluated for any areas of depression, as in a depressed skull fracture. Does the nose appear broken? Are there any broken teeth? Is there any clear, watery discharge from the nose or ear, suggestive of a leakage of cerebrospinal fluid?

The *respiratory pattern* should be evaluated. Central neurogenic hyperventilation is seen in lesions of the midbrain or pons. This type of respiration consists of rapid, deep, regular breathing. *Cheyne-Stokes* breathing is characterized by rhythmic changes in the breathing pattern. Periods of rapid breathing are separated by periods of apnea. Cheyne-Stokes breathing is associated with brain-stem compression or bilateral cerebral dysfunction.

---

*Commonly related to phenytoin (Dilantin) therapy.

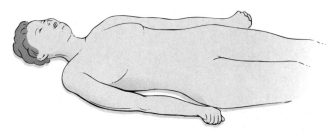

Decerebrate posture

Figure 21-60 Postures of comatose patients.

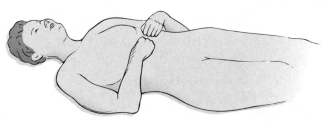

Decorticate posture

The neurologic examination of the comatose patient is largely based on pupillary size and light reflexes. The pupils are small and reactive in bilateral cerebral dysfunction. They are dilated after an overdose of hallucinogenic agents or central nervous system stimulants. A unilateral fixed and dilated pupil is suggestive of pressure on the ipsilateral oculomotor nerve. Pupillary dilatation precedes paralysis of the extraocular muscles; this is because the pupillary nerve fibers are superficial to the fibers innervating the extraocular muscles and are more vulnerable to extrinsic stresses. This is an important sign of uncal herniation. In the presence of normally reactive pupils with absence of corneal reflexes and absence of extra-ocular movement, a metabolic abnormality may be the cause of the coma.

The fundus of the eye may provide a clue as to the cause of the coma.

If there is no evidence of a fracture of the cervical spine, *oculocephalic reflexes* should be tested. If a comatose patient's head is rapidly turned to one side while the eyelids are held open, the eyes should move conjugately to the other side. This is the *doll's eyes reflex*. In a patient with a lesion in the brain stem, the doll's eyes reflex is absent. The doll's eyes reflex can be elicited only in a comatose patient because alert individuals fixate on an object and override this reflex.

Caloric stimulation is used to enhance the doll's eyes reflex or to test movements in an individual with a fractured cervical spine. The patient should be placed with the head flexed at 30°. This orients the semicircular canal in a horizontal position. A large-bore syringe is filled with 20 to 30 mL of ice water, and the water is squeezed into one of the external auditory canals. The normal response is the development of nystagmus. Slowly the eyes move conjugately to the ipsilateral side and then move rapidly (nystagmus) back to the midline. The use of cold water causes nystagmus to the opposite side. If warm water is used, the eyes move rapidly toward the side being irrigated. This can easily be remembered by using the mnemonic COWS, which stands for "cold opposite, warm same."

An absence of the caloric response is seen in patients with a disruption of the connections between the vestibular nuclei and the sixth cranial nerve nucleus at the level of the brain stem.

As was indicated earlier in the chapter, headache is an important symptom of neurologic disease. Table 21-2 provides a differential diagnosis of headaches.

The correct assessment of a patient's motor activity can help localize the site of a lesion. The term *extrapyramidal* refers to those parts of the motor system that are not directly involved with the pyramidal tracts. The extrapyramidal system is composed of the basal ganglia, nuclei of the midbrain and reticular formation, and cerebellum. Table 21-3 lists the major areas and the specific motor problems associated with lesions of the lower motor neuron, the pyramidal tract, and the extrapyramidal tract. Table 21-4 summarizes the important signs and symptoms in five common chronic neurologic disorders.

Table 21-2 Differential Diagnosis of Headache

Type	Epidemiology	Location	Signs and Symptoms
Migraine	Family history Young adults Female	Bifrontal	Nausea Vomiting Possible neurologic deficits
Cluster	Adolescent male	Orbitofrontal Unilateral	Unilateral nasal congestion Lacrimation
Tension	Female	Bilateral Generalized or occipital	
Hypertensive	Family history	Variable	Hypertensive retinopathy Possible papilledema
Increased intracranial pressure		Variable	Nausea Vomiting Papilledema
Meningitis		Bilateral Often occipital	Nuchal rigidity Fever
Temporal arteritis*	Older adults	Unilateral Over temporal artery	Tender temporal artery Loss of vision in ipsilateral eye

*See Chapter 25, The Geriatric Patient.

A comparison of the effects of upper and lower motor neuron lesions is shown in Table 21-5.

Paraplegia and *quadriplegia* are upper motor neuron defects. They can also involve lower motor neurons. Injury of the spinal cord can produce partial or complete paralysis. In patients with cervical or thoracic lesions, spasticity is present below the level of the lesion, and flaccidity is present in all muscles supplied from reflex arcs at the level of the lesion. In the presence of sacral lesions, a flaccid paralysis results. Table 21-6 summarizes motor involvement in spinal cord lesions.

Often a patient may complain of a decreased ability to perform a task. Physical examination may reveal decreased motor strength. Table 21-7 summarizes the major actions of the more common muscles and their corresponding cord segments.

Table 21-3 Effects of Various Lesions

Feature	Lower Motor Neuron	Pyramidal Tract	Extrapyramidal Tract
Major effect	Flaccid paralysis	Spastic paralysis Hyperactive reflexes	No paralysis
Muscle appearance	Atrophy Fasciculations	Mild atrophy from disuse	Rest tremor
Muscle tone	Decreased	Increased	Increased
Muscle strength	Decreased or absent	Decreased or absent	Normal
Coordination	Absent or poor	Absent or poor	Slowed

Table 21–4 Common Neurologic Conditions and Their Signs and Symptoms

Condition	Age at Onset (Year)	Sex	Signs and Symptoms
Multiple sclerosis	30-35	Female	Nystagmus Diplopia Slurring of speech Muscular weakness Paresthesias Poor coordination Bowel and bladder dysfunction
Amyotrophic lateral sclerosis	50-80	Male	Irregular twitching of involved muscles Muscular weakness Muscle atrophy* Absence of sensory or mental deficits
Parkinson's disease	60-80	Male	Rigidity Slowing of movements Involuntary tremor Difficulty swallowing Tremor in upper extremities Jerky, "cogwheel" motions Slow, shuffling gait with loss of arm swing Masklike facial expression Body in moderate flexion Excessive salivation
Myasthenia gravis	20-50	Female	Generalized muscular fatigue Bilateral ptosis* Diplopia Difficulty swallowing Voice weakness
Huntington's disease	35-50	Both sexes	Choreiform movements Dementia Rapid movements Facial grimacing Dysarthria Personality change

*See Figure 21-21.
†See Figure 10-16.

Table 21–5 Comparison of Effects of Upper and Lower Motor Neuron Lesions

Effect	Upper Motor Neuron Lesion	Lower Motor Neuron Lesion
Voluntary control	Lost	Lost
Muscle tone	Spastic, increased	Flaccid, decreased
Reflex arcs	Present	Absent
Pathologic reflexes	Present	Not present
Muscle atrophy	Little or none	Significant

Table 21–6 Motor Involvement in Spinal Cord Lesions

Affected Cord Segment	Motor Involvement
C1–C4	Paralysis of neck, diaphragm, intercostals, and all four extremities
C5	Spastic paralysis of trunk, arms, and legs; partial shoulder control
C6, C7	Spastic paralysis of trunk and legs; upper arm control; partial lower arm control
C8	Spastic paralysis of trunk and legs; hand weakness only
T1–T10	Spastic paralysis of trunk and legs
T11–T12	Spastic paralysis of legs
L1–S1	Flaccid paralysis of legs
S2–S5	Flaccid paralysis of lower legs; bowel, bladder, and sexual function affected

Table 21–7 Motor Function According to Cord Segments

Area of Body	Action Tested	Cord Segment
Shoulder	Flexion, extension, or rotation of neck	C1–C4
Arm	Adduction of arm	C5–T1
	Abduction of arm	C4–C6
	Flexion of forearm	C5–C6
	Extension of forearm	C6–C8
	Supination of forearm	C5–C7
	Pronation of forearm	C6–C7
Hand	Extension of hand	C6–C8
	Flexion of hand	C7–C8, T1
Finger	Abduction of thumb	C7–C8, T1
	Adduction of thumb	C8, T1
	Abduction of little finger	C8, T1
	Opposition of thumb	C8, T1
Hip	Flexion of hip	L1–L3
	Extension of leg	L2–L4
	Flexion of leg	L4–L5, S1–S2
	Adduction of thigh	L2–L4
	Abduction of thigh	L4–L5, S1–S2
	Medial rotation of thigh	L4–L5, S1
	Lateral rotation of thigh	L4–L5, S1–S2
	Flexion of thigh	L4–L5
Foot	Dorsiflexion of foot	L4–L5, S1
	Plantar flexion of foot	L5, S1–S2
Toe	Extension of great toe	L4–L5, S1
	Flexion of great toe	L5, S1–S2
	Spreading of toes	S1–S2

Useful Vocabulary

Listed here are the specific roots that are important for understanding the terminology related to neurologic diseases.

Root	Pertaining to	Example	Definition
esthe-	feeling	an***esthe***sia	Loss of feeling
-gnosia	recognition	ag***nosia***	Loss of the power to recognize sensory stimuli
myelo-	spinal cord	***myelo***gram	Radiographic study of the spinal cord
-paresis	weakness	hemi***paresis***	Muscular weakness affecting half the body
-plegia	paralysis	ophthalmo***plegia***	Paralysis of the eye muscles
radicul(o)-	spinal nerve root	***radiculo***pathy	Disease of a spinal nerve root

Writing Up the Physical Examination

Listed here are examples of the write-up for the examination of the neurologic system.

- The patient is oriented to person, time, and place. Cranial nerves II to XII are intact. Motor examination reveals normal gait, normal heel-to-toe movement, and normal strength bilaterally. Reflexes are equal bilaterally and are within normal limits. The sensory examination results are normal, with pain, light touch, and stereognosis intact. Cerebellar function is normal.
- The mental status examination results are within normal limits. There is a marked weakness of the lower half of the right side of the face. The right nasolabial fold is flat, and the mouth droops downward on the right. There is no other cranial nerve abnormality. The motor and sensory examination results are within normal limits. Reflexes are normal. Romberg test result is negative.
- The patient has an expressive aphasia and a right hemiplegia with ipsilateral trigeminal hemiplegia. Reflexes in the right lower extremity are hyperactive in comparison with the left. Sensory examination is difficult to assess. Babinski's sign is present on the right side.
- Mental status is within normal limits. Motor examination results and reflexes are equal bilaterally. There is a sensory level at L2 on the right and at L4 on the left. Vibration sense is impaired more on the right than on the left, as is position sense. Romberg test result is positive.

Bibliography

American Heart Association: 2000 Heart and Stroke Update, Dallas, American Heart Association, 2000.

Davenport R: Diagnosing acute headache. Clin Med 4:108, 2004.

Diener HC, Limmroth V: Medication-overuse headache: A worldwide problem. Lancet Neurol 3:475, 2004.

Froehling DA, Silverman MD, Mohr DN, et al: Does this dizzy patient have a serious form of vertigo? JAMA 271:385, 1994.

Goetz CG, Pappert EJ: Textbook of Clinical Neurology. Philadelphia, WB Saunders, 1998.

Goldstein LB, Matchar DB: Clinical assessment of stroke. JAMA 271:1114, 1994.

Maizels M: The patient with daily headaches. Am Fam Physician 70:2299, 2004.

Murphy SL: Deaths: Final Data for 1998. Natl Vital Stat Rep 48(11):1, 2000.

Ryan RE, Pearlman SH: Common headache misdiagnoses. Prim Care Clin Office Pract 31:395, 2004.

Williams AC, Davies D: Essential Clinical Neurology. Philadelphia, Churchill Livingstone, 2001.

CHAPTER 22

Putting the Examination Together

A physician is not only a scientist or a good technician. He must be more than that—he must have good human qualities. He has to have a personal understanding and sympathy for the suffering of human beings.

Albert Einstein   (1879–1955)

The Techniques

The previous chapters dealt with the individual organ systems and the history and physical examinations related to each of them. The purpose of this chapter is to help the student assimilate each of the individual examinations into one complete and smoothly performed examination.

Ideally, a complete examination is performed in an orderly, thorough manner with as few movements as possible required of the patient. Most errors in performing a physical examination result from a lack of organization and thoroughness, not from a lack of knowledge. Evaluate each part of the examination carefully before moving on to the next part. The most common errors in performing the physical examination are related to the following:

- Technique
- Omission
- Detection
- Interpretation
- Recording

Errors in *technique* are related to lack of order and organization during the examination, faulty equipment, and poor bedside etiquette. Errors of *omission* are common in examinations of the eye and nose; auscultation of the neck vessels, chest, and heart; palpation of the spleen; rectal and genital examinations; and the neurologic examination. Errors of *detection* are those in which the examiner fails to find abnormalities that are present. The most common errors of this type involve thyroid nodules, tracheal deviation, abnormal breath sounds, diastolic murmurs, hernias, and abnormalities of the extraocular muscles. Errors in *interpretation* of findings occur most commonly with tracheal deviation, venous pulses, systolic murmurs, fremitus changes, abdominal tenderness, liver size, eye findings, and reflexes. The most common types of *recording* errors are related to descriptions of heart size and murmurs, improper terminology, and obscure abbreviations.

The following examination sequence is the one the author uses and is demonstrated in the DVD-ROM enclosed with this book. There is no right or wrong sequence. Develop your own approach. Just be sure that at the end of whichever technique you use, a complete examination has been performed.

In most situations, the patient will be lying in bed when you arrive. After introducing yourself and documenting a complete history, you should inform the patient that you are ready to begin the physical examination. Always start by washing your hands.

The reader is advised now to watch the video presentation on the DVD-ROM to review the complete physical examination of the man and the breast and pelvic examinations of the woman. The DVD-ROM will help you put the examination together.

Patient Lying Supine in Bed

General Appearance
Inspect the patient's facial expression (see Chapters 13, The Chest; 14, The Heart; and 17, The Abdomen).

Vital Signs (Chapter 14, The Heart)
1. Palpate blood pressure in right arm.
2. Auscultate blood pressure in right arm.
3. Auscultate blood pressure in left arm.*

Have Patient Sit Up in Bed

Vital Signs
Check for orthostatic changes in left arm (see Chapter 14, The Heart).

Have Patient Turn and Sit with Legs Dangling off Side of Bed

Vital Signs
1. Palpate radial pulse for rate and regularity (see Chapter 15, The Peripheral Vascular System).
2. Determine respiratory rate and pattern (see Chapter 13, The Chest).

Head (Chapter 9, The Head and Neck)
1. Inspect cranium.
2. Inspect scalp.
3. Palpate cranium.

Face (Chapters 8, The Skin, and 9, The Head and Neck)
1. Inspect face.
2. Inspect skin on face.

Eyes (Chapter 10, The Eye)
1. Assess visual acuity, both eyes.
2. Check visual fields, both eyes.
3. Determine eye alignment, both eyes.
4. Test extraocular muscle function, both eyes.
5. Check pupillary response to light, both eyes.
6. Test for convergence.
7. Inspect external eye structures, both eyes.
8. Perform ophthalmoscopic examination, both eyes.

Nose (Chapter 11, The Ear and Nose)
1. Inspect nose.
2. Palpate nasal skeleton.

---

*If the blood pressure is elevated in the upper extremity, blood pressure in the lower extremity must be assessed to exclude coarctation of the aorta. The patient is asked to lie prone, and blood pressure by auscultation is determined (see Chapter 14, The Heart).

3. Palpate sinuses (frontal, maxillary), both sides.
4. Inspect nasal septum, both sides.
5. Inspect turbinates, both sides.

Ears (Chapter 11, The Ear and Nose)
1. Inspect external ear structures, both sides.
2. Palpate external ear structures, both sides.
3. Evaluate auditory acuity, both sides.
4. Perform Rinne test, both sides.
5. Perform Weber test.
6. Perform otoscopic examination, both sides.
7. Inspect external canal, both sides.
8. Inspect tympanic membrane, both sides.

Mouth (Chapter 12, The Oral Cavity and Pharynx)
1. Inspect outer and inner surfaces of lips.
2. Inspect buccal mucosa.
3. Inspect gingivae.
4. Inspect teeth.
5. Observe Stensen's and Wharton's ducts, both sides.
6. Inspect hard palate.
7. Inspect soft palate.
8. Inspect tongue.
9. Test hypoglossal nerve function (see Chapter 21, The Nervous System).
10. Palpate tongue.
11. Inspect floor of mouth.
12. Palpate floor of mouth.
13. Inspect tonsils, both sides.
14. Inspect posterior pharyngeal wall.
15. Observe uvula as patient says "Ah" (see Chapter 21, The Nervous System).
16. Test gag reflex (see Chapter 21, The Nervous System).

Neck (Chapter 9, The Head and Neck)
1. Inspect neck, both sides.
2. Palpate neck, both sides.
3. Palpate lymph nodes of head and neck, both sides.
4. Palpate thyroid gland by anterior approach.
5. Evaluate position of trachea (see Chapter 13, The Chest).

Neck Vessels (Chapter 14, The Heart)
Inspect height of jugular venous pulsation, right side.

Neck* (Chapter 9, The Head and Neck)
1. Palpate thyroid gland by posterior approach.
2. Palpate for supraclavicular lymph nodes, both sides.

Posterior Chest (Chapter 13, The Chest)
1. Inspect back, both sides.
2. Palpate back for tenderness, both sides.
3. Evaluate chest excursion, both sides.
4. Palpate for tactile fremitus, both sides.
5. Percuss back, both sides.
6. Evaluate diaphragmatic excursion, right side.
7. Auscultate back, both sides.
8. Palpate for costovertebral angle tenderness, both sides (see Chapter 17, The Abdomen).

---

*The examiner should now go to the back of the patient while the patient remains seated with legs dangling off the side of the bed.

Sacrum (Chapter 14, The Heart)
Test for edema.

Anterior Chest* (Chapter 13, The Chest)
1. Inspect patient's posture.
2. Inspect configuration of chest.
3. Inspect chest, both sides.
4. Palpate chest for tactile fremitus, both sides.

Female Breast (Chapter 16, The Breast)
1. Inspect breast, both sides.
2. Inspect breast during maneuvers to tense pectoral muscles, both sides.

Heart (Chapter 14, The Heart)
1. Inspect for abnormal chest movements.
2. Palpate for point of maximum impulse.
3. Auscultate for heart sounds, all four positions.

Axilla (Chapter 16, The Breast)
1. Inspect axilla, both sides.
2. Palpate axilla, both sides.
3. Palpate for epitrochlear nodes, both sides (see Chapter 15, The Peripheral Vascular System).

Have Patient Lean Forward

Heart (Chapter 14, The Heart)
Auscultate with diaphragm at cardiac base.

Have Patient Lie Supine with Head of Bed Elevated About 30°

Neck Vessels (Chapter 14, The Heart)
1. Inspect jugular venous wave form, right side.
2. Auscultate carotid artery, both sides.
3. Palpate carotid artery, each side separately.

Breasts, Male and Female (Chapter 16, The Breast)
1. Inspect breast, both sides.
2. Palpate breast, both sides.
3. Palpate subareolar area, both sides.
4. Palpate nipple, both sides.

Chest (Chapter 13, The Chest)
1. Inspect chest, both sides.
2. Evaluate chest excursion, both sides.
3. Palpate for tactile fremitus, both sides.
4. Percuss chest, both sides.
5. Auscultate breath sounds, both sides.

Heart (Chapter 14, The Heart)
1. Inspect for movements.
2. Palpate for localized motion, all four positions.
3. Palpate for generalized motion, all four positions.
4. Palpate for thrills, all four positions.
5. Auscultate heart sounds, all four positions.
6. Time heart sounds to carotid pulse.

---

*The examiner should now go to the front of the patient while the patient remains seated with legs dangling off the side of the bed.

Have Patient Turn on Left Side

Heart (Chapter 14, The Heart)
Auscultate with bell at cardiac apex.

Have Patient Lie Supine with Bed Flat

Abdomen (Chapter 17, The Abdomen)
1. Inspect contour of abdomen.
2. Inspect skin of abdomen.
3. Inspect for hernias.
4. Auscultate abdomen for bowel sounds, one quadrant.
5. Auscultate abdomen for bruits, both sides.
6. Palpate abdomen lightly, all quadrants.
7. Palpate abdomen deeply, all quadrants.
8. Percuss abdomen, all quadrants.
9. Percuss liver.
10. Percuss spleen.
11. Test superficial abdominal reflex (see Chapter 21, The Nervous System).
12. Check for rebound tenderness.
13. Check for hepatic tenderness.
14. Evaluate hepatojugular reflux (see Chapter 14, The Heart).
15. Palpate liver.
16. Palpate spleen.
17. Palpate aorta.
18. Check for shifting dullness if ascites is suspected.

Pulses (Chapter 15, The Peripheral Vascular System)
1. Palpate radial pulse, both sides.
2. Palpate brachial pulse, both sides.
3. Palpate femoral pulse, both sides.
4. Palpate popliteal pulse, both sides.
5. Palpate dorsalis pedis pulse, both sides.
6. Palpate posterior tibial pulse, both sides.
7. Time radial and femoral pulses, right side.
8. Perform heel-to-knee test (part of neurologic examination; see Chapter 21, The Nervous System).

Male Genitalia (Chapter 18, Male Genitalia and Hernias)
1. Inspect skin and hair distribution.
2. Instruct patient to bear down, and observe inguinal area.
3. Inspect penis.
4. Inspect scrotum.
5. Palpate for inguinal nodes, both sides.
6. Elevate scrotum and inspect perineum.

Have Male Patient Stand in Front of Seated Examiner

Male Genitalia (Chapter 18, Male Genitalia and Hernias)
1. Inspect penis.
2. Inspect external urethral meatus.
3. Palpate shaft of penis.
4. Palpate urethra.
5. Inspect scrotum.
6. Palpate testicle, both sides.
7. Palpate epididymis and vas deferens, both sides.
8. Instruct patient to bear down, and observe inguinal area.
9. Test superficial cremasteric reflex (see Chapter 21, The Nervous System).
10. Transilluminate any masses.
11. Palpate for hernias, both sides.

Have Male Patient Turn Around and Bend over Bed

Rectum (Chapter 17, The Abdomen)
1. Inspect anus.
2. Inspect anus while patient strains.
3. Palpate anal sphincter.
4. Palpate rectal walls.
5. Palpate prostate gland.
6. Test stool for occult blood.

Help Female Patient to Lithotomy Position

Female Genitalia (Chapter 19, Female Genitalia)
1. Inspect skin and hair distribution.
2. Inspect labia majora.
3. Palpate labia majora.
4. Inspect labia minora, clitoris, urethral meatus, and introitus.
5. Inspect area of Bartholin's glands, both sides.
6. Inspect perineum.
7. Test for pelvic relaxation.
8. Perform speculum examination.
9. Inspect cervix.
10. Obtain Pap smear.
11. Inspect vaginal walls.
12. Perform bimanual examination.
13. Palpate cervix and uterine body.
14. Palpate adnexa, both sides.
15. Palpate rectovaginal septum.
16. Test stool for occult blood.

Have Patient Sit on Bed with Legs off Side

Mental Status
Ask routine questions (see Chapters 1, The Interviewer's Questions; 21, The Nervous System; and 25, The Geriatric Patient).

Face (Chapter 21, The Nervous System)
1. Test motor function of trigeminal nerve, both sides.
2. Test sensory function of trigeminal nerve, both sides.
3. Test corneal reflex, both eyes.
4. Test facial nerve, both sides.
5. Test spinal accessory nerve, both sides.
6. Test double simultaneous stimulation, both sides.
7. Perform finger-to-nose test.

Neck
Test range of motion (see Chapter 20, The Musculoskeletal System).

Hands and Wrists (Chapters 20, The Musculoskeletal System, and 21, The Nervous System)
1. Inspect hand and wrist, both sides.
2. Inspect nails, both sides (see Chapter 8, The Skin).
3. Palpate shoulder joint, both sides.
4. Palpate interphalangeal joints, both sides.
5. Palpate metacarpophalangeal joints, both sides.
6. Test light touch sensation, both sides.
7. Test vibration sense, both sides.
8. Test position sense, both sides.
9. Test object identification, both sides.

10. Test graphesthesia, both sides.
11. Test two-point discrimination, both sides.
12. Assess rapid alternating movements, both sides.

Elbows (Chapter 20, The Musculoskeletal System)
1. Inspect elbow, both sides.
2. Test range of motion, both sides.
3. Palpate elbow, both sides.
4. Test upper extremity strength, both sides.
5. Test biceps tendon reflex, both sides (see Chapter 21, The Nervous System).
6. Test triceps tendon reflex, both sides (see Chapter 21, The Nervous System).

Shoulders (Chapter 20, The Musculoskeletal System)
1. Inspect shoulder, both sides.
2. Test range of motion, both sides.
3. Palpate shoulder joint, both sides.

Shins
1. Inspect skin, both sides.
2. Test for edema, both sides (see Chapter 14, The Heart).

Feet and Ankles (Chapters 20, The Musculoskeletal System, and 21, The Nervous System)
1. Inspect feet and ankles.
2. Test range of motion, both sides.
3. Palpate Achilles tendon, both sides.
4. Palpate metatarsophalangeal joints, both sides.
5. Palpate metatarsal heads, both sides.
6. Palpate ankle and foot joints, both sides.
7. Test light touch sensation, both sides.
8. Test vibration sense, both sides.
9. Test position sense, both sides.
10. Test lower extremity strength, both sides.
11. Test ankle reflex, both sides.
12. Test plantar response, both sides.

Knees (Chapters 20, The Musculoskeletal System, and 21, The Nervous System)
1. Inspect knee, both sides.
2. Test range of motion, both sides.
3. Palpate patella, both sides.
4. Perform ballottement of patella if effusion is suspected.
5. Test patellar reflex, both sides.

Have Patient Stand with Back to Examiner

Hips (Chapter 20, The Musculoskeletal System)
1. Inspect hips.
2. Test range of motion.

Spine (Chapters 20, The Musculoskeletal System, and 21, The Nervous System)
1. Inspect spine.
2. Palpate spine.
3. Test range of motion.
4. Assess gait.
5. Perform Romberg test.

The Written Physical Examination

After the examination has been completed, the examiner must be able to record objectively all the findings of inspection, palpation, percussion, and auscultation. Be precise in stating locations of abnormalities. Small drawings may be useful to describe a shape or location better. When describing the size of a finding, state the size in millimeters or centimeters rather than comparing it with a fruit or nut, for example, because these can vary greatly in size. It is best not to use most abbreviations because they may mean different things to different readers. However, the abbreviations used in the following examples are standard and may be used. Finally, do not make diagnostic statements in the write-up; save them for the summary at the end. For example, it is better to state that "a grade III/VI holosystolic murmur at the apex with radiation to the axilla" is present rather than "a murmur of mitral insufficiency."

Patient: John Henry*

General appearance: The patient is a 65-year-old white man who is lying in bed on two pillows and is in no acute distress. He is well developed and thin and appears slightly older than his stated age. The patient is well groomed, alert, and cooperative.

Vital signs: Blood pressure (BP), 185/65/55 right arm (lying), 180/60/50 left arm (lying), 175/65/50 left arm (sitting); heart rate, 90 and regular; respirations, 16.

Skin: Pink, with small hyperkeratotic papules over the face; nail beds slightly dusky; hair thin on head; hair absent on lower portion of lower extremities; normal male escutcheon (distribution of pubic hair).

Head: Normocephalic without evidence of trauma; no tenderness present.

Eyes: Visual acuity with glasses using near card: right eye (OD), 20/60, left eye (OS) 20/40; visual fields full bilaterally; extraocular movements (EOMs) intact; PERRLA [pupils are equal, round, and reactive to light and to accommodation] xanthelasma present bilaterally, L > R; eyebrows normal; bilateral arcus senilis present; conjunctivae without injection; opacities present in both lenses, R > L; left disc sharp with normal cup–disc ratio; normal arteriovenous (AV) ratio OS; no AV nicking present OS; there is a flame-shaped hemorrhage at the 6 o'clock position OS; several cotton-wool spots are also present at the 1 and 5 o'clock positions OS; right fundus not well visualized as a result of lenticular opacity.

Ears: Pinnae in normal position; no tenderness present; small amount of cerumen in left external canal; canals without injection or discharge; Rinne test, BC > AC right ear, AC > BC left ear; Weber test, lateralization to the right ear; both tympanic membranes are gray without injection; normal landmarks seen bilaterally.

Nose: Nose straight without masses; patent bilaterally; mucosa pink with a clear discharge present; inferior turbinate on the right slightly edematous.

Sinuses: No tenderness detected over frontal and maxillary sinuses.

Throat: Lips slightly cyanotic without lesions; patient wears an upper denture; buccal mucosa pink without injection; all lower teeth are present and are in fair condition; no obvious caries; gingivae normal; tongue midline without fasciculations; no lesions seen or palpated on tongue; mild injection of posterior pharynx with yellowish-white discharge present on posterior pharynx and tonsils; tonsils minimally enlarged; uvula elevates in midline; gag reflex intact.

Neck: Supple with full range of motion; trachea midline; small (1- to 2-cm) lymph nodes are present in superficial cervical and tonsillar node chains; thyroid borders palpable; no thyroid nodules or enlargement noted; no abnormal neck vein distention present; neck veins flat while patient is sitting upright.

Chest: Anteroposterior (AP) diameter increased; symmetric excursion bilaterally; tactile fremitus normal bilaterally; chest resonant bilaterally; vesicular breath sounds bilaterally; coarse breath sounds with occasional crackles present at the bases.

Breasts: Mild gynecomastia, L > R; no masses or discharge present.

Heart: Point of maximum impulse, sixth intercostal space (PMI 6ICS) 2 cm lateral to midclavicular line (MCL); normal physiologic splitting present; no heaves or thrills are present; S_1 and S_2 distant; a grade II/VI high-pitched holodiastolic murmur is heard at the 2ICS at the right upper sternal border; a grade I/VI medium-pitched systolic crescendo-decrescendo murmur is heard in the aortic area; the systolic murmur is midpeaking (Fig. 22-1).

Vascular: A carotid bruit is present on the right; no bruits are heard over the left carotid, renal, femoral, or abdominal arteries; lower extremities are slightly cool in comparison with upper extremities; 1+ pretibial edema is present on the right lower extremity; 2+ pretibial edema is present on the left; mild venous varicosities are present from midthigh to calf bilaterally; no ulceration or stasis changes are present; no calf tenderness is present.

---

*This name is fictitious. Any similarity to any person living or dead with this name is purely coincidental.

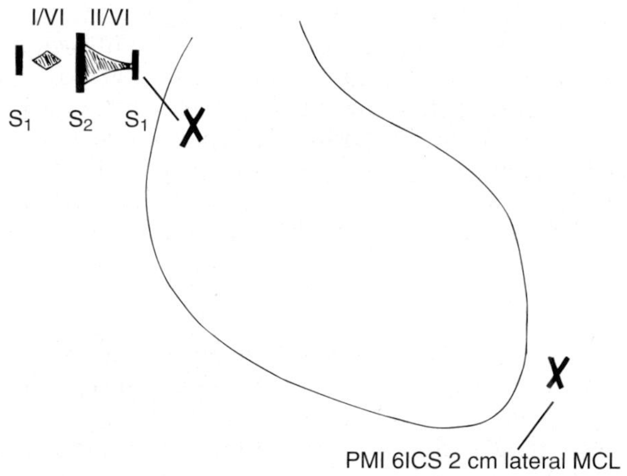

Figure 22–1 Location of cardiac physical signs.

Abdomen: The abdomen is scaphoid; a right lower quadrant (RLQ) appendectomy scar and a left lower quadrant (LLQ) herniorrhaphy scar are present; both scars are well healed; a 3×3 cm mass is seen in the RLQ after coughing or straining; no guarding, rigidity, or tenderness is present; no visible pulsations are present; bowel sounds are present; percussion note is tympanitic throughout the abdomen except over the suprapubic region, where the percussion note is dull; liver span is 10 cm from top to bottom in the MCL; spleen percussed in left upper quadrant but not palpated; kidneys not felt; no costovertebral angle tenderness (CVAT) present; an easily reducible right indirect inguinal hernia is felt at the external ring.

Rectal: Anal sphincter normal; no hemorrhoids present; nontender prostate enlarged symmetrically; prostate firm without nodules felt; no luminal masses felt in rectum; stool negative for blood.

Genitalia: Circumcised man with normal genitalia; penis without induration; left hemiscrotum 4 to 5 cm below the right; palpation of left hemiscrotum reveals dilatation of the pampiniform plexus; soft testes $2 \times 3 \times 1$ cm bilaterally.

Lymphatic: Nodes in anterior triangle chains already noted; two firm, 1- to 2-cm, rubbery, freely mobile nodes in left femoral area; no epitrochlear, axillary, or supraclavicular nodes felt.

Musculoskeletal: Distal interphalangeal joint enlargement on both hands, causing pain on making a fist, L > R; no tenderness or erythema present; proximal joints normal; neck, arms, hips, knees, and ankles with full range of active and passive motion; muscles appear symmetric; mild kyphosis present.

Neurologic: Oriented to person, place, and time; cranial nerves I to XII intact; gross sensory and motor strength intact; cerebellar function normal; plantar reflexes down; gait normal; deep tendon reflexes as shown in Table 22-1.

Summary: Mr. Henry is a 65-year-old man in no acute distress. Physical examination reveals systolic hypertension, retinal changes suggestive of sustained hypertension, a mild cataract in his right eye, a conductive hearing loss in his right ear, tonsillopharyngitis, and gynecomastia. Cardiac examination reveals aortic insufficiency. Peripheral vascular examination reveals possible atherosclerotic disease of the right carotid artery and mild venous disease of the lower extremities. The patient has a right, easily reducible inguinal hernia. A left-sided varicocele is present. Mild osteoarthritis of the hands is also present.

Table 22–1 Deep Tendon Reflexes of Patient John Henry

Side	Biceps	Triceps	Knee	Achilles
Right	1+	0	2+	1+
Left	2+	1+	3+	2+

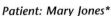

*Patient: Mary Jones**

General appearance: The patient is a 51-year-old African-American woman who is sitting up in bed in mild respiratory distress. She is obese and appears to be her stated age. She is well groomed and alert, but she constantly complains about her shortness of breath.

Vital signs: BP, 130/80/75 right arm (lying), 125/75/70 left arm (lying), 120/75/70 (sitting); heart rate, 100 and regular; respirations, 20.

Skin: Upper extremities slightly dusky in comparison with lower extremities; good tissue turgor; patient is wearing a wig to cover her marked total baldness; normal female escutcheon.

Head: Normocephalic without evidence of trauma; face appears edematous; no tenderness noted.

Eyes: Visual acuity using near card: OD, 20/40, OS, 20/30; visual fields full bilaterally; EOMs intact; PERRLA; eyebrows thin bilaterally; conjunctivae red bilaterally with injection present; lenses clear; both discs appear sharp with some nasal blurring; the cup–disc ratio is 1:3 bilaterally, and the cups are symmetric; the retinal veins appear dilated bilaterally.

Ears: Pinnae in normal position; no mastoid or external canal tenderness; canals without injection or discharge; Rinne test, AC > BC bilaterally; Weber test, no lateralization; both tympanic membranes clearly visualized; normal landmarks seen bilaterally.

Nose: Straight without deviation; mucosa reddish-pink; inferior turbinates within normal limits.

Sinuses: No tenderness detected.

Throat: Lips cyanotic; all teeth present except for all third molars, which have been extracted; occlusion normal; no caries seen; gingivae normal; tongue midline with markedly dilated tortuous veins on undersurface; no fasciculations of tongue noted; posterior pharynx appears within normal limits; uvula midline and elevates normally; gag reflex intact.

Neck: Full with normal range of motion; trachea midline; neck veins distended to angle of jaw while sitting upright; no adenopathy of neck noted.

Chest: AP diameter normal; symmetric excursion bilaterally; increased tactile fremitus at right base posteriorly corresponds to area of bronchial breath sounds; percussion note in this area is dull, all other chest areas are resonant; bronchophony and egophony present in area of bronchial breath sounds; crackles and wheezes present in area at right posterior base.

Breasts: Left mastectomy scar; right breast without masses, dimpling, or discharge.

Heart: PMI 5ICS MCL; normal physiologic splitting present; no heaves or thrills present; S_1 and S_2 within normal limits; no murmurs, gallops, or rubs present.

Vascular: There are no bruits present over the carotid, renal, femoral, or abdominal arteries; the extremities are without clubbing or edema.

Abdomen: The abdomen is obese without guarding, rigidity, or tenderness; no visible pulsations are present; bowel sounds are normal; percussion note is tympanitic throughout the abdomen; liver span is 15 cm in the MCL; spleen not percussed or palpated; kidneys not palpated; no CVAT present.

Rectal: Refused.

Pelvic: Deferred until patient more stable.

Lymphatic: No adenopathy felt in the neck chains or in the epitrochlear, axillary, supra-clavicular, or femoral regions.

Musculoskeletal: Marked edema of both upper extremities, L > R; neck, arms, knees, and ankles with full range of active and passive motion; muscles appear symmetric except for upper extremities.

Neurologic: Oriented to person, place, and time; cranial nerves I to XII intact; gross sensory and motor strength intact; cerebellar function normal; plantar reflex down bilaterally; deep tendon reflexes as shown in Table 22-2.

Table 22–2 Deep Tendon Reflexes of Patient Mary Jones

Side	Biceps	Triceps	Knee	Achilles
Right	2+	2+	2+	1+
Left	2+	1+	2+	2+

*This name is fictitious. Any similarity to any person living or dead with this name is purely coincidental.

Summary: Ms. Jones is a 51-year-old African-American woman, status post left mastectomy, in respiratory distress. She is cyanotic and has evidence of vascular engorgement of the upper half of her body. Her trachea is fixed to the mediastinum. Chest examination reveals evidence of consolidation of the right lower lobe of her lung.

Bibliography

Corbett EC, Payne NJ, Bradley EB, et al: Enhancing clinical skills education: University of Virginia School of Medicine's Clerkship Clinical Skills Workshop Program. Acad Med 82:690, 2007.

DeMaria AN: Wither the cardiac physical examination? J Am Coll Cardiol 48:2156, 2006.

Fletcher FK, Stern DT, White C, et al: The physical examination of patients with abdominal pain: The long-term effect of adding standardized patients and small-group feedback to a lecture presentation. Teach Learn Med 16:171, 2004.

Goldstein EA, MacLaren CF, Smith S, et al: Promoting fundamental clinical skills: A competency-based college approach at the University of Washington. Acad Med 80:423, 2005.

March SK, Bedynek JL, Chizner MA: Teaching cardiac auscultation: Effectiveness of a patient-centered teaching conference on improving cardiac auscultatory skills. Mayo Clin Proc 80:1443, 2005.

Ortiz-Neu C, Walters CA, Tenenbaum J, et al: Error patterns of 3rd-year medical students on the cardiovascular physical examination. Teach Learn Med 13:161, 2001.

Vukanovic-Criley JM, Criley S, Warde CM, et al. Competency in cardiac examination skills in medical students, trainees, physicians, and faculty: A multicenter study. Arch Intern Med 166:610, 2006.

Wiener S, Nathanson M: Physical examination: Frequently observed errors. JAMA 236:852, 1976.

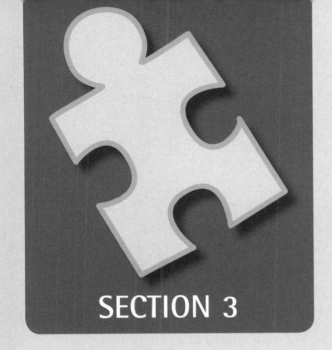

SECTION 3

Evaluation of Specific Patients

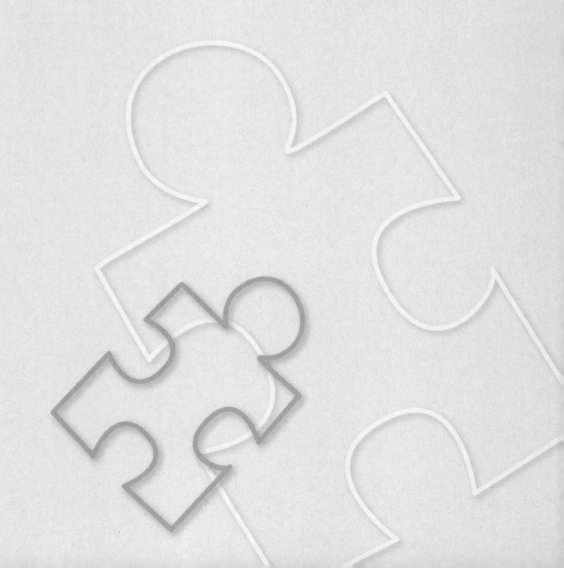

CHAPTER 23

The Pregnant Patient

It was the best of times, it was the worst of times....

Charles Dickens   (1812–1870)

General Considerations

As of 2007, the average birth rate for the world is 20.3 live births per year per 1000 total population, which for a world population of 6.6 billion amounts to 134 million babies born per year. In 2007, in the United States, the birth rate was 14.16 per 1000 total population. The lower birth rate in the United States reflects primarily the current smaller proportion of women of childbearing age as baby boomers age and Americans are living longer.

The lowest birth rates worldwide, less than 8.5 per 1000, were recorded in Japan, Germany, Singapore, Hong Kong and Macao. The highest birth rates, 49.0 or more per 1000, were recorded in Niger, Liberia, Guinea-Bissau, and Democratic Republic of the Congo.

Childbearing among teenagers has been on a long-term decline in the United States since the late 1950s, except for a brief, but steep, upward climb in the late 1980s through 1991. The 2004 birth rate (41.2 births per 1000 teenagers from 15 to 19 years of age) is 1% lower than in 2002 and 33% lower than the most recent peak in 1991.

The birth rate for African-American teenagers in 2004 was down 46% to 62.9 per 1000 teenagers from a high of 115.5 in 1991. The birth rate for Hispanic teenagers in 2004 was down 23% to 82.6 per 1000 teenagers from a high of 106.8 in 1993. More than 25% of all children were delivered by cesarean section; the total cesarean delivery rate was 26.1%, the highest ever reported in the United States.

The average age of mothers at first birth has increased steadily since the mid-1970s, to 25.1 years in 2002, an all-time high for the nation. In 2002, by state, the average age of mothers at first birth ranged from 23 years to 28 years. Mothers living in northeastern states were the oldest at first birth; mothers living in Arkansas, Louisiana, Mississippi, New Mexico, Oklahoma, and Wyoming were the youngest.

Slightly more than 1 per 10 women smoked during pregnancy in 2002, a decline of 42% since these data were first collected in 1989.

The risk of death from complications of pregnancy has decreased approximately 99% during the 20th century. However, since 1982, there has been no further decrease in the maternal mortality rate. Racial disparity in pregnancy-related mortality persists: The mortality rate among African-American mothers is at least three to four times higher than that among white mothers. In a 2003 study, the Centers for Disease Control and Prevention reviewed the pregnancy-related mortality rate in the United States from 1991 to 1999. During this period, there were 4200 deaths from pregnancy-related conditions. The overall pregnancy-related mortality rate was 11.8 deaths per 100,000 live births for the 9-year surveillance period. In comparison with pregnancy-related mortality rates among white women, excess risk for African-American women increased significantly with age and was most evident at ages older than 39 years. The most frequent pregnancy outcome associated with a pregnancy-related death was live birth (60%), followed by undelivered pregnancy (10%) and stillbirth (7%). The leading causes of pregnancy-related death were embolism (19.6%), hemorrhage (17.2%), pregnancy-induced hypertension (15.7%), infection (12.6%), cardiomyopathy (8.3%), stroke (5.0%), and anesthesia (1.6%).

Any woman in the reproductive age group who is sexually active and misses her menstrual period should be considered pregnant until proven otherwise. Even if she presents with symptoms not directly related to the abdomen, she should be evaluated for pregnancy. A sexually active woman in the reproductive age group may have a history of 2 years of amenorrhea (loss of menstrual periods) but can be pregnant nonetheless. Whatever the cause of the amenorrhea was 2 years ago, it may be different now. "Think pregnancy" should be your motto in the evaluation of such patients. This is extremely important because the diagnosis or treatment of a woman's medical or surgical problem may be deleterious to the developing fetus if she is pregnant. As discussed later in this chapter, many of the symptoms of pregnancy are nonspecific and can be interpreted erroneously if the pregnancy is not recognized. For example, the urinary frequency that is common in early pregnancy might easily be mistaken for cystitis. The patient might then receive an antibacterial agent such as a sulfonamide or a quinolone, which is potentially toxic to the developing fetus. When the urinary symptoms fail to respond to the medication, the patient might then be referred for intravenous pyelography, which adds the risk of radiation to an early pregnancy.

Structure and Physiology

The anatomy and the physiologic changes related to the menstrual cycle that occur in the nonpregnant woman have already been discussed. This chapter reviews the physiologic alterations resulting from pregnancy and the functional pelvic anatomy.

Basic Physiology of Reproduction

When semen is deposited in the vagina, sperm travel through the cervix and uterus and into the fallopian tubes, where fertilization may occur if an ovum is present. The majority of sperm deposited in the vagina die within 1 to 2 hours because of the normal acidic environment. The sperm are aided in their travel into the fallopian tubes by uterine and tubal contractions and favorable mucous conditions.

The fertilized ovum, or zygote, remains in the fallopian tube for about 3 days. While in the tube, the fertilized ovum divides repeatedly to form a round mass of cells called the *morula*. If there is an obstruction in the fallopian tube, the fertilized ovum may become trapped in the tube and attach itself to the lining of the tube, giving rise to an *ectopic*, or *tubal, pregnancy*. In a normal pregnancy, approximately 6 to 8 days after fertilization, the morula becomes a *blastocyst*, which migrates through the tube into the uterus, where it attaches itself to the endometrium (*implantation*), with the inner cell mass adjacent to the endometrial surface. Substances that destroy the surface epithelial cells are released, allowing the blastocyst to burrow into the endometrium. The endometrium then grows over the invading blastocyst.

The primitive *chorion*, the combination of *trophoblast* and primitive *mesoderm*, secretes a luteinizing hormone known as *human chorionic gonadotropin* (hCG), which controls the corpus luteum and inhibits pituitary gonadotropic activity. Quickly thereafter, as the invasion proceeds, maternal venous blood vessels are tapped to form lakes of blood, and *chorionic villi* develop. These can be identified as early as the 12th day after fertilization. These villi develop a leafy appearance and are called the *chorion frondosum*. By the 15th day after fertilization, the maternal arterial vessels are tapped, and by the 17th to 18th day, a functioning placental circulation is established. At term, the uteroplacental blood flow is estimated to be about 550 to 705 mL/minute. Figure 23-1*A* illustrates the path of sperm, fertilization, and implantation.

Decidua is the name given to the endometrium of pregnancy. There are three types, distinguished by location with regard to the growing embryo. The *decidua capsularis* is the

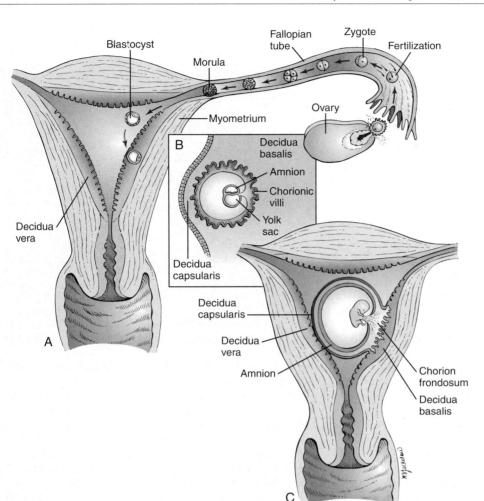

Figure 23–1 *A,* Fertilization and implantation. *B* and *C,* Cross-sectional view through the uterus of a pregnant woman at approximately 8 days and 20 days, respectively.

overlying endothelium that covers the conceptus, and the *decidua basalis* is the decidual tissue lying between the blastocyst and the myometrium. The decidua of the remainder of the endometrial cavity is the *decidua vera*. A cross section through the uterus of a pregnant woman and the different types of decidua in early pregnancy are illustrated in Figure 23-1*B* and *C*.

One of the first placental hormones produced by the developing trophoblastic tissue is hCG. This hormone is present as early as the 8th day after fertilization has taken place. The titers increase to a maximal level by about the 60th to 70th days after fertilization and then decrease. The primary function of hCG is to maintain the corpus luteum during the first 2 months of pregnancy until the placenta can produce enough progesterone by itself. Other hormones, such as human placental lactogen, human chorionic thyrotropin, and adrenocorticotropic hormone, and estrogens are also produced by the placenta. It is beyond the scope of this book to discuss the actions of these hormones; the reader is referred to the references at the end of this chapter for further information.

Functional Anatomy of Birth

The pelvic cavity is bounded above by the plane of the *brim* (the inner sacral promontory to the upper and inner borders of the symphysis pubis), below by the plane of the *outlet* (the lower and inner borders of the symphysis pubis to the end of the sacrum or coccyx), posteriorly by

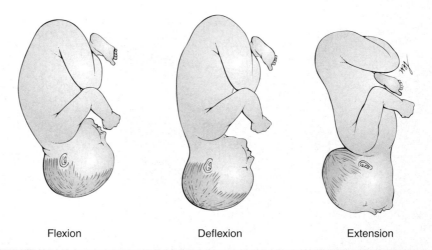

| Flexion | Deflexion | Extension |

Figure 23–2 Types of fetal positions.

the sacrum, laterally by the sacrosciatic ligaments and ischial bones, and anteriorly by the pubic rami.

The birth canal, through which the infant is delivered, may be thought of as a cylindric passage with walls composed partially of hard parts (the bony pelvis) and partially of soft parts (the muscles of the pelvic floor and the pelvic ligaments). The cross section of the cylinder is oval, rather than circular, to accommodate the oval cross section of the entering fetal part (e.g., the head) as it descends through the pelvis as a result of the expulsive effect of uterine contractions.

This mechanism for delivery and its corresponding anatomy would be easily understood were it not for the fact that the long axis of the schematic oval, which lies transversely at the entrance to the pelvis, comes to lie in the anteroposterior axis in the midpelvis. The entering fetal part must therefore descend in a spiral path as it progresses through the birth canal.

The process of birth varies greatly, depending on the relationships—lie, presentation, attitude, and position—of the fetus to the maternal anatomy. It is important to define these relationships accurately to understand the birth process.

The term *lie* refers to the relation of the long axis of the fetus to that of the mother. In more than 99% of full-term pregnancies, the lie is in the same plane as or parallel to the long axis of the mother; this is called a *longitudinal lie*. In rare instances, the long axis of the fetus is perpendicular to the maternal pelvis; this is called a *transverse lie*.

The term *presentation* refers to the part of the fetus in the lower pole of the uterus overlying the pelvic brim (e.g., cephalic, vertex, breech) that can be felt through the cervix. Usually the fetus's head is flexed so that the chin is in contact with the chest. In this case, the occipital fontanelle is the *presenting part*, and the presentation is referred to as a *vertex presentation*. The fetus is in the occiput or vertex presentation in approximately 95% of all labors.

The *attitude*, or *habitus*, of the fetus is the posture of the fetus: flexion, deflexion, or extension. Figure 23-2 illustrates these postures. In most cases, the fetus becomes bent over so that the back is convex, the head is sharply flexed on the chest, the thighs are flexed over the abdomen, and the legs are bent at the knees. This is the description of the fetal attitude of flexion.

The *position* is the relationship of an arbitrarily chosen portion of the presenting part of the fetus to the maternal pelvis. For example, in a vertex presentation, the chosen portion is the fetal *occiput;* in a breech presentation, it is the *sacrum;* and in a face presentation, it is the chin, termed the *mentum.* The maternal pelvis is divided into eight parts for the purpose of further defining position. These divisions are shown in Figure 23-3.

Because the arbitrarily chosen portion of the presenting part may be either left or right, the portion can be described as left occiput (LO), right occiput (RO), left sacral (LS), right sacral (RS), left mental (LM), or right mental (RM). This part is also directed anteriorly (A), posteriorly (P), or transversely (T). For each of the three presentations (vertex, breech, and face), there are therefore six varieties of position. For example, in a vertex presentation, if the

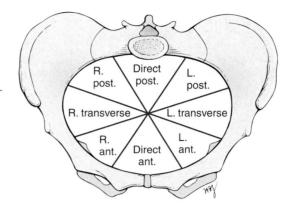

Figure 23–3 Divisions of maternal pelvis as seen from above. Ant., anterior; L., left; post., posterior; R., right.

occiput is in the left anterior segment of the maternal pelvis, the position is described as *left occiput anterior* (LOA), which is the most common of all vertex presentations. The common clinical vertex positions are illustrated in Figure 23-4. "Left" and "right" always denote the side of the mother. Likewise, "anterior," "posterior," and "transverse" refer to the mother's pelvis.

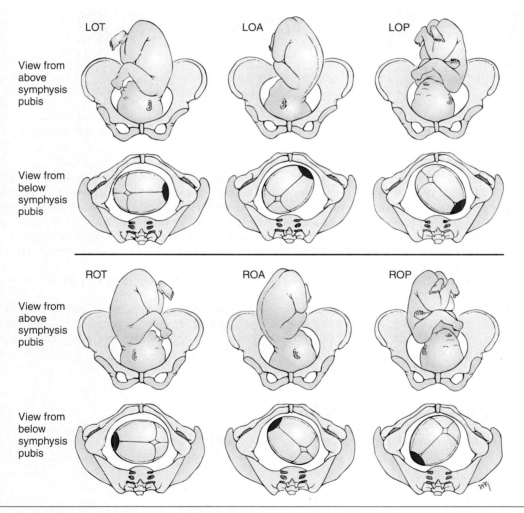

Figure 23–4 Common clinical vertex positions. For each position shown, the top diagram is the view from above the symphysis pubis; the bottom is the view from below the symphysis pubis. "Right" and "left" refer to the mother's side. "Anterior," "posterior," and "transverse" refer to the maternal pelvis. Red area is the fetal occiput. LOA, left occiput anterior; LOP, left occiput posterior; LOT, left occiput transverse; ROA, right occiput anterior; ROP, right occiput posterior; ROT, right occiput transverse.

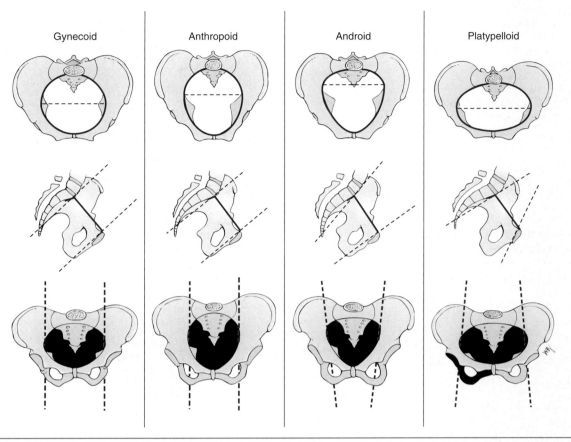

| Gynecoid | Anthropoid | Android | Platypelloid |

Figure 23–5 Basic types of pelvic anatomy. *Top view* is from above, looking down at inlet; *middle view* is from the side; *bottom view* is from the front.

The term *station* characterizes the level of descent of the presenting part of the fetus; "0 station" signifies that the fetal occiput has reached the level of the maternal ischial spines and that the widest transverse part of the infant's head (*biparietal diameter*) is at the level of the pelvic brim. This is also known as *engagement*. If the vertex is at "−1 station," it means that the fetal occiput is at a plane 1 cm above the level of the maternal ischial spines (and that the biparietal diameter is therefore 1 cm above the pelvic brim), and the infant's head is therefore not engaged.

The cardinal movements of labor are engagement, descent, flexion, internal rotation, extension, external rotation, and expulsion.

There are four basic pelvic configurations: *gynecoid, anthropoid, android,* and *platypelloid.* These are based on the shape of the brim, midpelvis, and outlet. Any pelvis is likely to combine features of more than one configuration. Figure 23-5 illustrates these basic types and summarizes the differences in pelvic anatomy.

Review of Specific Symptoms

The most common symptoms of pregnancy are the following:

- Amenorrhea
- Nausea
- Breast changes
- Heartburn
- Backache
- Abdominal enlargement
- Quickening
- Skin changes

- Disturbances in urination
- Vaginal discharge
- Fatigue

Amenorrhea

Amenorrhea results from the high levels of estrogen, progesterone, and hCG, which increase and alter [decidualize] the uterine endometrium and do not allow the endometrium to slough as in menstrual bleeding.

Nausea

Nausea, with or without vomiting, is the so-called *morning sickness of pregnancy*. As the name implies, the symptom is usually worse during the early part of the day and usually passes in a few hours, although it may last longer. More than 50% of all pregnant women in their first trimester have gastrointestinal symptoms. Although the cause is unknown, high levels of estrogen and hCG have been implicated in its development. Pregnant women are also hypersensitive to odors, and they may experience alterations in taste. Morning sickness usually improves after 12 to 16 weeks, when the hCG levels fall. Severe vomiting may occur, resulting in dehydration and ketosis, but this is uncommon, occurring in fewer than 2% of pregnancies.

Breast Changes

Several changes in the breast occur with pregnancy. One of the earliest symptoms is an increase in the vascularity of the breast, associated with a sensation of heaviness, almost pain. This occurs at about the 6th week. By the 8th week, the nipple and areola have become more pigmented, and the nipple becomes more erectile. The Montgomery tubercles become prominent as raised pinkish-red nodules on the areola. By the 16th week, a clear fluid called *colostrum* is secreted and may be expressed from the nipple. By the 20th week, further pigmentation and mottling of the areola have developed. Figure 23-6 illustrates the changes in the nipple and areola.

Heartburn

Heartburn in pregnancy occurs because progesterone causes relaxation of the gastroesophageal sphincter. Another cause of heartburn in the third trimester is the pushing upward of the enlarged uterus. This upward displacement exerts pressure on the stomach. There is a decrease in gastric motility, as well as a decrease in gastric acid secretion, which delays digestion.

Backache

As a result of secretion of estrogen and progesterone, the pelvic joints relax, and the increased uterine weight accentuates lordosis. The abdominal muscles stretch and lose tone.

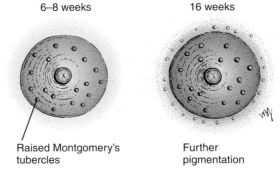

Figure 23–6 Nipple and areola changes during pregnancy.

6–8 weeks   16 weeks

Raised Montgomery's tubercles   Further pigmentation

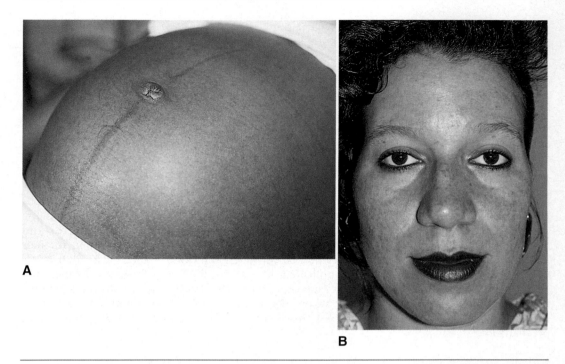

Figure 23–7 Skin changes resulting from high levels of ovarian, placental, and pituitary hormones. *A,* Linea nigra. *B,* Chloasma.

Abdominal Enlargement

The uterus rises out of the pelvis and into the abdomen by the 12th week of gestation, and an increase in abdominal girth is usually apparent by the 15th week. This enlargement is usually more apparent earlier in multiparous women, whose abdominal muscles have lost some of their tone during previous pregnancies.

Quickening

Quickening is the sensation of fetal movement. It is a faint sensation initially. Quickening usually begins at 20 weeks in the primigravida but is usually felt 2 to 3 weeks earlier in the multipara. Although an important symptom, quickening is not a reliable sign of pregnancy because a woman can convince herself of its presence.

Skin Changes

In addition to the skin changes of the breast already discussed, hyperpigmentation is common, especially in women with dark hair and a dark complexion. The linea alba darkens to become the *linea nigra,* as shown in Figure 23-7*A.* Areas prone to friction (e.g., medial thighs, axilla) also tend to darken. New pigmentation on the face, called *chloasma,* also commonly develops on the cheeks, forehead, nose, and chin. These skin changes are caused by the presence of high levels of ovarian, placental, and pituitary hormones. A woman with chloasma appears in Figure 23-7*B.*

"Stretch marks," or *striae gravidarum,* are irregular, linear, pinkish-purple lesions that develop on the abdomen, breasts, upper arms, buttocks, and thighs. They are caused by tears in the connective tissue below the stratum corneum. Figures 23-8 and 23-9 show striae gravidarum of the abdomen and breasts, respectively. The linea nigra is also present on the patient in Figure 23-8. Figure 23-10 illustrates the common skin changes seen in pregnancy.

Transverse grooving, as well as increased brittleness or softening, of the nails may occur. Eccrine sweating progressively increases throughout pregnancy, whereas apocrine gland

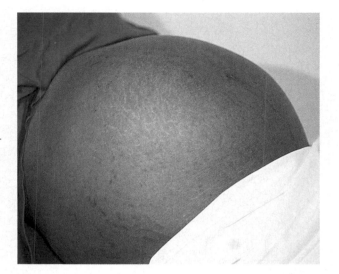

Figure 23–8 Striae gravidarum of the abdomen. Note also the linea nigra.

activity decreases. Hirsutism, caused by increased androgen secretion, may also occur on the face, arms, legs, and back.

Disturbances in Urination

Beginning at the 6th week, urinary bladder symptoms are common. Increased frequency of urination is thought to be caused by increased vascularity of the bladder, as well as by pressure of the enlarging uterus on the bladder. As the uterus rises above the pelvis, the symptoms tend to remit. Near term, however, urinary symptoms recur as the fetal head settles into the maternal pelvis and impinges on the volume capacity of the urinary bladder.

Vaginal Discharge

An asymptomatic, white, milky vaginal discharge is common as the elevated estrogen levels increase the production of cervical mucus and secretions from the vaginal walls.

Fatigue

Easy fatigability is common during early pregnancy. Some physicians believe that progesterone has a soporific effect and is the cause of the fatigue.

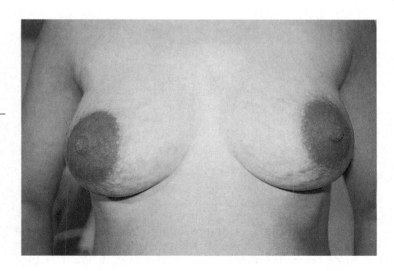

Figure 23–9 Striae gravidarum of the breasts. Note also the marked pigmentation of the areolae.

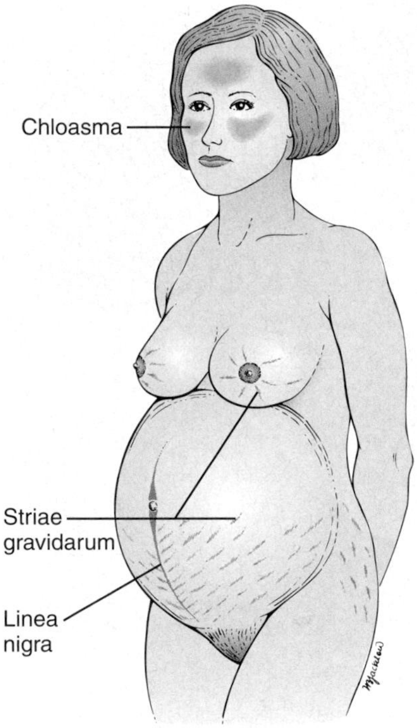

Figure 23–10 Common skin changes during pregnancy.

Other Symptoms

Several other symptoms are common in pregnant women. These include varicose veins, headache, leg cramps, swelling of the legs and hands, constipation, bleeding gums, nosebleeds, insomnia, and "dizziness."

Obstetric Risk Assessment

Documentation of the medical history of the pregnant woman is similar to that of the nonpregnant woman. In addition, the interviewer must assess obstetric risk. The following major risk factors must be evaluated:

- Age
- Parity
- Height
- Pregnancy weight
- Diabetes, hypertension, and renal disease
- Hemoglobinopathy and isoimmunization
- History of previous pregnancies
- Sexually transmitted infections
- Other infections
- Tobacco, alcohol, and drug use

Age

Older women have an increased risk of conceiving fetuses with chromosomal abnormalities. The chance of having a chromosomally abnormal child is about 1 per 200 at age 35 years and reaches about 1 per 20 at age 44 years. Women younger than 20 years generally give birth to more premature infants and to infants with lower birth weights than do women aged 25 to 35 years.

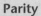

Parity

Women who have had more than five children are at increased risk of *placenta previa* and *placenta accreta*, possibly because of scarring of the endometrium. Postpartum hemorrhage and uterine rupture are also more common in this group of women.

Height

Women who are less than 5 feet (152.5 cm) tall usually have small pelves and therefore may be prone to *cephalopelvic disproportion** and may require cesarean sections.

Pregnancy Weight

Perinatal mortality rate is increased among women whose initial prepregnancy weight is less than 120 pounds, especially if their weight gain during pregnancy is less than 11 pounds. Being overweight or obese also puts the mother and her fetus at increased risk of obstetric complications, including early miscarriage. gestational hypertension, preeclampsia, gestational diabetes, fetal macrosomia, cesarean delivery, and operative complications such as increased operative time, increased blood loss, infection, and anesthetic complications. Therefore, women who are significantly underweight or overweight should undergo medical and nutritional evaluation, counseling, and therapy before becoming pregnant.

Diabetes, Hypertension, or Renal Disease

In women with diabetes, hypertension, or renal disease, there is an increased risk of fetal intrauterine growth retardation, premature labor, toxemia, and abruptio placentae. Diabetes mellitus occurs in 2% to 3% of all pregnancies and is thus the most common medical complication of pregnancy. Screening for gestational diabetes is now routine, because the rate of gestational diabetes may be as high as 30% of births.

Hemoglobinopathy and Isoimmunization

Determine the presence of any hemoglobinopathy, because pregnancy can precipitate an exacerbation of the anemia. Women who are Rh-negative must be monitored closely throughout pregnancy if they have Rh antibodies from isoimmunization, because severe hemolytic anemia may develop in the fetus before delivery.

History of Previous Pregnancies

A history of traumatic or second trimester fetal loss increases the possibility of cervical injury and subsequent incompetence of the cervix, an often preventable cause of second trimester miscarriage. A history of premature delivery (newborn's weight <2500 g) or immature delivery (< 1000 g) increases the probability of recurrent early delivery. These patients require particularly close surveillance. A history of unexplained pregnancy loss in the third trimester should alert the clinician to undiagnosed medical problems in the mother, such as gestational diabetes or systemic lupus erythematosus. For women who have undergone previous cesarean section, there must be exact information about the reason for the procedure and the type of uterine incision used, so that it can be determined whether the patient is a candidate for a vaginal birth.

Sexually Transmitted Infections

Because medical therapy for a human immunodeficiency virus (HIV)–positive mother can reduce transmission of the infection to the fetus by more than two thirds, it is obvious that identification of HIV-positive mothers is essential. Although HIV testing cannot be required of

---

*Disparity between the size of the maternal pelvis and the fetal head, which precludes vaginal delivery.

the mother, it is mandatory that she be counseled about the value of testing. Screening for HIV is routinely offered and is usually (90%) accepted. A history of genital herpes simplex necessitates screening for recurrences near the time of delivery, because cesarean delivery may be necessary to prevent transmission to the neonate. Screening for gonorrhea is performed in high-risk populations.

Other Infections

Questioning regarding exposure to rubella, chickenpox, and parvovirus (fifth disease) is critical. It may be necessary to determine antibody titers. Screening for syphilis, chlamydia, hepatitis B surface antigen, and group B streptococcus in the third trimester is now routine. Screening for tuberculosis is performed in high-risk populations.

Tobacco, Alcohol, and Drug Use

Tobacco, alcohol, and drug use; exposure to toxic substances in the workplace or at home; and exposure to other teratogenic agents must be determined. Women who smoke cigarettes place their fetuses at a higher risk of complications and should be encouraged to stop smoking. The fetus is more likely to exhibit intrauterine growth retardation and to become hypoxic during labor as a result of a reduction in placental exchange. Special note must be made of *any* drugs taken during pregnancy. Ideally, this issue should be discussed before the woman conceives so that she can be properly counseled.

Any of these hazards may increase the risk of maternal or fetal morbidity and mortality and should be evaluated.

Calculation of Due Date

A question that most women have after being told that they are pregnant is "When am I due?" To calculate the expected date of confinement (EDC), first determine the date of the onset of the last menstrual period (LMP) and then calculate the EDC as follows:

LMP	12/29/07
Go back 3 months	9/29/07
Add 1 year	9/29/08
Add 7 days	10/06/08 = EDC

Alternatively, the EDC can be calculated by adding 9 months and 7 days to the first day of the LMP. This calculation is based on a gestation of 280 days and is known as *Nägele's rule*. By knowing the EDC, the examiner can predict the size of the uterus on physical examination, provided that the LMP is correct and that conception actually occurred at that time. If the size of the uterus differs significantly from that expected according to the EDC, the causes must be determined. Ultrasonography and other diagnostic tests can be helpful in dating a pregnancy.

Impact of Pregnancy on the Patient

Pregnancy can be one of the most exciting times in a woman's life or one of the worst. Even a woman who experiences joy from becoming pregnant may suffer anxiety during her pregnancy. "Will the baby be normal?" "How will I tolerate labor?" "How will the baby change my life?" "I've put on so much weight. Will I ever be able to take it off?" These are just a few of the many questions commonly asked by pregnant women, and these issues cause much of their anxiety. Anxiety over body image is common as pregnancy progresses.

Pregnancy may worsen an existing psychiatric illness, and pregnancy and the postpartum period can be stressful enough to induce a psychiatric illness. It has been estimated that one per five pregnant women experiences some sort of mental health problem during pregnancy. In addition, a severe psychotic episode occurs in 1 to 2 women per 1000 live births.

Depression is common during pregnancy; almost 15% of all pregnant women suffer some degree of depression during pregnancy, and 8% suffer depression during the postpartum period. Postpartum depression, or the *postpartum blues*, may be related to the diminishing of excitement after delivery, the loss of sleep during labor, anxiety about the ability to care for the child, perineal pain, feeding difficulties, and concern about appearance. Fortunately, postpartum depression is usually self-limited and remits within a week. Women at greatest risk for the development of postpartum depression are those with an unwanted pregnancy and those with marital difficulties. Sympathetic reassurance and support can help a woman return to her baseline state.

In previously psychotic patients, depression or schizophrenia is likely to occur during the postpartum period. Confusion, paranoid delusions, and disorientation may result. An important symptom is an aversion to the infant. Because child abuse by this group of patients is common, their symptoms must be identified quickly.

Physical Examination

The equipment necessary for the examination of the pregnant woman is the same as for the nonpregnant woman. In addition, specialized instruments such as an ultrasonic Doppler scanner or fetoscope may be used to listen to the fetal heart. The ultrasonic scanner can detect the fetal heartbeat as early as gestational weeks 6 to 7; an ultrasonic Doppler scanner is used at about week 10; and a fetoscope or stethoscope can be used after the 20th week to auscultate the fetal heartbeat.

Always try to make the patient as comfortable as possible. She should be examined in comfortable surroundings, with attention to privacy. Discuss with her all the procedures that you will perform. The patient's gown should open in the front for ease of examination. The patient is draped in the same way as discussed in previous chapters and as shown in Figure 19-26. If the patient is in advanced pregnancy, avoid having her lie for a long period on her back, because the gravid uterus diminishes venous return and produces supine hypotension. It is useful for the woman to urinate before the pelvic examination. As always, wash your hands before beginning the examination. Make sure that your hands are warm and dry.

Because the examination of the pregnant woman is identical to the examinations described in the other chapters of this book, only special techniques and modifications for pregnancy are discussed here.

Initial Comprehensive Evaluation

There are three main goals to the initial evaluation:

1. Determine the health of the mother and fetus.
2. Determine the gestational age of the fetus.
3. Initiate a plan for continuing care.

The physical examination must include the following:

- Determination of height and weight
- Assessment of blood pressure
- Inspection of the teeth and gums
- Palpation of the thyroid gland
- Auscultation of the heart and lungs
- Examination of the breasts and nipples
- Examination of the abdomen
- Examination of the legs for varicosities and edema
- Inspection of the vulva, vagina, and cervix
- Cytologic study (Pap smear)
- Swab for *Chlamydia* organisms and gonorrhea
- Palpation of the cervix, uterus, and adnexa, including physical assessment of uterine size in terms of gestational age

Whenever possible, ultrasonography should be performed at the first prenatal visit in order to verify the presence of an intrauterine pregnancy with a fetal heartbeat, to confirm or adjust the gestational age, and to check for multiple fetuses. Another sonographic examination is usually performed at about 16 to 20 weeks to confirm that the pregnancy is progressing normally and to recognize any major abnormality.

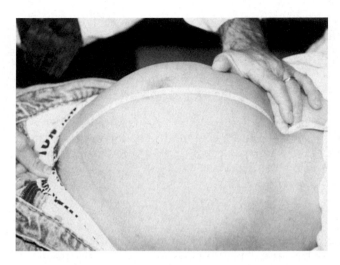

Figure 23–11 Technique for measuring fundal height.

Head, Eyes, Ears, Nose, Throat, and Neck

Inspect the face. Is chloasma present? What is the texture of the hair and skin? Inspect the mouth. What is the condition of the teeth and gums? Palpate the thyroid. Is it enlarged symmetrically?

Chest

Inspect, palpate, and auscultate the chest. Is there any evidence of labored breathing?

Heart

Palpate for the point of maximum impulse. Is it displaced laterally? During the later stages of pregnancy, the gravid uterus pushes up on the diaphragm, and the point of maximum impulse is displaced laterally. Auscultate the heart. Systolic ejection murmurs are common during pregnancy as a result of the hyperdynamic state. Diastolic murmurs are always pathologic.

Breasts

Inspect the breasts. Are they symmetric? Notice the presence of vascular engorgement and pigmentary changes. Are the nipples everted? An inverted nipple may interfere with a woman's plans to breast-feed. Palpate the breasts. The normal nodularity of breast tissue is accentuated during pregnancy, but *any discrete mass should be considered pathologic until proved otherwise*.

Abdomen

Inspect for the linea nigra and striae gravidarum. Notice the contour of the abdomen. Palpate the abdomen. Fetal movement may be felt by the examiner after 24 weeks. Are there uterine contractions? Hold your hand on the abdomen as the uterus relaxes.

Use a tape measure to assess the fundal height. The measurement should be taken from the top of the symphysis pubis in a straight line to the top of the fundus, with the bladder empty. The technique is demonstrated in Figure 23-11. Between 20 and 32 weeks, the superior-inferior measurement in centimeters should equal the number of weeks of gestation. The uterus rises up and enters the abdomen at 12 weeks. It reaches the umbilicus at about 20 weeks and is just under the costal margin by 36 weeks. The reduction in fundal height that usually occurs between the 38th and 40th weeks is called *lightening* and results from the descent of the fetus into the pelvis, or "dropping." Figure 23-12 illustrates the approximate size of the uterus by weeks.

Auscultate the fetal heart and determine the *fetal heart rate* (FHR), and note its location. Throughout pregnancy, the FHR is approximately 120 to 160 beats per minute. From weeks 12 to 18, the FHR is usually detected in the midline of the mother's lower abdomen. After 30 weeks, the FHR is best heard over the fetal chest or back. Knowing the location of the fetal back is helpful in determining where to listen for the FHR.

Genitalia

Inspect the mother's external genitalia. Are any lesions present? Inspect the anus. Are varicosities present?

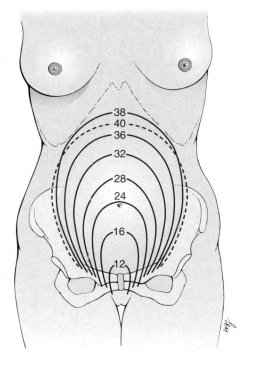

Figure 23–12 Approximate uterine size by week.

With gloves on, perform a speculum examination as described in Chapter 19, Female Genitalia. Inspect the cervix. A dusky blue color is characteristic of pregnancy and occurs by weeks 6 to 8. Is the cervix dilated? If so, fetal membranes may be seen within. Note the character of the vaginal secretions. Obtain cytologic studies for a Pap test and a swab for *Chlamydia* organisms and gonorrhea. As the speculum is removed, inspect the vaginal walls. The vaginal walls are commonly violaceous in pregnancy. Withdraw the speculum carefully.

Perform a digital bimanual examination, paying special attention to the consistency, length, and dilation of the cervix; the fetal presenting part (in advanced pregnancy); the structure of the pelvis; and any abnormalities of the vagina and perineum. Is the cervix closed? A nulliparous cervix should be closed, whereas a multiparous cervix may allow the tip of a finger through the external os. Estimate the length of the cervix by palpating the lateral side of the cervix from the cervical tip to the lateral fornix. Only at term should the cervix shorten, or efface. The normal length of the palpable (vaginal) portion of the cervix is 1.5 to 2 cm.

Palpate the uterus for size, consistency, and position. An early sign of pregnancy, at about 6 to 12 weeks, is the softening of the entire isthmus of the cervix; this is known as *Hegar's sign.* During the bimanual examination of the uterus, the examiner will notice an extreme softening of the lower uterine segment. This produces a sensation of the close proximity of the fingers of the hand in the vagina (internal) and that in the abdomen (external). The technique for evaluating the presence of Hegar's sign is illustrated in Figure 23-13. Bimanual palpation of the uterus is useful up to about 12 to 14 weeks' pregnancy. After that, the uterus can be palpated abdominally. Fetal parts are usually palpated from about 26 to 28 weeks' gestation by abdominal examination (described later).

Palpate the adnexa. Early in pregnancy, the corpus luteum may be palpable as a cystic mass on one ovary. As you withdraw your hand from the vagina, evaluate the pelvic muscles.

A rectovaginal examination is not indicated unless the woman has a retroverted, retroflexed uterus and needed information cannot be obtained by other means.

Extremities

Inspect for varicosities. Is edema present?

This completes the routine initial examination.

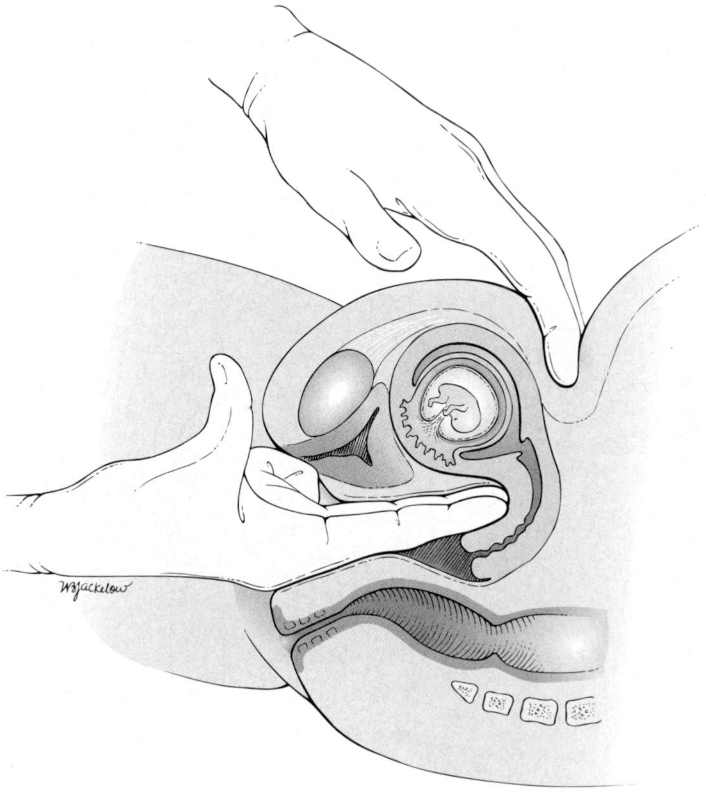

Figure 23–13 Technique for evaluating the presence of Hegar's sign.

Subsequent Antenatal Examinations

Subsequent antenatal examinations are important for screening for impaired fetal growth, malpresentation, anemia, preeclampsia, and other problems. In the absence of specific complaints by the patient or of abnormal findings on the initial examination or initial laboratory and sonographic studies, only a few parts of the physical examination just outlined are routinely performed during each visit. These include weight, blood pressure, and examination of the abdomen. This section concerns the abdominal examination.

The physical examination should confirm that fetal growth is consistent with gestational age. Attention should then be given to assessing the lie and presentation of the fetus. From the 28th week of gestation to term, the following four maneuvers, known as *Leopold's maneuvers*, provide vital information for the examiner about these important questions. The patient lies supine for these maneuvers.

The *first maneuver* is used to evaluate the upper pole and defines the fetal part in the fundus of the uterus. Stand facing the patient at her side, and gently palpate the upper uterine fundus with your fingers to ascertain which fetal pole is present. This technique is demonstrated in Figure 23-14. Usually, the fetal buttocks are felt at the upper pole. They feel firm but irregular. In a breech presentation, the head is at the upper pole. The head feels hard and round and is usually movable.

The *second maneuver* is used to locate the position of the fetal back. Standing in the same place as in the first maneuver, place the palms of your hands on either side of her abdomen, and apply gentle pressure to the uterus to identify the fetal back and limbs, as shown in Figure 23-15. On one side, the fetal back is felt: rounded, smooth, and hard. On the other side are the limbs, which are nodular or bumpy, and kicking may be felt.

The *third maneuver* is to palpate the lower pole of the fetus. From the same position as in the first two maneuvers, use your thumb and fingers of one hand to grasp the lower portion of the maternal abdomen just above the symphysis pubis. This maneuver is illustrated in Figure 23-16. If the presenting portion is not engaged, a movable part, usually the head of the fetus, is felt. If the presenting portion is engaged, this maneuver indicates that the lower pole of the fetus is fixed in the pelvis.

The *fourth maneuver* is performed to confirm the presenting portion and to locate the side of the fetus's cephalic prominence. You should now stand beside the patient, facing

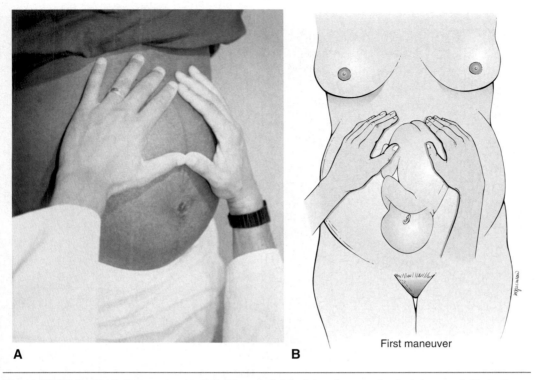

A **B**

First maneuver

Figure 23–14 Leopold's first maneuver. *A,* Position of clinician's hands on mother's abdomen. *B,* Illustration of relationship of clinician's hands and fetus.

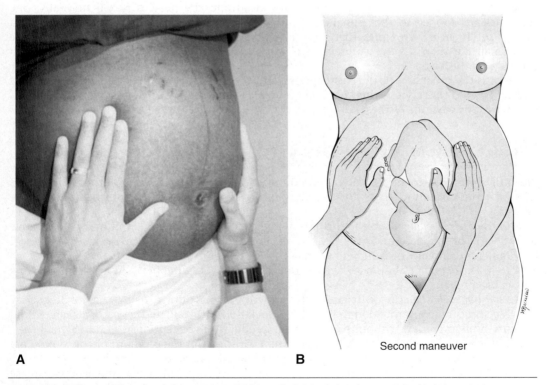

A **B**

Second maneuver

Figure 23–15 Leopold's second maneuver. *A,* Position of clinician's hands on mother's abdomen. *B,* Illustration of relationship of clinician's hands and fetus.

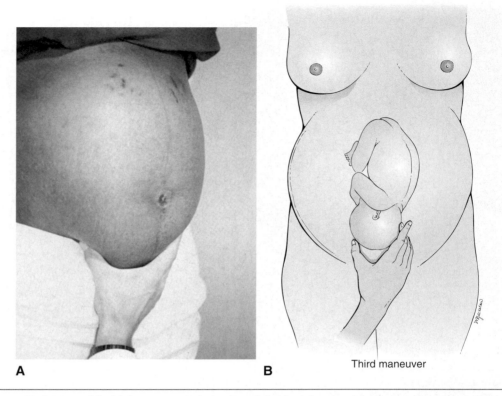

A   B   Third maneuver

Figure 23–16 Leopold's third maneuver. Relationship of clinician's hand and fetal presenting part. *A,* Position of clinician's hand on mother's abdomen. *B,* Illustration of relationship of clinician's hand and fetus.

her feet. Place your hands on either side of her lower abdomen. With the tips of your fingers, exert a deep pressure in the direction of the pelvic inlet, as indicated in Figure 23-17. If the presenting portion is the head and the head is flexed normally, one hand will be stopped by the cephalic prominence as the other hand descends farther down on the pelvis. In a vertex presentation, the cephalic prominence is on the same side as the fetal small parts. In a vertex presentation with the head extended, the prominence is on the side of the back.

Labor is the process of birth. The diagnosis and the mechanism of labor are complex topics and are beyond the scope of this book. The reader is referred to the references at the end of this chapter for discussions of these topics.

Clinicopathologic Correlations

Bleeding during pregnancy is fairly common but is not considered to be normal. The causes may be benign or serious and vary according to the stage of pregnancy and the nature of the bleeding.

First trimester bleeding may be indicative of implantation of the ovum, or it may be indicative of cervicitis or vaginal varicosities. More seriously, it could be indicative of a threatened, inevitable, incomplete, or complete abortion.

A *threatened abortion* should always be considered when vaginal bleeding occurs in the first 20 weeks of pregnancy.

An *inevitable abortion* can be diagnosed if a patient presents during the first half of pregnancy with bleeding and crampy abdominal pain in association with a dilated cervix or a gush of fluid (rupture of membranes) without passing of the products of conception.

An *incomplete* or *complete abortion* occurs when part or all of the products of conception are extruded through the cervix and into the vagina and are passed out of the body.

Second or *third trimester bleeding* occurs in about 3% of all pregnancies. About 60% of these bleeding episodes result from placenta previa or abruptio placentae. Both of these conditions may gravely endanger the mother and fetus.

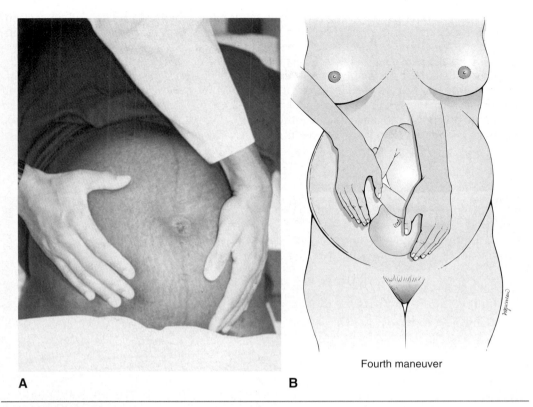

A   **B**

Fourth maneuver

Figure 23–17 Leopold's fourth maneuver. Relationship of clinician's hands and fetal presenting part. *A,* Position of clinician's hands on mother's abdomen. *B,* Illustration of relationship of clinician's hands and fetus. Note that the examiner's right hand is stopped higher by the fetus's cephalic prominence.

The incidence of *placenta previa* is about 1 per 250 deliveries and is more common among multiparas than among primigravidas. Placenta previa is characterized by painless vaginal bleeding in association with a soft, nontender uterus. The hemorrhage usually does not occur until the end of the second trimester or later. Although there are several types of placenta previa, the symptoms arise from the abnormal location of the placenta over or near the internal os of the cervix. Ninety percent of all patients with placenta previa have at least one antepartum hemorrhage. There is also a 20% incidence of premature delivery because of hemorrhage.

Abruptio placentae is the premature separation of a normally situated placenta. It also has an incidence of 1 per 75 to 225 deliveries. The symptoms include mild to severe pain with or without external bleeding in association with increasing uterine tone and tenderness. Fetal distress may or may not occur. The incidence of abruptio placentae is higher among women with high parity. It is also more common among African-American women than among white or Latino women. Hypertension is, by far, the most commonly associated condition. Cigarette smoking and cocaine abuse have also been linked to an increased risk of abruptio placentae. Women with a history of abruptio placentae are at significant risk of recurrence in subsequent pregnancies.

Vasa praevia is another serious but rare condition in which some of the fetal vessels in the membranes cross the region of the internal os. These vessels occupy a position in front of the presenting portion of the fetus. Rupture of the membranes may be accompanied by rupture of the fetal vessel, causing fetal blood loss and possible exsanguination.

Postpartum hemorrhage (PPH) is the most common cause of serious bleeding in obstetric patients and one of the leading causes of maternal death. It is sometimes defined as blood loss in excess of 500 mL during the first 24 hours after delivery, although the estimation of blood loss is notoriously inaccurate, and the loss of 500 mL after vaginal delivery or 1000 mL after cesarean delivery is quite common. The most common causes of PPH are uterine atony and laceration of the vagina or cervix. There are many causes for uterine atony: complications of general anesthesia, overdistention of the uterus by a large fetus or multiple fetuses, prolonged labor, rapid labor, augmented labor, high parity, retained products of conception, coagulation defects, sepsis, ruptured uterus, chorioamnionitis, and drugs such as aspirin, nonsteroidal anti-inflammatory agents, and magnesium sulfate. It has been estimated that postpartum hemorrhage occurs in 1% to 5% of all deliveries, depending on the definition used.

Pseudocyesis, or false pregnancy, is said to occur in 1 per 5000 putative pregnancies. In this condition, nonpregnant women present with many of the classic symptoms of pregnancy and often report fetal movement. They may exhibit weight gain and amenorrhea. Many of these patients are psychotic and may be schizophrenic. They are fixated on their alleged pregnancies. Aggressive psychiatric help is usually required.

Useful Vocabulary

Listed here are the specific roots that are important for understanding the terminology related to the pregnant patient.

Root	Pertaining to	Example	Definition
-par(ere)	parity	multi***para***	A woman who has had two or more pregnancies that resulted in viable offspring
-gravid	pregnancy	primi***gravida***	A woman pregnant for the first time
part-	partus	***part***urient	Giving birth; a woman in labor
puer-	puerperium	***puer***pera	A woman who has just given birth
-cyesis	pregnancy	pseudo***cyesis***	False pregnancy
-tocia	labor	dys***tocia***	Abnormal labor
-natal	birth	pre***natal***	Before birth
lochi-	postpartum	***lochi***orrhea	Abnormally profuse discharge of vaginal lochia

Writing Up the Physical Examination

Listed here are examples of the write-up for the assessment of the pregnant patient.

- Patient is a 32-year-old white woman, para 2-0-0-2 (see Chapter 19, Female Genitalia). Her larger infant weighed 7 pounds 4 ounces. Both deliveries were normal, spontaneous, and vaginal. LMP = 8/1/08. EDC = 5/8/09. Blood pressure is 125/80. Findings of examination of the head, eye, ear, nose, throat, and neck are unremarkable except for presence of chloasma. Breasts are symmetrically enlarged with venous pattern visible. Colostrum expressed. Chest is clear to percussion and auscultation. Heart rate is 100 and regular.

Heart sounds are normal. A grade II/VI midsystolic murmur is heard at the aortic area. No gallops are present. Examination of the abdomen reveals a 32-week gestation and is appropriate for dates. There are reddish, slightly depressed streaks on the lower abdomen. 1+ pretibial edema is present bilaterally. Movement of the fetus is felt. The fetus is in a longitudinal lie in a vertex presentation, with its back to the left. Fetal heart rate is 150 and is heard through the back of the fetus, 2 cm to the left of midline in the lower left quadrant.

- Patient is a 29-year-old African-American woman, para 2-1-1-3. Her first pregnancy was full term, delivered by cesarean section because of a double footling breech presentation; weight, 7 pounds 2 ounces. Her next two pregnancies were vaginal deliveries after cesarean section. The first infant weighed 7 pounds 7 ounces, and the second one weighed 5 pounds 6 ounces. Patient had one elective termination of pregnancy at 8 weeks between her first and second children. LMP = 9/3/07. EDC = 6/10/08. Blood pressure is 135/75. Thyroid is mildly enlarged symmetrically without nodularity. Multiple spider angiomas are present over the face, neck, upper chest, and arms. Breasts are symmetrically enlarged, with increased pigmentation of the areolae present. Striae gravidarum are present on the breasts. Chest is clear to percussion and auscultation. Heart rate is 90 and regular. S_1 and S_2 are normal. No murmurs, gallops, or rubs are heard. Uterus is felt in the abdomen at about a 16-week gestation, which is consistent with dates. Fetal heart rate is 160 with ultrasonic Doppler scan and is located in the midline of the lower abdomen. Bimanual examination reveals a soft lower uterine segment. External os admits a fingertip. Cervix is approximately 2 cm in length. Uterus is globular and smooth. Adnexa is unremarkable. Rectovaginal examination not performed. No edema present. Mild varicosities of both lower extremities are present.

Bibliography

ACOG Committee: ACOG Practice Bulletin. Clinical Management Guidelines for Obstetrician-Gynecologists. Number 64, July 2005 (Replaces Committee Opinion Number 238, July 2000): Hemoglobinopathies in pregnancy. Obstet Gynecol 106:203, 2005.

ACOG Committee on Practice Bulletins: ACOG Practice Bulletin. Clinical Management Guidelines for Obstetrician-Gynecologists. Number 60, March 2005. Pregestational diabetes mellitus. Obstet Gynecol 105:675, 2005.

American College of Obstetricians and Gynecologists: ACOG Committee Opinion. Number 315, September 2005. Obesity in pregnancy. Obstet Gynecol 106:671, 2005.

American College of Obstetricians and Gynecologists: ACOG Committee Opinion. Number 316, October 2005. Smoking cessation during pregnancy. Obstet Gynecol 106:883, 2005.

American College of Obstetricians and Gynecologists Committee on Health Care for Underserved Women: ACOG Committee Opinion No. 343: Psychosocial risk factors: Perinatal screening and intervention. Obstet Gynecol 108:469, 2006.

Centers for Disease Control, National Center for Health Statistics, National Vital Statistics Reports 54(8), 2005.

Chang J, Elam-Evans LD, Berg CJ, et al: Pregnancy-related mortality surveillance: United States, 1991–1999. MMWR Morb Mortal Wkly Rep 52(SS1-2):1, 2003.

Committee on Adolescent Health Care, ACOG Working Group on Immunization: ACOG Committee Opinion No. 344: Human papillomavirus vaccination. Obstet Gynecol 108:699, 2006.

Committee on Genetics, American College of Obstetricians and Gynecologists: ACOG Committee Opinion. Number 325, December 2005. Update on carrier screening for cystic fibrosis. Obstet Gynecol 106:1465, 2005.

Dawes MC, Ashurst H: Routine weighing in pregnancy. BMJ 304:487, 1992.

Floyd LR, O'Connor MJ, Sokol RJ, et al: Recognition and prevention of fetal alcohol syndrome. Obstet Gynecol 106:1059, 2005.

Herbert WNP, Bruninghaus HM, Barefoot AB, et al: Clinical aspects of fetal heart auscultation. Obstet Gynecol 69:574, 1987.

Johnson K, Posner SF, Biermann J, et al: Recommendations to improve preconception health and health care—United States. A report of the CDC/ATSDR Preconception Care Work Group and the Select Panel on Preconception Care. MMWR Recomm Rep 55(RR-06):1, 2006.

National Center for Health Statistics, National Vital Statistics Reports 53(9), 2004.

Santelli JS, Lindberg LD, Finer LB, et al: Recent declines in adolescent pregnancy in the United States: More abstinence or better contraceptive use? Am J Pub Health 97(1):150, 2007.

Santelli JS, Lyon MOM, Rogers J, et al: Abstinence and abstinence-only education: A review of US policies and programs. J Adolesc Health 38:83, 2006.

Santelli JS, Abma J, Ventura S, et al: Can changes in sexual behaviors among high school students explain the decline in teen pregnancy rates in the 1990s? J Adolesc Health 35:80, 2004.

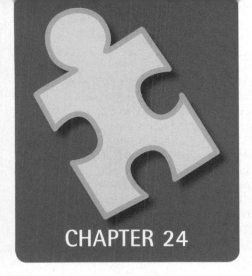

CHAPTER 24

The Pediatric Patient

Children are not like men nor women; they are almost as different creatures, in many respects, as if they never were to be the one or the other; they are as unlike as buds are unlike flowers, and almost as blossoms are unlike fruits.

Walter Savage Landor (1775–1864)

General Considerations

Since the late 1920s, awareness of the importance of child health care has increased. Along with better control of infectious disease and great strides in nutrition and technology has come the recognition of the importance of the behavioral and social aspects of a child's health. Despite the many advances and the marked reduction in infant mortality rates, the neonatal period remains a time of very high risk.[*] In 2004, a total of 27,936 deaths occurred in children younger than 1 year, an infant mortality rate of 6.8 per 1000 live births; 70% of these deaths occurred in the first month after birth, almost all of those in the first week.[†] The three leading causes of neonatal death were congenital malformations, deformations, and chromosomal abnormalities (20%); disorders related to short gestation and low birth weight (16%); and maternal complications of pregnancy that affected newborns (5.4%).

Unintentional injury and *sudden infant death syndrome* (SIDS) are the leading causes of infant mortality after the first month of life. SIDS is the leading cause of death among infants aged 1 to 12 months and is the third leading cause overall of infant mortality in the United States. Although the overall rate of SIDS in the United States has declined by more than 50% since 1990, thanks to the "Back to Sleep" campaign, rates have declined less among non-Hispanic African-American and American Indian/Alaska Native infants. SIDS is defined as the sudden death of a healthy infant younger than 1 year that cannot be explained after a thorough investigation is conducted, including a complete autopsy, examination of the death scene, and review of the clinical history. Preventing SIDS remains an important public health priority. Several risk factors have been associated with SIDS, including prone sleeping, sleeping on soft

---

[*]Centers for Disease Control and Prevention and National Center for Health Statistics at *www.cdc.gov/ VitalStats*.
[†]Data from National Center for Health Statistics, 3700 East-West Highway, Hyattsville, Md 20782.

This chapter was written in collaboration with Margaret Clark Golden, MD, and Robert W. Marion, MD. Dr. Clark Golden is Clinical Associate Professor of Pediatrics and Director of the Third Year Pediatric Clerkship at the State University of New York (SUNY) Downstate College of Medicine, Brooklyn, NY. Dr. Marion is Professor of Pediatrics & Obstetrics and Gynecology and the Ruth L. Gottesman Professor of Developmental Pediatrics at Albert Einstein College of Medicine. He is also the Director of the Center for Congenital Disorders, Children's Hospital at Montefiore Hospital, Bronx, NY.

surfaces, loose bedding, overheating as a result of overdressing, smoking in the home, maternal smoking during pregnancy, bed sharing, and prematurity or low birth weight. In a small portion of cases, SIDS seems to be caused by a mutation in a gene that leads to a cardiac channelopathy, resulting in prolonged QT interval and other arrhythmogenic states.

Unintentional injury remains the top killer of children aged 1 to 14 years,* ahead of cancer and birth defects. More than 5300 children in the United States died in 2004 from unintentional injuries—an average of 15 children each day. Motor vehicle occupant injury is the leading cause of injury-related death among all children after infancy. Death from airway obstruction is the leading cause of injury death for children younger than 1 year, and drowning follows motor vehicle injuries for children aged 1 to 14 years. Poverty is the primary predictor of fatal injury; male sex and race are additional factors. Native American and African-American children are the groups at highest risk; they are about twice as susceptible to fatal injury as are white children.

Previous chapters discussed the history and physical examination as they relate to adult patients. This chapter discusses the differences related to physical diagnosis in the pediatric age group. The field of pediatrics is broad and encompasses birth through adolescence, often defined as up to age 22. During this period, there are enormous changes in children's emotional, social, cognitive, and physical development, all of which must be discussed thoroughly.

This chapter is organized somewhat differently from the previous chapters. The first section is devoted to the pediatric history, which is similar in most pediatric age groups but differs in important ways from the adult history. The sections that follow are devoted to the physical examinations of the following age groups:

- Neonatal period (birth to 1 week of age)
- Infancy (1 week to 1 year of age)
- Toddler and early childhood (1 to 5 years of age)
- Late childhood (6 to 12 years of age)
- Adolescence (12 to 22 years of age)

Most of this chapter is devoted to the first three groups because the order and techniques of examining children 6 to 22 years of age are similar to those for adults.

The reader is advised to watch the video presentation on the DVD-ROM attached to this book to review the physical examinations of the newborn and the toddler, as well as specific pointers about the neurologic assessment at these ages. The DVD-ROM also contains a demonstration of an adolescent history with a standardized patient.

The Pediatric History

The pediatric history, like the adult history, is obtained before the examination is performed. During this period, the child can get accustomed to the clinician. Unlike the adult history, however, much of the pediatric history is taken from the parent or guardian. If the child is old enough, interview the child as well.

Good communication with the child is the key to a successful work-up, just as with an adult. An infant communicates by crying and, in so doing, indicates that something is wrong. Although older children can communicate through language, they also often use crying as a response to pain or to express emotional unrest. This mode of communication merits attention. Newborns can also communicate by cooing and babbling, which indicates contentment.

In infancy, children use sounds to mimic words, as well as using gestures to communicate. At about 10 to 12 months of age, children usually speak their first word, usually "dada" or "mama." By 15 months of age, children are expected to say between 3 and 10 words, and by 2 years of age, their vocabulary may contain more than 200 words; it is at this age that we expect children to be able to put 2 or more words together in a phrase, such as "Juice gone" or "Up me!" By 3 years of age, children are able to put together sentences of 5 or 6 words from a 1500-word vocabulary, and should be 50% intelligible to an adult who does not know the child. By the time they are 6 years of age, they are able to communicate in longer sentences, with a vocabulary of several thousand words, and use most of the grammar of their native language. Three-year-olds can give the clinician a good idea of what hurts, where, and how it feels. The 6-year-old can give some idea of how and when the complaint started. The examiner must pay attention to everything the child says, because the words used may give insight into the child's physical, emotional, and developmental state, as well as his or her home situation and other factors in his or her environment.

---

*See www.cdc.gov/WISQARS.

A good relationship with a child begins by making friends with him or her. Not wearing a white coat may alleviate some of the child's fears, but there are other ways as well. Start by admiring the child's shoes or toy; his possessions are more neutral topics for the child to talk about at first than his or her own body or behavior. One of the best ways to make a child feel comfortable is through praise. When talking to a child, it is useful to say, "Thank you for holding still. That makes the examination easier." The use of "You're a good boy" or "You are such a sweet girl" may produce embarrassment. Therefore, praise should be given for a child's behavior and not for his or her personality. Sharing a book with the child (e.g., as part of the "Reach Out and Read" program*) is another useful way to engage the toddler or preschooler.

It is important not to talk down to children. The examiner must assess the developmental level of the child and choose words that are appropriate to that child's level of understanding. This is especially important in dealing with a preteenage child; in fact, when interviewing such a child, the interviewer may gain more cooperation from the child by treating him or her as a bit older than his or her actual age, rather than younger.

Although most of the history is obtained from the parent or guardian, some questions are asked of the child. There are two simple rules in asking questions of children:

1. Use simple language.
2. Do not ask too many questions too quickly.

Interviewers are often amazed by how well a child can respond to questions phrased according to these rules. School-aged children can respond to *structured*, open-ended questions. Asking "How do you like school?" may elicit only a shrug. Asking "What do you like best about school?" is likely to get the child talking. It is useful to spend time observing the child at play while interviewing a parent. It is also rewarding to allow a toddler to play with a stethoscope, tongue blade, or penlight to "make friends" with the equipment that will be used later in the physical examination.

The pediatric history consists of the following:

- Chief complaint
- History of the present illness
- Birth history
- Past medical history
- Nutrition
- Growth and development
- Immunizations
- Social and environmental history
- Family history
- Review of systems

The *chief complaint* and the *history of the present illness* are obtained in the same manner as with the adult patient. The history should identify the informant, and the interviewer should try to establish whether and where the child has a regular source of medical care. The history of the present illness should always include information about the effect of an acute illness on the child's oral intake, activity level, hydration status, and ability to sleep. For a chronic problem, the examiner should look for effects on the child's growth and development.

Birth History

The *past medical history* section begins with the *birth history*. An opening with the mother such as "How was your pregnancy?" may be all that is needed to start this part of the medical history. Determine any maternal problems, medications taken, illnesses, bleeding, whether x-ray films were taken during the pregnancy, and whether the child was born "on time." Ask the following questions:

"How old were you at the time of your child's delivery? How old was the baby's father?"

"How many times have you been pregnant? Have you had any miscarriages or children who died in infancy?" If yes, *"Do you know the cause? Were any of your children born too early?"* (Box 24-1 contains an explanation of the shorthand notation for this information.)

---

*See *www.reachoutandread.org* (accessed June 26, 2008). "Reach Out and Read" is a national nonprofit organization that promotes early literacy by giving new books to children in pediatric examination rooms.

Box 24–1 Shorthand Notation for Birth History

Most centers use some variation of the following shorthand notation to summarize a woman's pregnancies and their outcomes: G3 P2-0-0-2. The "G" stands for "gravida" and is the number of pregnancies. The "P" stands for "para," for the number of birth/pregnancy outcomes; each of the four numbers after the "P" stands for a different outcome:

- The first place is the number of *f*ull-term births
- The second place is the number of *p*reterm births
- The third place is the number of *a*bortions/miscarriages
- The fourth place is the number of *l*iving children

(A mnemonic for remembering this notation is FPAL: *FiliPino AirLines*.)

In this example, this woman who is described as being G3 P2-0-0-2 is currently pregnant for the third time; she has delivered two full-term infants, she has had no preterm births and no miscarriages, and both her children are living.

By convention, in the case of a newborn, the notation for the mother reflects the notation when she was pregnant but had not yet delivered this child. For instance, in the case of a first-born child, the mother would be described as G1 P0-0-0-0.

Here's a quiz: Suppose a woman is described as G1 P2-0-0-2. How is that possible?*

*Answer: She has been pregnant once with twins, who were delivered at term and both of whom are living.

"When did you start prenatal care?" If prenatal care was started late, inquire tactfully about why by asking, "What is the reason you have not seen a doctor earlier?"

"Did you have any illnesses during your pregnancy?" If yes, ask the mother to describe them, and find out when during the pregnancy they occurred. Be sure to ask about chronic illnesses, such as diabetes, hypertension, asthma, or epilepsy, because these can have an effect on the health of the fetus. Also, inquire about any rashes that developed during pregnancy.

"How much weight did you gain during your pregnancy?"

"During your pregnancy, did you take any drugs, recreational or otherwise? Any herbal products? Drink alcohol? Smoke cigarettes? Have any 'x-rays'? Have any abnormal bleeding?" In asking these questions, the concern is whether the fetus has been exposed to any agents, known as teratogens, that can cause birth defects. Although concerns about teratogens are real, many women who have taken innocuous medications during pregnancy feel guilt that their ingestion may have somehow harmed their child; in these cases, reassurance that the agent was safe may relieve a great deal of maternal anxiety.

"Were you told during your pregnancy that you had high blood pressure? diabetes? protein in your urine?"

"What were the results of your blood tests? Were you tested for Group B strep or any other infections?" Standard prenatal care includes testing for maternal blood group, hepatitis B surface antigen, syphilis, chlamydial infection, and, in the last trimester, group B streptococcal vaginal colonization. Testing for gestational diabetes is also becoming more prevalent.

Although testing for human immunodeficiency virus (HIV) infection is not automatic, most women also accept it, because therapy with antiretroviral drugs in the last trimester can reduce rates of congenital infection from 25% to less than 2%.

"Did you have any special testing during the pregnancy? ultrasound examinations? amniocentesis or chorionic villus sampling (CVS)?" If yes, *"What were the results?"* Amniocentesis should be offered to all pregnant women aged 35 years and older. Inquire about the reasons for any special testing.

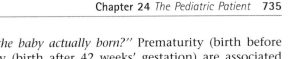

"What was your due date? When was the baby actually born?" Prematurity (birth before 37 weeks' gestation), and postmaturity (birth after 42 weeks' gestation) are associated with increased risk of early mortality and with specific clinical syndromes.

"When did you first feel the baby move? Was the baby active throughout pregnancy?" If this is not the first pregnancy, ask the mother to compare this fetus's activity with her other pregnancies.

"How long was your labor? Were there any unusual problems with it?"

"What type of delivery did you have, vaginal or cesarean?" If cesarean, ask for the reason. Was it because of a previous cesarean birth or a problem related to this pregnancy?*

"Did the baby come out head first or feet first?"

"How long were your membranes ruptured before the child was born?" If the membranes have been ruptured more than 18 hours, the risk of infection ascending from birth canal to the baby increases rapidly.

"What was the child's birth weight?"

"Were you told of any abnormalities at birth?"

"Were you told the Apgar† scores?" If the parents don't know, ask, "Did he cry right away? Or did the doctors need to do something to help him start breathing?"

"Did the child experience any problems in the newborn nursery, such as breathing difficulties? Jaundice? Feeding problems?"

"Did the child receive oxygen in the nursery? antibiotics? phototherapy?"

"After delivery, how long did the baby remain in the hospital?"

"Did the child go home with you?" If not, ask why not.

"Were you told that any problems were found on the newborn screening tests?"‡ If yes, "What were they? Was follow-up testing performed?"

Note the order of these questions: they begin with the **prenatal course,** then focus on the actual **birth,** and then turn to the **postnatal course**. See the sample write-up of a newborn's history at the end of this chapter. The amount of detail needed in the birth history depends on the age of the child and the clinical situation. Most of this information is pertinent for an infant; for a teenager, it is probably enough to know whether the child was born full term and whether there were any problems in the neonatal period.

Past Medical History

As with the adult, the *past medical history* should include details of any hospitalizations, injuries, and surgeries, as well as any medications taken on a regular basis. Ask, "Does your child have any chronic health problems?" Common chronic health problems in children include asthma, seizure disorders, eczema, recurrent ear infections or urinary tract infections, sickle cell disease, cystic fibrosis, diabetes, gastroesophageal reflux disease, and cerebral palsy. If the child was born before term, ask about late effects of preterm birth, such as chronic lung disease, nutritional problems, developmental difficulties, and sensory deficits.

It is important to identify *allergies* to medication (including penicillin), foods, or other substances. The most common problem associated with medications is the development of a rash. Rashes, however, are common in children and may have occurred coincidentally at the time a medication was prescribed. Therefore, try to determine whether the medication was the

---

*In 2007, fewer than 5% of births in the United States involved the use of forceps or a "vacuum extractor" to assist in vaginal delivery of a baby. In previous decades, use of such tools was much more common, and cesarean delivery was less common; see *www.cdc.gov/nchs/VitalStats.htm* (accessed June 26, 2008).
†A rapid determination of the child's cardiopulmonary status at birth. This is discussed later in the chapter.
‡All states collect a small amount of blood from the newborn to screen for a variety of inborn errors of metabolism (up to 40 different disorders, most of them quite rare). In addition, most states screen newborns for hearing loss by using special equipment.

cause of the rash. Certain viral states "sensitize" a patient to a medication. The medication may be given at other times without any problems. Whenever a parent describes a "medication allergy," ask the following questions:

> *"How do you know the child is allergic to . . . ?"*
>
> *"What was the rash like?"* A hivelike or urticarial rash is likely to be a true allergy.
>
> *"Did the child have any problems other than the rash?"*
>
> *"How long after the child started the medication* did the rash appear?"*
>
> *"After the medication was stopped, how long did the rash last?"*
>
> *"Has the child ever taken the medication again with recurrence of the rash?"*

Nutrition

Nutrition is central to the child's well-being. Getting a complete *nutritional history* not only helps you monitor the child's health but may also help you make the diagnosis of an acute problem. Ask the following questions:

> *"Is the child being breast-fed?"* If yes, *"How often? For how long at each feeding? Is vitamin D or supplemental fluoride being given?"*
>
> *"How many ounces of formula†️ is the baby given a day? What kind of formula do you feed? How do you prepare it?"*
>
> *"When did you introduce solid foods, such as cereals?"*
>
> *"Has the child ever had a problem with vomiting? diarrhea? constipation? colic? Would you describe the child as 'a fussy eater'?"*

For infants, differentiate diarrhea from normal liquid stools. If the child is breast-fed, the stools are usually a yellow or mustard-colored liquid and may follow each feeding. If the child is formula-fed, the stools are more likely to be yellowish-tan and firmer. Infants frequently have green, brown, or grayish stools, and normal stools may be loose or liquid in consistency. With diarrhea, the stools are more frequent and all liquid, and watery rings stain the infant's diaper. Minor changes in the stool are common. Normal infants may have several bowel movements a day but may go 1 or more days without a bowel movement. Small, hard, pebble-like stools indicate constipation.

Until an infant is 1 year of age, breast milk or infant formula should be his or her main food. Cow's milk may be fine for older children, but it may irritate the infant's digestive system, which is not fully developed. There are some major differences between cow's milk and breast milk or formula: Cow's milk has too much protein and sodium and too little iron, vitamin C, copper, and zinc for developing infants; also, the type of fat in cow's milk is poorly absorbed by infants.

For a toddler or older child, determine how many ounces of milk and juice the child drinks. Inquire about the daily consumption of vegetables, fruit, protein, and "junk foods." Does the child take a vitamin supplement? It is also valuable to ask about the meal pattern: Does he or she eat breakfast, lunch, dinner, and snacks? Where does he or she eat? With whom? Older children and adolescents eat many meals away from home; such patients are your best source of information about their eating patterns.

Growth and Development

Ask about the child's pattern of growth. As is discussed later, the height, weight, and head circumference of children should be plotted on appropriate growth curves. Has the child's growth been consistent, or has he or she crossed percentile lines on the growth chart? Is the mother concerned about her child's growth?

---

*The typical ampicillin rash occurs about 7 to 8 days after the drug is started and is not considered a penicillin allergy.
†️The normal newborn can take 15 to 20 ounces a day.

Ask, "How has the child been growing? Are you concerned about his or her weight gain or about his or her linear growth?" Asking about how quickly the child outgrows shoes and clothes may give you an indication of his or her growth rate.

The *child's characteristics* or *temperament during infancy* may be predictive of early developmental progress and of how he or she will respond to new experiences in years to come.

Ask, "Would you describe your child as active, average, or quiet?" If this is not the mother's first child, it is appropriate to ask how this infant compares with the family's other children: Is this child slower, faster, or about the same in development?

> *"When did the child first sleep through the night?"*
>
> *"Do you have any concerns about the child's development?* If yes, *"What are they?"*
>
> *"Has the child ever failed to make progress or ever lost any ability he or she once had?"*
>
> *"Does the child have difficulty keeping up with other children?"*

After asking general questions about the child's development, you need to get information about specific *developmental milestones* that reflect the child's ability in four areas: gross motor, language, fine motor, and personal/social development. The following questions should be asked:

> *"At what age did the child roll over for the first time? sit without support? point at objects? wave 'bye-bye'? recognize objects by name? stand holding on? walk without support? say his or her first words? walk up and down stairs without support? learn to dress himself or herself? learn to tie shoes? put two words together? speak in full sentences?"*
>
> *"At what age was the child toilet-trained?"*
>
> *"How old do you think your child acts now?"*
>
> *"How often does your child have tantrums?"*

The *Denver Developmental Screening Test*, shown in Figure 24-1, was developed to detect developmental delays in the first 6 years of a child's life, with special emphasis on the first 2 years. It is standardized on the basis of findings from a large group of children in the Denver, Colorado, area and tests the four main areas of development indicated previously. A line is drawn from top to bottom of the sheet according to the age of the child. Each of the milestones crossed by this line is tested. Each milestone has a bar that indicates the percentage of the "standard" population that should be able to perform this task. Failure to perform an item passed by 90% of children is significant. Two failures in any of the four main areas indicate a developmental delay. This test is a screening device for developmental delays; it is not an intelligence test.

For the school-aged child, the child's social, motor, and language development, as well as emotional maturation, are reflected in current behavior. A nice way to broach this topic is to ask, "How would you describe your child as a person?" Follow up with some or all of these questions:

> *"What do you enjoy the most about your child? the least?"*
>
> *"Does your child usually complete what he or she starts?"*
>
> *"How does your child get along with other children his or her age?"*
>
> *"How many hours of sleep does your child get each night?"*
>
> *"Does the child have any recurrent nightmares?"*
>
> *"Does the child have temper tantrums?"* Whereas tantrums in toddlers and preschoolers are not unusual at those ages, tantrums in a school-aged child are unusual and may indicate potentially serious problems.
>
> *"What type of responsibility can he or she be given?"*
>
> *"How old was your child when he or she started school?"*
>
> *"In what grade is he or she now?"*

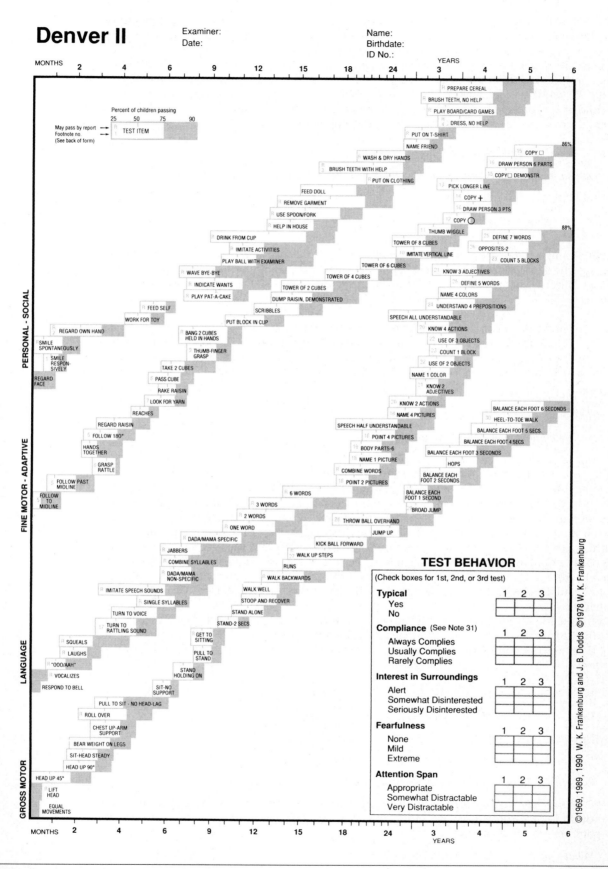

Figure 24–1 Denver Developmental Screening Test. (Reprinted with permission from William K. Frankenburg, MD, Denver Developmental Materials, Inc., Denver, Colo.)

DIRECTIONS FOR ADMINISTRATION

1. Try to get child to smile by smiling, talking, or waving. Do not touch him/her.
2. Child must stare at hand several seconds.
3. Parent may help guide toothbrush and put toothpaste on brush.
4. Child does not have to be able to tie shoes or button/zip in the back.
5. Move yarn slowly in an arc from one side to the other, about 8" above child's face.
6. Pass if child grasps rattle when it is touched to the backs or tips of fingers.
7. Pass if child tries to see where yarn went. Yarn should be dropped quickly from sight from tester's hand without arm movement.
8. Child must transfer cube from hand to hand without help of body, mouth, or table.
9. Pass if child picks up raisin with any part of thumb and finger.
10. Line can vary only 30 degrees or less from tester's line. ∕
11. Make a fist with thumb pointing upward and wiggle only the thumb. Pass if child imitates and does not move any fingers other than the thumb.

 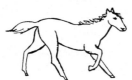 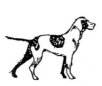

12. Pass any enclosed form. Fail continuous round motions.
13. Which line is longer? (Not bigger.) Turn paper upside down and repeat. (pass 3 of 3 or 5 of 6)
14. Pass any lines crossing near midpoint.
15. Have child copy first. If failed, demonstrate.

When giving items 12, 14, and 15, do not name the forms. Do not demonstrate 12 and 14.

16. When scoring, each pair (2 arms, 2 legs, etc.) counts as one part.
17. Place one cube in cup and shake gently near child's ear, but out of sight. Repeat for other ear.
18. Point to picture and have child name it. (No credit is given for sounds only.)
    If less than 4 pictures are named correctly, have child point to picture as each is named by tester.

   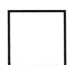 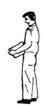

19. Using doll, tell child: Show me the nose, eyes, ears, mouth, hands, feet, tummy, hair. Pass 6 of 8.
20. Using pictures, ask child: Which one flies?... says meow?... talks?... barks?... gallops? Pass 2 of 5, 4 of 5.
21. Ask child: What do you do when you are cold?... tired?... hungry? Pass 2 of 3, 3 of 3.
22. Ask child: What do you do with a cup? What is a chair used for? What is a pencil used for?
    Action words must be included in answers.
23. Pass if child correctly places <u>and</u> says how many blocks are on paper. (1, 5).
24. Tell child: Put block **on** table; **under** table; **in front of** me, **behind** me. Pass 4 of 4.
    (Do not help child by pointing, moving head or eyes.)
25. Ask child: What is a ball?... lake?... desk?... house?... banana?... curtain?... fence?... ceiling? Pass if defined in terms of use, shape, what it is made of, or general category (such as banana is fruit, not just yellow). Pass 5 of 8, 7 of 8.
26. Ask child: If a horse is big, a mouse is __? If fire is hot, ice is __? If the sun shines during the day, the moon shines during the __? Pass 2 of 3.
27. Child may use wall or rail only, not person. May not crawl.
28. Child must throw ball overhand 3 feet to within arm's reach of tester.
29. Child must perform standing broad jump over width of test sheet (8 1/2 inches).
30. Tell child to walk forward, ⚬⚬⚬⚬➤ heel within 1 inch of toe. Tester may demonstrate.
    Child must walk 4 consecutive steps.
31. In the second year, half of normal children are non-compliant.

OBSERVATIONS:

Figure 24–1 cont'd

"How is he or she doing in school?"

"Has he or she ever been left back?"

"Has your child's teacher ever told you that he or she suspects a problem?" If yes, *"What is the problem?"*

"What is your child's grade level for reading? math?"

"What does your child enjoy doing during his or her free time?"

"What kinds of things scare him or her?"

"How does the child get along with his or her brothers and sisters?"

"How much time does your child spend watching TV? playing video games? on the computer?"

"Does he or she have a TV in his or her room?"

It is useful to ask whether the child has any disturbing habits. This question allows the parent or guardian to vent any previously unexpressed concerns. This may be asked as follows:

"Is there anything about the child's behavior that worries you or that is different from that of other children?"

In 2007, because of striking increase in the prevalence of autism and autistic spectrum disorders, the American Academy of Pediatrics recommended screening all children for the following behaviors:

- Not turning when the parent says the baby's name
- Not turning to look when the parent points and says "Look at . . . ," and not pointing themselves to show parents an interesting object or event
- Lack of back-and-forth babbling
- Smiling late
- Failure to make eye contact with people

Because it is clear that early intervention can significantly improve the outcome for children with autism and autistic spectrum disorders, the Academy recommends that this screening be performed at least twice during the first 2 years of life.

Immunization History

The pediatric history contains detailed information about *immunizations*. The current recommended immunization schedule, as of October 2008, is shown in Table 24-1. Because the

Table 24–1 Table of Vaccines by Age Group

2, 4, and 6 months	DTaP IPV Hep B HIB PCV Rotavirus
6 months–5 years	Annual influenza vaccine
12 months	MMR VAR Hep A
12-18 months	Booster doses of DTaP, HIB, PCV Hep A, second dose (IPV, Hep B*)
4-6 years	DTap, fifth dose MMR, second dose VAR
11 years and up	Tdap MCV4 HPV4

Note: The vaccine schedule changes frequently. Also, new combination vaccines become available; please refer to the *www.cdc.gov/nip* immunization web site (accessed June 26, 2008) for the latest indications, and refer to the package inserts for individual vaccine products.
DTaP, diphtheria and tetanus toxoids and acellular pertussis vaccine; Hep A, hepatitis A vaccine; Hep B, hepatitis B vaccine; HIB, *Hemophilus influenzae* type B vaccine; HPV4, human papillomavirus vaccine (as of 2008, licensed only for girls and women); IPV, inactivated poliovirus vaccine; MCV4, conjugated meningococcal vaccine; MMR, live attenuated measles, mumps, and rubella; VAR, varicella vaccine; PCV, pneumococcal conjugate vaccine; Rotavirus, oral, live attenuated rotavirus vaccine; Tdap, tetanus, reduced-dose diphtheria toxoids, and acellular pertussis vaccine.
*The third doses of these two vaccines can be given as early as 6 months, but should be given by 18 months if not given earlier.

immunization schedule is updated every 6 months, please refer to the Centers for Disease Control and Prevention web site at *www.cdc.gov/nip* (accessed June 26, 2008).

Vaccines are one of the major successes of 20th century medicine; clinicians are unlikely to ever see many of the vaccine-preventable diseases such as polio or diphtheria, and if an immunized child does have one of these diseases, that child may have an immune deficiency. However, if the child is missing one or more vaccines, you should consider the possibility the child is suffering from a vaccine-preventable illness.

As the schedule of vaccines has become rather complex, many parents are unsure about the exact vaccines given to the child. Ask to see the immunization record, which many parents carry with them. Also, many localities have centralized vaccine registries where health-care providers can access the record of a particular child.

You can partially reconstruct the child's vaccine history, if necessary, with the following questions:

"How many sets of vaccines has your child had?" (The primary series is given at 2, 4, and 6 months of age.)

"How many injections did the child get each time?" (Most schedules will have 2 or more injections per visit.)

"Did the child get shots right after his or her first birthday? How many?"

"How about at 15 to 18 months?"

"What shots did he or she get before kindergarten?"

For the child 11 or older, ask, "Has she gotten any vaccines recently? How many?" Recent additions to the vaccine schedule provide adolescents with protection against pertussis, meningococcal disease, hepatitis A, and, for girls, human papillomavirus, the leading cause of cervical cancer. Also ask, "Did your child have a reaction to any of the shots?"

For an older child, ask "Has he or she ever had chickenpox?" See the Clinicopathologic Correlations section at the end of this chapter for a detailed description of this disease, whose incidence is decreasing.

Social and Environmental History

The *social and environmental history* should include the parents' ages and occupations, as well as the current living conditions. Ask these questions:

"How many rooms do you live in?"

"Who lives in your home?"

"Are there any pets?"

"Does anyone in the household smoke? Are there carpets? Is dust a problem? Are there problems with cockroaches or other environmental contaminants?"

"Does the child sleep in his or her own room? Does the child sleep in a crib or a bed? Does the child sleep in the parents' bed?"

"Is the child cared for in any other house?"

"Who supervises the child during the day?"

"How does the family have fun together?"

"Do both the child's parents share in family life?"

"What is the condition of the paint and plaster in your home?"

"Has the child had any known exposure to lead?"

Dust and chips from deteriorating lead-based paint are the most common sources of lead exposure in young children. Although the rates and severity of pediatric lead poisoning have declined in the United States, childhood lead poisoning remains a problem throughout the world. The effects of lead poisoning are more pervasive and longer lasting in children than previously believed, and they occur at levels once thought safe. Prenatal exposure and exposure in children 2 to 3 years of age are of particular concern. In 2006, elevated blood lead levels were found in 39,000 children* on screening blood tests. Children who are younger than 6 years, especially 1- and 2-year-olds, are at greatest risk because of normal hand-to-mouth activity. Although pica (a morbid craving to ingest nonfood substances such as chalk or coal) has been implicated in lead poisoning, children more commonly ingest lead-containing dust through normal hand-to-mouth activity. Ask the parent or guardian the following:

> *"Does the child live in or visit a home that was built before 1960?"*
>
> *"Has any renovation been done in your home recently?"*
>
> *"Does the child have a sibling, house mate, or friend with an elevated blood level of lead?"*
>
> *"Has the child visited other countries for substantial periods of time?"*
>
> *"Does the child live near a heavily traveled major highway, bridge, or elevated train?"*
>
> *"Does the family use ceramic pottery from another country?"*
>
> *"Does the child come in contact with an adult whose job or hobby involves exposure to lead?"*

If the answer to any of these questions is yes, the child should be tested with a direct blood lead test.

Other questions related to safety in and around the home concern the presence of smoke detectors and window guards in the home, use of a crib with the child sleeping on his or her back, supervision and hot water temperature during baths, and use of car seats and bicycle helmets.

Family History

The pediatric *family history* is basically the same as in the adult history but may play a more significant role in identifying genetic disorders and inborn errors of metabolism. When taking the family history of a pediatric patient, it is worthwhile to construct a *pedigree* or *genogram*, a graphic representation of the family history. As illustrated in Figure 24-2, in a pedigree, boys and men are represented by squares; girls and women are represented by circles; the patient, or

*See *www.cdc.gov/nchs/lead/surv/stats.htm*.

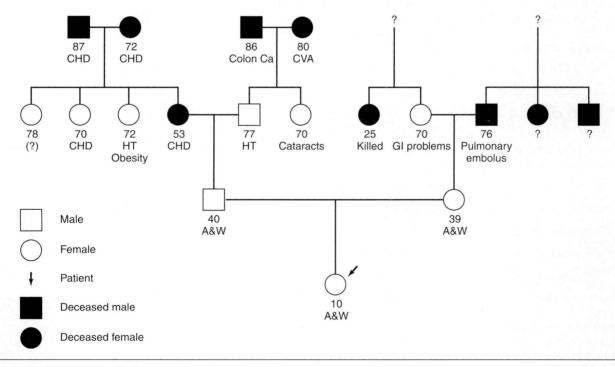

Figure 24–2 Pedigree (family tree). A&W, alive and well; Ca, cancer; CHD, coronary heart disease; CVA, cerebrovascular accident; GI, gastrointestinal; HT, hypertension.

proband, is illustrated with an arrow; and for individuals who are deceased, the shape is black, or a line is drawn through the circle or square. Information about three generations should be obtained: that is, the child and his or her siblings; the parents and their siblings; and the grandparents. For each individual, the following information should be obtained:

- If alive, name and current age
- Presence of any illnesses, such as diabetes, asthma, coronary artery disease, hypertension, stroke, and cancer
- Presence of birth defects or genetic disorders such as sickle cell disease, hemophilia, cystic fibrosis and Tay-Sachs disease; if known, each individual's carrier status for any of these conditions should be noted as well
- Any miscarriages or children who died in infancy or later
- If deceased, age at and cause of death
- Presence of consanguinity

By analyzing the pedigree, the examiner can gain insight into the child's risk for having specific diseases in the future.

Review of Systems

The *review of systems* needs to be age-appropriate, and so it is described along with the approach to the physical examination in the following sections.

The Adolescent Interview

The adolescent interview can present a number of special challenges, as well as its own special delights.

Adolescents, aged 13 to 22 years, make up 15% of the U.S. population. Too old to be considered children but too young to be considered adults, adolescents may avoid health care because they do not feel comfortable either at the pediatrician's office or at an internist's office. On the other hand, mortality rates are almost five times higher among 15- to 24-year-olds than among 5- to 14-year-olds, and adolescents experience considerable morbidity. Perhaps 20% of adolescents have a chronic health condition, and many suffer consequences of engaging in adult behaviors: sexual activity, drug and alcohol use, driving, paid employment, and competitive sports. Adolescents' limited life experience and their psychologic stage (described as "adolescent egocentrism") magnify the risks of these exposures. The rapid physical changes in a teenager's body come at a time when the psychologic process of forming a body image is at its strongest; the mismatch between the actual and the desired physique can be a serious source of distress for a teenager. Major mental illness, from depression to schizophrenia, can manifest in this age range as well.

Until ages 11 to 12 years, the pediatric history is usually obtained from the child and parent together. Both sources continue to be important, but it is essential to give an adolescent private time with the doctor. In fact, laws in most states entitle adolescents to *confidential care* for sexually transmitted diseases, pregnancy, and drug use.

Early in the visit, it is vital to establish the ground rules about confidentiality with both the parent and the teenager, as well as to support the parent's role in their son's or daughter's health care. For instance, the clinician may say something like, "For someone your son's age, it's very important for him to have a private visit with his doctor, just as it would be for you with your doctor. I will keep what he and I talk about confidential unless something comes up that is acutely life-threatening. While it's crucial that *I* keep what he tells me confidential, I also encourage my teenaged patients to share with their parents what they have told me."

The HEADS mnemonic is a useful tool for remembering the main topics for the private adolescent interview. Beginning with more neutral questions about home, education, and activities can promote the teenager's comfort, and the teenager can see how you respond to disclosures. For "**H**ome," you might ask the following questions:

"How are things at home?'

"What are your responsibilities?"

"What are the rules that you have to follow?"

"Do you have brothers or sisters? How do you get along? What sort of things do you argue about?"

If the situation warrants it, you might need to ask, "Do you feel safe at home?"
For "**E**ducation," you can ask the following questions:

"How is school going?"

"What grade are you in?"

"What school do you go to?"

"What subjects are you taking?"

"What do you like best? least?"

"What are your future plans?"

"Do you feel safe at school?"

If indicated, you might need to ask the following questions:

"Have you been involved in any fights?"

"Have you ever been suspended? What was that about?"

"**A**" can stand for "activities" or "alcohol." Some questions about activities are as follows:

"Are you involved in any clubs or sports?"

"What do you do after school?"

"What do you like to do with your friends?"

"Are your friends mostly girls? mostly boys? both?"

Asking about alcohol use broaches a potentially sensitive subject, and there are many ways to introduce it; for instance:

"Do any of your friends use alcohol? Have you ever tried it?"

"Lots of kids your age are curious about drinking. How about you?"

"You mentioned that you like to go to clubs with your friends. Are any of you served alcohol there? How about you?"

If the teenager does report drinking, then you need to explore how much, how often, and whether there have been negative consequences: for example, losing consciousness, a "driving while intoxicated" (DWI) offense, or a suspension from school.

"**D**" stands for "drugs" or "depression." Drug use can be asked about in the same way as alcohol. Remember that nicotine and other chemicals in tobacco are drugs. Screening for depression merits special emphasis. Suicide is one of the top three causes of death among teenagers, and at least 50% of teenagers who complete suicide had visited a physician in the preceding 2 weeks. Therefore, at every visit with a teenager, ask something like:

"How has your mood been?"

"Do you ever find yourself feeling down and sad for more than a few hours?"

If the teenager admits to a depressed mood, then you need to probe further:

"How would you describe your mood?"

Thoughts of suicide on the part of a teenager are a clear-cut indication to violate confidentiality. You must involve the parent or another responsible adult in getting the adolescent prompt mental health care.

The "**S**" stands for "safety" and "sex." Safety refers not only to personal safety practices, such as using a seat belt or wearing a bike helmet, but also to the risk of violence in interpersonal relations: at home, with an intimate partner, at school, or in the community.

Almost 50% of students in 9th through 12th grades have initiated sexual activity, 6% of them before age 13 (2005 Youth Risk Behavior Survey).* Half of the new cases of sexually transmitted diseases occur in people aged 15 to 24 years, and almost 1 million girls aged 15 to 19 years become pregnant each year.

There are many ways to introduce the topic of sexual activity. For instance, you can *normalize* the questions: "I know that lots of people your age are thinking about having sex. How about you?" It may also be very helpful to explain your "need to know": "In order to understand what is causing your pain, I need to know something about your sexual experiences." However or whenever you bring it up, it is useful to be explicit: Something like "Have you ever had sex?" is more likely to tell you what you need to know than "Are you sexually active?" The teenager may answer no to the second question because he or she has not had sex in 2 weeks. It is also important to consider the possibility that your patient is having sex with someone of the same gender and to phrase your questions with as little heterosexual bias as possible.

It can be challenging to maintain your composure when a teenager discloses high-risk behavior to you. You need to help the teenager appreciate the risk that he or she is incurring at the same time that you support your relationship with your patient. One way to handle this is to invite the teenager to reflect on his or her own behavior:

> *"You decided to get a ride home with Jason after he put away several beers. How are you feeling about that decision now?"*

> *"I think we were both worried that you might have gotten pregnant last weekend, when you had sex without a condom. How do you think you could have handled that situation differently?"*

A large number of teenagers who are sexually promiscuous turn out to have been victims of incest or sexual abuse as children. In more than 80% of all cases of sexual abuse, the molester is not a stranger. All children should be told that their bodies are private and that no one has the right to touch them in a way that makes them feel uncomfortable. Children need to know that there are different types of touch: *Good* touches are hugs, kisses, and pats; *confusing* touch is tickling or rubbing; *bad* touch is hitting, hurting, spanking, or touching or fondling the "private parts" of their bodies. Listen carefully to a child who describes any type of sexual abuse. Children do not confabulate sexually explicit stories. If the clinical circumstances warrant, a child older than 3 years of age can be asked the following:

> *"Has anyone touched your body in any way that made you feel uncomfortable or confused?"*

A child who has been sexually or physically abused may exhibit behavior such as aggression, moodiness, irritability, withdrawal, regression, memory loss, insecurity, and clinging. In addition, the child may exhibit some of the following physical changes: torn or bloody clothing, bruises or other suspect injuries, difficulty in walking or sitting, loss of appetite, stomach problems, genital soreness or burning sensation, difficulty in urination, vaginal or penile discharge, excessive bathing, or a desire not to bathe at all. An older child in school may exhibit a drop in academic performance, prevarication, stealing, or even running away from home.

Adolescents and even younger children now spend a great deal of time exploring the Internet, which is both a boon and a source of concern. Ask the youngster about the family's rules about using the Internet. Specifically, ask the following:

> *"How much time each day do you spend online?"*

> *"Do you have a page on MySpace or FaceBook or something similar?"*

> *"Have you ever been a victim of 'cyber-bullying'? Have you ever gone out with someone you met online?"*

The American Academy of Pediatrics has published guidelines for youngsters and families to minimize the hazards of Internet use.[†]

---

*CDC Youth Behavior Surveillance—US, 2005. MMWR Surveill Summ 55(55-S), June 9, 2006.
[†]See *http://safetynet.aap.org* (accessed June 27, 2008).

Table 24–2 Apgar Scale

Sign	Score		
	0	**1**	**2**
Color	Blue pale	Pink body with blue extremities	Completely pink
Heart rate	Absent	Below 100	Over 100
Reflex irritability*	No response	Grimace	Sneeze or cough
Muscle tone	Flaccid	Some flexion of the extremities	Good flexion of the extremities
Respiratory effort	Absent	Weak, irregular	Good, crying

The acronym *APGAR* is useful for remembering the examinations of the Apgar test: **A**ppearance, or color; **P**ulse, or heart rate; **G**rimace, or reflex irritability; **A**ctivity, or muscle tone; **R**espiratory effort.

Examination of the Newborn

When examining the newborn, you are trying to answer three questions:

1. How well is this infant making the transition to extrauterine life?
2. Is there any evidence of birth trauma?
3. Does this infant have any evidence of congenital malformations?

The newborn is assessed in the delivery room immediately after birth to determine the integrity of the cardiopulmonary system. The infant is dried with a towel and placed on a warming table, where the initial examination is conducted. Gloves are worn for this initial examination, because the newborn is coated with the mother's vaginal secretions and blood.

The initial examination consists of the evaluation of five signs:

1. Color
2. Heart rate
3. Reflex irritability*
4. Muscle tone
5. Respiratory effort

Dr. Virginia Apgar developed a scale for rating these signs 1 and 5 minutes after birth. The *Apgar scale* is shown in Table 24-2. Each of the signs is scored from 0 to 2. At 1 minute, a total score of 3 to 4 indicates severe cardiopulmonary depression, and the infant requires immediate resuscitative measures; a score from 5 to 6 indicates mild depression. The tests are repeated at 5 minutes; a score of 8 or more indicates grossly normal findings of the cardiopulmonary examination.

General Assessment

After the Apgar score has been determined, the *gestational age* should be assessed. Because gestational age based on menstrual dates is frequently inaccurate, it is important to make an objective determination of the gestational age, which is an indicator of the maturity of the newborn. Gestational age has important implications for the challenges of adaptation the infant will face in the coming hours and days. Experienced clinicians can make a fairly accurate assessment of gestational age in the delivery room. A more formal assessment is then performed in the nursery; it should be done in the first 24 hours after the infant's birth. The standardized system for assessing gestational age is the *Ballard Clinical Assessment*. This is based on 10 neurologic signs and 11 external signs such as skin texture, breast size, and genital development. The neurologic scoring system is shown in Figure 24-3, and the external criteria are shown in Table 24-3.

The total scores of the neurologic and external signs are summed. The sum is then correlated with the gestational age, according to the graph shown in Figure 24-4. A sum between 46 and 60 is associated with a gestational age of 37 to 41 weeks. A child with a gestational age from 37 to 41 weeks is denoted a *term infant*, although some authorities believe that a gestational age of

*Passage of a small catheter through the external nares to the pharynx, which is done to determine "reflex irritability," can also determine patency of the internal nasal choanae. See later discussion under "Nose."

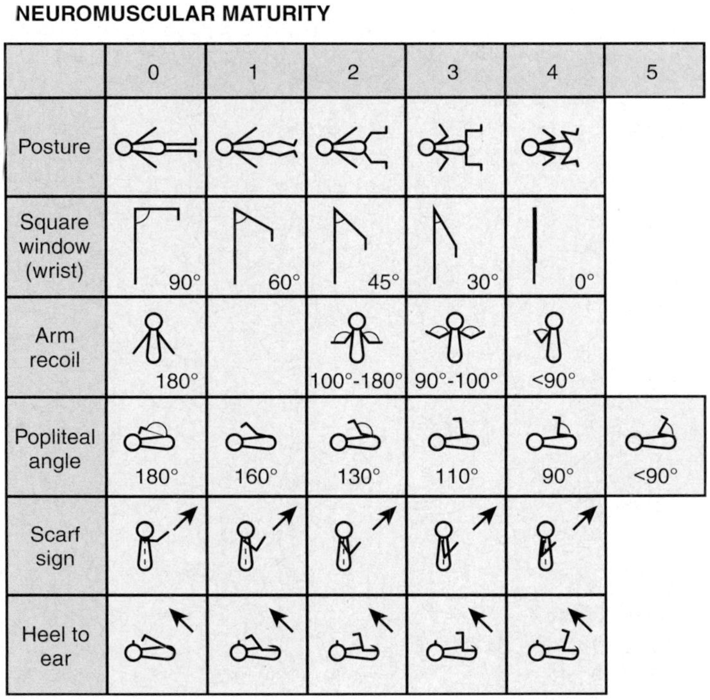

NEUROMUSCULAR MATURITY

Figure 24–3 Ballard Clinical Assessment. (Reprinted with permission from Ballard J, Novak K, Driver M: A simplified score for assessment of fetal maturation of newly born infants. J Pediatr 95:769, 1979.) Following are some notes on techniques for assessing the neurologic criteria:

Posture: Observed with infant quiet and in supine position. Score 0, arms and legs extended; 1, beginning of flexion of hips and knees, arms extended; 2, stronger flexion of legs, arms extended; 3, arms slightly flexed, legs flexed and abducted; 4, full flexion of arms and legs.

Square window: The hand is flexed on the forearm between the thumb and index finger of the examiner. Enough pressure is applied to get as full a flexion as possible, and the angle between the hypothenar eminence and the ventral aspect of the forearm is measured and graded according to the diagram. (Care is taken not to rotate the infant's wrist while performing this maneuver.)

Arm recoil: With the infant in the supine position, the forearms are first flexed for 5 seconds, then fully extended by pulling on the hands, and then released. The sign is fully positive if the arms return briskly to full flexion (score 2). If the arms return to incomplete flexion or the response is sluggish, it is scored as 1. If they remain extended or show only random movements, the score is 0.

Popliteal angle: With the infant supine and the pelvis flat on the examining couch, the thigh is held in the knee-to-chest position, with the examiner's left index finger and thumb supporting the knee. The leg is then extended by gentle pressure from the examiner's right index finger behind the ankle, and the popliteal angle is measured.

Scarf sign: With the infant supine, the examiner takes the infant's hand and tries to put it around the neck and as far posteriorly as possible around the opposite shoulder. This maneuver is assisted by lifting the elbow across the body. How far the elbow goes across is measured and graded according to the illustrations. Score 0, elbow reaches opposite axillary line; 1, elbow reaches between midline and opposite axillary line; 2, elbow reaches midline; 3, elbow does not reach midline.

Heel-to-ear maneuver: With the infant supine, the examiner draws the infant's foot as near to the head as it will go without forcing it. The examiner observes the distance between the foot and the head, as well as the degree of extension at the knee, and grades according to the diagram. Note that the knee is left free and may draw down alongside the abdomen.

38 to 42 weeks defines a term infant (see Fig. 24-4). A child with a gestational age of less than 37 weeks is *preterm;* one with a gestational age of more than 41 weeks (or 42 weeks) is *post-term.*

The newborn infant is also weighed, but weight alone does not determine maturational age. The birth weight is correlated with gestational age according to the standard classification of Battaglia and Lubchenco, which is shown in Figure 24-5. By this method, the infant is classified as being small, appropriate, or large for gestational age. If the birth weight is between the 10th and 90th percentiles, the infant is *appropriate for gestational age* (AGA). If the birth weight is lower than the 10th percentile on the intrauterine growth curve, the newborn is classified *small for gestational age* (SGA). If the birth weight is higher than the 90th percentile, the newborn is called *large for gestational age* (LGA).

The value of the weight for gestational age determination lies in its ability to predict certain risk groups. Many babies who are LGA are infants of diabetic mothers. Such infants are at risk for a number of complications, both in the immediate neonatal period and later in life.

Table 24–3 Scoring System for External Criteria of Ballard Clinical Assessment

External Sign			Score			
	0	**1**	**2**	**3**	**4**	**5**
Skin	Gelatinous red, transparent	Smooth, pink, visible veins	Superficial peeling and/or rash, few veins	Cracking pale area, rare veins	Parchment deep cracking, no vessels	Leathery, cracked, wrinkled
Lanugo	None	Abundant	Thinning	Bald areas	Mostly bald	
Plantar creases	No crease	Faint red marks	Anterior transverse crease only	Creases anterior 2/3	Creases cover entire sole	
Breast	Barely perceptible	Flat areola, no bud	Stippled areola, 1-2 mm bud	Raised areola, 3-4 mm bud	Full areola, 5-10 mm bud	
Ear	Pinna flat, stays folded	Sl. curved pinna; soft c̄ slow recoil	Well-curv. pinna; soft but ready recoil	Formed and firm c̄ instant recoil	Thick cartilage ear stiff	
Genitals (male)	Scrotum empty, no rugae		Testes descending, few rugae	Testes down, good rugae	Testes pendulous, deep rugae	
Genitals (female)	Prominent clitoris and labia minora		Majora and minora equally prominent	Majora large, minora small	Clitoris and minora completely covered	

Maturity Rating

Score	Weeks
5	26
10	28
15	30
20	32
25	34
30	36
35	38
40	40
45	42
50	44

Reprinted with permission from Ballard J, Novak K, Driver M: A simplified score for assessment of fetal maturation of newly born infants. J Pediatr 95:769, 1979.

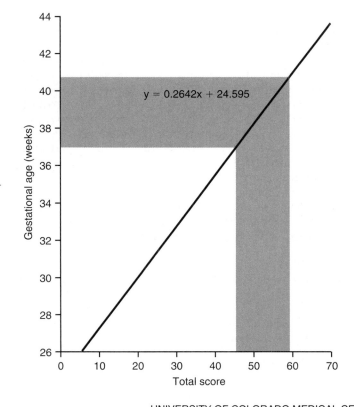

Figure 24–4 Graph for determining gestational age on the basis of neurologic criteria and external signs.

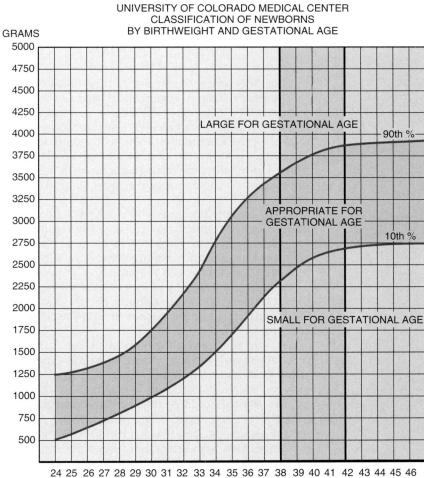

Figure 24–5 Classification of newborns by birth weight and gestational age.

These infants must be carefully monitored for hypoglycemia and polycythemia; they are more likely to have hyperbilirubinemia in the first 3 days after birth, and they are three to five times more likely to have a congenital malformation than are infants in the general population. In infants who are SGA, major considerations include the presence of a chromosomal abnormality, such as trisomy 13 or trisomy 18, or exposure to a teratogenic agent, such as alcohol or a congenital infection during gestation. Children who were SGA must also be monitored for hypoglycemia during the immediate neonatal period. Also, all preterm newborns, even if they do not have *low birth weight* (<2500 g), are at risk for respiratory distress secondary to surfactant deficiency, for hypoglycemia, and for hypocalcemia.

The remainder of the examination is usually performed in the warmed environment of the nursery, often within 24 hours after birth. Before examining the child, review some key historical facts with the mother and the nurses:

"How is the child feeding? Is there any coughing or choking during feedings? How much weight has the baby lost?" (Newborns often lose weight, up to 10% of birth weight, in the first week. They should regain birth weight by the end of the second week.)

"Has the child vomited?" If so, *"What has the child vomited?"*

"Is there any drooling?" Drooling in the newborn can be a sign of esophageal atresia.

"Has there been any respiratory distress, noisy breathing, or cyanosis?"

"Has the child voided?" Failure to void within 48 hours of birth may signify renal failure or urinary tract obstruction.

"Has there been any abdominal distention?"

"Has the child passed meconium?" Failure to pass meconium (the first material to be evacuated from the bowels) by 48 hours of age may indicate bowel obstruction, meconium ileus (seen in cystic fibrosis), or Hirschsprung's disease.

"Have there been any tremors or seizure-like activity?" Tremors may indicate hypoglycemia or hypocalcemia, either of which necessitates prompt attention.

Thus, this review of systems for a newborn is brief but significant.

The comprehensive examination begins with inspection. If the infant has achieved temperature stability, then he or she should be undressed except for the diaper. Is there evidence of respiratory distress or cyanosis? (If so, immediate intervention is indicated. If not, proceed with the rest of the examination.) The following description of the examination is in a head-to-toe sequence. However, the examiner must usually vary the order when actually performing the examination, using the infant's quiet state to listen to the heart and lungs, catching glimpses of the eyes when the infant opens them, and taking advantage of crying spells to examine the mouth.

The *respiratory rate* and degree of *respiratory effort* are carefully assessed while the infant is undressed. The respiratory rate of a newborn usually averages from 30 to 50 breaths per minute. Observe the respiratory rate for 1 to 2 minutes, because periods of apnea and periodic breathing are common, especially among preterm infants. Look for grunting respirations and for chest retractions, each of which is evidence of respiratory distress.

Determine the *pulse* by auscultation of the heart. The average heart rate of a newborn ranges from 120 to 140 beats per minute. There are wide fluctuations; the rate increases to as fast as 190 during crying and decreases to as low as 90 during sleep. A heart rate lower than 90 is of concern.

Measure the *temperature* by using a rectal thermometer. The infant is placed in a prone position on an examining table or in the examiner's lap. The infant's buttocks are spread, and a well-lubricated thermometer is inserted slowly through the anal sphincter to approximately 1 inch (2.5 cm). Note that this also establishes that the anus is patent, thereby ruling out the existence of imperforate anus. After 1 minute, the temperature may be read. Newborn infants often have relative thermal instability, and for this reason the ambient temperature should also be determined. Achieving temperature stability is one of the early adaptational challenges for a term infant and takes much longer for preterm infants. (Note that the nursing staff usually measures the newborn's temperature.)

Basic *measurements* are taken next. The infant's length is measured from the top of the head to the bottom of the feet; the length is usually between 18.5 and 20.5 inches (47 and 52 cm).

The head is measured at its greatest circumference around the occipitofrontal area. In general, three measurements are taken, the largest of which is recorded. The head circumference is usually 13.5 to 14.5 inches (34 to 37 cm). The chest circumference is normally smaller than the head circumference by 0.75 to 1.20 inches (2 to 3 cm). The chest measurement is taken at the level of the nipples midway between inspiration and expiration. By the time the child is 1 year of age, the chest circumference exceeds the head circumference. These and all other measurements performed during the physical examination should be plotted on appropriate growth curves, correcting for the gestational age.

Note the *posture.* A normal term newborn keeps the arms and legs symmetrically flexed. Relaxation of the limbs is suggestive of neurologic depression and necessitates further evaluation. The finding of one side flexed while the other side is relaxed is abnormal; such posture is suggestive of an injury, either neurologic or musculoskeletal, that occurred before or during the birthing process.

Note the *movements.* Normally, all four limbs should be moving in a random and asymmetric manner. Fine movements of the face and fingers are usually present. Abnormal movements include jerky, symmetric, coarse movements. All extremities should be moving, with full range of motion seen at some time. Injury to the *brachial plexus* may cause paralysis of the upper arm. This injury may result from lateral traction on the head and neck during delivery of the shoulder. *Erb's palsy* produces an inability to spontaneously abduct the arm at the shoulder, rotate the arm externally, flex the elbow, and supinate the forearm. This injury to the fifth and sixth cervical nerves results in a characteristic position of arm adduction, with elbow extension, forearm pronation, and arm internal rotation. The grasp reflex is usually preserved. *Klumpke's paralysis* results from injury to the seventh and eighth cervical nerves, producing paralysis of the hand and forearm. The grasp reflex is absent. Involvement of the first thoracic nerve with Klumpke's paralysis may also result in ipsilateral ptosis and miosis, or *Horner's syndrome.* The prognosis of any brachial plexus palsy depends on whether the nerve or nerves were lacerated or only bruised. If the palsy is related only to edema of the nerve fibers and not to actual injury, function usually returns within a few months.

Skin

Skin color in newborns is related partially to the amount of fat present. Preterm infants generally appear redder because they have less subcutaneous fat than do term infants.

The newborn has vasomotor instability, and the color of the skin may vary greatly from moment to moment and from one area of the body to another. It is often noted that when the infant is lying on one side for a time, a sharp color demarcation appears: The lower half of the body becomes red, and the upper half is pale. Seen more commonly in preterm than in term infants, this has been termed the *harlequin color change* and is benign. The episodes may persist from 30 seconds to 30 minutes.

Inspect for cyanosis or acrocyanosis. *Acrocyanosis* is a benign condition in which the hands and feet are cyanotic and cool but the trunk is pink and warm. This condition is common among newborns. In central *cyanosis,* the tongue and gums are also blue. Persistent central cyanosis can be suggestive of respiratory abnormalities or the presence of cyanotic congenital heart disease.

Is *plethora* present? Plethora is a condition marked by an excess of blood and a marked redness of the complexion. Plethora in the newborn usually indicates high levels of hemoglobin.

Is *pallor* present? Pallor may be associated with anemia or, more commonly, with cold stress and peripheral vasoconstriction. Pallor may also reflect asphyxia, shock, sepsis, or edema. It should be recognized that the presence of pallor may mask cyanosis in a newborn with circulatory failure.

Are there any skin findings from *birth trauma,* manifested by petechiae, ecchymoses, or lacerations?

Physiologic jaundice is found in almost 50% of all term newborns by the third or fourth day after birth. This finding, which is even more prevalent among preterm infants, results from delay in the maturation of enzymatic processes in the liver. In most cases, jaundice is a self-limited condition, resolving after 96 hours of age. However, very high levels of bilirubin in the newborn's serum can lead to a condition known as *kernicterus,* in which permanent neurologic damage may occur. As such, it is important to monitor the serum bilirubin level and to treat elevated levels with phototherapy.

Icterus appearing before the third day may indicate a pathologic condition. Disorders that must be considered are hemolytic anemia, caused by blood group incompatibility or by

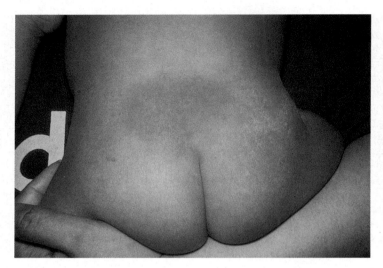

Figure 24–6 Mongolian spot.

bacterial or viral infections, and galactosemia, an inborn error of galactose metabolism. Visible jaundice in newborns does not appear until the serum bilirubin is approximately 5 mg/dL. When the level exceeds this threshold, the jaundice spreads in an orderly manner, from the top of the head to the soles of the feet. When the soles become yellow, the serum bilirubin level has usually reached 12 mg/dL. Many centers now use a transcutaneous bilirubinometer to facilitate recognizing potentially dangerous levels of jaundice.

Observe the *pigmentation*. Large, slate-blue, well-demarcated areas of pigmentation in the sacrogluteal area or elsewhere are called *mongolian spots* and are normal variants. Ninety percent of all mongolian spots are in the buttock area. These spots fade and disappear by 5 to 6 years of age in 98% of children who have them. Mongolian spots are present in more than 90% of African-American newborns and 70% of Asian-American newborns but in fewer than 10% of white newborns. Figure 24-6 shows a classic mongolian spot.

Telangiectases on the eyelids, glabella, or nape of the neck are common and frequently disappear during the first few years of life. They are often referred to as "stork bites" or "angel kisses."

Vascular nevi may be isolated defects or part of a syndrome and can be classified as malformations or hemangiomas. Hemangiomas are the most common tumors of infancy. They may be flat and are commonly caused by dilated capillaries, or they may be mass lesions and consist of large, blood-filled cavities. The *port wine stain*, also known as the *nevus flammeus*, consists of dilated capillaries and appears as a pink to purple macular lesion of variable size. It can be as large as half the body. It manifests at birth and represents a permanent defect. Figure 24-7 shows a port wine stain involving the ophthalmic division of the trigeminal nerve. Often, children with port wine stains in this area have associated capillary hemangiomas of the ipsilateral meninges and occipital portion of the cerebral cortex, a condition known as *Sturge-Weber syndrome*. Mental retardation, seizures, hemiparesis, contralateral hemianopsia, and glaucoma are often seen in the first few years of life. Figure 24-8 shows a child with Sturge-Weber syndrome (see also Fig. 10-24).

The *strawberry nevus*, or *capillary hemangioma*, is a bright red, protuberant lesion seen commonly on the face, scalp, back, or anogenital area. It may be present at birth, but it more commonly develops within the first 2 months of life. Girls are affected more often than boys. The lesion may expand rapidly, reach a stationary period, and then regress. More than 60% of capillary hemangiomas become involuted by the time the child is 5 years of age, and 95% become involuted by 9 years of age. Figure 24-9 shows a strawberry nevus.

The *cavernous hemangioma* is more deeply situated and is a cystic, often compressible lesion that is more diffuse and ill defined than the capillary hemangioma. The overlying skin may appear normal in color or may have a bluish hue. Like the capillary hemangioma, the cavernous hemangioma has a growth phase followed by a period of involution. If it is located near the trachea, life-threatening compression may result when the hemangioma enlarges. The child pictured in Figure 24-10 has a combination of a strawberry nevus and a cavernous hemangioma. The strawberry lesion overlies the cavernous hemangioma. The child pictured in Figure 24-11 has a mixed hemangioma; it has both superficial capillary and deep

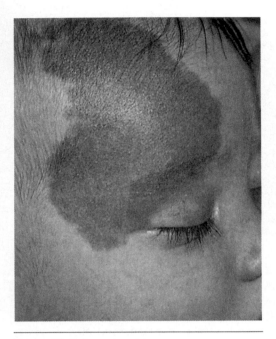

Figure 24–7 Port wine stain.

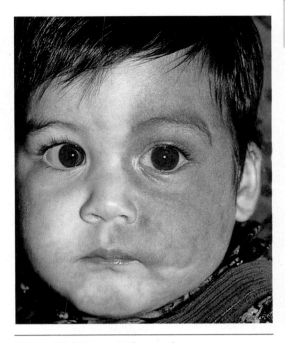

Figure 24–8 Sturge-Weber syndrome.

cavernous components. This lesion involuted by the child's third year of life. Although these lesions usually resolve by the seventh year of life, they may leave scarring, loose skin, and telangiectases. Also, as part of the Klippel-Trénaunay syndrome, they may be associated with overgrowth of a portion of the body (a complete side, an arm, a leg, or a smaller portion.)

Other birthmarks that may suggest the presence of an underlying genetic disorder include *café au lait spots* (see Fig. 8-44) and *hypopigmented macules*. One or two café au lait spots, the color of coffee with milk, are not uncommon in the newborn. In dark-skinned individuals, the macule is darker than the surrounding skin and should be described as "café sans lait" (coffee without milk). The presence of more than six of these spots, measuring greater than 0.5 cm,

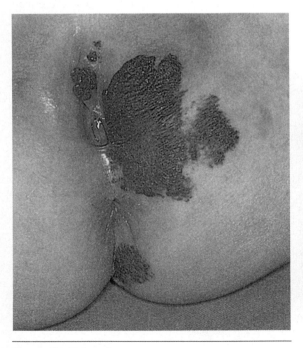

Figure 24–9 Strawberry nevus.

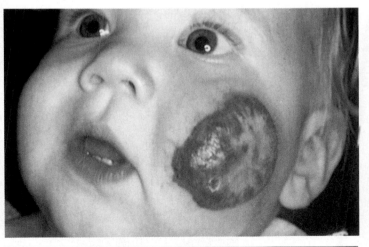

Figure 24–10 Strawberry hemangioma overlying cavernous hemangioma.

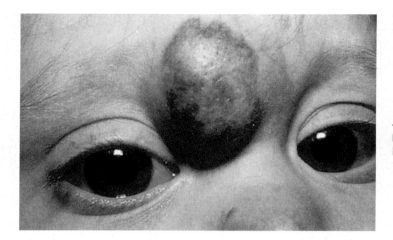

Figure 24–11 Mixed hemangioma.

is the hallmark of *neurofibromatosis type I*, an autosomal dominantly inherited condition that combines café au lait spots, axillary or inguinal freckles (see Fig. 8-47), pigmented hamartomas in the iris (*Lisch nodules*), and bony abnormalities such as scoliosis and pseudarthrosis with benign tumors of the Schwann cells called *neurofibromas*. In this condition, multiple café au lait spots are frequently the presenting feature.

The presence of *hypopigmented macules* suggests a condition known as *tuberous sclerosis complex*. In this disorder, the hypomelanotic macules (Fig. 24-12) are often described as ash-leaf shaped, with one side smooth and the other side jagged, and are associated with other dermatologic manifestations (facial angiofibromas known as *adenoma sebaceum*, and shagreen patches, as seen in Fig. 24-13), the presence of benign tumors in the brain (cortical "tubers," subependymal nodules), kidney (angiomyolipomas and cysts), and heart (rhabdomyomas), seizures, and mental retardation. Because of the significance of some of these findings, the presence of multiple hypomelanotic ash-leaf spots noted during an initial evaluation should trigger a full evaluation for associated features.

Is a *rash* present? Bullous lesions may be present at birth. One or two blisters on the lips or hands may represent "sucking blisters." Widespread blisters, many of them ruptured and leaving a collarette of scale with underlying pigmentation, represent *transient neonatal pustular melanosis*, which is benign. This condition, present at birth, is of unknown origin and is most commonly found on the trunk and extremities. It is seen in 5% of African-American newborns and in 0.5% of white newborns. Figure 24-14 shows transient neonatal pustular melanosis in a newborn. Notice the intact pustule and the ruptured pustule with a collarette of scale. The vesicopustules last 48 to 72 hours, and the pigmented macules may last 3 weeks to 3 months.

Erythema toxicum is a common rash among newborns. It is a self-limited, benign eruption of unknown cause, consisting of erythematous macules, papules, and pustules. The condition is

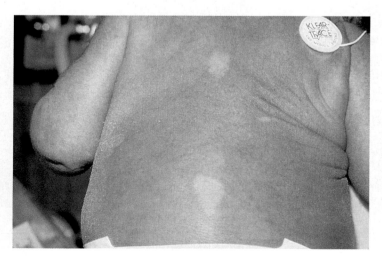

Figure 24–12 Hypopigmented macules in a newborn in whom a cardiac rhabdomyoma was diagnosed.

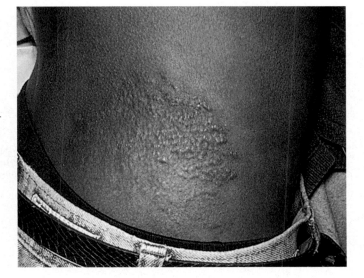

Figure 24–13 Shagreen patch.

seen in 40% of otherwise healthy term newborns; it is not seen in premature newborns. The lesions may appear anywhere on the body except on the palms and soles and have the appearance of flea bites. It is most commonly seen during the first 3 to 4 days after birth but may be present at birth. The lesions may last 2 to 3 weeks. Erythema toxicum is pictured in Figure 24-15.

Milia on the face are seen in almost 50% of all newborns. Milia appear as tiny whitish papules on the cheeks, nose, chin, and forehead and usually disappear by 3 weeks of age.

Blisters which first appear at 3 to 4 days of life may be *staphylococcal pustulosis*, which manifests as pustular or bullous skin lesions found mainly around the groin and umbilicus. The vesicular lesions of herpes simplex also usually appear after the third day after birth, up to the third week.

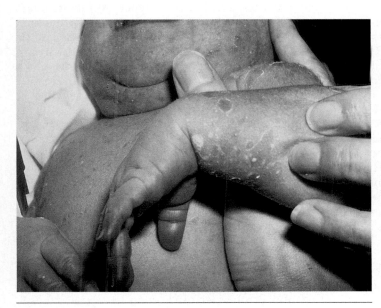

Figure 24–14 Transient neonatal pustular melanosis.

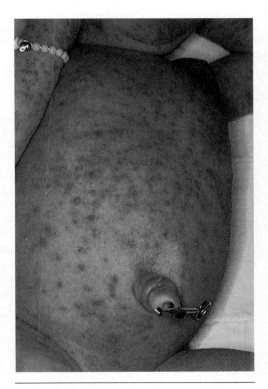

Figure 24–15 Erythema toxicum.

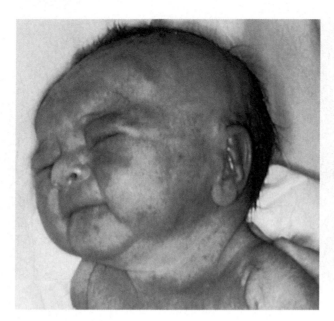

Figure 24–16 Congenital rubella with a blueberry muffin rash.

Prenatal or transplacental infections of the fetus may manifest with cutaneous symptoms. If a pregnant woman contracts rubella in the first trimester, there is a 20% chance that the infant may have the congenital rubella syndrome. A cutaneous sign of congenital rubella is the *blueberry muffin* lesion. Such lesions, which represent sites of extramedullary hematopoiesis, are bluish-red macular/papular lesions ranging in size from 2 to 8 mm. They are noted at birth or within the first 24 hours and appear on the face, neck, trunk, or extremities. Other features of the congenital rubella syndrome include eye defects, cardiac defects such as ventriculoseptal defects and valvular defects, deafness, bone lesions, hepatosplenomegaly, jaundice, thrombocytopenia, interstitial pneumonitis, and, later, mental retardation. Figure 24-16 shows a child with the classic blueberry muffin rash of congenital rubella.

Congenital syphilis may present as an erythematous maculopapular rash that later turns brown or becomes a hemorrhagic vesicular rash. This is a rash that commonly affects the palms and soles.

Is *hair* present? A newborn's skin may be covered with fine, soft, immature hair, known as *lanugo hair*. Lanugo hair frequently covers the scalp and brow in premature infants but is usually absent in term infants, except perhaps on the ears and shoulders. Inspect the lumbosacral area for tufts of hair. Tufts of hair (hypertrichosis) in this area are suggestive of the presence of an occult spina bifida or a sinus tract, anomalies that may be an external sign of tethering of the spinal cord. Figure 24-17 shows sacral hypertrichosis in a child who had a tethered spinal cord. Examine the *fingernails*. In a post-term infant, the fingernails are long and may be stained yellow if meconium was present in the amniotic fluid. Hypoplastic fingernails may be a marker for fetal alcohol syndrome.

Examine the *dermatoglyphics* of the fingers, palms, and soles. In addition to their value for identification purposes, these patterns are important indicators of genetic abnormalities. Normal finger dermatoglyphic patterns are the loop, whorl, and arch. The loop is normally the most prevalent pattern. The arch is the least prevalent pattern, and the presence of more than four arches is usually abnormal, often signaling the presence of congenital abnormalities. A single transverse palmar crease, known as a *simian crease*, is found in more than 50% of individuals with chromosomal abnormalities such as trisomy 21; however, simian creases are present in 10% of individuals who are normal.

Head

Examination of the head involves a thorough assessment of its shape, symmetry, and fontanelles. The skull may be *molded*, especially if the labor was prolonged and the head was engaged for a long period. The skull of a child born by cesarean section has a characteristic roundness.

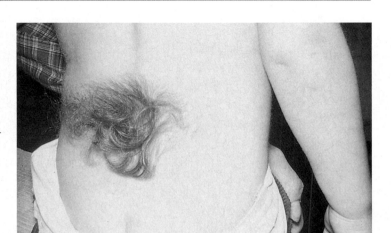

Figure 24–17 Sacral hypertrichosis.

In the newborn, the *sutures* are frequently felt as ridges as a result of the overriding of the cranial bones by molding as the skull passes through the vaginal canal. Palpate the fontanelles, or "soft spots." The *anterior fontanelle* is located at the junction of the sagittal and coronal sutures, is usually 1.5 to 2.5 inches (4 to 6 cm) in diameter, and appears diamond-shaped. The triangular *posterior fontanelle* is located at the junction of the sagittal and lambdoid sutures and measures 0.4 to 0.8 inch (1 to 2 cm) in diameter. Normally, the fontanelles are flat. A bulging fontanelle may be indicative of increased intracranial pressure; a depressed fontanelle may be seen in dehydration. Normally during crying, the fontanelles bulge. Pulsations of the fontanelles reflect the pulse. The anterior fontanelle normally closes by 18 months of age, but there is a wide range of normality; the posterior fontanelle should be closed by 2 months of age and may already be closed in the neonatal period. The locations of the fontanelles are shown in Figure 24-18.

Caput succedaneum is edema of the soft tissues over the vertex of the skull that is related to the birth process during a vertex delivery. The normal movement of the fetal head through the birth canal produces a marked molding of the very soft fetal skull and scalp edema. This swelling, which is present at delivery, crosses the sutures and resolves in the first few days. In a face presentation, there can be diffuse swelling, discoloration, and swelling of the newborn's face.

Caput succedaneum should be differentiated from a *cephalohematoma*, which is a subperiosteal hemorrhage limited to one cranial bone, often the parietal. There is no discoloration of the overlying scalp, and the swelling does not cross the suture line. The swelling is usually not visible until several hours or days after birth, inasmuch as subperiosteal bleeding is generally a slow process. About 15% of cephalohematomas are bilateral, and each is palpably distinct from the other side. No treatment is required for cephalohematomas, which are generally resorbed by 2 to 12 weeks, depending on the size. Figure 24-19 shows a newborn with a caput

Figure 24–18 Location of the fontanelles.

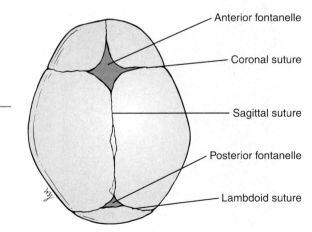

Anterior fontanelle

Coronal suture

Sagittal suture

Posterior fontanelle

Lambdoid suture

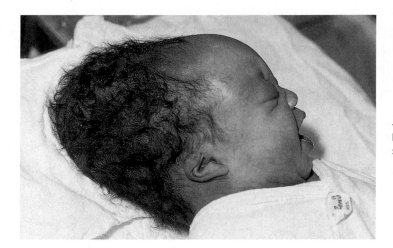

Figure 24–19 Caput succedaneum.

succedaneum; Figure 24-20 shows a child with a cephalohematoma. Note in Figure 24-20 that the swelling stops in the midline at the sagittal suture; this is characteristic of a cephalohematoma, and the extravasated blood may contribute to jaundice.

A few days after delivery, the head shape should return to normal. An unusual head shape may be due to *craniosynostosis*, premature closure of the sutures of the skull, or may represent a *deformational process*, caused by unusual forces acting on the otherwise normal skull. The latter condition, termed *plagiocephaly*, may become worse during the first few months of life because the infant will prefer to rest his or her head on one side. This position of comfort dictates which side of the occiput is more prominent. After 6 months, when the infant is able to sit unassisted, the plagiocephaly caused by intrauterine deformation gradually resolves.

Craniosynostosis is a malformation caused by sutural closure at an unusually early age. Closure of the coronal sutures leads to *brachycephaly*, in which the head is short in the anteroposterior diameter and wider laterally. This is the opposite of the head shape that results from premature closure of the sagittal suture, a head that is long in the anteroposterior diameter and narrow laterally (a skull shape known as *dolichocephalic*). Premature closure of one lambdoid suture leads to posterior plagiocephaly that does not resolve on its own.

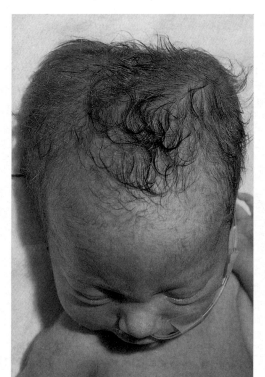

Figure 24–20 Cephalohematoma.

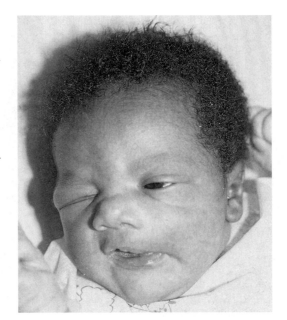

Figure 24–21 Traumatic facial palsy, left.

Inspect the skull for *symmetry*.

Inspect the scalp for lesions from *fetal scalp electrodes*, used for monitoring fetal well-being during difficult labors, and for areas of alopecia. A 0.4- to 0.8-inch (1- to 2-cm) well-demarcated area of smooth shiny skin with no hair may represent *aplasia cutis congenita*, an abnormality of fetal development of unknown cause. Usually an isolated finding in an otherwise well newborn, aplasia cutis also occurs commonly in trisomy 13.

Inspect the *face* for symmetry. The eye creases should be equal. Observe the infant as he or she sucks or cries. The mouth should remain on a level plane. If it is asymmetric, suspect a facial paralysis or a congenital anomaly of one or more facial muscles, a condition known as *asymmetric crying facies syndrome*. Figure 24-21 shows a 2-day-old neonate born by forceps extraction with a traumatic peripheral facial nerve palsy.* Notice the involvement of the entire left side of the face with failure of the left eye to close and the drooping of the corner of the left side of the mouth. Failure of eye closure on the affected side is usually the first noticeable sign of a peripheral facial palsy. During labor and delivery, the peripheral portion of the facial nerve may be compressed over the stylomastoid foramen through which the nerve emerges, or where the nerve traverses the ramus of the mandible.

The face may reveal abnormal features such as *epicanthal folds, widely spaced eyes,* or *low-set ears,* each of which may be associated with congenital defects.

Eyes

Several attempts to evaluate the eyes of the newborn may be necessary. Eyelid edema related to the birth process, medications, or infection makes this part of the examination difficult.

Inspect the eyes for *symmetry*. The eyes should be the same size and should be at the same depth in the orbits. Bulging eyes may be a sign of congenital glaucoma. Microcornea may result from congenital rubella.

Assess whether the eyes are normal distance from one another. If there is a concern about the eyes being too close together (*hypotelorism*) or too far apart (*hypertelorism*), careful measurements should be taken. These include inner canthal distance (distance between the inner canthi), outer canthal distance (distance between the outer canthi), and interpupil distance (distance between the pupils). Each of these measurements should be plotted on an appropriate growth curve. Such growth curves can be found in reference texts, such as *Smith's Recognizable Patterns of Human Malformations* (Jones, 2005). Hypotelorism (all measurements less than the fifth percentile) may be associated with midline defects of the brain, such as alobar holoprosencephaly; hypertelorism can be part of a number of multiple malformation syndromes, such as cleidocranial dysplasia and Aarskog's syndrome.

*As noted earlier, forceps are now rarely used in the United States.

Inspect the *eyelids* for evidence of trauma. Use a soft cloth gently to remove the vernix caseosa and any conjunctival exudate. Newborns rarely have eyebrows, but long eyelashes are frequently present. Medial epicanthal folds, flaps of skin covering the inner canthus of the eye, are seen frequently in individuals with midface hypoplasia. This condition occurs in a number of disorders, including trisomy 21 and fetal alcohol syndrome, but may be seen in normal individuals as well.

The best method of evaluating the eyes of a newborn is to hold the infant upright at arm's length while slowly rotating him or her in one direction. The infant's eyes usually open spontaneously.

Inspect the *sclerae*. In newborns, the sclerae may be icteric as a result of physiologic jaundice (described earlier). When icterus is absent, the sclerae of a young infant may appear bluish. During the first 6 months, the connective tissue of the sclera becomes thicker, leading to the normal white color expected in an adult. Persistence of blue color of the sclera after 6 months of age is suggestive of the presence of a connective tissue disorder, such as *osteogenesis imperfecta* or *Ehlers-Danlos syndrome* (see Fig. 10-48).

Inspect the *cornea*. The cornea should be clear. Cloudiness or a corneal diameter that is greater than 0.4 inch (1 cm) may be indicative of congenital glaucoma.

Inspect the *iris*. The iris of a newborn may be pale because full pigmentation does not occur before 10 to 12 months of life. Is an abnormal ventral cleft present in the iris? This cleft, known as a *coloboma*, is associated with defects in the iris and retina (see Figs. 10-62 and 10-140). A coloboma is commonly associated with chromosomal abnormalities such as trisomy 13 or 18 and the syndrome of *c*oloboma, *h*eart disease, *a*tresia choanae, *r*etardation of growth or development, *g*enitourinary tract anomalies, and *e*ar anomalies (CHARGE). In rare cases, the irides are absent; this condition is associated with the susceptibility to development of Wilms' tumor. Is there a ring of whitish dots at the periphery of the iris? These dots are best seen in a slit-lamp examination by an ophthalmologist, but the ring is sometimes visible to the naked eye. These dots, called *Brushfield's spots*, may be associated with trisomy 21 or may be normal.

Inspect the *conjunctivae*. Small subconjunctival hemorrhages are common, a result of the forces involved in the birth process. They heal without any effect on the child's vision. As a result of the erythromycin drops* instilled at birth, there may be some inflammation of the conjunctivae, as well as edema of the eyelids.

The *pupils* of neonates are usually constricted until about the third week after birth. Pupillary reflexes are present but hard to interpret in this age group.

Rotate the infant slowly to one side. The eyes should turn in the direction to which he or she is being turned. At the end of the motion, the eyes should quickly look back in the opposite direction after a few quick, nonsustained nystagmoid movements. This is termed the *rotational response*, and its presence establishes that the motor control of the eyes is intact.

Place the infant back on his or her back.

To test for *visual acuity* in the newborn, the examiner must rely on indirect methods such as the response to a bright light, known as the *optical blink reflex*. This reflex is normally observed when a bright light is shined on each eye: the newborn blinks and dorsiflexes the head. The visual acuity of newborns has been estimated to be approximately 20/100 to 20/150, according to their ability to fixate on and imitate the adult face.

In all newborns, the presence of the *red reflex* bilaterally suggests grossly normal eyes and the absence of glaucoma, cataract, or intraocular disorders. Determine the presence of the red reflex by holding the ophthalmoscope 10 to 12 inches (25 to 30.5 cm) away from the infant's eyes. The presence of the red reflex indicates that there is no serious obstruction to light between the cornea and the retina. If a red reflex is absent, funduscopic examination is required at this time. A funduscopic examination by an ophthalmologist is also indicated if you suspect any of the intrauterine infections associated with chorioretinitis, such as toxoplasmosis, congenital rubella, or cytomegalovirus infection.

Ears

Inspect the *external ear*. An imaginary line from the inner and outer canthus of the eye toward the vertex should be at or below the level of the superior attachment of the ear. Low-set ears are often associated with congenital kidney defects or chromosomal disorders. Frequently, the ears are misshapen as a result of intrauterine positioning. Such misshaping usually resolves within 1 to 2 days after birth. In rare instances, one ear is malformed and reduced in size.

---

*As prophylaxis against gonorrheal conjunctivitis, also known as ophthalmia neonatorum.

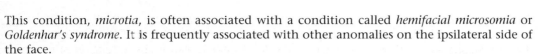

This condition, *microtia*, is often associated with a condition called *hemifacial microsomia* or *Goldenhar's syndrome*. It is frequently associated with other anomalies on the ipsilateral side of the face.

Are any *skin tags* present? A skin tag or cleft in front of the tragus often represents a remnant of the first branchial cleft and may be an isolated anomaly or part of a more widespread group of malformations, such as Treacher Collins syndrome or the aforementioned hemifacial microsomia.

Hearing in newborns may be tested by using the *primitive acoustic blink* reflex. Blinking in response to snapping of the fingers or a loud noise indicates that the newborn can hear. This is a crude test with low sensitivity. A negative response should be further tested with a specific pure-tone screening device. Most states now mandate neonatal hearing screening before discharge from the birth hospital. The parents of a child who passes the screen can be told with confidence that their child has normal hearing at birth. (Some congenital causes of deafness may cause progressive hearing loss over the first 2 years of life.) Only a fraction of children who fail the screen do in fact have hearing deficits.

The *external canal* should be inspected. Hold the otoscope (as indicated in Chapter 11, The Ear and Nose) by bracing it against the newborn's head. Insert the otoscope by pulling the pinna gently downward. The external canal is usually filled with vernix caseosa, and so the tympanic membrane may not be seen. If the tympanic membrane can be seen, usually only the most superior portion is visualized. The tympanic membrane may appear to be bulging, with amniotic fluid behind it. This is a normal condition. Rotation of the tympanic membrane to the adult position occurs within 6 to 12 weeks.

Nose

If this has not already been done in the delivery room, patency of the nasopharynx is determined by passing a soft, sterile, 6-French catheter through each external naris and advancing it into the posterior nasopharynx. This test rules out the presence of unilateral or bilateral *choanal atresia*, which is a cause of severe respiratory distress in newborns. Newborns are nasal breathers, and obstruction to nasal flow can cause considerable distress; the infant with nasal obstruction is cyanotic and distressed at rest, but the cyanosis diminishes when he or she cries. Choanal atresia may occur as an isolated anomaly (in which case, more than 90% of affected individuals are female), or it may be part of the *CHARGE syndrome*, which was mentioned in the discussion of iris colobomas.

Mouth and Pharynx

Assess the lips and philtrum. Is there a cleft of the lip? This may be to the left or the right of the midline and may be unilateral or bilateral. Is the philtrum well formed, with normal architecture? Flattening of the philtrum is seen in infants with fetal alcohol syndrome.

Test the *sucking reflex*. Put on a glove, and insert your index finger into the newborn's mouth. A strong sucking reflex should be present. The sucking reflex is usually strong by 34 weeks' gestation and disappears at 9 to 12 months of age. Feel for any clefts in the palate.

Inspect the *gingivae*. The gums should be raised, smooth, and pink.

Inspect the *tongue*. The normal frenulum may be short or may extend almost to the tip of the tongue. Because the production of saliva is limited in the first few months of life, the presence of excessive saliva in the mouth is suggestive of *esophageal atresia*.

Inspect the *palate*. Is there a *cleft palate* (see Fig. 12-32)? A *bifid uvula* may be associated with a submucosal cleft palate. Is the palate *high-arched?* Petechiae are commonly found on the hard and soft palates. Pinhead, whitish-yellow, rounded lesions on either side of the raphe on the hard palate are *Epstein's pearls*. These are mucous retention cysts and disappear within the first few weeks after birth. Similar cysts may be present on the gingivae. Inspect for *neonatal teeth*. These teeth have poor root systems and may have to be removed to prevent accidental aspiration.

Inspect the *oropharynx*. This can be performed while the infant is crying. Tonsillar tissue is not visible in the newborn. Small ulcers or clusters of small, whitish-yellow follicles on an erythematous base are sometimes seen on the anterior tonsillar pillars and are known as *Bednar's aphthae*. The cause is unknown, and they disappear within the first week after birth.

Listen to the child's *cry*. Evaluate the cry for its nature, pitch, intensity, and effort. A healthy child has a strong cry, indicative of normally functioning airways. The cry varies in intensity with breathing. The cry is high-pitched and shrill in diseases associated with increased intracranial pressure. Children born to drug-addicted mothers often have high-pitched cries.

A low-pitched, hoarse cry that is infrequent and low in intensity is often associated with hypothyroidism, hypocalcemic tetany, or Williams' syndrome. A sound that resembles a cat mewing suggests a condition known as *cri du chat syndrome*, caused by a deletion of the short arm of chromosome 5 (del 5p). Absence of crying is suggestive of severe illness or mental dysfunction.

Assess the *mandible*. Is it hypoplastic, small, and recessed? Occurring in isolation or in association with a U-shaped cleft of the palate in the Pierre Robin malformation sequence, micrognathia may be associated with life-threatening obstructive apnea, a medical emergency that necessitates immediate attention. To assess for obstructive apnea in such infants, the examiner listens with the stethoscope for air movement through the nose. Lack of audible air movement in the presence of appropriate movements of the chest is diagnostic of obstructive (as opposed to central) apnea. Such children should immediately be placed prone; with their face down, gravity pulls the tongue away from the posterior pharynx and enables air flow.

Neck

The neck of a newborn appears relatively short. Is the neck *symmetric* with regard to the midline? Rotate the infant's head. Normally, the infant's head should be easily rotated to either side so that the chin can touch either shoulder. *Torticollis* is a condition in which the head is tilted to one side while the chin is rotated to the other shoulder. In the newborn, a hematoma of the sternocleidomastoid muscle as a result of a birth injury may produce this condition. Palpate for a mass in the area of the sternocleidomastoid muscle if torticollis is present.

Palpate for *masses*. A midline mass may be a thyroglossal cyst or thyromegaly. A lateral mass may be a cystic hygroma or branchial cleft cyst.

Is *webbing* of the neck present? Webbing is a feature of *Turner's syndrome, Noonan's syndrome,* and other congenital abnormalities.

Palpate the *clavicles* to rule out a fracture. You should feel for the crepitus of a fractured clavicle. Clavicular fractures as a result of a birth injury usually occur at the junction of the middle and outer thirds of the bone. Decreased motion in the upper extremity may be associated with a clavicular fracture. Clavicular fracture is a rather common injury even during uneventful births and usually heals without any sequelae.

Chest

Observe the *respiratory rate* while the infant is undisturbed. At several hours after birth, the rate may vary from 20 to 80 breaths per minute, with an average of 30 to 40. Because of the wide variation, respirations should be counted for 1 to 2 minutes.

Inspect the *respiratory pattern*. The breathing pattern of newborns is almost entirely diaphragmatic. Irregular, shallow respirations are common in newborns. *Periodic breathing* is characterized by periods of apnea lasting 5 to 15 seconds and is not associated with bradycardia. *True apnea* has a duration of more than 20 seconds and is associated with bradycardia. The latter is more commonly found in premature infants with pulmonary disease. Infants with true apnea are thought to be at higher risk for *sudden infant death syndrome* (SIDS). The presence of an *expiratory grunt, retractions* of the chest, or *flaring* of the nostrils is indicative of respiratory distress.

Inspect for *deformities*. The most important chest deformity in newborns is asymmetry owing to unequal chest expansion on one side. Other deformities seen in adults, such as pectus excavatum and pectus carinatum, are rarely seen in newborns.

Auscultate the chest with either the bell or the small diaphragm of the stethoscope. Bronchovesicular breath sounds should be easily heard throughout the lung fields and are higher in pitch than those in adults. Absence of breath sounds on one side may be indicative of pneumothorax or a diaphragmatic hernia. Pneumothorax is relatively common in newborns as a result of the large transpulmonary pressures involved in inflating the lungs for the first time.

If respiratory distress is present, percuss the chest by using either one finger to tap the chest or using the method discussed for adults (see Chapter 13, The Chest). Normally, the thorax of a newborn is hyperresonant throughout. Dullness may indicate an effusion or consolidation.

Breast

Inspect the breasts. The breasts of both male and female newborns are enlarged. A milky discharge from the nipple, known as *witch's milk*, may be present. This is the effect of maternal estrogen and is present for 1 to 2 weeks after birth.

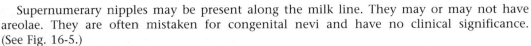

Supernumerary nipples may be present along the milk line. They may or may not have areolae. They are often mistaken for congenital nevi and have no clinical significance. (See Fig. 16-5.)

Asymmetry of the chest wall may be a normal variant or may represent hypoplasia of the pectoralis minor and major muscles. The latter condition, when associated with deficiency of the ipsilateral hand, may be part of the *Poland malformation sequence*.

Heart

Inspect the patient for *cyanosis*. If central cyanosis is present within the first hours or days after birth, suspect atresia of one of the right heart valves, transposition of the great vessels, or persistent fetal circulation.

Inspect for evidence of *congestive heart failure*. In newborns, the most important signs of heart failure are poor feeding, persistent tachycardia of up to 200 beats per minute, tachypnea, pallor, and an enlarged liver. Crackles are not sensitive indicators of heart failure in newborns. Heart failure during the first few days after birth is frequently caused by hypoplastic left heart syndrome.

Palpate for the *point of maximum impulse*. In newborns younger than 48 hours old, the point of maximum impulse is often in the xiphoid region. After this period and for several years, the point of maximum impulse should be in the fourth left intercostal space just lateral to the midclavicular line. A right-sided point of maximum impulse is suggestive of *dextrocardia*, a left-sided pneumothorax, or a diaphragmatic hernia (which is usually on the left side, so that the herniated abdominal contents displace the heart to the right.)

Auscultate the heart in the same locations as in adults by using the small diaphragm and bell of the stethoscope. Because the respiratory rate is so rapid in newborns, it is often difficult to distinguish respiratory from cardiac events. Sometimes occluding the nares for a few seconds may help to elucidate the sounds. Auscultation in newborns has a low degree of sensitivity in detecting congenital heart disease. Many "normal" murmurs heard in the early neonatal period are related to the marked changes in circulation after birth. It has been suggested that there is less than a 1 in 10 chance that a murmur heard in the neonatal period is the consequence of actual congenital heart disease. A systolic murmur at the upper left sternal border from a *patent ductus arteriosus* is commonly heard at birth but disappears by the second or third day after birth as the ductus spontaneously closes. In contrast, many severe congenital heart lesions, such as transposition of the great vessels, produce no murmur in the neonatal period. If any murmurs are present, they should be noted and described as indicated in Chapter 14, The Heart.

Pulses

Palpate the femoral pulses, at the midpoint of the inguinal ligament. Spend enough time to be sure you are feeling the arterial pulsations and not the movement of the abdominal wall with respiration. Weak femoral pulses should raise the suspicion of coarctation of the aorta. In hypoplastic left heart syndrome or preductal coarctation of the aorta, the femoral pulses may be present for the first 24 to 48 hours and disappear as the ductus closes. Repeated examinations of the newborn are important to be sure that the femoral pulses remain strong after ductal closure.

Abdomen

Inspect the abdomen. The abdomen of a newborn is protuberant as a result of the poor development of the abdominal musculature. If the abdomen is scaphoid, there should be a high index of suspicion that a diaphragmatic hernia is present and that the abdominal organs may be located in the chest.

Is an *umbilical hernia* present? The abdominal wall is relatively weak in newborns, especially in premature infants. Umbilical hernias are common in African-American infants. An umbilical hernia in a non–African-American child may be an indication of hypothyroidism.

Although uncommon, two major defects in the abdominal wall are well known. *Omphaloceles* are severe umbilical hernias in which some of the abdominal contents are located outside the body. Omphaloceles, which always involve the umbilicus and, as such, are always in the midline, may be isolated anomalies or may be associated with additional anomalies, such as in the *Beckwith-Wiedemann syndrome*. *Gastroschisis*, which results from an embryonic vascular deficiency, is similar to omphalocele in that abdominal contents are located outside the abdominal cavity. However, gastroschisis is never midline, is never covered by a membrane, and usually is located in the right upper quadrant. Gastroschisis may be associated with intestinal atresias, a condition known as *apple peel bowel*.

Inspect the *umbilical cord stump*. Is there evidence of yellow staining by meconium as a result of fetal distress? The normal umbilical cord contains two thick-walled arteries and one thin-walled vein. This examination needs to be performed in the delivery room, before the cord is treated with triple dye for antisepsis. Newborns with a single artery may have congenital abnormalities of the kidneys and spine. Drainage of a clear discharge from the umbilicus is suggestive of the presence of a patent urachus* or possibly an omphalomesenteric duct.

Auscultate the abdomen. The abdomen of a newborn infant is tympanitic, with metallic tinkling sounds being heard every 15 to 20 seconds.

Palpate the abdomen. To relax the abdomen, use your left hand to hold the infant's hips and knees in a flexed position while the child is sucking, and palpate with your right hand. In general, the liver edge may be felt as much as 0.75 inch (2 cm) below the right costal margin in the newborn. A liver edge more than 1.2 inches (3 cm) below the right costal margin is suggestive of hepatomegaly. The liver span can be measured by percussion, and this measurement is more accurate than abdominal measurements because respiratory conditions could hyperinflate the lungs and push a normal liver down into the abdominal cavity. Palpation of the spleen tip is less common.

Palpate the *kidneys*. Place your left hand under the right side of the child's back, and lift upward. At the same time, place your right hand in the child's right upper quadrant, and palpate for the right kidney. Reverse hands to palpate the left kidney.

Unless it is clinically indicated, the *rectum* is not examined. However, in infant girls especially, the patency of the anus should be determined by inspection while spreading the buttocks. In infants with *imperforate anus*, a blind dimple may be present; in infant girls, a rectovaginal fistula may allow passage of stool vaginally. In infant boys, an imperforate anus may be associated with a rectovesical fistula and no passage of meconium. Note that patency of the anus is established when the infant's temperature is taken rectally, as described previously. The presence of an imperforate anus may be the first evidence that the child has a condition known as VATER or VACTERL association—*v*ertebral *a*nomaly, *c*ardiac defect, *t*racheo-*e*sophageal fistula, *r*enal defects, and *l*imb defect (specifically, an anomaly of the thumb or radius)—a group of congenital anomalies that occur more commonly together than would be expected by chance.

Genitalia

Inspect the external genitalia for *ambiguity*.

In the term male infant, the scrotum is relatively large and rugate. The foreskin of the penis is tight and adherent to the glans penis. Inspect the glans for the location of the external urethral meatus. *Hypospadias* is a condition in which the meatus is located in an abnormal ventral position, anywhere from the lower glans of the penis to the scrotum. It is important to detect hypospadias in the neonatal period because it represents a contraindication to circumcision; indeed, the penis may look partially circumcised, because in this defect, the foreskin usually does not cover the entire glans. Penile erections are common, often preceding the voiding of urine. The testicles should be descended into the scrotum or the inguinal canals. Palpate the testicles by a downward movement, which counteracts the active cremasteric reflex. Are any masses present? *Hydroceles* or *hernias* are common in newborns. A hydrocele, which can be transilluminated, should be monitored until the child is 6 months of age. If it is still present then, the hydrocele usually must be repaired. A hernia should be repaired as soon as possible.

In the term female infant, the labia majora should cover the labia minora and clitoris. There should be a fingertip space between the vagina and the anus. If not, the possibility of sexual ambiguity exists. A whitish vaginal discharge is common during the first few days after birth and is an effect of estrogen; the discharge may become bloody later in the first week from withdrawal of maternal estrogen. The examiner should inspect the *urethral meatus* and *vaginal orifice* by placing a gloved thumb and index finger on the child's perineum while pressing downward and laterally on the buttocks.

Sexual ambiguity in the newborn is both a psychologic emergency for the parents and possibly a medical emergency for the child. The most common cause is *congenital adrenal hyperplasia* resulting from 21-hydroxylase deficiency in a female infant. Affected children have a large clitoris or phallus and possibly fused labia but no palpable gonads in the *labioscrotal folds*. The child should be assessed immediately with appropriate blood tests, because many infants with 21-hydroxylase deficiency manifest *salt loss* and can go into shock and die in the first week or two after birth.

---

*A canal in the fetus that connects the urinary bladder to the allantois.

In a male or female infant born vàginally after a breech presentation, the external genitalia are often erythematous and edematous as a result of the trauma related to the birth process.

Musculoskeletal Examination

The purpose of the musculoskeletal examination of the newborn is to detect gross abnormalities. The appearance of the extremities at birth usually reflects the positioning of the child within the uterus, known as *intrauterine packing*.

Inspect the *extremities* and *digits*. Are all four extremities and 20 digits present? Polydactyly, the presence of one or more extra digits, is fairly common. It may be inherited as an autosomal dominant trait or may be part of a more complex multiple malformation syndrome. Most polydactyly is postaxial (on the small digit side of the hand or foot), and the extra digit is represented by a skin tag (called a *postminimus*). Hypodactyly, the absence of one or more digits, is never considered a normal variant. The absence of digits should always trigger an evaluation for associated anomalies.

Palpate the *clavicle* if this has not already been done. An area of crepitus over the distal third is suggestive of a fractured clavicle. Decreased motion in the upper extremity may also be associated with a clavicular fracture.

Check for a *brachial palsy*, which has been discussed earlier.

The most important part of the musculoskeletal examination of the newborn is the evaluation of the lower extremities. The *hips* are examined for the possibility of developmental dysplasia, in which a hip either is dislocated from the acetabulum or can be dislocated. Inspect the contours of the legs while the child is lying prone. The presence of asymmetric skin folds on the medial aspect of the thigh is suggestive of a proximally dislocated femur. The perineum should not be visible when the child is in this position, because the normal position of the thighs should cover most of it. If the perineum is visible, you must suspect *bilateral* hip dislocations.

With the child lying supine, place the infant's feet side by side with the soles on the examination table, allowing the hips and knees to flex. Observe the relative height of the knees. If one knee is at a lower level, you should suspect that the shortness of that knee is secondary to a dislocation of the hip on that side, a congenitally short femur, or both. This is known as *Galeazzi's sign*. If both knees are at the same height, either both hips are normal or both hips are dislocated.

After inspection of the knee heights, each hip is examined to determine joint stability. Two maneuvers are useful in detecting hip instability. First perform *Barlow's maneuver*. Flex the newborn's legs 90° at the hip and 90° at the knee. Hold the legs by placing your thumbs over the midthigh medially and your index fingers over the greater trochanters, as shown in Figure 24-22 (*right*). Bring the knee to midline and gently press *back* toward the examination table. Feel for a "clunk" as an unstable femoral head slips past the posterior rim of the acetabulum and dislocates from the socket. Now perform *Ortolani's maneuver*, which is a sign of

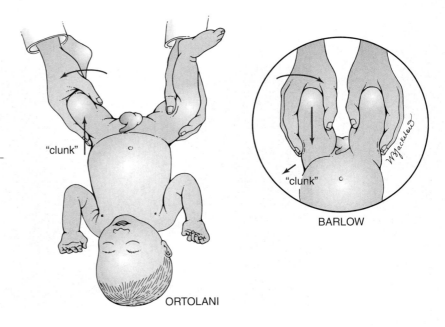

Figure 24–22 Ortolani's (*left*) and Barlow's (*right*) maneuvers.

"clunk"

"clunk"

BARLOW

ORTOLANI

relocating the femoral head into the acetabulum. Abduct the hip (knee goes *o*utward) while you apply gentle upward pressure over the greater trochanter and push the femoral head anteriorly, as shown in Figure 24-22 (*left*). A "clunk" indicates that the hip is relocating in the socket. Repeat with the other leg. If you feel a clunk in either hip, avoid repeat examinations of the hip until an expert examination can be done: movement of the femoral head in and out of the socket can damage the articular cartilage. It is common to feel clicks under your examining fingers; when in doubt, ask for expert evaluation. These tests should be performed on a relaxed infant. After the neonatal period, Ortolani's maneuver may yield a false-negative result.

Inspect the *feet*. Observe the foot at the sole. An imaginary line from the center of the heel through the center of the metatarsal-tarsal line should bisect either the second toe or the space between the second and third toes. If the line crosses more laterally, the forefoot is adducted (turned inward) in relation to the hindfoot. This is the common condition known as *metatarsus adductus* and is often the result of intrauterine packing. This condition may resolve spontaneously within the first few years of life, but early casting or exercises for passive correction may be required.

The most serious foot deformity at birth is the *clubfoot*, also known as *talipes equinovarus*. The entire foot is deviated toward the midline. There is forefoot adduction, fixed inversion of the hindfoot, and fixed plantar flexion. The Achilles tendon is foreshortened, and the foot assumes the position of a horse's hoof, hence the prefix "equino-." The calf muscles on the affected side are also smaller than those on the unaffected side. Therapy should begin within the first few days after birth. Manipulation is vital. If the deformity is not corrected by retention casting or splinting, surgical release may be necessary at a later date. The 3-week-old infant pictured in Figure 24-23 was born with bilateral clubfoot and bilateral hip dislocations. Multiple musculoskeletal deformities may be a clue to a neuromuscular problem in utero.

Neurologic Examination

Careful inspection is the most important aspect of the neonatal neurologic examination. The inspection should include the following:

- Posture
- Symmetry of extremities
- Spontaneous movements
- Facial expressions and symmetry
- Eye movements and symmetry

Notice the *position* of the newborn. Is hyperextension of the neck present? This sign is frequently found in infants with severe meningeal or brain-stem irritation. What is the position of the thumb? The *cerebral thumb sign* is the finding of the thumb curled under the flexed fingers. It is associated with many cerebral abnormalities, although it may be present intermittently in normal newborns.

The *motor* examination consists of testing the *range of motion* of all joints. Assess muscle tone and compare one side with the other. Compare the muscle sizes and strengths. Compare the resistance to passive stretch.

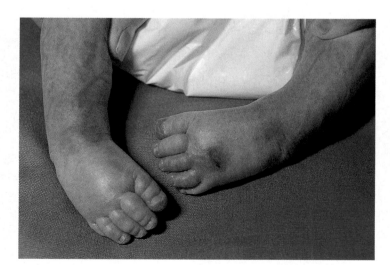

Figure 24–23 Talipes equinovarus.

The *sensory* examination is performed only if a nerve palsy or spina bifida is suspected. Usually pain is the only sensation tested; the object is to elicit a grimace or cry, which indicates cortical perception of pain, and not just withdrawal of the limb, which can be a spinal reflex. Testing the *cranial nerves* is also difficult in newborns, but the presence of facial symmetry and of the *rotational response* indicate that cranial nerves III, IV, VI, and VII are grossly intact. Observing a feeding for coordination of sucking, swallowing, and breathing is a good test of nerves IX and X. A simple test for cranial nerve XII consists of pinching the nostrils of the newborn. A reflex opening of the mouth with extension and elevation of the tongue in the midline is the normal response. Deviation of the tongue to one side indicates a lesion of the nerve on that side.

Because the corticospinal tracts are not fully developed in newborns, the response to testing of the deep tendon reflexes is variable and is neither sensitive nor specific. *Babinski's reflex* is usually present in newborns and is tested as in adults. Babinski's reflex may be present in normal children until the first birthday.

Test for *infantile automatisms*. These are primitive reflex phenomena that may be present at birth, depending on gestational age, but disappear soon thereafter. There are many automatisms, and not all have to be tested. The most important ones are as follows:

- Rooting response
- Plantar grasp
- Palmar grasp
- Moro's reflex
- Galant's reflex
- Perez's reflex
- Placing response
- Stepping response

The rotational response, optical blinking reflex, acoustic blink response, and sucking response are also automatisms and are discussed earlier in this chapter.

The following reflexes are elicited while the newborn infant is lying supine on the examination table.

The *rooting response* is elicited by having the infant lie in a quiet state with hands held against the chest. The examiner then touches the corner of the infant's mouth or cheek. The normal response is turning of the head to the same side and opening of the mouth to grasp the finger. If only the upper lip is touched, the head normally retroflexes; if only the lower lip is touched, the jaw normally drops. The rooting response is present by 32 weeks' gestation and usually disappears after 3 to 4 months after birth. This primitive response facilitates nursing. It is absent in infants with severe central nervous system disease.

The *plantar grasp* is elicited by flexing the leg at the hip and knee. Dorsiflex the infant's foot with your hand. The normal response is plantar flexion of the toes over the hand. This response disappears by 9 to 12 months.

The *palmar grasp* is elicited by stabilizing the infant's head in the midline. Place your index finger into the newborn's palm from the ulnar side. The normal response is flexion of all the fingers to grasp the index finger. If the reflex is sluggish, allow the child to suck, which normally facilitates the grasp response. The palmar grasp is usually established by 32 weeks' gestation and usually disappears after 3 to 5 months after birth. The absence of this response in a newborn or its persistence after 5 months is suggestive of cerebral disease. The newborn commonly holds the hand in a fist. After 2 months, however, the presence of this sign might suggest neurologic disease.

The infant is now picked up and held supine in the examiner's hands.

Moro's reflex, or the *startle reflex*, is elicited by supporting the infant's body in the right hand and supporting the head with the left hand. The head is suddenly allowed to drop a few centimeters, with immediate re-support by the examiner's hand. The Moro reflex consists of symmetric abduction of the upper extremities at the shoulders and extension of the fingers. Adduction of the arm at the shoulder completes the reflex. The infant usually then emits a loud cry. Moro's reflex is one of the most important motor automatisms. The normal response, which appears in an incomplete form at 28 weeks' gestation, indicates an intact central nervous system. The reflex normally disappears by 3 to 5 months of age. Persistence past 6 months may indicate neurologic disease.

The infant is now turned over and held in the prone position in one of the examiner's hands.

Galant's reflex is elicited by stroking one side of the back along a paravertebral line 2 to 3 cm from the midline going from the shoulder to the buttocks. The normal response is lateral curvature of the trunk toward the stimulated side, with the shoulder and hip moving toward the side stroked. Galant's reflex normally disappears after 2 to 3 months. This reflex is absent in newborns with transverse spinal cord lesions.

Perez's reflex is elicited by placing your thumb at the infant's sacrum and rubbing it firmly along the spine toward the infant's head. The normal response is extension of the head and spine with flexion of the knees. Frequently, the newborn also urinates. This reflex is normally present until 2 to 3 months of age. Its absence suggests severe neurologic disease of the cerebrum or cervical spinal cord or a myopathy.

The child is now laid down on the examination table and then picked up by the examiner, who holds the infant upright. The examiner's hands should be under the arms around the infant's chest, with the head supported by the fingers extended up the infant's back.

The *placing response* is elicited by allowing the dorsum of one of the infant's feet to touch the undersurface of a tabletop lightly. The normal placing response is for the infant to flex the knee and hip, then place the stimulated foot on top of the table. This response is then tested with the other foot. Placement of the soles of both feet on top of a table should elicit the *stepping response*, which is the alternating movements of both legs. Both these responses are best observed after 4 to 5 days after birth and disappear after 2 to 5 months. If paresis of the lower extremities is present, these responses are absent.

Examination of the Infant

Infants 1 week to 6 months of age can be examined on the examination table with a parent standing nearby. It may be easier to perform part of the examination while the infant is in the parent's arms or lap. Infants 6 months to 1 year of age are best examined on the parent's lap. The examiner should also be seated, at the child's level.

The more difficult portions of the examination, such as the evaluation of the pharynx and the otoscopic examination, should be performed last. To listen to the lungs and heart, take advantage of any time when the infant is quiet. Observation is a key element of the examination; the most meaningful assessments of the child's respiratory state, or use of arms and legs, are often obtained when the child is unaware of being observed.

The information for the **review of systems** for an infant comes entirely from the parent or another adult. Children this age cannot tell you that they have pain except by crying or being irritable; thus, a major challenge in examining a child of this age is to localize the pain.

Inquire about the following:

General: fever, activity level, sleeping, feeding.

Head, eyes, ears, nose, and throat (HEENT): bulging or sunken fontanelle, nasal discharge, stuffiness, drooling, ear pulling or rubbing, ear discharge. Does child see? hear? have crossed eyes? Is there excessive or decreased tearing?

Heart: history of murmur, cyanosis; trouble feeding, sweating during feedings, squatting (in older infants and toddlers: this is a symptom in children with tetralogy of Fallot, because squatting increases peripheral resistance and decreases the right-to-left shunting across the ventricular septal defect).

Respiratory: cough, difficulty breathing (fast or effortful breathing); noisy breathing, hoarseness.

Abdomen: Feeding pattern, stool pattern, diarrhea, distention, mass, jaundice, crying and drawing up legs (characteristic of *intussusception*).

Genitourinary: frequency of voids/wet diapers; strength of urinary stream; crying with voiding, vaginal discharge, skin irritation in diaper area. In the older infant, there should be periods when the diaper is dry, indicating the development of an increased bladder capacity.

Skin: Is there a rash? itching? easy bruising? change in birth marks?

Musculoskeletal: Is there equal use of both hands? of both legs? Is there pain or deformity of an extremity?

Neurologic: Is there any seizure activity or other abnormal movements? How is the child's developmental progress (described previously)? Has there been loss of previously attained milestones?

Before starting the examination, wash your hands in warm water.

General Assessment

Observe the infant's activity, alertness, and social responsiveness.

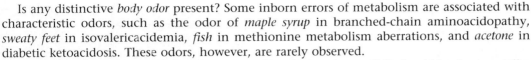

Is any distinctive *body odor* present? Some inborn errors of metabolism are associated with characteristic odors, such as the odor of *maple syrup* in branched-chain aminoacidopathy, *sweaty feet* in isovalericacidemia, *fish* in methionine metabolism aberrations, and *acetone* in diabetic ketoacidosis. These odors, however, are rarely observed.

The infant's temperature is usually measured by the nursing staff. It should be done rectally, as described for the newborn, until the child is at least 6 months of age.* After that, there are a number of devices for estimating the child's temperature in a less invasive way. For the first 3 months after birth, a temperature of 100.4° F, or 38° C, is considered elevated and may indicate that the child has a serious bacterial infection.

The average heart rate of a child during the first 6 months of life is 130 beats per minute, with a range of 80 to 160 at rest. The average resting heart rate during the second 6 months of life is 110 beats per minute, with a range of 70 to 150. The normal respiratory rate varies from 20 to 40 breaths per minute. Blood pressure is difficult to assess in this age group but may be determined by the *flush method*. In this technique, the arm is elevated while the uninflated *infant cuff* is applied to the arm. The examiner then presses on the arm from the fingers to the elbow so that blanching is noted. The cuff is inflated to just beyond an estimated blood pressure. The pale arm is then placed at the infant's side, and the cuff pressure is allowed to fall slowly. A sudden flush of color occurs at a level slightly lower than the true systolic pressure. The systolic blood pressure of a 1-day-old infant determined by the flush method is 50 mm Hg. By the second week after birth, the systolic blood pressure has risen to 80 mm Hg. By the end of the first year, the systolic blood pressure is 95 mm Hg. A more accurate Doppler blood pressure assessment is available for critical determinations.

Determine the infant's *length* and *weight*. Plot these measurements on the standard growth charts. Growth charts are used to determine whether a child is growing according to a group of standards. More important than a single value is the use of these charts to follow the rate of change at subsequent examinations. The National Center for Health Statistics publishes a variety of growth charts for boys and girls in two age groups: birth to 36 months and 2 to 20 years. Examples of these charts are shown in Figures 24-24 and 24-25, and the charts are available at the web site of the Centers for Disease Control and Prevention, *www.cdc.gov* (accessed June 26, 2008). Note that the current growth charts also include a chart for body mass index (BMI), which varies by age; specifically, preschool children have much lower BMI than do infants or older children. Growth charts are now available for children with trisomy 21, achondroplasia, and Turner's syndrome. For children with these syndromes, growth should be plotted on the disease-specific curves whenever possible.

Somatic growth is one of the most important parts of the pediatric examination. These parameters must be determined at every visit. Deviations from the standard curves are often early sensitive indicators of a pathologic process

Skin

Inspect for dermatologic conditions. *Seborrheic dermatitis* is the most common rash seen in the first month of life; it begins at 2 to 4 weeks of age and subsides after 3 to 4 months of age. An initial manifestation is often a crusting of the scalp known as *cradle cap*, as shown in Figure 24-26. The greasy, salmon-colored, nonpruritic, sharply delimited oval scales involve the scalp and face, especially the forehead, eyebrows, nasolabial folds, and retroauricular folds. Figure 24-27 shows seborrheic dermatitis in another patient. Notice the greasy papular eruption on the face of this 3-week-old infant. Seborrheic dermatitis may be differentiated from *atopic dermatitis* by its early onset, lack of pruritus, and absence of vesicles.

Atopic dermatitis, also known as infantile eczema, is very common in infants and begins at about 6 to 8 weeks of age. It is characterized by dryness of the skin, pruritus, erythematous papules and vesicles, serous discharge, and crusting. The usual site in children 6 months of age is the face (Fig. 24-28), with the nose commonly spared (the *headlight sign*). The extensor surfaces of the arms and legs are the most common sites in 8- to 10-month-old infants, as seen in Figure 24-29. Notice the exudative lesions on the lower extremity. Patients with atopic dermatitis tend to have an extra groove of the lower eyelid, called the *atopic pleat*. This feature is shown in the 6-month-old child with atopic dermatitis in Figure 24-30.

Are any *vascular lesions* present?

Palpate the skin and assess *skin elasticity*. Pull up 1 to 2 inches (2.5 to 5 cm) of skin over the abdomen and release it. It should quickly return to its former position. A decreased response is termed *tenting* and is suggestive of dehydration or malnutrition. Skin that seems

---

*There is evidence that even under 6 months of age, other means of measurement may be valid.

Text continued on p. 777

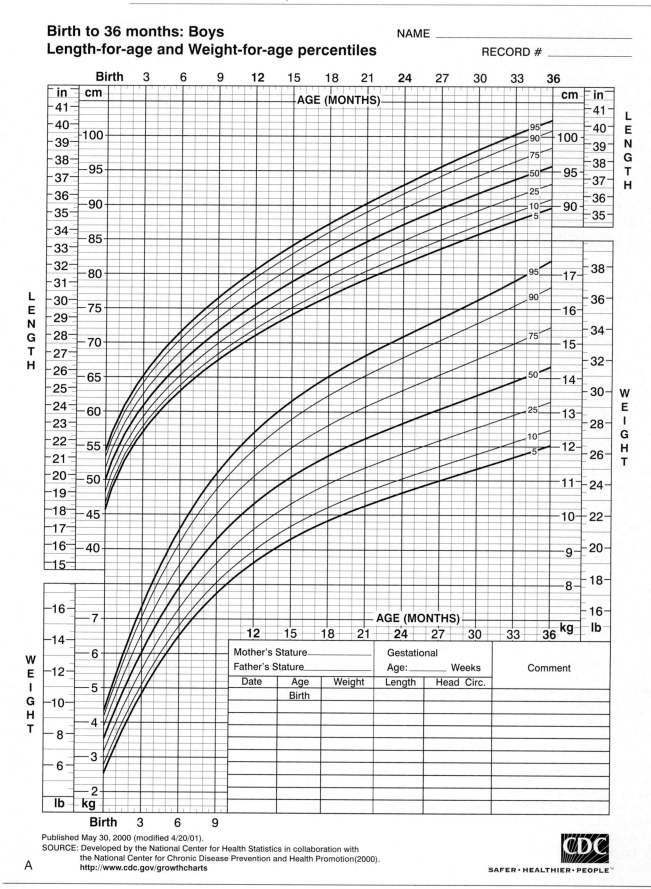

Published May 30, 2000 (modified 4/20/01).
SOURCE: Developed by the National Center for Health Statistics in collaboration with
the National Center for Chronic Disease Prevention and Health Promotion(2000).
http://www.cdc.gov/growthcharts

Figure 24–24 National Center for Health Statistics (NCHS) growth charts, birth to 36 months of age. *A,* NCHS percentiles for boys.

**Birth to 36 months: Boys
Head circumference-for-age and
Weight-for-length percentiles**

NAME _____

RECORD # _____

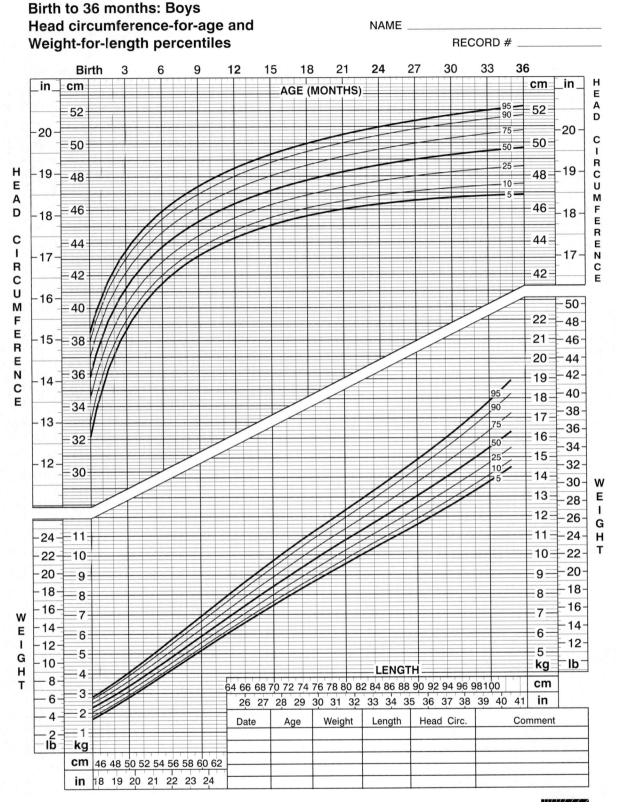

Published May 30, 2000 (modified 10/16/00).
SOURCE: Developed by the National Center for Health Statistics in collaboration with
the National Center for Chronic Disease Prevention and Health Promotion (2000).
http://www.cdc.gov/growthcharts

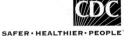

A

Figure 24–24 *A, cont'd.*

Birth to 36 months: Girls
Length-for-age and Weight-for-age percentiles

NAME _____

RECORD # _____

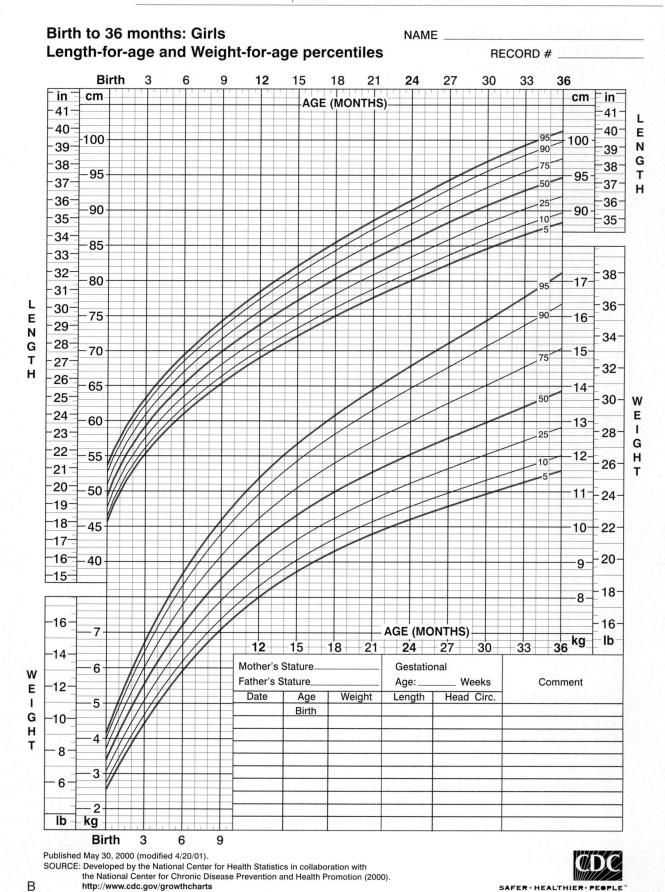

Published May 30, 2000 (modified 4/20/01).
SOURCE: Developed by the National Center for Health Statistics in collaboration with
   the National Center for Chronic Disease Prevention and Health Promotion (2000).
   http://www.cdc.gov/growthcharts

B

SAFER · HEALTHIER · PEOPLE™

Figure 24–24 *B,* NCHS percentiles for girls.

Birth to 36 months: Girls
Head circumference-for-age and
Weight-for-length percentiles

NAME _____

RECORD # _____

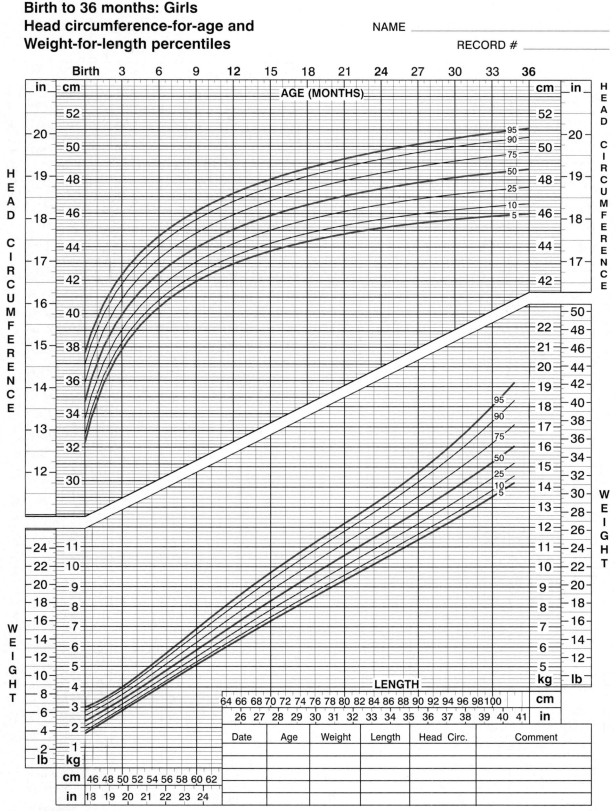

Published May 30, 2000 (modified 10/16/00).
SOURCE: Developed by the National Center for Health Statistics in collaboration with
the National Center for Chronic Disease Prevention and Health Promotion (2000).
http://www.cdc.gov/growthcharts

B

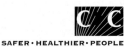

SAFER·HEALTHIER·PEOPLE™

Figure 24–24 B, cont'd.

2 to 20 years: Boys
Stature-for-age and Weight-for-age percentiles

NAME _____

RECORD # _____

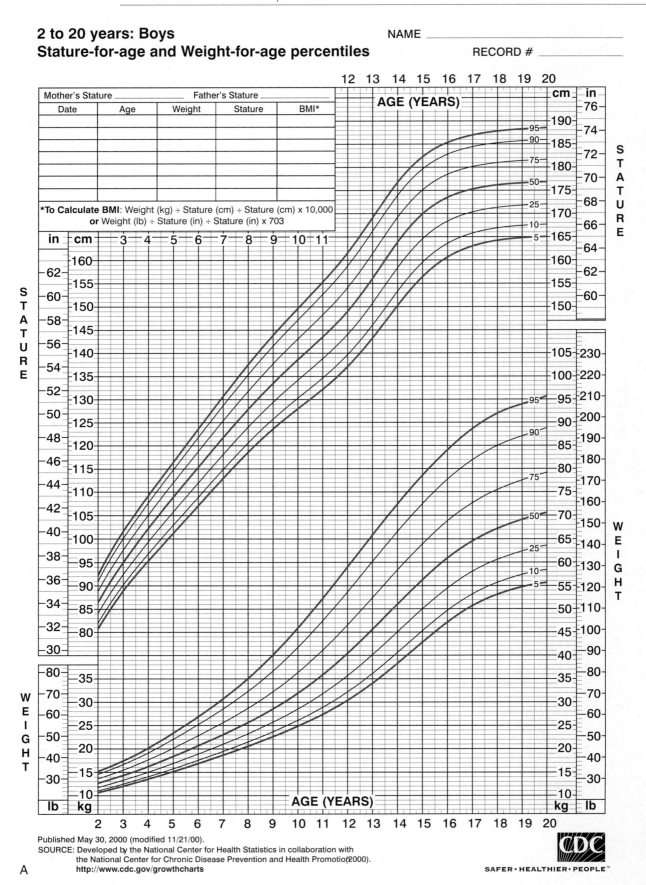

*To Calculate BMI: Weight (kg) ÷ Stature (cm) ÷ Stature (cm) x 10,000
or Weight (lb) ÷ Stature (in) ÷ Stature (in) x 703

Published May 30, 2000 (modified 11/21/00).
SOURCE: Developed by the National Center for Health Statistics in collaboration with
the National Center for Chronic Disease Prevention and Health Promotion (2000).
http://www.cdc.gov/growthcharts

A

Figure 24–25 National Center for Health Statistics (NCHS) growth charts, 2 to 20 years of age. *A,* NCHS percentiles for boys.

2 to 20 years: Girls
Stature-for-age and Weight-for-age percentiles

NAME _____

RECORD # _____

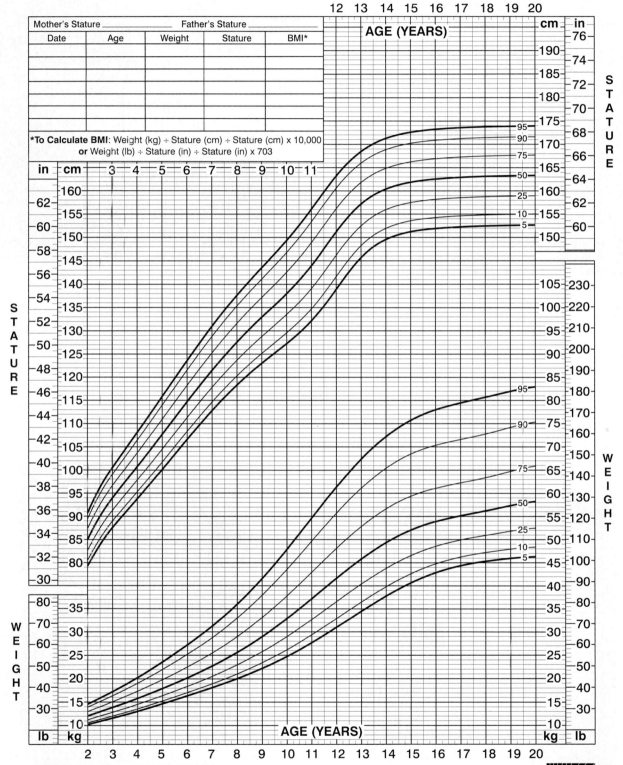

Mother's Stature _____ Father's Stature _____

Date	Age	Weight	Stature	BMI*

*To Calculate BMI: Weight (kg) ÷ Stature (cm) ÷ Stature (cm) x 10,000
or Weight (lb) ÷ Stature (in) ÷ Stature (in) x 703

AGE (YEARS)

Published May 30, 2000 (modified 11/21/00).
SOURCE: Developed by the National Center for Health Statistics in collaboration with
the National Center for Chronic Disease Prevention and Health Promotion (2000).
http://www.cdc.gov/growthcharts

CDC
SAFER · HEALTHIER · PEOPLE™

B

Figure 24–25 *B,* NCHS percentiles for girls.

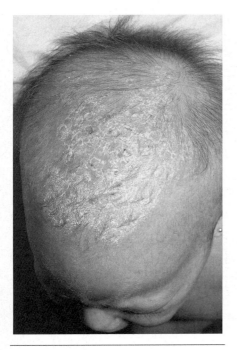

Figure 24–26 Seborrheic dermatitis, or cradle cap.

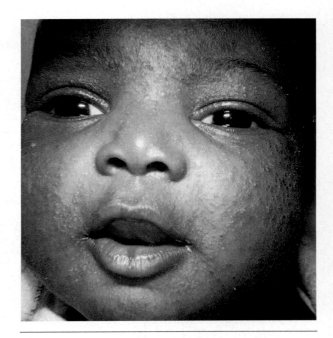

Figure 24–27 Seborrheic dermatitis.

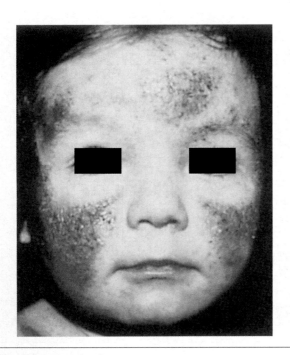

Figure 24–28 Infantile eczema.

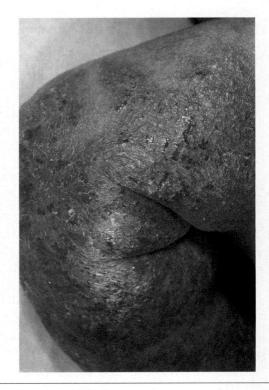

Figure 24–29 Atopic dermatitis.

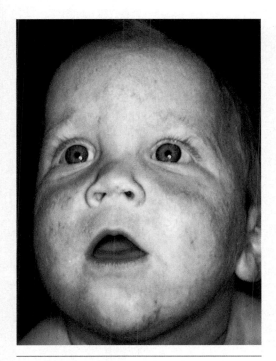

Figure 24–30 Atopic pleat.

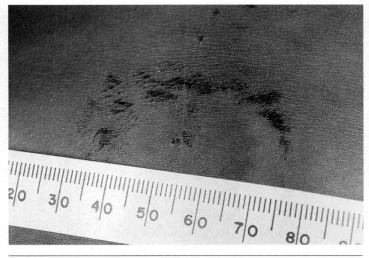

Figure 24–31 Human bite wound.

excessively stretchy may be an indication of *Ehlers-Danlos syndrome*, which is a combination of hyperelasticity of skin with joint laxity and easy dislocation and with easy bruisability. Most forms of Ehlers-Danlos syndrome are inherited through autosomal dominance. Therefore, when these features are found in the infant, both parents should be examined.

Is there any evidence of physical *child abuse?* Are any bruises, welts, lacerations, or unusual scars present? Inspect the buttocks and lower back for evidence of bruises. Paired, crescent-shaped bruises facing each other on any part of the body may represent human bite marks. Bite marks should be suspected when ecchymosis, lacerations, or abrasions are found in any oval shape. Tooth marks by the canine teeth are the most prominent part of a bite. Bites made by animals tear the flesh; bites made by humans crush the flesh. The distance between the maxillary canine teeth in a child is less than 1.2 inches (3 cm); in an adult, it is greater. Figure 24-31 shows a human bite wound. Notice that the intercanine distance is greater than 3 cm.

Is there evidence of traumatic alopecia from pulling out of the hair? The damaged hair is broken at various lengths. Are small, circular, punched-out lesions of uniform size present? These may represent cigarette burns. A large circular-type burn on the buttocks and thighs may result from the infant's immersion in scalding water. Inflicted tap water scalds are the most common type of nonaccidental burn injury. The most common sites include the perineum or extremities. The child pictured in Figure 24-32 has first- and second-degree burns on the penis, thighs, and inguinal and suprapubic areas. The buttocks and sacrum were spared. These burns were caused by holding the child under hot water from the faucet. Burns by a hot object are the second most common type of inflicted burns. A well-circumscribed affected area with the outline of the hot object used is commonly seen. Figure 24-33 shows the typical appearance of specific types of burns. The diagnosis of physical child abuse is especially important in the first 6 months of life because the risk of a fatal outcome is very high if the diagnosis is missed. In a case of suspected child abuse, the clinician must consider possible organic or accidental causes for the findings, such as platelet deficiency with an unusual number of bruises. However, if child abuse is suspected, health authorities must be notified.

Head

Measure the *occipitofrontal* head circumference, as indicated previously, and chart it on the standard growth charts (see Fig. 24-24). A head that is growing too rapidly should be evaluated for *hydrocephaly*. *Microcephaly* is a defect in which the head size is three standard deviations below the normal mean and is related to a defect in brain growth. Check for asymmetry.

Is the *face* symmetric? An easy way to detect facial paralysis is to observe the child when he or she cries. The weakened or paralyzed side appears expressionless in comparison with the normal side.

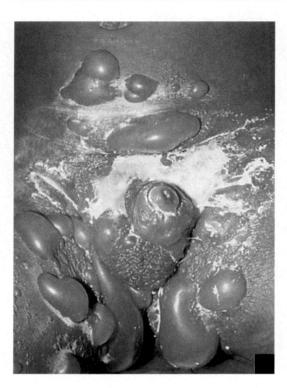

Figure 24-32 Hot water immersion burns.

As mentioned previously, asymmetry of the skull and face may be the result of a deformational process: that is, environmental forces acting on normal tissue. It has been found that infants who are put to sleep on their backs are less prone to SIDS. However, sleeping in the same position may cause the skull to become lopsided, or plagiocephalic; this shift in head shape also causes an asymmetry of the facial structures. This asymmetry is self-limited, however, and resolves soon after the infant begins to sit upright.

Eyes

In an infant older than 3 weeks of age, check the *pupillary responses*. A sluggishly reacting pupil is suggestive of congenital glaucoma.

The production of tears during crying begins at about 2 to 3 months of age, but the nasolacrimal duct is not fully patent until 5 to 7 months of age. If chronic tearing is present, the nasolacrimal duct may not be patent. In this case, massaging over the nasolacrimal sac may yield a purulent or mucoid discharge, which is suggestive of nasolacrimal obstruction.

Visual acuity is assessed by qualitative observations. By 4 weeks of age, the infant's eyes should be able to fixate on and follow a target through a brief arc. By 8 weeks of age, the child

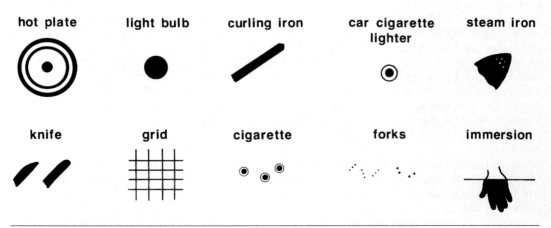

Figure 24-33 Appearance of specific types of burns.

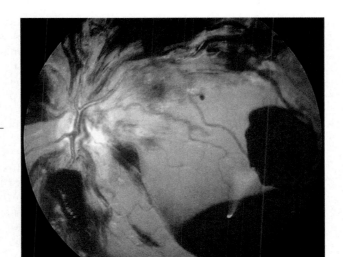

Figure 24–34 Retina of shaken infant. Note the massive hemorrhages.

should be able to visually follow an object past the midline, coordinating eye movements with head turning. At 4 months of age, the normal infant can visually follow an object in all directions. Convergence is also present by this time. The presence of *optokinetic nystagmus* indicates a complete pathway from the retina to the occipital visual cortex. This response can best be elicited in children 3 months of age and older by using a long, striped cloth and passing it rapidly from one side to the other in the child's view. The development of nystagmus as the child attempts to maintain fixation on a stripe is the normal response, indicating normal visual pathways. At 5 to 6 months of age, the child should be able to focus on objects but is farsighted. The child should be able to reach out for an object and grasp it. Recognition of objects and faces by 4 to 6 months of age is suggestive of normal visual acuity.

Observe *ocular motility* in a child 3 months of age or older. Have the child visually follow an object into the various positions of gaze. Alignment of the eyes is best determined by the symmetry of the *corneal light reflex* and the *alternate cover test*, which were described in Chapter 10, The Eye. The child is most susceptible to *amblyopia* within the first 2 years of life, although the risk is present until 6 to 7 years of age.

If there is a suspicion of child abuse, examine the retina. Although examination of the retina is not routine in this age group, visualization of the retina may reveal evidence of child abuse. A shaken child may have characteristic retinal hemorrhages, as shown in Figure 24-34.

Funduscopy is not useful for detecting papilledema in an infant with an open fontanelle, because an increase in intracranial pressure produces a bulging of the fontanelle, and even separation of the cranial sutures, before papilledema.

Nose
Elevate the tip of the nose to view the nasal septum, floor of the nose, and turbinates. Are any masses or *foreign bodies* present? A foreign body should be suspected in any child with a chronic unilateral nasal discharge, especially if it is foul-smelling.

Neck
Palpate for lymphadenopathy in the same areas as in the adult.

Any child with an acute febrile illness with irritability should be examined for *nuchal rigidity*, resulting from meningeal irritation, although these may be late findings in a young infant with meningitis. The Brudzinski and Kernig tests are described in Chapter 21, The Nervous System. Nuchal rigidity can sometimes be detected by encouraging the child to look at something below him or her; the natural tendency is to flex the neck, but such a movement is avoided with meningeal irritation.

Chest
The examination of the chest is best performed while the infant is either sleeping or being held by a parent.

Often the tracheal breath sounds, or even nasal and pharyngeal sounds, are transmitted down to the chest. Do not misinterpret these sounds as crackles, and do not interpret the accompanying tactile sensation of "rattling" as abnormal fremitus.

Is the child in *respiratory distress?* The most important signs of distress are tachypnea, the use of accessory muscles, head bobbing, and flaring of the nasal alae. Intercostal retractions are also commonly present. Does the child have *stridor*, a high-pitched noise on inspiration? Stridor is indicative of tracheal narrowing, as in *croup*.

Auscultate the lung fields. Percuss if you hear any focal abnormalities in the lungs.

Heart

Inspect for *cyanosis*. If cyanosis develops within the first few days to weeks of life, there is probably a serious anatomic anomaly such as tetralogy of Fallot.*

Inspect for evidence of *congestive heart failure*. The most important signs are persistent tachycardia, tachypnea, and an enlarged liver. A persistent tachycardia of more than 200 beats per minute in newborns or more than 150 beats per minute in children up to 1 year of age should alert the examiner. Feeding problems are often the first sign that an infant has heart failure. Such infants take a long time to feed, often more than an hour to take 2 or 3 ounces. The parent describes the child becoming "tired" or "out of breath" during feeding and as having to stop to catch his or her breath after every two or three sucks. Persistent *diaphoresis* and failure to thrive are also important signs associated with congestive heart failure. Observing a feeding may be extremely useful if heart failure is suspected. If heart failure develops within the first week or two, a structural defect such as a ventricular septal defect, patent ductus arteriosus, or coarctation of the aorta should be suspected. A truncus arteriosus also produces heart failure during this period, often with minimal cyanosis.

Palpate for the point of maximum impulse.

Auscultate as in newborns. S_3 and S_4 may be normal in this age group. As previously noted, the clinical significance of a murmur, especially in the first few weeks of life, must be carefully assessed. (A summary of pathologic murmurs heard in the pediatric age group is given in Table 24-4 later in this chapter.)

Palpate for the femoral pulses as discussed above.

Abdomen

Observe the abdomen for any masses. An umbilical hernia is common in this age group, especially in darker skinned children. Large peristaltic waves moving from the left to the right in the upper abdomen are occasionally present in infants with *pyloric stenosis*. These are especially easy to note during or after a feeding.

Inspect the *umbilicus*. In healthy children, the umbilical cord stump falls off before the end of the second week after birth. Persistence of the stump past this period suggests the presence of white cell adhesion defect or a patent urachus. After the umbilical cord stump has fallen off, the examiner must check for an *umbilical granuloma*, which if present should be cauterized with silver nitrate.

Auscultate, percuss, and palpate the abdomen, using light and deep palpation. Are any masses present?

Palpate for the *liver, spleen*, and *kidneys*. The estimated liver span of a 6-month-old infant varies from 1 to 1.2 inches (2.5 to 3 cm). At 1 year of age, the span is approximately 1.2 inches (3 cm).

Genitalia

Inspect the external genitalia. Check for *ambiguous genitalia*. Is diaper rash present?

The foreskin is not fully retractable until 3 years of age or later. If you do manage to retract it, be sure you return it to its original location; otherwise you may cause *paraphimosis*, a situation in which the retracted foreskin impedes venous drainage of the glans and results in progressive edema and pain. Diaper rash can cause *balanitis*, which is an acute inflammation of the glans penis. In boys who are uncircumcised, *phimosis*, the pathologic inability to retract the foreskin, may develop after balanitis.

Observe the position of the *urethral meatus*.

---

*Tetralogy of Fallot consists of pulmonic stenosis, an overriding aorta, a ventricular septal defect, and right ventricular hypertrophy; these conditions arise from an abnormal septation of the truncus arteriosus.

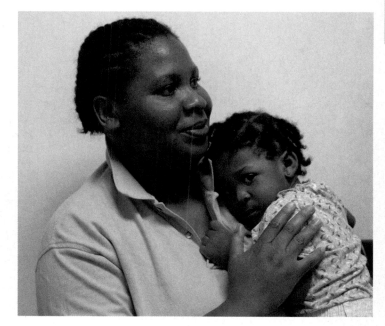

Figure 24–35 Positioning of child for otoscopic examination. There are many ways to position the child in parent's lap, which provides the child with some security. The child should be upright so that the examiner can brace the child's head against the parent's chest. The parent needs to hold the child's hands so that he or she does not grab the otoscope. If necessary, the child's legs can be scissored between the parent's legs.

Inspect the *scrotum*. Is unilateral swelling present? Enlargement may represent a hernia or a hydrocele. Inspect any mass by transillumination. Remember that hydroceles can be transilluminated, but hernias usually cannot. Auscultate the mass. Listening to a bowel-containing hernia may reveal bowel sounds.

Palpate the testes. Are both in the scrotum? Can an undescended testicle be palpated in the inguinal canal? If not, then while the infant is lying on the examination table, press on the abdomen while trying to palpate the undescended testicle in the inguinal canal with the other hand.

In the infant girl, is a vaginal *discharge* present? There is commonly a whitish, often blood-tinged discharge lasting up to 1 month after birth. This is related to the placental transfer of maternal hormones.

Musculoskeletal Examination

Palpate the *clavicle*. At 1 month of age, the presence of a callus formation is suggestive of a healing clavicular fracture.

The *hips* must be reexamined for dislocation at every routine visit for the first year of life. The technique is described in the section on Examination of the Newborn. After 4 months of age, a dislocated hip can no longer move in and out of the socket, and so Barlow's and Ortolani's tests will yield negative results. Instead, the examiner finds that the hip does not fully abduct.

Neurologic Examination

By the fourth month, when the supine infant is pulled into a sitting position, no head lag should be present. Many other infantile reflexes have disappeared by 4 months, most notably the Moro reflex. By the eighth month, the infant should be able to sit without support.

Coordination of the hands begins at about 5 months, when infants can reach and grasp objects. By 7 months, they can transfer these objects from hand to hand. At 8 to 9 months, they should be able to use a pincer grip to pick up small objects.

Ears

Otoscopy is one of the most difficult skills to learn to perform in infants and toddlers, and it is also one of the most important because these are the ages when *otitis media* is most prevalent.

The child can either be placed prone on the examination table or held by a parent. Figure 24-35 demonstrates how to position the child in the parent's lap. To examine the ear, use one hand to pull the pinna out, back, and up* as your other hand holds the otoscope firmly; your hands should be braced against the child's head, so that if the child's head moves, the

---

*The pinna is pulled down until a child is about 4 to 6 months of age; afterwards, pulling up, as in adults, usually provides the best visualization.

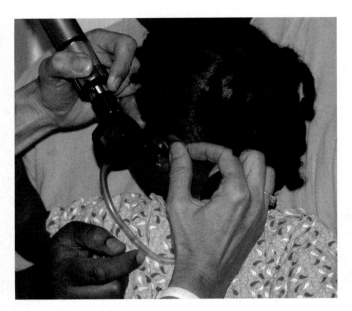

Figure 24–36 Positioning of examiner's hands for otoscopic examination. Note that the little finger of the hand holding the otoscope is braced against the child's head. (The examiner is left-handed.) The first two fingers of the other hand retract the pinna, while the remaining fingers are wrapped around the bulb of the insufflator, prepared to squeeze the bulb if the examination warrants.

examiner's hands and otoscope move as a unit, and there is less risk of inserting the speculum too far into the canal. Always use the largest speculum possible, which should be introduced slowly into the external canal. Figure 24-36 demonstrates the positioning of the examiner's hands. Notice how the hands are braced against the child's head, as well as the correct position for holding the pneumatic bulb. The *tympanic membrane* should be easily visualized unless cerumen is present. Any cerumen should be removed by someone experienced in doing so.

Is the tympanic membrane erythematous? Is it bulging? Check for a light reflex. Its presence, however, does not rule out otitis media. Are air-fluid levels visible behind the drum? These signs are suggestive of fluid in the middle ear.

Pneumatic otoscopy (see Chapter 11, The Ear and Nose) is an important skill for detecting mobility of the ear drum. In many young children, the ear drum may be red from crying or fever without middle ear infection. Decreased mobility is indicative of middle ear fluid, which is characteristic of otitis media; the presence of pus behind an immobile ear drum (opaque yellow fluid) is the best evidence of bacterial otitis (see Fig. 11-29). Figure 24-37 shows the ear specula designed to facilitate pneumatic otoscopy; the flared portion near the tip is coated with soft rubber to provide a seal without traumatizing the ear canal. The speculum on the left is the regular one; the one on the right is used for pneumatic otoscopy.

Mouth and Pharynx
The examination of the mouth and pharynx is the last part of the examination in this age group.

The child should be seated on the parent's lap, with the parent holding the child's head. It is usually possible to examine a crying infant without using the tongue depressor. A frightened

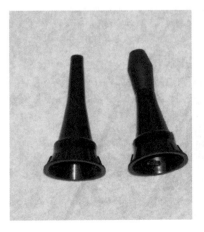

Figure 24–37 Ear specula designed to facilitate pneumatic otoscopy. A comfortable but tight seal in the ear canal is important for insufflation to be effective. Both of these reusable specula have the same internal diameter. Note that the one on the right is flared at the tip (with a coating of soft rubber) to provide a seal.

child who is holding his or her mouth firmly closed can be examined if you occlude the nares; this will make the child open the mouth. Enlist the parent as the nose-holder if you must use this technique. The tongue depressor can then be slipped between the teeth and over the tongue.

Inspect the *gingivae*. Gingival ulceration is frequently the result of *primary* herpetic infection. Small, discrete, whitish vesicles are also present before ulceration. They are found on the buccal mucosa, palate, and tongue. Severe cases can produce external lesions around the mouth; see Figure 24-54.

Are any *teeth* present? The first teeth to erupt are the lower central incisors, at about 6 months. These are followed by the lower lateral incisors at 7 months and the upper central teeth at 7 to 8 months. The upper lateral teeth begin to erupt at about 9 months. Salivation is temporarily increased with the eruption of new teeth. (A summary of the chronology of dentition is given in Table 24-5 at the end of the chapter.)

Review of Systems and Examination of the Young Child

A child 1 to 5 years of age is becoming verbal and, if in pain, can tell you where it hurts. They may start to report nausea, sore throat, chest pain, fatigue, or headache. Note that headache in a preschool child is unusual and probably indicates a serious intracranial pathologic process. Other questions to add to the infants' review of systems include questions about snoring and loss of bowel or bladder control in a child who has been toilet trained. Most children have achieved daytime control by 4 years of age, although only about half of children are dry at night by then. Restless sleep, including nightmares, night terrors, and sleep walking are not uncommon at this age.

For an adequate examination, the child needs to be relaxed. With children in this age group, it is important that you speak softly and demonstrate the parts of the examination on dolls or toy animals, on yourself, or on the parent. Allowing the child to hold the stethoscope or penlight often distracts him or her enough so that other parts of the examination can be performed. The child soon learns that the light and stethoscope need not be feared. Play with the child. Have the child "blow out" the light. Let the child use the stethoscope as a telephone. Above all, *talk* to the child. It is amazing how easily an examination can be performed while telling a young child a simple fantasy about imaginary animals. Ask the child questions about these characters. A reassuring voice goes a long way in making the child comfortable. As you proceed with the examination, describe to the child what is being done, such as "Now I'm going to listen to your heart beating." Children also seem to be reassured by conversations with their parents during the examination. Children younger than 3 years of age are best examined on the parent's lap; do your best to stay at the child's level.

The child should be completely undressed for the examination. If the child is modest, provide a gown or remove only the clothing that is necessary for each part of the examination. Re-cover that area before moving on. Modesty varies greatly among children in this age group. Respect the child's modesty.

Start the examination by washing your hands in warm water. Warm hands are more comfortable for the child. If the child is on an examination table, have the parent stand at the child's feet. Any child in respiratory distress is easiest to examine in the position of most comfort, usually sitting.

Gently tell the child what to do. It is better to say, "Please turn on your back" instead of "Would you please turn on your back?" Frame requests in the positive ("Hold still like a statue") instead of in the negative ("Don't move"). The child may not hear the negation of "move."

In a child who appears to be *apprehensive*, auscultation of the heart and lungs should be performed *first* because this requires the child's cooperation and should be performed early when the child may be more cooperative. Because the sight of medical instruments is likely to frighten a child, use them last. Proceed with the examination in the following order for a cooperative older child (past the second birthday):

- Take measurements and vital signs (this is often done by a nurse or assistant before the clinician begins his or her encounter with the child)
- Observe the child's behavior (this is your most important source of information about his or her neurologic and musculoskeletal systems)
- Inspect the skin
- Examine the head and neck
- Examine the chest

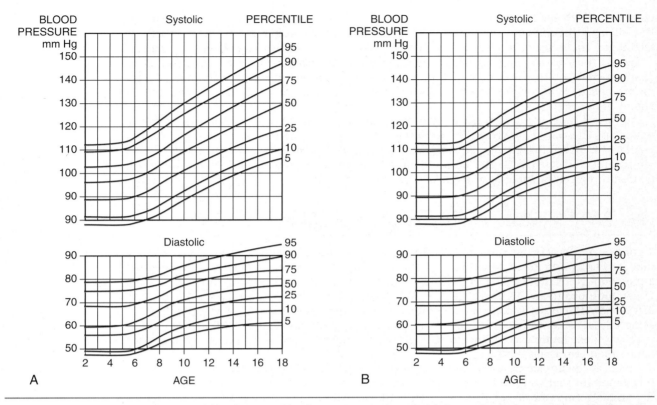

Figure 24–38 National Heart, Lung, and Blood Institute blood pressure measurements. *A,* Percentiles for boys. *B,* Percentiles for girls.

- Examine the heart
- Examine the abdomen
- Examine the genitalia
- Examine the extremities
- Examine the deep tendon reflexes if indicated
- Examine the eyes
- Examine the nose
- Examine the ears
- Examine the mouth and pharynx

General Assessment

As mentioned before, there are a variety of ways of measuring temperature in a child older than 6 months. The heart rate of a child aged 1 to 5 years ranges from 80 to 140 beats per minute; the average rate is 100. The respiratory rate varies from 24 to 40 breaths per minute at 1 year of age and decreases to 20 to 24 by 5 years of age. Blood pressure assessment by auscultation is usually possible with children at least 3 to 4 years of age and should be performed on all children. Inform the child that the cuff will get tight for a few moments. The size of the cuff is important. The cuff must cover two thirds of the distance between the antecubital fossa and the shoulder. A cuff that is too small yields falsely high readings; conversely, a cuff that is too large yields falsely low readings. The techniques of palpatory and auscultatory blood pressure determination are the same as those used in adults. The National Heart, Lung, and Blood Institute has published standards of blood pressure measurements in boys and girls from 2 to 18 years of age. Figure 24-38 shows these percentile charts for boys and girls, taken in the right arm with the child seated.

Determine the *height, weight,* and *body mass index* for all children, and *head circumference up to age 3.** Plot these values on the standard growth charts (see Figs. 24-24 and 24-25).

---

*Head circumference should be measured in older children if there is any reason to suspect abnormal head growth.

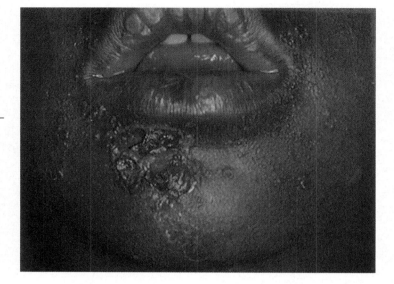

Figure 24–39 Impetigo.

Skin

The examination of the skin is the same for children as for adults.

Careful descriptions of the numerous rashes seen in this age group are paramount for diagnosis. There are many exanthematous diseases of childhood. These rashes may consist of macules, papules, vesicles, pustules, or petechiae. (A summary of important viral and bacterial exanthems is given in Table 24-6 at the end of the chapter.)

Impetigo is one of the most common skin conditions of children in this age group. It is a highly contagious, superficial skin infection caused by a group A beta-hemolytic streptococcus, *Staphylococcus aureus*, or both, and is more common in summer. The primary lesion is a vesicopustule; once it has ruptured, it produces a honey-colored crust surrounded by a rim of erythema. The lesions may be seen on any part of the body, but the face is a common location. The child pictured in Figure 24-39 has the classic weeping, encrusted lesions of impetigo. Figure 24-40 shows the lesions of impetigo in another child.

Examine the spine. Tufts of hair along the spine, especially over the sacrum, may mark the location of a *spina bifida occulta* or other spinal dysraphism (see Fig. 24-17).

Is there evidence of *trauma* or *child abuse?* The signs of physical child abuse are discussed in the previous section.

Head

Examine the *lymph nodes*. All the chains (as indicated in Chapter 9, The Head and Neck) must be examined. Small (0.75- to 1.5-inch [2- to 4-mm]), movable, nontender, discrete nodes are commonly found. Warm, tender nodes are usually indicative of infection.

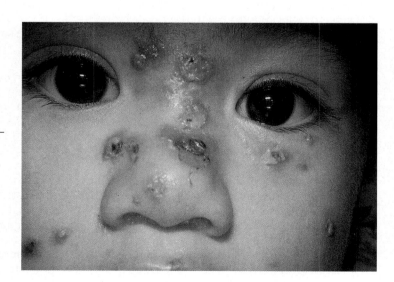

Figure 24–40 Impetigo.

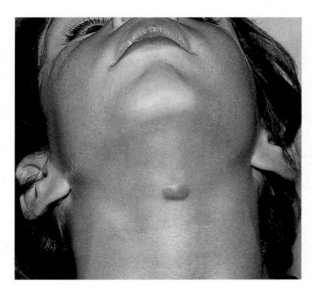

Figure 24–41 Thyroglossal cyst.

Inspect the shape of the head.

Palpate the *sutures* in the 1- to 3-year-old child. Check for the fontanelles. The posterior fontanelle frequently closes soon after the neonatal period. The anterior fontanelle may close as early as 8 months of age or may remain open until 2 years of age. Persistence of the anterior fontanelle past 2 years of age may be a sign of an underlying disorder. The most common problem associated with failure of the anterior fontanelle to close is hypothyroidism; increased intracranial pressure must also be considered in these children.

Palpate over the *maxillary sinuses* in children older than 2 years. Tenderness may indicate sinusitis.

Inspect the area of the *parotid glands*. Localized swelling can best be detected by telling the child to look up to the ceiling while he or she is seated. Note any swelling below the angle of the jaw. Palpate the area. An enlarged parotid gland often pushes the lobe of the ear away from the side of the head; this can be seen when the child is observed from behind.

Inspect the size and shape of the neck. Check for a *thyroglossal duct cyst*. The child in Figure 24-41 has a midline thyroglossal duct cyst.

Palpate the anterior and posterior triangles for lymphadenopathy as in adults. Anterior cervical adenopathy is associated with inflammation of the sinuses, ears, teeth, or pharynx. Group A beta-hemolytic streptococcus is an important cause of pharyngitis in children aged 3 years and older, and can lead to rheumatic fever or postinfectious glomerulonephritis. In predicting a positive bacterial throat culture, the most important diagnostic sign is reported to be tender anterior cervical lymphadenopathy.

Palpate the sternocleidomastoid muscle.

Inspect the location of the *trachea*. Is it midline?

Palpate the *thyroid gland*. This is usually best done by using your thumb and index finger to feel for the gland while the child is in a supine position.

Chest

Inspect the shape of the chest.

Determine the *respiratory rate*. The respiratory rate of a 6-year-old child is 16 to 20 breaths per minute.

Palpate the chest for tactile fremitus, as described in Chapter 13, The Chest. Tactile fremitus has low sensitivity and specificity in childhood.

Auscultation needs to be done systematically, but it can be difficult, and patience is required. If you tell a child to "take a deep breath," the child frequently holds the breath; instead, tell the child to imitate you taking deep breaths. Alternatively, you can ask the child to "blow out the birthday candles." Are the breath sounds normal? Are there any adventitious sounds? Breath sounds in children sound louder than those in adults as a result of the chest configuration.

Percuss the chest, using the same technique as in adults. Because the chest wall is thinner in children than in adults, the percussion notes are more resonant in children. Percuss gently, because overly vigorous percussion may produce vibrations over a large area and obscure an area of dullness.

Heart

In the cardiac examination of a young child, follow these procedures:

1. Inspect the precordium.
2. Palpate for any lifts, heaves, or thrills.
3. Auscultate in the same areas described in Chapter 14, The Heart. Describe any murmurs or abnormal sounds.
4. Palpate the femoral pulses.

Abdomen

The examination of the abdomen is often one of the earlier parts of the examination of a young child because this requires no instruments other than the stethoscope and is usually painless. An anxious child 2 or 3 years of age can be examined in the parent's lap: By leaning back in the chair, the parent acts as the examining table, with the supine child semireclined against the parent's chest and abdomen. An adequate abdominal examination on a child may require repeated "visits" to that part of the examination, until the child is relaxed with the process.

Inspect the abdomen. As children grow older, the protuberant abdomen becomes more scaphoid, except in children who are obese.

Inspect the *umbilicus*. Tell the child to cough. Are there any bulging masses at the umbilicus?

Auscultate for peristaltic sounds. Are any *bruits* present? The presence of an abdominal bruit may be suggestive of coarctation, especially in the presence of upper extremity hypertension and reduced or delayed femoral pulses. Use the stethoscope to listen over the kidneys posteriorly. The presence of a bruit in this location is suggestive of renal artery stenosis.

Percuss the abdomen for abnormal dullness.

Light palpation is performed as described in the adult examination. Is tenderness noted? Observe the patient's face while palpating. Facial expressions are more useful than asking the child, "Does this hurt?" Children are often very ticklish; if you sandwich the child's hand between your two hands as you examine, the child's tendency to giggle diminishes. Alternatively, light palpation can be done with the stethoscope after listening to the bowel sounds.

Deep palpation is also performed as in adults.

Palpate the *liver* and *spleen* as described in Chapter 17, The Abdomen. The liver span of a 3-year-old is approximately 1.5 inches (4 cm). By 5 years of age, the span has increased to 2 inches (5 cm). Begin palpation for organomegaly well down in the lower abdomen, and work your way up. Otherwise, you risk missing the edge of a markedly enlarged liver or spleen.

The *kidneys* may be palpable by ballottement in children up to 5 to 6 years of age. Place your left hand under the right costal margin at the costovertebral angle. Your right hand is placed over the midposition of the right abdomen. Tap firmly on the abdomen to try to feel the size of the kidney. The hands should be reversed to feel the left kidney.

Palpate the *femoral pulses*. Place the tips of your fingers along the inguinal ligament, midway between the symphysis pubis and the iliac crest. Time the pulse with the radial pulse; they should peak at the same time.

Palpate the femoral *lymph nodes*. It is common to find several 0.2 to 0.4-inch (0.5- to 1-cm) nodes.

Inspect the *anus*. Is diaper rash present in a child who is not yet toilet trained? Is there evidence of excoriations? Pinworm infestation commonly causes pruritus and excoriations.

Rectal examination is usually not part of the standard examination in this age group. Only children with abdominal pain or symptoms referable to the lower gastrointestinal tract require a rectal examination. Instruct the child to lie on his or her side, knees drawn up, facing the parent at the side of the table. Tell the child that the examination will be like "taking your temperature." You should use your fifth finger, gloved and well lubricated, for the examination. Tenderness and sphincter tone are determined, as well as the presence of a mass.

Genitalia

If the child is male, inspect the *penis*. If you have occasion to retract the foreskin, return it to its normal position.

Inspect the urethral meatus.

Inspect the *scrotum*. Is there any unilateral enlargement present? Suspect a hydrocele or hernia if the scrotum appears large. Use transillumination, and auscultate any scrotal mass.

Palpate the *testicles*. Are both present in the scrotum? In this age group, the testicles can often become retracted into the inguinal canal. If one or both testicles are not felt in the scrotum, try manipulating the testicle from the inguinal area into the scrotum. If that maneuver fails, tell the child to sit on a chair with his feet on the seat. Instruct him to grab his knees. Repeat the palpation. This additional abdominal pressure may force a retracted or undescended testicle into the scrotum. Warm hands and a warm room often aid in this procedure.

Another useful maneuver to counteract an active cremasteric reflex is to have the child lie down supine and flex his leg at the knee, placing his foot on the opposite leg. This "tailor position" brings the tendon of the sartorius muscle over the inguinal canal and prevents an active reflex from retracting the testicle.

Palpation for an *inguinal hernia* can usually be performed in children 4 years of age and older. The procedure is the same as in adults and should be performed with the child standing.

If the child is female, inspect the *vaginal area*. Is a *rash* present? Rashes may be related to bubble baths. Is a *discharge* present? A discharge in girls aged 2 to 6 years may be related to a foreign body in the vagina. A nasal speculum can be used by an experienced examiner to inspect the vagina for the cause of the discharge. Look for an intact hymen and a smooth vaginal opening. Be on the lookout for sexual abuse. The most important signs of abuse include difficulty walking, vaginal or anal infections, genital irritation or swelling, torn or stained underclothes, vaginal or anal bleeding, and bruises. Most children who have been sexually abused, however, exhibit no physical findings.

Musculoskeletal Examination

Observe the *gait* by telling the child to walk back and forth with shoes or socks on. Having the child walk on a cold floor without socks or shoes may distort the gait. "In-toeing" and "out-toeing" are common in children. Most such gaits are physiologic variants that arise from in utero positioning and resolve spontaneously during the active growing period.

Tell the child to stand in front of you, and inspect the legs. Is bowing present? Commonly, a child may appear bowlegged (*genu varum*) for 1 to 2 years after starting to walk. Knock-knees (*genu valgum*) frequently follow bowing and are seen in children 2 to 4 years of age. The normal gait of a child 2 to 4 years of age is wide-based, with a prominent lumbar lordosis.

In a child with a *limp*, the entire lower extremity from the toes to the hip should be examined for evidence of trauma or localized bone tenderness. Children with abnormalities of the hip frequently localize the area of discomfort to the knee. Any child complaining of knee pain must have his or her hips fully assessed. The presence of a limp and knee pain in a child 3 to 8 years of age, especially a boy, is suggestive of *Legg-Calvé-Perthes disease*, which is aseptic necrosis of the femoral head. The *irritable hip* syndrome, or toxic synovitis, is another cause of limp in this age group. This condition affects both sexes equally.

Inspect the child's shoes. Is there evidence of abnormal wear?

Neurologic Examination

The development of speech and the ability to manipulate small objects, throw a ball, feed and dress oneself, and understand simple directions are the best indicators of a normally developing nervous system.

Deep tendon reflexes are usually not tested unless there is reason to suspect a developmental abnormality or an acute insult to the central nervous system (infection or trauma). If they are tested, use the same techniques as described in Chapter 21, The Nervous System.

Eyes

Visual acuity in children aged 1 to 3 years is assessed by their ability to identify brightly colored objects and to circumnavigate the examining room. Routine visual acuity testing should begin when the child is about 4 years of age, with an appropriate Snellen eye chart. Pediatric eye charts use pictures or the "illiterate E." Average visual acuity for a 3-year-old child is 20/40; at age 4 to 5 years, it is 20/30.

Confrontation visual field testing is performed only in children older than 4 years of age in whom there is a suspicion of decreased acuity or an intracranial mass. The test is conducted as in adults, except that a small toy is used instead of finger counting. The toy is brought in from the periphery of the child's vision, and the child is instructed to tell the examiner when he or she sees it.

Check *ocular motility*. Are the eyes straight? Be aware that a child with large epicanthal folds that partially cover the globe may be thought to have strabismus. The eyes should be parallel in all fields of gaze. Shine a light from 2 feet (61 cm) away, and have the child look at it. The light should fall in the center of both pupils. Hold the patient's head, and turn it to the right and then to the left while the position of the light is maintained. Is the corneal reflection symmetric in both eyes as the head is turned? If there is asymmetry, perform the *cover test* as described in Chapter 10, The Eye.

Is the conjunctiva red? One of the most common eye problems in this age group is *red eye*. The causes are numerous and include conjunctivitis, obstruction of the nasolacrimal duct, chalazion, local trauma, allergy, and toxin exposure.

Nose

Inspect the nostrils. Is *flaring* of the nostrils present? Flaring occurs in any type of respiratory distress.

Inspect the tip of the nose. Is there a permanent transverse crease near the lower part of the nose directing the tip upward? This is commonly seen in allergy sufferers. This unmistakable sign is caused by the *allergic salute:* using a palm or an extended forefinger to rub the nose upward and outward.

Elevate the tip of the nose and inspect the nasal mucosa. Are secretions present? Purulent secretions from above and below the middle turbinate may be suggestive of sinusitis. Watery discharge may be indicative of allergy or viral upper respiratory infection. Epistaxis is usually caused by local trauma and is quite common in preschool- and school-aged children. In children with head trauma, the presence of a clear discharge from the nose is suggestive of cerebrospinal fluid leakage.

Check for *nasal polyps*. These may be associated with allergies or cystic fibrosis.

Ears

Is any *discharge* present? Purulent discharge may be related to bacterial infection. Eczema may cause flaking and cracking behind the ears. A bloody discharge may be caused by irritation, injury, a foreign body, or a basilar skull fracture.

Use the otoscope to inspect the *external canal* and *tympanic membrane*. A cooperative 2- to 3-year-old child may be either sitting or lying prone on the examination table with the head turned to one side. An uncooperative child can be held upright or prone in a parent's arms. The otoscope should be held as indicated previously. Use the largest speculum possible. Insert the speculum tip to only 1/2 inch (1.2 cm).

Inspect the tympanic membrane. Redness is commonly seen and may be caused by infection, trauma, or even crying. In suppurative otitis media, the drum bulges outward and becomes diffusely erythematous or even opaque yellow, hearing is decreased, and the light reflex may be lost. Is the tympanic membrane perforated? Does the tympanic membrane move with insufflation? An immobile drum is present in suppurative or serous otitis media (see previous discussion and Fig. 11-29).

Palpate the *mastoid tip*. Is it tender? Tenderness is suggestive of mastoiditis, which may be associated with redness of the mastoid and forward displacement of the pinna, most obvious when the child is viewed from behind.

Are *posterior auricular lymph nodes* present? These nodes are classically found in children with rubella. They are also found in children with measles, roseola, chickenpox, or inflammations of the scalp.

Check *hearing*. Hearing is necessary for the normal development of language. As a screening test, occlude one ear, and whisper a number into the child's other ear. Ask the child what number he or she heard. Repeat the test with the other ear. If hearing loss is suspected, or the child has language delay, the child should be scheduled for audiometric testing as soon as possible.

Mouth and Pharynx

The evaluation of the mouth and pharynx is usually the last part of the examination of the small child.

Inspect the *lips* for any lesions and color.

Tell the child, "Open your mouth. I am going to count your teeth." Inspect the *teeth* for number and caries. The first lower molars erupt at about 1 year of age. These are followed by

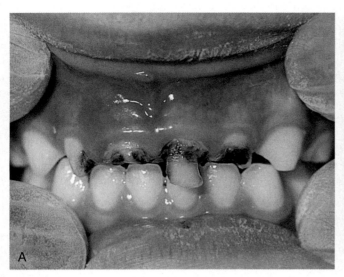
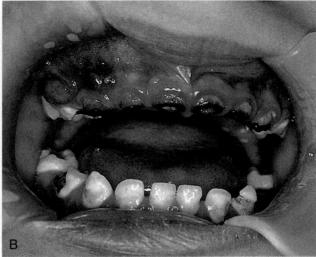

Figure 24–42 *A,* Milk caries. *B,* Periapical abcesses secondary to carious destruction.

the first upper molars at 14 months, lower canines (cuspids) at 16 months, upper canines at 18 months, second lower molars at 20 months, and second upper molars at 2 years. These complete the primary dentition of 20 teeth. Flattened edges are seen in children who grind their teeth. (Table 24-5 at the end of this chapter summarizes the ages at tooth eruption.)

Multiple caries, especially of the upper incisors, are often an indication of *milk caries,* also known as *nursing bottle caries.* They are caused by the child's going to sleep with a bottle of milk or juice in the mouth. Cariogenic fluids such as milk or sweetened beverages that constantly bathe the teeth while the infant is asleep are the cause of nursing bottle carries. The interaction of *Streptococcus mutans* and other microorganisms in the mouth and fermentable carbohydrates results in acid demineralization of the susceptible tooth enamel. Untreated carious destruction progresses through the enamel, dentin, and pulp, producing *periapical abscesses.* The maxillary anterior teeth are the first to be affected. The mandibular teeth are the least affected. Figure 24-42*A* shows severe milk caries that necessitated removal of all the child's primary dentition. Always look for a small pimple in the alveolar ridge above a damaged tooth; this is evidence of a *periapical abscess* and necessitates urgent referral for dental treatment. The child pictured in Figure 24-42*B* had periapical abscesses of all her upper teeth and severe decay of her mandibular teeth.

Inspect the *bite.* Slight maxillary protrusion is termed *overbite* and is the normal position; mandibular protrusion is termed *underbite.*

Have the child bite down while you inspect the occlusion. Normally, the upper teeth override the lower teeth.

Inspect the *gingivae* for any lesions.

Inspect the *buccal mucosa.* In measles, on the second or third day of the disease, pinpoint white spots are often seen on the buccal mucosa opposite the lower molars. These spots are called *Koplik's spots* and are pathognomonic for measles. Vesicles on an erythematous base are suggestive of *herpes simplex* infection. Similar vesicles on the soft palate and tonsillar pillars are suggestive of *herpangina* caused by coxsackievirus infections. Dusky red 1- to 3-mm spots on the buccal mucosa and palate are an early sign of rubella. These diffusely scattered oral lesions, known as *Forschheimer's spots,* appear on the posterior hard and soft palates and develop at the end of the prodromal stage or at the beginning of the cutaneous eruption. Figure 24-43 shows Forschheimer's spots of rubella.

Inspect the *tongue.* Geographic tongue is a normal variation (see Fig. 12-25*A*). Dryness is seen in dehydration and in chronic mouth breathers. Strawberry tongue is indicative of scarlet fever.

The child should be seated during this part of the examination for best visualization of the posterior pharynx. Tell the youngster that you are going to look in his or her throat and that he or she should open the mouth as widely as possible. If the child is extremely uncooperative, have the child lie on his or her back on the examination table. The parent should stand at the head of the table, raise the child's hands over the head, and squeeze the child's elbows against

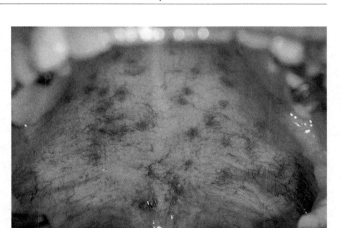

Figure 24–43 Forschheimer's spots of rubella.

the head so that the head does not move. The examiner can then lean over the child, holding a tongue blade in one hand and a light in the other.

Inspect the *posterior pharynx*. Inspect the size of the *tonsils*. Tonsillar size is estimated on a scale from 1+ to 4+, whereby 4+ indicates that the tonsils meet in the midline. "Kissing" tonsils (see Fig. 12-41) may be indicative of obstructive apnea. Is a purulent exudate present? Is a membrane present? Membranes are seen in diphtheria and *Candida* infections.

Are *petechiae* present? Streptococcal pharyngitis is often associated with petechiae.

Inspect the *posterior pharyngeal wall*. A cobblestone appearance is suggestive of chronic postnasal drip.

Review of Systems and Examination of the Older Child

School-aged children may have chronic somatic complaints such as headaches, stomach pain, or leg pains which often have a partly emotional basis. A good history of the circumstances in which these complaints occur can help you tease out the triggers. Other items to add to the *review of systems* for children aged 6 to 12 years include persistent sneezing and nasal itching, itchy eyes, snoring, disturbed sleep, daytime somnolence, chest pain, exercise-induced cough or wheezing, nocturnal cough, palpitations, polyuria, polydipsia, syncope, persistent sadness or worry, sports injuries, and concussion.

It is usually easy to examine children 6 to 12 years of age. They understand the purpose of the examination and rarely present any problems. It is often helpful to engage the child in conversation regarding school, friends, or hobbies. Conversation helps relax the child even if he or she does not appear apprehensive.

Allow the child to wear a gown or drape.

The order of the examination is essentially the same as in adults. If the child is complaining of pain in a certain area, that area should be examined last.

As with younger children, brief explanations about each part of the examination should be given to older children.

Wash your hands with soap and warm water before beginning the examination.

General Assessment

In children 6 to 12 years of age, the *temperature* may be taken orally. The pulse of an average child in this age group varies from 75 to 125 beats per minute, and the respirations vary from 15 to 20 breaths per minute.

Blood pressure should be obtained in all children in this age group by the methods described in Chapter 14, The Heart. Use the correct cuff size.

Measure the child's height and weight, and chart these on the child's record.

Skin

Inspect the skin for any evidence of fungal disease, especially between the toes.

Are any *rashes* present? Persistent dandruff may be *tinea capitis* and not seborrhea. Seborrhea is most commonly seen in infancy and adolescence. Eczema, on the other hand, is very common at this age and is often most noticeable in the antecubital and popliteal fossae.

Eyes

The examination of the eyes is essentially the same as in adults, with emphasis on *visual acuity*. A test with a standard Snellen eye chart is necessary.

Ears

The examination of the ears is the same as in adults, with emphasis on *auditory acuity*. Audiometric testing should be performed on all school-aged children.

Nose

The examination of the nose is essentially the same as in adults.

Mouth and Pharynx

The *teeth* should be examined with regard to their condition and spacing. Have the child bite down, and observe the *bite*. (See Table 24-5 at the end of this chapter, which summarizes the ages at which shedding of the primary teeth occurs, as well as the ages of secondary tooth eruption.)

Inspect the *tongue* for dryness, size, and lesions. Deep furrows are common and have no clinical significance.

Inspect the *palate* for petechiae.

Inspect the *tonsils* for enlargement, injection, and exudation.

Neck

Palpate the *thyroid* for nodules. The thyroid is rarely palpable in normal children in this age group.

Palpate for *lymphadenopathy*. Anterior cervical nodes are seen in association with upper respiratory infections and dental infections. Posterior adenopathy is seen with infections of the middle ear and scalp. Generalized adenopathy is seen in viral diseases such as infectious mononucleosis, measles, and rubella.

Is the *trachea* midline?

Chest

The examination of the chest is the same as in adults. Breast development may be noticed in normal girls as young as 8 years. See the discussion of Tanner staging in the Genitalia section.

Heart

The examination of the heart is the same as in adults.

Abdomen

The order of the abdominal examination is the same as in adults. The span of the liver at 8 years of age is 2 to 2.2 inches (5 to 5.5 cm); at 12 years of age, the span is approximately 2.2 to 2.6 inches (5.5 to 6.5 cm).

Genitalia

The age of development of secondary sexual characteristics varies greatly. As indicated in Chapter 16, The Breast, development of the breasts in girls may begin as early as 8 years of age and continues for the next 5 years. The development of pubic hair in girls occurs at around the same time. Testicular development in boys begins somewhat later, at about 9 to 10 years of age. Pubic hair starts to develop in boys at about 12 years of age and continues to develop until 15 years of age. The growth of the penis begins about a year after the beginning of testicular enlargement, at 10 to 11 years of age. In boys with Klinefelter syndrome (karyotype 47,XXY), this normal relationship between appearance of pubic hair, development of testes, and growth of the penis is disturbed; the hallmark of this syndrome is the presence of prepuberty-sized testes with normal pubic hair and penile length growth. Whereas the growth spurt in girls occurs at about 12 years of age, early in their pubertal development, this spurt is not seen until around 14 years of age in boys, when the genital changes are fairly well advanced.

Sex maturity ratings for boys and girls were established by J. M. Tanner in 1962. In the boy, the growth of pubic hair and the development of the penis, testes, and scrotum are used to assign a sex maturity rating from 1 to 5. The examiner should record two ratings: one for the pubic hair and one for the genitalia. If the development of the penis differs from that of the testes and scrotum, the two ratings should be averaged. The Tanner sex maturity ratings for genital development in boys are illustrated and summarized in Figure 24-44.

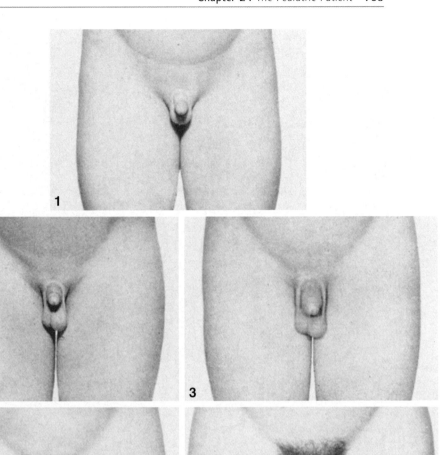

Figure 24–44 Tanner's Stages of Development. Genital development in boys. Numbers indicate sex maturity ratings.

Stage	Characteristics
1	Prepubertal; testes, scrotum, and penis are about the same size and proportion as in early childhood
2	Enlargement of the testes and scrotum; reddening and coarsening of scrotal skin; little change in size of penis
3	Enlargement of penis, which occurs mainly in length; further growth of testes and scrotum
4	Further enlargement of penis with growth in width and length; enlargement of glans penis; darkening of scrotal skin
5	Adult genitalia

The Tanner sex maturity ratings for pubic hair development in boys and girls are illustrated and summarized in Figure 24-45.

The Tanner sex maturity ratings for girls are based on the growth of pubic hair and the development of the breasts. Five stages are observed for each. The examiner should record two ratings: one for the breasts and one for the pubic hair. The sex maturity ratings for breast development in girls are illustrated and summarized in Figure 24-46.

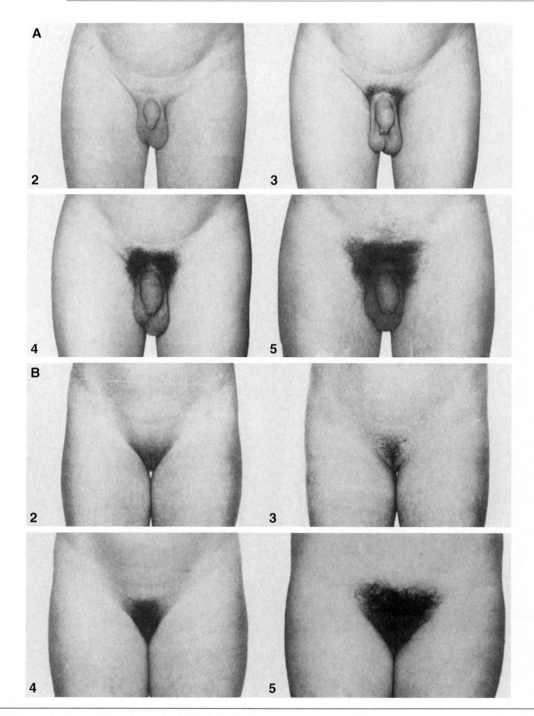

Figure 24–45 Tanner's Stages of Development. Pubic hair development. Numbers indicate sex maturity ratings. *A,* Development in boys. *B,* Development in girls.

Stage	Characteristics
1	Prepuberal; no true pubic hair
2	Sparse growth of slightly pigmented, downy hair; only slightly curled; hair mainly at base of penis or along labia
3	Increase in hair, which is becoming coarser, curled, and darker
4	Adult-type hair, but limited in area; no spread to medial surface of thighs
5	Adult-type hair with spread to thighs

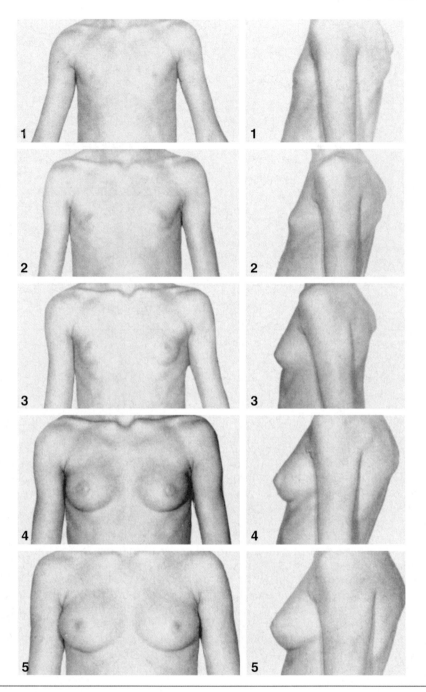

Figure 24–46 Tanner's Stages of Development. Breast development in girls. Numbers indicate sex maturity ratings.

Stage	Characteristics
1	Prepubertal; elevation of papilla only
2	Breast bud stage: elevation of breast and papilla as a small mound; enlargement of diameter of areola
3	Further enlargement of breast and areola with no separation of contours
4*	Areola projected above level of breast as a secondary mound
5	Mature stage: recession of areola mound to the general contour of the breast; projection of papilla only

*This stage is absent in approximately 25% of girls. Conversely, this stage may persist throughout life.

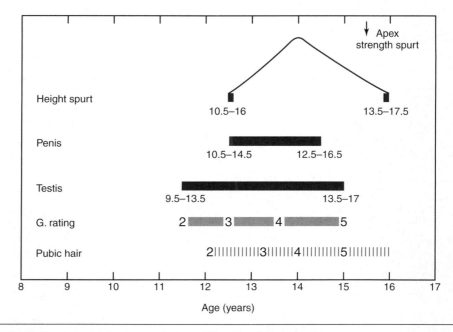

Figure 24–47 Developmental sequence in boys. "G. rating," genital rating.

A summary of the developmental sequence for boys is diagrammed in Figure 24-47; a summary for girls is diagrammed in Figure 24-48.

The youngster should be given a gown to avoid embarrassment in front of a parent.

Inspect the *external genitalia*. Is *pubic hair* present? What are the *sex maturity ratings?* Are any lesions present? Is there evidence of sexual abuse?

Palpate the testes. Is an *inguinal hernia* present?

Pelvic examinations are not routine in this age group unless clinically indicated and should be performed by an experienced examiner. Vaginal bleeding in girls younger than 9 years of age is a result of infection from foreign objects in more than 66% of cases. Trauma accounts for an additional 16%.

Musculoskeletal Examination

An important goal of the musculoskeletal examination of children aged 6 to 12 years is to detect *scoliosis*. Scoliosis is the most common spinal deformity, especially in pubertal girls. Have the patient stand stripped to the waist. Inspect the back. Are the shoulders, or scapulae, at the same height? Is the occiput aligned over the intergluteal cleft? Ask the child to bend down and try to touch the toes, allowing the arms to hang freely. A unilateral elevation of the lower ribs is seen in patients with scoliosis. This is shown in Figure 24-49. Another method for detecting scoliosis is for you to mark the spinous processes with a pen while the child is standing in front of you. Then ask the child to bend forward from the waist. A deviation of the marks to either side suggests scoliosis. Unfortunately, none of the methods for detecting scoliosis has adequate sensitivity or specificity.

Neurologic Examination

The neurologic examination is essentially the same as outlined in Chapter 21, The Nervous System. However, in children in this age group, the complete neurologic examination is indicated only when there is evidence of developmental abnormalities, an acute insult to the central nervous system, or a complaint such as headache.

Review of Systems and Examination of the Adolescent

The *review of systems* for the adolescent is almost the same as for the adult. Of note, questions about menstruation, including menstrual cramps or premenstrual symptoms; about sexual function and symptoms of sexually transmitted disease; and about sports injuries, mood disorders, and thought disorders become relevant with the teenaged patient. The examination of adolescents is also exactly the same as that of adults. It is appropriate for the examiner to ask

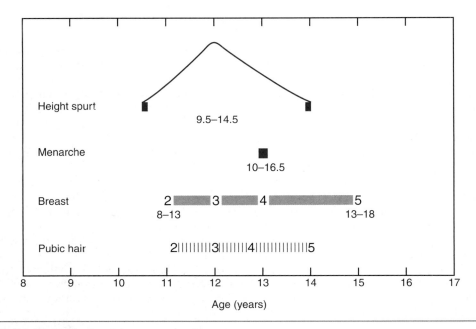

Figure 24–48 Developmental sequence in girls.

the parent to leave during the examination. However, some younger adolescents prefer to have their parent present for the examination; therefore, ask the patient his or her preference.

Because the examination is so similar to that of adults, only the dissimilarities are described in this section.

General Assessment

The average *heart rate* of the adolescent is 60 to 100 beats per minute. The respiratory rate varies from 12 to 18 breaths per minute at 16 years of age.

Blood pressure is important to determine by the methods discussed in Chapter 14, The Heart.

Skin

Examination of the skin of adolescents usually reveals evidence of *pubertal changes*. These include acne, areolar pigmentation, functioning of the apocrine sweat glands, pigmentation of the external genitalia, and development of axillary and pubic hair.

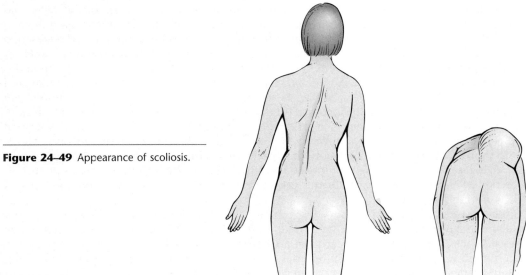

Figure 24–49 Appearance of scoliosis.

Breasts

Determine the *Tanner sex maturity rating* of the breasts in girls.

Breast development occurs in both boys and girls. A boy with unilateral gynecomastia who is at Tanner stage 3 or 4 can be reassured that this change is part of normal puberty and will be transient.

Asymmetric breast development in girls is common. Reassure the patient that puberty is progressing normally.

Abdomen

The abdominal examination is the same as in adults. The liver span of a 16-year-old varies from 2.4 to 2.8 inches (6 to 7 cm).

Genitalia

Determine the *sex maturity ratings* of the pubic hair and genitalia for male patients. Determine the sex maturity rating of the pubic hair for female patients.

The examiner should evaluate the patient and try to explain to him or her about the body changes that are related to normal puberty.

If an internal pelvic examination is necessary for a female adolescent, an extremely gentle approach is required. Use of a Pedersen speculum often renders the examination less uncomfortable. If the examiner is a man, a female nurse must be present; if the examiner is a woman, it is ideal if a female nurse is present.

Musculoskeletal Examination

Knee pain in an adolescent is usually the result of trauma. Partial avulsion of the tibial tubercle associated with a painful swelling in that area is called *Osgood-Schlatter disease*. This common condition is seen more frequently in pubertal boys and is usually self-limited. Knee pain may also be referred from the hip and result from a *slipped capital femoral epiphysis* (SCFE). Movement of the hip into external rotation as the leg is flexed at knee and hip is very suggestive of SCFE. SCFE is fairly common during the pubertal growth spurt and is especially common in obese adolescents.

Scoliosis often progresses rapidly during the pubertal growth spurt.

If the adolescent is seeking medical clearance for competitive sports, it is worth performing a comprehensive musculoskeletal screening examination to detect, among other things, incompletely rehabilitated sports injuries. One such screening examination was well described by Foster and colleagues (2006).

Clinicopathologic Correlations

Viral exanthematous diseases of childhood are extremely common. There are now immunizations for many of the classic childhood exanthems. In the early years of the 20th century, pediatricians frequently referred to many childhood diseases by number. Scarlet fever and measles were numbers one and two, respectively; rubella became known as the third disease; fourth disease was probably a combination of scarlet fever and rubella and did not represent a distinct entity; the fifth disease was *erythema infectiosum;* and the sixth disease was *roseola*.

Rubella, or *German measles*, is a common communicable disease caused by a togavirus and is characterized by mild constitutional symptoms, a rash, and generalized enlargement and tenderness of the lymph nodes of the head and neck. It is transmitted by respiratory droplets. The lymphadenopathy precedes the rash, which consists of red or pink macules or papules, starting first on the face and then spreading to the extremities. Intraoral lesions—Forschheimer's spots—are often observed before development of the rash. Figure 24-43 shows Forschheimer's spots on the palate of a child with rubella. Rubella is now extremely rare as a result of the widespread use of the rubella vaccine, but it remains important to recognize this disease because of the risk to the fetus if a nonimmune woman contracts rubella during pregnancy.

Fifth disease was linked in 1983 to human parvovirus B19. Erythema infectiosum is a moderately contagious disease affecting school-aged children. It produces an asymptomatic "slapped cheek" erythema on the face and an erythematous maculopapular, lacy, serpiginous, blanching rash on the trunk and extremities. The rash, sometimes pruritic, lasts 2 to 40 days, with an average duration of 11 days. There is no gender predilection. Fever is usually absent or low grade. Figure 24-50 shows the classic "slapped cheek" rash on a child with fifth disease.

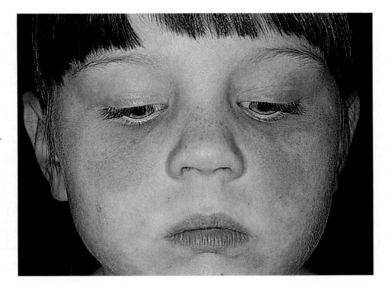

Figure 24–50 "Slapped cheek" rash of fifth disease.

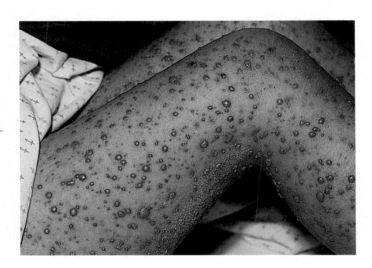

Figure 24–51 Chickenpox.

Chickenpox, or *varicella*, is caused by the varicella-zoster DNA virus belonging to the Herpesviridae family. The illness is extremely contagious over several days preceding the development of the rash. Before the introduction of the vaccine in 1995, it was estimated that more than 3 to 4 million cases occurred each year. The vesicular eruption begins on the trunk, and the vesicular lesions are described as "a dewdrop on a rose," progressing to pustular lesions that then crust over in 3 to 5 days. New lesions appear as older ones are crusting. Mild fever, malaise, pruritus, anorexia, and listlessness accompany the rash. The vesicular rash of chickenpox is pictured in Figure 24-51. The distribution is shown on another child in Figure 24-52, and a close-up photograph of the vesicular lesions is shown in Figure 24-53. Although it is usually a mild, self-limited illness in healthy children, varicella can be fatal in someone who is immunocompromised. Like rubella, varicella is teratogenic, causing birth defects in approximately 10% of fetuses exposed during the 5th to 14th weeks of gestation.

Herpes simplex virus is a common cause of painful oral lesions in children, especially toddlers and school-aged children. Figure 24-54 shows herpetic gingivostomatitis in a 6-year-old boy. Extensive perioral vesicles, pustules, and erosions are common. The gingivae become markedly edematous and erythematous and bleed easily. Fever, irritability, and cervical and submaxillary lymphadenopathy are common. The acute phase lasts 4 to 9 days and is self-limited, although affected children are at risk for significant dehydration during this phase because oral intake is so painful. The vesicles rupture and become encrusted. Desquamation and healing are usually complete in 10 to 14 days.

Kawasaki's disease, or mucocutaneous lymph node syndrome, is an acute febrile illness of young children. Almost all affected children are younger than 5 years, and most are younger

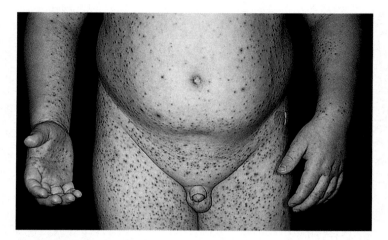

Figure 24–52 Chickenpox.

than 3 years. The cause is unknown, although a viral or rickettsial agent is suspected. The male–female incidence ratio is 2.5:1, and the overall frequency is highest among Asians. Kawasaki's disease is the most frequent cause of acquired heart disease in children from 1 to 5 years of age. The histopathologic condition is a vasculitis with a predilection to aneurysmal disease of the coronary arteries. This coronary thromboarteritis occurs in 25% to 30% of untreated cases of Kawasaki's disease. The annual incidence in the United States is estimated to range from 4.5 per 100,000 children to 8.5 per 100,000 children. The illness occurs most commonly during winter and spring.

High fever, around 40° C, is usually the first sign and lasts for at least 5 days. Within a few days, an irregular, morbilliform, macular eruption develops over the trunk and legs. Figure 24-55 shows the typical rash in a patient with Kawasaki's disease. Erythema multiforme can also be seen (Fig. 24-56). Palm, sole, and fingertip desquamation occurs 10 to 18 days after the onset of fever; this is one of the most characteristic features of the disease. Figure 24-57 shows this desquamation on the hands of a child with Kawasaki's disease. Desquamation also commonly occurs in the inguinal and perineal area, and may precede the extremity changes. The conjunctiva becomes injected, and punctate redness of the palate and strawberry tongue develop, as shown in Figure 24-58. Peripheral edema and asymmetric cervical lymphadenopathy are seen early in the disease in 75% of patients. Arthritis is present in 40% of cases. Although most individuals recover without sequelae, death occurs in approximately 2% of patients as a result of coronary arteritis. The diagnostic criteria for Kawasaki's disease are as follows:

Fever for at least 5 days

Presence of four of the following:

- Bilateral nonpurulent conjunctival injection
- Changes in the mucosa of the oropharynx

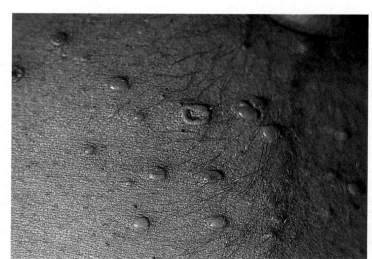

Figure 24–53 Close-up of chickenpox vesicles.

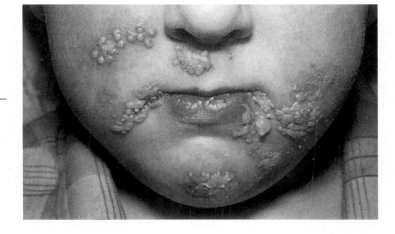

Figure 24–54 Herpetic gingivostomatitis.

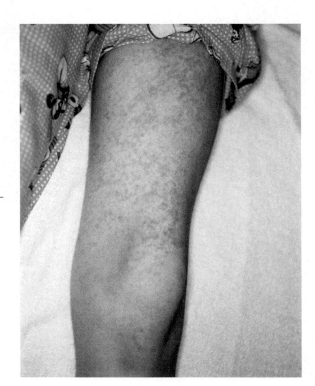

Figure 24–55 Rash in a patient with Kawasaki's disease.

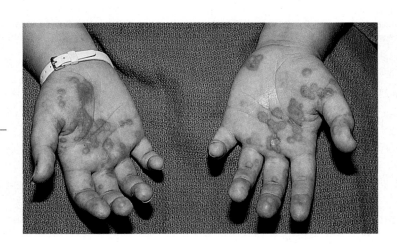

Figure 24–56 Erythema multiforme in a patient with Kawasaki's disease.

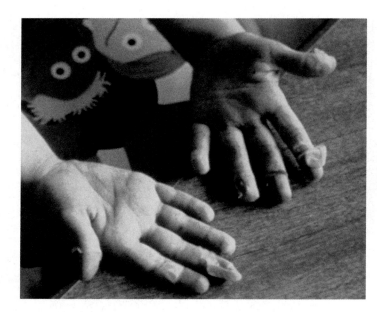

Figure 24–57 Desquamation on the hands of a child with Kawasaki's disease.

Table 24–4 Cardiovascular Murmurs of Childhood

Condition	Cycle	Location	Radiation	Pitch	Other Signs
Ventricular septal effect	Pansystolic	Left sternal border at the fourth or fifth intercostal space	Over the precordium; in rare cases, to the axilla	High	Thrill at left lower sternal border
Mitral insufficiency	Pansystolic	Apex	Axilla	High	S_1 decreased S_3
Pulmonic stenosis	Systolic ejection	Left second or third intercostal space	Left shoulder	Medium	Widely split S_2 Right-sided S_4 Ejection click
Patent ductus arteriosus	Continuous	Left second intercostal space	Left clavicle	Medium	Machinery-like, harsh sound Thrill
Venous hum	Continuous	Medial third of clavicles, often on the right	First and second intercostal spaces	Low	Can be obliterated by pressure on the jugular veins

Table 24–5 Chronology of Dentition

Tooth Type	Deciduous Teeth				Permanent Teeth Eruption	
	Eruption Maxillary (Months)	Eruption Mandibular (Months)	Shedding Maxillary (Years)	Shedding Mandibular (Years)	Maxillary (Years)	Mandibular (Years)
Central incisors	6-8	5-7	7-8	6-7	7-8	6-7
Lateral incisors	8-11	7-10	8-9	7-8	8-9	6-7
Canines (cuspids)	16-20	16-20	11-12	9-11	11-12	9-11
First premolars (bicuspids)	—	—	—	—	10-11	10-12
Second premolars	—	—	—	—	10-12	11-13
First molars	10-16	10-16	10-11	10-12	6-7	6-7
Second molars	20-30	20-30	10-12	11-13	12-13	12-13
Third molars	—	—	—	—	17-22	17-22

Table 24–6 Exanthematous Diseases of Childhood

Disease	Cutaneous Lesion	Location	Mucous Membranes Affected	Systemic Components
Chickenpox (varicella) (see Figs. 24-51, 24-52, and 24-53)	Maculopapular, "tear-drop" vesicles on an erythematous base	Trunk, face, and scalp; centrifugal* spread	Yes	Mild febrile disorder; malaise; rash preceded by a 24-hour prodrome of headache and malaise; all stages and sizes of lesions found at the same time and in the same area; pruritus
Measles (rubeola)	Erythematous, maculopapular, purplish-red	Scalp, hairline, forehead, behind ears, upper neck; rash starts on head and spreads rapidly to upper extremities and then to lower extremities; rash often slightly hemorrhagic; as rash fades, brown discoloration occurs and then disappears within 7-10 days	Yes[†]	Three- to 4-day prodrome of high fever, chills, headache, malaise, cough, photophobia, conjunctivitis; 2 days before the rash develops, Koplik's spots[†] may be seen
Rubella (German measles)	Rose-pink, small, irregular macules and papules[‡]; rash is the first evidence of the disease	Hairline, face, neck, trunk, extremities; centripetal[§] spread; rapidly involves body in 24 hours and tends to fade as it spreads	Yes[‡]	Mild fever, if any; headache, sore throat, mild upper respiratory infection; presence of suboccipital and posterior auricular lymph nodes
Erythema infectiosum (fifth disease; see Fig. 24-50)	Erythematous malar blush	Face, upper arm, thighs; sudden rash in an asymptomatic child, in a "slapped cheek" appearance; maculopapular rash on upper extremities the next day; several days later, a lacy rash on proximal extremities	No	Mild fever, mild pruritus
Roseola infantum (exanthema subitum)	Rose pink, 2- to 3-mm macules; rash appears at end of febrile period; duration of rash only 24 hours	Trunk	Rarely	Sudden onset; high fever
Scarlet fever	Fine punctate, erythematous lesions that blanch on pressure	Face, along skinfolds, buttocks, sternum, between scapulae	Yes[¶]	Disease results from toxin produced by group A streptococci as a result of pharyngeal infection[¶]: abrupt onset of fever, headache, sore throat, vomiting; 12-48 hours later, rash appears

*Moving outward from the center.
[†]Koplik's spots are highly diagnostic; these appear on the buccal mucosa opposite the first molar teeth; they often appear as bluish-white, pinpoint papules on an erythematous base.
[‡]Forschheimer's sign consists of petechiae or reddish spots on the soft palate during the first day of the illness (see Fig. 24-43).
[§]Moving toward the center.
[¶]Bright red lesions, often on tonsils and soft palate.

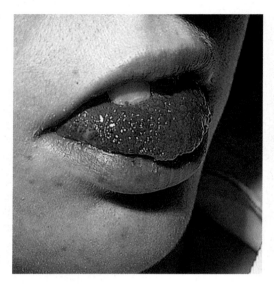

Figure 24–58 Strawberry tongue in a child with Kawasaki's disease.

- Changes of the extremities (e.g., edema, erythema, or desquamation)
- Rash (not vesicular), primarily truncal
- Cervical adenopathy

Early involvement of the cardiovascular system is manifested by tachycardia and often an S_3 gallop. Early intervention with intravenous gamma globulin and antiplatelet therapy has been shown to significantly reduce coronary abnormalities.

Heart murmurs are common in the pediatric age group. Some are serious, but many normal preschool children have a short, musical systolic murmur at the lower left sternal border. Table 24-4 summarizes the more common murmurs and associated findings. Table 24-5 lists N.B. the chronology of dentition. Table 24-6 lists the more common exanthematous diseases of childhood.

Review the DVD-ROM included with this book, which demonstrates a telephone consultation with a parent as well as a history and physical examination of a newborn and toddler.

Sample Write-Up of a Newborn's History

This 2830-g female infant was born at 38 2/7 weeks to a 47-year-old G1 P0-0-0-0 mother by NSVD (normal spontaneous vaginal delivery) at 1:35 AM on 1/16/2008. The pregnancy was complicated by chronic hypertension, for which the mother was treated with Aldomet (methyldopa). The mother is O+ and hepatitis B surface antigen, syphilis, HIV, and Chlamydia negative. Amniocentesis at 14 weeks revealed a 47,XX trisomy 21 karyotype. The mother continued the pregnancy, despite the amniocentesis results, explaining that she "wanted to know what I would be facing beforehand." At 36 weeks, a vaginal culture for group B streptococcus was negative. Mother went into labor at 38+ weeks; she developed malignant hypertension unresponsive to magnesium sulfate, so a C-section (cesarean section) was performed under general anesthesia after 17 hours of labor. Rupture of membranes was at delivery. The baby's Apgar scores were 5 and 8, with points off for tone, reflex, respiratory effort, and color at 1 minute. Baby was transferred to the NICU (neonatal intensive care unit) for observation for Down's syndrome and hypermagnesemia.

Bibliography

American Academy of Pediatrics: Task Force on Sudden Infant Death Syndrome. The changing concept of sudden infant death syndrome: Diagnostic coding shifts, controversies regarding the sleeping environment, and new variables to consider in reducing risk. Pediatrics 116:1245, 2005.

Anderson RN, Smith BL: Deaths: Leading Causes for 2001. Natl Vital Stat Rep 52(9):1, 2003.

Baron J, Rothrock S, Brennan J, et al: Pediatric Emergency Medicine. Philadelphia, Elsevier, 2008.

Beckwith JB: Defining the sudden infant death syndrome. Arch Pediatr Adolesc Med 157:286, 2003.

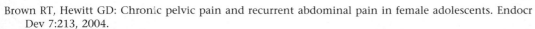

Brown RT, Hewitt GD: Chronic pelvic pain and recurrent abdominal pain in female adolescents. Endocr Dev 7:213, 2004.

Centers for Disease Control and Prevention: Recommended immunization schedules for persons aged 0-18 years—United States, 2007. MMWR 55(51&52):Q1, 2006. Available at: *www.cdc.gov/mmwr/preview/mmwrhtml/mm5551a7.htm*; accessed June 29, 2008.

Committee on Environmental Health, 1997–1998, American Academy of Pediatrics: Screening for elevated blood lead levels. Pediatrics 101:1072, 1998.

Coupey SM: Primary Care for the Sexually Active Adolescent Female. St. Louis, Mosby, 2000.

De Jonste JC, Shields MD: Chronic cough in children. Thorax 58:1715, 2003.

Dixon SD, Stein MT: Encounters with Children: Pediatric Behavior and Development, 3rd ed. St. Louis, Mosby, 2000.

Foster HE, Kay LJ, Friswell M, et al: Musculoskeletal Screening Examination (pGALS) for school-age children based on the adult GALS screen. Arthritis Rheum 55:709, 2006.

Goldenring JM, Cohen E: Getting into adolescent heads. Contemp Pediatr 5:75, 1988.

Greene WB: Essentials of Musculoskeletal Care, 2nd ed. Rosemont, Ill, American Academy of Orthopaedic Surgeons/American Academy of Pediatrics, 2001.

Hurwitz S: Clinical Pediatric Dermatology, 2nd ed. Philadelphia, WB Saunders, 1993.

Johnson CF: Inflicted injury versus accidental injury. Pediatr Clin North Am 37:807, 1990.

Jones KL (ed): Smith's Recognizable Patterns of Human Malformation, 5th ed. Philadelphia, WB Saunders, 1997.

Kaltman J, Shah M: Evaluation of the child with an arrhythmia. Pediatr Clin North Am 51:1537, 2004.

Kochanek KD, Murphy SL, Anderson RN, et al: Deaths: Final data for 2002. Natl Vital Stat Rep 53(5):1, 2004.

Kohli R, Li BK: Differential diagnosis of recurrent abdominal pain: New considerations. Pediatr Ann 33:113, 2004.

Krous HF, Beckwith JB, Byard RW, et al: Sudden infant death syndrome and unclassified sudden infant deaths: A definitional and diagnostic approach. Pediatrics 114:234, 2004.

Marshall WA, Tanner JM: Variations in the pattern of pubertal changes in boys. Arch Dis Child 45:22, 1970.

McIsaac WJ, Kellner JD, Aufricht P, et al: Empirical validation of guidelines for the management of pharyngitis in children and adults. JAMA 291:1587, 2004.

Pinkham JR, Casamassimo PS, Fields HW Jr, et al (eds): Pediatric Dentistry: Infancy Through Adolescence, 3rd ed. Philadelphia, WB Saunders, 1999.

Ross EM, Candy DCA, Davies EG: Clinical Pediatrics. Philadelphia, WB Saunders, 2000.

Sargent JD, DiFranza JR: Tobacco control for clinicians who treat adolescents. CA Cancer J Clin 53:102, 2003.

Shah BR, Laude TA: Atlas of Pediatric Clinical Diagnosis. Philadelphia, WB Saunders, 2000.

Slap GB: Menstrual disorders in adolescence: Best practices and research. Clin Obstet Gynecol 17:75, 2003.

Tanner JM: Growth at Adolescence, 2nd ed. Oxford, UK, Blackwell Scientific, 1962.

Wallis AL, Cody BE, Mickalide AD: Report to the Nation: Trends in Unintentional Childhood Injury Mortality, 1987-2000, Washington, DC, National SAFE KIDS Campaign, 2003.

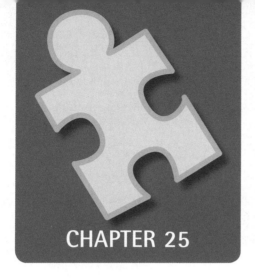

CHAPTER 25

The Geriatric Patient

Old age isn't so bad when you consider the alternative.

Maurice Chevalier (1888–1972)

General Considerations

The geriatric patient is an individual 65 years of age or older. Among such individuals, there is considerable variation in general health, mental status, functional ability, personal and social resources, marital status, living arrangements, creativity, and social integration. The age range of this rapidly growing population spans more than 40 years. The world's geriatric population is currently increasing at a rate of 2.5% per year—significantly faster than the total population. Between 1900 and 2000, the number of Americans older than 65 years increased from a little more than 3 million to 35 million. Since 1960, the geriatric population has grown 107%, in comparison with 50% for the U.S. population as a whole. From 2000 to 2040, in the United States, the number of people 65 years of age or older is projected to increase from 34.8 million to 77.2 million. It is estimated that in the developed nations of the world, there are 146 million people 65 years of age and older. This group will increase to 232 million by the year 2020.

A decreasing rate of mortality, especially from heart disease and stroke, and a reduction in risk factors such as smoking, high blood pressure, and high serum cholesterol levels have contributed to this increased survival.

The population older than 85 years of age represents the fastest-growing segment of the U.S. population. This "graying of America" is expected to continue. By the year 2020, one fifth of the population will be older than 65 years of age. These statistics are extremely important in view of the cost of medical care for this population. Currently, 32% of all health-care dollars is spent on the geriatric population, which constitutes only 12% of the total population.

Some other statistics are important. Eighty-nine percent of the elderly are white. Elderly women outnumber elderly men 1.5:1 overall and 3:1 among individuals 95 years of age and older. African Americans constitute 12% of the total U.S. population but only 8% of the older age groups. In 1986, most older men (77%) were married, whereas most older women (52%) were widows. Fifteen percent of older men live alone, in comparison with 40% of women. Nursing home residents account for 5% of the population older than 65 years. Approximately 12% of the population older than 65 years of age continue to work; 25% are self-employed, in comparison with 10% of the total population. Five percent of the geriatric population—nearly 1 million individuals—are victimized by abuse or neglect. The U.S. Bureau of the Census estimates that 1 million Americans will be 100 years of age or older by the year 2050 and that nearly 2 million will be that age by the year 2080.

Falls are the leading cause of death from injury in individuals 65 years of age and older. Two thirds of reported injury-related deaths in patients 85 years of age and older are caused by falls. Falls are a leading cause of traumatic brain injuries. Approximately 3% to 5% of falls in older

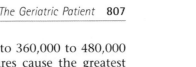

adults cause fractures. On the basis of the 2000 census, this translates to 360,000 to 480,000 fall-related fractures each year. Of all fall-related fractures, hip fractures cause the greatest number of deaths and lead to the most severe health problems and reductions in quality of life. In 1991, Medicare costs for hip fractures were estimated to be $2.9 billion. A fear of falling is also common; 50% to 60% of all patients older than 65 years of age have this fear.

Structure and Physiology

This section covers some of the anatomic and physiologic changes that are attributed to aging, as well as some of the physical findings that result.

Skin

There is atrophy of the epidermis, hair follicles, and sweat glands, which results in thinning skin. The skin becomes fragile and discolored. Wrinkling and dryness result from reduced skin turgor. In addition, the nails become thin and brittle, with marked ridging. There is decreased vascularity of the dermis, which contributes to prolonged healing time. There are common pigmentary changes, such as the development of *senile lentigines,* or "liver spots." These brown macules are commonly found on the backs of the hands, forearms, and face. They are caused by localized mild epidermal hyperplasia, in association with increased numbers of melanocytes and increased melanin production. Figure 25-1 shows senile lentigines on the hand of an 87-year-old woman.

Another common skin change is *senile (solar) keratosis,* which is a well-defined, raised papule or plaque of epidermal hyperkeratosis. The surface scale varies in color from yellow to brown. These lesions are common on the face, neck, trunk, and hands. Figure 25-2 shows several senile keratoses on an 82-year-old man.

There is commonly a degeneration of the elastic fibers and collagen of the skin, resulting in a loss of elasticity and the development of *senile purpura.* These purple macules, commonly seen on the backs of the hands or on the forearms, result from blood that has extravasated through capillaries that have lost their elastic support. Figure 25-3 shows senile purpura on the forearm of a 90-year-old woman.

Sebaceous gland hyperplasia, especially on the forehead and nose, is common. These yellowish glands range in size from 1 to 3 mm and have a central pore. It is important to differentiate these benign lesions from basal cell carcinomas.

Hair loses its pigment, which commonly results in *"graying" of the hair.* With the reduction in the number of hair follicles, there is *hair loss* all over the body: head, axilla, pubic area, and extremities. With the reduction in estrogens, an increase in hair may actually develop in many older women, especially on the chin and upper lip. Chin hairs on a 79-year-old woman are shown in Figure 25-4.

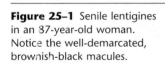
Figure 25–1 Senile lentigines in an 87-year-old woman. Notice the well-demarcated, brownish-black macules.

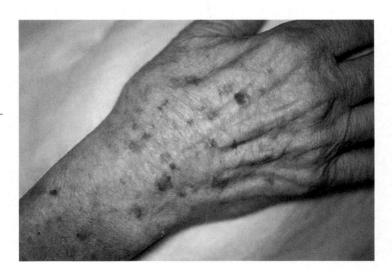

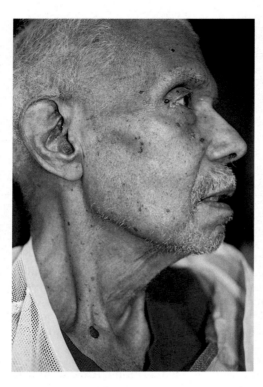

Figure 25–2 Raised senile keratoses on the face and neck of an 82-year-old man.

As a result of the reduction in subcutaneous tissue, there is less insulation and less padding over bony surfaces. This predisposes older people to hypothermia and the development of *pressure sores*, or *decubitus ulcers*. Figure 25-5 shows a pressure sore that developed on an 85-year-old man within 1 week. The man had been seen 1 week earlier when a small, intact erythematous area was noticed over his sacral area. He was brought back to the emergency department 7 days later with the decubitus ulcer seen in the figure. The ulceration eroded through the skin and muscle, into the sacrum, and into the bowel, with the development of a rectovesicular fistula.

Eyes

As a result of a reduction of orbital fat, the eyes appear sunken. Laxity of the eyelids, or *senile ptosis*, often develops. *Ectropion* or *entropion* may develop, caused by the lower eyelid's falling away or falling inward, respectively. There may also be a clogging of the lacrimal duct, resulting in *epiphora*, or tearing. Fatty deposits in the cornea may produce an *arcus senilis*, seen in Figures 10-53 and 10-54. Inadequate production of mucous tears by the conjunctiva may predispose persons to *corneal ulcers, exposure keratitis,* or *dry eye syndrome*.

An accumulation of yellow pigment in the lens alters color perception. A loss of elasticity in the lens results in *presbyopia*. Nuclear sclerosis of the lens develops into *cataract* formation.

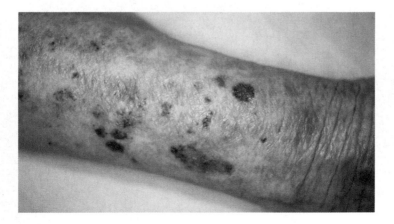

Figure 25–3 Senile purpura on the forearm of a 90-year-old woman. Note the red macules and the loss of turgidity of the skin.

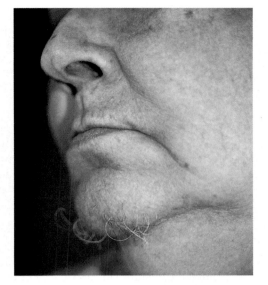

Figure 25–4 Chin hairs on a 79-year-old woman.

Patients experience a decrease in visual acuity and commonly complain of sensitivity to glare from interior lights, sunlight, or reflection from floors.

Degenerative changes in the iris, vitreous humor, and retina may impair visual acuity, reduce the fields of vision, and lead to the development of floaters (*muscae volitantes*). *Senile macular degeneration* (see Figs. 10-121 to 10-123) and *retinal hemorrhages* are other medically significant causes of decreases in visual acuity.

Ears

Degeneration of the organ of Corti may result in *presbycusis*, an impaired sensitivity to high-frequency tones. Patients experience a slowly progressive hearing loss with a consistent pattern of pure tone loss. *Otosclerosis* may produce *conductive deafness*, as does the excessive cerumen accumulation so commonly seen in older individuals. A degeneration of the hair cells in the semicircular canals may produce *vertigo*.

Nose and Throat

Atrophic changes occur in the mucosa of the nose and throat. Taste and especially smell may be altered, particularly in institutionalized individuals. A decrease in mucus production predisposes older patients to upper respiratory infections. A loss of elasticity in the laryngeal muscles may produce tremulousness and high pitch of the voice.

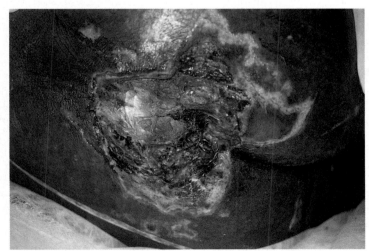

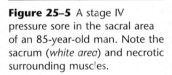

Figure 25–5 A stage IV pressure sore in the sacral area of an 85-year-old man. Note the sacrum (*white area*) and necrotic surrounding muscles.

Mouth

Loss of teeth from dental caries or periodontal disease is common. *Gingival recession* may produce problems with dentures and a malalignment of bite. Atrophic changes in the salivary glands cause dryness of the mouth, known as *xerostomia*, a common complaint among the elderly.

Lungs

A loss of elasticity in the pulmonary septa and atrophy of the alveoli cause a coalescence of the alveoli, with a reduction in vital capacity and oxygen diffusion. There are decreases in forced vital capacity and expiratory flow rate. A degeneration of bronchial epithelium and mucous glands increases the susceptibility to infections. Skeletal changes also contribute to a decrease in vital capacity.

Cardiovascular System

A loss of elasticity of the aorta may cause aortic dilation. The semilunar and atrioventricular valves may degenerate and become regurgitant. Alternatively, these valves may become sclerotic, which causes stenosis of the valves. Degeneration or calcification of the conducting system may cause *heart block* or *arrhythmias*.

Noncompliance of the peripheral arteries may cause *hypertension* with a *widened pulse pressure*. Systolic blood pressure rises progressively with age, whereas diastolic pressure levels off in the sixth decade of life; these developments lead to an increased prevalence of isolated systolic hypertension. Coronary atherosclerosis may produce angina, *myocardial infarction*, or nonspecific symptoms such as confusion or tiredness.

There are also decreases in plasma volume, ventricular filling time, and baroreflex sensitivity.

Breasts

The amount of glandular tissue decreases, and the tissue is replaced by fatty deposits. As a result of a loss of elastic tissue, the breasts become pendulous, and the ducts may be more palpable.

In men, *gynecomastia* may result from a change in the metabolism of sex hormones by the liver (see Fig. 16-21).

Gastrointestinal System

Atrophy of the gastrointestinal mucosa occurs with a reduction in the number of stomach and intestinal glands, causing alterations in secretion, motility, and absorption. Changes in elastic tissue and colonic pressures may result in diverticulosis, which can lead to diverticulitis. Pancreatic acinar atrophy is common, as are decreases in hepatic mass, hepatic blood flow, and microsomal enzyme activity. These decreases result in an increased half-life of lipid-soluble drugs.

Genitourinary System

There is a decrease in the number of glomeruli and a thickening of the basement membrane in Bowman's capsule, resulting in a reduction in renal function. Degenerative changes occur in the renal tubules, which themselves are reduced in number. Renal blood flow is reduced to half by 75 years of age. Vascular changes may also contribute to a reduced glomerular filtration rate.

In men, *prostatic atrophy* or *prostatic hypertrophy* develops. Benign prostatic hypertrophy is present in 80% of all men older than 80 years. The penis decreases in size, and the testicles hang lower in the scrotum.

In postmenopausal women, the reduction in estrogen is associated with an increase in susceptibility to *osteoporosis*. The labia and clitoris are reduced in size, and the vaginal mucosa becomes thin and dry. The uterus and ovaries also decrease in size.

As discussed previously, pubic hair decreases in amount and becomes gray.

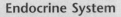

Endocrine System

There is decreased metabolism of thyroxine and decreased conversion of thyroxine to triiodo-thyronine. Because of a reduction in pancreatic beta cell secretion, *hyperglycemia* may result. The hypothalamus and the pituitary gland secrete reduced amounts of hormones. An increase in the secretion of antidiuretic hormone and atrial natriuretic hormone may alter fluid balance. There are also increased levels of norepinephrine.

Musculoskeletal System

There is general atrophy of muscles, causing a decline in strength. *Muscle wasting* is seen most commonly in the distal extremities, especially in the dorsal interosseous muscles.

Osteoclastic activity is greater than osteoblastic activity. An enlargement of the cancellous bone spaces and a thinning of the trabeculae result in osteoporosis. *Kyphosis* and a loss of height are common (see Fig. 13-6). Degenerative changes and a loss of elastic tissue occur in joints, ligaments, and tendons. This frequently results in *joint stiffness*. Degenerative changes in bone may result in bone cysts and erosions, making these bones prone to *fracture*. *Osteoarthritis* is common. Thinning of cartilage and synovial thickening produce joint stiffness and pain. Range of motion is also reduced, perhaps because of pain. Figure 20-59 shows Heberden's and Bouchard's nodes in an 86-year-old woman with osteoarthritis.

Nervous System

Changes in brain function may adversely affect memory and intelligence, although other skills such as language and sustained attention may remain. Significant variability exists among individuals, and many elderly individuals continue to perform at levels that are comparable with or exceed those of much younger people.

Brain weight is frequently reduced 5% to 7% as a result of atrophy of selected areas. There is a decrease in blood flow to the brain by 10% to 15%. Vascular changes of atherosclerosis can result in *multiple infarcts* or *transient ischemic attacks*.

Reflexes are commonly reduced; the gag reflex is frequently absent. The Achilles tendon reflex is often symmetrically reduced or absent. Primitive reflexes, such as snout or palmo-mental, may be present in *normal* elderly persons.

Hematopoietic System

There is an increase in the amount of marrow fat and a decrease in the amount of active bone marrow.

Immune System

There is a decreased number of newly formed T lymphocytes and a reduced capability of T lymphocytes to proliferate in response to mitogens or antigens. Humoral immunity is impaired, and suppressor T lymphocytes are decreased in number.

Basic Principles of Geriatric Medicine

Whereas in the younger population the goal of medicine is to cure, the ultimate goal in the geriatric population is to preserve the patient's quality of life. The health-care professional must strive to maintain function and relieve the symptoms that can be relieved. This often involves moving from a doctor-patient relationship alone to a doctor-family or doctor-caregiver relationship. In the event of terminal illness, you should ensure as little mental and physical distress as possible and provide appropriate emotional support to the patient and family. There are a few basic principles of geriatric medicine.

First, there is an *altered manifestation of disease*. The actual symptom may not be a symptom of the organ system involved with the disease. For example, if a person in his or her 50s were to have a heart attack, the individual, unless diabetic, would usually suffer from chest pain. This is not the case in the geriatric age group. It is well documented that 70% of nondiabetic individuals older than 70 years of age do not have chest pain with a myocardial infarction. Such patients may present instead with breathlessness, falling, confusion, or palpitations.

Another illustration of this alteration in symptoms is the geriatric patient with diabetes mellitus. Ordinarily, because of lack of insulin, younger patients become acidotic and ketotic, with a smell of ketones on their breath. They may also exhibit shallow, rapid respirations. Older patients with uncontrolled diabetes mellitus may not become ketotic and acidotic. Instead, the syndrome of hyperosmolar, nonketotic coma may ensue. These patients, who do not have the smell of ketones on their breath and are not acidotic, are hyperosmolar and may have serum glucose levels in excess of 600 to 700 mg/dL. They may even present in coma.

A third example is a patient with hyperthyroidism. A geriatric patient with hyperthyroidism might not present with the tachycardia, sweats, or anxiety states that are seen in younger individuals with increased thyroid activity. The geriatric patient may instead appear depressed and apathetic.

An older patient with acute appendicitis might not suffer from abdominal pain, and an older patient with pneumonia might not have shortness of breath; confusion may be the only symptom.

A second principle in geriatric medicine is the *nonspecific manifestation of disease*. When an elderly person becomes ill, a family member commonly reports that the patient "just hasn't gotten out of bed." The patient may go to bed and stay there. The patient may not want to eat and may have only nonspecific complaints.

A third principle is the *underreporting of illness*. When an interviewer asks a geriatric patient about various symptoms, the patient may fail to report blindness caused by a cataract, deafness caused by otosclerosis, pain in the legs at night, urinary incontinence, constipation, confusion, and so forth. The geriatric patient may believe that these symptoms are normal for a 75- or 80-year-old person. Abdominal pain and other gastrointestinal complaints such as increased gas are commonly mistaken by geriatric patients as a normal part of aging. Sometimes a patient may say, "Nothing can be done about it, so I don't want to bother anyone by mentioning it."

A fourth principle is the recognition that *multiple pathologic conditions may be present* in a geriatric patient. Such a patient may have been given multiple medications or therapies. One medicine may have deleterious effects on a patient if some other condition exists. Of course, this can occur with any patient, but it is more likely to occur in older patients who probably have several pathologic conditions.

A fifth principle is *polypharmacy*, which is defined as the administration of three or more medicines. It is critical that the interviewer see and know about all the medications being taken by the patient. Instruct the patient or family to bring in all medications, both prescription and nonprescription, and ask the patient how he or she is taking them. There is commonly a significant discrepancy between the written prescription and the dosage that the patient actually takes.

Americans older than 65 years of age use about 25% of all prescription medications consumed in the United States, and at any one time, the average geriatric patient uses 4.5 prescription medications. The average nursing home resident consumes the most medications, averaging eight medications at any one time. The use of mood-altering drugs is common in the geriatric population. Approximately 7% of nursing home residents are taking three or more psychoactive drugs.

Finally, what is the patient's *chief complaint?* This is sometimes referred to as "the myth of the chief complaint." Many geriatric patients do not have a single complaint. There may be several problems related to their many conditions. In fact, as already discussed, if a chief complaint is given, it may bear no relationship to the organ system involved. *Be careful in the evaluation of the chief complaint when dealing with older patients.*

Advance directives are critical for all patients, especially those in the geriatric age group. Advance directives used in the United States take two forms: the living will and the health proxy. The living will is a treatment directive listing interventions that the patient wishes or does not wish to be performed in the event that he or she becomes unable to make such decisions. The health proxy, also known as *the durable power of attorney for health care*, assigns a surrogate decision maker whom the patient trusts to make decisions for him or her in the event he or she cannot make them. By law, that person cannot be the patient's physician. These important documents provide an avenue of communication between the physician and the patient on the patient's end-of-life care. If these documents have not been filed, all too often there may be uncertainty about the patient's wishes, and the physician and family are left in the dark. Review the DVD-ROM included with this book, which demonstrates how to ask about advance directives.

The Geriatric History

The main components of the medical history are basically the same for geriatric patients as for younger patients, except for the chief complaint and the family history. With the exception of a family history of Alzheimer's disease, the family history is less important for geriatric patients than for younger patients. For example, the fact that a family member died of a myocardial infarction at 60 years of age is relatively unimportant for a patient who is already in his or her 80s. It is also often difficult for an older patient to remember how and when relatives died.

Before beginning the history, determine whether there is an impairment of hearing, vision, or cognition. A quick check of these three functions is mandatory. Ask the patient whether he or she uses any assistive devices (e.g., hearing aid, glasses, cane, walker, wheelchair). If so, evaluate the condition of the device. Is the patient using the device properly? Ask the patient how the device was obtained; often these devices have been given to the patient by friends or family members or have been left by deceased spouses.

If there is a hearing impairment, sit facing the patient, as close as possible and at ear level with the patient. Make sure that the patient is wearing, if required, the hearing aid or other assistive device. Try to minimize both audible and visual distractions. Speak in a slow, low-pitched, and moderately loud voice. Allow the patient to observe your lips as you talk. Finally, confirm with the patient that he or she is being understood by repeating portions of the history.

Because many older patients have memory deficits or dementia, it is frequently necessary to obtain a confirming history from a family member or caregiver.

All support systems must be evaluated. These include family, friends, and professional services.

Ascertain diet because many older patients have poorly balanced diets.

A *comprehensive geriatric assessment* is an essential component of the history. It ensures that the patient's many complex health-care needs are evaluated and met. Every geriatric history must include a comprehensive assessment of activities. Measures of the patient's ability to perform basic activities, called *activities of daily living* (ADL), must be gathered. These activities include bathing, dressing, toileting, continence, feeding, and transferring in and out of bed or on and off a chair. The ability to perform more complex tasks, called *instrumental activities of daily living* (IADL), is also assessed. These tasks include food preparation, shopping, housekeeping, laundry, financial management, medicine management, use of transportation, and use of the telephone.

Other areas that must be evaluated for all geriatric patients are the following:

- Abuse and neglect
- Affective disorders
- Caregiver stress
- Cognitive impairment
- Decubitus ulcers
- Dental impairment
- Discussion of advance directives*
- Falls
- Feeding impairment
- Gait abnormalities
- Health maintenance
- Hearing impairment
- Incontinence (fecal and urinary)
- Infections (recurrent)
- Nutritional assessment
- Osteoporosis
- Podiatric disorders
- Polypharmacy
- Preoperative evaluation, if appropriate
- Rehabilitation needs
- Sleep disorders
- Visual impairment

---

*These include living wills, "do not resuscitate" orders, and proxy appointments.

Certain questionnaires and scales have been validated with elderly persons and may be used to *screen patients for affective disorders* such as depression or dementia. An example is the Yesavage Geriatric Depression Scale, which consists of 30 items (Table 25-1). Each of the patient's answers that matches the score sheet is scored 1 point. A total score from 0 to 9 is indicative of no depression; from 10 to 19, mild depression; and from 20 to 30, severe depression.

The presentation of depression is not always classic, especially in older individuals. Symptoms suggestive of psychomotor retardation, such as listlessness, decreased appetite, cognitive impairment, and decreased energy, may be important clues.

Finally, an *assessment of mental status* is required for all older patients. Memory deficits and decreased intellectual functioning influence the reliability of the medical history; therefore, evaluate mental status early in your assessment. Casual conversation is rarely sufficient for detecting cognitive impairment in elderly patients. All older patients should be screened with the use of a validated instrument such as the Folstein Mini-Mental State Examination.* This test evaluates five areas of mental status: *orientation, registration, attention and calculation, recall,* and *language*. Scores of 1 point are given for each correct patient response. In the domain of orientation, knowledge of the *date, day, month, year,* and *season* would score 5 points. The maximum score for the complete test is 30. Scores greater than 24 are indicative of no cognitive impairment; patients with scores of 20 to 24 need further testing. Scores lower than 20 are indicative of cognitive impairment.

Impact of Growing Old on the Patient

Growing old can bring great joy and satisfaction: free time to start new hobbies or new occupations; time to travel; time to meet new friends; time to write about lifelong experiences; time to become creative; time to impart wisdom to younger generations; time to enjoy grandparenthood, great-grandparenthood, or even great-great-grandparenthood. Among individuals older than 65 years of age, 94% are grandparents and 46% are great-grandparents. Becoming a grandparent can give an older person a new lease on life and allow him or her to relive the memories of earlier years. Old age can allow the individual to use the knowledge attained throughout life to pursue goals that, perhaps because of time or financial constraints, could not be achieved earlier. All this is true if the patient's health permits it. The physical and mental health of the person may, however, limit enjoyment of this period of life.

As already discussed, many physical changes occur with aging. Specific disabilities, such as locomotor afflictions, may be particularly handicapping in the presence of normal cognitive functioning. Loss of vision or hearing can lead to social isolation. These physical changes can have a profound effect on the emotional health of the individual. The loss of friends and loved ones may take its toll on the patient as well.

Of the 35 million Americans older than 65 years, it is estimated that 12% to 15% suffer from some functional psychiatric disorder, ranging from anxiety and depression to severe delirium and other psychotic states. Depression may result from loss, which is common among geriatric patients: loss of health, friends, spouses, and relatives, or loss of status or participation in society. These losses and others can be devastating to the older patient.

The patient may feel trapped within an aged body. Grief, a sense of helplessness, or a sense of emptiness can develop. Guilt feelings may also develop: "Why did I outlive... ?" In older individuals, as in children, being left alone provokes terror and anger because of a sense of vulnerability. Depression and loss of self-esteem may contribute to suicide, with rates being highest among white men in their 80s.

Finally, concerns and fears related to their own death are important. It is interesting to note that most older individuals fear death less than younger persons do. What older persons fear is not when they will die but *how* they will die. Will they be in pain? Will they be alone? The health-care provider must address these questions directly so that the anxiety and depression so commonly related to these issues can be allayed.

Physical Examination

The physical examination of the geriatric patient is no different from that already described in Section 2 of this book. Special attention, however, should be given to the following areas.

---

*Psychological Assessment Resources, Inc.; (800) 331-8378.

Table 25–1 Yesavage Geriatric Depression Scale

1. Are you basically satisfied with your life?	yes/no
2. Have you dropped many of your activities and interests?	yes/no
3. Do you feel that your life is empty?	yes/no
4. Do you often get bored?	yes/no
5. Are you hopeful about the future?	yes/no
6. Are you bothered by thoughts you can't get out of your head?	yes/no
7. Are you in good spirits most of the time?	yes/no
8. Are you afraid that something bad is going to happen to you?	yes/no
9. Do you feel happy most of the time?	yes/no
10. Do you often feel helpless?	yes/no
11. Do you often get restless and fidgety?	yes/no
12. Do you prefer to stay at home, rather than going out and doing new things?	yes/no
13. Do you frequently worry about the future?	yes/no
14. Do you feel you have more problems with memory than most?	yes/no
15. Do you think it is wonderful to be alive now?	yes/no
16. Do you often feel downhearted and blue?	yes/no
17. Do you feel pretty worthless the way you are now?	yes/no
18. Do you worry a lot about the past?	yes/no
19. Do you find life gets very exciting?	yes/no
20. Is it hard for you to get started on new projects?	yes/no
21. Do you feel full of energy?	yes/no
22. Do you feel that your situation is hopeless?	yes/no
23. Do you think that most people are better off than you are?	yes/no
24. Do you frequently get upset over little things?	yes/no
25. Do you frequently feel like crying?	yes/no
26. Do you have trouble concentrating?	yes/no
27. Do you enjoy getting up in the morning?	yes/no
28. Do you prefer to avoid social gatherings?	yes/no
29. Is it easy for you to make decisions?	yes/no
30. Is your mind as clear as it used to be?	yes/no

Score Sheet*

1. No	2. Yes	3. Yes	4. Yes	5. No
6. Yes	7. No	8. Yes	9. No	10. Yes
11. Yes	12. Yes	13. Yes	14. Yes	15. No
16. Yes	17. Yes	18. Yes	19. No	20. Yes
21. No	22. Yes	23. Yes	24. Yes	25. Yes
26. Yes	27. No	28. Yes	29. No	30. No

*See text for interpretation.

Reprinted from Yesavage JA, Brink TL, Rose TL, et al: Development and validation of a geriatric depression rating scale: A preliminary report. J Psychiatr Res 17:37, 1983. Copyright 1983, with permission from Pergamon Press Ltd., Headington Hill Hall, Oxford OX3 OBW, UK.

Disrobing may be embarrassing for the older patient, especially because the examiner may be much younger than the patient. Modesty must be respected. Make sure that only the area being examined is exposed. Try to make sure that the room is warm; older individuals tend to become chilled easily. Finally, remember that putting on a robe or gown may not present any difficulty for a younger patient, but for an older patient who may have difficulty moving, perhaps because of arthritis, it can be a real problem.

Assessment of Vital Signs

Perform a routine evaluation, including orthostatic changes in pulse and blood pressure. Be careful if the patient complains of dizziness or chest discomfort. If this occurs, have the patient lie down immediately. Obtain body temperature. If the patient is hypometabolic, as happens in hypothyroidism or in exposure hypothermia, the temperature may be less than 36°C. In the geriatric population, a normal temperature is commonly found in patients with severe infections. Accurate weights should be documented and observed over time.

Skin

Observe the skin for any malignant changes, pressure sores, evidence of pruritus, and ecchymoses suggestive of falls or abuse.

Head, Eyes, Ears, Nose, Throat, and Neck

Evaluate the patient for any evidence of skull trauma. Palpate the superficial temporal arteries, which are located anterosuperior to the tragus. In patients who complain of visual symptoms, headaches, or polymyalgic symptoms, polymyalgia rheumatica or temporal (giant cell) arteritis should be suspected (see the Clinicopathologic Correlations section at the end of this chapter).

Is entropion (see Fig. 10-19) or ectropion (see Fig. 10-20) present? Determine visual acuity, if this was not already tested. Eye movement should be checked for gaze palsies. The ability to gaze upward declines with increasing age. Are cataracts present (see Figs. 10-67 and 10-68)? Examine the retina, if a cataract does not exist. Is macular degeneration present (see Figs. 10-120 to 10-122)?

Is cerumen impacted in the external canal (see Fig. 11-4)? Evaluate auditory acuity, if this was not already done.

Ask the patient to remove any dentures, if present. Examine the mouth for dryness, lesions (see Figs. 12-16, 12-17, and 12-20), condition of teeth, oral ulcers (see Fig. 12-45), and malignancies (see Figs. 12-50 and 12-52 to 12-54). Poor-fitting dentures may cause difficulty eating and chewing, which may lead to weight loss. Examine the tongue for malignancy (see Fig. 12-52).

Auscultate the neck. Are carotid bruits present? Palpate the thyroid. Are nodules present? Is the thyroid diffusely enlarged?

Breasts

Examine the breasts for dimpling, discharge, and masses. The incidence of breast cancer increases with advancing age. The incidence is highest among women 85 years of age and older (see Fig. 16-6).

Chest

Inspect the shape of the chest. Is kyphoscoliosis present? Auscultate the chest. Are any adventitious sounds present?

Cardiovascular System

Evaluate the point of maximum impulse. Is it displaced laterally? Auscultate the heart in the four main positions. Are any murmurs, rubs, or gallops heard? Systolic murmurs are heard in 55% of all older adults.

Are the peripheral pulses present? Loss of peripheral pulses is common and may have little clinical significance, especially if the patient does not complain of intermittent claudication. Is there evidence of peripheral vascular disease?

Abdomen

Perform routine palpation and percussion of the abdomen. Is the bladder enlarged? Is a pulsatile abdominal mass present? Palpate for inguinal and femoral hernias. Is there evidence of urine leakage on the undergarments? Perform a rectal examination. Examine the stool for blood. In a man, is the prostate enlarged?

Musculoskeletal Examination

Examine the joints. Ask the patient to stand up from a seated position, and observe for any difficulties. Can the patient lift the hands over the head to brush his or her hair?

The extremities should be examined for arthritis, impaired range of motion, and deformities. The feet should be inspected for nail care (see Fig. 20-70), calluses, deformities (see Figs. 20-52 and 20-53), and ulceration (see Figs. 20-71 and 20-72). Evaluate the peripheral pulses.

Neurologic Examination

Evaluate mental status, if this was not already done. Check vibration sense. Lack of vibration sense is the most common deficit in otherwise healthy elderly individuals. Test reflexes; asymmetry is suggestive of stroke, myelopathy, or root compression. Evaluate for rigidity. Cogwheel rigidity is suggestive of Parkinson's disease. Perform the Romberg test. Evaluate gait.

Any patient presenting with a change in function must be evaluated for dementia, depression, and Parkinson's disease.

Evaluate motor strength, tone, and rapid alternating movements.

Clinicopathologic Correlations

Many organ system problems are seen in the geriatric age group. This section covers several disorders and functional states that are especially common among older individuals and are not discussed in other chapters of this book.

Senile macular degeneration occurs in nearly 10% of the geriatric population, affecting more women than men. It represents the most common cause of legal blindness in the United States. There is painless and progressive loss of central vision. The patient frequently complains of difficulty reading. Because only the macula is involved, peripheral vision is spared, and complete blindness does not result. See Figures 10-121 to 10-123.

Temporal arteritis and *polymyalgia rheumatica* are unique to the geriatric age group and probably are manifestations of a condition known as *giant cell arteritis*. Polymyalgia rheumatica is estimated to occur in 40% to 50% of patients with temporal arteritis. Both of these conditions are threefold to fourfold more frequent among women than among men.

The symptoms of temporal arteritis include headache, which is frequently associated with scalp tenderness; the temporal artery may also be tender. There are several generalized symptoms as well, such as fever, weight loss, anorexia, and fatigue. Visual disturbances include loss of vision, blurred vision, diplopia, and amaurosis fugax. Sometimes patients may also complain of pain on chewing food. The diagnosis is made from temporal artery biopsy, which has a sensitivity of 90% and a specificity of 100%.

Many patients with polymyalgia rheumatica complain of symmetric pain, especially in the morning, and stiffness of the neck, shoulders, lower back, and pelvic girdle. They often find it difficult to brush their hair. The proximal muscle groups of the upper extremities and pelvic girdle are commonly affected.

Pressure sores, or *decubitus ulcers*, are serious problems that can lead to pain, a longer hospital stay, and a slower recovery. They are caused by unrelieved pressure that results in damage to underlying tissue. They affect up to 3 million individuals yearly. The annual health-care expenditures for these lesions are in excess of $5 billion. It has been estimated that the cost to heal one decubitus ulcer ranges from $5,000 to $50,000. In long-term health-care facilities, the prevalence of decubitus ulcers is 15% to 25%, whereas the prevalence in the community is 5% to 15%. There are thousands of legal cases each year as a result of the development of pressure sores and the related morbidity and mortality. Bacteremia is common, and osteomyelitis occurs in more than 25% of all patients with nonhealing decubitus ulcers.

Decubitus ulcers result from prolonged pressure over bony prominences. A pressure ulcer starts as reddened skin but gets progressively worse, forming a blister, then an open sore, and finally a crater. The most common places for pressure ulcers are over bony prominences (bones close to the skin) such as the elbows, heels, hips, ankles, shoulders, back, sacrum, and back of the head. It is thought that this pressure causes a decrease in perfusion to the area, leading to the accumulation of toxic products, with subsequent necrosis of skin, muscle, subcutaneous tissue, and bone. Moisture, caused by fecal or urinary incontinence or by perspiration, is also implicated because it causes maceration of the epidermis and allows tissue necrosis to occur. Shearing force is also a factor. Shear is generated when the head of a bed is elevated, causing the torso to slide down and transmit pressure to the sacrum. Poor nutritional status and delayed wound healing are other widespread contributing factors.

Pressure ulcers are staged to classify the degree of damage observed. The four clinical stages of decubitus ulcers are as follows:

Stage I: Nonblanching erythema of intact skin; the heralding lesion of skin ulceration
Stage II: Partial-thickness skin loss involving epidermis or dermis; ulcer extending up to subcutaneous fat

Stage III: Full-thickness skin loss involving damage or necrosis of subcutaneous tissue without involving muscle or bone

Stage IV: Full-thickness skin loss with extensive destruction, tissue necrosis, or damage to underlying muscle, bone, or supporting structures

Ulcers covered by superficial necrosis must undergo débridement before they can be staged. The patient in Figure 25-5 presented with a stage I pressure sore, and 1 week later, when this photograph was taken, the sore had rapidly advanced to a stage IV lesion. The patient died of sepsis 4 days after the photograph was taken.

Prevention of decubitus ulcers is extremely important in the care of bedridden or chair-bound patients. Repositioning or rotating the patient at least every 2 hours, minimizing moisture, practicing basic skin care, and improving the nutritional state are important. Skin should be cleansed at the time of soiling and at routine intervals. Care should be used to minimize the force and friction applied to the skin.

Urinary incontinence is an important problem in the geriatric age group. It occurs in 15% to 30% of community-dwelling individuals 65 years of age and older. Among institutionalized patients, the prevalence is 40% to 60%. About 12 million adults in the United States have urinary incontinence. It is most common in women older than 50 years. In 2000, the total cost of health care for urinary incontinence was more than $15 billion.

There are many causes of urinary incontinence, including decreased bladder capacity, increased residual volume, medications, diabetes, and pelvic relaxation. In women, thinning and drying of the skin in the vagina or urethra may cause urinary incontinence; in men, an enlarged prostate gland or prostate surgery can cause urinary incontinence. The major transient causes of urinary incontinence can be remembered by the mnemonic "DIAPPERS":

D: Delirium or dementia
I: Infections (urinary)
A: Atrophic vaginitis or urethritis; atonic bladder
P: Psychologic causes such as depression; prostatitis
P: Pharmacologic agents such as anticholinergics, psychotropics, alcohol, diuretics, opiates, and alpha-adrenergic agents
E: Endocrine abnormalities such as diabetes and hypercalcemia
R: Restricted mobility
S: Stool impaction

There are four types of urinary incontinence: stress, urge, overflow, and functional. In *stress incontinence*, urine leaks because of sudden pressure on the lower abdominal muscles, as during coughing, laughing, or lifting a heavy object. It is very common in women. *Urge incontinence* occurs when the need to urinate comes on too fast—before the patient can get to a toilet. Urge incontinence is most common in elderly persons and may be a sign of an infection in the kidneys or bladder. *Overflow incontinence* is a constant dripping of urine caused by an overfilled bladder. This type of urinary incontinence often occurs in men and can be caused by an enlarged prostate gland or tumor. Diabetes or certain medicines may also cause this problem. *Functional incontinence* occurs when the patient has normal urine control but has trouble getting to the bathroom in time because of arthritis or other conditions that make it hard to ambulate.

Dementia, according to criteria contained in the American Psychiatric Association's (1994) *Diagnostic and Statistical Manual of Mental Disorders* (4th edition, text revision), is characterized by an acquired and persistent impairment in short- and long-term memory and other disturbances, such as impairment in language (e.g., reading, writing, fluency, naming, repetition), concentration ability, visuospatial function (e.g., drawing, copying), emotions, and personality, despite a state of clear consciousness. A diagnosis of dementia requires evidence of decline from previous levels of functioning and impairment in multiple cognitive domains. The prevalence of dementia in the general population 65 years of age is estimated to be 5% to 10%, and the incidence doubles with every additional 5 years. In chronic care facilities, the prevalence is higher than 50% of all hospitalized patients. Despite its prevalence, dementia is often unrecognized in its early stages.

The most common causes of dementia are strokes and Alzheimer's disease. The onset and course of the symptoms often provide clues to the cause of dementia. A sudden onset is almost always related to a cerebrovascular accident. A subacute, insidious course may be related to tumor, Jakob-Creutzfeldt disease, or Alzheimer's disease. Dementia with rigidity and brady-kinesia is strongly suggestive of Parkinson's disease. Dementia in association with urinary

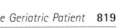

incontinence and a spastic, magnetic gait is seen in hydrocephalus. The development of dementia after a fall should raise suspicion of a subdural hematoma.

Some of the symptoms that may be indicative of dementia are difficulty in the following areas:

- Learning and retention of new information
- Handling of complex tasks
- Reasoning ability
- Spatial ability and orientation
- Language
- Behavior

Falls are a common problem in the geriatric age group. More than 30% of adults 65 years of age and older fall each year. Of those who fall, two thirds fall again within 6 months. Falls are the leading cause of injury-related deaths among people aged 65 years or older and are the most common cause of nonfatal injuries and hospital admissions for trauma. In 2004, the most recent year statistics are available, almost 15,000 people in this age group died from falls, and about 1.9 million were treated for injuries in emergency rooms. The elderly account for 75% of deaths from falls. More than half of all fatal falls involve people aged 75 years or older—only 4% of the total population. Among people aged 65 to 69 years, 1 of every 200 falls results in a hip fracture, and among those aged 85 years or older, 1 fall per 10 results in a hip fracture. One fourth of those who fracture a hip die within 6 months of the injury.

The most profound effect of falling is the loss of independent functioning. Of persons who fracture a hip, 25% require life-long nursing care, and approximately 50% of the elderly who sustain a fall-related injury are discharged to a nursing home instead of returning home.

In 2001, more than 1.6 million older adults were treated in emergency departments for all fall-related injuries, nearly 388,000 were hospitalized, and 11,600 people 65 years of age and older died from fall-related injuries. Falls are the result of a decline in vision, balance, sensory perception, strength, and coordination and are often precipitated by medication ingestion. Most falls are sustained by patients who have taken long-acting sedative-hypnotic agents, antidepressants, or major tranquilizers. *Whenever possible, try to reduce the number of medications that a patient is taking.*

Several modifiable risk factors have been identified with falling. These include lower body weakness, problems with walking and balance, and taking four or more medications or any psychoactive medications. The health-care provider should try to encourage elderly patients to improve lower body strength and balance through regular physical activity. Tai chi is one exercise program that has been shown to be very effective. In one study, tai chi reduced the number of falls by 47%. All health-care providers must also review carefully all of a given patient's medications to reduce side effects and interactions. Eye examinations to check vision are needed at least once a year.

Approximately half to two thirds of all falls occur in and around the home. Therefore, it makes sense to reduce potential home hazards. To make living areas safer, elderly persons should (1) remove tripping hazards such as throw rugs, (2) use nonslip mats in the bathtub, (3) have grab rails installed next to the toilet and in tub, (4) have handrails installed on both sides of stairways, and (5) improve lighting throughout the home.

Review the DVD-ROM included with this book, which demonstrates how to perform a screening mental status examination on a geriatric patient.

Bibliography

Allman RM: Pressure ulcers among the elderly. N Engl J Med 320:850, 1989.

American Psychiatric Association: Diagnostic and Statistical Manual of Mental Disorders, 4th ed, text rev. Washington, DC, American Psychiatric Association, 1994.

Baker DI, Gottschalk M, Bianco LM: Step by step: Integrating evidence-based fall-risk management into senior centers. Gerontologist 47:548, 2007.

Bell AJ, Talbot-Stern JK, Hennessy A: Characteristics and outcomes of older patients presenting to the emergency department after a fall: A retrospective analysis. Med J Aust 173:176, 2000.

Brillhart B: Pressure sore and skin tear prevention and treatment during a 10-month program. Rehabil Nurs 30(3):85, 2005.

Butler RN, Lewis M, Sunderland T: Aging and Mental Health: Positive Psychosocial and Biomedical Approaches. New York, Macmillan, 1991.

Cassel CK, Cohen HJ, Larson EB, et al (eds): Geriatric Medicine, 3rd ed. New York, Springer-Verlag, 1997.

Centers for Disease Control and Prevention: Incidence and costs to Medicare of fractures among Medicare beneficiaries aged > or = 65 years—United States, July 1991–June 1992. MMWR Morb Mortal Wkly Rep 45:877, 1996.

Centers for Disease Control and Prevention: Web-based Injury Statistics Query and Reporting System (WISQARS). National Center for Injury Prevention and Control, Centers for Disease Control and Prevention, 2003. Available at *www.cdc.gov/ncipc/wisqars*; accessed July 1, 2008.

Choi H, Palmer MH, Park J: Meta-analysis of pelvic floor muscle training: Randomized controlled trials in incontinent women. Nurs Res 56:226, 2007.

Cigolle CT, Langa KM, Kabeto MU, et al: Geriatric conditions and disability: The Health and Retirement Study. Ann Intern Med 147:156, 2007.

Cleeland CS: Pain and its treatment in outpatients with metastatic cancer. N Engl J Med 330:592, 1994.

Covinsky KE: Dementia, prognosis, and the needs of patients and caregivers. Ann Intern Med 140:573, 2004.

de Laat EH, Scholte op Reimer WJ, van Achterberg T: Pressure ulcers: Diagnostics and interventions aimed at wound-related complaints: A review of the literature. J Clin Nurs 14:464, 2005.

Donald IP, Bulpitt CJ: The prognosis of falls in elderly people living at home. Age Ageing 28:121, 1999.

Ferri FF, Fretwell MD: Practical Guide to the Care of the Geriatric Patient. St. Louis, Mosby–Year Book, 1992.

Field MJ, Cassel CK (eds): Approaching Death: Improving Care at the End of Life. Washington, DC, National Academy Press, 1997.

Folstein MF, Folstein SE, McHugh PR: "Mini-Mental State": A practical method for grading the cognitive state of patients for the clinician. J Psychiatr Res 12:189, 1975.

Freedman VA, Martin LG, Schoeni RF: Disability in old age decreased in recent years. JAMA 288:3137, 2002.

Ganz DA, Bao Y, Shekelle PG, et al: Will my patient fall? JAMA 297:77, 2007.

Gill TM, Williams CS, Robison JT, et al: A population-based study of environmental hazards in the homes of older persons. Am J Public Health 89:553, 1999.

Guideline for the prevention of falls in older persons. American Geriatrics Society, British Geriatrics Society, and American Academy of Orthopaedic Surgeons Panel on Falls Prevention. J Am Geriatr Soc 50:664, 2001.

Hall SE, Williams JA, Senior JA, et al: Hip fracture outcomes: Quality of life and functional status in older adults living in the community. Aust N Z J Med 30:327, 2000.

Hausdorff JM, Rios DA, Edelber HK: Gait variability and fall risk in community-living older adults: A 1-year prospective study. Arch Phys Med Rehabil 82:1050, 2001.

Jager TE, Weiss HB, Coben JH, et al: Traumatic brain injuries evaluated in U.S. emergency departments, 1992–1994. Acad Emerg Med 7:134, 2000.

Katz S, Stroud MW III: Functional assessment in geriatrics: A review of progress and directions. J Am Geriatr Soc 37:267, 1989.

Krach CA, Velkoff V: Centenarians in the United States, 1990. P23-199RV. Washington, DC, Bureau of the Census, 1999.

Leipzig RM: Update in geriatric medicine. Ann Intern Med 139:1003, 2003.

Lim MR, Huang RC, Wu A, et al: Evaluation of the elderly patient with an abnormal gait. J Am Acad Orthop Surg 15:107, 2007.

Lord SR, Dayhew J: Visual risk factors for falls in older people. J Am Geriatr Soc 49:508, 2001.

Luggen AS: Wrinkles and beyond: skin problems in older adults. Adv Nurs Pract 11:55, 2003.

Magaziner J, Hawkes W, Hebel JR, et al: Recovery from hip fracture in eight areas of function. J Gerontol Med Sci 55A:M498, 2000.

Meier D, Morrison RS: Old age and care near the end of life. Generations 23:6, 1999.

Morrison RS, Siu AL: Survival in end-stage dementia following acute illness. JAMA 284:47, 2000.

Murphy SL: Deaths: Final Data for 1998. Natl Vital Stat Rep 48(11):1, 2000.

Qaseem A, Snow V, Shekelle P, et al: Evidence-based interventions to improve the palliative care of pain, dyspnea, and depression at the end of life: A clinical practice guideline from the American College of Physicians. Ann Intern Med 148:141, 2008.

Rummans TA, Bostwick JM, Clark MM: Maintaining quality of life at the end of life. Mayo Clin Proc 75:1305, 2000.

SUPPORT Principal Investigators: A controlled trial to improve care for seriously ill hospitalized patients. The Study to Understand Prognoses and Preferences for Outcomes and Risks of Treatment (SUPPORT). JAMA 274:1591, 1995.

Tinetti ME: Preventing falls in elderly persons. N Engl J Med 348:42, 2003.

U.S. Bureau of the Census: Population Projections Program, Population Division, Washington, DC, 2002. Available at *www.census.gov/population/www/projections/popproj.html*; accessed July 1, 2008.

Wilkins K: Health care consequences of falls for seniors. Health Rep 10(4):47, 1999.

Wolf RS: Elder abuse: Ten years later. J Am Geriatr Soc 36:758, 1988.

Wolf SL, Barnhart HX, Kutner NG, et al: Reducing frailty and falls in older persons: An investigation of tai chi and computerized balance training. Atlanta FICSIT Group. Frailty and Injuries: Cooperative Studies of Intervention Techniques. J Am Geriatr Soc 44:489, 1996.

Wolinsky FD, Fitzgerald JF, Stump TE: The effect of hip fracture on mortality, hospitalization, and functional status: A prospective study. Am J Public Health 87:398, 1997.

Yesavage JA, Brink TL, Rose TL, et al: Development and validation of a geriatric depression rating scale: A preliminary report. J Psychiatr Res 17:37, 1983.

CHAPTER 26

The Acutely Ill Patient

Ther is no thing more precious here than tyme.

Saint Bernard (1090–1153)

The objective of this chapter is to provide a practical approach to acutely ill patients. The emphasis is on diagnosis, not on therapy. In the assessment of acutely ill patients, time is a critical factor. Unlike the assessment of stable patients, the evaluation of acutely ill patients involves not achieving a specific diagnosis but rather identifying a pathophysiologic abnormality that may be identical for several diagnoses. In the evaluation of acutely ill patients, always ask yourself, "What is the most serious threat to life, and have I ruled it out?" Remember, also, that *your* health is important. Exposure to body substances places you at risk. The minimum isolation precaution for an emergency response is the wearing of latex gloves.

When delivering health care in the field, and perhaps even in the hospital, as you approach the apparent patient, always perform a brief evaluation to determine whether you are in a safe environment; if not, protect yourself and your patient to limit exposure to possible injury. This may be a rare situation, but in circumstances in which it is likely that the rescuer could be injured or killed while rendering care, the rescuer should wait until the situation can be made safe. For example, in an automobile accident, a patient trapped in a car in a busy traffic lane should *not* be given first aid until safety flares or cones can be placed to prevent secondary accidents.

During this evaluation, search for other injured persons who may be hidden from view as you approach the scene of the accident. You should also try to determine the mechanisms of injury and attempt to memorize the scene for later reconsideration in the emergency department and perhaps as a witness for the injured party.

The task for the clinician in approaching most, if not all, patients in acute situations is, first, to ascertain that they are not in cardiopulmonary arrest and do not have major perturbations of their vital signs to the point that their continued viability is threatened. The general approach to these acute, undefined encounters is to consider the patient unstable until you can confirm, through a series of diagnostic steps, that the patient is well enough for you to take the time to perform a more rigorous and complete physical examination and document a complete history.

This strategy involves moving through a series of simple algorithms, which are grouped into two categories termed the *primary* and *secondary surveys*. The primary survey is a check for conditions that are an immediate threat to the patient's life. This initial assessment should take no longer than 30 seconds. The primary survey is subdivided into a *cardiopulmonary resuscitation* (CPR) *survey* and a *key vital functions assessment*. The algorithms for the primary survey are shown in Figures 26-1 and 26-2. The secondary survey is a check for conditions that could become life-threatening problems if not recognized and attended to.

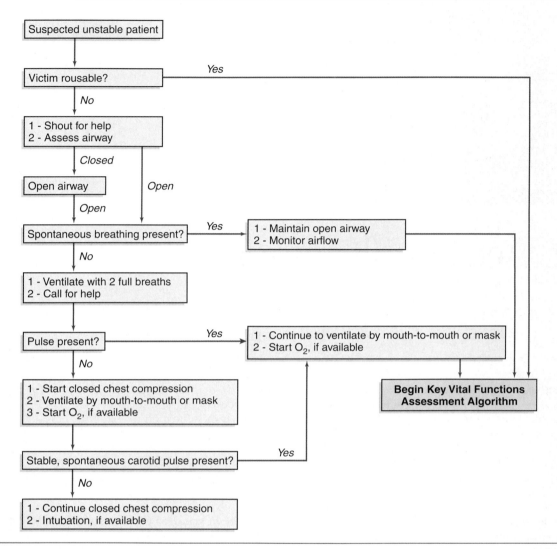

Figure 26–1 Cardiopulmonary resuscitation (CPR) survey algorithm.

The primary and secondary surveys are used for both adult and pediatric patients, as well as for medical and injury-related problems. The treatment process is integrated into the diagnostic process. For example, if the patient is not breathing, ventilations are begun immediately, before you move on to the next diagnostic step in the algorithm.

The first task is to recognize when a patient is acutely ill. An unusual appearance or behavior may be the only sign. These include breathing difficulties, clutching the chest or throat, slurring of speech, confusion, unusual odor to the breath, sweating for no apparent reason, or uncharacteristic skin color (e.g., pale, flushed, or bluish).

Remember that an acutely ill patient is anxious and frightened; a calm and reassuring voice can go a long way toward comforting the patient. It is always easier to care for a relaxed patient than for an anxious one.

Primary Survey

Cardiopulmonary Resuscitation Survey

It should not be assumed that any patient who is not obviously interacting with his or her environment is simply sleeping. For the purpose of this approach, the patient is in cardiopulmonary arrest until it is proved otherwise. As you approach the patient, observe the patient closely, looking for spontaneous breathing or movements. If these are not discernible, stimulate the patient by talking loudly to him or her. If necessary, shout "ARE YOU OKAY?"

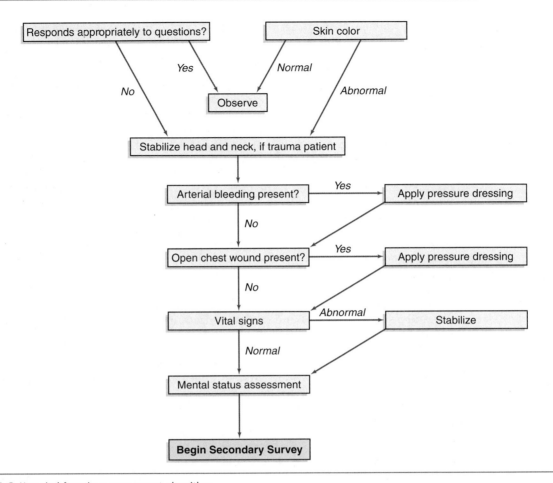

Figure 26-2 Key vital functions assessment algorithm.

If there is no response, obtain an open airway by the chin-lift/head-tilt maneuver and look, listen, and feel (feel air movement against your cheek) for breathing. To open an unconscious victim's airway, hyperextend the head and lift the patient's chin; place one hand on the patient's forehead and the other behind the patient's occiput, and tilt his or her head backward. This maneuver moves the tongue away from the back of the throat, allowing air to pass around the tongue and into the trachea. Caution should be exercised with any patient who has a suspected neck injury. With such a patient, try to open the airway by lifting the chin without tilting the head backward; grasp the lower teeth and pull the mandible forward. If necessary, tilt the head back very slightly. If a patient is wearing dentures, remove them only if they occlude the airway.

If there is no evidence of spontaneous breathing, deliver two full breaths by using mouth-to-mouth ventilation. Next, call for help in any way you can without leaving the patient; it is unlikely that you can manage the entire resuscitation by yourself.

Determine whether there is spontaneous cardiac function by feeling for a carotid pulse or, in an infant, by palpating the precordium for a cardiac impulse. If there is no pulse, begin external chest compressions and intersperse them with ventilations; in other words, begin CPR. Current guidelines (Hazinski et al, 2005) are 30 chest compressions for every two rescue breaths for five cycles (2 minutes). Recheck breathing after every five cycles. The 30:2 ratio is the same for CPR that a single rescuer provides for adults, children, and infants (except newborns). The only exception to this guideline is when two rescuers perform CPR on a child or infant (except newborns), in which they should provide 15 compressions for every two rescue breaths.

Key Vital Functions Assessment Survey

Once it has been determined that the patient does not need CPR or the patient has recovered spontaneous cardiopulmonary activity, ascertain whether key life-sustaining functions are adequate and stable or whether augmentation or other supportive measures are necessary.

In the initial overview of the patient, two observations can save a great deal of time and help avoid unnecessary or untimely interventions. First, if the patient's central nervous system is functioning, as manifested by the patient's ability to respond appropriately to questions, it is unlikely that key vital functions are so deranged as to necessitate immediate intervention. Second, if the patient's skin is warm, dry, and of normal color, it is likely that oxygenation and flow of blood to the periphery are adequate. In shock, peripheral blood flow is shunted centrally; thus, skin changes are early indicators of hypovolemic or cardiogenic (low cardiac output) shock. The key diagnostic skin signs associated with these major acute cardiopulmonary derangements are gray, mottled, or cyanotic color; cold skin temperature; and markedly sweaty skin. The last sign, termed *diaphoresis*, is caused by activation of the sympathetic nervous system by any major threat to homeostasis.

At this point in the algorithm, if the patient has sustained a possible head injury, immobilize the patient's head and neck by using boards, tape, bulky dressings, or towels or by assigning someone to hold the head immobile. Once the evaluation is complete and imaging studies are performed, if necessary, these restrictions to movement can be removed. However, once a patient is immobilized, removal of these measures requires careful decision-making.

The next two orders of priority are the search for and the management of arterial bleeding and open chest injuries. The latter are termed *sucking chest wounds* because they allow air to enter the pleural space, leading to collapse of the underlying lung (pneumothorax). Arterial bleeding and a sucking chest wound can cause death in a short time, and both are treated by application of a pressure dressing to occlude the area.

At this point in the algorithm, the patient has been stabilized to the point at which formal vital signs can be obtained. In the field, these include the patient's mental status, respiratory rate and pattern, pulse, blood pressure, and, in some circumstances, body temperature. Mental status can be assessed according to the *AVPU* system (more traditionally categorized as alert, lethargic, stuporous, or comatose). The AVPU mnemonic for level of consciousness is as follows:

A: patient is *a*lert

V: patient responds to a *v*erbal stimulus

P: patient responds to a *p*ainful stimulus

U: patient is *u*nresponsive

The blood pressure can be estimated by the pulse wave fullness and by assessing which pulses are palpable. If the radial pulse at the wrist is palpable, the systolic blood pressure is at least 80 mm Hg. If the radial pulse is impalpable and only the femoral pulse is perceptible, the systolic blood pressure is 60 to 70 mm Hg. If a vital sign is abnormal, treat the abnormality to bring it back to normal. For example, if the patient is breathing spontaneously at a rate of only five breaths per minute, augment and assist the patient's breathing so that the depth and rate of breathing are normalized. This can be accomplished by applying interspersed mouth-to-mouth ventilations, using a self-inflating bag-valve-mask device, or performing endotracheal intubation and placing the patient on a ventilator. In a similar manner, the blood pressure can be supported by raising the legs, thus emptying the blood stored in the venous system back into the central circulation.

A trauma victim should have a cardiopulmonary examination as well. You are seeking to rule in or rule out a tension pneumothorax (shift of the heart away from the tension, increased breath sounds over the side with the tension pneumothorax, distended neck veins, subcutaneous emphysema), cardiac tamponade (distended neck veins, distant heart sounds, hypotension, pulsus paradoxus, normal breath sounds), and chest wall disruption (paradoxical movement of a flail segment).

Secondary Survey

In the secondary survey, document a history from the patient, the patient's relatives, emergency department personnel, or bystanders. The secondary survey is a systematic method for determining whether other conditions or injuries are present and necessitate attention.

This survey consists of a rapid interview, a check of the vital signs, and a focused physical examination. The mnemonic *AMPLE* can be helpful in gathering pertinent information:

A: *a*llergies

M: *m*edications currently being taken

P: *p*ast medical history

L: *l*ast meal

E: *e*vents preceding the medical event

A critical piece of information in dealing with a trauma patient is the mechanism of injury. Did the patient sustain blunt trauma, or was a weapon used to cause a penetrating injury? In the case of a vehicular accident, ascertain whether the patient was ejected from the car or was wearing a seat belt and whether there were other injuries or fatalities in the accident. In addition, trauma victims must have all their bones and joints—including the rib cage, pelvis, facial bones, and skull—palpated and gently compressed to determine whether there is a fracture step-off or crepitation; also check for stability of structure and for function. A screening neurologic examination is necessary to determine whether there are focal cranial nerve, motor, or sensory findings. Most patients with multisystem trauma require a rectal examination to determine the presence of blood, tenderness, or upward displacement of the prostate. The latter is a sign of urethral injury.

If alert, an injured patient can direct you to the appropriate body areas to be evaluated during the physical examination. The assessment of the patient involves examination of three main regions: the head and neck, the torso, and the extremities. Can the patient move the neck? Ask the patient to move the neck *slowly*. Can the shoulders be moved? Ask the patient to take a deep breath and then blow it out. Does this elicit any pain? Is the patient able to move the fingers? Can the arms be bent? Can the patient move the toes? ankles? Can the patient bend the legs? If the patient can move all extremities without experiencing pain, help the patient up to a sitting position slowly. If the patient cannot move a body part or can do so only with pain, reassess the airway, breathing, and circulation, and get immediate assistance. Continue to observe the patient's level of consciousness, breathing, and skin color.

Head and Neck

Look at the victim's face. Evaluate skin color and temperature. Is there evidence of *raccoon eyes* or *Battle's sign?* A patient with raccoon eyes is shown in Figure 10-28. Periorbital ecchymoses, or raccoon eyes, are seen 6 to 12 hours after a fracture of the base of the skull. Battle's sign is ecchymosis behind the ear caused by basilar skull or temporal bone fractures; this sign may take 24 to 36 hours to develop. Palpate the head.

Examine the eyes for pupillary size and responsiveness to light. Are the pupils equal? Are the pupils pinpoint? Is there a unilateral dilated pupil? Are the pupils fixed? Table 26-1 reviews the eye signs in a comatose patient.

Is there a discharge from the ears, nose, or mouth?

Inspect the neck. Is the trachea deviated? Suspect a chest injury, such as a tension pneumothorax, if the trachea is not midline. Palpate the neck for crepitus, which is indicative of air under the skin from rupture of the lung.

Abdomen

Inspect the abdomen. Is abdominal distention present? Is there evidence of blunt abdominal trauma, such as an ecchymosis, an abrasion, or an abdominal wound? *Cullen's sign* is a bluish discoloration around the umbilicus indicative of intra-abdominal bleeding or trauma. *Grey Turner's sign* is ecchymotic discoloration around the flanks, which is suggestive of retroperitoneal bleeding. Swelling or ecchymosis often occurs late; therefore, its presence is extremely important.

Gently palpate the abdomen, noting the presence of tenderness. If the patient is a woman of childbearing age, always consider the possibility that she may be pregnant.

Inspect the anus and the perineum. Inspect the urethral meatus for blood.

Table 26–1 Eye Signs in a Comatose Patient*

Eye Sign	Possible Causes
Pupils reactive, eyes directed straight ahead, normal oculocephalic reflex (OCR)[†]	Toxic/metabolic cause
Pinpoint pupils	Narcotic poisoning (OCR intact) Pontine or cerebellar hemorrhage (OCR absent) Thalamic hemorrhage Miotic eye drops
Disconjugate deviation of eyes	Structural brain-stem lesion
Conjugate lateral deviation of eyes	Ipsilateral pontine infarction Contralateral frontal hemispheric infarction
Unilateral dilated, fixed pupil with no consensual responses	Supratentorial mass lesion Impending brain herniation Posterior communicating aneurysm
Bilateral midposition pupils, fixed pupils	Midbrain lesion Impending brain herniation
Raccoon eyes (periorbital ecchymoses), Battle sign	Fracture of the base of the skull

*Eye signs are difficult to evaluate in patients with artificial lenses, prosthetic eyes, contact lenses, or cataracts or after cataract surgery.
[†]"Doll's eyes": Rotate the head quickly but gently from side to side. In an unconscious patient with an intact brain stem, the eyes move conjugately in a direction opposite the head turning.

Perform a rectal examination to assess anal sphincter tone, to determine whether blood is present, and to verify that the prostate is in its normal position.

Pelvis

Use the heels of your hands to apply gentle downward pressure on the anterior superior iliac spine and on the symphysis pubis. Is tenderness present? If so, there may be a fracture of the pelvic ring.

Extremities

Inspect and palpate all extremities for evidence of injury. Try to determine whether the patient can move all extremities. Palpate all peripheral pulses.

Back

Inspect the back, looking for obvious signs of injury. This can be done by gently insinuating your hands beneath the back and neck without moving the patient. If this cannot be done, the patient should be gently "log-rolled" onto the side. To do this, you need at least four assistants: one to control the head and neck, two to roll the patient onto the side, and one to cautiously move the lower extremities. Figure 26-3 shows this log-roll procedure.

Vital Signs

Reassess vital signs.

Documenting the history from an acutely ill patient conforms closely to documentation of the standard history, but it is abbreviated to allow rapid diagnostic and management decisions to be made. The physical examination of an acutely ill nontrauma patient includes cardiopulmonary and abdominal examinations and evaluation of the peripheral pulses.

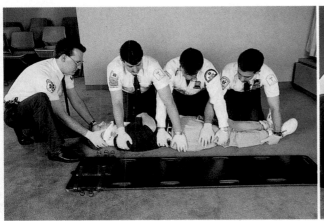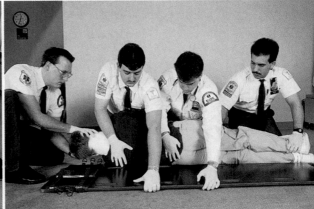

A **B**

Figure 26-3 Log-roll procedure. *A,* Positioning for log-rolling. (1) Apply a cervical spine immobilization device and place the patient's arms at the side. Note that one emergency management technician (EMT) maintains cervical immobilization manually throughout this procedure. (2) Three EMTs can be positioned at the side of the patient at the level of the chest, hips, and lower extremities while the long spine board is positioned on one side of the patient. (3) Check the patient's arm on the side of the EMTs for injury before log-rolling the patient, and then align the lower extremities. Note: The EMT at the lower extremities holds the patient's lower leg and thigh region; the EMT at the hips holds the patient's lower legs and places the other hand on top of the patient's buttocks; and the EMT at the chest holds the patient's arms against the body and at the level of the lower buttocks. *B,* Log-rolling the patient. (4) On command from the EMT at the head, all EMTs rotate the patient toward themselves, keeping the body in alignment. (5) The EMTs then reach across with one hand and pull the board beneath the patient's arm. (6) On command from the EMT at the head, they gently roll the patient onto the board and then roll the board to the ground. (7) Strap the patient's torso and extremities securely to the board, and immobilize the head.

The Pediatric Emergency

When assessing an acutely ill child, always consider the similarities and differences between the pediatric age group and adult patients; approach the pediatric emergency as you would an emergency in an adult, but recognize the smaller size of the patient and the difference in the physiologic responses to acute illness and injury. The primary assessment of a child is the same as that of an adult.

The most dangerous life-threatening pediatric emergency is *respiratory distress*. Respiratory distress in a pediatric patient may arise from a variety of conditions that result from upper or lower airway disease. Common pediatric respiratory problems of the upper airway include croup (laryngotracheobronchitis), epiglottitis, foreign bodies, and bacterial tracheitis. Lower airway obstruction may result from asthma, pneumonia, bronchiolitis, and foreign bodies.

The hallmarks of respiratory distress are tachypnea, nasal flaring, retractions, stridor, cyanosis, head bobbing, prolonged expiration, and grunting. Children with upper airway disease almost always exhibit stridor. In a child with stridor, distinguish between croup and epiglottitis; a child with epiglottitis may have a rapid progression to respiratory failure. Fortunately, the incidence of epiglottitis has decreased, presumably because of the *Haemophilus influenzae* type B (HIB) vaccine. **If epiglottitis is suspected, do not examine the airway without being prepared to provide airway stabilization on an emergency basis**. Manipulation of the child's airway can lead to complete airway obstruction. Table 26-2 compares some of the important differences between epiglottitis and croup.

The peak time for foreign body aspiration is 1 to 2 years of age. In a child, consider relief of airway obstruction in the following situations:

- Choking is present
- The cough becomes ineffective
- Breathing becomes stridorous
- There is loss of consciousness
- The child becomes cyanotic

Table 26–2 Differentiation Between Epiglottitis and Croup

Characteristics	Epiglottitis	Croup
Cause	*Haemophilus influenzae* type B	Viral, usually parainfluenza virus
Age of child	Any age (peak, 3-7 years)	3 months–3 years
Clinical appearance	Extremely ill ("toxic")	Not extremely ill
Season	No seasonal predominance	Autumn and winter
Clinical onset	Rapid	Insidious
Upper respiratory tract infection	Rare	Common
Fever	>104° F (40° C)	<103° F (39.5° C)
Sore throat	Severe	Variable
Cough	Not "barking"; throughout the day	"Barking"; during the night
Drooling	Prominent	None
Stridor	On inspiration	On inspiration and expiration
Position	Sitting forward with neck extended and mouth open	Variable
Epiglottis	Bright red	Normal

Immediately place the child face down, with the head lower than the torso, over your arm, which is placed on your thigh. Support the child's head by holding his or her jaw. Deliver five forceful back blows with the heel of your other hand between the child's scapulae. Turn the child onto the back while holding the child's head. Place two fingertips on the middle portion of the sternum, one fingerbreadth below the nipples. Depress the sternum 1 inch. Repeat this maneuver up to five times. Attempt to remove any visible material from the pharynx. Repeat the back blows and chest thrusts until the object is dislodged.

If the child becomes unconscious, check the mouth for a foreign body, and then perform mouth-to-mouth breathing. Gently tilt the child's head back while placing the other fingers under the jaw at the chin, and lift the chin upward. Seal the child's mouth and nose with your mouth. Deliver two breaths, watching the chest rise. Repeat the back blows and chest thrusts. Have someone call for help.

Dehydration is another important pediatric emergency. The most common causes are vomiting and diarrhea. In a child with mild dehydration (<5%), there may be only a slight decrease in mucous membrane moisture. In severe dehydration (15%), the following are commonly found:

- Parched mucous membranes; no tears
- Markedly decreased skin turgor
- Sunken fontanelles
- Sunken eyeballs
- Tachypnea
- Capillary refill* longer than 2 seconds
- Cool and clammy skin
- Orthostatic hypotension: systolic pressure less than 80 mm Hg
- Tachycardia: faster than 130 beats per minute

Immediate intravenous infusion of isotonic fluids should be started in children with severe dehydration.

The secondary assessment outlined earlier and the AVPU mnemonic are just as important for children as for adults. Table 26-3 provides a useful reference for CPR.

---

*Capillary refill is an assessment of perfusion. It is the time required for a patient's skin color to return to normal after the nail bed has been pressed. The normal refill time is less than 2 seconds.

Table 26–3 Cardiopulmonary Resuscitation Reference Chart

Action	Infant (<1 Year of Age)	Child (>1 Year of Age)	Adult
If victim has a pulse, give one breath:	Every 3 seconds	Every 3 seconds	Every 5-6 seconds
If victim has no pulse, locate compression landmark:	1 fingerbreadth below the nipple line	Same as in adult	One finger on sternum
Compressions are performed with:	Two or three fingers on sternum	Heel of hand on sternum	Two hands stacked, with heel of one hand on sternum
Rate of compressions per minute:	>100	100	80-100
Compression depth:	1/3 to 1/2 depth of chest	1/3 to 1/2 depth of chest	1 to 1 1/2 inches (2.5-3.8 cm)
Ratio of compressions to breaths with:			
One rescuer	30:2*	30:2	30:2
Two rescuers	15:2*	15:2	30:2

*3:1 in neonates.

Bibliography

Barkin RM, Rosen P (eds): Emergency Pediatrics: A Guide to Ambulatory Care, 5th ed. St. Louis, Mosby, 1999.

Capehorn DMW, Swain AH, Goldsworthy LL (eds): A Handbook of Paediatric Accident and Emergency Medicine: A Symptom-Based Guide. Philadelphia, WB Saunders, 1998.

Hazinski MF, Nadkarni VM, Hickey RW, et al: Major changes in the 2005 AHA guidelines for CPR and ECC: Reaching the tipping point for change. Circulation 112(Suppl I):IV-206, 2005.

Henry MC, Stapleton ER (eds): EMT Prehospital Care, 2nd ed. Philadelphia, WB Saunders, 1997.

Howell JM, Altieri M, Jagoda AS, et al (eds): Emergency Medicine. Philadelphia, WB Saunders, 1997.

McSwain NE, White RD, Paturas JL, et al: The Basic EMT: Comprehensive Prehospital Patient Care. St. Louis, Mosby Lifeline, 1997.

Revere C, Hasty R: Diagnostic and characteristic signs of illness and injury. J Emerg Nurs 19:2, 1993.

Thomas H, O'Connor RE, Hoffmann GL, et al: Emergency Medicine: Self Assessment and Review, 4th ed. St. Louis, Mosby, 1999.

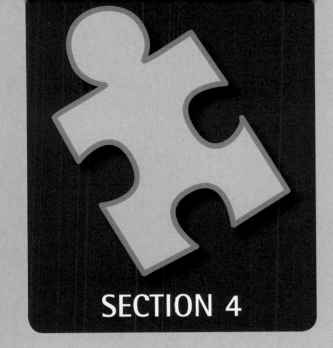

SECTION 4

Putting the Data to Work

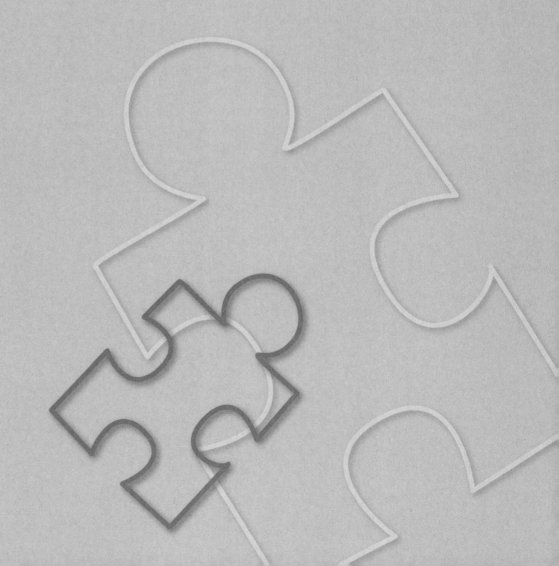

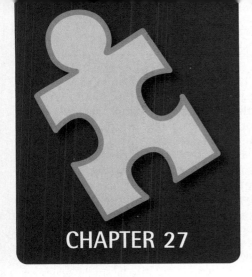

CHAPTER 27

Diagnostic Reasoning in Physical Diagnosis

Medicine is a science of uncertainty and an art of probability. One of the chief reasons for this uncertainty is the increasing variability in the manifestations of any one disease.

Sir William Osler   (1849–1919)

Art, Science, and Observation

This is one of the most important chapters of the book, because it considers the methods and concepts of evaluating the signs and symptoms involved in diagnostic reasoning. The previous chapters discuss the "science" of medicine by explaining the techniques for interviewing and performing the physical examination. The ability to make the "best" decision in the presence of uncertainty is the "art" of medicine. But there are rules and standards for the practice of this art, and these are the focus of this chapter.

The primary steps in this process involve the following:

- Data collection
- Data processing
- Problem list development

Data collection is the product of the history and the physical examination. These can be augmented with laboratory and other test results such as blood chemistry profiles, complete blood cell counts, bacterial cultures, electrocardiograms, and chest radiographs. The history, which is the most important element of the database, accounts for more than 70% of the problem list. The physical examination findings contribute an additional 20% to 25% of the database; less than 10% of the database is related to laboratory and other test results.

Data processing is the clustering of data obtained from the history, physical examination, and laboratory and imaging studies. It is rare for patients to have a solitary symptom or sign of a disease. They more commonly complain of multiple symptoms, and the examiner may find several related signs during the physical examination. It is the job of the astute observer to fit as many of these clues together into a meaningful pathophysiologic relationship. This is data processing.

This chapter was written in collaboration with Jerry A. Colliver, PhD, and Ethan D. Fried, MD. Dr. Colliver is the former Director of Statistics and Research Consulting (1981–2007) and Professor of Medical Education at Southern Illinois University School of Medicine, Springfield, IL. Dr. Fried is Assistant Professor of Clinical Medicine at Columbia College of Physicians and Surgeons, New York, NY.

For example, suppose the interviewer obtains a history of dyspnea, cough, earache, and hemoptysis. Dyspnea, cough, and hemoptysis can be grouped together as symptoms suggestive of cardiopulmonary disease. Earache does not fit with the other three symptoms and may be indicative of another problem. For another patient who complains of epigastric burning relieved by eating and whose stool is found to contain blood, this symptom and this sign should be studied together. These data suggest an abnormality of the gastrointestinal tract, possibly a duodenal ulcer. Although patients usually have multiple symptoms or signs from a pathologic condition, they may not always manifest all the symptoms or signs of the disease being considered. For instance, the presence of polyuria and polydipsia in a patient with a family history of diabetes is adequate to raise the suspicion that a lateral rectus palsy may be related to diabetes, even if diabetes has not previously been diagnosed in this patient. In another patient, a 30-pound weight loss, anorexia, jaundice, and a left supraclavicular lymph node are suggestive of gastric carcinoma with liver metastasis to the porta hepatis. This illustrates the concept of data-processing multiple symptoms into a single diagnosis. The process has sometimes been likened to the rule of *Occam's razor:* The simplest theory is preferable—in this case, that all the symptoms can be explained by one diagnosis. Although it is a useful rule to keep in mind, it is not always applicable.

Problem list development results in a summary of the physical, mental, social, and personal conditions affecting the patient's health. The problem list may contain an actual diagnosis or only a symptom or sign that cannot be clustered with other bits of data. The date on which each problem developed is noted. This list reflects the clinician's level of understanding of the patient's problems, which should be listed in order of importance. Table 27-1 is an example of a problem list.

The presence of a symptom or sign related to a specific problem is a *pertinent positive finding.* For example, a history of gout and increased uric acid level are pertinent positive findings in a man suffering from excruciating back pain radiating to his testicle. This patient may be suffering from renal colic secondary to a uric acid kidney stone. The absence of a symptom or sign that, if present, would be suggestive of a diagnosis is a *pertinent negative finding.* A pertinent negative finding may be just as important as a pertinent positive finding; the fact that a key finding is not present may help rule out a certain diagnosis. For example, the absence of tachycardia in a woman with weight loss and a tremor makes the existence of hyperthyroidism less than likely; the presence of tachycardia would strengthen the likelihood of hyperthyroidism.

An important consideration in any database is the patient's demographic information: *sex, age, ethnicity*, and *area of residence*. A *man* with a bleeding disorder dating from birth is likely to have hemophilia. A *65-year-old* person with exertional chest pain is probably suffering, statistically, from coronary artery disease. An *African-American* patient with episodes of severe bone pain may be suffering from sickle cell anemia. A person living in the *San Joaquin Valley* who has pulmonary symptoms may have coccidioidomycosis. This information is often suggestive of a unifying diagnosis, but the absence of a "usual" finding should never totally exclude a diagnosis.

It has been said, "Common diseases are common." This apparently simplistic statement has great merit because it underlines the fact that the observer should not assume an exotic diagnosis if a common one accurately explains the clinical state. (In contrast, if a common diagnosis cannot account for all the symptoms, the observer should look for another, less

Table 27–1 Example of a Problem List

Problem	Date	Resolved
1. Chest pain	6/28/08	
2. Acute inferior myocardial infarction	1/30/06	2/15/06
3. Colon cancer	4/30/04	6/3/04
4. Diabetes mellitus	1999	
5. Hypertension	1993	
6. "Red urine"	6/10/05	
7. Distress over son's drug abuse	1/05	

common diagnosis.) It is also true that "Uncommon signs of common diseases are more common than common signs of uncommon diseases."

Finally, "A rare disease is *not* rare for the patient who has the disease." If a patient's symptoms and signs are suggestive of an uncommon condition, that patient may be the 1 in 10,000 with the disease. Nevertheless, statistics based on population groups provide a useful guide in approaching clinical decision-making for individual patients.

Diagnostic Reasoning from Signs and Symptoms

Unfortunately, decisions in medicine can rarely be made with 100% certainty. Probability weights the decision. Only if the cluster of symptoms, signs, and test results is unequivocal can the clinician be certain of a diagnosis. This does not occur often. How, then, can the clinician make the "best" decision—best in light of current knowledge and research?

Laboratory tests immediately come to mind. But signs and symptoms obtained from the patient's history and physical examination perform the same function as laboratory tests, and the information and results obtained from signs, symptoms, and tests are evaluated in the same way and are subject to the same rules and standards of evidence for diagnostic reasoning. Also, signs and symptoms actually account for more (90%) of the developing problem list than do laboratory test results (<10%).

Sensitivity and Specificity

Throughout this text, signs and symptoms have been described according to their *operating characteristics:* sensitivity and specificity. These operating characteristics, which also apply to laboratory tests, indicate the usefulness of the sign, symptom, or test to the clinician in making a diagnosis. *Sensitivity* is equal to the true-positive rate, or the proportion of positive test results in individuals with a disease. Sensitivity, therefore, is based solely on patients with the disease. *Specificity* is equal to the true-negative rate, or the proportion of negative test results in individuals without a disease. Specificity, therefore, is based only on individuals without the disease. A *false-positive* finding refers to a positive test result in an individual without the disease or condition. Thus, a sign, symptom, or test with 90% specificity can correctly identify a condition in 90 of 100 normal individuals; findings in the other 10 individuals are false positive, and the false-positive rate is 10%. If a test result or observation is negative in a person with the disease, the result is termed *false negative*.

The *2 × 2 table* is useful for representing the relationship of a test, symptom, or sign to a disease. D+ indicates the presence of the disease; D− indicates the absence of the disease; T+ is a positive test result, or the presence of a symptom or sign; T− is the absence of a positive test result, or the absence of a symptom or sign. Each of the cells of the table represents a set of patients. Consider the following 2 × 2 table:

	With Disease D+	Without Disease D−
Test Positive T+	True Positive (TP)	False Positive (FP)
Test Negative T−	False Negative (FN)	True Negative (TN)

Sensitivity is defined as the number of true positive results (TP) divided by the number with disease (i.e., the total of the true positive and the false negative results [FN]):

$$\text{Sensitivity} = \text{TP}/(\text{number with disease}) = \text{TP}/(\text{TP} + \text{FN})$$

Specificity is defined as the number of true negative results (TN) divided by the number without disease (i.e., the total of false positive results [FP] and true negatives):

$$\text{Specificity} = \text{TN}/(\text{number without disease}) = \text{TN}/(\text{FP} + \text{TN})$$

Substituting numbers:

	D+	D−
T+	65 (65%) (TP)	100 (10%) (FP)
T−	35 (35%) (FN)	900 (90%) (TN)
	100	1000

The upper left cell of the 2×2 table indicates that 65 of 100 patients with a certain disease (65%) had a certain positive test result or symptom or sign. Thus, the test has a true-positive rate of .65, or a sensitivity of 65%.

The true-negative rate is .90, as indicated in the lower right cell; this means that 900 of 1000 individuals without the disease (90%) did not have a positive test result or symptom or sign. Therefore, the specificity of the test is 90%.

The false-positive rate is .10, meaning that 100 of 1000 in the normal population (10%) had the finding for some reason, without having the disease in question. This is shown in the upper right cell.

Finally, the lower left cell indicates that the test result, symptom, or sign is absent in 35 of 100 patients with the disease. Thus, the false-negative rate is 35%.

Note that the true-positive rate plus the false-negative rate equals 1.0; the false-positive rate plus the true-negative rate also equals 1.0. If the disease is aortic stenosis and the symptom is syncope, then according to the preceding table, 65% of patients with aortic stenosis have syncope, and 35% do not; 90% of individuals without aortic stenosis do not have syncope, and 10% do.

Likelihood Ratio

Because sensitivity and specificity are used to measure different properties, a symptom, sign, or test has both sensitivity and specificity values: high sensitivity and high specificity, low sensitivity and low specificity, high sensitivity and low specificity, or low sensitivity and high specificity. Sensitivity and specificity are often combined to form the likelihood ratio (LR), which provides a unitary measure of the operating characteristics of a sign, symptom, or test. The LR is defined as the ratio of the true-positive rate to the false-positive rate:

$$\text{LR} = \text{sensitivity}/(1 - \text{specificity}) = \text{TP rate}/\text{FP rate}$$

Thus, the LR indicates the proportion of accurate to inaccurate positive test results. In the preceding example of syncope and aortic stenosis, where sensitivity = TP rate = .65, and 1 − specificity = FP rate = .10, the LR would be equal to .65/.10, or 6.5. In other words, a positive sign, symptom, or test result is 6.5 times more likely in patients with disease than in individuals without disease. In the example, the occurrence of syncope would be 6.5 times greater in patients with aortic stenosis than in individuals without it. Tests or signs with LRs greater than 10 are generally highly useful because they provide considerable confidence in diagnostic reasoning.

Ruling In and Ruling Out Disease

Sensitivity and specificity (and the LR) refer to properties of the symptom, sign, or test result that are invariant across different populations. This is true even though particular populations may differ with regard to the prevalence of the disease or condition in question. Sensitivity is based solely on patients with disease, and specificity is based solely on individuals without disease. Thus, the relative sizes of the two groups—with disease and without disease—in the population of concern, which is the basis for the computation of prevalence, play no role in the computation of sensitivity and specificity. Sensitivity and specificity are simply the operating characteristics of the test and as such provide general information about the usefulness of the test for diagnostic reasoning *with any population of patients*. But in actual clinical practice, the clinician is concerned with the individual patient and whether that patient's test results are predictive of disease. How certain can the clinician be that a patient has a disease if the test result is positive or if a symptom or sign is present? How certain can a clinician be that a person is healthy if a test result is negative or if a symptom or sign is absent? Typically, these questions are answered by computing the positive and negative predictive values, which are based on sensitivity and specificity but also take into account the prevalence of disease in the population of which the patient is a member.

First, however, consider two special cases of diagnostic reasoning in which clinical decisions can be based on only a knowledge of sensitivity and specificity. If the sensitivity of a given symptom, sign, or test is quite high, 90% or greater, and the patient has a negative result, the clinician can somewhat confidently rule out disease because so few patients with disease have a negative test result (<10%). Sackett (1992) devised the following acronym for this special case: **Sen**sitive signs when **N**egative help rule **out** the disease (**SnNout**). In the absence of a highly sensitive sign, a person is most likely not to have the disease. The second special case occurs if the specificity of a given test, symptom, or sign is quite high, 90% or greater, and the patient has a positive result. The clinician can then somewhat confidently rule in disease because so few individuals without disease have a positive test result (<10%). Sackett's acronym for this case is **Sp**ecific signs when **P**ositive help rule **in** the disease (**SpPin**). In the presence of a highly specific sign, a person is most likely to have the disease.

Positive and Negative Predictive Values

SnNout and SpPin are quite useful in those two special cases, but usually the clinician wants to predict the actual probability of disease for a patient with a positive result or the probability of no disease for an individual with a negative result. The former is estimated by the *positive predictive value* (PV+), which is equal to the number of true positive findings divided by the total number of positive result findings in the population of which the patient is a member (the true positive findings plus the false positive findings):

$$PV+ = TP/\text{all positive findings} = TP/(TP + FP)$$

The positive predictive value is the *frequency of disease* among patients with positive test results. Stated another way, it is the probability that a patient with a positive test result actually has the disease. The *negative predictive value* (PV−) is equal to the number of true negative results divided by the total number of negative results in the patient's population (the true negative findings plus the false negative findings):

$$PV- = TN/\text{all negative findings} = TN/(TN + FN)$$

The negative predictive value is the *frequency of nondisease* in individuals with negative test results. Stated another way, it is the probability of not having the disease if the test result is negative or if the symptom or sign is absent.

For example, assume that the 2×2 table discussed earlier represents the entire population of interest to the clinician. The PV+ is calculated as follows:

$$PV+ = 65/(65 + 100)$$
$$= .39$$

and the PV− is as follows:

$$PV- = 900/(35 + 900)$$
$$= .96$$

Thus, the predicted probability that a person with a positive result in fact has the disease is 39%. The predicted probability that a person with a negative result does not have the disease is 96%. In the hypothetical example, the probability that a patient with syncope actually has aortic stenosis is only 39%, whereas the probability that a person without syncope does not have aortic stenosis is 96%. The high PV− of 96% is consistent with the high test specificity of 90%.

Prevalence

Clearly, the sensitivity and specificity of a sign, symptom, or test are important factors in predicting the probability of disease, given the test results. So too is the prevalence of the disease in the population of which the patient is a member. The *prevalence of disease* refers to the proportion with disease in the population of interest. In a 2×2 table that represents the entire population (or a representative sample), prevalence is equal to the number with disease (TP + FN) divided by the total number in the population (TP + FP + FN + TN). Again, assuming that the preceding 2×2 table represents the entire population of concern, prevalence is calculated as follows:

$$\text{Prevalence} = (65 + 35)/(65 + 100 + 35 + 900)$$
$$= 100/1100$$
$$= .09$$

Among this population, 9% have the disease in question.

Two intuitive examples illustrate the role of prevalence in predicting the probability of disease. Consider the value of the symptom of chest pain for predicting the probability of coronary artery disease. The first patient is a 65-year-old man with chest pain. The prevalence of coronary artery disease in the population of 65-year-old men is high. Therefore, the presence of chest pain has a high positive predictive value for this patient, and it is probable that coronary artery disease exists in this patient. However, the absence of chest pain has a low negative predictive value, indicating that, because the prevalence is high, coronary artery disease may exist even in the absence of symptoms.

In contrast, consider the positive predictive value of chest pain in a 20-year-old woman. Among women in this age group, the prevalence of coronary artery disease is low, so the probability that this patient's chest pain represents coronary artery disease is low. The presence of chest pain in a 20-year-old woman has a low positive predictive value. However, the absence of chest pain has a high negative predictive value, indicating that coronary artery disease is unlikely to be present.

Figure 27-1 illustrates how changes in disease prevalence affect predictive values. The most significant increase in the positive predictive value of a sign, symptom, or tests occurs when the disease is less common. At this end of the curve, small changes in prevalence produce great changes in the positive predictive value. Conversely, the most significant increase in the negative predictive value occurs when the disease is most prevalent. Slight decreases in the prevalence of common diseases produce significant increases in the negative predictive value. The higher the prevalence is, the higher the positive predictive value is and the lower the negative predictive value is.

Differences in prevalence rates may be related either to the clinical setting in which the patient is seen or to the specific demographic characteristics of the patient. For example, a clinician performing routine examinations in an outpatient clinic will find a prevalence of disease different from that found by a clinician working only with inpatients in a hospital specializing in that disease. The *demographic characteristics* of the patient refer to age, gender, and race, and these characteristics play a major role in the prevalence of many diseases.

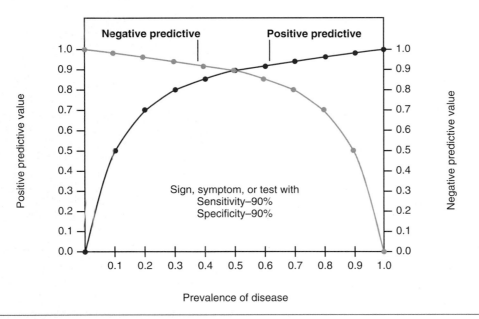

Figure 27–1 Effect of changing disease prevalence on predictive values.

Both the clinical setting and the characteristics of the patient help determine the usefulness of the sign, symptom, or laboratory test because they affect both the positive and the negative predictive values of the finding.

Bayes' Theorem

The formulas for PV+ and PV− are appropriate only if data in the 2 × 2 table are for the entire population or a representative sample of that population, in which case the prevalence of disease in the population is accurately reflected in the table. More typically, the sensitivity and specificity of the test, sign, or symptom are determined independently of the prevalence of disease, which must be ascertained by the clinician for the specific patient in question (e.g., prevalence of disease for the patient's gender, age group, or ethnic group, or for inpatients versus outpatients). Thus, the positive and negative predictive values are typically computed with Bayes' theorem, which expresses PV+ and PV− as functions of sensitivity, specificity, and prevalence. To understand Bayes' theorem, consider the tree diagram in Figure 27-2.

Consider again the example of syncope in patients with aortic stenosis, using the data in the 2 × 2 table. This time, do *not* assume that the data represent the entire population; assume that the data for the diseased and nondiseased groups were obtained separately, meaning that the prevalence of disease cannot be determined from the table, although sensitivity and specificity can be. Now assume that the prevalence of aortic stenosis is 80% in a given patient population. The sensitivity of syncope related to aortic stenosis remains 65% and the specificity 90%, as indicated in the table. Using Bayes' theorem, calculate the PV+ and PV− as follows:

$$PV+ = \frac{(.80)(.65)}{(.80)(.65) + (1 - .80)(1 - .90)}$$

$$= 96\%$$

$$PV- = \frac{(1 - .80)(.90)}{(.80)(1 - .65) + (1 - .80)(.90)}$$

$$= 39\%$$

Thus, a positive finding of syncope would increase the probability that the patient has aortic stenosis from 80% (the prevalence, or unconditional probability, of aortic stenosis in the general population) to 96% (the conditional probability of aortic stenosis in the presence of syncope). A negative finding for syncope would increase the probability of absence of stenosis from 20% (1 − prevalence in the general population) to 39% (the conditional probability of no stenosis in the absence of syncope). The absence of syncope in this patient has reduced the probability of aortic stenosis from 80% to 61% (100% − 39%).

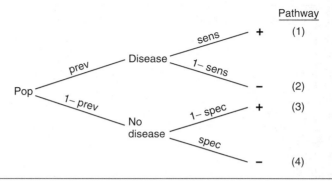

Figure 27–2 Tree diagram.

- Starting on the left, the diagram shows that the population consists of those with disease and those without disease. Prev is the proportion with disease; $1 - $ prev is the proportion without disease.
- Moving to the right, the diagram shows that patients with disease can have positive or negative results, and those without disease can also have positive or negative results. Sens is the proportion of diseased patients with positive results; $1 - $ sens is the proportion of diseased patients with negative results. Spec is the proportion of nondiseased patients with negative results; $1 - $ spec is the proportion of nondiseased patients with positive results.
- PV+ refers in general to patients with positive results, which is represented in the diagram by pathways (1) and (3). PV+ refers particularly to patients with positive test results who also have disease, which is represented in the diagram by pathway (1). PV+ specifically is the proportion of patients with positive test results who also have disease. This can be obtained by dividing the term represented by pathway (1) by the sum of the terms represented by pathways (1) and (3):

$$PV+ = \frac{(1)}{(1)+(3)} = \frac{\text{prev} \times \text{sens}}{(\text{prev} \times \text{sens}) + (1-\text{prev})(1-\text{spec})}$$

- PV− can be obtained by dividing the term represented by pathway (4) by the sum of the terms represented by pathways (2) and (4):

$$PV- = \frac{(4)}{(2)+(4)} = \frac{(1-\text{prev})(\text{spec})}{(\text{prev})(1-\text{sens}) + (1-\text{prev})(\text{spec})}$$

Pursuing this example, now assume that the prevalence of aortic stenosis is only 20% in another patient population but that sensitivity and specificity remain at 65% and 90%, respectively. Bayes' theorem now shows the PV+ and the PV− are as follows:

$$PV+ = \frac{(.20)(.65)}{(.20)(.65)+(1-.20)(1-.90)}$$

$$= 62\%$$

$$PV- = \frac{(1-.20)(.90)}{(.20)(1-.65)+(1-.20)(.90)}$$

$$= 91\%$$

Notice that the PV+ has fallen from 96% (when prevalence was 80%) to 62% (with prevalence reduced to 20%). When the prevalence of a disease is quite low, the positive predictive value of a sign, symptom, or test is extremely low, even if the sensitivity and specificity are high. Also, notice that PV− has increased from 39% (when prevalence was 80%) to 91% (with prevalence reduced to 20%). Low prevalence of disease implies high negative predictive value. In general, with more disease (Prev ↑), more people with positive results will have the disease (PV+ ↑), and more people with negative results will have the disease (and fewer will not have the disease [PV− ↓]). In brief, as Prev ↑, PV+ ↑ but PV− ↓.

Nomogram

To simplify matters, a Bayes nomogram is given in Figure 27-3, which can be copied and used in the clinic or office. The nomogram provides the predictive values without requiring the calculations of Bayes' theorem. To use the nomogram, first locate on the relevant axes the points that correspond to (1) the prevalence of disease for the patient's population and (2) the LR for the sign, symptom, or test. Recall that the LR is the ratio of the TP rate (sensitivity) to the FP rate (1 − specificity). Next, place a straight edge on the nomogram to connect the points. The PV+ is given by the point at which the straight edge intersects the predictive value axis. For example, if prevalence = .80 and LR = .65/.10 = 6.50, the PV+ = .96, as computed earlier with Bayes' theorem. To determine the PV−, use 1 − prevalence and TN rate/FN rate instead of prevalence and the LR.

Multiple Signs and Symptoms

Typically, diagnostic reasoning is based on multiple signs and symptoms and possibly on laboratory test results. These multiple findings must be combined to evaluate a diagnostic possibility. For example, consider the following clinical situation: A 21-year-old asymptomatic woman finds a thyroid nodule on self-examination, and she is referred to an endocrinologist

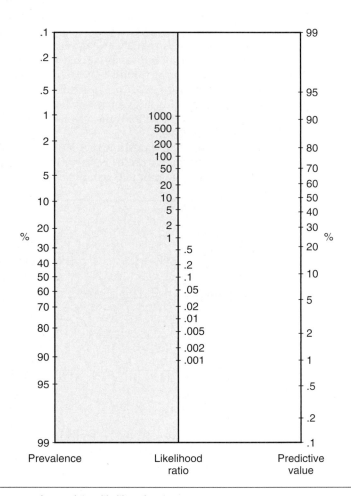

Figure 27–3 Nomogram for applying likelihood ratios.

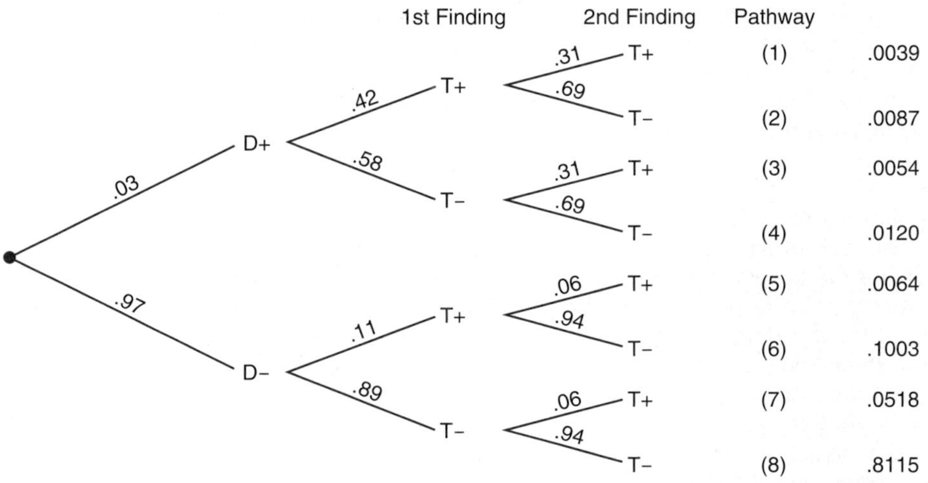

Figure 27–4 Extended tree diagram. D+, with disease; D–, without disease; T+, positive test result; T–, negative test result.

for evaluation. The clinician describes the thyroid nodule as hard to palpation and fixed to the surrounding tissue. In this clinician's practice, the prevalence of thyroid cancer is 3%. What is the chance that this nodule is cancerous?

To start, you can consider each finding separately. First, evaluate the predictive value of the presence of a palpable hard nodule. The sensitivity and specificity of this finding are 42% and 89%, respectively. With a prevalence of malignancy of 3%, Bayes' theorem (or the nomogram) shows that the PV+ = 11% and the PV– = 98%. For the second finding, fixation of the nodule to the surrounding tissue, sensitivity is 31% and specificity is 94%. Again, with a prevalence equal to 3%, Bayes' theorem (or the nomogram) shows that PV + = 14% and PV– = 98%.

But what about the presence of both: a hard nodule that is fixed to the surrounding tissue? What about the presence of either a hard or a fixed nodule? Or the presence of neither? What are the predictive values of these combined findings? If it is assumed that the multiple signs, symptoms, and tests are independent (i.e., their findings are unrelated), the predictive values of these combined findings can be determined by extending the Bayesian tree diagram and adding a second finding, as shown in Figure 27-4.

Thus, Bayes' theorem can be used to compute the positive predictive values of the combined findings by calculating the product of the probabilities for each pathway (presented in parentheses to the right of the tree) and summing the products as follows:

PV+

$$\text{p (Disease, given both findings)} = \frac{(1)}{(1) + (5)} = \frac{.0039}{.0039 + .0064} = .38$$

$$\text{p (Disease, given either finding)} = \frac{(2) + (3)}{(2) + (3) + (6) + (7)}$$
$$= \frac{.0087 + .0054}{.0087 + .0054 + .1003 + .0518} = .08$$

$$\text{p (Disease, given neither finding)} = \frac{(4)}{(4) + (8)} = \frac{.0120}{.0120 + .8115} = .01$$

PV–

$$\text{p (No disease, given neither finding)} = \frac{(8)}{(4) + (8)} = \frac{.8115}{.0120 + .8115} = .99$$

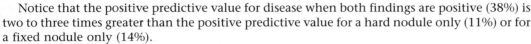

Notice that the positive predictive value for disease when both findings are positive (38%) is two to three times greater than the positive predictive value for a hard nodule only (11%) or for a fixed nodule only (14%).

In practice, multiple signs, symptoms, and test findings are typically not independent, because the presence of one finding increases the probability of the presence of another finding. Of course, the opposite is also possible, in that the second finding may be less likely in the presence of the first. Either way, the assumption of independence is violated, and the practice of calculating products of sensitivities in compound Bayesian trees (e.g., .42 × .31 in first pathway) does not produce accurate predictive values. Instead, the sensitivity and specificity for the actual compound finding must be known, such as the probability of the combined finding of a hard and fixed nodule. At present, this information is limited in the clinical research literature, but studies of compound findings with their sensitivities and specificities are increasing. It is hoped that this information will soon be available for clinical practice.

Decision Analysis

Diagnostic reasoning is only the first step in clinical decision-making. After reaching a decision about a diagnosis, the clinician must decide on a plan of treatment and management for the particular patient. These decisions must take into account the probability and utility (i.e., worth or value) of each possible outcome of the treatment or management plan, given the patient's population (gender, age, ethnicity, inpatient or outpatient, and so forth). Similarly, the clinician may need to decide whether to order laboratory tests to confirm a diagnosis only suggested by the signs and symptoms elicited during the clinical examination. These test-ordering decisions must be based on the probability and utility of the possible outcomes of the test (possibly invasive and costly), and the patient's population must again be taken into account. The purpose of this section is to extend the discussion of clinical decision-making to include making decisions about test ordering, treatment, and management.

Typically, a decision tree is used to represent the various alternatives, with probabilities assigned to the alternatives and utilities attached to the possible outcomes. Sackett and colleagues (1991) presented an excellent, detailed discussion of clinical decision-making. The following discussion relies on their test-ordering, decision-making example.

Their example involves "a 35 year old man with 'heartburn' for several years, no coronary risk factors, and a 6-week history of nonexertional, squeezing chest pain deep in his lower sternum and epigastrium, usually radiating straight through to his back and most likely to occur when he lies down after a heavy meal. He has a negative physical exam."

The clinician in the example concludes that esophageal spasm is the best diagnosis and that significant coronary stenosis is very unlikely, perhaps 5% at most for this patient's population. To address the latter possibility (serious, although unlikely), the clinician considers ordering exercise electrocardiography (E-ECG) just to be on the safe side, knowing that for greater than 70% stenosis, the sensitivity and specificity of E-ECG are 60% and 91%, respectively. According to this information and Bayes' theorem (or the nomogram), PV+ = .26 and PV− = .98.

Construct Decision Tree

To decide whether to test with E-ECG, the clinician performs a decision analysis, first by constructing the decision tree in Figure 27-5, which depicts the decision-making situation. The clinician will decide whether to order E-ECG, as indicated on the left by the branching at the box-shaped "decision" node. If the clinician orders E-ECG, the results can be positive or negative, as shown by the next branching from the circular "chance" node; in either case, the patient can be found to have or not to have coronary stenosis, as shown by the branchings at the next two "chance" nodes. If the clinician decides not to order E-ECG, it is unknown whether the patient has the disease, as shown by the branching at the lower right "chance" node.

Assign Probabilities

Next, a probability is assigned to each branch in the tree, as shown in Figure 27-6. Ideally, probabilities should be based on strong clinical research studies. The proportions of patients with positive and negative E-ECG results are known to be 12% and 88%, respectively. Of those with positive results, 26% have stenosis and 74% do not. Notice that this first probability is the positive predictive value (PV+), which shows the proportion of individuals with a positive test result who do in fact have stenosis; the second proportion is 1 − PV+. Of those with negative results, the probabilities are 2% and 98%, respectively. The second probability here is the

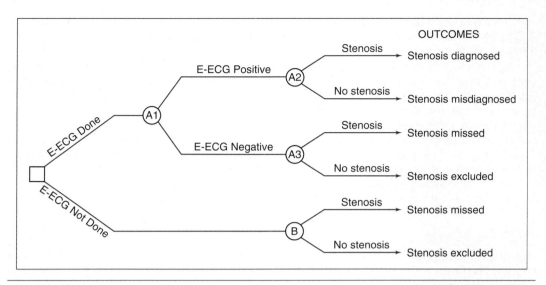

Figure 27–5 Decision tree for exercise electrocardiography (E-ECG).

negative predictive value (PV−), and the first is 1 − PV−. In the general population not undergoing E-ECG, 5% have stenosis and 95% do not.

Attach Utilities

A utility is then attached to each of the possible outcomes, which are represented by the pathways through the tree. The utility refers to the worth, or value, of the outcome. Utilities may be objective, stated in monetary terms or expected years of life, or subjective, stated in relative terms of anticipated value to the patient or society. In the example, there are six outcomes (pathways through the tree), with a description or label for each outcome at the right of the pathway. A positive E-ECG result for a patient with stenosis, for example, is labeled "Stenosis diagnosed." To the right of these labels are the utilities assigned by Sackett and colleagues (1991). These utilities are subjective, but they clearly show the relative worth of each of the outcomes: Stenosis excluded (1.00, most valuable), Stenosis misdiagnosed (.75), Stenosis diagnosed (.50), Stenosis missed (.25, least valuable). The exact numerical value of each subjective utility is arbitrary, but the ordering of outcomes given by the utilities is not;

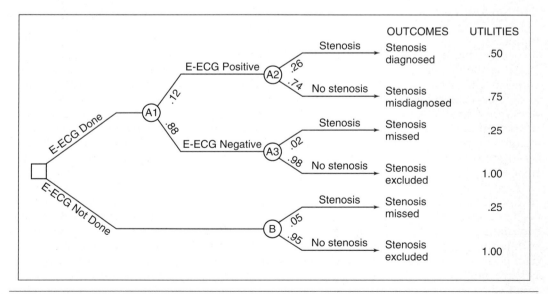

Figure 27–6 Decision tree for exercise electrocardiography (E-ECG) with probabilities and utilities added.

that is, the same decision would be reached had the utilities been, say, 4, 3, 2, and 1, respectively. Of course, if the value of one outcome is much greater than that of a second, and the value of the second is similar to those of the third and fourth (e.g., 1.00, .50, .45, .40), the difference between the utilities for the first and second outcomes should be much greater than that between the second outcome and the third and fourth outcomes. This assignment of utilities could affect the decision reached.

Compute Expected Values

The expected value for each pathway through the tree is equal to the product of the probabilities and the utility for that outcome. For the first pathway, the expected value is given by $.12 \times .26 \times .50 = .0156$. The expected values for all six pathways, therefore, are .0156, .0666, .0044, .8622, .0125, and .9500. The expected value for each decision node is computed by summing the expected values for the outcomes originating from that node. For the decision to order E-ECG, the expected value is the sum of the expected values for the first four outcomes: $.0156 + .0666 + .0044 + .8624 = .9490$. For the decision not to order an E-ECG, the expected value is the sum of the last two outcomes: $.0125 + .9500 = .9625$.

Make a Decision

The expected value of the decision not to order E-ECG (.9625) is greater than that for ordering one (.9490). The decision analysis shows that the "best" decision for this patient is not to test. The decision would have been the same had the utilities been 4, 3, 2, 1 rather than 1.00, .75, .50, .25; the expected values for testing versus not testing would have been 3.796 and 3.850. Had the utilities been 1.00, .50, .45, and .40, the expected values would have been .928 and .970.

Clearly, the utilities, particularly subjective utilities, are the Achilles' heel of decision analysis, although even objective utilities can be somewhat arbitrary. The expected values of the decision are affected by the utilities chosen for the analysis, and different utilities may lead to different decisions. Also, the probabilities assigned to the branches of the tree affect the outcome of the decision analysis, but the probabilities are typically less subjective than the utilities, being based on actual values such as sensitivities, specificities, and positive and negative predictive values obtained from the clinical research literature. Because the variability in the utilities and probabilities can affect the conclusion of the decision analysis, it has been suggested that the decision-maker systematically vary the utilities and probabilities within the reasonable range for the patient in question. This tests the vulnerability of the decision to reasonable variation in the utilities and probabilities. This is called a *sensitivity analysis* (although *vulnerability analysis* might be a better term, to avoid confusion with conventional test sensitivity). If the decision to test or not to test is consistent over these variations in utilities and probabilities, the clinician can be more confident in the decision. Otherwise, the decision is reduced to a toss-up between the alternatives.

In Sackett and colleagues' example, the expected values for the decisions to test or not to test were quite close (.949 and .962), but they seem informative, at least intuitively, possibly because, surprisingly, they show a greater value for not testing. At the very least, the decision analysis shows that testing this patient is no better than not testing him. But what if the results were reversed, with the expected values for testing or not testing equal to .962 and .949, or with expected values for surgery or no surgery at .962 and .949? Close values such as these are not uncommon in decision analysis, and they illustrate the need to think clearly about the subjective meaning of the utility scale, which is given in terms of the nature of the outcomes to which the utilities are attached. For example, consider a four-point scale in which 4 represents stenosis excluded, 3 represents stenosis misdiagnosed, and so forth; the expected values for testing and not testing of 3.796 and 3.850, respectively, differ by only .054 of the unit distance between stenosis excluded (4) and stenosis misdiagnosed (3). The two decisions are closely valued. Nevertheless, in the absence of any other information, the "best" decision is not to test, which means simply that in the long run, with close-call decisions like this, there is a slight advantage to acting in accordance with the decision analysis.

The Rational Clinical Examination

In 1992, the *Journal of the American Medical Association* initiated a series of articles on the *rational clinical examination*. This series underscores the points made in this chapter: namely, that signs and symptoms provide critical information in diagnostic reasoning and that the operating characteristics (sensitivity and specificity) of the signs and symptoms must be considered in the reasoning process, as must the prevalence of the disease in question. In other words, the clinical examination can and should be more rational, based on empirical evidence of the predictive value of signs and symptoms used in diagnostic reasoning. A listing of the JAMA articles on The Rational Clinical Examination since 1998 can be found in Appendix D.

The rational clinical examination is part of a broader movement called *evidence-based medicine*, which "de-emphasizes intuition, unsystematic clinical experience, and pathophysiologic rationale as sufficient grounds for clinical decision-making and stresses the examination of evidence from clinical research." The evidence-based approach to the practice of clinical medicine has its origins in clinical research generated within the relatively new field of *clinical epidemiology*. In the past, epidemiology was concerned with the causes of diseases, and hence the interest was in establishing that exposure to certain risk factors caused certain diseases. Thus, classic epidemiology has been characterized as the study of the distribution of disease across time, place, and peoples. Clinical epidemiology has expanded this focus to encompass the study of the entire clinical process, including diagnosis, treatment, prognosis, prevention, evaluation of health-care services, and risk-benefit analysis. Evidence from clinical research in these areas will probably be used to provide an empirical base for rational clinical practice, including diagnostic reasoning, as the "art" of clinical decision-making becomes more of a science.

Bibliography

Bowen JL: Educational strategies to promote clinical diagnostic reasoning. N Engl J Med 355:2217, 2006.

Bradley CP: Can we avoid bias? BMJ 330:784, 2005.

Brorsson B, Wall S: Assessment of Medical Technology: Problems and Methods. Stockholm, Swedish Medical Research Council, 1985.

Cutler P: Problem Solving in Clinical Medicine: From Data to Diagnosis, 2nd ed. Baltimore, Williams & Wilkins, 1985.

Elstein AS, Schwarz A: Evidence base of clinical diagnosis: Clinical problem solving and diagnostic decision making: Selective review of the cognitive literature. BMJ 324:729, 2002.

Hunink M, Glasziou P, Siegel J, et al: Decision Making in Health and Medicine: Integrating Evidence and Values. New York, Cambridge University Press, 2001.

Kassirer JP: Diagnostic reasoning. Ann Intern Med 110:893, 1989.

Lau AYS, Coiera EW: Do people experience cognitive biases while searching for information? J Am Med Inform Assoc 14:599, 2007.

Sackett DL: A primer on the precision and accuracy of the clinical examination. JAMA 267:2638, 1992.

Sackett DL, Haynes RB, Guyatt GH, et al: Clinical Epidemiology: A Basic Science for Clinical Medicine, 2nd ed. Boston, Little, Brown, 1991.

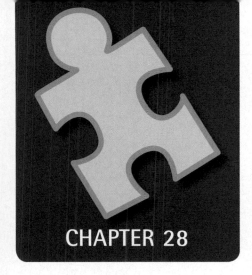

CHAPTER 28

The Clinical Record

May I never forget that the patient is a fellow human creature in pain. May I never consider the patient merely a vessel of disease.

From Oath of Maimonides   (1135–1204)

Putting the History and Physical Examination Together

Until this point, this book has dealt separately with the history and the physical examination. Chapters 1 to 6 give an in-depth analysis of history-taking techniques. Chapters 7 to 21 discuss the many elements of the physical examination, and Chapter 22 suggests an approach to performing the complete physical examination and its write-up. Chapters 23 to 26 cover the evaluation of specific patients. Chapter 27 discusses data gathering and data analysis. This chapter suggests how the history and the physical examination can be integrated into one succinct statement about the patient.

In writing up the history and the physical examination, the examiner should follow several rules:

- Record all pertinent data
- Avoid extraneous data
- Use common terms
- Avoid nonstandard abbreviations
- Be objective
- Use diagrams when indicated

The patient's medical record is a legal document. Comments regarding the patient's behavior and attitudes should *not* be part of the record unless they are important from a medical or scientific standpoint. Describe all parts of the examination that you performed and indicate those that you did not perform. A statement such as "the examination of the eye is normal" is much less accurate than "the fundus is normal." In the first case, it is not clear whether the examiner actually attempted to look at the fundus. If a part of the examination was not performed, state that it was "deferred" for whatever reason. Finally, it is not necessary to state all the possible abnormalities if they are not present. It is acceptable to state that "the pharynx was normal" instead of "the pharynx was not injected, and there was no evidence of discharge, erosion, masses, or other lesions." It is clear from the first statement that the examiner inspected the pharynx and believed that it was normal.

Now consider again the patient Mr. John Doe, whose interview was recorded in Chapter 6, Putting the History Together. The following text describes the complete history and physical examination of this patient.

Patient: John Doe
Date: July 19, 2009

History
Source
Self, reliable.

Chief Complaint
"Chest pain for the past 6 months."

History of Present Illness
This is the first St. Catherine's Hospital admission for this 42-year-old lawyer with athero-sclerotic coronary artery disease. The patient's history of chest pain began 4 years before admission. He described the pain as a "dull ache" in the retrosternal area, with radiation to his left arm. The pain was provoked by exertion and emotions. On July 15, 2008, Mr. Doe suffered his first heart attack while playing tennis. He had an uneventful hospitalization in Kings Hospital in New York City. After 3 weeks in the hospital and 3 weeks at home, he returned to work. The patient suffered a second heart attack 6 months later (January 9, 2009), again while playing tennis. The patient was hospitalized in Kings Hospital, during which time he was told of an "irregularity" in his heart rate. Since then, the patient has not experienced any palpitations, nor has he been told of any further irregularities.

Over the past 6 months, Mr. Doe has noted an increase in the frequency of his chest pain. The pain now occurs four to five times a day and is relieved within 5 minutes with one or two nitroglycerin tablets under his tongue. The pain is produced by exercise, emotions, and sexual intercourse. The patient also describes one-block dyspnea on exertion. The patient relates that 6 months ago, he could walk two or three blocks before becoming short of breath.

Although the patient shows significant denial of his illness, he is anxious and depressed.
The patient has currently been admitted for elective cardiac catheterization.

Past Medical History
General: Good.
Past illnesses: History of untreated hypertension for years (blood pressure not known); no history of measles, chickenpox, mumps, diphtheria, or whooping cough.
Injuries: None.
Hospitalizations: Appendectomy, age 15 years, Booth Memorial Hospital in Rochester, New York (Dr. Meyers, surgeon).
Surgery: See Hospitalizations.
Allergies: None.
Immunizations: Salk vaccine for polio, tetanus vaccine, both as a child; no adverse reactions remembered.
Substance abuse: A 40-pack-year (2 packs a day for 20 years) history of smoking; stopped smoking after first heart attack; marijuana on rare occasions in past; drinks alcohol "socially" but also admits to feeling the need for a drink as the day goes on (CAGE score, 1); denies use of other street drugs.
Diet: Mostly red meat, with little fish in diet; three cups of coffee a day; recent decrease in appetite, with a 10-pound weight loss in past 3 months.
Sleep patterns: Recently, falls asleep normally but awakens around 3 AM and cannot go back to sleep.

Current medications:

Atenolol, 50 mg once daily

Isosorbide dinitrate, 10 mg qid

Nitroglycerin, 1/150 grains prn

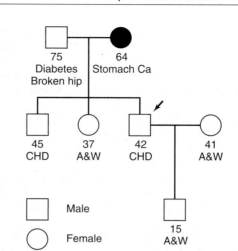

Figure 28–1 Family tree of patient John Doe. A&W, alive and well; Ca, cancer; CHD, coronary heart disease.

Chlor-Trimeton, for colds

Aspirin, for headaches

Multivitamins with iron, daily

Family History (Fig. 28-1)

Father, 75, diabetes, broken hip

Mother died, 64, stomach cancer

Brother, 45, heart attack at age 40

Sister, 37, alive and well

Son, 15, alive and well

Wife, 41, alive and well

There is no family history of congenital disease. No other history of diabetes or cardiac disease. No history of renal, hepatic, or neurologic disease. No history of mental illness.

Psychosocial History
"Type A" personality; born and raised in Middletown, New York; family moved to Rochester, New York, when Mr. Doe was 13 years of age; patient moved to New York City after high school; college and law school in New York City; he is now a senior partner of a law firm for which he has worked for the past 17 years; married to Emily for the past 13 years; was an active tennis player before second heart attack; before 6 months ago, enjoyed the theater and reading.

Sexual, Reproductive, and Gynecologic History
Patient is male, exclusively heterosexual, with one partner, his wife. He has one son, age 15 years. Recently, because of angina, the patient has stopped having sexual relations. He has noted that for the past 2 years his erections have been "less hard."

Review of Systems
General: Depressed for the past 6 months as a result of his ill health.
  Skin: No rashes or other changes.
  Head: No history of head injury.

Eyes: Wears glasses for reading; no changes in vision recently; saw ophthalmologist 1 year ago for routine examination; no history of eye pain, tearing, discharge, or seeing halos around lights.

Ears: Patient not aware of any problem hearing; no dizziness, discharge, or pain present.

Nose: Occasional upper respiratory infection, two or three times a year, lasting 3 to 5 days; no hay fever, sinus symptoms.

Mouth and throat: Occasional sore throats and canker sores associated with colds; no difficulty in chewing or eating; brushes and flosses twice a day; sees dentist twice a year; no gingival bleeding.

Neck: No masses or tenderness.

Chest: History of occasional blood-tinged sputum and cough in the morning when patient was smoking, but not recently; last chest x-ray film 1 year ago, was told it was normal; one-block dyspnea on exertion (as noted in History of Present Illness); no history of wheezing, asthma, bronchitis, or tuberculosis.

Breasts: No masses or nipple discharge noted.

Cardiac: As noted in History of Present Illness.

Vascular: No history of cerebrovascular accidents or claudication.

Gastrointestinal: Recent decrease in appetite with 10-pound weight loss in past few months; uses no laxatives; no history of diarrhea, constipation, nausea, or vomiting; no bleeding noted.

Genitourinary: Urinates four to five times a day; urine is light yellow in color, never red; nocturia X1; no change in stream; no history of urinary infections; no sexual intercourse in past 6 months, owing to angina during sex; no history of venereal disease.

Musculoskeletal: No joint or bone symptoms; no weakness; no history of back problems or gout.

Neurologic: No history of seizures or difficulties in walking or balance; no history of motor or sensory symptoms.

Endocrine: No known thyroid nodules; no history of temperature intolerance; no hair changes; no history of polydipsia or polyuria.

Psychiatric: Depressed and very anxious about his ill health; also anxious about the results of the upcoming cardiac catheterization; asked, "What's going to happen to me?"

Physical Examination

General appearance: The patient is a 42-year-old, slightly obese white man who is lying in bed. He appears slightly older than his stated age. He is in no acute distress but is very nervous. He is well groomed, cooperative, and alert.

Vital signs: Blood pressure (BP), 175/95/80 right arm (supine), 175/90/85 left arm (supine), 170/90/80 left arm (sitting), 185/95/85 right leg (prone); heart rate, 100 and regular; respirations, 14.

Skin: Pink; no cyanosis present; five to seven nevi (each 0.5 to 1.5 cm in diameter) on back, most with hair; normal male escutcheon.

Head: Normocephalic, without signs of trauma.

Eyes: Visual acuity with reading glasses using near card: right eye (OD) 20/40, left eye (OS) 20/30; confrontation visual fields full bilaterally; extraocular movements (EOMs) intact; pupils are equal, round, and reactive to light (PERRL); eyebrows normal; conjunctivae pink; discs sharp; marked arteriovenous (AV) nicking present bilaterally; copper wiring present bilaterally; a cotton-wool spot is present at 1 o'clock position (superior nasal) in the right eye and at 5 o'clock position (inferior temporal) in the left eye; no hemorrhages are present.

Ears: Normal position; no tenderness present; external canals normal; Rinne test, air conduction > bone conduction (AC > BC) bilaterally; Weber test, no lateralization; both tympanic membranes appear normal, with normal landmarks clearly seen.

Nose: Straight, without masses; patent bilaterally; mucosa pink, without discharge; inferior turbinates appear normal.

Sinuses: No tenderness present over frontal or maxillary sinuses.

Mouth and throat: Lips pink; buccal mucosa pink; all teeth in good condition, without obvious caries; gingivae normal, without bleeding; tongue midline and without masses; uvula elevates in midline; gag reflex intact; posterior pharynx normal.

Neck: Supple, with full range of motion; trachea midline and freely mobile; no adenopathy present; thyroid not felt; prominent "a" wave seen in neck veins while lying at 45°; neck veins flat while sitting upright.

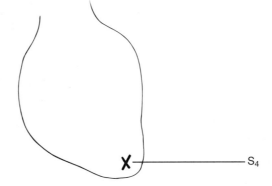

Figure 28–2 Diagram showing location of abnormal cardiac findings in patient John Doe.

Chest: Normal anteroposterior (AP) diameter; symmetric excursion bilaterally; normal tactile fremitus bilaterally; chest resonant bilaterally; clear on percussion and auscultation.

Breasts: Normal male, without masses, gynecomastia, or discharge.

Heart: Point of maximum impulse (PMI), fifth intercostal space, midclavicular line (5ICS-MCL); S_1 and S_2 normal; normal physiologic splitting present; a loud S_4 is present at the cardiac apex; no murmurs or rubs are heard (Fig. 28-2).

Vascular: Pulses are present and symmetric down to the dorsalis pedis bilaterally; no bruits are present over the carotid or femoral arteries; no abdominal bruits are present; no edema is present.

Abdomen: A well-healed appendectomy scar is present in the right lower quadrant (RLQ); the abdomen is slightly obese; no masses are present; no tenderness, guarding, rigidity, or rebound is present.

Rectal: Anal sphincter normal; no hemorrhoids present; prostate slightly enlarged and soft; no prostatic masses felt; no stool in ampulla.

Genitalia: Circumcised man with normal genitalia; penis normal without induration; testicles, $4 \times 3 \times 2$ cm (right) and $3 \times 6 \times 4$ cm (left) with normal consistency.

Lymphatic: No adenopathy noted.

Musculoskeletal: There are several stony-hard, slightly yellowish, nontender masses over the extensor tendons on the patient's hands; normal range of motion of neck, spine, and major joints of upper and lower extremities.

Neurologic: Oriented to person, place, and time; cranial nerves II to XII intact (cranial nerve I not tested); gross sensory and motor function normal; cerebellar function normal; plantar reflexes down; gait normal; deep tendon reflexes as in Table 28-1.

Summary

Mr. Doe is a "type A" 42-year-old man with a history of two myocardial infarctions, whose current admission is for elective cardiac catheterization. His risk factors for coronary artery disease are untreated hypertension and a long history of cigarette smoking. The patient has a brother who suffered a myocardial infarction at the age of 40 years.

Physical examination reveals a slightly obese man with hypertension and its associated early to intermediate funduscopic changes. Cardiac examination reveals a loud fourth heart sound, suggestive of a noncompliant (stiff) ventricle. This may be a manifestation of ischemic heart disease or ventricular hypertrophy secondary to the hypertension. Although the patient is not aware of any lipid abnormalities, numerous tendinous xanthomata on the hands are present, which are strongly suggestive of hypercholesterolemia, an additional risk factor for premature coronary artery disease.

Table 28–1 Deep Tendon Reflexes of Patient John Doe

Side	Biceps	Triceps	Knee	Achilles
Right	2+	2+	2+	1+
Left	2+	2+	1+	1+

Reflex scoring: 2+, normal; 1+, diminished.

Table 28–2 Problem List for Patient John Doe

Problem	Date	Resolved
1. Chest pain	2004	
2. Myocardial infarction	July 15, 2008	3 weeks later
3. Myocardial infarction	January 9, 2009	6 weeks later
4. Hypertension	Years	
5. Smoking	1984	July 15, 2008
6. Tendinous xanthomata	?	
7. S4 gallop		
8. Dyspnea on exertion	6 months ago	
9. Depression	3 months ago	
10. Weight loss	3 months ago	
11. Sleeping abnormality	3 months ago	
12. Diet modification	3 months ago	
13. Appendectomy	1982	

The problem list containing all Mr. Doe's health problems, identified with their dates of recognition and resolution, might look like Table 28-2. This list is used each time the patient is seen and examined. For each problem, the clinician should develop a strategy for its ultimate resolution. Each problem should have the following four components:

- **S**ubjective data
- **O**bjective data
- **A**ssessment
- **P**lan

This is the SOAP format (Weed, 1967), which contains an update of the subjective and objective data, as well as the assessment of the problem and the plan for its resolution. The *heading* of the progress note should include the date, the time, the name of the person who is writing the note, and the service the patient is using. It is very helpful to list the antibiotics and what day of the course of antibiotics at the top of the progress note, as well as other medications and doses. If the patient has undergone surgery, indicate postoperative time on the top as well (e.g., "Postop Day #3").

Subjective information is what patients tell you. How are they feeling? What are their symptoms? What are they eating? If their food status is NPO (nothing by mouth), note it here. How are they sleeping—well? How are they ambulating, urinating, defecating, and so forth?

If a patient tells you that he or she is "not doing well," you should not write this in your note, because this may be misinterpreted as your assessment. Instead, obtain a description of *the reason* the patient feels he or she is not doing well.

Objective information is what you gather from your physical examination, laboratory tests, and radiographic studies. Always include the vital signs and total fluid input and output over the last shift if the patient is NPO or on a diuretic regimen. If daily weights are being recorded, they should be included here as well. Your physical examination write-up should include only pertinent positive and negative findings and any changes.

The **assessment** is your impression of the patient's problem or level of progress; it is a summary of how the patient is doing and what has changed from the previous day.

The **plan** is what you are going to do about each problem. It may include continuing, starting, or discontinuing a medication, laboratory tests to order, test results to obtain, consults to be called, and individual or family education.

The SOAP note is not supposed to be as complete as an admit note. Complete sentences are not necessary, and abbreviations are common. Remember that abbreviations, however, differ for each specialty! *PND* generally is an abbreviation for paroxysmal nocturnal dyspnea for most

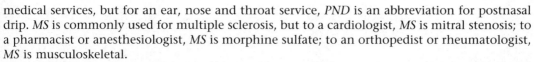

medical services, but for an ear, nose and throat service, *PND* is an abbreviation for postnasal drip. *MS* is commonly used for multiple sclerosis, but to a cardiologist, *MS* is mitral stenosis; to a pharmacist or anesthesiologist, *MS* is morphine sulfate; to an orthopedist or rheumatologist, *MS* is musculoskeletal.

The length of the note differs for each specialty as well. In general, medical notes tend to be long and surgical notes are short, but you will have to get a sense of what to do from the house staff team. Typically, medical students' notes are more detailed than the house staff note.

Always remember that the chart is a legal document. You should be confident in your presentations, but be conservative in the chart and present the facts clearly. Do not discuss other clinicians' opinions. Let the chart speak for itself.

The Human Dimension

The practice of medicine is an extraordinary profession. The thrill of interviewing and examining your first patient should always stay in your mind. Clinicians must remember that even during the most trying times, they have been granted the enormous responsibility of caring for a patient. Common courtesy, kindness, respect, and attentiveness to the patient go a long way in establishing the so-called bedside manner, which has become less evident in the past few decades. Imagine yourself in the patient's situation. How would you like to be treated? Each student in medical school has the potential to develop into a devoted and compassionate clinician.

Always strive for precision and accuracy. Be strict in your approach to the history and physical examination. Always follow the same basic routines. Do not take shortcuts. It takes time to develop the skills of inspection, palpation, percussion, and auscultation. Only with experience can the clinician master physical diagnosis. This textbook is only the introduction to a lifetime of learning about patients and their problems and diseases. As students, you will learn much from your patients. Even seasoned diagnosticians learn daily from their patients. Just as no two individuals have the same face or body appearance, no two individuals will react the same way to the same disease. This is one of the most exciting things about medicine: Every day offers new patients, new problems, new solutions.

Bibliography

Cameron S, Turtle-Song I: Learning to write case notes using the SOAP format. J Couns Dev 80:286, 2002.

Weed LL: Medical records that guide and teach. N Engl J Med 278:593, 1968.

Weed LJ: The problem oriented record as a basic tool in medical education, patient care, and research. Ann Clin Res 3:131, 1971.

CHAPTER 29

Focusing on the Focused History and Physical Examination

All we know is still infinitely less than all that still remains unknown.

William Harvey   (1578–1657)

General Considerations

The focused history and physical examination constitute a modality that is important to master in order to explore a patient's need and to educate the patient within a short period of time. It is a great skill and takes time to master. Only after becoming comfortable and confident with the complete history and physical examination can the clinician master the focused history and physical examination, because it relies on extracting the components that are most relevant.

It would be wonderful if clinicians were able to spend 45 minutes to 1 hour with each new patient, but time restraints generally allow the health care provider only about 10 to 15 minutes for each new patient encounter at most. Thus, taking a focused history and performing a focused physical examination are critical skills. It is extremely important to learn to become focused and efficient in documenting a medical history and in performing the physical examination, despite the fact that most medical schools do not teach these focused clinical skills.

Always start with open-ended questions and determine why the patient sought medical attention *today.* At some point in the interview, it would be helpful to ask the patient, "What do you think is going on?" There may be conflict or hidden anxiety, and this question may help the patient to open up to the actual problem. Let the patient speak without interruption, if possible. Always avoid leading or biased questions.

The focused history and physical examination is a complex activity comprising several different skills. It is, however, difficult to teach. Scientific knowledge must be integrated with excellent communication and hypothetical-deductive reasoning to produce a series of pertinent questions about the health of the patient.

As discussed in Chapter 27, Diagnostic Reasoning in Physical Diagnosis, most of the time, the diagnosis is not clear-cut; the history is often not that of a 70-year-old man with a history of hypertension and hypercholesterolemia who presents with crushing chest pain, or that of a 43-year-old obese woman who presents with severe right upper quadrant pain and nausea. In most cases, there exists uncertainty as to the diagnosis, and the health-care provider must assess the relative chance that the patient is or is not suffering from a particular medical problem. There are elements of uncertainty in almost every case you will see. Despite the technology of the 21st century, physicians still must use their judgment when making clinical decisions. The hard part of practicing medicine lies in knowing when it is acceptable to be cost conscious with the use of further testing and when this technology must be used. Codifying the way in which health-care providers logically approach medical problems and deal with uncertainty is a difficult task. Good medicine is playing the odds after having obtained the important data. The focused history starts with uncovering the major details of the current medical problem or the reason the patient has sought medical attention at this time.

In documenting a focused history and performing a focused physical examination, you need to explore the chief complaint, the history of the present illness, the past medical history, medications and allergies, the family history and social history, the occupational history, and the sexual history that are relevant to that specific patient. **It is important to recognize that *focused* does not mean making one diagnosis and skipping the differential diagnosis**. In the focused physical examination, you need to examine specifically the body part or system directly involved with the medical problem when there is no time to perform a head-to-toe examination. Remember, however, that other organ systems may need to be evaluated as well! A patient with chest pain requires a full cardiac examination, in addition to examination of the legs for peripheral pulses and edema, carotid artery auscultation and palpation, evaluation of liver size, and evaluation of the retina for related vascular changes.

After your clinical evaluation, tests should be obtained *only* to corroborate your clinical impression or if the result will in some way affect your decision-making. Remember that common things are common. Uncommon symptoms are more likely to represent an uncommon manifestation associated with a common condition than with a totally uncommon illness.

Illustrative Case

Now consider as an example the case of Mr. Roger Stern. Mr. Stern is a 29-year-old man who has come to the emergency room with a chief complaint of "diarrhea and abdominal pain." What possible diagnoses are you thinking about? What pathologic conditions may be involved? Acute problems? Chronic problems? Some possibilities include genetic disorders, infectious diseases, diseases of immunity, neoplastic diseases, environmental problems, nutritional pathologic processes, vascular disorders, or traumatic conditions. Now try to narrow down the possible diagnoses by starting the interview:

Where is the pain in your abdomen?

Right here (pointing to his lower abdomen)

How long have you been having the abdominal pain?

I have been having diarrhea and abdominal pain for the past 3 months.

What was the reason you came in today?

I saw some blood mixed in the stools, and I got very scared.

I can understand your concern. I am glad you came in today. We will do everything possible to help you …. Can you describe the pain?

It's crampy and comes in waves. I also have this bloating sensation in my abdomen all the time . . . it's as if gas is always there.

What makes the pain better?

It's hard to say . . . not much.

What makes it worse?

I don't really know . . . perhaps anxiety?

Has there been a change in your life that has created more anxiety?

I guess my job has been rather stressful. I don't get along well with my bosses.

What type of work do you do?'

I am a legal assistant.

On a scale of 1 to 10, with 10 being the worst, how would you describe the pain?

I guess the pain is about 5 to 7.

How does the pain affect your lifestyle?

I do go to work, but it's tough getting up all the time to go to the bathroom and making excuses.

When you have the pain in your abdomen, do you have pain in any other area of your body at the same time?

No, I don't think so.

Have you noticed that the pain is worse when you're hungry . . . or after meals?

No, it just comes and goes and is not related to eating.

Now let's talk about the diarrhea. Can you describe it for me?

The stool is very loose and sometimes watery. And today there was *blood* in it.

Was there blood in the toilet bowl?

No. It was kind of wrapped with the stool.

How many times did you see blood with your stool?

Three times!

Is there mucus in the stool?

Yes, often. It's kind of stringy.

Is the stool formed?

Not really.

About how many bowel movements do you have a day?

About 8 to 10 for the past week.

Does the stool float?

No.

Does it smell strange?'

No. [*pause*] Doc, do you think I have cancer?

Mr. Stern, it's really too early to say. I need to ask you some more questions, perform a physical examination, and do some other tests. When we have all the tests back, I will be in a better position to advise you. At this time, however, there are many things that it could be. Let me ask you a few more questions. Have you had a fever?

No. I don't think so.

Have you noticed that milk or milk products make the diarrhea worse?

No.

Have you noticed that wheat, oat, barley, or rye products make the diarrhea worse?

No. I love bread and wheat products. They don't seem to make things worse.

Do you drink alcohol?

Not really. Maybe one beer over the weekend at most.

Have you had abdominal pain in the past?

I first noticed abdominal pain with watery diarrhea about 15 months ago.

What happened then?

I was traveling with a friend to Central America.

Did you see a doctor?

No.

Did you take any medications?

My friend gave me some Pepto-Bismol and Imodium for the pain and diarrhea.

Did it help you?

The pain persisted on and off for about 3 weeks and then disappeared.

Do you take other medications?

No. I have been in good health otherwise. I have no other problems.

Have you had other episodes of abdominal pain?

The pain and diarrhea returned about 3 months ago, but the diarrhea was no longer watery. The stool was just very loose.

Have you seen any doctor about this problem?

Yes, I saw a local doc about 3 weeks ago who gave me some antibiotic for it.

Do you remember the name of the antibiotic?

It was Flagyl.

Did it help you?

No. In fact, it seemed to make it worse, so I stopped taking it after 5 or 6 days.

Do you have nausea?

Not really.

Any vomiting?

No.

How's your diet?

I think okay, but recently I'm not too hungry because of the abdominal pain and diarrhea.

Has there been any change in your weight?

I've lost maybe about 5 pounds in the past month.

Does anyone else in your family have a similar problem?

No.

Have you ever had surgery?

No.

Tell me about your parents' health.

My Mom is 54, and she's fine. My Dad died about 15 months ago from a sudden heart attack. He was 56. I miss him a lot.

I am sorry to hear about your father.

Thanks.

Do you have any siblings?

Yeah, I have an older brother who's fine. He's 31.

Do you use any recreational drugs?

Marijuana about once or twice a month.

Anything else?

No.

Do you have any allergies?

No.

Are you sexually active?

Yeah.

Are your partners male, female, or both?

Only women. I've got a great relationship going on now. I've been living with my girl-friend for the past 8 months. I sure hope it continues.

Do you use protection?

Condoms . . . all the time!

Mr. Stern, I just have a few more general questions before I begin the physical examination. Have you ever had a problem with your eyes?

Eyes . . . yeah. When I was 19 years old in college, I had iritis in my right eye.

Tell me more about that.

I had real bad pain in my right eye, and it got real red. I saw the eye doc, who gave me steroids to take for about 4 weeks. I also remember that I had to wear sunglasses most of the time because the light really bothered me. I got better in about 3 weeks. I took all the meds because I didn't want that to come back again! Thank God it never came back!

Any history of back problems?

Yeah, I've had low back pain for several years since, I guess, I was 21. I think it's from too much bowling.

Did you ever see a doctor about it?

No. I just take some aspirin or Tylenol, which helps it.

Have you had any oral ulcers?

Not really.

Any urinary problems?

Nope.

Any rashes?

No.

Any chest pain?

No.

Any shortness of breath?

No.

In summary, Mr. Stern is a 29-year-old man who is seeking evaluation for a history of abdominal pain and diarrhea. The patient describes the first episode of pain about 15 months ago while on a trip in Central America. The pain disappeared and returned about 3 months ago. Today, the patient noticed red blood mixed with his stool and has sought medical evaluation. The patient describes the pain as crampy in nature and is relieved with defecation. He feels the pain mostly in his lower abdomen. He describes the pain as about a 5 or 7 on a scale of 10. He also has a bloating sensation in his abdomen most of the time. He does not have any nausea or vomiting. He denies being febrile. He has had a 5-pound weight loss in the past month. He saw a local physician about 3 weeks ago who gave him some antibiotic, which seemed to make things worse, and so he stopped taking the medication after 5 or 6 days. The symptoms have still persisted. He has had about 8 to 10 bowel movements a day for the past week. There has been some stringy mucus mixed in with the stool. The stools do not float. There is no lactose sensitivity. There is no apparent sensitivity to gluten (wheat, oat, barley, or rye products).

He is not taking any medications. He does not have any known allergies.

He is single and lives with his girlfriend of 8 months and always uses condoms for sexual protection. He uses marijuana about one or twice a month. He does not use any other recreational drugs. He works now as a legal clerk.

His mother is 54 years old and is in good health. His father died at age 56 from a sudden heart attack about 15 months ago. He has an older brother, age 31, who is in good health.

His review of systems is pertinent in that when he was 19 years old, he had iritis in his right eye, which was treated with steroids for 4 weeks and sunglasses. It improved in about 3 weeks. He also has a history of low back pain, which he attributes to bowling. The pain is intermittent and started when he was about 21 years old.

Diagnostic Evaluation

In speaking with Mr. Stern, there appear to be several important diagnoses. Inflammatory bowel disease (IBD), irritable bowel syndrome, traveler's diarrhea, pseudomembranous colitis, celiac disease, and giardiasis are certainly in the differential diagnosis. The history of iritis and low back pain makes the diagnosis of IBD a strong possibility. IBD, consisting of Crohn's disease and ulcerative colitis, is very common, with an annual incidence in the United States of approximately 3 to 10 new cases per 100,000 people. Extraintestinal inflammatory manifestations are common. Ocular manifestations occur in 5% of patients with IBD, and ankylosing spondylitis, in 5% to 10%. The most common extraintestinal manifestation is a peripheral, large-joint, asymmetric, nondeforming arthritis; this occurs in 20% of patients with IBD. Mr. Stern does not have a history of this type of arthritis. Genetic disorders seem unlikely, inasmuch as the appearance of this patient's problem started at age 27 or 28. Viral or bacterial gastroenteritis also seems unlikely, because of the apparent chronicity of the problem despite the travel history 15 months ago to Central America. *Salmonella, Shigella,* and *Campylobacter* enterocolitis are generally associated also with fever and are short-lived infections, lasting from 3 to 6 days, although *Campylobacter* infection may cause a more protracted diarrheal illness. Antibiotic-associated colitis (pseudomembranous colitis) is unlikely, inasmuch as most of the symptoms antedated the use of the recently prescribed antibiotics. Colorectal carcinoma is unlikely because of the history and this patient's age. Giardiasis is still a possibility, but it is low on the list of differential diagnoses: Most patients with giardiasis exhibit a malabsorptive diarrhea, and lactase deficiency occurs frequently, in 20% to 24% of patients; Mr. Stern denies milk intolerance. The regular use of condoms by a man who has sex only with women makes the diarrheal illness less likely to be related to acquired immunodeficiency syndrome (AIDS). Diarrheal illnesses and malabsorptive syndromes can occur in as many at 50% of AIDS patients. Malabsorption syndromes are common. They are characterized by defective adsorption of fats, fat-soluble and other vitamins, carbohydrates, electrolytes, minerals, and water. Although chronic diarrhea and flatulence are common in malabsorption syndromes, the hallmark of malabsorption is excessive fecal fat content, or steatorrhea. Mr. Stern denies floating stools, a symptom of steatorrhea. Celiac disease is a chronic disease, but this patient's lack of sensitivity to gluten makes this diagnosis less likely. Vascular disorders are unlikely because of the age of the patient and the lack of other medical conditions.

On the basis of the history, the focused physical examination of Mr. Stern should include the following:

- General appearance for signs of wasting, jaundice
- Inspection of skin for rashes
- Inspection of the mouth for oral ulcers
- Inspection of the abdomen
- Light palpation of the abdomen in all four quadrants after auscultation
- Deep palpation of all four quadrants
- Percussion of the abdomen
- Evaluation of liver size
- Rectal examination and evaluation for fecal occult blood
- Evaluation of sacroiliac joints for tenderness

After performing these physical examination maneuvers, you should be able to narrow down and/or confirm the most likely diagnosis. Always obtain as much information as possible. You can always narrow down your differential diagnosis.

The reader should review the DVD-ROM included with this book to see how this history and physical exam is performed.

It is a difficult task to obtain a good focused history and perform a good focused physical examination. It requires an excellent knowledge of physical diagnosis, pathophysiologic processes, and epidemiologic data in order to home in on the important aspects of the patient's medical problem.

Bibliography

Alaedidni A, Green PH: Narrative review: Celiac disease. Understanding a complex disease. Ann Intern Med 142:289, 2005.

Bowen JL: Educational strategies to promote clinical diagnostic reasoning. N Engl J Med 355:2217, 2006.

Bradley CP: Can we avoid bias? BMJ 330:784, 2005.

Drossman DA: Functional abdominal pain syndrome. Clin Gastroenterol Hepatol 2:353, 2004.

Gandhi TK, Kachalia A, Thomas EJ, et al: Missed and delayed diagnoses in the ambulatory setting: A study of closed malpractice claims. Ann Intern Med 145:488, 2006.

Heller RF, Sandars JE, Patterson L, et al: GPs' and physicians' interpretation of risks, benefits and diagnostic test results. Fam Pract 21:155, 2004.

Jason H: Becoming a truly helpful teacher: Considerably more challenging, and potentially more fun, than merely doing business as usual. Adv Physiol Educ 31:312, 2007.

King DB, Dickinson JA, Boulton MR, et al: Clinical skills textbooks fail evidence-based examination. Evid Based Med 10:131, 2005.

Lau AYS, Coiera EW: Do people experience cognitive biases while searching for information? J Am Med Inform Assoc 14:599, 2007.

Lembo A, Ameen VZ, Drossman DA: Irritable bowel syndrome: Toward an understanding of severity. Clin Gastroenterol Hepatol 3:717, 2005.

Manning-Dimmitt LL, Dimmitt SG, Wilson GR: Diagnosis of gastrointestinal bleeding in adults. Am Fam Phys 71:1339, 2005.

Peltier D, Regan-Smith M, Wofford J, et al: Teaching focused histories and physical exams in ambulatory care: A multi-institutional randomized trial. Teach Learn Med 19:244, 2007.

Westbrook JI, Gosling AS, Coiera EW: The impact of an online evidence system on confidence in decision making in a controlled setting. Med Decis Making 25:178, 2005.

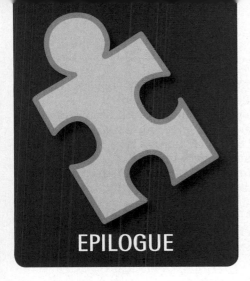

Epilogue

I will use treatment to help the sick according to my ability and judgment, but never with a view to injury and wrongdoing. And whatsoever I shall see or hear in the course of my profession in my discourse with others, ... I will never divulge, holding such things to be holy secrets.

From *The Physician's Oath*, Hippocrates (460–377) BCE

Ethical Challenges

Since the mid-1960s, there has been an increased awareness of and interest in medical ethics. With the first human heart transplant operation by Dr. Christiaan Barnard in 1967, the U.S. Supreme Court's declaration in 1973 that state laws prohibiting abortion were unconstitutional, and the controversy in 1975 over removing the respirator from a patient with irreversible brain damage in the case of Karen Ann Quinlan, modern medical ethics was born. Touching on three key issues—organ transplantation, abortion, and the standards of death—these landmarks set the stage for current thoughts about the ethical dimensions of health care.

Since then, there have been many other ethical challenges to the health-care system. In 1978, the first baby to be conceived in a test tube, Louise Brown, was born. In 1982, Dr. Barney Clark was the first person to receive a mechanical artificial heart, the Jarvik-7. In 1984, the infant Baby Fae received a heart transplanted from a baboon. In 1988, the Baby M case involved the ethical issues of Mary Beth Whitehead's "surrogate motherhood" for William Stern. From 2003 to 2005, legal and political conflict raged around the maintenance of life support (tube feedings) for Terri Schiavo, a severely brain-damaged woman who had been kept alive for 15 years.

As clinicians in the 21st century, you will be faced with many ethical issues: standards of brain death, physician-assisted suicide, in vitro fertilization, autonomy, informed consent, "do-not-resuscitate" orders, surrogate motherhood, euthanasia versus letting-die issues, rights of disabled persons, confidentiality, coerced surgery, abortion, "Baby Doe" regulations, interracial transplantation, surrogacy arrangements, allocation of scarce medical resources, whistle-blowing on unethical colleagues, use of patients as research subjects, mandatory

This Epilogue was written in collaboration with Talia H. Swartz, MD, PhD, Department of Internal Medicine, Mount Sinai Medical Center, New York, New York.

testing for acquired immunodeficiency syndrome (AIDS), and genetic manipulation. One of the first ethical issues you may face is the use of patients as "teaching tools."

A current ethical issue is the mandatory testing for human immunodeficiency virus (HIV). Should an HIV test be required as part of premarital testing, preadmission to hospitals, pre-insurance examinations, or preemployment testing? Several arguments have been made in its favor, including a person's right to donate blood, the tracing of potential infected contacts, determination of the incidence and rate of spread of HIV, quarantine of infected persons, and tattooing of infected persons. Some of the arguments against mandatory testing concern discrimination, "social purification," violation of a person's privacy, false-positive test results, and health insurance difficulties.

An ethical problem is one in which two or more norms or principles create a challenge about what to do. There are many types of ethical problems. These problems can be divided into four main groups:

1. *Ethical distress:* An individual knows the course of action, but a barrier prevents its accomplishment.
2. *Ethical dilemma:* There exist two or more courses of action, each of which is right or wrong, and selecting one will compromise the end result.
3. *Distributive justice:* Benefits are given to several individuals, but not to everyone. On what basis should the distribution be made?
4. *Locus of authority:* There are two or more authorities, all believing that they know which outcome will best benefit the patient, but only one will prevail.

Consider the following examples of contemporary issues in medical ethics:

- Avia and Hal are newlyweds. They want to have children, but each is from a family with a known inherited illness. Any or all of their children may be affected. Genetic alteration may be an option. Is it right for such couples to endeavor to change their future children's genetic makeup? Is modification of natural biology a human right?
- Florence is 31 years of age. When Florence became pregnant, she was overjoyed. She is now in her second month of pregnancy. Recently she developed fever, tender lymphadenopathy, rash, and sore throat. Rubella was diagnosed. Although Florence dreads the thought of giving birth to a retarded, blind, or congenitally malformed child, her religion does not allow abortion. Nonetheless, she questions whether it is right to bear a child that she knows will live a life of suffering.
- Baby John is born with significant birth defects. As his condition continues to deteriorate, is there a point when aggressive therapy should be discontinued?
- Natalie and Marshall have been unsuccessful in conceiving a child, and evaluation indicates that Natalie is unable to bear a child. The couple decides on a surrogate pregnancy with Marshall's sperm. They meet the surrogate mother, whom they like, and she conceives their child. During a conversation in her second trimester, the surrogate mother-to-be indicates that she would be unwilling to undergo a cesarean section if the child's life were in jeopardy. Who has the right to make that decision?
- Sam, a major benefactor to the hospital, is 76 years of age. He has Parkinson's disease and diabetes mellitus. Sam is in the emergency department complaining of severe chest pain. Brittany is a 41-year-old nurse with a history of angina who is also in the emergency department complaining of severe chest pain. There is only one bed left in the coronary intensive care unit. Who should get the bed?
- Jack is a 42-year-old man who has sex with only men and is HIV-positive. Although counseled about his promiscuous sexual behavior, he is unwilling to curb his unprotected sexual encounters, posing a threat to his partners and to the community at large. What is your role as his physician as it relates to confidentiality and the "politics" of disease?
- Maria is 20 years of age and is the single mother of two children. She is in the first trimester of her third pregnancy. Recent symptoms of severe weakness and gingival bleeding brought her to medical attention. A work-up revealed acute monomyelocytic leukemia and anemia with a hemoglobin measurement of 7.8 g/dL. Therapy for the leukemia would be a great risk to the life of the fetus, but the patient refuses to terminate her pregnancy. To complicate the issue, her fiancé, a Jehovah's Witness, has persuaded the patient to refuse any transfusion of blood or blood products. How do you, as her physician, handle this situation?
- Lynn is a 62-year-old woman with a 2-year history of lung cancer. Because of severe back pain for the past 3 months, she is evaluated, and it is determined that she has

multiple metastases to her spine impinging on nerve roots. Despite analgesic therapy, she continues to have debilitating, unrelenting pain. She now consults you, requesting physician-assisted suicide.

Unethical Labeling of Patients

One of the significant problems currently seen in health care is the unethical labeling of patients. Terms such as "gomer" ("*get out of my emergency room*"), "albatross," "turkey," and "slug" are examples of disrespect. Health-care providers who use such terms are often reacting negatively to certain social and personal traits of their patients, as well as to certain medical conditions. This is particularly evident with illnesses that are usually incurable, are self-inflicted, or that challenge the health-care provider's faith in the "science" of medicine. Often, these patients have illnesses that defy medical intervention, thus frustrating the health-care provider. A patient who is of low socioeconomic class, has an illness engendering fear or disgust, is uncooperative, or is psychologically dysfunctional is at the greatest risk of being labeled in this derogatory manner.

Health-care providers may use these negative terms as "safety valves" for the emotionally charged environment in which they work, but this only further distances them from their patients. Each provider must recognize and come to grips with his or her anxieties about dealing with illness and treating patients and must not allow these destructive attitudes to interfere with the care of the sick. Remember the quotation from Francis Weld Peabody that introduces this book: "the secret in the care *of* the patient is in caring *for* the patient."

Health-Care Proxy

A **health-care proxy form** is an extremely important document that every patient should have in order to serve as protection of his or her wishes at a time when he or she might be incapacitated. A health-care proxy is a person who is appointed to make decisions on behalf of the patient if the patient is unable to do so. This health-care proxy is anyone whom the patient designates as someone he or she trusts: for example, a family member or close friend. Once this health-care proxy is designated, that person is authorized to make health-care decisions for the patient should the patient lose the ability to make decisions for himself or herself. It is not necessary to have a lawyer fill out this health-care proxy form; it is a form that can be completed by the patient with understanding on the part of the health-care proxy of this designation and the signatures of two witnesses. This becomes hospital record and can be used in the future as necessary. Any adult, 18 years of age or older, may be the health-care proxy. It is important that once the proxy is designated, the patient discuss wishes about advanced directives if such a situation should arise: the desire to be maintained on artificial nutrition, mechanical ventilation, renal replacement, or organ/tissue donation. Knowledge of the patient's viewpoints of these measures will help improve the ability of the health-care proxy to make decisions that best reflect the patient's wishes. The patient may even give the health-care proxy specific instructions to follow, and this may be documented in the health-care proxy form, but this is not required.

Even though the patient has signed this health-care proxy form, he or she still has the right to make health-care decisions for himself or herself as long as he or she is able to do so. Treatment cannot be given to the patient or stopped if the patient objects, and the proxy has no power to object. The patient may also cancel the authority given to the health-care proxy by telling him or her orally or in writing.

Appointing a health-care proxy is voluntary. No one can require a patient to appoint one. Copies of the health-care proxy form should be given to the proxy, the physician, family members, an attorney, and close friends. A copy should also be kept in the patient's wallet. If the patient is hospitalized, the form should be brought in and included in the medical record.

It is important to understand the difference between a **living will** and a health-care proxy form. A living will is a document that provides specific instructions about health-care decisions. A patient may put such instructions on his or her health-care proxy form. Unlike a living will, a health-care proxy form does not require that a patient knows in advance all the decisions that may arise. Instead, the health-care proxy can interpret a patient's wishes as medical circumstances change and can make decisions that a patient could not have known would have to be made.

Health Care Proxy Form

YOUR BIRTH DATE

_____/_____/_____

(1) I, _____ , residing at _____
(PRINT your name)

_____
(Street)   (City or Town)   (State)

appoint _____
(Name of person you choose as Agent/Proxy)

of _____
(Street)   (City/town)   (State)   (Phone)

as my health care agent to make any and all health care decisions for me, except to the extent that I state otherwise. This proxy shall take effect only when and if I become unable to make my own health care decisions.

(2) Optional: Alternate Agent/Proxy

If my Agent is unwilling or unable to serve, then I appoint as my Alternate Agent:
_____ , of
(Name of person you choose as Alternate Agent)

_____ .
(Street)   (City/town)   (State)   (Phone)

as my health care agent to make any and all health care decisions for me, except to the extent that I state otherwise.

(3)

Unless I revoke it or state an expiration date or circumstances under which it will expire, this proxy shall remain in effect indefinitely. (*Optional: If you want this proxy to expire, state the date or conditions here.*) This proxy shall expire (*specify date or conditions*):

_____

_____

_____

(4) Optional:

I direct my health care agent to make health care decisions according to my wishes and limitations, as he or she knows or as stated below. (*If you want to limit your agent's authority to make health care decisions for you or to give specific instructions, you may state your wishes or limitations here.*) I direct my health care agent to make health care decisions in accordance with the following limitations and/or instructions (*attach additional pages as necessary*):

_____

_____

In order for your agent to make health care decisions for you about artificial nutrition and hydration (*nourishment and water provided by feeding tube and intravenous line*), your agent must reasonably know your wishes. You can either tell your agent what your wishes are or include them in this section.

(5) Your Identification (please print)

Your Name _____

Your Signature_____ Date_____

Your Address_____

(6) Optional: Organ and/or Tissue Donation

I hereby make an anatomical gift, to be effective upon my death, of: (*check any that apply*)
☐ Any needed organs and/or tissues
☐ The following organs and/or tissues_____

_____

☐ Limitations_____

If you do not state your wishes or instructions about organ and/or tissue donation on this form, it will not be taken to mean that you do not wish to make a donation or prevent a person, who is otherwise authorized by law, to consent to a donation on your behalf.

Your signature _____ Date _____

(7) Statement by Witnesses

(*Witnesses must be 18 years of age or older and cannot be the health care agent or alternate.*)
I declare that the person who signed this document is personally known to me and appears to be of sound mind and acting of his or her own free will. He or she signed (or asked another to sign for him or her) this document in my presence.

Date _____   Date _____
Name of Witness 1 (*print*)   Name of Witness 2 (*print*)

Signature _____   Signature _____

Address_____   Address_____

Adapted from the New York State Health Proxy Form.

The structure of the health-care proxy form may differ from state to state, but the common elements all include the following:

- Name and address of the agent/proxy
- Name and address of an alternative agent
- Duration of the proxy (not indicating a duration means it is valid unless stated otherwise)
- Special instructions: these can broaden or limit the powers of the agent. If the patient does not want to be sustained by feeding tubes no matter what, this can be stated here. If there are certain treatments that the patient does not want to receive, such as blood transfusion, then they must be indicated. However, if the patient wants to give the agent more flexibility with some or no restriction, this too must be written.
- Name, date, and signature of the primary individual
- Instructions about tissue or organ donation
- Signatures of two adult witnesses, stating that they have witnessed this agreement and that both parties appear to be competent. The witnesses must be 18 years of age or older. The agent and primary individual do not qualify as witnesses.

A copy of a sample proxy form is shown on the previous page. You should copy this form and give it to all your patients if they have not already designated a health-care proxy.

Health-care proxy forms have become increasingly important today as a result of conflicts among relatives of the primary individual. The Terri Schiavo case is a famous modern-day example that lasted for 15 years of court battles (1990–2005). The patient was an American woman who suffered brain damage and became dependent for survival on a feeding tube. Her husband wanted to remove her feeding tube, but her parents opposed this action. This resulted in lengthy court battles that raised many moral, political, and medical issues. The whole controversy may have been avoided had the patient designated either her parents or her husband as her health-care proxy. Without a health-care proxy, a surrogate that follows next of kin becomes designated; however, the decision-making capacity of a surrogate is much more limited and varies by state. Therefore, if any individual can designate a health-care proxy while he or she is in good health, much agonizing and conflict can be avoided if a situation warrants this need in the future.

The reader should review the DVD-ROM included with this book for an example of discussing a health-care proxy with a patient.

Concluding Thoughts

As a health-care professional, you will be faced with many types of problems that involve complex decision-making. Always treat your patients and colleagues with fairness, respect, and dignity. Your medical training may be harsh at times; however it is important to maintain the enthusiasm that sparked your desire to join this profession. I wish you the best of luck in dedicating your career to caring for your patients.

Bibliography

Freeman JM, McDonnell K: Tough Decisions: Cases in Medical Ethics, 2nd ed. New York, Oxford University Press, 2001.

Glannon W: Biomedical Ethics. New York, Oxford University Press, 2004.

Jonsen AR, Siegler M, Winslade WJ: Clinical Ethics: A Practical Approach to Ethical Decisions in Clinical Medicine. New York, McGraw-Hill Medical, 2002.

Kurland G: My Own Medicine: A Doctor's Life as a Patient, New York, Henry Holt & Company, 2002.

Lynne D: Terri's Story: The Court-Ordered Death of an American Woman. Nashville, Tenn, Cumberland House, 2005.

Pellegrino ED, Thomasma DC: The Virtues in Medical Practice. New York, Oxford University Press, 1993.

Pence GE: Classic Cases in Medical Ethics: Accounts of the Cases That Have Shaped Medical Ethics, with Philosophical, Legal, and Historical Backgrounds, 4th ed. New York, McGraw-Hill, 2003.

Petrinovich L: Living and Dying Well. New York, Plenum Press, 1996.

Rosner F: Modern Medicine and Jewish Ethics, 2nd ed. New York, Yeshiva University Press, 1991.

Weisman J: As I Live and Breathe: Notes of a Patient-Doctor. New York, Farrar, Straus and Giroux, 2003.

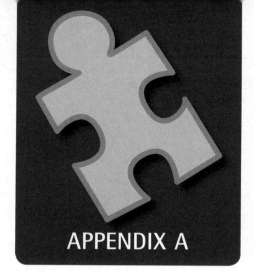

APPENDIX A

Commonly Abused Drugs

Drug	Street Name	How Used	Symptoms and Signs
Marijuana, hashish	*Pot, grass, reefer, weed, hash, sinsemilla, joint*	Smoked Ingested	Loss of initiative Recent memory loss Dry mouth and throat Mood changes Increased appetite
Alcohol	*Booze, brew, hooch*	Ingested	Impaired coordination Impaired judgment
Nicotine	*Smoke, butt, coffin nail*	Smoked Chewed	Tobacco smell Stained teeth
Amphetamines	*Speed, uppers, pep pills, bennies, dexies, black beauties, meth, crystal*	Ingested Injected Sniffed	Dilated pupils Increased energy Irritability Nervousness Needle marks
Cocaine	*Coke, crack, snow, white lady, toot*	Snorted Injected Ingested Smoked	Dilated pupils Increased energy Restlessness Intense anxiety Paranoid behavior Needle marks
Barbiturates	*Downers, barbs, yellow jackets, red devils, blue devils, double trouble*	Injected Ingested	Constricted pupils Confusion Impaired judgment Drowsiness Slurring of speech Needle marks
Methaqualone	*Ludes, sopors, quaaludes*	Ingested	Slurring of speech Drowsiness Impaired judgment Euphoria Seizures

Drug	Street Name	How Used	Symptoms and Signs
Heroin, morphine	*Junk, scag, dope, horse, smack, dreamer*	Injected Smoked Sniffed "Skin popped" (injected subcutaneously)	Constricted pupils Needle marks Drowsiness Mental clouding
Codeine	*School boy*	Ingested Sniffed	Constricted pupils Drowsiness
Demerol		Ingested Injected	Constricted pupils
Methadone		Ingested	Drowsiness
Percodan		Ingested	Mental clouding
Pentazocine		Injected	Needle marks
PCP (phencyclidine)	*Angel dust, hog, killer weed, supergrass*	Smoked Snorted Injected Ingested	Dilated pupils Slurring of speech Hallucinations Blurring of vision Lack of coordination Agitation Confusion Aggressive behavior
LSD (lysergic acid diethylamide)	*Acid, cubes, purple haze*	Ingested Injected	Dilated pupils Hallucinations Mood swings Increased alertness Acute panic reactions
Mescaline	*Mesc, cactus*	Ingested	Dilated pupils Hallucinations Mood swings
Psilocybin	*Magic mushrooms*	Ingested	Dilated pupils Hallucinations Mood swings
Airplane glue, paint thinner*		Inhaled Sniffed	Poor motor coordination Impaired vision Violent behavior
Nitrous oxide	*Laughing gas, whippets*	Inhaled Sniffed	Hilarity Euphoria Lightheadedness
Amyl nitrite	*Poppers, rush, locker room, snappers, amies*	Inhaled Sniffed	Hilarity Dizziness Headache Impaired thought

*The active agent in airplane glue and paint thinner is toluene. Naphtha, methyl ethyl ketone, and gasoline may produce similar symptoms.

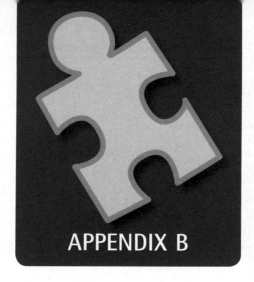

APPENDIX B

Signs and Symptoms in Deficiency States

Deficiency	Signs	Symptoms
Vitamin A (see Fig. 5-6)	Hyperkeratinization of the skin Keratinizing metaplasia in the linings of the respiratory, gastrointestinal, and genitourinary tracts Metaplasia of the endocrine, salivary, sebaceous, and lacrimal glands	Night blindness Retarded growth (children) Xerophthalmia Xeroderma
Vitamin D (rickets, osteomalacia)	Craniotabes Rachitic rosary* Bowing of the legs Knock-knee Pigeon chest deformity Harrison's grooves† Scoliosis Compression of affected vertebrae Carpopedal spasms Generalized spasticity Convulsive seizures	Irritability Restlessness Dental problems Coughing Pulmonary infections Seizures
Thiamine (beriberi)	Bilateral, symmetric peripheral neuropathy (distal parts of lower extremities first) Decreased perception of light touch Calf muscle tenderness Loss of vibration sense Loss of normal reflexes Motor weakness Secondary muscle atrophy Cardiac enlargement Congestive heart failure Wide pulse pressure Arrhythmias Polyneuropathy	Lack of initiative Anorexia Mental depression Irritability Poor memory Easy fatigability Inability to concentrate Vague abdominal problems Paresthesias of the toes Burning sensation in the lower extremities Dyspnea Palpitations Peripheral edema

Deficiency	Signs	Symptoms
Niacin (pellagra) (see Fig. 5-10)	Extensive dermatitis (common on parts of body exposed to sunlight or mechanical trauma; often bilateral and symmetric) Glossitis Stomatitis Chronic hypertrophy with induration of skin Pigmentation on pressure points Skin fissuring Atrophic skin changes Scaling of skin	Skin rashes Swollen tongue Increased salivation Burning sensation in mouth Poor digestion Diarrhea (often foul smelling; sometimes bloody) Gaseous distention Eructation Vomiting Disorientation Confusion Hallucinations Delirium Paranoia Depression
Riboflavin	Cheilosis Angular stomatitis Glossitis Seborrheic dermatitis, especially in the nasolabial region, around the eyes, behind the ears, and on the scrotum Ocular manifestations	Photophobia Burning sensation in eyes Itching of eyes Skin rashes Fissuring of mouth
Vitamin C (scurvy) (see Figs. 5-7 and 5-8)	Defective collagen formation Ecchymoses Subperiosteal hematomas Follicular hyperkeratoses Petechial hemorrhages (lower extremities) Gingival hemorrhages Hemarthroses Hemorrhages Anemia Scorbutic rosary[‡]	Impaired wound healing Failure to thrive, irritability, and frequent crying (children) Bleeding tendencies Painful joints Weight loss Nonspecific aches and pains Brown pigmentation Curling of hair Keratoconjunctivitis sicca[§] Emotional changes
Protein-calorie (kwashiorkor) (see Fig. 5-5)	Retarded growth Edema Hyperpigmentation of skin Depigmentation of skin Hepatomegaly Severe tissue wasting Loss of subcutaneous fat Functional dehydration	Apathy Anorexia Edema Changes in hair color and consistency Changes in skin color Abdominal enlargement Diarrhea Steatorrhea
Folate (see Fig. 5-9)	Anemia Stomatitis Glossitis	Pallor Weakness Diarrhea
Calcium	Osteoporosis Osteomalacia	Bone fractures
Iron	Anemia Koilonychia[¶] Glossitis	Pallor Weakness Fatigability Dyspnea on exertion Headache Palpitations Fissuring at corners of mouth Painful tongue

*Beading of the ribs at the costochondral junction.
[†]Lateral thoracic depressions at the sites of attachment of the diaphragm.
[‡]Beading of the ribs at the costochondral junction.
[§]A condition of marked hyperemia of the conjunctiva, lacrimal deficiency, thickening of the corneal epithelium, itching and burning of the eye, and reduced visual acuity.
[¶]Spoon nail.

Continued

Deficiency	Signs	Symptoms

Iodine	Goiter	Swelling of neck
		Hypothyroid symptoms
		    (see Chapter 9, The Head
		    and Neck)

Zinc (see Fig. 5-11)	Growth retardation Hypogonadism Delayed sexual maturation Seborrheic dermatitis	Loss of taste Anorexia Behavioral problems Skin rashes Hair loss Decreased libido Decreased fertility Diarrhea
Magnesium	Vertical nystagmus	Muscle tremor Choreiform movements Convulsions Weakness Paralysis Dysphagia
Potassium	Arrhythmias	Diarrhea Weakness Nervous irritability Disorientation Palpitations
Sodium	Dehydration signs	Confusion Coma Vomiting Lethargy Anorexia Nausea Headache Obtundation Seizures

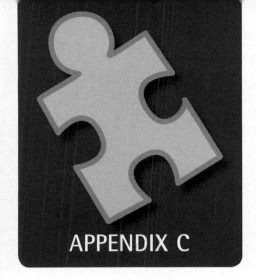

APPENDIX C

Conversion Tables

Temperature*

Centigrade	Fahrenheit	Centigrade	Fahrenheit
33.0	91.4	37.8	100.0
33.2	91.8	38.0	100.4
33.4	92.1	38.2	100.7
33.6	92.5	38.4	101.1
33.8	92.8	38.6	101.4
34.0	93.2	38.8	101.8
34.2	93.6	39.0	102.2
34.4	93.9	39.2	102.5
34.6	94.3	39.4	102.9
34.8	94.6	39.6	103.2
35.0	95.0	39.8	103.6
35.2	95.4	40.0	104.0
35.4	95.7	40.2	104.3
35.6	96.1	40.4	104.7
35.8	96.4	40.6	105.1
36.0	96.8	40.8	105.4
36.2	97.1	41.0	105.8
36.4	97.5	41.2	106.1
36.6	97.8	41.4	106.5
36.8	98.2	41.6	106.8
37.0	98.6	41.8	107.2
37.2	98.9	42.0	107.6
37.4	99.3	42.2	108.0
37.6	99.6	42.4	108.3

*To convert centigrade to Fahrenheit: (9/5 × centigrade temperature) + 32. To convert Fahrenheit to centigrade: 5/9 × (Fahrenheit temperature − 32).

Weight*

Pound	Kilogram	Kilogram	Pound
1	0.5	1	2.2
2	0.9	2	4.4
4	1.8	3	6.6
6	2.7	4	8.8
8	3.6	5	11.0
10	4.5	6	13.2
20	9.1	8	17.6
30	13.6	10	22
40	18.2	20	44
50	22.7	30	66
60	27.3	40	88
70	31.8	50	110
80	36.4	60	132
90	40.9	70	154
100	45.4	80	176
150	68.1	90	198
200	90.8	100	220

*To convert pounds to kilograms: pounds × 0.454 kilogram. To convert kilograms to pounds: kilograms × 2.204 pounds. Measurements in table are rounded to the nearest first decimal place.

Length*

Inch	Centimeter	Centimeter	Inch
1	2.54	1	0.4
2	5.08	2	0.8
4	10.16	3	1.2
6	15.24	4	1.6
8	20.32	5	2.0
10	25.40	6	2.4
20	50.80	8	3.1
30	76.20	10	3.9
40	101.60	20	7.9
50	127.00	30	11.8
60	152.40	40	15.7
70	177.80	50	19.7
80	203.20	60	23.6
90	228.60	70	27.6
100	254.00	80	31.5
150	381.00	90	35.4
200	508.00	100	39.4

*To convert inches to centimeters: inches × 2.54 centimeters. To convert centimeters to inches: centimeters × 0.3937 inch. Measurements in centimeters calculated from inches are rounded to the nearest second decimal place; those in inches calculated from centimeters, to the nearest first decimal place.

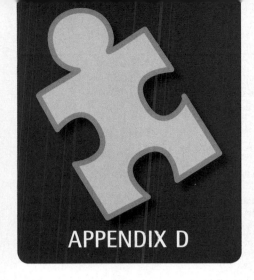

APPENDIX D

The Rational Clinical Examination: Additional References

Akshay B, Thavendiranathan P, Detsky AS: Does this patient have hearing impairment? JAMA 295:416-428, 2006.

Anand SS, Wells PS, Hunt D, et al: Does this patient have deep vein thrombosis? JAMA 279:1094-1099, 1998.

Anderson MR, Klink K, Cohrssen A: Evaluation of vaginal complaints. JAMA 291:1368-1379, 2004.

Attia J, Hatala R, Cook DJ, et al: Does this adult patient have acute meningitis? JAMA 282:175-181, 1999.

Barton MB, Harris R, Fletcher SW: Does this patient have breast cancer? The screening clinical breast examination: should it be done? How? JAMA 282:1270-1280, 1999.

Bastian LA, Smith CM, Nanda K: Is this woman perimenopausal? JAMA 289:895-902, 2003.

Bent S, Nallamothu BK, Simel DL, et al: Does this woman have an acute uncomplicated urinary tract infection? JAMA 287:2701-2710, 2002.

Booth CM, Boone RH, Tomlinson G, et al: Is this patient dead, vegetative, or severely neurologically impaired? Assessing outcome for comatose survivors of cardiac arrest. JAMA 291:870-879, 2004.

Bundy DG, Byerley JS, Liles EA, et al: Does this child have appendicitis? JAMA 298:438-451, 2007.

Butalia S, Palda VA, Sargeant RJ, et al: Does this patient with diabetes have osteomyelitis of the lower extremity? JAMA 299:806-813, 2008.

Call SA, Vollenweider MA, Hornung CA: Does this patient have influenza? JAMA 293:987-997, 2005.

Choudhry NK, Etchells EE: Does this patient have aortic regurgitation? JAMA 281:2231-2238, 1999.

Chunilal SD, Eikelboom JW, Attia J, et al: Does this patient have pulmonary embolism? JAMA 290:2849-2858, 2003.

D'Arcy CA, McGee S: Does this patient have carpal tunnel syndrome? JAMA 283:3110-3117, 2000.

Ebell MH, Smith MA, Barry HC, et al: Does this patient have strep throat? JAMA 284:2912-2918, 2000.

Ganz DA, Bao Y, Shekelle PG, et al: Will my patient fall? JAMA 297:77-86, 2007.

Goldstein LB, Simel DL: Is this patient having a stroke? JAMA 293:2391-2402, 2005.

Green AD, Colón-Emeric CS, Bastian L, et al: Does this woman have osteoporosis? JAMA 292:2890-2900, 2004.

Holroyd-Leduc JM, Tannenbaum C, Thorpe KE, et al: What type of urinary incontinence does this woman have? JAMA 299:1446-1456, 2008.

Holsinger T, Deveau J, Boustani M, et al: Does this patient have dementia? JAMA 297:2391-2404, 2007.

Khan NA, Rahim SA, Anand S, et al: Does the clinical examination predict lower extremity peripheral arterial disease? JAMA 295:536-546, 2006.

Klompas M: Does this patient have acute thoracic aortic dissection? JAMA 287:2262-2272, 2002.

Klompas M: Does this patient have ventilator-associated pneumonia? JAMA 297:1583-1593, 2007.

Lederle FA, Simel DL: Does this patient have abdominal aortic aneurysm? JAMA 281:77-82, 1999.

Luime JJ, Verhagen AP, Miedema HS, et al: Does this patient have an instability of the shoulder or a labrum lesion? JAMA 292:1989-1999, 2004.

Margaretten ME, Kohlwes J, Moore D, et al: Does this adult patient have septic arthritis? JAMA 297:1478-1488, 2007.

Margolis P, Gadomski A: Does this infant have pneumonia? JAMA 279:308-313, 1998.

McGee S, Abernethy WB, Simel DL: Is this patient hypovolemic? JAMA 281:1022-1029, 1999.

Moayyedi P, Talley NJ, Fennerty MB, et al: Can the clinical history distinguish between organic and functional dyspepsia? JAMA 295:1566-1576, 2006.

Murff HJ, Spigel DR, Syngal S: Does this patient have a family history of cancer?: An evidence-based analysis of the accuracy of family cancer history. JAMA 292:1480-1489, 2004.

Myers KA, Farquhar DRE: Does this patient have clubbing? JAMA 286:341-347, 2001.

Panju AA, Hemmelgarn BR, Guyatt GH, et al: Is this patient having a myocardial infarction? JAMA 280:1256-1263, 1998.

Rao G, Fisch L, Srinivasan S, et al: Does this patient have Parkinson disease? JAMA 289:347-353, 2003.

Rothman R, Owens T, Simel DL: Does this child have acute otitis media? JAMA 290:1633-1640, 2003.

Roy CL, Minor MA, Brookhart MA, et al: Does this patient with a pericardial effusion have cardiac tamponade? JAMA 297:1810-1818, 2007.

Salkind AR, Cuddy PG, Foxworth JW: Is this patient allergic to penicillin? An evidence-based analysis of the likelihood of penicillin allergy. JAMA 285:2498-2505, 2001.

Scherer K, Bedlack RS, Simel DL: Does this patient have myasthenia gravis? JAMA 293:1906-1914, 2005.

Shaikh N, Morone NE, Lopez J, et al: Does this child have a urinary tract infection? JAMA 298:2895-2904, 2007.

Smetana GW, Shmerling RH: Does this patient have temporal arteritis? JAMA 287:92-101, 2002.

Solomon DH, Simel DL, Bates DW, et al: Does this patient have a torn meniscus or ligament of the knee? Value of the physical examination. JAMA 286:1610-1620, 2001.

Steiner MJ, DeWalt DA, Vyerley JS: Is this child dehydrated? JAMA 291:1368-1379, 2004.

Straus SE, Thorpe KE, Holroyd-Leduc J: How do I perform a lumbar puncture and analyze the results to diagnose bacterial meningitis? JAMA 296:2012-2022, 2006.

Sumant RR, Goldman LE, Simel DL, et al: Do opiates affect the clinical evaluation of patients with acute abdominal pain? JAMA 296:1764-1774, 2006.

Tibbles CD, Edlow JA: Does this patient have erythema migrans? JAMA 297:2617-2627, 2007.

Trowbridge RL, Rutkowski NK, Shojania KG: Does this patient have acute cholecystitis? JAMA 289:80-86, 2003.

Whited JD, Grichnik JM: Does this patient have a mole or a melanoma? JAMA 279:696-701, 1998.

Williams JW, Noël PH, Cordes JA, et al: Is this patient clinically depressed? JAMA 287:1160-1170, 2002.

Wong CL, Holroyd-Leduc JM, Thorpe KE, et al: Does this patient have bacterial peritonitis or portal hypertension? How do I perform a paracentesis and analyze the results? JAMA 299:1166-1178, 2008.

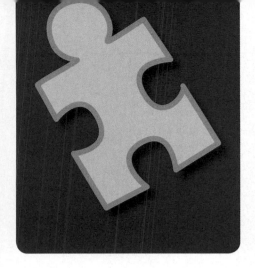

Index